Rob & Smith's
Operative Surgery

Orthopaedics

Fourth Edition

General Editors

David C. Carter MD, FRCS(Ed), FRCS(Glas)
Regius Professor of Clinical Surgery, Royal Infirmary, Edinburgh, UK

R. C. G. Russell MS, FRCS
Consultant Surgeon, Middlesex Hospital and Royal National Throat, Nose and Ear Hospital, London, UK

Consulting Editor

Hugh Dudley CBE, ChM, FRCS(Ed), FRACS, FRCS
Emeritus Professor, St Mary's Hospital, London, UK

Art Editor

Gillian Lee FMAA, HonFIMI, AMI, RMIP
15 Little Plucketts Way, Buckhurst Hill, Essex, UK

Other volumes available in the series

Cardiac Surgery 4th Edition
Stuart W. Jamieson and Norman E. Shumway

The Ear 4th Edition
John C. Ballantyne and Andrew Morrison

General Principles, Breast and Extracranial Endocrines 4th Edition
Hugh Dudley and Walter J. Pories

Genitourinary Surgery 5th Edition
Hugh N. Whitfield

Gynaecology and Obstetrics 4th Edition
J. M. Monaghan

The Hand 4th Edition
Rolfe Birch and Donal Brooks

Head and Neck 4th Edition
Ian A. McGregor and David J. Howard

Neurosurgery 4th Edition
Lindsay Symon, David G. T. Thomas and Kemp Clark

Nose and Throat 4th Edition
John C. Ballantyne and D. F. N. Harrison

Ophthalmic Surgery 4th Edition
Thomas A. Rice, Ronald G. Michels and Walter W. J. Stark

Paediatric Surgery 4th Edition
L. Spitz and H. Homewood Nixon

Plastic Surgery 4th Edition
T. L. Barclay and Desmond A. Kernahan

Surgery of the Colon, Rectum and Anus 5th Edition
L. P. Fielding and S. M. Goldberg

Thoracic Surgery 4th Edition
The late J. W. Jackson and D. K. C. Cooper

Trauma Surgery 4th Edition
Howard R. Champion, John V. Robbs and Donald D. Trunkey

Rob & Smith's
Operative Surgery

Orthopaedics

Edited by

George Bentley ChM, FRCS
Professor of Orthopaedic Surgery, The Institute of Orthopaedics, University of London; Honorary Consultant Orthopaedic Surgeon, The Royal National Orthopaedic Hospital, Stanmore, Middlesex and the Middlesex Hospital, London, UK

Robert B. Greer III MD, FACS
Professor and Chairman of Orthopaedic Surgery, Pennsylvania State University College of Medicine, Hershey, Pennsylvania 17033, USA

Fourth Edition

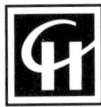

CHAPMAN & HALL MEDICAL
London · Glasgow · Weinheim · New York · Tokyo · Melbourne · Madras

Published by Chapman & Hall, 2-6 Boundary Row, London SE1 8HN, UK

Chapman & Hall, 2-6 Boundary Row, London SE1 8HN, UK

Blackie Academic & Professional, Wester Cleddens Road, Bishopbriggs, Glasgow G64 2NZ, UK

Chapman & Hall GmbH, Pappelallee 3, 69469 Weinheim, Germany

Chapman & Hall Inc., One Penn Plaza, 41st Floor, New York, NY10119, USA

Chapman & Hall Japan, Thomson Publishing Japan, Hirakawacho Nemoto Building, 6F, 1-7-11 Hirakawa-cho, Chiyoda-ku, Tokyo 102, Japan

Chapman & Hall Australia, Thomas Nelson Australia, 102 Dodds Street, South Melbourne, Victoria 3205, Australia

Chapman & Hall India, R. Seshadri, 32 Second Main Road, CIT East, Madras 600 035, India

First edition 1957
Second edition 1969
Third edition 1979
Fourth edition 1991
First published as a paperback edition 1993
Reprinted 1994

© 1993 Chapman & Hall

Composition by Genesis Typesetting, Laser Quay, Rochester, Kent
Printed and bound in Great Britain by the Alden Press Ltd, Oxford

ISBN 0 412 53790 7

Apart from any fair dealing for the purposes of research or private study, or criticism or review, as permitted under the UK Copyright Designs and Patents Act, 1988, this publication may not be reproduced, stored, or transmitted, in any form or by any means, without the prior permission in writing of the publishers, or in the case of reprographic reproduction only in accordance with the terms of the licences issued by the Copyright Licensing Agency in the UK, or in accordance with the terms of licences issued by the appropriate Reproduction Rights Organization outside the UK. Enquiries concerning reproduction outside the terms stated here should be sent to the publishers at the London address printed on this page.

The publisher makes no representation, express or implied, with regard to the accuracy of the information contained in this book and cannot accept any legal responsibility or liability for any errors or omissions that may be made.

A Catalogue record for this book is available from the British Library

Library of Congress Cataloging-in-Publication Data

Rob & Smith's operative surgery.
    Rev. ed. of: Operative surgery. 3rd ed. 1979
    Includes bibliographies and index.
    Contents: Alimentary tract and abdominal wall.
    1. General principles, oesophagus, stomach, duodenum, small intestine, abdominal wall, hernia/edited by Hugh Dudley—[13] Orthopaedics/[edited by] George Bentley, Robert B. Greer III.
        1. Surgery, Operative. I. Rob, Charles.
II. Dudley, Hugh A.F. (Hugh Arnold Freeman).
III. Pories, Walter J. IV. Carter, David C. (David Craig). V. Operative surgery. [DNLM: 1. Surgery, Operative. I. Smith of Marlow, Rodney Smith, Baron, 1914-   .WO 500 061 1982]
    RD32.06   1983   617'.91   83-14465

Contributors

C. E. Ackroyd MA, FRCS
Consultant Orthopaedic Surgeon, Southmead Hospital, Bristol, UK

J. Crawford Adams MD, MS, FRCS
Consulting Orthopaedic Surgeon, St Mary's Hospital, London, UK

Paul Aichroth MS, FRCS
Consultant Orthopaedic Surgeon, Westminster Hospital and Westminster Children's Hospital, London and Queen Mary's Hospital, Roehampton, UK

Peter C. Amadio MD
Assistant Professor of Clinical Orthopaedics, SUNY, Stony Brook, and Active Staff, St. John's Episcopal Hospital, Smithtown, New York, USA

J. C. Angel FRCS
Consultant Orthopaedic Surgeon, Royal National Orthopaedic and Edgware General Hospitals, Middlesex, UK

G. C. Bannister MChOrth, FRCS
Consultant Senior Lecturer, Southmead Hospital, Bristol, UK

N. J. Barton FRCS
Consultant Hand Surgeon, Nottingham University Hospital and Harlow Wood Orthopaedic Hospital, Mansfield, Nottinghamshire, UK

E. H. Bates FRCS, FRACS
Chairman, Section of Orthopaedics, Prince of Wales Children's Hospital, Sydney, Australia

J. I. L. Bayley FRCS
Consultant Orthopaedic Surgeon, Royal National Orthopaedic Hospital, Stanmore, Middlesex, UK

Sir George Bedbrook OBE, OStJ, MS(Melb), HonMD(WA), HonFRCS(Ed), HonDTech(Wait), FRCS, FRACS, DPRM(Syd), FCRM(Hon)
Emeritus Consultant Orthopaedic Surgeon and Spinal Surgeon, Royal Perth Hospital and Spinal Unit, Royal Perth Rehabilitation Hospital, Western Australia

George Bentley ChM, FRCS
Professor of Orthopaedic Surgery, The Institute of Orthopaedics, University of London; Honorary Consultant Orthopaedic Surgeon, The Royal National Orthopaedic Hospital, Stanmore, Middlesex, and the Middlesex Hospital, London, UK

Rolfe Birch MChir, FRCS
Consultant Orthopaedic Surgeon, St. Mary's Hospital, London and The Royal National Orthopaedic Hospital, Stanmore, Middlesex, UK

M. D. Brough MA, FRCS
Consultant Plastic Surgeon, University College Hospital, Royal Free Hospital, Whittington Hospital and Royal Northern Hospital, London, UK

Paul T. Calvert MA, FRCS
Consultant Orthopaedic Surgeon, St George's Hospital, Blackshaw Road, London, UK

A. Catterall MChir, FRCS
Consultant Orthopaedic Surgeon, Charing Cross Hospital, London, and Royal National Orthopaedic Hospital, Stanmore, Middlesex, UK

The late Sir John Charnley CBE, FRS, FRCS, FACS
Formerly Emeritus Professor of Orthopaedic Surgery, University of Manchester; Honorary Orthopaedic Surgeon, Centre for Hip Surgery, Wrightington Hospital, Wigan; Consultant Orthopaedic Surgeon, King Edward VII Hospital, Midhurst, Sussex, UK

S. C. Chen FRCS
Consultant Orthopaedic Surgeon, Enfield Group of Hospitals, Middlesex, UK

Neil Citron MChir, FRCS
Consultant Orthopaedic Surgeon, St Helier's Hospital, Carshalton, Surrey, UK

C. L. Colton FRCS, FRCS(Ed)
Consultant Orthopaedic Surgeon, University Hospital, Queen's Medical Centre, Nottingham, UK

H. V. Crock AO, MD, MS, FRCS, FRACS
Honorary Consultant, Royal Postgraduate Medical School, Hammersmith Hospital, London, UK

H. Alan Crockard FRCS, FRCS(Ed)
Consultant Neurosurgeon, The National Hospitals for Nervous Diseases, Maida Vale, London, UK

James E. Culver MD
Head, Section of Hand Surgery, Department of Orthopaedic Surgery, Cleveland Clinic Foundation, Cleveland, Ohio, USA

J. C. Dorgan MCh Orth, FRCS
Consultant Orthopaedic Surgeon, Royal Liverpool Childrens Hospital and Royal Liverpool Hospital, Liverpool, UK

G. S. E. Dowd MD, MChOrth, FRCS
Consultant Orthopaedic Surgeon, St Bartholomew's and Homerton Hospitals, London, UK

R. B. Duthie CBE, MA, ChM, FRCS
Nuffield Professor of Orthopaedic Surgery, Nuffield Department of Orthopaedic Surgery, University of Oxford, UK

Michael Edgar MChir, FRCS
Consultant Orthopaedic Surgeon, The Middlesex Hospital, London, and The Royal National Orthopaedic Hospital, Stanmore, Middlesex, UK

Philip M. Faris MD
Clinical Associate Professor, Department of Orthopaedic Surgery, Louisiana State University Medical Center, USA

Malcolm W. Fidler MS, FRCS
Consultant Orthopaedic Surgeon, Onze Lieve Vrouwe Gasthuis and Netherlands Cancer Institute, Amsterdam, The Netherlands

J. A. Fixsen MChir, FRCS
Consultant Orthopaedic Surgeon, The Hospital for Sick Children, Great Ormond Street and St Bartholomew's Hospital, London, UK

Anthony J. B. Fogg FRCS
Consultant Orthopaedic Surgeon, Princess Margaret Hospital, Swindon, UK

Mark C. Gebhardt MD
Assistant Professor of Orthopaedic Surgery, Harvard Medical School, Massachusetts General Hospital and the Children's Hospital, Boston, Massachusetts, USA

William N. Gilmour FRCS, FRACS
Emeritus Consultant Surgeon, Royal Perth Hospital and Princess Margaret Hospital for Children, Perth, Australia

M. J. Griffith MChOrth, FRCS, FRCS(Ed)
Consultant Orthopaedic Surgeon, West Wales General Hospital, Carmarthen, UK

David L. Hamblen PhD, FRCS
Professor of Orthopaedic Surgery, Western Infirmary, Glasgow, UK

Philip H. Hardcastle FRCS(Ed), FRACS
Consultant Surgeon, Spinal Unit, Royal Perth Rehabilitation Hospital, Perth, Western Australia

Kevin Hardinge MChOrth, FRCS
Hunterian Professor, Royal College of Surgeons of England; Honorary Lecturer, Victoria University of Manchester; Consultant Orthopaedic Surgeon, Centre for Hip Surgery, Wrightington Hospital, Wigan, UK

Michael H. Heckman MD
Consultant Surgeon, South Texas Sports Medicine and Orthopaedics, Corpus Christi, Texas; and Department of Orthopaedic Surgery, University of Texas Health Science Center, San Antonio, Texas, USA

B. Helal MChOrth, FRCS
Honorary Consultant Orthopaedic Surgeon, The Royal London Hospital and the Royal National Orthopaedic Hospital, London, and Enfield Group of Hospitals, Middlesex, UK

Adrian N. Henry MCh, FRCS, FRCSI
Formerly Senior Consultant Orthopaedic Surgeon, Guy's Hospital, London, UK

Sean P. F. Hughes MS, FRCS
Professor of Orthopaedic Surgery, University of Edinburgh; Clinical Research Unit, Princess Margaret Rose Orthopaedic Hospital, Edinburgh, UK

James M. Hunter MD
Clinical Professor of Orthopaedic Surgery, Thomas Jefferson University and Chief, Hand Surgery Service, Department of Orthopaedics, Thomas Jefferson Hospital, Philadelphia, Pennsylvania, USA

John N. Insall MD
Professor of Orthopaedic Surgery, Cornell University Medical College and Director, The Knee Service, The Hospital for Special Surgery, New York, USA

Andrew M. Jackson FRCS
Consultant Orthopaedic Surgeon, University College Hospital and The Hospital for Sick Children, Great Ormond Street, London, UK

J. P. Jackson FRCS
Emeritus Orthopaedic Surgeon, University Hospital, Nottingham and Harlow Wood Orthopaedic Hospital, Mansfield, Nottinghamshire, UK

Robert W. Jackson MD, MS(Tor), FRCS(C)
Chief of Staff/Surgery, Orthopaedic and Arthritic Hospital, 43 Wellesley Street East, Toronto and Professor of Surgery, University of Toronto, Toronto, Canada

Julian Jessop FRCS
Lecturer, University Department of Orthopaedic Surgery, The Institute of Orthopaedics, Royal National Orthopaedic Hospital, Stanmore, Middlesex, UK

H. B. S. Kemp MS, FRCS
Consultant Orthopaedic Surgeon, The Middlesex Hospital, London and The Royal National Orthopaedic Hospital, Stanmore, Middlesex, UK

J. Kenwright FRCS
Consultant Orthopaedic Surgeon, The Nuffield Orthopaedic Centre, Oxford, UK

Kevin King FRCS, FRACS
Director, Department of Orthopaedic Surgery, The Royal Melbourne Hospital, Victoria, Australia

E. O'Gorman Kirwan FRCS, FRCS(Ed)
Consultant Orthopaedic Surgeon, University College Hospital, and Royal National Orthopaedic Hospital, London, UK

Leslie Klenerman ChM, FRCS
Professor and Head of University Department of Orthopaedic and Accident Surgery, Royal Liverpool Hospital, Liverpool, UK

Sanford S. Kunkel MD
Orthopaedic Surgeon, Methodist Hospital, Indiana, USA

V. G. Langkamer FRCS
Orthopaedic Registrar, Southmead Hospital, Bristol, UK

R. J. Langstaff
Honorary Senior Registrar, University Hospital, Queen's Medical Centre, Nottingham, UK; Senior Specialist (Orthopaedics), Royal Air Force Medical Services

Robert D. Leffert MD
Associate Professor of Orthopaedic Surgery, Harvard Medical School; Chief of Surgical Upper Extremity Rehabilitation Unit and Department of Rehabilitation Medicine, White 10, Massachusetts General Hospital, Boston, Massachusetts 02114, USA

John C. Y. Leong FRCS, FRCS(Ed), FRACS
Professor of Orthopaedic Surgery, University of Hong Kong

I. J. Leslie MChOrth, FRCS
Department of Orthopaedic and Traumatic Surgery, Bristol Royal Infirmary, Bristol, UK

E. Letournel MD
Professor of Orthopaedic Surgery and Traumatology, Centre Medico-Chirurgical de la Porte de Choisy, Paris, France

Alan Lettin MS, FRCS
Consultant Orthopaedic Surgeon, St Bartholomew's Hospital, London and Royal National Orthopaedic Hospital, Stanmore, Middlesex, UK

P. S. London MBE, FRCS, MFOM, FACEM(Hon)
Formerly Surgeon, Birmingham Accident Hospital, Birmingham, UK

J. S. P. Lumley MS, FRCS, FMAA(Hon), FGA
Professor of Vascular Surgery, St Bartholomew's Hospital, London, UK

M. F. Macnicol FRCS, MCh, FRCS Ed(Orth)
Consultant Orthopaedic Surgeon, Princess Margaret Rose Orthopaedic Hospital, Edinburgh, UK

Henry J. Mankin MD
Edith M. Ashley Professor of Orthopaedic Surgery, Harvard Medical School; Chief, Orthopaedic Service, Massachusetts General Hospital, Boston, Massachusetts, USA

R. A. B. Mollan MD, FRCS(Ed), FRCSI
Professor of Orthopaedic Surgery, Queen's University of Belfast, UK

T. R. Morley FRCS
Consultant Orthopaedic Surgeon, The Hospital for Sick Children, Great Ormond Street, London, and The Royal National Orthopaedic Hospital, Stanmore, Middlesex, UK

I. W. Nelson MA, FRCS
Clinical Lecturer, Nuffield Department of Orthopaedic Surgery, University of Oxford, UK

J. P. O'Brien PhD, FRCS(Ed), FACS, FRACS
Consultant Surgeon in Spinal Disorders, 149 Harley Street, London, UK

The late Sir Henry Osmond-Clarke KCVO, CBE, FRCS(I), FRCS
Former Orthopaedic Surgeon to Her Majesty Queen Elizabeth II; Consulting Orthopaedic Surgeon, The Royal London Hospital, London and Robert Jones and Agnes Hunt Orthopaedic Hospital, Oswestry, UK

H. Piggott FRCS
Consultant Orthopaedic Surgeon, United Birmingham Hospitals, Royal Orthopaedic Hospital, Birmingham, and Warwickshire Orthopaedic Hospital, Coleshill, Warwickshire, UK

Andrew O. Ransford FRCS
Consultant Orthopaedic Surgeon, Royal National Orthopaedic Hospital, London, UK

Harold J. Richards FRCS
Formerly Consultant in the Surgery of Orthopaedics and Trauma, University Hospital of Wales and Prince of Wales Orthopaedic Hospital, Cardiff, UK

John T. Scales OBE, FRCS, CIMechE
Emeritus Professor of Biomedical Engineering, The Royal National Orhtopaedic Hospital, Stanmore, Middlesex, UK

Thomas P. Sculco MD
The Hospital for Special Surgery, 535 East 70th Street, New York, NY 10021, USA

Campbell Semple FRCS
Consultant Hand Surgeon, Western Infirmary, Glasgow, UK

W. J. W. Sharrard MD, ChM, FRCS
Emeritus Consultant Orthopaedic Surgeon, Royal Hallamshire Hospital and Children's Hospital, Sheffield; Professor of Orthopaedic Surgery, University of Sheffield, UK

E. W. Somerville FRCS(Ed), FRCS
Emeritus Consultant Orthopaedic Surgeon, Nuffield Orthopaedic Centre, Oxford, UK

W. M. Steel FRCS(Ed)
Consultant Orthopaedic Surgeon, Department of Postgraduate Medicine, University of Keele, Hartshill, Stoke-on-Trent, UK

John D. M. Stewart MA, FRCS
Consultant Orthopaedic Surgeon, Chichester District Health Authority, West Sussex, UK

Ian Stother FRCS(Ed), FRCS(Glas)
Consultant Orthopaedic Surgeon, Glasgow Royal Infirmary and The Glasgow Nuffield Hospital, Glasgow, UK

Michael Sullivan FRCS
Consultant Orthopaedic Surgeon, Royal National Orthopaedic Hospital, London, UK

John P. W. Varian FRCS, FRACS(Orth)
Consultant Hand Surgeon, Blackrock Clinic, Dublin, Ireland

William Angus Wallace FRCS(Ed), FRCS(Ed)Orth
Professor of Orthopaedic and Accident Surgery, University of Nottingham, Queen's Medical Centre, Nottingham, UK

W. Waugh MChir, FRCS
Emeritus Professor of Orthopaedic and Accident Surgery, University of Nottingham; Honorary Consultant Orthopaedic Surgeon, Harlow Wood Orthopaedic Hospital, Mansfield, Nottinghamshire, UK

Paul C. Weaver MD, FRCS, FRCS(Ed)
Consultant Surgeon (Surgical Oncology), Portsmouth and South East Hampshire Group of Hospitals, Portsmouth; Clinical Teacher, University of Southampton, UK

J. K. Webb FRCS
Consultant Orthopaedic Surgeon, University Hospital, Queen's Medical Centre, Nottingham, UK

P. J. Webb FRCS
Consultant Orthopaedic Surgeon, The Hospital For Sick Children, Great Ormond Street, London, and The Royal National Orthopaedic Hospital, Stanmore, Middlesex, UK

Thomas E. Whitesides Jr MD
Professor of Orthopaedics, Department of Orthopaedic Surgery, Emory University School of Medicine, Atlanta, Georgia, USA

Alan H. Wilde MD
Chairman, Department of Orthopaedic Surgery and Head, Section of Rheumatoid Surgery, Cleveland Clinic Foundation, Cleveland, Ohio, USA

Russell E. Windsor MD
Assistant Professor, Department of Orthopaedic Surgery, Cornell University Medical College; Assistant Attending Orthopaedic Surgeon, The Hospital for Special Surgery and The New York Hospital, New York, USA

Robert E. Zickel MD
Clinical Professor of Orthopaedic Surgery, Columbia University, New York, USA

Contributing Medical Artists

G. Bartlett

L. Butler
Medical Illustrator, 46 Selworthy House, Battersea Church Road, London SW11 3NG, UK

Laurel L. Cook
Medical Illustrator, Medical Graphics, 69 Revere Street, Boston, Massachusetts 02 114, USA

Michael J. Courtney

Peter Cox MMAA, AIMI, RDD
Medical Illustrator/Graphic Designer, 2 Frome Villas, Frenchay, Bristol BS16 1LT, UK

Laura Pardi Duprey
146 H. Union Avenue, Rutherford, New Jersey 07070, USA

Patrick Elliott BA(Hons) ATC, AIMI
Senior Medical Artist, Department of Medical Illustration, Royal Hallamshire Hospital, Glossop Road, Sheffield S10 3QX, UK

D. Howat
Medical Illustrator, 688 Orrang Road, Toorak, Victoria, Australia

Mark Iley
Illustrator, 12 High Street, Great Missenden, Bucks HP16 9AB, UK

Donn Johnson
Veterans Administration Medical Center, Atlanta, Georgia, USA

T. King

The late Robert Lane
Medical Illustrator, Studio 19A, Edith Grove, London SW10, UK

Gillian Lee FMAA, AIMI, AMI, RMIP
Medical Illustrator, 15 Little Plucketts Way, Buckhurst Hill, Essex IG9 5QU, UK

Geoffrey Lyth FA, BA, FMAA
Abbey View, Sneaton, Nr Whitby, North Yorkshire YO22 5HS, UK

Gillian Oliver MMAA, AIMI, FTF
Freelance Medical Illustrator, 15 Bramble Road, Hatfield, Hertfordshire AL10 9RZ, UK

J. A. Pangrace AMI
Medical Illustrator, 9500 Euclid Avenue, Cleveland, Ohio 44195, USA

R. C. Pearson
Medical Illustrator, Department of Photography and Medical Illustration, Robert Jones and Agnes Hunt Orthopaedic Hospital, Oswestry, Shropshire, UK

F. Price

Paul Richardson
6 Crofton Road, Orpington, Kent BR6 8AF, UK

Adrian Shaw
Medical Illustrator, 138 Penylan Road, Cardiff CF2 5RE, UK

William Thackeray
Medical Illustrator, 117 Oliphant Avenue, Dobbs Ferry, New York 10522, USA

Philip Wilson FMAA, AIMI, FTF
Freelance Medical Artist, 23 Normanhurst Road, St Paul's Cray, Orpington, Kent BR5 3AL, UK

Anthony C. S. Yiu
Medical Illustration Unit, University of Hong Kong, Pokfulam, Hong Kong

Department of Medical Illustration
Western Infirmary, Glasgow, UK

Contents

	Preface	xxi
Repair of musculoskeletal tissues	Emergency skin cover in orthopaedics M. D. Brough	1
	Tendon repair, replacement and transfer B. Helal S. C. Chen	16
	Repair of divided peripheral nerves Rolfe Birch	24
	Vascular injury and repair J. S. P. Lumley	39
Infections	Surgical management of acute bone and joint infections M. F. Macnicol	54
	Chronic infections of bone and joint R. A. B. Mollan	61
Arthropathies	Swanson arthroplasty of the metacarpophalangeal joint for rheumatoid disease James E. Culver	68
	Synovectomy of the elbow for rheumatoid disease Alan H. Wilde	73
	Surgical procedures in haemophilia R. B. Duthie I. W. Nelson	77
Bone biopsy	Techniques of bone biopsy Mark C. Gebhardt Henry J. Mankin	91
Fracture treatment	Principles of fracture management C. E. Ackroyd	100

	Traction treatment of fractures John D. M. Stewart	123
	External skeletal fixation J. Kenwright	145
Upper limb fractures	**Fractures of the long bones of the upper limb** Paul T. Calvert	153
	Fractures at the elbow in adults G. S. E. Dowd	165
	Operative treatment of fractures of the hand N. J. Barton	175
	Primary treatment of the acutely injured hand Campbell Semple	188
Lower limb fractures	**Intracapsular fractures of the neck of the femur** C. E. Ackroyd G. C. Bannister V. G. Langkamer	199
	Trochanteric fractures of the femur G. C. Bannister C. E. Ackroyd V. G. Langkamer	209
	Subtrochanteric fractures of the femur: Zickel nail fixation Robert E. Zickel	216
	Küntscher's closed intramedullary nailing technique for the treatment of femoral shaft fractures Kevin F. King	223
	Supracondylar fractures of the femur C. E. Ackroyd	242
	Fractures of the patella V. G. Langkamer C. E. Ackroyd	252
	Tibial plateau fractures J. K. Webb	256
	Management of tibial shaft fractures J. K. Webb R. J. Langstaff	268
	Fractures of the ankle C. L. Colton C. E. Ackroyd	284

	Recognition and treatment of compartment compression syndromes Thomas E. Whitesides Jr Michael H. Heckman	295
	Fractures and dislocations in the foot P. S. London	309
Pelvis and acetabulum	**Displays, correction and fixation of stove-in hip joints** E. Letournel	321
	Replacement and fixation of the posterior lip of the acetabulum E. Letournel	339
	Exposure and fixation of disrupted pubic symphysis E. Letournel	346
Fractures in children	**Operative treatment of children's fractures** I. J. Leslie	351
Delayed union, non-union and malunion	**Delayed union, non-union and malunion of long-bone fractures** G. S. E. Dowd George Bentley	369
Metastatic disease	**Metastatic bone disease in the limb** Malcolm W. Fidler	384
Amputations	**General principles of amputation surgery** J. C. Angel	397
	Amputation through the upper limb J. C. Angel	402
	Forequarter amputation Paul C. Weaver	409
	Hindquarter amputation Paul C. Weaver	414
	Disarticulation of the hip J. C. Angel	419
	Above-knee amputation J. C. Angel	422
	Disarticulation at the knee J. C. Angel	427

	Below-knee amputation J. C. Angel	431
	Syme's amputation J. C. Angel	437
	Transmetatarsal amputation J. C. Angel	441
	Amputation of the toes J. C. Angel	444
Cervical spine	**Axillary approach for thoracic outlet syndrome** Robert D. Leffert	447
	Transoral approach to the cervical spine H. Alan Crockard Andrew O. Ransford	453
	Anterior fusion of the cervical spine David L. Hamblen	463
	Posterior fusions of the cervical spine David L. Hamblen	471
Thoracic and lumbar spine	**Halofemoral traction** J. C. Dorgan	482
	The halo–body cast Sean P. F. Hughes	486
	Posterior procedures for idiopathic scoliosis Michael Edgar	491
	Anterior procedures for spinal deformity T. R. Morley P. J. Webb	504
	Luque instrumentation for neuromuscular scoliosis George Bentley Julian Jessop	512
	Surgical management of lumbar disc prolapses H. V. Crock	517
	Chemonucleolysis for herniated intervertebral disc Michael Sullivan	530
	Posterior decompression for spinal stenosis Michael Sullivan	534
	Posterior lumbar spinal fusion E. O'Gorman Kirwan	539

	Intertransverse fusion for spondylolisthesis and lumbar instability E. O'Gorman Kirwan	545
	Surgical reduction of severe spondylolisthesis J. P. O'Brien	549
	Operations for infections of the spine John C. Y. Leong	559
	Metastatic bone disease of the spine Malcolm W. Fidler	571
	Approaches to the spine J. K. Webb	597
	Spinal injuries Sir George Bedbrook Philip H. Hardcastle	624
Shoulder	**Recurrent anterior dislocation of the shoulder** William Angus Wallace	671
	Injuries of the acromioclavicular joint William Angus Wallace	686
	Arthroscopy of the shoulder J. I. L. Bayley	692
	Rotator cuff repair J. I. L. Bayley	697
	Operations for Erb's palsy B. Helal S. C. Chen	705
	Rupture of the biceps B. Helal S. C. Chen	709
	Arthroplasty of the shoulder Alan Lettin	713
	Arthrodesis of the shoulder The late Sir Henry Osmond-Clarke	721
Elbow	**Prosthetic replacement of the elbow** Thomas P. Sculco Philip M. Faris	729
	Tendon replacement to restore elbow flexion B. Helal S. C. Chen	736

Forearm, wrist and hand

Tendon reconstruction in the forearm B. Helal S. C. Chen	745
Surgery of the wrist I. J. Leslie	765
Tendon transfer for mobile radial deviation of the wrist B. Helal S. C. Chen	805
Tendon injuries in the hand John P. W. Varian	808
Primary repair of the divided digital flexor tendon Harold J. Richards	828
Two-stage tendon reconstruction using gliding tendon implants James M. Hunter Peter C. Amadio	836
Dupuytren's contracture W. M. Steel	855
Trigger finger and thumb Neil Citron	865

Pelvis and hip

Operations for congenital dislocation of the hip A. Catterall	870
Innominate osteotomy A. Catterall	893
High femoral osteotomy in childhood E. W. Somerville	900
Slipped upper femoral epiphysis M. J. Griffith	909
Correction of flexion contracture of the hip B. Helal S. C. Chen	921
Adductor release (with or without partial anterior obturator neurectomy) W. J. W. Sharrard	926
Hip flexor release: iliofemoral approach W. J. W. Sharrard	931
Iliopsoas tendon lengthening or recession: medial (Ludloff) approach W. J. W. Sharrard	936

	Proximal hamstring release W. J. W. Sharrard	940
	Total hip replacement arthroplasty Kevin Hardinge	943
	Girdlestone's pseudarthrosis of the hip E. W. Somerville	965
	Arthrodesis of the hip J. Crawford Adams	970
Thigh and knee	**Distal hamstring release** W. J. W. Sharrard	981
	Transfer of the hamstrings to the quadriceps in the adult J. A. Fixsen	985
	Proximal gastrocnemius release W. J. W. Sharrard	989
	Supracondylar osteotomy of the femur J. A. Fixsen	992
	Rupture of the quadriceps mechanism B. Helal S. C. Chen	995
	Quadricepsplasty in the adult J. A. Fixsen	1003
	Diagnostic arthroscopy of the knee George Bentley Anthony J. B. Fogg	1007
	Arthroscopic surgical procedures Ian Stother	1019
	Arthroscopic meniscectomy Ian Stother	1043
	Arthroscopic meniscal repair Robert W. Jackson Sanford S. Kunkel	1056
	Open meniscectomy of the knee Adrian N. Henry	1062
	Loose bodies in the knee Paul Aichroth	1073
	Repair and reconstruction of knee ligament injury Paul Aichroth	1079

	Recurrent dislocation of the patella Paul Aichroth	**1102**
	Synovectomy of the knee W. Waugh	**1109**
	Tibial osteotomy for arthritis of the knee J. P. Jackson	**1113**
	Arthroplasty of the knee Russell E. Windsor John N. Insall	**1119**
	Compression arthrodesis of the knee The late Sir John Charnley	**1131**
	Massive replacement for tumours of the lower limb H. B. S. Kemp John T. Scales	**1137**
Leg and foot	**Treatment of leg length inequality** Andrew M. Jackson	**1152**
	Distal gastrocnemius release W. J. W. Sharrard	**1169**
	Lengthening and repair of the tendo Achillis B. Helal S. C. Chen	**1172**
	Transfer of tibialis posterior tendon to the dorsum of the foot B. Helal S. C. Chen	**1184**
	Multiple tendon transfers into the heel E. W. Somerville	**1187**
	Arthrodeses of the ankle E. W. Somerville	**1191**
	Arthrodeses of the foot E. W. Somerville	**1199**
	Wedge tarsectomy E. W. Somerville	**1208**
	Operations for flat foot and pes cavus Leslie Klenerman	**1211**
	Operations for congenital talipes equinovarus E. H. Bates	**1220**

The Robert Jones operation for clawing of hallux B. Helal S. C. Chen	**1227**
Flexor to extensor transfer for clawing of the lateral four toes (Girdlestone's operation) B. Helal S. C. Chen	**1230**
Forefoot reconstruction B. Helal S. C. Chen	**1232**
Hallux valgus and hallux rigidus H. Piggott	**1244**
Dorsal nerve transfer for plantar digital neuroma (Morton's metatarsalgia) W. N. Gilmour	**1255**
Hammer and mallet toe H. Piggott	**1259**
Subluxation of the lesser metatarsophalangeal joints H. Piggott	**1263**
Dorsally displaced fifth toe H. Piggott	**1267**
Ingrowing toe-nail H. Piggott	**1270**
Index	**1273**

Preface

The 10 years that have elapsed since the publication of the third edition of *Orthopaedics* have seen the most exciting developments in the applied science of operative surgery. This new edition aims to reflect these changes and to present in a concise manner the indications for operative treatment of all common orthopaedic conditions that face the contemporary practising surgeon. New procedures are described to reflect the speed of change in the subject where these are considered to be established. Important non-operative techniques such as traction methods are covered also.

All the chapters have been rewritten and 31 new chapters have been added: seven on important general subjects such as musculoskeletal infections, management of primary and secondary tumours and arthritis, nine on the spine, six on the upper limb and hand, three on the knee, three on foot surgery, and three on fracture management. A few classic procedures such as arthrodesis of the shoulder and knee are retained because of their international importance and the principles they embody. Each author has presented his subject in his personal style but the form of illustrations has been standardized and improved.

The needs of the orthopaedic trainee and young consultants in practice have been foremost in preparing this edition; but the experienced surgeon will find much useful information, especially when faced with some of the less common procedures that occur in any busy practice.

The restructuring of this edition has involved many colleagues to whom we are deeply indebted. In particular Chris Russell, Julian Jessop and Chris Lavy have provided invaluable help. Mary Bramwell made the completion of the task possible. As before the staff of Butterworth–Heinemann provided their expertise and have been unfailingly helpful.

George Bentley
Robert B. Greer III

Illustrations by Gillian Oliver

Emergency skin cover in orthopaedics

M. D. Brough MA, FRCS
Consultant Plastic Surgeon, University College Hospital, Royal Free Hospital, Whittington Hospital and Royal Northern Hospital, London, UK

Introduction

Closure of open wounds is required to retain the integrity of skin cover of the body. It will prevent penetration of infection and encourage early healing of the wound.

All open wounds should be treated as an emergency, cleaned and debrided. Simple wounds should be repaired primarily; but while immediate skin cover is usually desirable, only rarely is it essential. Vital structures such as nerves and vessels which are exposed must be covered; but provided adequate debridement is carried out, a simple clean dressing is often adequate and sometimes preferable in covering a compound wound for the first 24 or 48 hours. Definitive skin cover can then be provided in more favourable circumstances.

A careful history of the nature of the injury, together with a critical examination of the wound, will usually establish whether or not there has been skin loss. If significant skin loss has occurred a skin graft or skin flap, or both, will be required to obtain complete skin cover.

2 Repair of musculoskeletal tissues

Primary procedure

Debridement

1

All wounds must be cleaned before closure. Simple uncontaminated lacerations may require only washing and irrigation with a simple detergent. Many wounds are contaminated with foreign bodies and these must be removed. Ingrained dirt or gravel in the skin must be removed, using a scrubbing brush if necessary, as it may cause permanent tattooing which can be difficult to remove later. All necrotic tissue and tissue of doubtful viability should be excised. Irregular skin edges should be trimmed. When surgical debridement is complete the wound should be irrigated liberally with appropriate detergent or saline. All patients should have appropriate tetanus prophylaxis.

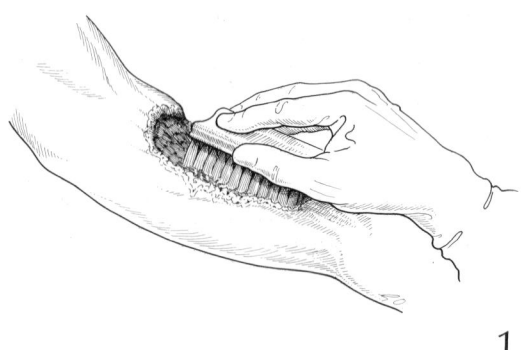

Sutures

2

Wounds should be closed in layers using interrupted absorbable sutures in the deep layers to obliterate any dead space. The skin should be closed with interrupted nylon sutures, although occasionally in clean wounds a subcuticular suture can be used to provide a better cosmetic result. Wounds should not be closed under tension in an emergency.

Drains

Vacuum drains should be used if there is concern about haemostasis. Plastic or rubber drains should be used if there is concern about infection.

LACERATIONS

Simple lacerations should be cleaned and examined carefully for damage to underlying structures which should be repaired. Irregular skin edges should be excised. Skin and subcutaneous fat should be undermined around the peripheral margin and the wound closed in layers.

CRUSH INJURIES

3

Damage caused by crush injuries is often difficult to assess. If there is any doubt, the wound should be cleaned and debrided and a simple dressing applied without inserting any sutures. The patient is returned to theatre after 24 or 48 hours and the wound reassessed. Viable tissue can now be sutured safely.

It has been common practice in the past to perform relieving incisions on the lower limbs in order to achieve skin closure over exposed bone. This procedure is mentioned only to be condemned as this may jeopardize the use of local flaps later.

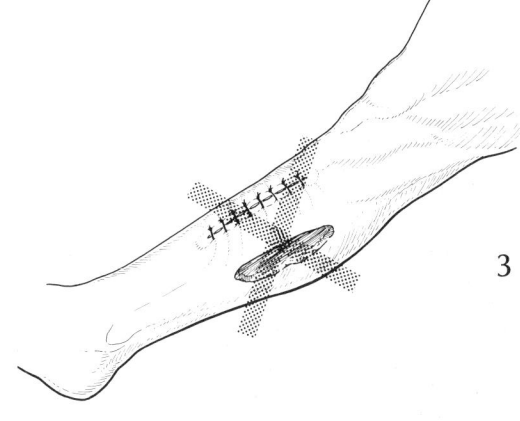

GUNSHOT INJURIES

4

These wounds are always very much more extensive than they appear. As a bullet penetrates tissue it slows down, dissipating heat which destroys local tissue. The extent of tissue damage may be considerable. Gunshot wounds should never be closed primarily and in most instances the track of the bullet should be laid open for several days. Damaged and necrotic tissue can then be debrided before wound closure.

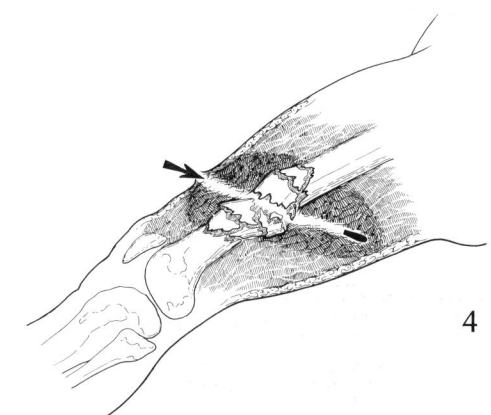

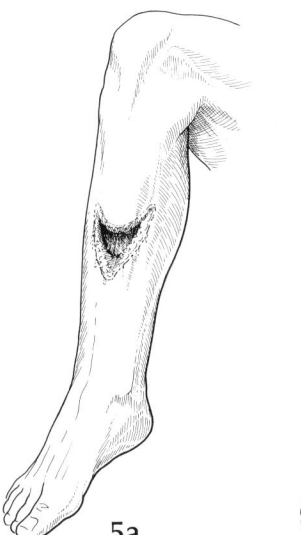
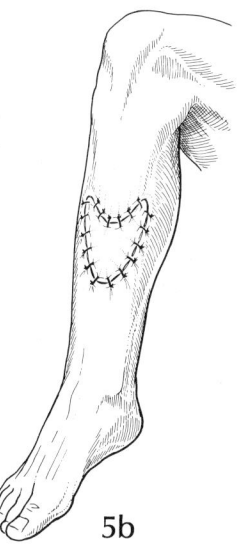

AVULSION FLAPS

5a & b

These are caused by a shearing force which is not at right angles to the skin. Usually a flap of skin and subcutaneous tissue, often triangular in shape, is elevated from the underlying deep fascia. A common site for this injury is the front of the leg. Survival of the flap may depend on several factors, including the extent of associated damage, the length of the flap related to the base, the age and nutritional state of the patient, and the previous use of steroids. If the flap is viable it should be carefully resutured but if non-viable tissue is evident this must be excised and the residual defect grafted. A mesh graft is often suitable. If the patient is elderly and debilitated it is worth considering treating the wound conservatively, with dressings after debridement.

DEGLOVING INJURIES

6

These injuries commonly occur from a shearing force of a large wheel on a limb at a relatively low velocity. The skin is sheared away from the deep fascia and loses its blood supply. The extent of tissue necrosis is notoriously difficult to assess at the primary procedure. An injection of fluorescein may be useful; but if in doubt, all undermined skin should be excised and the defect grafted. Alternatively, only obviously devitalized skin is excised primarily and the wound dressed. The patient is returned to theatre 24 hours later when a further assessment of the residual skin is made and debridement and grafting are then performed.

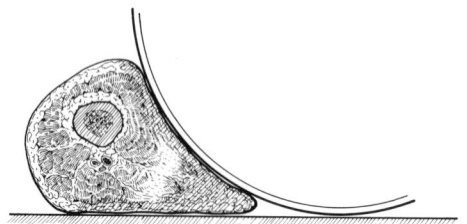

SPECIAL AREAS

Face

Debridement must be conservative but all foreign bodies must be removed as tattooing from dirt may be very disfiguring later. All structures must be replaced meticulously in their original places. Fine sutures are used for the skin and removed within four days. If skin loss is evident, expert advice should be sought.

Hand

Primary skin cover in the hand is required more often than elsewhere, particularly when deep structures such as tendons have been exposed or repaired. Skin grafts and local flaps can be used for small defects but regional or free flaps may be needed for extensive skin loss.

Sole of the foot

Debridement of this highly specialized skin should be conservative in the primary procedure.

Skin loss

When skin loss has occurred to an extent that primary closure of the wound is not possible, the defect should normally be covered with a split-skin graft. Full-thickness skin grafts are seldom used except on the face, as these require closure of the donor defect and are less reliable in taking. Skin flaps which take their blood supply with them are used for covering bone without periosteum, tendon without paratenon, exposed nerves and vessels and open joints.

SPLIT-SKIN GRAFTS

7

Split-skin grafts are usually taken from the thigh. Here a large area of skin is available from which a graft is readily harvested. The inner aspect of the thigh is usually used in young people so that the donor site is inconspicuous. The outer aspect of the thigh is used in the elderly where a slow healing wound is more easily managed.

To harvest a graft the assistant supports the thigh from beneath and compresses the soft tissues to put the skin under tension. The donor skin is put under further tension by stretching it with two boards held by the surgeon and the assistant respectively. The graft is then cut using a rapid shearing movement of the graft knife with slow advancement of the cutting edge. When sufficient skin has been obtained the donor site is covered with paraffin gauze, dressing gauze, wool and a crêpe bandage. The dressing can be reduced but not completely removed after 48 hours. The paraffin gauze should be soaked off at 10–14 days.

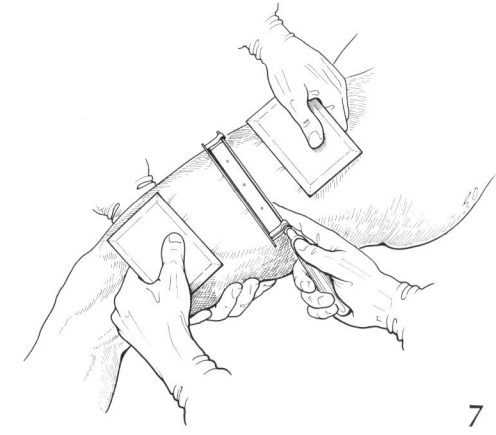

Application of skin grafts

The wound must be prepared by careful debridement and haemostasis. Muscle and fascia are well-vascularized and provide a good bed for a skin graft.

8a

The skin graft is stretched onto paraffin gauze with the epidermis against the gauze. The gauze is cut at the edge of the graft and applied in sheets to the defect. If the graft is on a convex surface, as on most parts of a limb, sutures may not be required, provided a bulky dressing is applied to immobilize the joints above and below. A plaster splint can be applied if desired. The dressing should be changed at one week.

8b

If the graft is in a concavity it should be sutured at its edges and the long suture ends should be tied together over a bolus of dressing to keep the graft applied to its bed.

Patients with skin grafts applied to the lower limb must be confined to bed for 10 days. If the limb is allowed to become dependent, the hydrostatic pressure in the limb will cause seromata to collect beneath the graft, with subsequent loss of the graft.

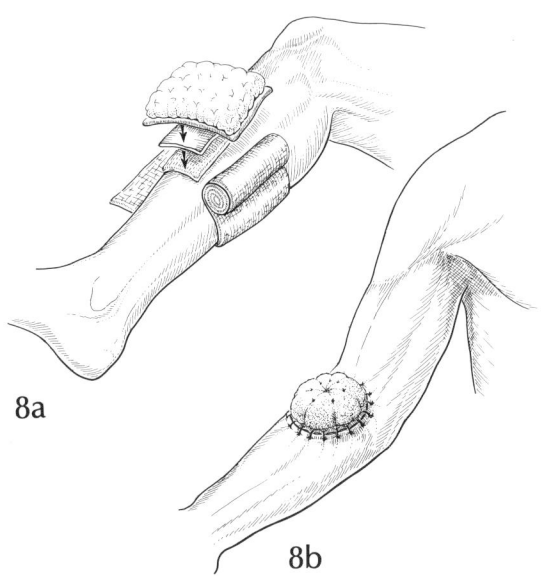

6 Repair of musculoskeletal tissues

Delayed grafting

Fat is poorly vascularized. If there is a large amount of fat at the site or if the wound has been contaminated, it should be packed with dressings of eusol and paraffin for a few days before the application of the split-skin graft.

The skin graft is harvested at the time of the primary procedure and stored at 4°C until the graft bed is ready. The graft is then applied as described above.

9

Occasionally the graft may be applied without a dressing if it is in a site which can be exposed without danger of incidental trauma, such as the front of the trunk. This has the advantage of allowing regular inspection to identify and aspirate any small seroma which may develop beneath the graft and avoids shearing forces of the dressing disturbing the graft.

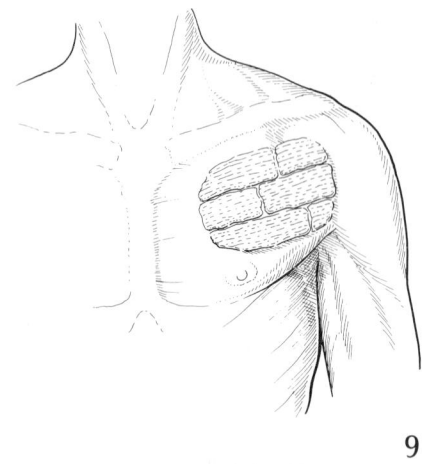

9

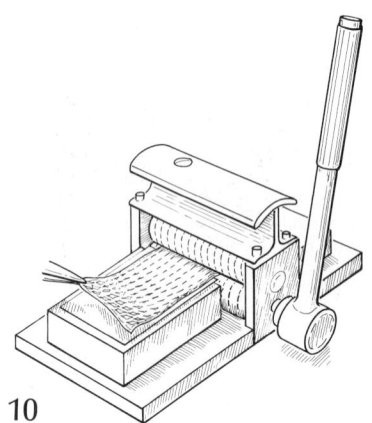

10

MESH GRAFTS

Mesh grafts are particularly useful for covering extensive defects where a limited donor site or graft is available. They are also useful in covering irregular surfaces and sites where serum may collect. Their principal disadvantage is the resultant cosmetic appearance although this does improve with time.

10

The split-skin graft is harvested in the normal way. It is then passed through the mesh dermatome. The graft is stretched over the defect and packed into any sulci to fit the irregular surface. Only rarely are sutures required and the graft is dressed as above.

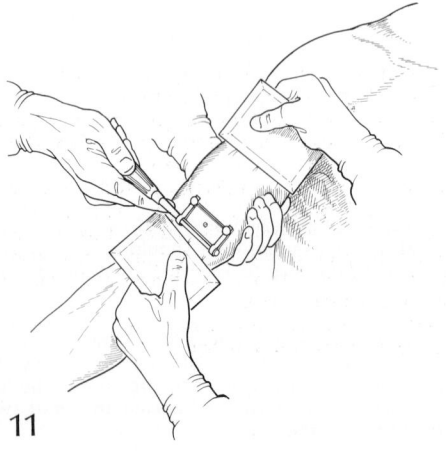

11

SMALL SPLIT-SKIN GRAFTS

11

Small split-skin grafts are often taken from the medial aspect of the arm with a Silvers knife. The donor site is covered with an appropriate smaller dressing. The forearm should not be used as a donor site as it may leave an unsightly scar.

FLAPS

12a & b

Flap tissue can be transposed from its original site to a new site provided its blood supply is retained in the pedicle by which it remains attached to the body. Skin flaps are used to cover vital structures and are not dependent on receiving a blood supply from their new bed initially, though this is often acquired later. Until recently most skin flaps used had a random-pattern blood supply; but with greater understanding of the blood supply to skin, the underlying fascia and the underlying muscles, there has been increased use of axial-pattern skin flaps, fasciocutaneous flaps, myocutaneous flaps and free flaps.

Principles of flaps

Skin flaps should be carefully planned preoperatively, particularly if a multi-staged procedure is envisaged. Care should be taken in raising the flap, and it should be remembered that flap movement is nearly always in three planes and not two. This is particularly important on limbs.

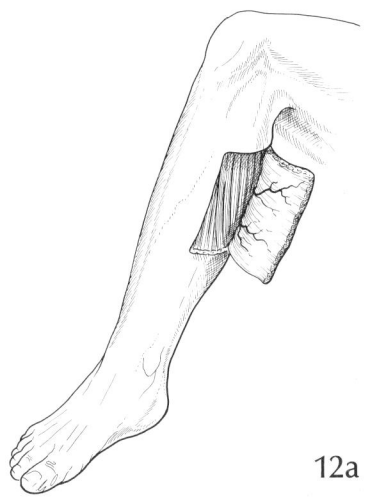

12a

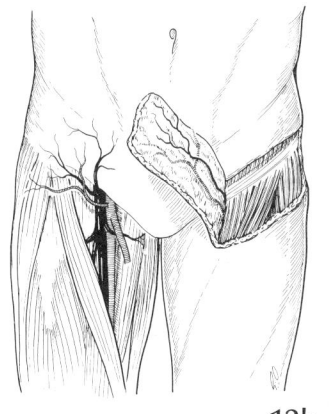

12b

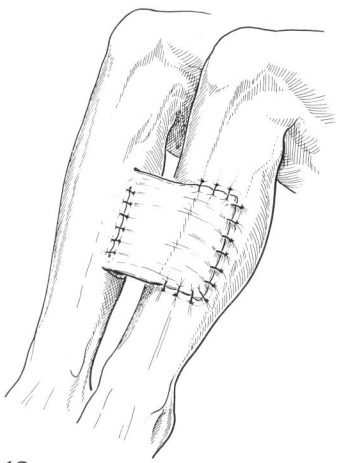

13

13

Care should be taken to avoid any adverse forces acting on the pedicle of the flap; the flap must lie comfortably without tension in its transposed position. As a general rule the defect must be increased to fit the flap. The flap must not be trimmed to fit the defect.

A delayed procedure consists of partially dividing the pedicle of the flap as well as dividing the axial vessel, if present, and then resuturing the wound. This deprivation of blood supply to the flap encourages increased blood flow to the flap from its new attachment and makes final division of the pedicle safer.

Bipolar coagulation must always be used to avoid damage to the vessels in the flap.

8 Repair of musculoskeletal tissues

LOCAL SKIN FLAPS

When treating a small defect it is often tempting to think that a small local flap can be used for cover; such procedure is hazardous for limb defects. Small local skin flaps are normally only safe in the head and neck region.

Regional and distant skin flaps

These are classified below and a description of one of each type of flap follows:

1. Abdominal tube pedicle flap
2. Cross-leg flap
3. Cutaneous axial-pattern flap
4. Fasciocutaneous flap
5. Muscle or myocutaneous flap
6. Free flap.

ABDOMINAL TUBE PEDICLE FLAP

Described first in 1917, this flap has been used extensively in reconstruction for most of this century. It is now rarely used due to the recent advent of other flaps but occasionally it is valuable when none of these are suitable.

14a–j

(a) A rectangular area of skin is marked out on the abdomen and an incision is made along the long sides, down to the deep fascia. The intervening tissue is undermined.
(b) The two skin edges are inverted and sutured together to form a tube. The secondary defect is closed primarily or grafted if necessary (see groin flap).
(c) A delayed procedure is carried out at one end after two weeks. A week later the same end is totally divided.
(d) A semicircular skin flap is raised on the contralateral wrist.
(e) It is reflected back to form a circular defect.
(f) The free end of the tube pedicle is sutured into the defect. The flap is protected with appropriate splinting.
(g) A delayed procedure is carried out weeks later at the residual abdominal attachment. A week after this, the abdominal end is detached completely and sutured to one margin of the defect to be reconstructed after the edges of both have been trimmed.
(h) A delayed procedure is carried out at the wrist at 2 weeks, and after a further week the wrist attachment is divided.
(i) This end of the tube pedicle is inserted into the opposite side of the defect to that shown in (g). The suture line of the tube must face the defect.
(j) After at least a further 3 weeks and preferably when the tube is soft, the suture line of the tube is opened and the flap sutured into the defect.

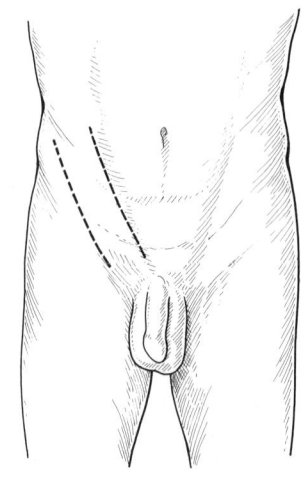

14a

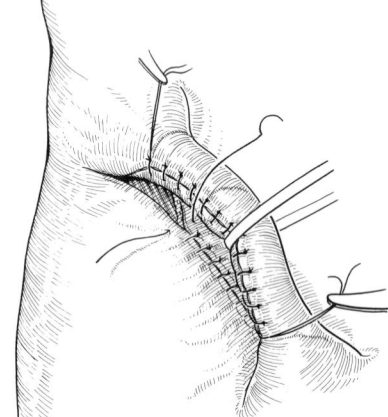

14b

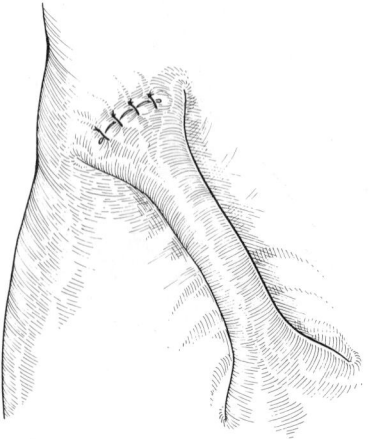

14c

Emergency skin cover in orthopaedics 9

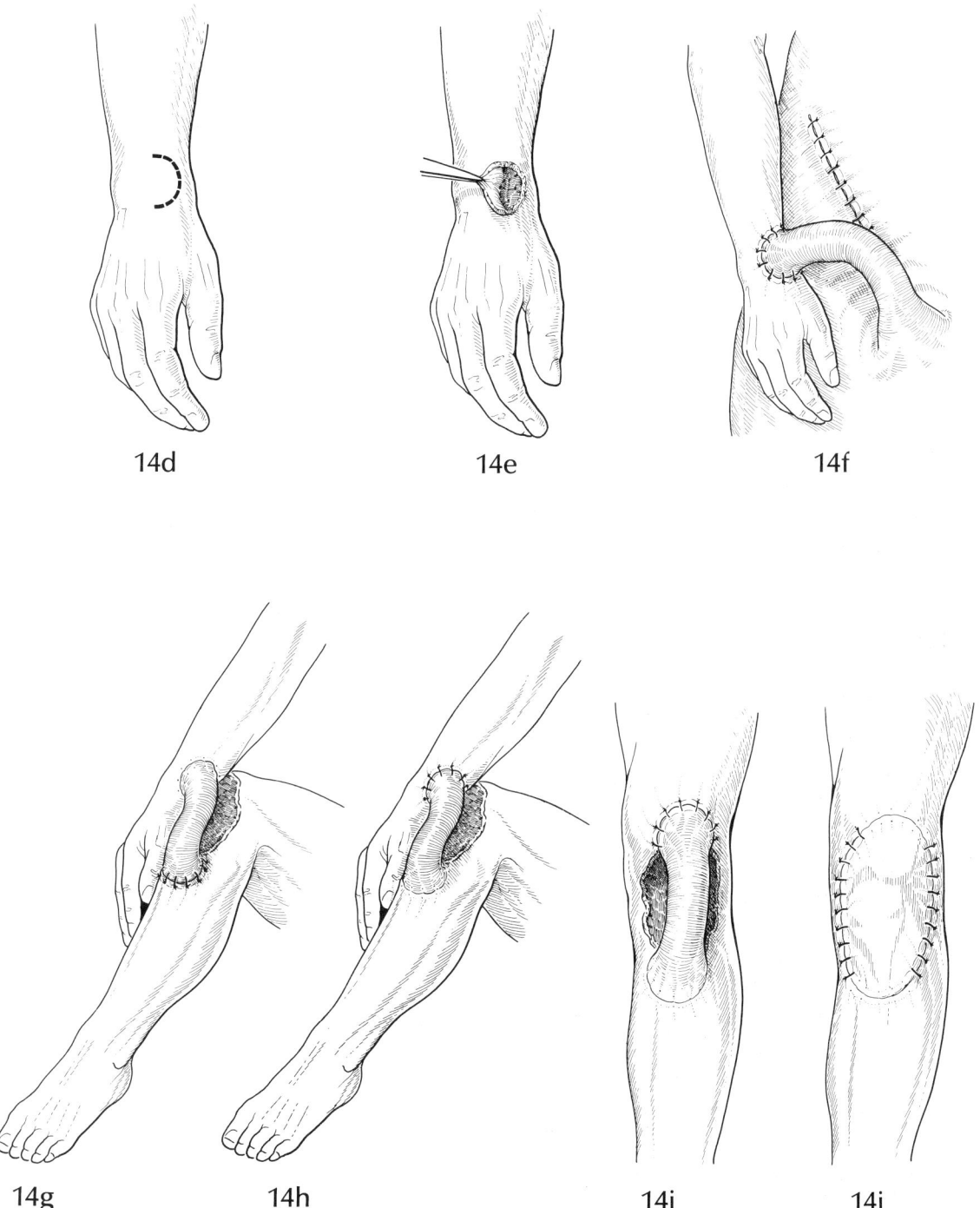

14d 14e 14f

14g 14h 14i 14j

10 Repair of musculoskeletal tissues

CROSS-LEG FLAP

15a–e

This flap used to be the standard flap for covering large defects of skin on the front of the tibia. Although it has been superseded by fasciocutaneous and myocutaneous flaps, it is still occasionally useful.

(a) Forty-eight hours before surgery the flap is planned and the patient's legs fixed in a bean bag in the planned postoperative position. This allows him to get used to this position prior to surgery and the postoperative discomfort and tendency to shift position is diminished.

(b) A rectangular flap on the back of the opposite calf is marked and elevated, together with the underlying fascia. The long saphenous vein should be preserved if possible. The defect on the recipient leg is enlarged to accommodate the flap. Split-skin grafts are used to cover the flap donor site and the under-surface of the skin bridge.

(c) The flap is sutured into the defect and the patient placed in the bean bag. Restraining bandages are applied initially, although with a cooperative patient these can be reduced and the bean bag removed temporarily after a few days to allow the wounds and grafts to be cleaned and redressed.

(d) A delayed procedure is performed at two weeks.

(e) The flap is divided and inset at three weeks.

Cross-arm and cross-thigh flaps can be designed on the same principles.

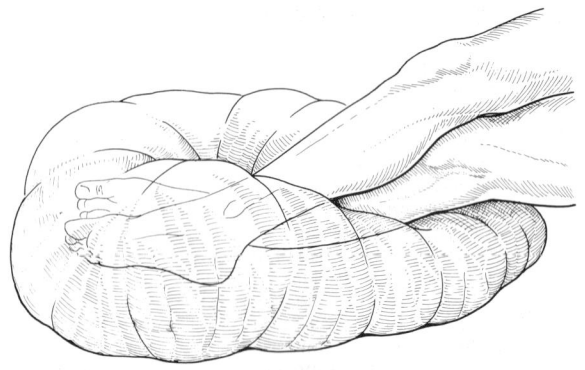

15a

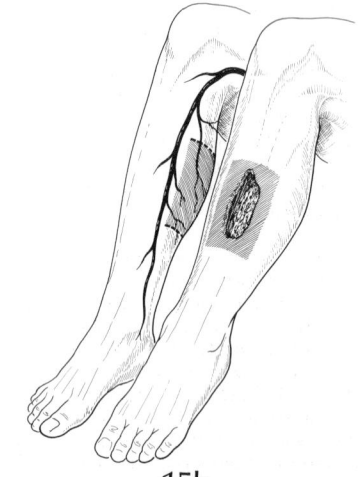

15b

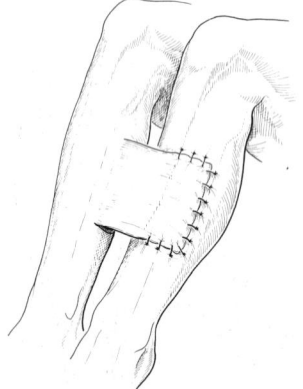

15c

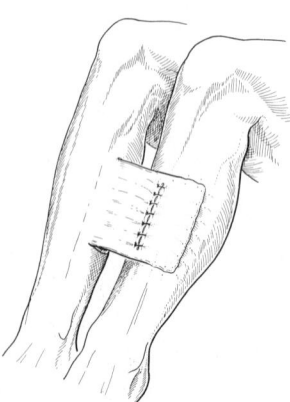

15d

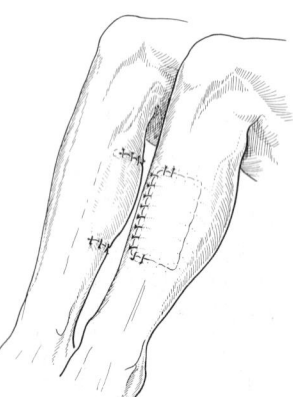

15e

CUTANEOUS AXIAL-PATTERN FLAP

16a–d

(a) If a flap of tissue is elevated with an arteriovenous system travelling along its main axis, the flap can be relatively long in relation to the width of its base. Long cutaneous flaps can be raised where a consistent arteriovenous system can be identified: one example of this is the groin flap. This flap is based on the superficial circumflex iliac artery and accompanying vein and is useful for defects of the hand, wrist and forearm. It can also be raised for transfer as a tube pedicle to the lower limb via the wrist, avoiding the first two stages of raising an abdominal tube pedicle flap. Other flaps of this type include the hypogastric flap based on the inferior epigastric vessels and the deltopectoral flap based on the first, second and third perforating vessels of the internal thoracic artery and accompanying veins.

(b) The flap is marked and elevated from its lateral extremity at the level of the deep fascia. The axial artery is identified in crossing sartorius where a perforating branch is given off. The flap is fully raised and the donor site is closed primarily provided the flap is less than 10 cm in width. The hip may have to be flexed to allow this.

(c) The recipient defect is enlarged to accept the flap, which is sutured into position. The intervening pedicle is sutured into a skin tube. The arm is fixed to the trunk by three adhesive bandages, one around the arm fixed to the chest and two on the forearm fixed to the lower trunk. A cooperative patient can be mobilized after a few days and the hip progressively extended from its flexed position.

(d) A delayed procedure is performed at 2 weeks and the flap divided and inset at 3 weeks. The pedicle is discarded and the groin wound closed.

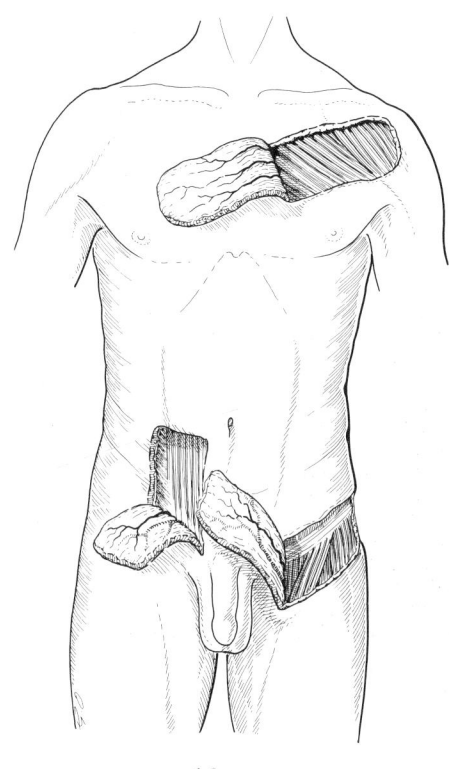

16a

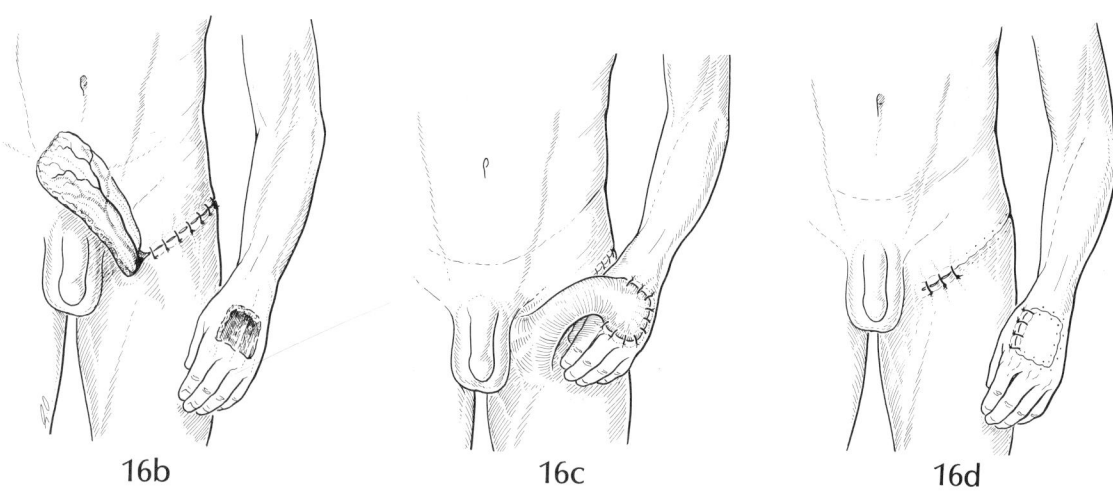

16b   16c   16d

FASCIOCUTANEOUS FLAP

17a & b

Recent research has demonstrated the rich vascular network of vessels lying on the deep fascia of the limbs. Inclusion of the fascia with a skin flap therefore makes its transfer safer and the flap can be made longer relative to its base. Fasciocutaneous flaps have been found to be particularly useful in the treatment of small lower limb defects.

(a) The dimensions of the defect are noted and a fasciocutaneous flap from adjacent healthy skin is planned allowing for the three-dimensional transfer.

(b) The flap is raised with the deep fascia and transposed into the defect. The donor site is covered with a split-skin graft which may be meshed if desired. The leg should be kept elevated for ten days to allow the graft to become stable.

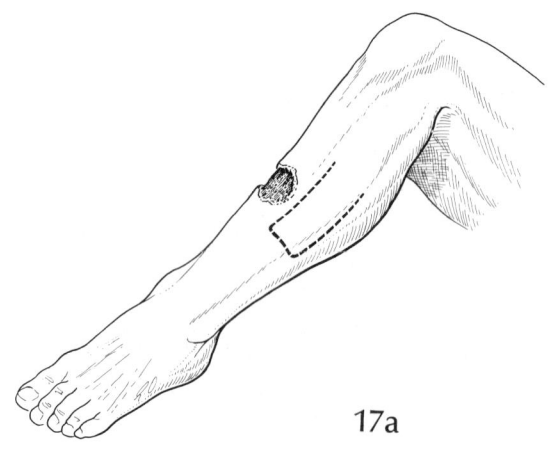

17a

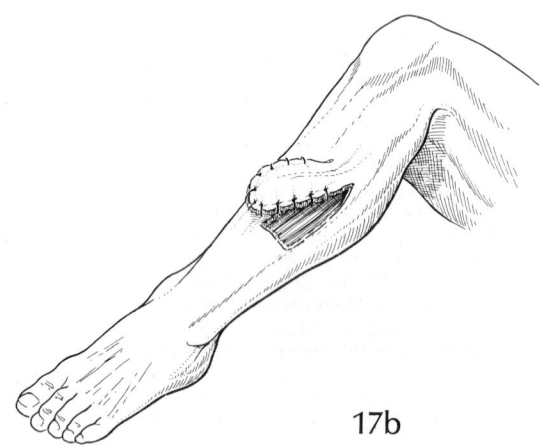

17b

Emergency skin cover in orthopaedics 13

MUSCLE OR MYOCUTANEOUS FLAP

Many superficial muscles have a vascular pedicle which is dominant. The vessel will supply not only the muscle but also, through many perforating vessels, the overlying skin and subcutaneous tissue. The composite tissue can therefore be transposed about the vascular pedicle on the axial flap principle. If the flap is bulky it may be possible to transfer the muscle alone and cover this with a split-skin graft.

In the lower limb, the most useful flaps for defects over and below the front of the knee joint are the two heads of gastrocnemius, using one of these at a time. These are usually more suitably transferred as simple muscle flaps rather than myocutaneous flaps.

18a–d

(a) The defect to be covered is first prepared. The patient is turned into the appropriate lateral position with the limb for surgery uppermost. A midline incision is made down the posterior aspect of the calf and through the deep fascia.
(b) An incision is made in the cleft between the two heads of the muscle and the head to be used is elevated. The incision between the heads is extended distally into the tendo Achillis and the hemitendon is transected, leaving 3 cm of tendon attached to the distal end of the muscle. The muscle is dissected free up to the distal end of the popliteal fossa where the main vascular pedicle enters the muscle.
(c) If appropriate, a subcutaneous tunnel to the defect is made. This is enlarged to allow transfer of the muscle. The tendon is sutured into a subcutaneous pocket created beyond the distal margin of the defect.
(d) The donor defect is closed in layers and a suction drain inserted. The exposed muscle is covered with a split-skin graft. The leg is splinted and elevated for ten days to allow the graft to consolidate and slow mobilization is instituted.

Many other muscle flaps can be used in a similar fashion though indications for these are not common. They include gracilis, rectus femoris, biceps femoris in the thigh, flexor hallucis, tibialis anterior and soleus in the leg, extensor digitorum brevis in the foot and extensor carporadialis and latissimus dorsi for the arm. The tensor fasciae latae flap is a mixed myocutaneous and fasciocutaneous flap and is used in the upper thigh and buttock region.

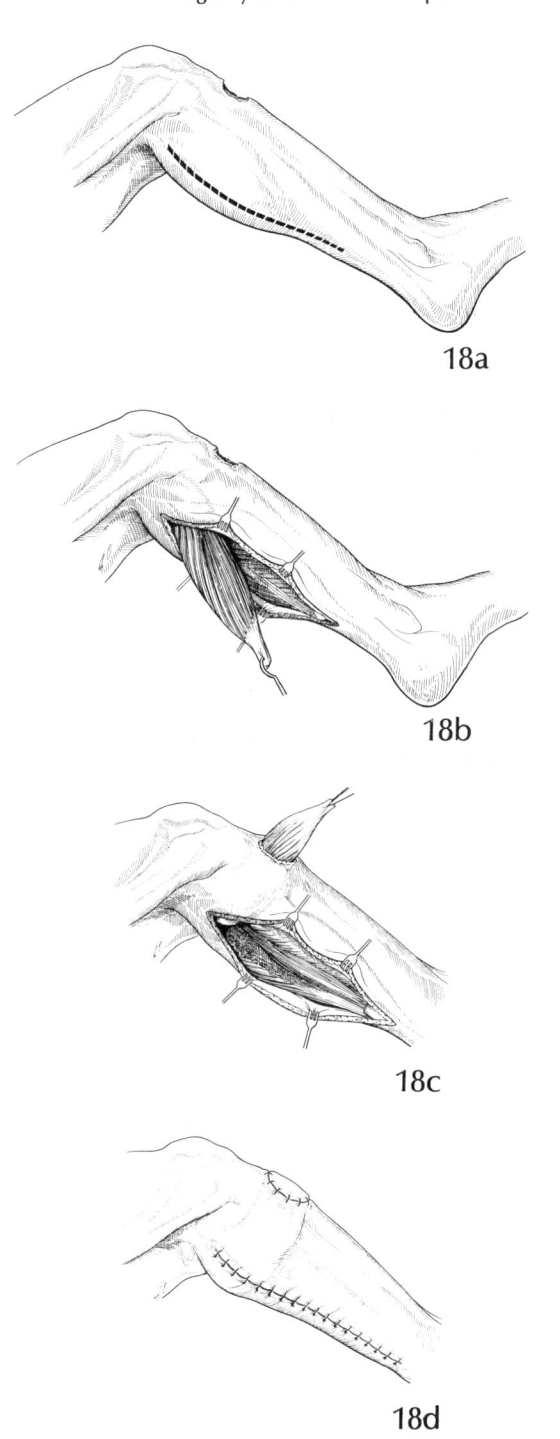

18a

18b

18c

18d

14   Repair of musculoskeletal tissues

FREE FLAPS

A free flap is an axial-pattern flap which is isolated and detached completely from the body, and after transfer to the recipient site has its axial vessels anastomosed to suitable adjacent vessels, allowing immediate vascular perfusion. The axial-pattern flap may consist of skin and subcutaneous tissue, muscle or bone or any combination of these. The potential in reconstruction is enormous and not only can a large skin defect be filled but an underlying bone defect can also be reconstructed at the same time. The surgery is highly specialized, requiring appropriate instruments and an operating microscope, and should only be undertaken in specialized units. A brief description of two flaps is given to indicate the scope of this surgery.

Free flap from latissimus dorsi muscle

19a–c

(a) The wound of a severe compound fracture of the right tibia and fibula is debrided. The fracture is reduced and stabilized with an external fixator. A large residual skin defect remains. A graft from the long saphenous vein is harvested from the left leg.
(b) The left latissimus dorsi muscle is elevated through an oblique incision and isolated from the thoracodorsal artery and vein. The vessels are divided and the flap transferred to the defect on the right leg, where it is sutured to the margins.
(c) The flap artery is sutured to the saphenous vein graft which is passed through a subcutaneous tunnel and in turn is sutured end-to-side to the superficial femoral artery in the thigh. The flap vein is sutured to the long saphenous vein after its division and mobilization. The latissimus dorsi muscle flap is then covered with a split-skin graft.

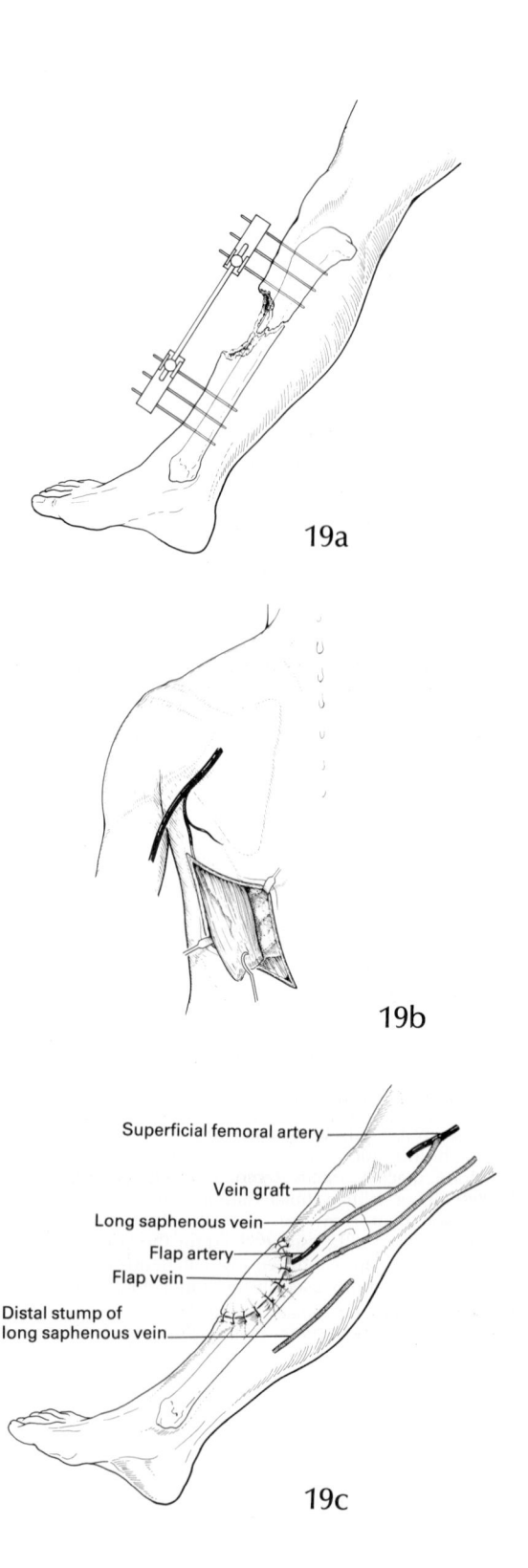

Fibular osseocutaneous free flap

20a–c

(a) A compound wound of the forearm with loss of a segment of radius is debrided. A graft of the long saphenous vein is harvested from the right leg.
(b) A fibular osseocutaneous flap is raised from the contralateral leg and isolated with the peroneal artery and one adjacent vena comitans.
(c) The flap is transferred and the bone segment fixed into the radial defect. The flap artery is anastomosed end-to-end to a segment of vein graft which in turn is sutured end-to-side to the brachial artery. Likewise the flap veins are anastomosed via segments of vein grafts to branches of the cephalic vein.

Free tissue transfer can be performed as an emergency procedure but in general, due to its complexity, is more safely and more reliably carried out as a planned procedure one or two days after the emergency.

Further reading

Barron JN, Saad MN. *Operative plastic and reconstructive surgery*, Vols 1–3, Edinburgh: Churchill Livingstone, 1981.

Converse JM. *Reconstructive plastic surgery: principles and procedures in correction, reconstruction and transplantation*, 2nd ed. Vols 1–7, Philadelphia: Saunders, 1977.

Grabb WC, Smith JW. *Plastic surgery*, 3rd ed. Boston: Little Brown, 1979.

McGregor IA. *Fundamental techniques of plastic surgery and their surgical applications*, 8th ed. Edinburgh: Churchill Livingstone, 1989.

Watson J, McCormack RM, eds. Rob and Smith's *Operative surgery: plastic surgery*, 3rd ed. London: Butterworths, 1979.

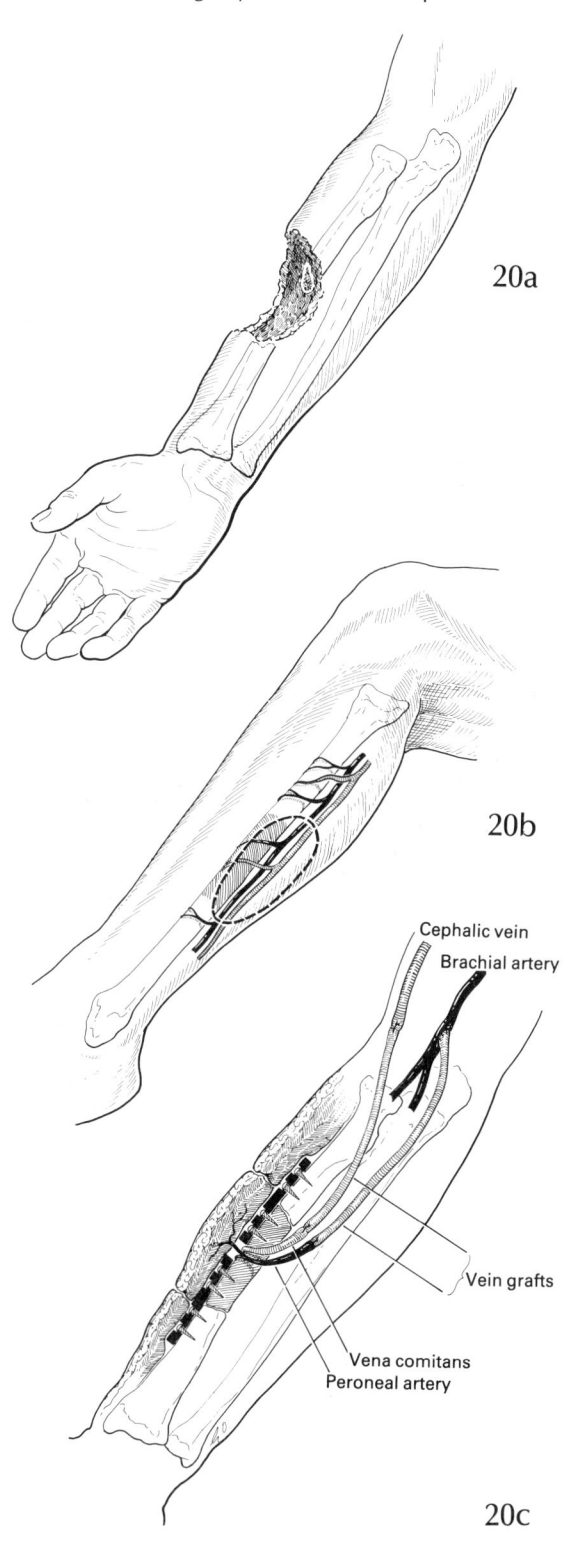

Illustrations by Gillian Oliver after B. Hyams

Tendon repair, replacement and transfer

B. Helal   MChOrth, FRCS
Honorary Consultant Orthopaedic Surgeon, The Royal London Hospital and The Royal National Orthopaedic Hospital, London, and Enfield Group of Hospitals, UK

S. C. Chen   FRCS
Consultant Orthopaedic Surgeon, Enfield Group of Hospitals, UK

Introduction

Damage to a tendon may be localized or extend over a distance. Apart from mechanical injury, the tendon can be injured from within by sharp fragments of bone or by avulsion, or from without by thermal agents such as severe burns or frostbite, by chemical agents and disease processes or radiation. When treating hand injuries it is important to know the occupation and hobbies of the patient, which hand is dominant and the time lapse since the injury.

Preoperative

Examination

A careful clinical examination should be made of every open wound, being constantly aware of the possibility of tendon injury. A tendon may appear to be intact in the depth of the wound but it may be cut some distance away, depending on whether the nearby joint or joints were flexed or extended at the time of injury. When in doubt, the wound should always be explored under regional or general anaesthesia.

Wound toilet

Preparation of the wound is important if primary healing is to take place. Dead and crushed tissues must be excised. Use of cleansing agents such as surgical spirits or iodine on exposed tendons can cause extensive chemical damage. Even a small puncture wound can take in fluid due to capillary action and involve, for instance, the whole flexor apparatus in a hand. Bland agents like Savlon (ICI Pharmaceuticals, UK) should be used. Physical scrubbing or jet lavage is necessary if the wound is grossly contaminated with dirt or mud.

Use of antibiotics

In contaminated wounds it is a wise precaution to use bacterial antibiotics in adequate dosage. A carefully planned and executed surgical operation can be ruined by infection.

Appropriate tetanus prophylaxis should be given in such cases.

PRIMARY TENDON REPAIR

Indications

Primary repair is the treatment of choice if:

1. damage to the tendon is localized;
2. there is good quality soft tissue cover;
3. the associated joints are mobile;
4. there are adequate surgical and anaesthetic skills; and
5. good theatre facilities are available.

It is permissible in certain situations to carry out a primary repair in the presence of more extensive damage to the tendon. The tendon can be lengthened locally by Z-shaped incisions or by advancement, using this technique more proximally, e.g. for extensor tendons of the hand and the tendon of the flexor pollicis longus. Conditions 2, 3 and 4 must be fulfilled.

Associated injuries

Fractures underlying tendon damage should be stabilized beforehand.

Other soft tissue injuries, for example to vessels and nerves damaged at the same level, may be repaired simultaneously. Cross-adhesions to nerves can be prevented by isolating the nerve and wrapping it in a silicone rubber membrane.

It must be emphasized that unless these criteria are adhered to, not only is the repair likely to fail, but the outcome of reconstructive measures at a later date will be prejudiced.

Contraindications

Primary repair is contraindicated when there is:

1. extensive tendon damage;
2. damage to overlying soft tissues;
3. severe contamination of the wound;
4. underlying fractures which cannot be stabilized because of the nature of the fracture or due to contamination;
5. damage to joints resulting in stiffness; or
6. lack of available surgical skill and operating facilities.

Timing

Primary repair is best carried out with a minimum of delay but, under certain circumstances, it may be postponed for 2 or 3 days for certain tendon repairs, for example the flexor apparatus of the hand, and for up to 2 weeks in other situations. After this period, there may be permanent retraction of the muscle belly.

Closure of the skin is mandatory if delay is anticipated.

Tendon sheath and pulleys

1

In primary tendon repair, the tendon sheath should be preserved and if possible repaired, as this reduces adhesion formation. In the hand, the flexor sheath consists of several parts, four annular pulleys and three criss-cross sections. It is important to preserve at least the A2 and A4 pulleys for efficient flexion of the fingers.

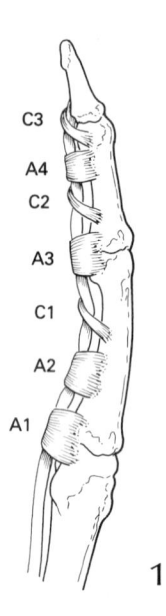

TENDON REPLACEMENT

This is indicated if the above criteria listed for primary repair cannot be met, or if there is paralysis of the muscle belly.

Contraindications

There are situations when even tendon replacement is neither possible nor advisable, for instance if there is extensive damage to other structures such as joints, nerves or vessels, when amputation might be the treatment of choice, or in the presence of extensive joint damage, when arthrodesis or tenodesis may be indicated.

Replacement tissues

Tendons may be replaced by:

1. transposition of a suitable tendon;
2. free tendon autografts;
3. fascial autografts;
4. muscle advancement;
5. two-stage tendon replacement by a temporary silicone rubber spacer followed by an autograft;
6. an autograft of tendons and sheath (whole flexor apparatus of a toe);
7. cadaver material – either free grafts or whole flexor apparatus; and
8. artificial tendons.

TENDON TRANSFER

A tendon transfer should only be performed when: associated injuries have been dealt with, e.g. fractures have been stabilized; when joints are supple; and when skin is in good order.

Essential criteria

In tendon transfers the following factors are important:

1. The tendon can be spared without significant loss of overall function of the limb.
2. The muscle of the tendon to be transferred is strong enough for the function needed. The muscle power of a transferred tendon loses strength by one MRC grade and therefore the muscle to be transferred should at least be Grade IV but ideally should be Grade V.
3. The tendon to be transferred is synergistic to the tendon to be replaced.
4. The amplitude of excursion of the tendon to be transferred is sufficient.
5. If possible the tendon to be transferred should have a straight-line pull in relation to the non-functioning muscle.
6. A donor tendon should never be attached to two recipient tendons with dissimilar functions.
7. If more than one tendon is to be given motive power, equal tension should be applied to each.
8. Joint or joints to be moved must be fully mobile with no contractures, and the tendon should be attached as distally as possible.

Operative technique

Suture materials

These should not cause any reaction as adhesions may form. Stainless steel wire or monofilament nylon are suitable materials. Polypropylene or Dacron (du Pont, UK) sutures can also be used.

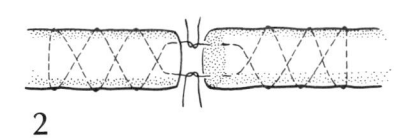

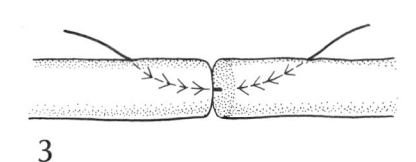

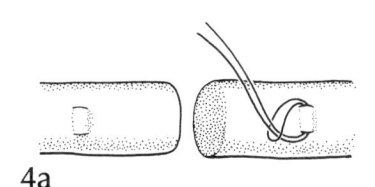

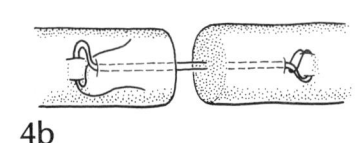

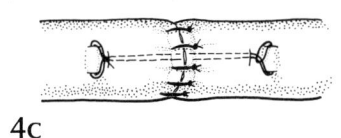

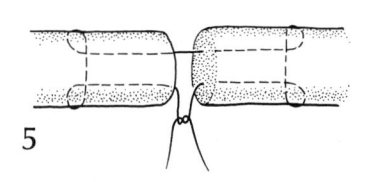

Suture technique

Many techniques have been described for attaching tendon to tendon. The handling must be gentle to cause minimal trauma. There are four methods for end-to-end anastomosis of tendons of equal girth.

Tendons of equal girth

2

The classic Bunnell criss-cross suture[1] tends to damage the tendons by a concertina action.

3

The Shaw barbed wire stitch[2] tends to fragment.

4a, b & c

Tsuge's looped suture method[3] for tendon repair is very attractive but the exposed sutures may cause adhesions. It is useful for extensor tendons where slight adhesions are not critical. A ring of 7/0 nylon interrupted sutures are placed peripherally around the cut ends of the tendon.

5

The Kessler grasping stitch[4] is preferable to the others as it is strong and simple. It is possible to insert this with one knot, which can be tied in the gap between the tendon ends.

20 Repair of musculoskeletal tissues

Tendons of unequal girth

6a, b & c

To join two tendons of unequal girth the following method is used. The smaller tendon is woven into the larger tendon through several stab incisions and these are anchored together with several sutures. The end of the larger tendon is split to enclose the smaller tendon like a 'fish-mouth'.

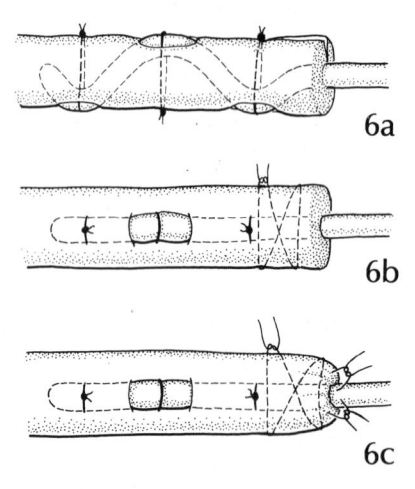

6a

6b

6c

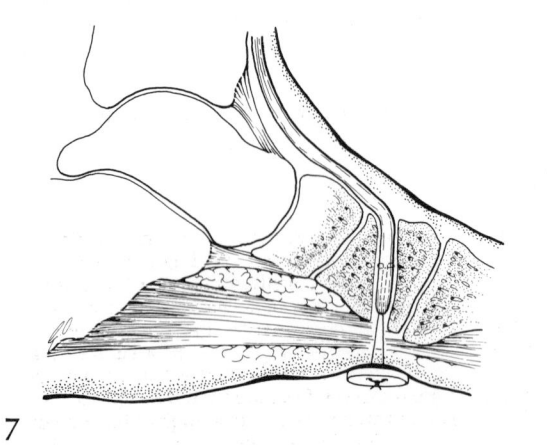

Anchorage of tendon

To bone

7

A drill hole is made in the bone to which the tendon is to be attached. the tendon is drawn into the hole by a pull-out stitch. The stitch is then tied over a button on the skin. After 3 weeks the pull-out stitch is removed.

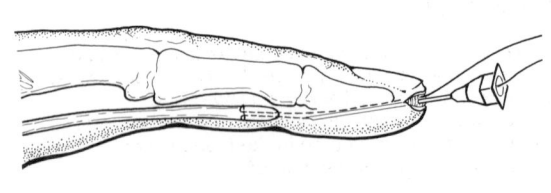

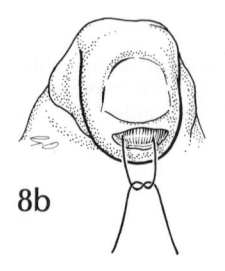

7

Apical suture

8a & b

Many techniques have been described for the distal attachment of the profundus tendon to the terminal phalanx. For ease of insertion and the least disturbance of soft tissue, the best technique is the apical suture on the palmar aspect of the terminal joint of the finger. The suture can be fed accurately into place by passing a hollow needle on either side of the tuft of the distal phalanx to the base of the phalanx and then passing the sutures through these hollow needles. A grove is made across the tuft of the distal phalanx through a transverse apical incision. The suture is tied across this groove and the skin incision closed.

8a

8b

Care of tendons during surgery

A tendon can be damaged very easily. Even a needle point or the tip of a fine forceps can cause damage resulting in adhesions. It is essential that handling of cut tendons or tendon grafts be reduced to a minimum. Gentle handling with moistened gloved fingers should be the rule. The cut tendon or tendon graft should always be kept moist with normal saline, and meticulous haemostasis should be carried out. Atraumatic needles and a non-reactive non-absorbable suture material, such as 4/0 nylon or stainless steel wire, should always be used for suturing a tendon. Tendon grafts should be smooth, and the surface undamaged. If the surface is covered with paratenon, any loose tags should be excised as these will encourage adhesions.

The tendon bed should also be treated with the utmost respect, for any damage to ligaments or periosteum can cause adhesions. If the tendon bed is already damaged, e.g. the bone is fractured and has been internally fixed, the repaired tendon should be protected by interposing a layer of synovial tissue or subcutaneous fat between it and the bone.

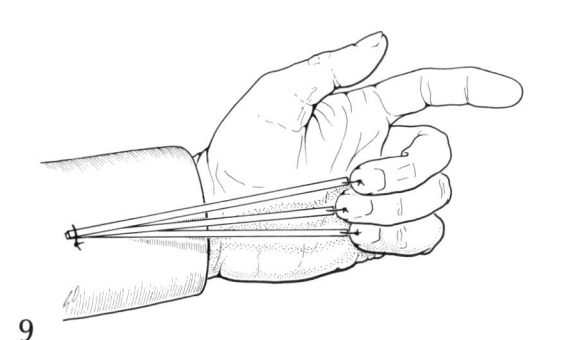

Protection of the repaired tendon

A repaired tendon takes about 3 weeks to heal. During the first week there is very little reaction. During the second week the repaired tendon is oedematous and weak and any tension during this stage will result in dehiscence of the tendon ends. During the third week the repaired tendon starts to heal by fibrous tissue crossing the approximated tendon ends. During the first 3 weeks of a tendon repair tension must be taken off the repair.

Protecting the suture line can be carried out by:

Plaster immobilization

This is preferred in hand injuries in children because it is the most immune to interference. The wrist and metacarpophalangeal joints are held in flexion, the plaster extending to the finger tips over the dorsal surface with the fingers kept straight.

After tendon repairs in other parts of the upper limb and in the lower limb, plaster immobilization for 3–6 weeks is essential.

Flexor tendon repair using the Kleinert technique[5]

9

This allows for early mobilization of the injured finger after a flexor tendon repair, thus avoiding the complication of joint stiffness. This method relies on the muscle actively relaxing when its antagonistic muscle is actively contracting. After the flexor tendon is repaired, a rubber band is attached from the finger nail by a suture to a plaster splint on the forearm. Limited extension against the elastic band is allowed from the start. It is important to include the other two unaffected ulnar digits when one of the three ulnar profundi have been repaired because this section of the muscle acts *en masse*.

Extensor tendon repair using the dynamic radial nerve palsy splint

When extensor tendons are repaired the same principle of reflex inhibition of antagonist muscles can be applied by the use of a dynamic radial nerve palsy splint.

Protection of the repaired extensor tendons is necessary for only 10 days when injured in the triangular expansion but requires 3 weeks at other sites[6].

22 Repair of musculoskeletal tissues

Immobilizing the motor tendon

This can be achieved in two ways.

10

A pull-out wire suture is placed into the tendon proximal to the suture line. The wire is anchored over a button on the skin.

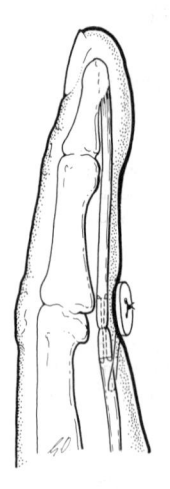

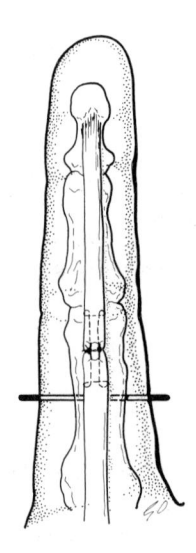

11

Alternatively, the tendon is transfixed proximal to the suture with a thin Kirschner wire which is brought out through the skin, enabling easy removal at the end of the third week.

Tension of tendon repair

It is important to judge the tension of tendon repair correctly. If the repair is too tight the joint under the influence of the repaired tendon cannot extend fully. If the repair is too lax, the muscle contractions cannot be fully transmitted to the tendon and therefore the joint will not have its full range of movement. Correct tension of tendon repair is critical in flexor tendon injuries of the hand. Too lax a tendon repair distally will produce relatively increased lumbrical tension on the extensor, and paradoxical extension of the finger will occur when flexion is attempted[7]. Division of the lumbrical tendon will abolish this.

Complications

Wrong tension of repair

Too tight or too loose a repair, unless very gross, can be compensated for by the muscle actively lengthening or shortening. If there is gross error in the tension, then the correct tension has to be achieved by lengthening or shortening the tendon surgically.

Adhesions

These may occur between tendon and sheath or skin. It is best to wait for about 6 months before a tenolysis is carried out. This is because an early tenolysis may give rise to further adhesions. Adhesions may also occur between a tendon and the overlying skin. Likewise it is best to wait for about the same period of 6 months before a dermolysis is carried out.

Bowstringing

It is important to leave pulleys, particularly the finger flexor pulleys, the extensor retinaculum of the wrist, and the superior extensor retinaculum of the ankle, to prevent bowstringing of tendons. Sometimes their removal is unavoidable and such structures may have to be sacrificed or they may have been damaged. Severe bowstringing can affect the efficiency of tendon function especially in the hand, and reconstruction of missing pulleys has to be undertaken.

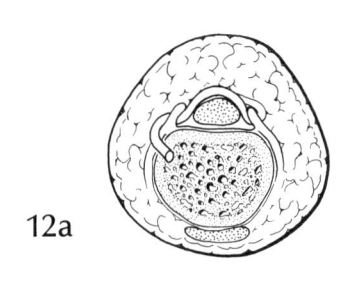

Technique of pulley reconstruction

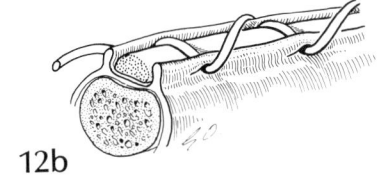

12a & b

Either a strip of fascia lata or the palmaris longus tendon can be used. It is woven through the sides of the gutter in the proximal phalanx from side to side like a shoe lace, over the flexor tendon or a silicone rubber rod. The ends are anchored with non-absorbable sutures.

References

1. Bunnell S. *Surgery of the hand*. 3rd ed. Philadelphia: Lippincott, 1956.
2. Shaw PC. A method of flexor tendon suture. *J Bone Joint Surg [Br]* 1968; 50-B: 578–87.
3. Tsuge K, Ikuta Y, Matsuishi Y. Intra-tendinous tendon suture in the hand: a new technique. *Hand* 1975; 7: 250–5.
4. Kessler I. The "grasping" technique for tendon repair. *Hand* 1973; 5: 253–5.
5. Kleinert HE, Kutz JE, Atasoy E, Stormo A. Primary repair of flexor tendons. *Orthop Clin North Am* 1973; 4: 865–9.
6. Stuart D. Duration of splinting after repair of extensor tendons in the hand. *J Bone Joint Surg [Br]* 1965; 47-B: 72.
7. Parkes AR. The "lumbrical plus" finger. *J Bone Joint Surg [Br]* 1971; 53-B: 236–9.

Illustrations by Philip Wilson

Repair of divided peripheral nerves

Rolfe Birch MChir, FRCS
Consultant Orthopaedic Surgeon, St Mary's Hospital, London and The Royal National Orthopaedic Hospital, Stanmore, UK

Introduction

The conducting elements of a peripheral nerve, the axons, are grouped into bundles each of which is enveloped in a tough cellular membrane, the perineurium. Numbers of bundles are held together by a loose connective tissue fabric, the epineurium, condensed on its surface as a recognizable sheath. An areolar connective tissue envelops the nerve trunks and segmental vascular pedicles enter along its course.

Primary repair is the suture of nerve stumps before neuroma formation. In clinical practice the time limit is between 7 and 10 days, although the earliest changes of proximal axonal sprouting and distal wallerian degeneration are detectable at 24 hours by electron microscopy.

Secondary repair is the suture of nerve stumps after resection of neuroma. It is performed when the initial wound has healed and oedema and joint stiffness have settled. Resection of nerve tissue is always required.

Grafting is indicated when sufficient nerve tissue has been lost that direct suture is impossible without undue tension. Grafting is necessary in the majority of delayed cases of nerve injury and it is inevitable where the nerve trunk has been ruptured from traction injury, or dislocation of a joint. Grafting may also be used in primary repair of such injuries.

Diagnosis

Open wounds

A surprising number of peripheral nerve injuries are missed on first presentation, even when there is a wound over the course of the nerve. Patients with complete division of the median nerve may admit only to distortion of sensation rather than complete loss of feeling. A typical response is that the hand feels 'wooden', like 'cotton-wool', or 'pins and needles'. There is wide variation in the area of total anaesthesia following division of the median or of the ulnar nerve. An important finding consistently present within 24 hours of complete division of either of these trunks is vasomotor and sudomotor paralysis. The denervated digits are red and dry. Division of one digital nerve to the finger or thumb may be missed as the area of total anaesthesia does not, typically, extend to the tip of the digits.

Difficult though examination of muscles may be with a distressed or a confused patient, it should be remembered that one intrinsic muscle of the hand consistently innervated by the median nerve is the abductor pollicis brevis. The abductor digiti minimi is the key to the superficial division of the ulnar nerve; the first dorsal interosseous, the key to the deep branch. The muscle bellies must be seen and felt to contract.

Particular difficulties arise with the uncooperative patient or the young child. Much can be learnt from the site of laceration and from evidence of associated injuries. Deep flexor tendon division must suggest median nerve injuries. Bleeding from the digital artery indicates injury of the more superficial digital nerve; bleeding from the ulnar artery suggests injury to the adjacent ulnar nerve.

Iatrogenic nerve injuries

A neural deficit following necessary surgical procedures to the injured limb, as for vascular injury or open reduction of fractures and dislocations, cannot be assumed to be simple contusion of the nerve. Unfortunately, the nerve may have been caught by suture material, compressed by an implant or even divided. Where the deficit is clear-cut and total, and where there was no such deficit preoperatively, the surgeon must in all conscience assume that there has been division of the nerve and act accordingly.

A recent review of complete transection of 68 major trunk nerves referred to the author's unit[1] showed that certain nerves, including the accessory, the upper trunk of the brachial plexus, and the common peroneal nerve, were particularly at risk during operations for lymph node biopsy, removal of swelling, or ligation of varicose veins. The radial and posterior interosseous nerve were particularly vulnerable during operations for fracture of the humerus or removal of metal implants. Delay in diagnosis ranged from instantaneous to 2 years. The mean interval between injury of the nerve and referral for repair was 6 months. The outcome following repair in the later cases was uniformly bad.

The diagnosis of neurapraxia is both unlikely and dangerous in such cases. When the surgeon finds that a nerve is not working and there is a wound over the course of that nerve, then he or she must assume that the nerve has been cut and that it will not get better until it is repaired.

Injuries of the terminal branches of the superficial radial nerve and of the medial cutaneous nerve of the forearm commonly lead to severe pain; repair of these slender cutaneous branches is difficult and often impossible. Prevention is the cure and surgeons are urged to be meticulous in protecting the sensory nerves during so-called minor operations for de Quervain's tenosynovitis, decompression of the ulnar nerve, and release of trigger finger.

Major vascular injuries

Open wounds of great vessels in the neck or axilla or in the thigh are usually associated with laceration of adjacent nerve trunks. Whilst repair of the artery and restoration of flow to the limb is of the greatest urgency, it should be remembered that compression from haematoma impairs the prognosis for recovery of divided nerves.

Ischaemia of limbs in closed injuries is common. Rupture of the axillary artery is a frequent complication of traction lesion of the infraclavicular brachial plexus and is usually associated with dislocation of the glenohumeral joint or fracture of the humeral shaft. Similarly, dislocation of the knee is commonly complicated by rupture or thrombosis of the popliteal artery. Failure to restore flow promptly leads to dense fibrosis of the muscles of the limb, with ischaemic injury of the trunk nerves. Late nerve repair in such neglected injuries is a waste of time. Wider decompression is an essential adjunct to the vascular repair; if this precaution is neglected then gangrene may result.

Impending Volkmann's ischaemic contracture

The features of this are well known: the patient, usually a child; the injury, usually a supracondylar fracture, although forearm fractures, tight plaster casts and dressings are other important causes. The incidence of this complication in the leg, from fractures of the tibia, is underestimated.

Tense tender swelling of muscles of the limb, diminution or absence of distal pulses, pain on passive extension of the fingers or toes, and increasing sensory disturbance or paresis indicate ischaemic injury to nerve and muscle. Any one of these features is a strong indication for exploration of the relevant artery and nerve trunk combined with fasciotomy to prevent irreversible loss or marring of function of the limb.

Closed injuries

It is widely assumed that the great majority of nerve lesions associated with closed fractures are of good prognosis. However, Seddon[2] pointed out that more than one third of radial nerve palsies associated with closed fractures of the humeral shaft did not recover, and he further pointed out that dislocation of the shoulder, the elbow, or of the knee joint frequently cause ruptures or entrapment of adjacent nerve trunks. My policy is as follows: where a fracture or dislocation was caused by more than a moderate degree of violence and where there has been wide displacement of the skeletal fragments, then absence of nerve function is assumed to be from rupture of that nerve trunk. Urgent exposure of the nerve, combined with internal fixation of the fracture, is recommended. Early recognition of such nerve injuries affords the surgeon the opportunity to go directly to primary repair by grafting, or to refer the patient to an interested colleague.

PRIMARY SUTURE

Indications

Many injuries of peripheral nerves in civilian practice are caused by clean cuts from a knife, glass or razor and these are suitable for primary suture. The most important proviso is that sufficient skill and facilities are available. It is far better to dress the wound or suture the skin carefully and go on to planned repair the following morning, or to refer the patient to an interested colleague, than it is to do an immediate but poor suture.

Contraindications

1. The general condition of the patient or associated injury to the head or viscera may dictate delay.
2. Compound or contaminated wounds or burns.
3. Traction injuries of the brachial plexus. Whilst primary repair by grafting is the favoured policy in our unit, it must be emphasized that this is difficult and time-consuming work. Experience in wide exposure and control and repair of injury to the major vessels is necessary.
4. Amputated limbs. There is no doubt that the prognosis for a successfully replanted hand is very much better following primary suture of the nerve than it is where suture is delayed for 2 or 3 months and this type of case is the exception that proves the rule!

Principles of the operation

Adjacent muscle and tendon injuries are repaired. It is important to repair the synovium over tendon suture lines, not only to reduce adhesions between the suture lines themselves but also, particularly, between them and the adjacent nerve trunks.

Divided vessels must be repaired – major vessels for obvious reasons, but the results of repair of digital and ulnar nerves are significantly improved by repair of corresponding arteries[3,4].

Instruments

1. Magnification. Loupes are certainly useful but the operating microscope is more comfortable and is a better light source.
2. Bipolar diathermy.
3. Fine instruments and sutures. A wide range of excellent micro-sutures is available and the quality of the needle is more important than that of the filament. The 8/0 nylon on a 6 mm needle (Ethicon W 2808, Edinburgh, UK) and the 9/0 nylon on a 4 mm needle (Ethicon W 2898) are very useful for epineurial sutures. Finer sutures are available for repair of bundles and we favour the 25 μm monofilament on a 4 mm, 70 μm needle (S & T – Chirurgicien Nadlen, 7893-Jestetten, Germany).
4. Nerve stimulator.

It is assumed that the operator is familiar with the use of these instruments.

Operation

This may be time-consuming and general anaesthesia is preferred. Neuromuscular blocking agents are to be avoided, at least during identification of the lesion, since they prevent or hamper the use of the stimulators. The limb is prepared and an occluding cuff is applied to the arm for more distal lesions. The cuff may be inflated after elevation of the limb for the preliminary phase of identification of the divided structure.

Incision

1a–e

Incisions should allow exposure, identification and control. In the fingers, lacerations should, where possible, be converted into volar zig-zag incisions. In the palm a laceration should be extended to follow the palmar creases; at the wrist the usual transverse wound can be extended proximally and distally with broadly based flaps. Decompression of the carpal tunnel is performed in major wrist lacerations.

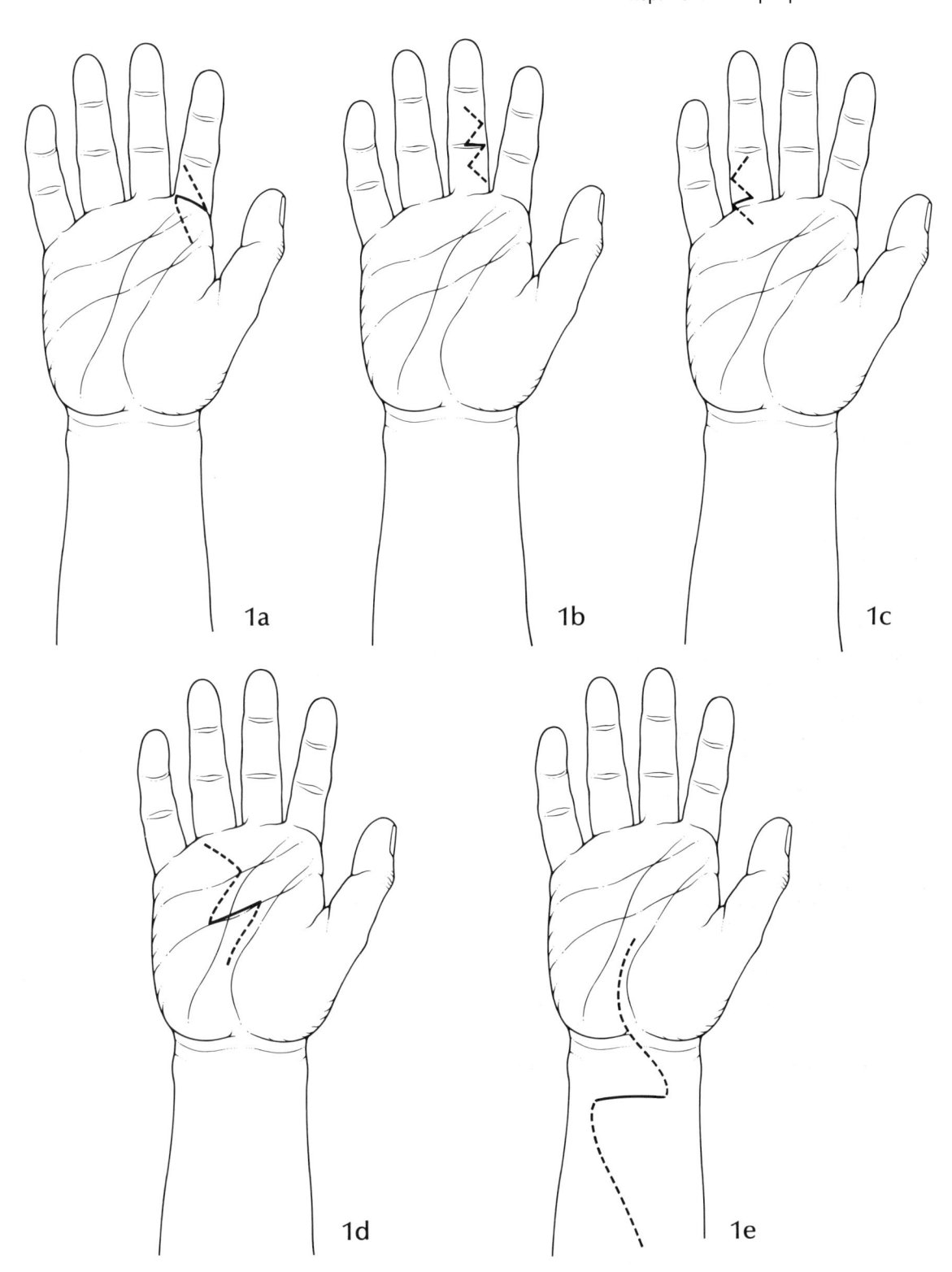

1a

1b

1c

1d

1e

Identification

2

Tendons retract within the synovial tunnels and nerve stumps may be hidden by blood clot or by blood-stained synovium. Flexion of the elbow and wrist assists in the presentation of tendons and nerves. Irrigation with warm saline aids identification. A divided nerve is very different from a divided tendon: the nerve is softer, the bundles are larger, and there is more bleeding from the cut face than in the case of the tendon.

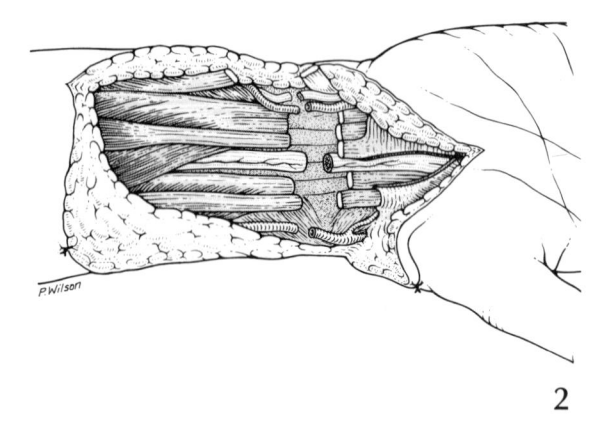

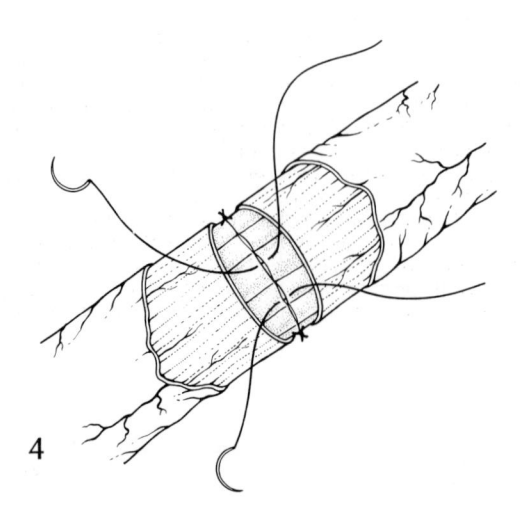

Adjacent repairs

Significant divided vessels are repaired. In clean lacerations direct end-to-end suture with 8/0 nylon is suitable for the ulnar and radial arteries, but 10/0 nylon sutures are used for digital arteries. Where there has been crushing of the vessel, damaged tissue is resected and an end-to-end or end-to-side reversed vein graft is used (see the chapter on 'Vascular injury and repair', pp. 39–53).

Tendons are repaired with a strong core suture, followed by a 6/0 nylon running suture for the epitenon. The synovium between deep and superficial flexor tendons is repaired with 3/0 polyglactin sutures (Vicryl, Ethicon, Edinburgh, UK); it is particularly important to seal the suture line of superficial tendon injuries from the overlying median nerve. If an occluding cuff has been used it should now be released and haemostasis secured. Longitudinal vessels coursing along and within the epineurium are a source of haematoma and disruption.

Nerve repair

3 & 4

The principle of nerve repair is to appose without tension and as accurately as possible the nerve faces and bundles. Orientation is determined by the longitudinal vessels, by the grouping of bundles in the nerve stump, particularly evident in the median nerve at the wrist, and by the varying size of the nerve bundles themselves. In clean lacerations no resection of the nerve faces is indicated. The anterior wall is repaired first. The areolar adventitia is swept back to prevent flapping into the suture line. The key sutures draw together matching bundles, evident by their size. The needle is passed through the perineurium; tension should be sufficient to appose the bundle without buckling.

5

Once correct orientation has been achieved and larger bundles have been accurately coapted, sutures taking a bite of epineurium as well as perineurium are placed, using 10/0 nylon sutures. Rotation of the limb allows slightly more than one half of the circumference of the nerve to be repaired.

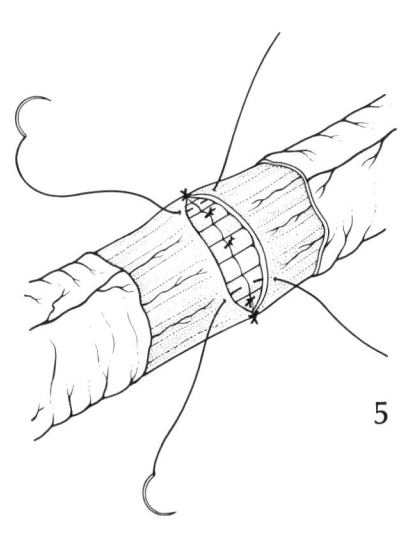

6

To rotate the nerve and so expose the posterior wall, I prefer gently rotating the nerve round on a saline-soaked dental roll, first from one side and then from the other. Fine skin hooks can be used to aid rotation of the nerve trunk. Stay sutures tend to pull out of the rather flimsy tissues of a freshly divided nerve and they may distort the nerve faces so preventing accurate matching. If stay sutures are used, 6/0 nylon passed through the epineurium only is chosen. Matching the posterior aspect of the nerve is more easily achieved after accurate repair of the anterior wall of the nerve. There is rarely any indication for suturing individual bundles deep within the nerve stump although this may aid matching in oblique lacerations.

With this technique between 18 and 25 sutures will be used to repair the ulnar nerve at the wrist and between 25 and 30 for the median nerve at the same level.

Where a proximal repair has been performed in the presence of a vascular injury, fasciotomy of the flexor muscles of the forearm should be done before wound closure. Where possible, the nerve suture line should be covered by a flap of synovium or by an undamaged muscle belly. Mobilization of the nerve is not necessary in primary repair where there has been no loss of nerve substance. Gentle flexion of wrist and elbow allows the nerve to be sutured without any tension. Where there has been damage of muscle bellies, a sealed vacuum drain is used but this should not be placed adjacent to the nerve suture for fear of disruption. The skin is closed with 4/0 nylon suture.

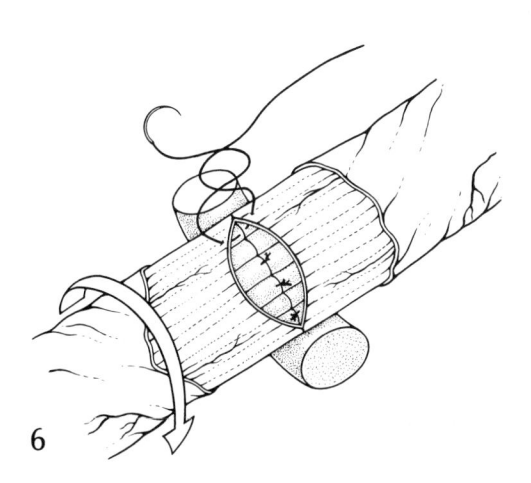

Postoperative management

7 & 8

The wound is dressed with dry gauze and copious loose cotton wool. Plaster of Paris splints are used to maintain the position of adjacent joints: a volar splint to support the wrist, a dorsal slab to maintain flexion of the wrist and the metacarpophalangeal joints. In injuries of the mid-forearm and more proximal levels, the elbow should be included in the splint. In children, inclusion of the elbow is advised.

Gentle active exercises of the fingers can be encouraged from the day after operation. The splint and dressings remain undisturbed for 3 weeks, at which time the wound is inspected and the sutures removed. Vigorous active exercises can now be encouraged for the fingers but hyperextension of the wrist or of the elbow should be prevented for a further 2 weeks. For lacerations at the level of the wrist a dorsal plaster of Paris splint should be worn for a further 2 weeks, preventing the wrist from extending beyond 20°.

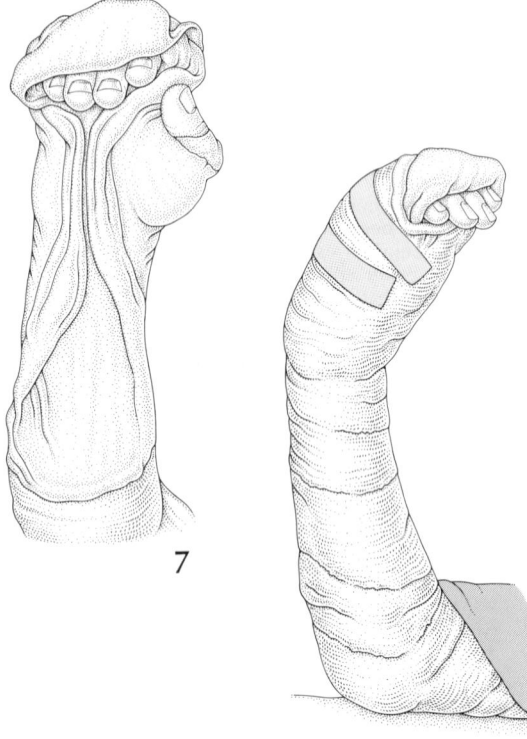

SECONDARY REPAIR

Indications

1. As an elective procedure, after the primary treatment of unsuitable wounds.
2. Where diagnosis is delayed.
3. The failed primary nerve repair.
4. Failure of recovery within the expected time, e.g. of radial nerve lesions associated with closed fractures of the humerus.

If after a properly executed primary repair, there is no evidence of recovery by 3 months, with a persistent Tinel sign at the level of the suture, then re-exploration should be advised. Electromyographic evidence of early muscle reinnervation precedes clinical activity by 4 to 6 weeks and for proximal motor nerves such investigation may be useful. However, the decision to explore in a late case must be a clinical one.

Contraindications

1. If the patient has adapted to the disability, as in many digital nerve lesions.
2. Where little worthwhile functional gain can be anticipated following repair of proximal lesions or after much delay. If the radial nerve has been injured in the axilla, or if the common peroneal division of the sciatic nerve has been injured at the hip, and if the delay is of the order of 12 months from the injury to repair, then the appropriate tendon transfer will give a surer functional improvement than nerve suture. Useful intrinsic muscular activity is rare following repair of ulnar and median nerves in the axilla and appropriate tendon transfers should be considered. However, useful recovery of sensation, sufficient to protect the hand from injury, may follow repair of median nerve lesions years after injury.
3. Severe ischaemic changes in the forearm and hand militate against any return of function and simple nerve suture alone in these cases is inadequate.
4. If the cosmetic and sensory loss following the taking of a graft are unacceptable to the patient. It is essential that the skeleton is stable, and that stiffness and contractures have been overcome prior to any delayed nerve repair. Good skin must be secured, if necessary with the full-thickness skin flaps.

Repair of divided peripheral nerves 31

Operation

Instruments and anaesthesia are as for primary repair.
The patient is warned of the possible need for taking a graft from the leg or arm and these limbs are included in the field.

Incision

9

Adequate exposure is essential. Incisions may be long. It is preferable to raise a flap, avoiding the previous scar overlying the site of nerve injury. The nerve trunk should be identified proximally and distally in healthy tissue; dissection proceeds from both ends towards the level of injury.

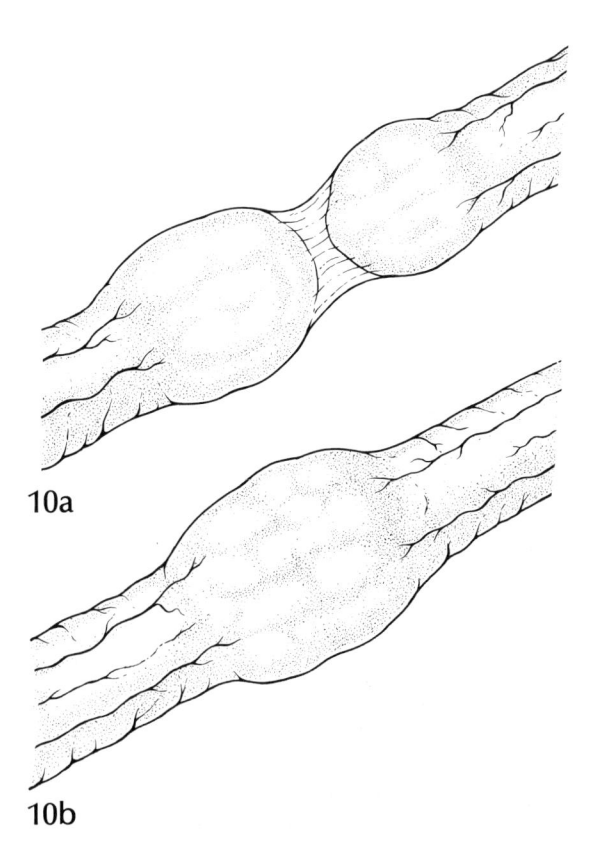

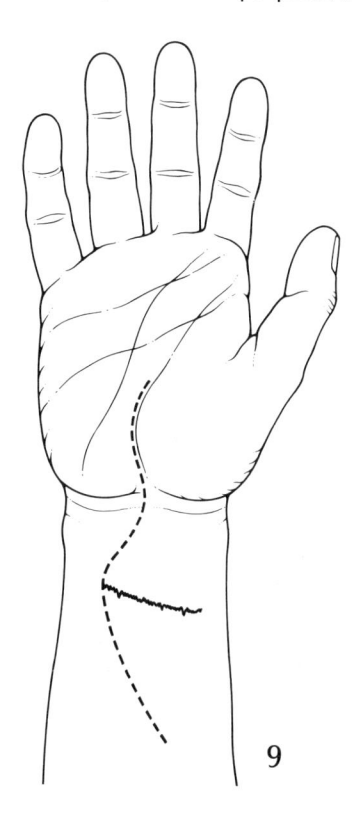

Findings

10a & b

The nerve may have been completely divided, with two nerve bulbs separated by a gap. Difficulties arise where there is a lesion in continuity. Where the neuroma is hard and where there is no conduction across it, resection and repair are indicated. Where the neuroma is soft and where there is evidence of conducting neural elements passing through it with muscle response distally on proximal stimulation, the nerve should be left.

Resection and biopsy

11, 12 & 13

The neuroma is resected back to healthy nerve faces. A fresh scalpel blade is used, for scissors crush. The first incision is made through the centre of the neuroma and serial slices about 1 mm in thickness are made proximally and distally until healthy pouting nerve bundles become evident. Palpation of the nerve trunks is most helpful in determining the final level of section and in distinguishing the firm, elastic quality of a healthy nerve from the fibrotic, hard, scarred segment. Biopsies are taken from the neuroma, the proximal nerve stump and the distal nerve stump. It is better to err on the side of resection than it is to leave a scarred face before suture. It is for this reason that the surgeon must be prepared to go on to repair by grafting if direct suture proves impossible.

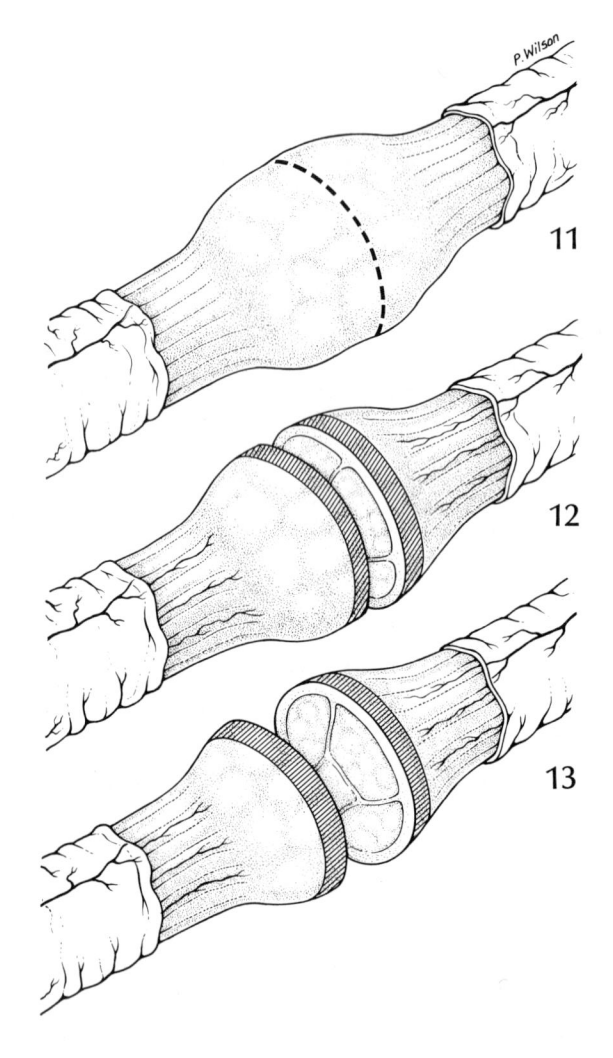

Mobilization

The gap will now be evident between the nerve faces. Mobilization of the nerve trunks may diminish this. It is possible to gain length for the median nerve at the elbow by dividing the lacertus fibrosus and also the deep origin of pronator teres. Anterior transposition of the ulnar nerve at the elbow allows gaps of up to 3 cm to be closed at that level. However, the gain from mobilization is limited. It is important to preserve vascular pedicles and proximal motor branches, and the stimulator is very helpful in such dissection.

I no longer practise extensive mobilization of nerve trunks. Indeed, I have found that anterior transposition of the ulnar nerve is followed by compression of the nerve trunk distal to the suture line from scar.

Secondary repair or graft?

Our present policy for median or ulnar nerves at the wrist or in the forearm is that secondary suture is performed only if the prepared nerve faces can be brought together without tension, with flexion of the wrist to no more than 30°. Mobilization is limited. In practice, this means that where more than about 1–1.5 cm of the nerve trunk has been resected, then nerve grafting is performed. Anterior transposition of the ulnar nerve is restricted for those cases where the nerve has been transected within the cubital tunnel or at the level of the medial epicondyle.

Different considerations apply where the divisions of the sciatic nerve have been injured at the knee or in the distal part of the thigh. Gaps of up to 4–5 cm may be treated by direct suture but the suture line is protected in serial splints for between 9 and 12 weeks.

Repair

14 & 15

The stiffness of the nerve with thickening of all connective tissue layers is a remarkable feature in secondary suture. Proliferation of the adventitia is more marked proximally and the thickened adventitia must be dissected away to expose the firm, white, crescentic margin of the epineurium. The bundles within do not pout as they do in primary repair. Orientation can be achieved by the grouping of bundles within the nerve face, by their variation in size, by the longitudinal blood vessels, and by the cross-section of the nerve which is often oval. However, the bundle of patterns will differ between the faces if more than a few millimetres of nerve trunk has been resected and in a late nerve repair the distal nerve stump will have shrunk.

Sutures of 8/0 nylon are passed through the epineurium to maintain apposition and to act as stay sutures. Sutures of 9/0 or 10/0 nylon are then passed through both the epineurium and the perineurium to secure coaptation of neural elements. The anterior wall repair is completed and the nerve is then rotated either with stay sutures or using a saline-soaked dental roll. The posterior repair is completed similarly.

As in primary repair haemostasis is secured after preparation of the nerve faces and in a late repair this may be a tedious business as bleeding from the scarred bed is often persistent, but it is better to endure this than risk disruption of repair by postoperative haematoma. The closure should be in layers. The skin is closed with 4/0 nylon.

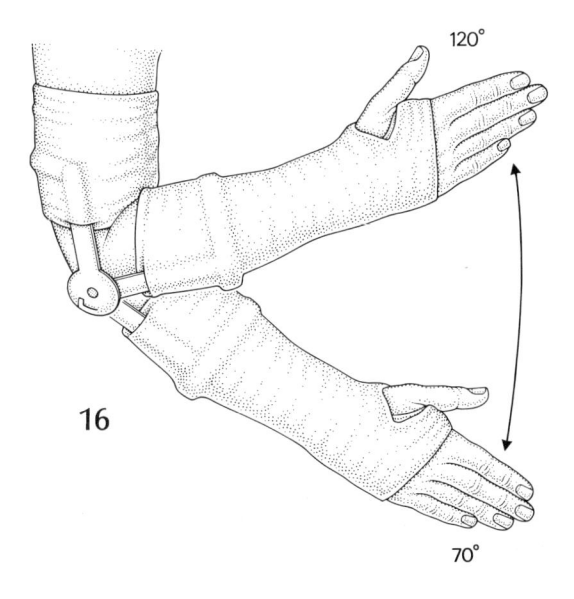

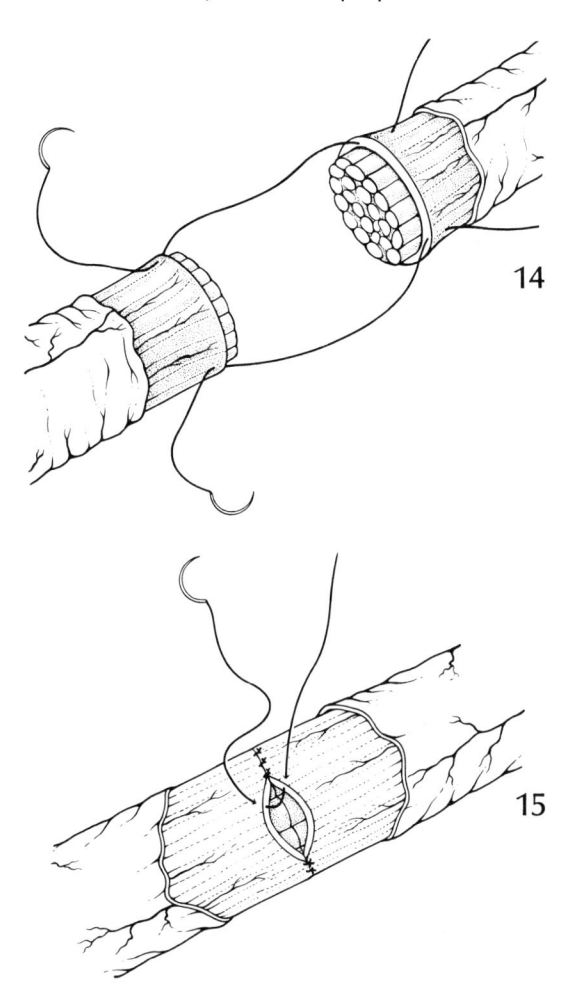

Postoperative management

16

Splinting is more prolonged than for primary repair. The wrist and elbow are immobilized in sufficient flexion to prevent tension at the suture line. These splints are left undisturbed for 3 weeks. A turnbuckle or hinge splint is then applied, allowing a staged increase in range of movement at the elbow joint over the course of the next 4 to 6 weeks. The wrist joint should be returned to neutral at 3 weeks to prevent flexion deformity.

GRAFTING

The old idea of bridging defects in trunk nerves by grafts taken from other nerves was proven in clinical practice by Seddon[5]. Millesi[6] has extended this work. Millesi points out that any tension is deleterious for nerve regeneration; he resects epineurium from proximal and distal nerve stumps and subdivides those trunks into clusters of bundles to allow accurate matching between proximal and distal faces.

Indications

Grafting is the most commonly employed technique in the repair of major trunk nerves in our unit. It is necessary when a segment of nerve has been lost, as in compound fractures or infected wounds, gunshot or missile injuries, ruptures from traction forces, and after a badly executed primary repair. Even in clean transections of nerve trunks within the brachial sheath, direct suture may be difficult without tension and grafting is commonly employed here.

The operation should be performed as early as possible after injury. As in all patients with nerve injuries, the necessary prerequisites are stability of the skeleton, correction of deformity, and healthy skin cover with a minimally scarred bed.

Donor nerve

The two most commonly used donor nerves are the sural nerve and the medial cutaneous nerve of the forearm. Up to 25 cm of the medial cutaneous nerve is available in adults and this is a bigger nerve than the sural nerve. A further advantage is that the graft is taken from the impaired limb. Up to 45 cm of the sural nerve can be elevated.

Operation

17 & 18

Incisions and isolation of the nerve follow the steps discussed above in secondary repair. After preparation of nerve faces adventitia and epineurium are resected for 3–4 mm from the edge of the cut nerve, displaying individual bundles or their aggregates surrounded by perineurium and a condensation of epineurium. The amount of graft required is estimated and the appropriate donor nerve displayed.

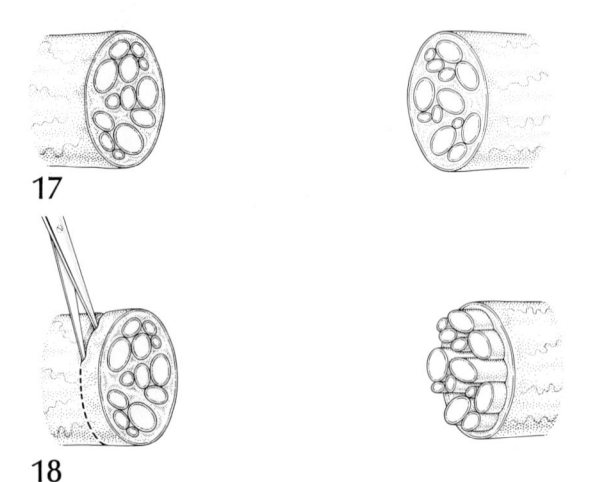

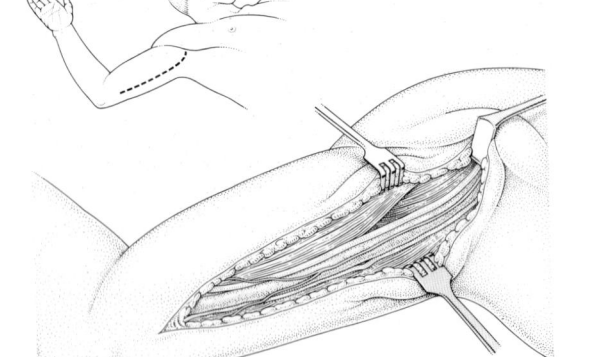

Medial cutaneous nerve of forearm

19

This is exposed through an incision along the brachial bundle, curving to the anterior axillary line. The nerve will be seen glistening through the brachial sheath closely applied to a brachial vein. It is between 2 and 3 mm in width and must be distinguished from the ulnar nerve. The axillary fat pad is swept down from the deep face of pectoralis major and this muscle is retracted by an assistant, allowing more proximal display of the nerve. The nerve pierces the brachial sheath about half-way down the arm and breaks up into two or three branches at this level, which are usually large enough to be used as grafts.

Sural nerve

20

This passes directly in the posterior midline of the calf and is closely applied to the short saphenous vein. It curves lateral to the tendo Achillis at the ankle. A longitudinal incision is necessary for adequate exposure, and gentle handling of the nerve. Lateral communicating branches are frequently encountered at the junction of the upper third and lower two-thirds of the leg.

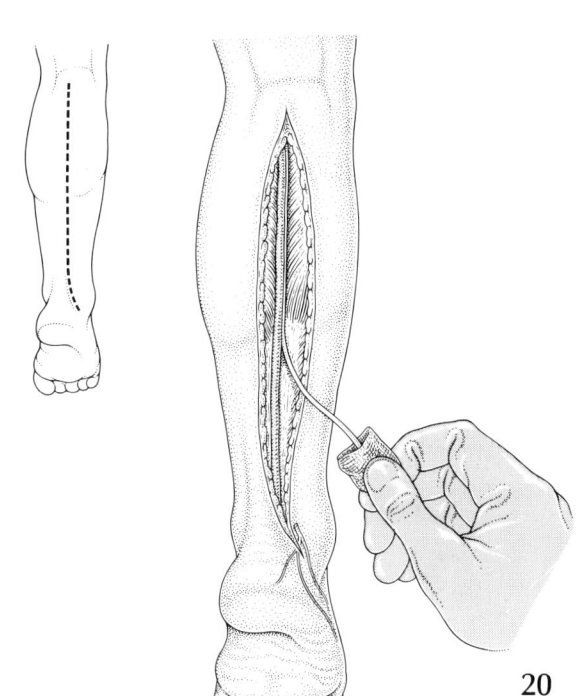

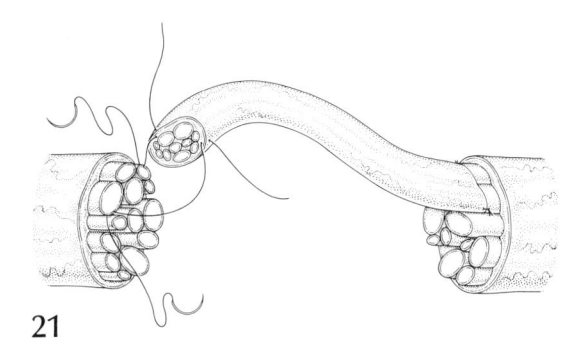

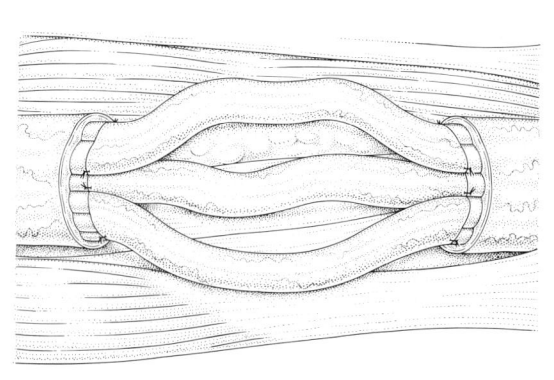

Repair

21 & 22

The gap between nerve stumps is measured with the elbow extended and the wrist in neutral. The graft is cut, with sharp microscissors, so that it lies slackly, in healthy tissue, without any tension whatsoever. Excision of scar from the bed of the graft is of fundamental importance. It may be necessary to run grafts in circuitous fashion over healthy muscle or fat. Grafts are held in place with one or two sutures of 9/0 or 10/0 nylon. The needle is passed through the epineurium of the graft and the perineurium of one of the bundles of the nerve stump.

Partial repair

After isolation of an injured nerve it may become apparent that the lesion is partial and that some bundles are intact. An attempt should be made to preserve these.

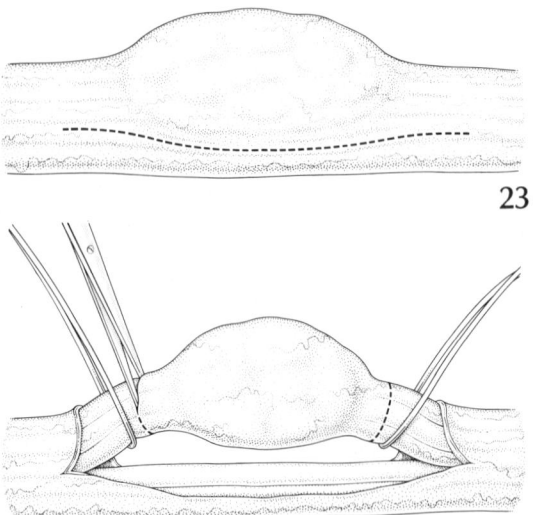

23 & 24

The epineurium is incised longitudinally and delicate dissection within the nerve trunk allows separation of intact bundles from those forming neuromas. Magnification of between 10 and 16 times is required for this.

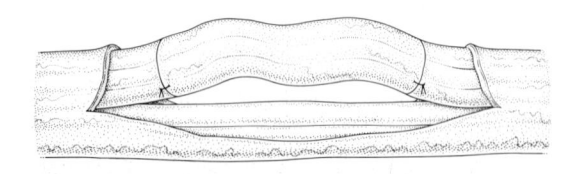

25

The injured portion of the nerve is resected and a graft inserted as already described.

Postoperative management

This is similar to the regime following primary repair of nerves. Gentle movements of the digits are encouraged from the outset, and splints are reduced to allow movement at adjacent joints at 3 weeks. A dorsal splint is applied to the wrist to prevent extension beyond 15° or 20° for a further 3 weeks and it may be necessary to control movement at the elbow for an equivalent length of time. If nerves in the axilla or in the arm have been grafted it is important to control extension of the elbow, and abduction and lateral rotation at the shoulder for 6 weeks. Until that time it is wise to restrict abduction at the shoulder to 45° and lateral rotation to 30°.

OTHER OPERATIONS

Epineural repair

Good results can be achieved following standard epineural repair without using the operating microscope. This technique is easy in delayed cases where the epineurium is thickened and the bundles less mobile within the nerve sheath. After exposing and, in late cases, preparing the nerve faces, the repair is performed using 6/0 nylon sutures, passing the needle through the epineurium only. The first two sutures are placed at the anterior 'corners' of the nerve and are left long to act as stay sutures and to roll the nerve over for exposure of the posterior wall. Gentle traction on these first sutures assists snatching of the cut nerve faces. Further epineurial sutures complete the repair.

External neurolysis

External neurolysis is the freeing of a nerve trunk from adjacent tendons, skin or muscle. It is occasionally useful in late exploration of nerves, where the gliding of tendons applies traction to the nerve or where scar is compressing the trunk. It is particularly indicated in late operative treatment of Volkmann's ischaemic contracture where the median nerve is compressed by the scarred flexor muscle (see chapter on 'Recognition and treatment of compartment compression syndromes', pp. 295–308).

Internal neurolysis

Internal neurolysis is dissection between bundles. The only indication for this operation in the repair of divided nerves is as a preparation for inlay grafting of partial division. Magnification is essential. Clumsily performed, the operation leads to increased neural deficit and significant pain. In my view the technique has no place at all in the treatment of compression neuropathy within the carpal tunnel or at the elbow.

Recent developments

Vascularized nerve grafts

Vascularized cutaneous nerve grafts have not proven themselves in clinical practice. On the other hand, maintaining blood supply to larger trunk nerves is worthwhile. The free vascularized ulnar nerve graft was a logical development of the nerve pedicle operation of Strange[7]. This technique does have a useful place in repair of severe injuries of the brachial plexus particularly when the gaps between nerve stumps are long, where the bed is scarred and where there is insufficient standard cutaneous nerve graft available. This technique has a definite although limited application in these serious injuries. A recent review of 63 patients showed that significant gain in function was achieved in two thirds and that results from the vascularized ulnar nerve graft were better than when an avascular strand of the nerve was used[8].

Nerve transfer

Seddon[2] described a patient in whom he with Yeoman had transferred intercostal nerves into the musculocutaneous nerve of a patient with a complete lesion of the brachial plexus. The operation of nerve transfer is now widely used for irreparable lesions of the brachial plexus where spinal nerves have been torn directly from the spinal cord. Narakas[9] has reviewed the indications for and the results of operations of nerve transfer for irreparable lesions of the brachial plexus.

In patients with irreparable injury to the fifth, sixth and seventh cervical nerves it is now our policy to transfer the accessory nerve to the suprascapular nerve, preserving branches to the upper fibres of trapezius and to transfer three or four intercostal nerves to the lateral cord. The operation is performed as soon as possible after injury.

Muscle autograft

Procedures for restoring function of the shoulder and the elbow, and some sensation in the hand and for relief of pain are surprisingly promising. Bridging gaps between nerve stumps with material other than nerve graft is an old idea. Recent work using muscle autograft which is frozen and then thawed appears to be promising[10,11]. Preliminary clinical trials suggest that this technique is particularly useful in the treatment of patients with painful neuromas of cutaneous nerves. Its use in patients with injuries to major trunk nerves must be subjected to the closest scrutiny before acceptance.

Fibrin glue

Young and Medawar[12] described the use of fibrin glue in repair of divided peripheral nerves in 1940. A commercial preparation is now available (Tisseel, Immuno Limited, Arctic House, Rye Lane, Dunton Green, Sevenoaks, Kent TN14 5HB). There is no doubt that fibrin glue considerably simplifies the technical difficulties of nerve grafting and of nerve transfer and Narakas (personal communication) has evidence suggesting that the quality of regeneration is improved.

Rehabilitation

The best rehabilitation is the early return of the patient to everyday tasks. It is the duty of the surgeon to direct the treatment of the patient towards that end. The prevention of fixed deformity, treatment of pain, and judicious transfers of tendons or muscles to improve function are complementary in this. Physiotherapy should be used for specific aims which include the prevention of deformity, securing a full range of active and of passive movements, and increasing strength. The surgeon who writes 'refer to physiotherapy', often for indefinite periods of intermittent treatment, is failing in his or her duty.

Prognosis

There are unalterable factors which determine the prognosis for a patient after repair of a divided nerve. These are well known: increasing age, increasing violence, infection, and more proximal lesions are all unfavourable. There are two factors which are within the control of the surgeon; these are the delay between injury and repair, and the skill and care with which that repair is effected. The evidence that delay is deleterious is incontrovertible. Inability to make an accurate diagnosis is the commonest cause of delay.

References

1. Dowell JK, Hollingdale J, Powell JM, Birch R. Iatrogenic peripheral nerve injuries of the upper and lower limbs. *J Bone Joint Surg [Br]* 1991; 73-B (in press)

2. Seddon HJ. *Surgical disorder of the peripheral nerves*, 2nd ed. Edinburgh: Churchill Livingstone, 1975.

3. Gelberman RH, Urbaniak JR, Bright DS, Levis LS. Digital sensibility following replantation. *J Hand Surg* 1978; 3: 313–9.

4. Leclercq DC, Carlier AJ, Khuc T, Depierreux L, Lejeune GN. Improvement in the results in 64 ulnar nerve sections associated with arterial repair. *J Hand Surg* 1985 Suppl; 10-A: 997–9.

5. Seddon HJ. Nerve grafting. *J Bone Joint Surg [Br]* 1963; 45-B: 447–61.

6. Millesi H. Interfasicular nerve grafting. *Orthop Clin North Am* 1981; 12: 287–301.

7. Strange FGStC. An operation for nerve pedicle grafting: preliminary communication. *Br J Surg* 1947; 34: 423–5.

8. Birch R, Dunkerton M, Bonney G, Jamieson AM. Experience with the free vascularized ulnar nerve graft in repair of supraclavicular lesions of the brachial plexus. *Clin Orthop* 1988; 237: 96–104.

9. Narakas AO, Hentz, VR. Neurotization in brachial plexus injuries: indications and results. *Clin Orthop* 1988; 237: 43–56.

10. Gattuso JM, Davies AH, Glasby MA, Gschmeissner SE, Huang CL-H. Peripheral nerve repair using muscle autograft: recovery of transmission in primates. *J Bone Joint Surg [Br]* 1988; 70-B: 524–9.

11. Norris RW, Glasby MA, Gattuso JM, Bowden REM. Peripheral nerve repair in humans using muscle autografts: a new technique. *J Bone Joint Surg [Br]* 1988; 70-B: 530–3.

12. Young JZ, Medawar PB. Fibrin suture of peripheral nerves: measurement of rate of regeneration. *Lancet* 1940; ii: 126–8.

Vascular injury and repair

J. S. P. Lumley MS, FRCS, FMAA(Hon), FGA
Professor of Vascular Surgery, St Bartholomew's Hospital, London, UK

EMERGENCY CONTROL OF HAEMORRHAGE

1

The emergency management of arterial haemorrhage is by compression of the main proximal artery on an adjacent bony surface, and local pressure on a swab (or any material available) over the bleeding point. In haemorrhage from the limbs, a tourniquet may be applied, particularly for transportation. As a tourniquet converts partial to complete distal ischaemia, the time and duration of application must be documented, and it must be removed as soon as possible. When a tourniquet is required for longer than 2 hours it should be released for a few minutes each hour, haemorrhage being controlled by local pressure during these periods. Venous haemorrhage of the limbs is reduced by elevation and controlled by a local compression bandage. Care must be taken to cover venous wounds in the neck to prevent air being drawn into the vascular tree during inspiration.

Where possible, the admitting hospital is forewarned to ensure that adequate personnel are available, and the radiology department and blood bank informed. On arrival, emergency control of haemorrhage is continued during assessment. An intravenous infusion is commenced through one or two wide-bore cannulae, and a plasma expander is administered while blood is being cross-matched. Antibiotics and tetanus prophylaxis are considered.

The signs of limb ischaemia include the six Ps (pallor, pulselessness, perishingly cold, pain, paralysis, and paraesthesia), but confusion may arise because of haemorrhage, shock, bruising, venous congestion, persistent pulses and peripheral nerve damage. Baseline measurements are made, and monitoring of pulse, blood pressure, urine output, central venous pressure, haemoglobin and arterial P_{O_2} commenced. A pulmonary artery line will provide additional information of oxygen utilization. Arteriography in the hypovolaemic patient requires optimal equipment and skilled personnel in order to provide useful imaging. It is helpful at some sites, such as the thoracic inlet, axilla, groin and knee, and for expanding haematomas and arteriovenous fistulae, but it must not delay necessary surgery. Satisfactory peroperative angiography is also dependent on the available apparatus and experience of the team. It can be of help in assessing injuries and monitoring vascular reconstruction.

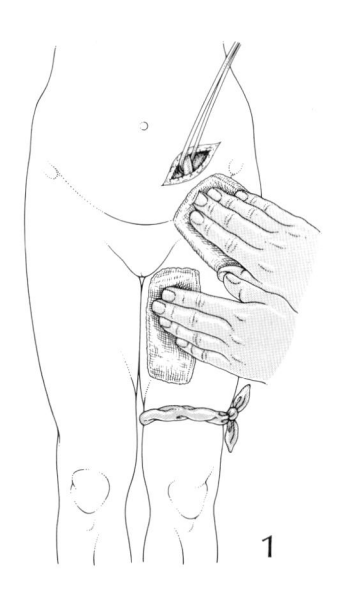

OPERATIVE CONTROL OF ARTERIAL HAEMORRHAGE

General anaesthesia is usually required for major vascular reconstruction. Lighting must be optimal and include spotlights or headlights for visualizing deeper structures. Magnification may be useful for smaller vessel reconstruction, using ocular loupes or an operating microscope.

Control of haemorrhage must continue during preparation, by compression or tourniquet. Skin preparation includes all areas that may require exposure, such as the abdomen in groin injuries and a normal leg when a length of vein may be required.

2

Incisions usually follow the line of an artery, dissecting around muscles and avoiding veins and lymphatics. Exposure must be such that normal artery is demonstrated on either side of the injury. It should be remembered that injuries are often more extensive than the external wound suggests. Intimal damage may not be obvious externally and pulsation can persist in a length of thrombosed artery.

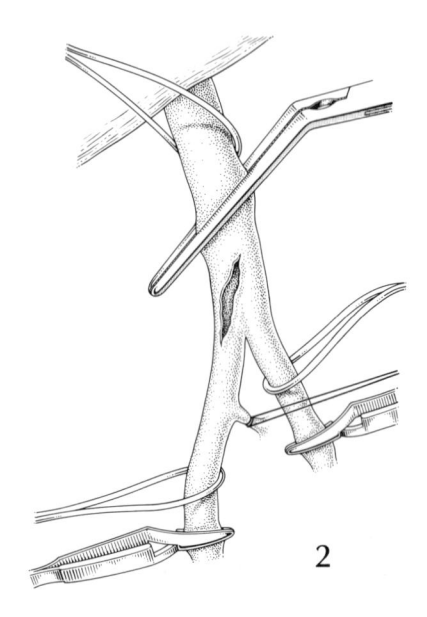

Identification of the bleeding point

An assistant maintains digital pressure over this site while the surgeon mobilizes normal proximal and distal artery. The vessel should be picked up by its adventitia, not by the full thickness of the wall, as this may damage the intima. Sharp dissection with a knife is preferred to blunt dissection during mobilization. A sling or 'sloop' (hollow or solid length of silicone) is drawn behind the vessel by a suture passer and then used to lift the artery clear of underlying tissue while it is being clamped.

Ligation of an artery

Arterial clamps include the bulldog and a number of named instruments with long light jaws with superficial serrations and a six- or seven-toothed ratchet. The pressure applied on closure is the minimum needed to control forward or back-bleeding. If a flat spine of atheroma is present, pressure should be applied across the back of the plaque, rather than crush it from side to side. For vessels of 1–3 mm diameter, a double loop of thread around them can be gently tightened to control the haemorrhage. The weight of an instrument attached to the end of the thread is usually enough to maintain it in position. The size of vascular clamps and other instruments should be appropriate to the vessels being operated on.

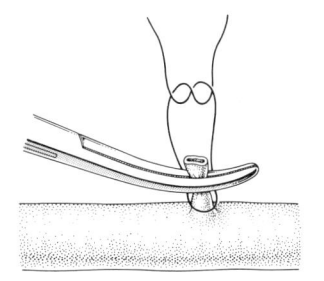

3a–d

Once the bleeding point has been identified and the haemorrhage controlled, a decision is made whether to ligate or reconstruct the vessel. Large arteries and those supplying essential organs are usually reconstructed or bypassed. Temporary shunting must be considered in some sites, e.g. the carotid arteries.

When ligating a vessel the damaged area must be clearly defined. It may then be possible to divide the ends and tie each over an applied haemostat (a) or the vessel may be tied in continuity on either side of the injury using an aneurysm needle to introduce the ligatures. The mouth of a small vessel which has retracted into the tissues may be oversewn (b), provided this does not put adjacent structures at risk. Large vessels are best doubly ligated (c) with or without transfixion of the second tie. Large atheromatous vessels may be difficult to control with one or more external ligatures and in these cases a continuous suture across the cut end (d) or within the lumen may be appropriate.

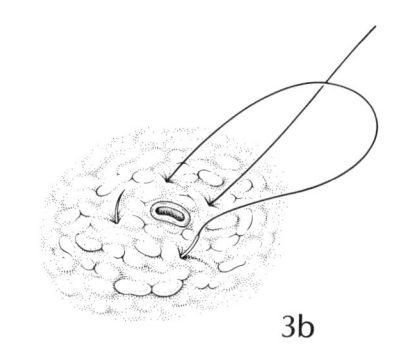

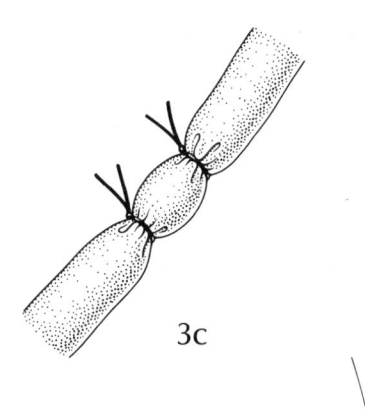

ARTERIAL RECONSTRUCTION

4a–e

When an artery is to be reconstructed the full length of injured vessel must be exposed. The injury usually needs enlargement using Pott's angled scissors to inspect the intima and to exclude intimal tears, subintimal haematomas and local thrombosis. An intact artery can be incised with longitudinal knife incisions, cutting through successive layers until the lumen is entered (a), the incision being enlarged with the angled scissors (b). Alternative means of entering the vessel are a knife stab-incision (c), cutting off a small branch adjacent to its origin (d) or the slice technique (e). Local debris is washed from the lumen with a stream of heparinized saline (1000 iu/300 ml saline solution). Systemic heparinization (100–150 iu/kg) may be appropriate but must be avoided in multiple injuries.

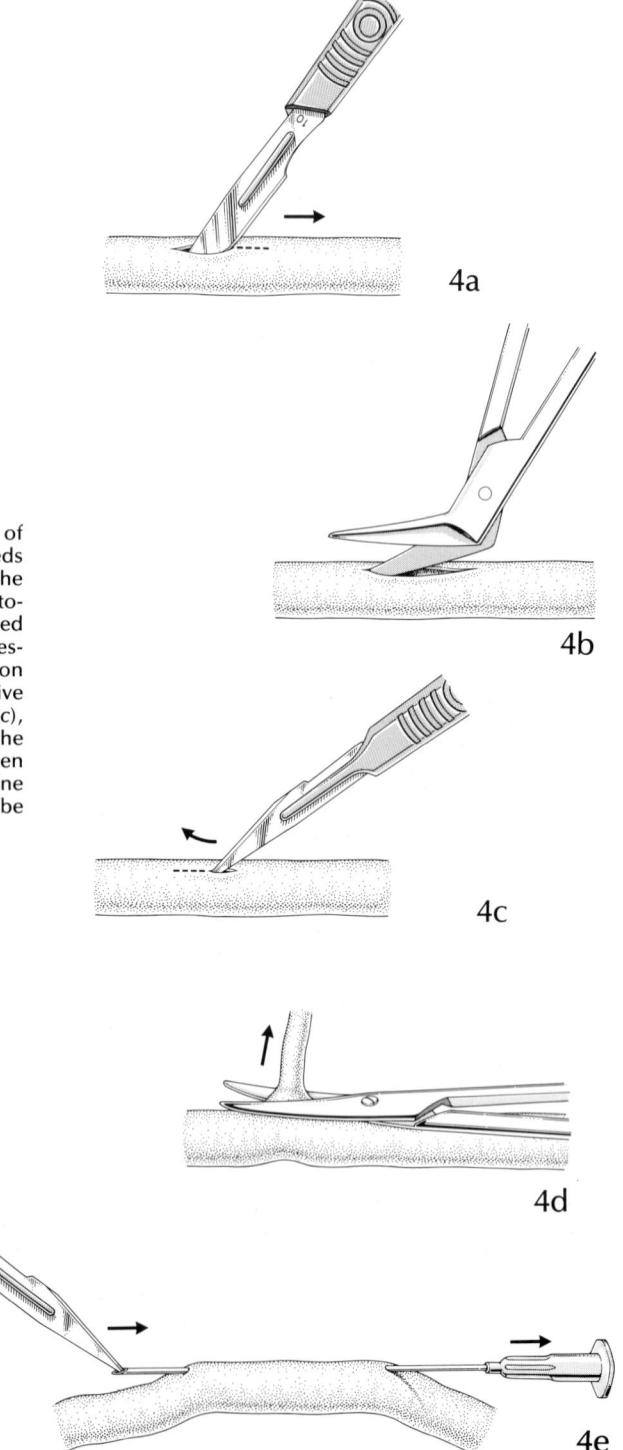

5

Forward and back-bleeding are next checked by temporary release of the proximal and distal clamps. A forceful forward flow (whoosh test) should be present and at least a trickle of back-bleeding. If either of these is absent wider exposure may be required to exclude further local injury, or a Fogarty catheter may be gently passed and withdrawn to remove local blood clot (for spasm, see p. 47. Heparinized saline may be flushed gently proximally and distally using a Tibbs adaptor which fits snugly into the lumen of the vessel. Great care must be taken not to flush debris proximally or distally where it might produce ischaemia of proximal or distal organs.

Management of the local injury may involve endarterectomy of loose or raised intima and pinning down the cut edge with a few interrupted vascular sutures placed from outside the lumen. Damaged arterial wall should be trimmed away. This and other reconstruction should be undertaken in a dry field, but the tissues must be kept moist and debris washed away with heparinized saline.

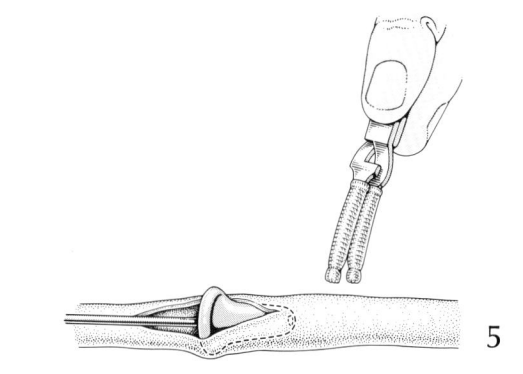

Direct suture

6

Vascular sutures are synthetic non-absorbable smooth-coated material with an atraumatic trocar or a round-bodied needle. Cutting needles are avoided as they can tear a vessel wall. Sutures may be double armed: 4/0 sutures are appropriate for 10–15 mm diameter vessels, 6/0 for 3 mm and 10/0 for microsurgery. A minimum of five throws is advised for each knot as the smooth coating allows a certain amount of slippage which could allow a knot to come undone in a pulsating vessel. A laceration or arteriotomy may be amenable to direct suture. The stitch includes all coats of the arterial wall, pinning down its intima. A continuous suture provides haemostasis. The depth of each bite is equivalent to half the distance between loops in a continuous suture. Interrupted sutures can be used for closure, but they are less haemostatic and take longer to insert. They are appropriate in children where they allow for subsequent growth.

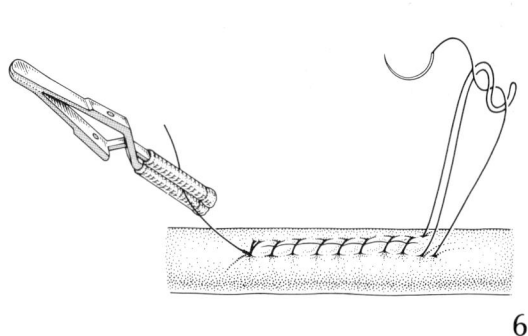

A bulldog or haemostat is applied to the end of a continuous suture to apply traction and keep it out of the operative field. However, the part of the suture involved in the closure must not be clamped or held with a forceps, as this can damage and weaken it with a risk of subsequent fracture. The handles of instruments in the operative field should be covered with a swab during a continuous stitch so that the loops do not get caught. As a continuous stitch reaches the end of an incision, forward and back flow are again checked and a Fogarty catheter passed if there is any change in bleeding status. Blood is then flushed from the clamped segment and the lumen filled with heparinized saline prior to completion of closure.

7

The free end of a continuous suture may be tied to the last loop or to a separate end-stitch. In the former, an additional bite should be made into normal vessel to avoid a corner leak. On completion of closure the low-pressure distal clamp is removed first and obvious leaks are oversewn with a mattress suture. The incision is then covered with a swab while the proximal clamp is removed and gentle pressure applied over the suture line for 2 to 3 minutes to allow needle holes to seal with fibrin. This routine is used on opening every reconstruction to ensure removal of all air bubbles and to reduce blood loss.

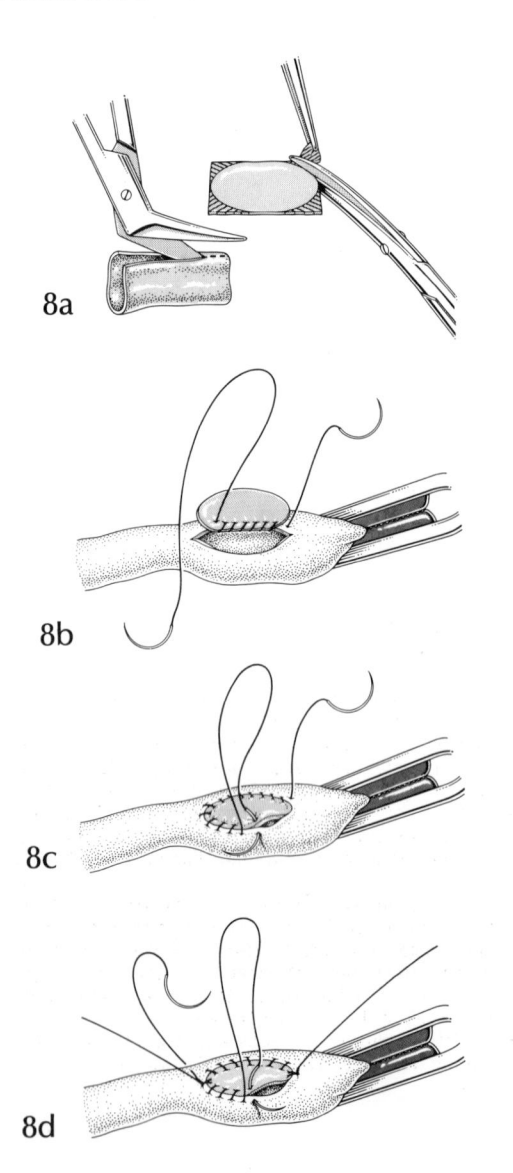

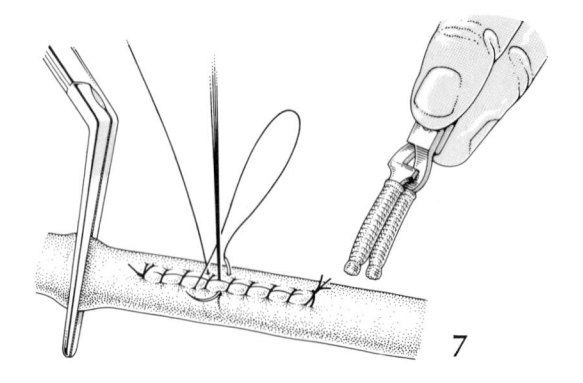

Patch

8a–d

If there has been loss of vessel wall, direct suture may narrow the lumen. An alternative form of reconstruction is then required, such as patching or resection.

If the wall defect is less than half the circumference of the vessel, it can be replaced by a vein patch. An appropriate length of superficial vein is obtained, if possible from the region of the operation site, provided it does not further markedly compromise venous return. A piece of lower leg or arm vein may also be obtained, avoiding the main long saphenous, which should be retained for longer bypasses at this time or in later life.

The vein segment is cut lengthways (a) and opened out. The required width is just more than that of the arterial defect: this allows for the depth of vessel and patch within the suture line. The ends of the patch are fashioned in elliptical form. The width and length of the required patch are best checked with a caliper and this should be available in all vascular instrument sets.

The patch can be stitched in from two end-stay sutures or from one side using a double-ended suture. Bites are taken first through the patch and then the artery (b), thus pulling the patch onto the artery when drawing the suture through. The intima of the patch and artery must be included within each bite. The patch and artery are best picked up as separate bites around narrow corners to ensure that the needle does not pick up the opposing wall. The loops should be laid radially around these corners (c, d).

End-to-end anastomosis

9a, b & c

It may be possible to excise a damaged segment of artery with end-to-end anastomosis. A gap of 1–2 cm can usually be compensated for by mobilizing the vessel on each side and dividing small branches. The ends are trimmed so that a well-defined edge is available for suture and excess adventitia is cut away. The two ends are matched as nearly as possible. Any disparity can be reduced by dividing the smaller end slightly obliquely (a) and taking wider bites of the larger vessel in the suture line. In an end-to-end anastomosis the cut ends must be brought together without tension. This is usually achieved by applying vascular clamps to each and drawing these instruments together to obtain approximation. This tension is maintained until completion of the anastomosis. Larger gaps have to be bridged by a vein graft.

End-to-end anastomoses are conveniently started with a stay suture on either side of the vessel. A continuous suture is placed across the front wall from one stay and tied to the non-needle end of the second (b). The stays are now used to rotate the anastomosis (c) to bring the back wall onto the front for closure. Forward and back flow are tested just before completion of the anastomosis, the clamped segment washed free of blood and debris, and then filled with heparinized saline to eliminate air bubbles. On completion of the anastomosis the low-pressure end is released first and obvious leaks oversewn with a mattress suture. A swab is then placed over the anastomosis before opening the proximal clamp.

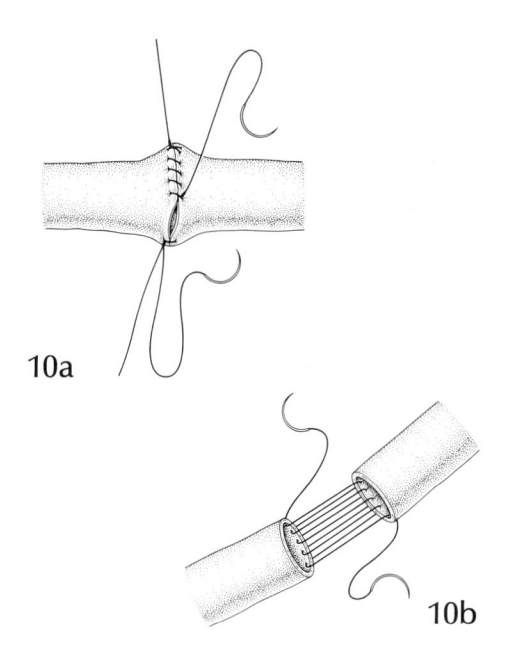

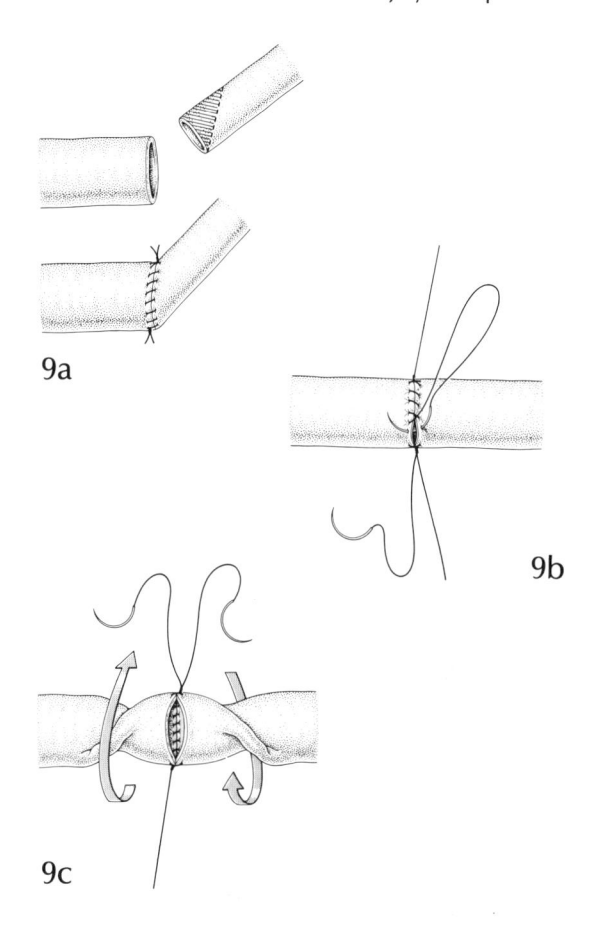

10a & b

In small vessels three stay sutures can be used and so keep the centre of the back wall pulled away, preventing it from being picked up by a suture placed in the front wall (a). Other alternatives are to use a double-ended suture placed first in the back wall and then proceeding in either direction around the anastomosis. Any knot is placed outside the lumen, but the back wall may be sutured either from within or outside the lumen as the stitch proceeds.

When using freely running suture materials such as Prolene (Ethicon, Edinburgh, UK), the parachute technique can be used in which the stitches on one side of the anastomosis are placed with the two vessel ends apart (b) and then gently tightened to bring the vessel ends together. During this manoeuvre a nerve hook can be used to tighten one or two loops at a time if the suture is not running freely, to avoid tearing the vessel wall.

46　Repair of musculoskeletal tissues

End-to-side anastomosis

11a, b & c

For an end-to-side anastomosis the side opening is made as already described for an arteriotomy (see p. 42) and the single end cut slightly obliquely, avoiding sharp corners. For narrow recipient vessels, the cut end may be spatulated (*a*) or sectioned in S-fashion as shown (*b*). A continuous suture may be placed from end-stay sutures (*c*), or by a double-ended technique as described for end-to-end anastomosis, care being taken on corner stitches, as described for patches. The opening procedure is as previously described.

Vein graft

12

If the cut ends of an artery cannot be approximated without tension, a vein segment may be needed for interposition, or a length of vein used for bypassing a damaged area. Longer lengths may require the use of the long saphenous vein and the non-injured leg should be prepared to allow this without further towelling (the use of the ipsilateral saphenous vein may further compromise venous return and increase postoperative oedema). The vein is exposed through a single or multiple shorter incisions and its branches tied with non-absorbable sutures; care is taken not to narrow the lumen or to leave a diverticulum. The vein and wound must be kept moist throughout.

After removal, the vein is gently distended with blood to check for leaks and used in the reversed state, so that the valves will not inhibit distal flow. One side of the vein is marked with Bonney's blue for orientation. Long grafts should be placed within normal tissues, if necessary tunnelling with fingers or long instruments to normal artery on either side of the injury. The anastomoses of grafts may be end-to-end or end-to-side, using the techniques described. The *in situ* technique, in which the vein is left in its bed and its valves destroyed, is not usually appropriate to trauma surgery.

Although synthetic material can be used for patching and bypass it should be avoided in limb trauma since a vein can usually be used without introducing marked disproportion. Foreign material in an infected bed can have the severe consequences of unresolved infection and anastomotic haemorrhage.

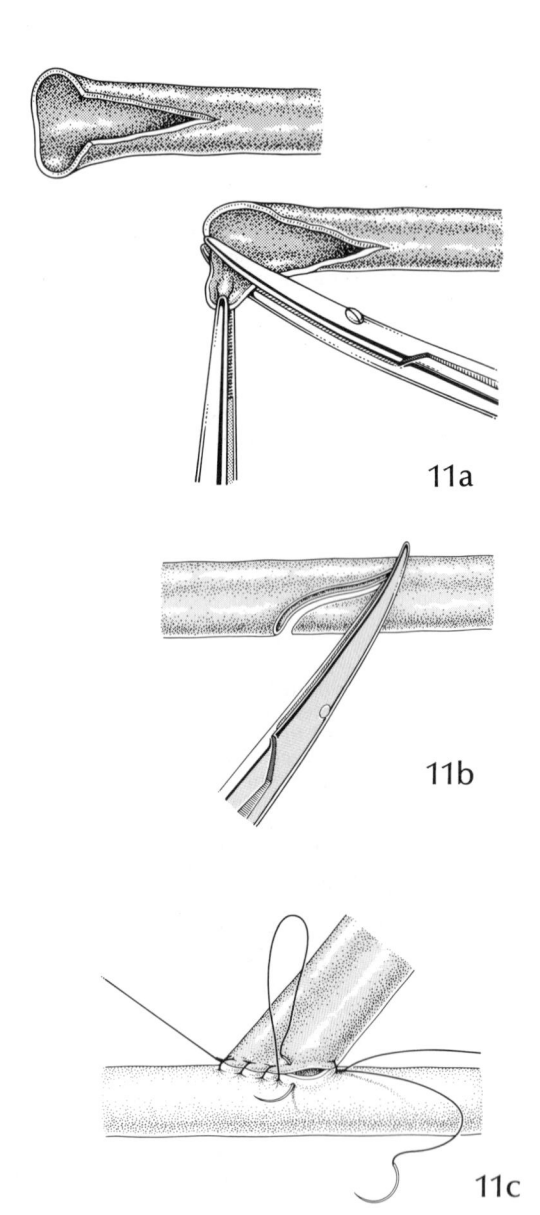

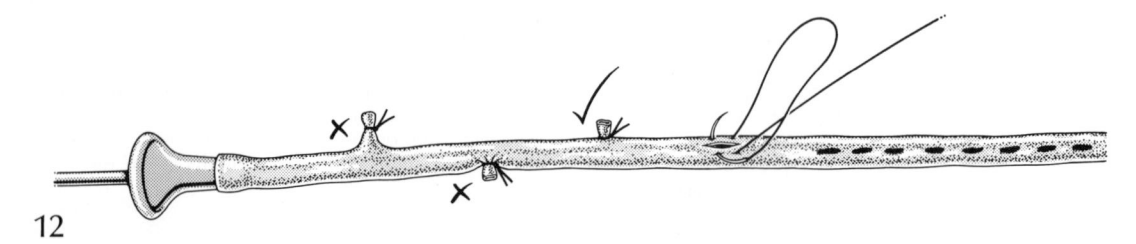

SPASM

13a & b

Spasm is frequently encountered following arterial injury in children, but is uncommon in older ages because of associated atheromatous change. At any age the aphorism 'spasm should be spelt CLOT' is worthy of note. The diagnosis should only be made after full exposure of the length of the injury or angiography has excluded intimal damage and thrombosis. The external application of warm saline or a vasodilator (papaverine; 1 per cent lignocaine) will slowly relieve spasm.

Other measures include intraluminal injection of 250 µg of sodium nitroprusside and blowing up a clamped segment of vessel with heparinized saline inserted into the lumen through a needle (a), or into an arteriotomy using a Tibbs adaptor. When an arteriotomy is present, graded dilatation can be undertaken with metal dilators (b) starting with the largest size that is freely admitted into the lumen and never dilating beyond the normal diameter of the vessel. A Fogarty catheter is valuable in removing clot and debris, but the balloon must never be forcibly distended and withdrawn as this will damage intima. Angioplasty catheters with balloons of appropriate diameter and length may be used to relieve spasm. Short catheters are available for peroperative access through an arteriotomy.

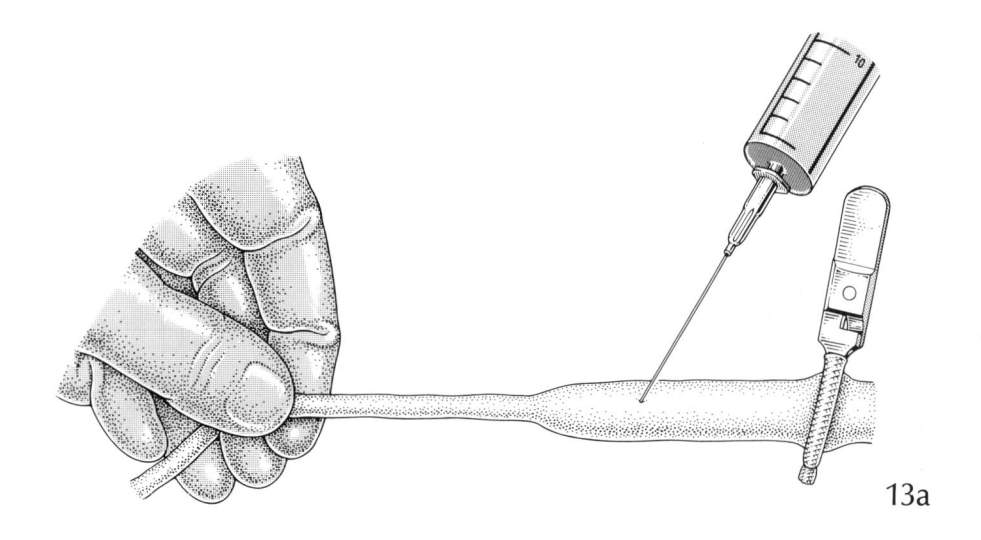

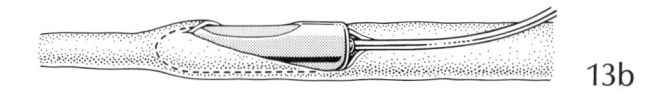

13a

13b

VENOUS INJURIES

Venous operative techniques are similar to those of arterial repair; however, veins are thin-walled, more fragile and more easily deformed. They also lack a firm wall and the pulsation which allows easy identification of an artery during dissection. Despite this, venous flow equates to that of an artery and blood loss can be extensive.

14

Digital pressure is applied to the bleeding point during exposure and then proximal and distal pressure on the vein prior to clamping. Tourniquets, where feasible, and digital pressure on either side of the bleeding point allow it to be precisely identified, clamped and ligated. Double ligatures and transfixion may be appropriate. Small vessels can be oversewn or compressed with metal (Weck) clips. Proximal and distal compression or control with vascular clamps allows venous lacerations to be examined in a bloodless field. They can be closed with a vascular suture, care being taken not to pick up the posterior wall as the consequent narrowing will increase distal venous pressure and accentuate bleeding.

Lack of venous outflow will give rise to distal oedema and compromise arterial reconstruction. Reconstruction of large veins is therefore desirable proximal to the knee and axilla. Operative and postoperative anticoagulation must be considered if there is not extensive injury, this being continued for 3 to 6 months postoperatively. When reconstructing small veins a distal arteriovenous anastomosis is needed to improve long-term patency.

WOUNDS

Contaminated wounds must be fully debrided. Viable skin is preserved, but radical excision is undertaken of all underlying dead tissue. A vascular reconstruction should be covered with viable muscle, where possible, and wounds closed secondarily at 3–5 days. Limbs should be elevated postoperatively to reduce oedema.

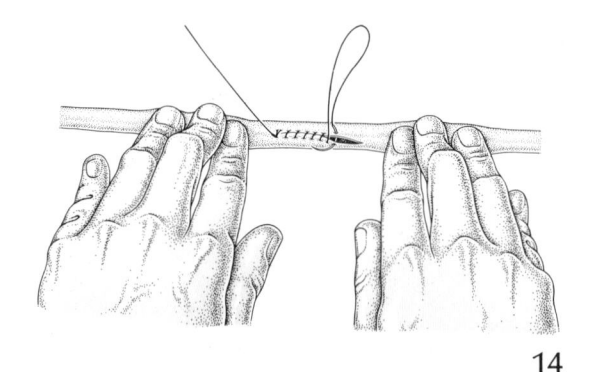

Muscle

Muscle is particularly susceptible to ischaemic changes, some persistent damage being expected after 6 hours. Total necrosis can be anticipated after 12 hours of absolute ischaemia. Revascularization of ischaemic muscle releases ischaemic metabolites which can produce acute renal failure requiring dialysis.

If the time of the injury is well-documented and ischaemia has been absolute for more than 12 hours, primary amputation must be considered as an alternative to revascularization. If ischaemia has only been partial, late revascularization after a number of days can be considered, the tissues being carefully examined at operation. Muscle viability can be difficult to determine immediately after revascularization. Yellowish muscle fibres may gradually improve over 12 hours. Some indication is obtained by colour, together with bleeding on incision and reaction to a nerve stimulator. If in doubt, the wound should be explored every 24 hours (depending on the general condition of the patient) until necrosis and putrefaction become obvious. Muscle fibres which fracture on digital pressure should be excised.

15a & b

Revascularization after 6 hours of ischaemia will produce marked muscle oedema and give rise to acute compartment syndromes. Pressure of more than 50 cm of water (or less in the hypovolaemic patient) is an indication for surgical fasciotomy. However, these measurements, even if available, are only rough guides and can change within an hour. Consequently, if a rise in pressure is suspected or anticipated on clinical grounds, immediate fasciotomy must be undertaken. Fasciotomy for trauma must include incision of skin and fascia throughout the length of each compartment: there is no place for subcutaneous fasciotomy.

In the lower limb all four compartments, anterior, superficial, deep posterior, and peroneal (a), should be decompressed. A single incision over the fibula, with subperiosteal excision of its middle third, does allow access to all compartments. However, this is a difficult procedure and a double incision is advised, the anterior and peroneal compartments being divided through an anterolateral incision (b), and the superficial and deep posterior compartments through a medial incision. As postoperative oozing can be marked, absorbent dressings are applied and fluid replaced as necessary.

The limb is elevated as high as possible using a roller towel for the upper limb and a calcaneal pin and traction for the lower. With maintained elevation, oedema gradually subsides over the next 10 to 12 days to allow skin closure. This is usually possible without grafting and is facilitated by pulling the edges together by skin strips or a skin traction device. Late sequelae of limb ischaemia include muscle fibrosis and contracture, cold sensitivity and neuralgia.

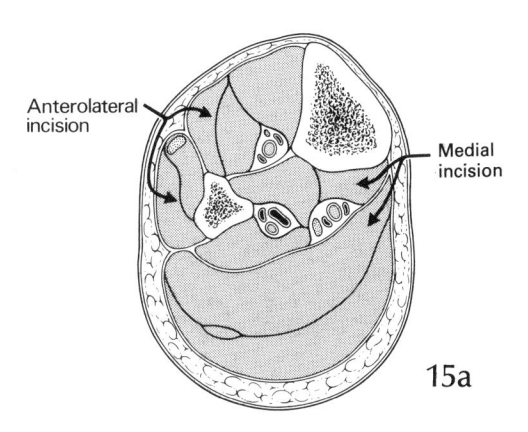

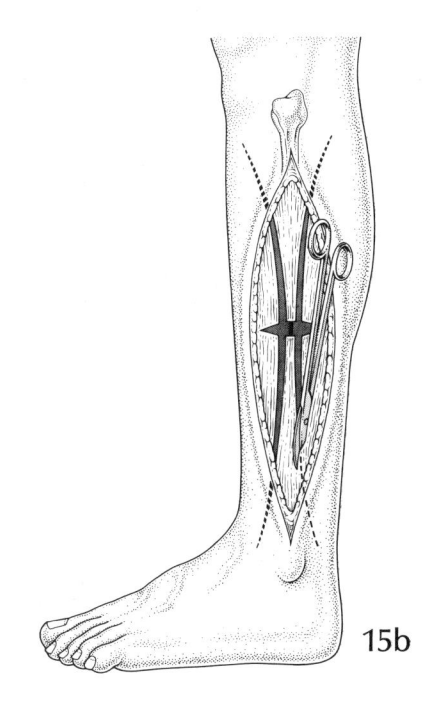

False aneurysm

16a–d

A false aneurysm (a) is often not obvious until the bruising of an injury has subsided. Once established it will usually enlarge and should be treated surgically as soon as the patient's condition permits, and before any tendency to rupture. Angiography may be needed to demonstrate the vessels involved, and the proximal and distal arterial tree. Adequate exposure and proximal and distal control of the damaged artery are desirable prior to dissection of the aneurysmal sac. If the sac is opened prior to clamping, Fogarty catheters may be passed proximally and distally and inflated to obtain haemostasis while the vessel is further dissected. Once the vessel has been mobilized, systemic heparinization is advisable prior to clamping.

It may be possible to perform direct suture of the defect in the wall (b); but if there is extensive damage, then patching (c), resection, end-to-end anastomosis or replacement of the damaged segment with vein (d) or synthetic material may be necessary. All clot and debris should be removed, but adherent parts of the sac wall can be left *in situ*, particularly over adjacent veins.

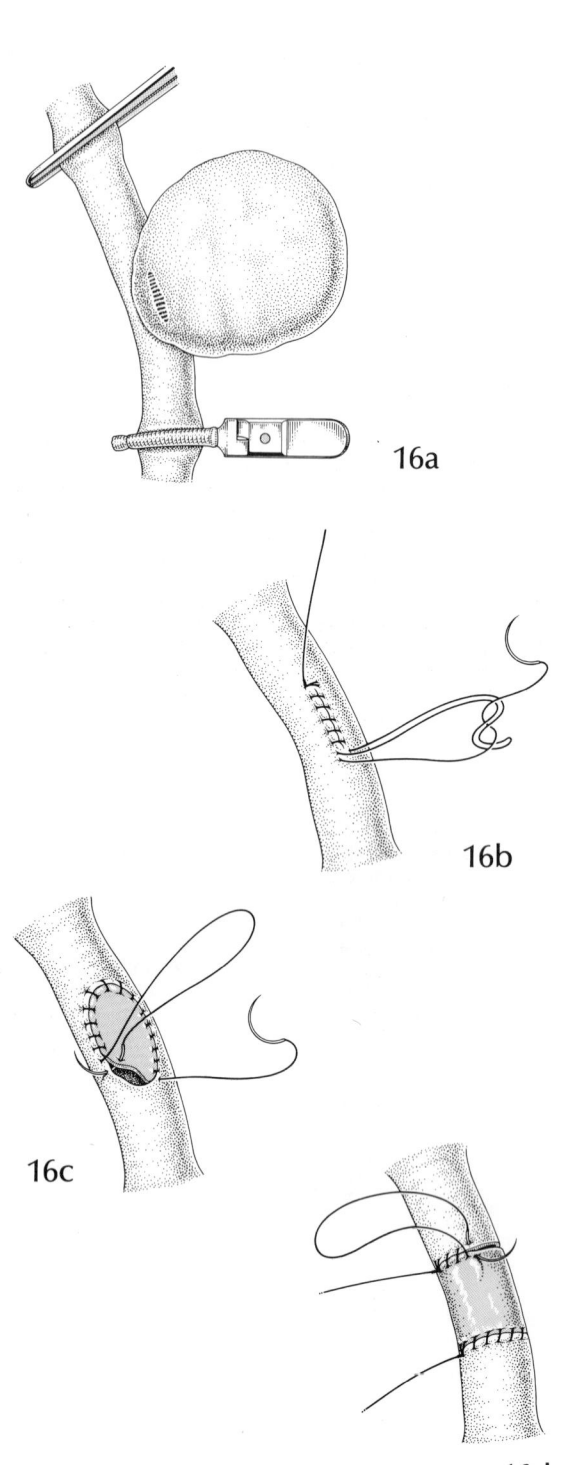

Vascular injury and repair 51

ARTERIOVENOUS FISTULA

The machinery murmur of a fistula is diagnostic once the condition has been suspected. Angiography may be desirable to identify the artery and veins involved and the precise site of the fistula: a rapid series of exposures is required to show early venous filling. Once established, fistulae tend to enlarge and should be treated surgically, as they may bleed and produce distal ischaemia. Large fistulae may carry sufficient blood flow to produce cardiac failure.

17a–d

As with false aneurysms, adequate exposure and proximal and distal control are desirable prior to dissection of the fistula site (a), systemic heparinization being instituted prior to clamping. Quadruple ligation (b) of the fistula is only advised for small vessels. In larger vessels it may be possible to do a direct suture of the artery (c) once the fistula has been taken down, or patch or resect and reconstruct the damaged segment. With large veins proximal to the knee and axilla, venous reconstruction must also be considered and the possible need for a distal arteriovenous fistula. When this is undertaken, a layer of muscle (d) or other tissue should be placed between the two reconstructed vessels.

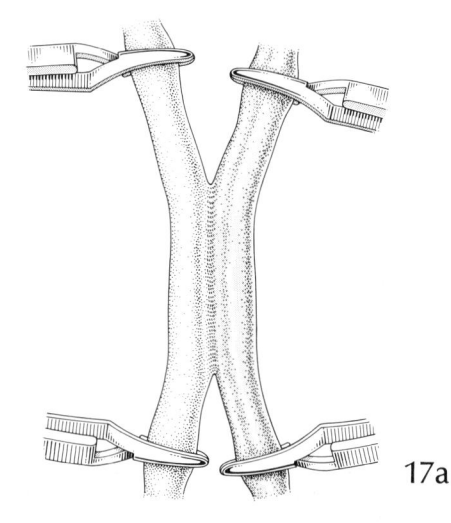

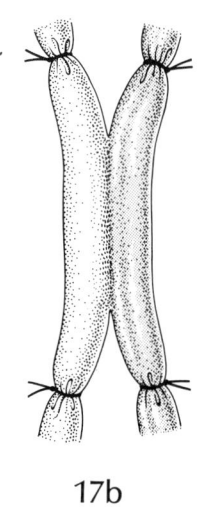

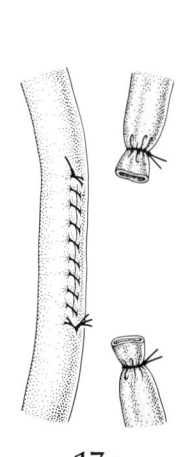

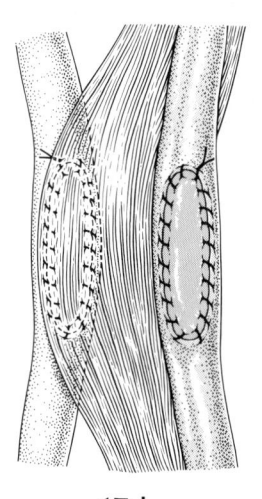

17a

17b

17c

17d

THORAX AND ABDOMEN

Deceleration aortic injuries are usually sited just distal to the left subclavian origin. They may also avulse the aortic root or be sited at the level of the diaphragm. If the lesion is not immediately fatal it may be diagnosed by mediastinal widening on radiography. The diagnosis must then be confirmed by aortography, repair usually being undertaken using cardiopulmonary bypass.

It has been aptly stated that the major hindrance in diagnosing abdominal injuries is the abdominal wall. Although needle aspiration, peritoneal lavage and laparoscopy can provide useful information in blunt abdominal trauma, penetrating injuries require laparotomy and full exploration of the abdominal cavity. This should include the lesser sac and retroperitoneum, with or without Kocherization of the duodenum. Two large intravenous cannulae should be *in situ* for fluid administration and two abdominal suckers available. Autotransfusion is useful if the surgical team has the necessary apparatus and experience in this technique.

18a, b & c

In massive haemorrhage, preliminary aortic clamping is advised. This may be: (a) in the chest through a left lower thoracotomy; (b) at the level of the diaphragm, dividing the lesser omentum between its vascular arcades, followed by transverse incision of the left crus of the diaphragm, to allow the application of the blades of a straight vascular clamp; (c) on the infrarenal aorta which is exposed by retracting the small gut to the patient's right side and dividing the peritoneum longitudinally over the aorta, just to its right, avoiding the inferior mesenteric artery; or by Taylor's wooden spoon which provides a useful temporary means of control by compressing the aorta onto the vertebral column.

Diffuse bleeding from the small vessels of the pelvis can be very difficult to control surgically and, when diagnosed clinically, may be more easily controlled by transvascular embolization.

Direct pressure is applied to a laceration of the inferior vena cava to obtain immediate local control. Proximal and distal pressure on either side of a laceration, together with good suction, can provide a bloodless field while repairing tears in the wall. Uncontrolled venous bleeding around the liver and in the pelvis present the rare occasions when temporary packing and abdominal closure are indicated. At re-exploration 24–48 hours later, haemorrhage is usually reduced and more easily manageable.

Proximal and distal ligation of the iliac veins is occasionally required in pelvic trauma. Exposure of the common iliac vein can be facilitated by clamping and dividing the overlying common iliac artery. End-to-end anastomosis of the artery is undertaken after the venous problems have been treated.

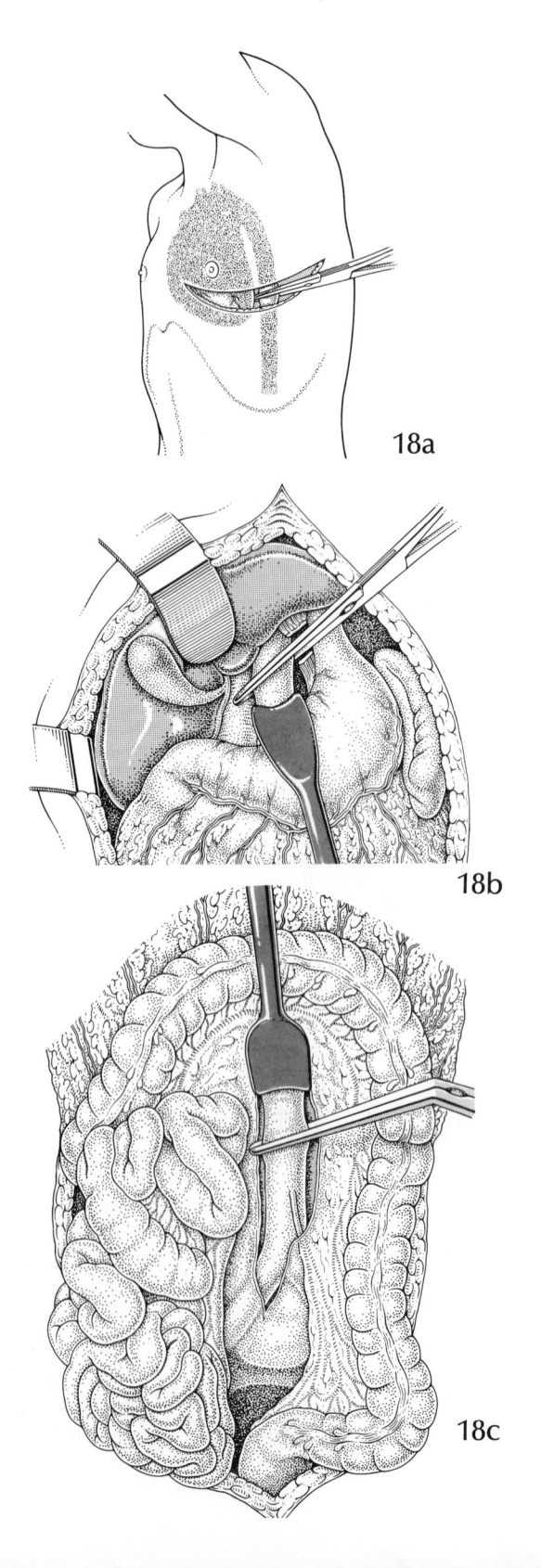

19a–d

Lumbar and intercostal vessels may be damaged during spinal fusion. (a) Pressure should initially be applied to the area over a swab for at least 5 minutes. The swab is left undisturbed after releasing the pressure for a few more minutes, and is then gently removed: if haemorrhage has stopped further action may be unnecessary. (b) If complete haemostasis is not obtained, damage of the lumbar and intercostal vessels away from the aorta and inferior vena cava can usually be controlled with ligation, transfixion or a Weck clip. (c) Avulsion of the vessels near their origin, with persistent haemorrhage, may be treated by a vertical mattress suture of 4/0 vascular material. (d) If this proves unsuccessful a dry field must be obtained by clamping or compressing the aorta or inferior vena cava proximally and distally in order to insert a mattress suture in a bloodless field.

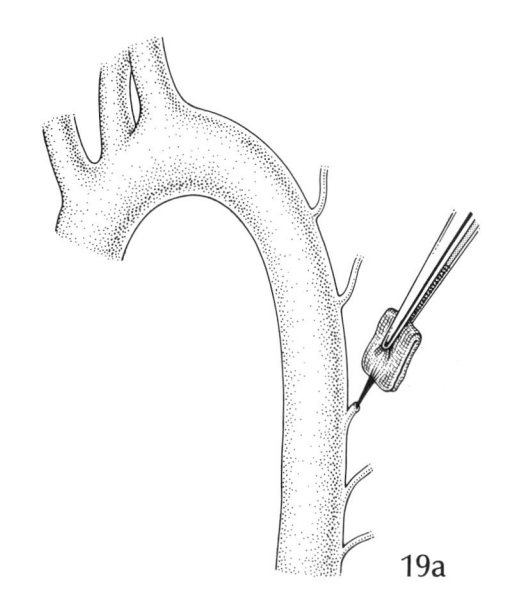

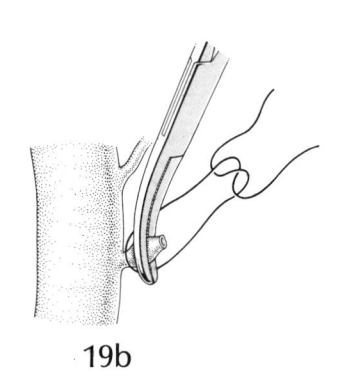

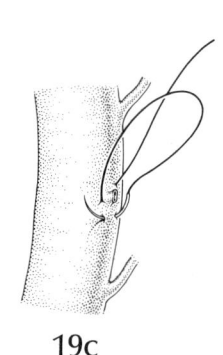

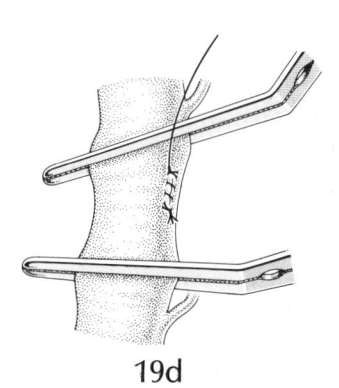

LIMB REPLACEMENT

Recovery after replacement of the major part of a limb is not usually complete, and rehabilitation may take 1–2 years. In view of this, great care must be taken in selecting individuals who are physically and mentally suited to this protracted programme. Grossly contaminated limbs, marked crushing and avulsion injuries are less suitable and prior vascular disease and general ill-health are bad prognostic signs.

Severed limbs should be placed in a sterile bag and stored in ice until required. Two teams are desirable to prepare the two damaged ends. Bone shortening and fixation are then undertaken followed by venous and arterial reconstruction. Usually two veins are anastomosed for each main artery. Nerves are brought together with one or two sutures and covered with a plastic cuff, secondary suture being undertaken after 3–4 weeks. Primary suture is only applicable in clean wounds.

Replacement of severed digits needs careful appraisal. Although revascularization and re-innervation are usually possible, they often result in a rigid finger which can hinder manual activity. Every attempt should, however, be made to retain the thumb and at least one digit to provide a pincer grip.

Illustrations by Mark Iley

Surgical management of acute bone and joint infections

M. F. Macnicol FRCS, MCh, FRCS Ed(Orth)
Consultant Orthopaedic Surgeon, Princess Margaret Rose Orthopaedic Hospital, Edinburgh, UK

Introduction

Pathology

Acute osteomyelitis is a blood-borne infection of bone, usually sited in the metaphysis. Septic arthritis may ensue if the metaphysis is intracapsular, as at the hip, knee, shoulder and elbow. Bacteria may also reach the joint by transgressing the epiphyseal growth-plate or by direct inoculation.

The sequestration and multiplication of infective organisms is the result of a complex interaction involving four factors.

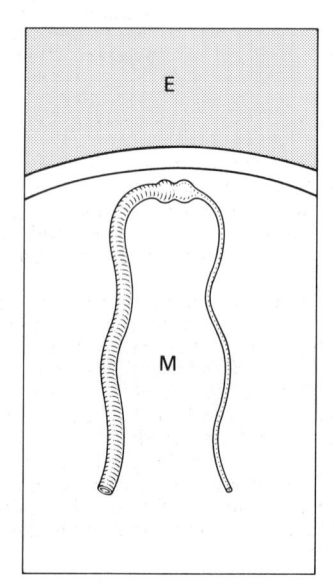

1

1. The vascular bed of the metaphysis, where the venous loops both allow blood flow to become sluggish and permit the permeation of bacteria into the extravascular space as the vessel wall lacks a basement membrane and cement substance. (M, metaphysis; E, epiphysis.)
2. Deficient phagocytosis secondary to both a paucity of local reticuloendothelial cells and probably a more generalized immunodeficiency of the patient.
3. Chemoattraction between the bacterial glycocalyx and larger collagen fibres of the growth-plate and articular cartilage.
4. The possibility of superimposed thrombosis secondary to local trauma, with the subsequent adherence of organisms to the entrapped red blood cells.

2

In the infant, pus erupts more readily into the surrounding periosteal or capsular space, whereas diaphysial spread (1) occurs in the older child with a more resistant cortex. The centrifugal direction of osseous circulation results in a gradual spread of infection into the subperiosteal space (2) with time, thus producing a clinically apparent abscess deep to the soft tissues. On rare occasions, the epiphysis may be primarily involved (3), particularly before it becomes substantially ossified.

The events that lead up to a subperiosteal abscess are therefore: (1) bacterial colonization; (2) bacterial multiplication; (3) collagen fibre fragmentation; (4) inflammatory cell reaction; (5) increased intraosseous pressure; (6) bone ischaemia; (7) bone necrosis; and (8) abscess formation.

Principles of treatment

The objectives of treatment are: (1) to reduce the multiplication of bacteria by the use of antibiotics; (2) to drain a subperiosteal abscess if it develops; and (3) to preserve articular cartilage and joint function.

Early diagnosis of acute osteomyelitis depends upon clinical suspicion and thorough examination of the child. The differential diagnosis includes juvenile chronic arthritis, acute rheumatic fever, neoplasm, haemophilia and Henoch–Schönlein purpura.

The presentation of osteomyelitis may be acute, subacute or recurrent, and in the immunodeficient child it may be multifocal. All modes of presentation may progress to chronic osteitis if early treatment is inadequate. The indications for surgical drainage are based upon a recognition that continuing sepsis will assuredly destroy a joint, and will affect the growth and structure of a long bone. Hence, operative treatment is mandatory if: (1) a clinically obvious abscess is present; (2) acute osteomyelitis fails to resolve after a 48-hour period of intravenous antibiotic treatment; or if (3) intra-articular suppuration occurs[1].

If the child is seriously ill from associated septicaemia there is a relative indication to explore bone and joints, although general anaesthesia may be considered to be inadvisable.

Microbiology

Both aerobic and anaerobic organisms may infect bones and joints (*Table 1*). The 'best guess' antibiotic for early treatment can only be expected to cover the more common bacteria, and the decision rests between flucloxacillin and ampicillin, fusidic acid and erythromycin, and a cephalosporin.

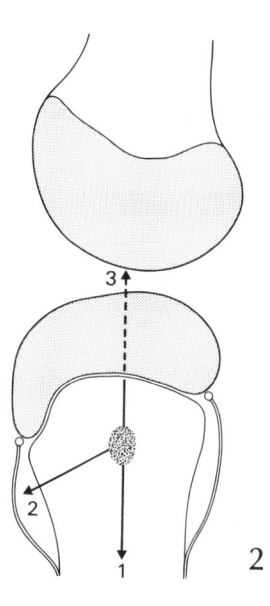

Table 1 Aerobic and anaerobic organisms causing acute bone and joint infection

Aerobic	Anaerobic
Staphylococcus aureus	*Peptococcus magnus*
Streptococcus pyogenes	*Peptococcus prevotii*
Haemophilus influenzae	*Peptococcus asaccharolyticus*
Streptococcus pneumoniae	*Peptococcus variabilis*
Staphylococcus albus	Other *Peptococcus* spp.
Escherichia coli	*Peptostreptococcus* spp.
Proteus spp.	*Veillonella alcalescens*
Klebsiella	*Bacteroides fragilis*
Pseudomonas	*Bacteroides melaninogenicus*
Salmonella	*Bacteroides* spp.
Brucella	*Fusobacterium naviforme*
Fungi	*Fusobacterium nucleatum*
Mycobacterium tuberculosis	*Propionibacterium acnes*
Meningococcus	*Eubacterium lentum*
Pneumococcus	*Clostridium* spp.

If a patient is allergic to the penicillins, clindamycin is of value when *Staphylococcus aureus* is cultured, with initial use of gentamicin if the patient is septicaemic. Chloramphenicol should be considered if *Haemophilus influenzae* is cultured, and vancomycin is effective against streptococci.

Direct sampling from subperiosteal, osseous or intrasynovial infections can be ensured by formal surgical drainage, arthroscopy and aspiration. Despite the use of immediate Gram- and Ziehl-Neelsen-staining, and rapid plating for both aerobic and anaerobic organisms, negative results do not exclude the presence of infection. Open biopsy undoubtedly yields the greatest chance of obtaining a positive culture, but the indiscriminate policy of operating upon every case of presumed osteomyelitis[2] cannot be recommended, and a rate of surgical drainage varying between 22 per cent[3] and 50 per cent[4] is more realistic.

Operations

SURGICAL DRAINAGE

A tourniquet is applied under general anaesthesia, and the affected limb is then cleansed and draped. Exsanguination with an Esmarch bandage should be avoided as it may disseminate the infection and may injure oedematous tissue.

Incision

3

The incision should allow unrestricted access to the bone or joint involved, and wider exposure is often necessary if anaerobic infection has produced a widespread myonecrosis. A tourniquet is contraindicated if sickle cell anaemia is suspected.

A longitudinal 5 cm incision is sufficient if the metaphysis is to be explored. The growth-plate should be avoided, and a minimal subperiosteal exposure usually suffices. Extension of the wound may be required, depending upon the findings.

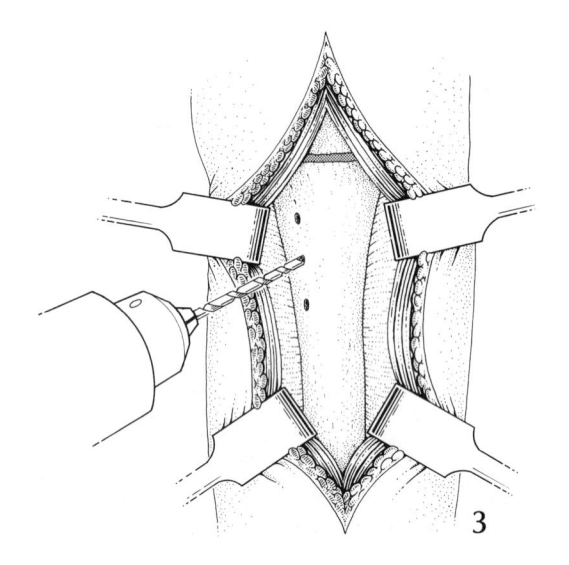

Drainage

Release of subperiosteal pus is all that is required, but if no pus is apparent the periosteum is gently elevated and three 4 mm drill holes are made in the cortex, parallel with the long axis of the bone. If a cortical window is considered to be advisable this can be achieved with a small osteotome or bone cutters.

Bacteriological specimens and a biopsy for histological examination should be obtained at this stage and sent immediately to the laboratory. Irrigation of the wound is advisable prior to loose apposition of the skin edges with interrupted sutures: 4/0 Ethilon or Prolene (Ethicon, UK) are ideal. There is no need to insert a drain, and closure of the periosteum or the subcutaneous tissues is inadvisable.

The affected limb is elevated after applying a compression dressing, and the tourniquet is released. Splintage with a rigid backshell will ensure that the relevant joints are rested, but the application of a full plaster is unnecessary.

Postoperative management

Antibiotics should be continued intravenously for a further 2 or 3 days, and orally for a minimum of 2 weeks. Resolution of the osteomyelitis is monitored by the clinical signs, the erythrocyte sedimentation rate, and serial radiographs in two planes. Isotope bone scanning may be advisable if there is concern about the vascularity of the bone, particularly the proximal femur.

ASPIRATION

4 & 5

Aspiration of a joint is recommended by some surgeons, and has a role to play in the earliest stages of the infection if clinical and radiographic features suggest an effusion. A needle can be inserted into the larger joints, but it should be remembered that a false-negative result may follow the bacteriological culture of an aspirate. Arthroscopy of the knee, shoulder and ankle allows access to these joints and may make formal arthrotomy unnecessary.

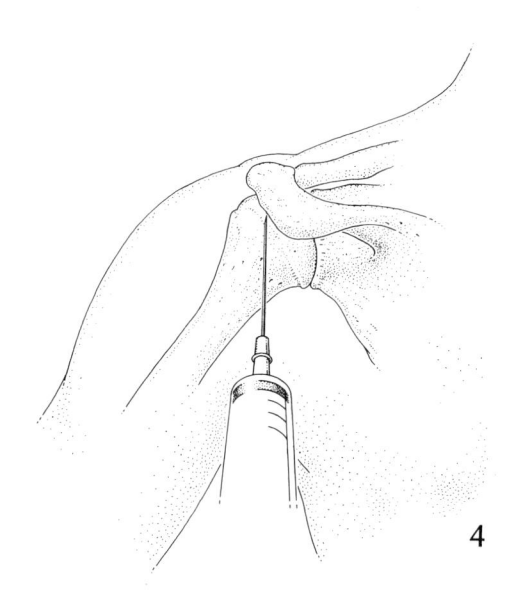

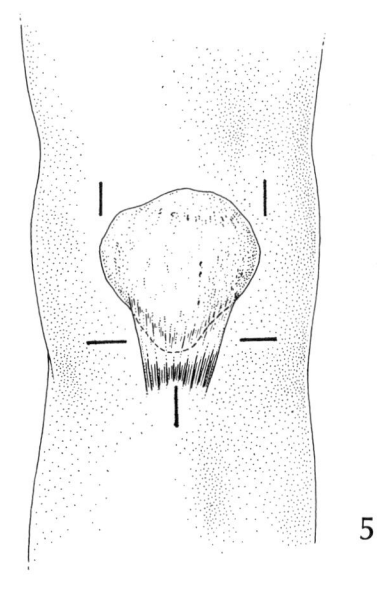

58 Infections

OTHER APPROACHES

Surgical approaches to the hip, shoulder, elbow, ankle and hindfoot are shown in *Illustrations 6–11*. The capsule should be opened by a cruciate incision or fenestration, allowing complete decompression and subsequent irrigation of the affected joint. Loose closure of the wound without a drain usually suffices at the end of the procedure, and the joint should be splinted initially in the position of function. The use of continuous passive motion is appropriate if there is no likelihood of subluxation and if the swelling of the soft tissues permits.

6

Individual anterolateral, lateral and posterior incisions allow satisfactory access to the hip joint.

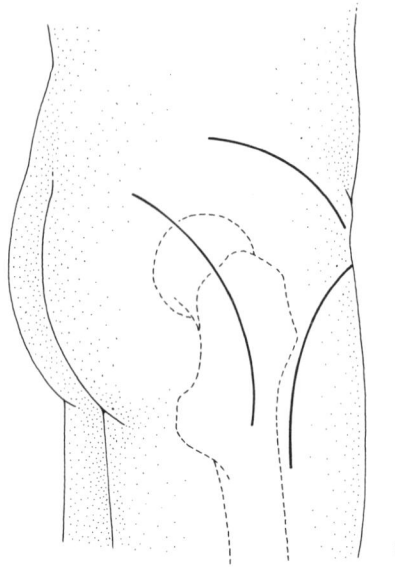

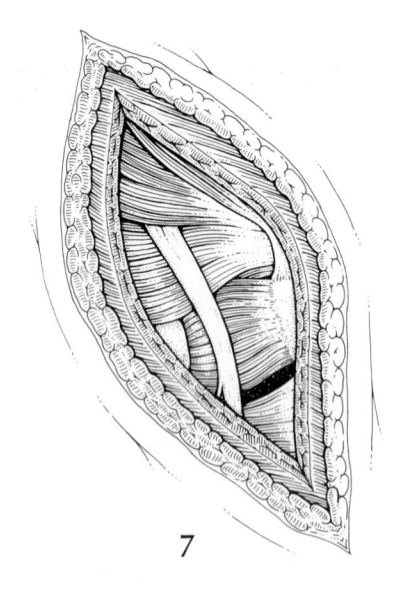

7

A posterior approach affords dependent drainage and gives excellent access if the sciatic nerve is protected, and the lateral rotators split in the line of their fibres.

Surgical management of acute bone and joint infections 59

8

The shoulder is exposed through an anterior incision.

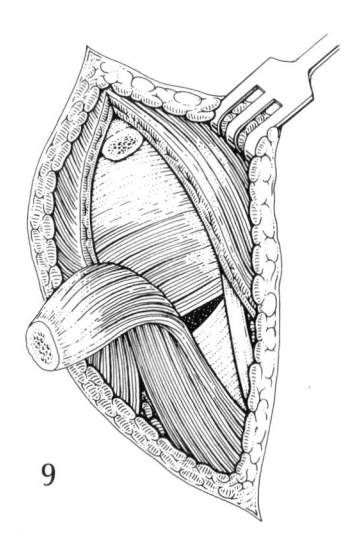

9

The fibres of subscapularis are exposed and split after reflecting the short head of biceps and coracobrachialis distally.

10

A lateral approach to the elbow is preferred.

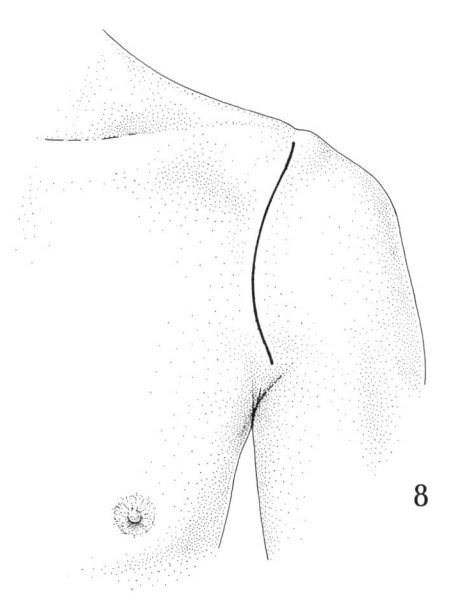

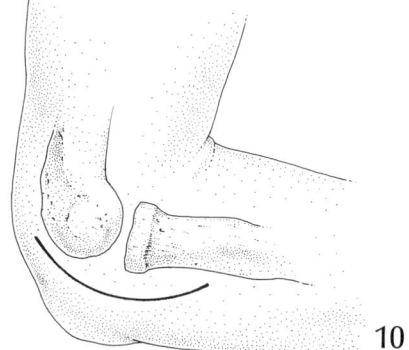

11a & b

Medial or posterior incisions provide satisfactory access to the ankle or subtalar joints.

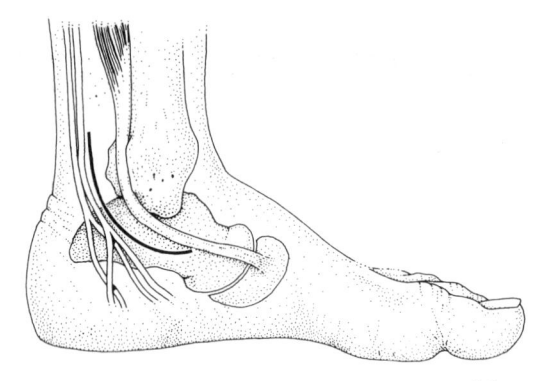

11a

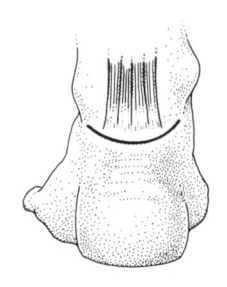

11b

References

1. Nade SML. Acute haematogenous osteomyelitis in infancy and childhood. *J Bone Joint Surg [Br]* 1983; 65-B: 109–19.

2. Mollan RAB, Piggot J. Acute osteomyelitis in children. *J Bone Joint Surg [Br]* 1975; 59-B: 2–7.

3. Cole WG, Dalziel RE, Leitl S. Treatment of acute osteomyelitis in childhood. *J Bone Joint Surg [Br]* 1982; 64-B: 218–23.

4. Blockey NJ, Watson JT. Acute osteomyelitis in children. *J Bone Joint Surg [Br]* 1970; 52-B: 77–87.

Further reading

Langer C. Ueber das Gefassystem der Rohrenknochen, mit Beitragen zur Keentniss des Baues und der Entwicklung des Knockengewebes. *S-B Akad Wiss Wien, math-nat KL* 1875; 1 Abt, 36: 1–40.

Lexer E. Experimental production of osteomyelitis foci. *Arch Klin Chir* 1894: 48: 181–200.

Koch W. Ueber Embolische knochennebrosen. *Langenbecks Arch Klin Chir* 1879; 23: 315–25.

Hobo T. Zur pathogenese der akuten haematogenen Osteomyelitis, mit Berucksichtigung der Vitalfarbungslehre. *Acta Sch Med Univ Kioto* 1921; 41: 1–29.

Starr CL. The acute haematogenous osteomyelitis. *Arch Surg* 1922; 4: 567–87.

Morrissey RT, Haynes DW, Nelson CL. Acute haematogenous osteomyelitis. The role of trauma in reproducible model. *Trans Orthop Res Soc* 1980; 26: 324.

Illustrations by Philip Wilson

Chronic infections of bone and joint

R. A. B. Mollan MD, FRCS(Ed), FRCSI
Professor of Orthopaedic Surgery, Queen's University of Belfast, UK

Chronic osteomyelitis presents a clinical spectrum of acute or chronic disease, a wide variety of infecting organisms and a variety of aetiological causes with, on occasion, underlying predisposing factors. Surgical treatment must be aimed at achieving a precise diagnosis of the pathological lesion, its extent and bacteriology, and at achieving a cure.

The disease may present as a chronic encapsulated pus cavity (Brodie's abscess) or as a persistent sinus and underlying area of purulent osteomyelitis.

62 Infections

BRODIE'S ABSCESS[1]

This is the localized and clinically quiescent type of osteomyelitis which develops in the metaphysis of the large tubular bones. Pain and localized signs of inflammation may be present for a considerable period before diagnosis is made. If the symptoms persist or there is radiographic evidence of advancing bone destruction, operative treatment is indicated.

In an even more chronic and very rare form, the sclerosing osteomyelitis of Garré, the whole shaft may be involved with multiple small abscesses surrounded by dense sclerotic bone.

Preoperative preparation

1

Radiographs reveal the benign cystic nature with surrounding dense sclerosis. Bone scan and tomography are helpful in finding the extent of the lesion and planning the extent of surgical decompression.

Antistaphylococcal treatment with flucloxacillin and fusidic acid is started a few days before surgery. When bacteriological samples are sent the laboratory must be informed of the prior treatment with antibiotics. A tourniquet is used if possible. A biopsy is essential to exclude Ewing's sarcoma.

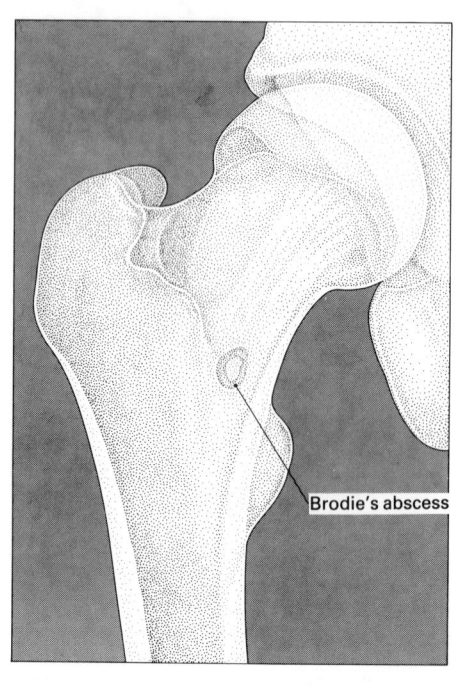

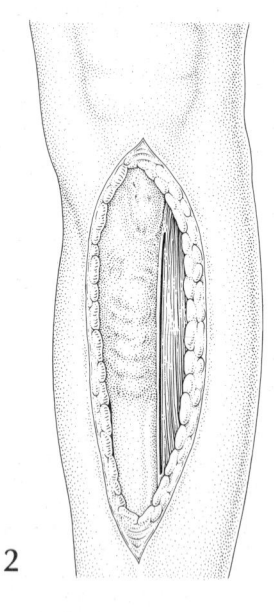

Surgical procedure

2

A direct approach onto the bone using fascial planes is atraumatic and prevents contamination and devascularization of soft tissues. Skin and fascia are incised in the same line and when bone is encountered the periosteum is incised longitudinally, stripped circumferentially and bone levers inserted on both sides to retract the soft tissues.

3

The abnormal bone is usually recognizable but if difficulty is encountered a peroperative radiograph will confirm the level. The roof of the abscess cavity is removed by drilling the cortex at 1 cm intervals with a 2.4 mm drill. A sharp chisel is used to join up the holes, gradually deepening the grooves until the cavity is entered. The whole thickness of the cortex is gradually and carefully transected and the roof elevated to reveal the cavity. Further removal of bone may be necessary to visualize the whole cavity.

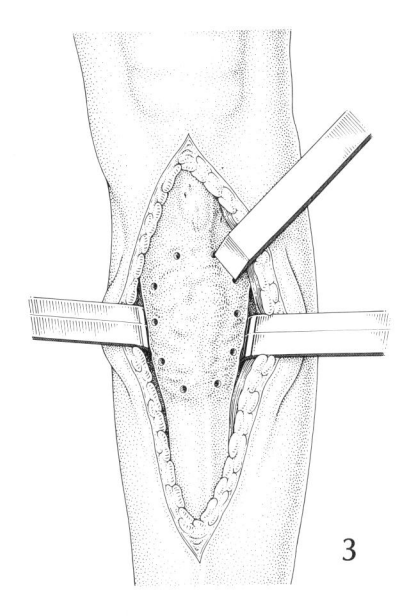

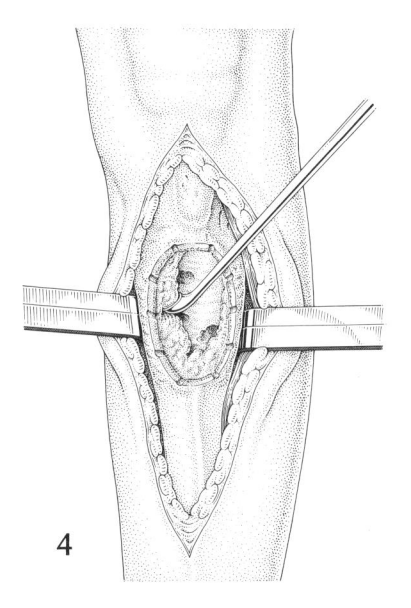

4

The contents of the cavity – pus and chronic inflammatory granulomata – and peripheral membrane are evacuated and sent for laboratory investigation. This should include direct Gram stain, aerobic and anaerobic culture and histology. The cavity is carefully curetted and all small cavities explored to ensure total evacuation of infected tissue. The cavity should be liberally flushed with saline or a suitable antiseptic solution such as hydrogen peroxide. If the defect is extensive, autogenous cancellous bone graft can be taken from the ilium to pack the cavity and the wound is then closed in layers. If any doubt exists as to whether all the infected tissue has been excised, then the cavity should be filled with antibiotic-loaded methacrylate beads and the skin closed. A second operation can be carried out in 2–3 weeks to remove the beads, to curette the cavity and fill it with bone graft.

Postoperative management

Antibiotic treatment will be dictated by the bacteriological results and combination chemotherapy with bacteriocidal agents should be continued for 6 weeks. Postoperatively the leg should be splinted with a split plaster of Paris cast until the removal of sutures after 12 days. A few days elevation and rest of the limb is beneficial.

Further splintage will depend on the size and site of the cavity, the bone involved, and the forces which would be expected during loading. It is essential to err on the safe side and the use of modern cast-bracing will preclude disuse osteoporosis, joint stiffness and muscle wasting.

CHRONIC SUPPURATIVE OSTEOMYELITIS

5

This is the likely end-result of poorly treated acute haematogenous osteomyelitis or infected fractures with or without internal fixation. In pathological terms the bone is infected with areas of abscess, dead bone (sequestra), dense sclerotic bone with doubtful blood supply, and sinuses. Attempts at healing result in areas of granulation tissue and periosteal reaction which forms an involucrum.

Stability of the bone is essential. In cases of haematogenous osteomyelitis, particularly in the infant, operative debridement should await restoration of the bone by the involucrum. In cases of infected non-union external fixation is used. It is important that the pin holes are predrilled slowly with sharp bits to prevent thermal necrosis which would inevitably lead to pin-tract infection and loosening.

Chronic multiple sinuses and previous surgery compound soft tissue scarring. Meticulous preoperative planning of the incision is essential and if necessary soft tissue flaps or vascularized grafts must be considered to achieve primary healing.

If this is not practicable then the wound will have to be left open and autogenous cancellous bone grafting is performed following the method of Papineau[2]. When granulation tissue has developed to cover the graft split-skin grafts can be used to achieve healing.

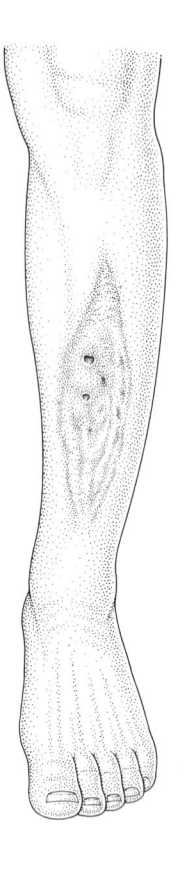

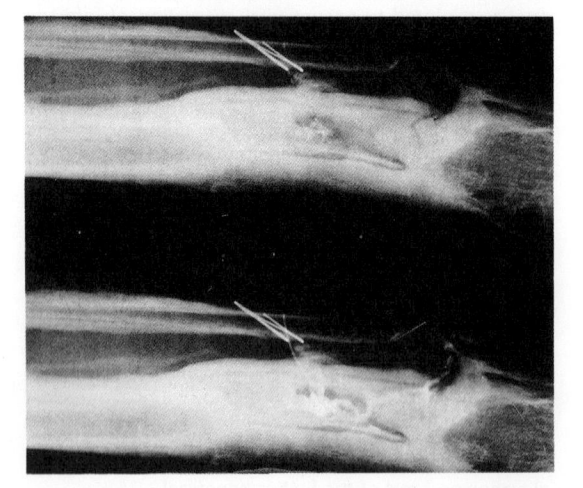

Preoperative preparation

6

Surgical treatment in a patient with toxaemia or septicaemia is dangerous and it is important to prepare the patient preoperatively. On admission, antistaphylococcal antibiotics, flucloxacillin and fusidic acid, should be commenced parenterally, preferably intravenously. Culture from sinus tracts will yield a variety of organisms which are likely to be secondary contaminants. Anaemia should be corrected well in advance of surgery, and liver and renal function checked. During the preparation phase of 7–10 days, a sinogram should be carried out to identify the track and source of discharge. Tomography is useful as multiple abscess cavities are often difficult to identify in the haphazard areas of sclerosis, sequestra and osteolysis.

Chronic infections of bone and joint 65

Surgical procedure

The stability of the limb is secured by an external fixator if non-union is present. The incision must take account of any plastic surgical procedure which may be necessary and further dissection of soft tissues will be dictated by the local blood supply to the flaps.

7

The sinus tracks must be totally excised by an elliptical incision around their mouths, then careful dissection and excision of the track down to the abscess cavity. Methylene blue injected into the sinus 24 hours before surgery will dye the scar and granulation tissue of the track and aid the total removal of sinus tracks.

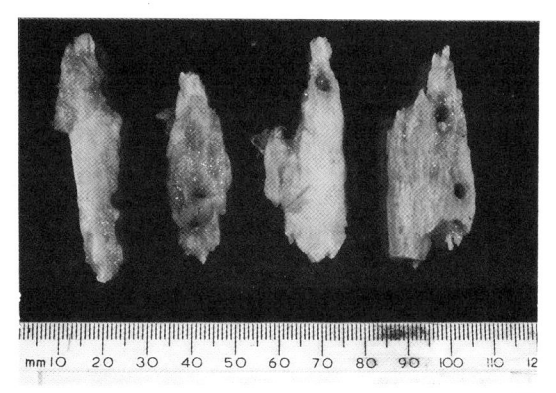

8

The bone is approached as directly as possible, the periosteum and fibrous tissue is stripped off and bone levers used to retract the tissue. The area of osteomyelitis is usually very obvious and the cavity should be deroofed carefully by predrilling to prevent extension of a fracture line.

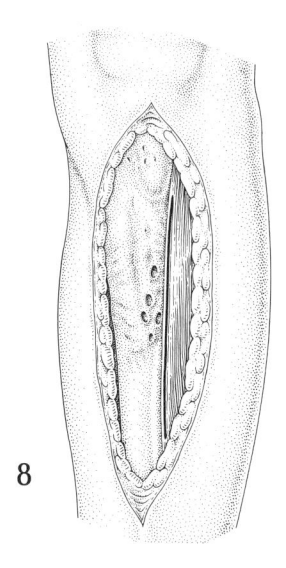

9

The whole infected cavity must be widely deroofed, resulting in the tubular bone having the appearance of a 'gutter'. Dense white bone should be chiselled away carefully to avoid fracture until punctate haemorrhage is seen. Sequestra, pyogenic membrane and granulation tissue must be radically excised by bone nibblers and sent for bacteriological examination. Direct microscopy and culture should be requested and the bacteriologist informed of current antibiotic therapy.

Deroofing should be continued until all cavities are explored and bleeding normal bone is visible at both extremities of the gutter. Extensive and careful curettage of the cavity should be supplemented by liberal flushing with saline or suitable antiseptic lotion.

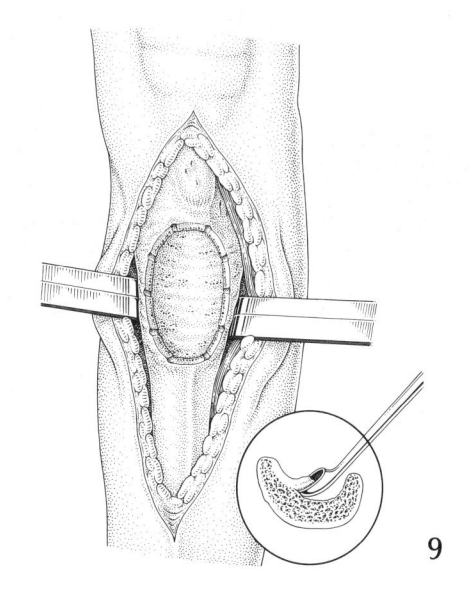

10 & 11

The cavity can then be filled with autogenous iliac bone grafts cut into small pieces and packed into the cavity. Alternatively, the cavity can be packed with antibiotic-loaded polymethylmethacrylate beads and a secondary bone grafting carried out at 2–3 weeks.

Skin closure with primary healing is preferable; but after a cancellous bone graft, a split-skin graft can be applied.

In particularly difficult or grossly infected cases a delayed bone graft is recommended. If thought necessary continuous irrigation with antibiotic fluids can be used for a period of days. This requires very careful and personal attention to detail to achieve efficient irrigation and to prevent contamination.

Postoperative management

The limb should be elevated and rested in a split plaster of Paris cast until skin healing occurs. Antibiotic therapy will be dictated by the result of the culture of the deep tissues. Parenteral antibiotics should be used until the patient is free of any postoperative nausea and sickness, and should be continued for at least 3 months.

Splintage will depend on the site and extent of bone damage and deficiency. Protection in traction may be required for some weeks prior to gentle mobilization in fracture braces. In the case of non-union, the limb must be held stable until union commences. The external fixator can then be removed and cast-bracing commenced to enhance union and bone strength.

THE TWO-STAGE PROCEDURE

This is a very safe method of dealing with infection. The use of gentamicin-loaded beads permits local elution of antibiotic treating Gram-negative organisms of a primary or secondary nature. The surgeon has an opportunity to reinspect the guttered bone to ensure that all infection has been eliminated.

The primary incision is reopened. The beads are removed and the dark granulations are curetted and removed to ensure that all visible bone has a good blood supply. Further removal of dense white bone may be necessary.

Autogenous cancellous iliac graft is taken and diced to small dimensions. It is gently packed to fill the defect. The wound is closed in layers; and sutures are removed at 12–14 days. Drains are not necessary.

PROBLEM BONE INFECTIONS

Osteomyelitis of the os calcis presents a difficult problem as the infection is in a predominantly cancellous matrix with little cortical bone. The weight-bearing ability of this bone is severely compromised. Because of the increase in antipersonnel explosives and the prevalence of chronic infection in developing countries, management of osteomyelitis in this bone deserves special mention.

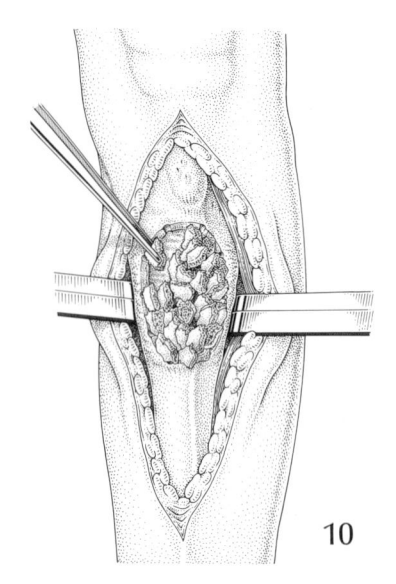

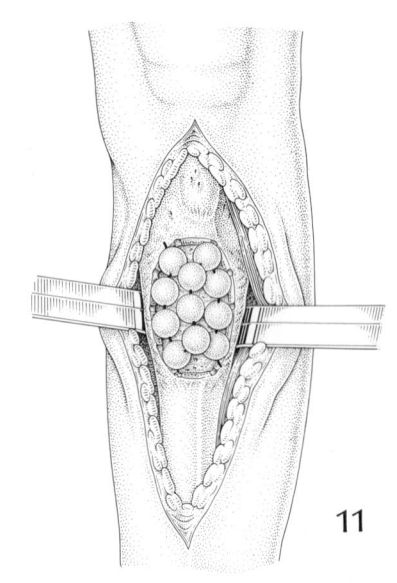

The heel pad is a very specialized structure. There is a tight honeycomb structure made up of small fascial compartments filled with fat which acts as a shock-absorber to both compression and shear. Scarring due to chronic infection or injudicious surgery compromises the structure; even if the osteomyelitis is healed, painful scars may lead to amputation. It is anatomically difficult and mechanically unsound to approach the heel from medial or lateral sides and thus the approach of Gaenslen[3] through the plantar surface is recommended.

Antibiotic treatment should start preoperatively with flucloxacillin and fusidic acid and later be modified by the culture results of deep swabs taken at surgery.

Surgical procedure

12

The patient should be prone with the leg slightly elevated. A midline incision is made from the insertion of the tendo Achillis to the midpoint of the plantar surface. The tendo Achillis is split medially for a few centimetres. The plantar aponeurosis is also split between abductor digiti minimi and flexor digitorum brevis. The lateral plantar artery and nerve are retracted medially. The flexor accessorius and long plantar ligament are split to reveal their insertions into the os calcis. The calcaneum is then split in the midline with a broad osteotome and the bone carefully prised apart to preserve its cortex and overall architecture.

Pus, granulations and sequestra are curetted, taking care to preserve normal bone. The cavity is irrigated and, if suitable, packed with autogenous cancellous bone. The halves of the os calcis should be approximated and the wound loosely packed.

Postoperative management

The leg should be encased in a split short-leg plaster of Paris cast with a window cut in the heel for dressings. The pack should be removed at 4 days and the wound dressed daily and allowed to heal by secondary intention. Partial weight-bearing should start at 6 weeks, gradually increasing as pain permits.

References

1. Brodie BC. An account of some cases of chronic abscess of the tibia. *Med-chir Trans* 1832; 17: 239–49.
2. Papineau L. L'excision – greffe avec fermeture retardée délibéreé dans l'ostéomyélite chronique. *Nouv Presse Med* 1973; 2: 2753–5.
3. Gaenslen FJ. Split-heel approach in osteomyelitis of the os calcis. *J Bone Joint Surg* 1931; 13: 759–72.

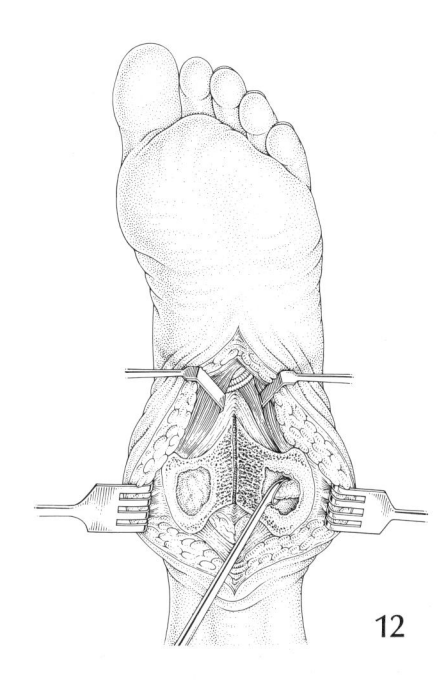

Further reading

Dombrowski ET, Dunn AW. Treatment of osteomyelitis by débridement and closed wound irrigation-suction. *Clin Orthop* 1965; 43: 215–31.

Kelly PJ. Infections of bones and joints in adult patients. *Am Acad Orthop Surg Instr Course Lect* 1977; 26: 3–13.

Launtenbach C. The treatment of bone infection with PMMA beads compared with local antibiotic instillation. *J Bone Joint Surg [Br]* 1980; 62-B: 275–6.

Roy-Camille R, Reignier B, Saillant G, Berteaux D. Resultats de l'intervention de Papineau: a propos de 46 cas. *Rev Chir Orthop* 1976; 62: 347–62.

Illustrations by J. A. Pangrace

Swanson arthroplasty of the metacarpophalangeal joint for rheumatoid disease

James E. Culver MD
Head, Section of Hand Surgery, Department of Orthopaedic Surgery, Cleveland Clinic Foundation, Cleveland, Ohio, USA

Introduction

Indications

Pain and/or deformity resulting in disability of the hand in the presence of articular damage are the primary indications for this procedure. Generally, the metacarpophalangeal joints of all four fingers are operated on at the same time.

Contraindications

1. A patient who is functioning well and has adapted to the deformity.
2. Inadequate bone stock, soft tissue structures that have been stretched and distorted beyond repair or reconstruction, or a rapidly progressive disease state.
3. An uncooperative patient.

Preoperative

Anaesthesia

Regional anaesthesia, such as an axillary block, is usually preferred for these patients with chronic disease.

Position and preparation of patient

The patient is placed supine with the arm extended on a side table. Care should be taken not to put undue stress on a diseased shoulder or elbow.

A tourniquet is essential for the operative procedure. It is applied unsterile high on the arm. The sterile drapes are placed over it.

Operation

Skin incision

1

A dorsal transverse incision[1] is made over the necks of the metacarpals. This exposes the bulging joint capsules of the metacarpophalangeal joints with the extensor tendons subluxed ulnarly. Alternatively, longitudinal incisions may be used in the midline over each of the metacarpophalangeal joints. Full-thickness skin flaps are mobilized with care to protect the veins and lymphatics that travel between the metacarpal heads.

Retinacular and capsular incisions

The retinaculum is incised on the radial side of each of the extensor tendons. A longitudinal capsular incision is made extending distally to the base of the proximal phalanx. Synovectomy is performed.

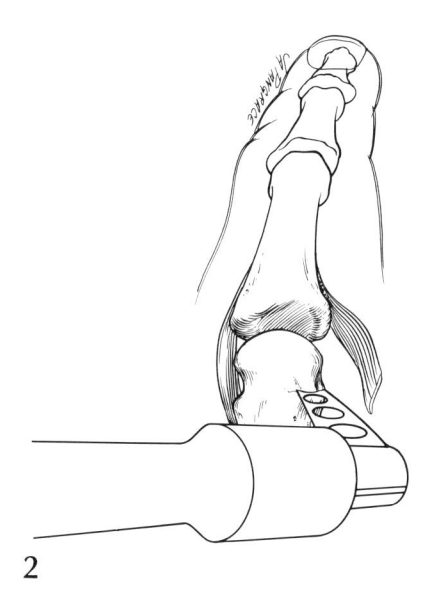

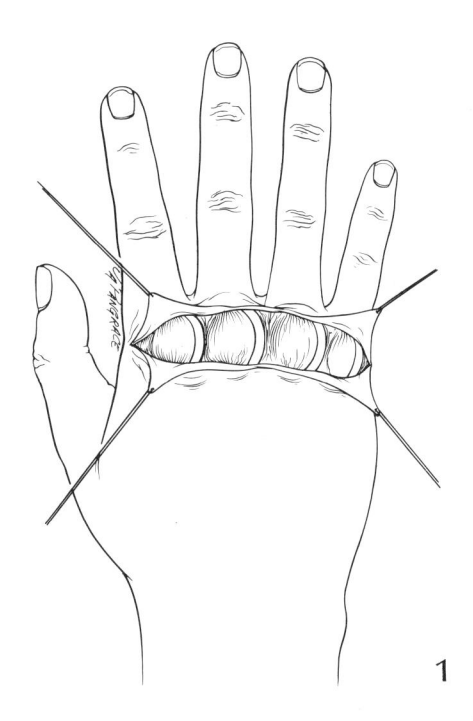

Resection of metacarpal head

2

The metacarpal head is excised with a power saw which provides a clean exact cut for removing the metacarpal heads. If there has not been significant contracture, the metacarpal head can be removed without completely detaching the collateral ligaments. In most cases the collateral ligaments can be preserved. If there has been an excessive amount of erosion of the metacarpal heads, or excessive soft tissue contracture has occurred, the collateral ligaments are released so more bone can be resected.

Preparation of base of the proximal phalanx

All articular cartilage is removed from the base of the proximal phalanx and any irregularities trimmed. If there has been excessive erosion on the dorsal cortex of the base of the proximal phalanx, more of the phalanx will need to be removed. In this case the collateral ligaments and volar plate are released and the proximal phalanx is shortened.

Preparation of medullary canals

3

Openings into the medullary canals of the metacarpals and proximal phalanges are made with a small awl. The opening into the canals must have a rectangular shape, matching the shape of the stems of the implant. Specially designed broaches and reamers are available which assist in accomplishing this. On occasion, power burrs with smooth tips are needed to ream the medullary canals. Trial implants are used to check the fit. The stems of the implant should easily piston in and out of the shafts and the central portion of the implant should fit flush against the bone. The largest implant that will accomplish this is chosen. The medullary canal of the metacarpal is sized first. It is important not to make the opening into the base of the proximal phalanx too large. There should be no buckling of the implant when the finger is extended. If there is, more bone is resected.

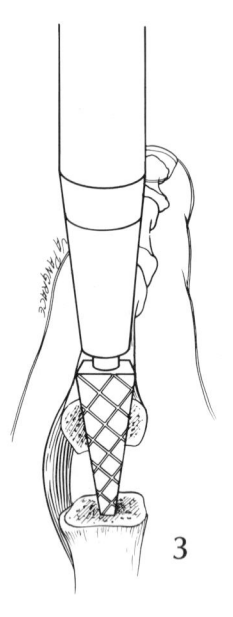

Inserting the final implant

4

The medullary canals are irrigated well with Ringer's solution and with neomycin solution. Because the Silastic (Dow Corning, UK) implants have an electrostatic charge, they pick up lint from the drapes and from the surgeon's gloves. Therefore it is important not to touch the implant except with forceps. Each implant stem is put in with the patient's finger flexed and then the finger is extended. The central portion of the implant should fit flush against the ends of the metacarpal and proximal phalanx. Alignment and stability are checked to be sure that the fingers are straight and not angulated or malrotated.

Closure

If the collateral ligaments were detached, the radial collateral ligament is reattached to the distal end of the metacarpal with a small non-absorbable suture placed through a drill hole. If the collateral ligaments have been detached from the proximal phalanx, the radial collateral ligaments will also need to be reattached. In the index finger, if the radial collateral ligament is inadequate, one half of the volar plate is split longitudinally, left attached distally and brought around the radial side of the joint and attached through a small drill hole. Capsular closure is accomplished with an absorbable suture. In the index finger the capsule can be used to pull the index finger into a slight amount of supination.

Centralization of extensor mechanism

5

The extensor tendons are centralized over the dorsum of the joints. The retinaculum on the ulnar side of the tendon may need to be released to accomplish this. The tendons are lapped over the radial retinaculum and secured with interrupted horizontal mattress sutures of a non-absorbable material. Each finger is tested for intrinsic tightness and, if present, the ulnar intrinsic to that digit is released. Small drains are placed in the wound after closure.

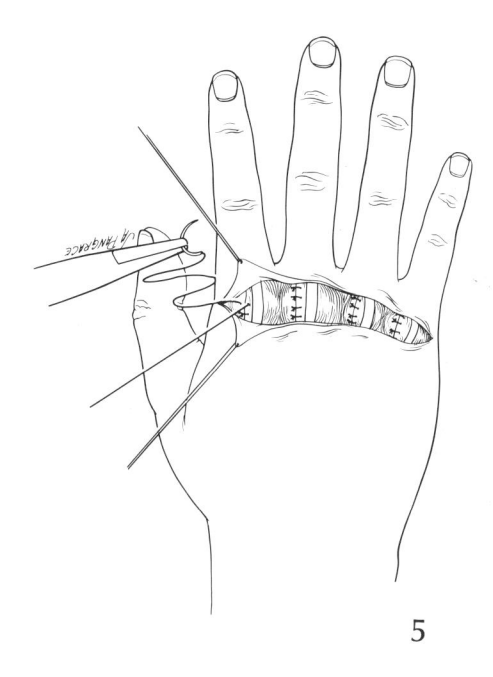

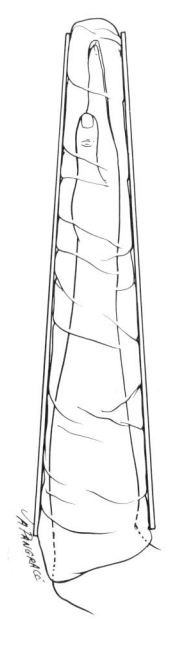

Dressings

6

A non-adherent gauze is placed over the incisions. Thick layers of polyester batting are placed on the volar and dorsal aspect of the hand, wrist and forearm, extending to the finger tips. Four-inch anterior and posterior plaster splints are applied extending to the finger tips and wrapped with a bias-cut stockinette. The bandage should be snug, but not constricting, giving gentle compression and immobilizing the metacarpophalangeal joints in a neutral position. Firm compression is applied by pressing the plaster splints firmly together, greatly reducing postoperative bleeding and preventing postoperative oedema.

Postoperative management

The hand is elevated at all times. Shoulder and elbow exercises are encouraged. In 3-5 days the dressing is removed and a light bandage is placed over the incision. The patient is then started on an intensive therapy programme including dynamic splinting, with a goal to gain a maximum amount of flexion and extension and to prevent recurrent ulnar deviation[2].

Complications

Superficial wound infections are uncommon and are usually due to necrosis of the skin edges. The infection responds well to antibiotics and local wound care. Generally, prophylactic antibiotics are given intravenously 30-45 minutes before inflation of the tourniquet and continued for 24 to 48 hours after surgery. Infection of the implant itself is rare. If an implant becomes infected, it should be removed and the wound irrigated well. The patient is covered with antibiotics and a new implant can be reinserted at the same time or at a later time.

Implant breakage may occur, but the incidence is low. Nothing need be done unless there is associated deformity, in which case the broken implant is replaced and the soft tissues reconstructed in order to maintain proper alignment.

Prolonged splinting and careful postoperative rehabilitation is imperative. In some patients, the range of movement may be quite limited. Dorsal capsulotomy may offer some improvement. Recurrent ulnar deviation may result from excessive use of the hand or due to inadequate soft tissues. If troublesome, implant revision may be done with special attention given to the soft tissue reconstruction and postoperative therapy.

References

1. Swanson AB. Flexible implant arthroplasty for arthritic finger joints: rationale, technique, and results of treatment. *J Bone Joint Surg [Am]* 1972; 54-A: 435-55.

2. Madden JW, De Vore G, Arem AJ. A rational postoperative management program for metacarpophalangeal joint implant arthroplasty. *J Hand Surg* 1977; 2: 358-66.

Illustrations by J. A. Pangrace

Synovectomy of the elbow for rheumatoid disease

Alan H. Wilde MD
Chairman, Department of Orthopaedic Surgery; Head, Section of Rheumatoid Surgery, Cleveland Clinic Foundation, Cleveland, Ohio, USA

Introduction

Indications for surgery

The diseases that are suitable for synovectomy of the elbow are adult rheumatoid arthritis, haemophilia, tuberculosis, coccidioidomycosis pigmented villonodular synovitis, and synovial osteochondromatosis.

In adult rheumatoid arthritis, synovectomy is indicated if the disease is predominantly synovial with few or no erosions and no major narrowing of the joint space, and persistent synovitis is unresponsive to medical treatment.

Tuberculosis can appear radiographically and is grossly similar to the early stages of rheumatoid arthritis.

In monoarticular arthritis of the elbow from whatever cause, synovectomy may provide the tissue necessary for the establishment of a diagnosis: not only should the synovium be submitted as a biopsy specimen but cultures should be obtained and analysed for aerobic and anaerobic bacteria, fungi and acid-fast organisms.

In juvenile rheumatoid arthritis, synovectomy of the elbow may be indicated in pauciarticular arthritis of long duration that has not responded to medical treatment. The radial head should not be resected if the growth-plates are still open.

Contraindications

Synovectomy of the elbow should not be performed in rheumatoid arthritis when there is severe pain accompanied by extensive joint destruction, instability or marked stiffness. In this situation, an unconstrained elbow replacement is a better choice of treatment.

Preoperative

Steroid preparations

A patient who has been on systemic steroids or who has taken steroids within 6 months of the operation should receive supplemental steroids at the time of surgery. The usual regimen is hydrocortisone sodium succinate 100 mg intramuscularly given on six separate occasions: the night before the operation, when the patient is sent to surgery, in the recovery room, twice on the first postoperative day and once on the second day. The patient's usual dose of cortisone is then resumed orally on the third postoperative day.

Anaesthesia and antibiotics

General or regional anaesthesia in the form of an axillary block of the brachial plexus is recommended.

Intravenous cephazolin 1 g every 6 hours is started at the induction of anaesthesia and is continued for 48 hours.

Position and preparation of the patient

The patient is positioned supine on the operating table with the involved arm on a hand table.

A properly calibrated pneumatic tourniquet should be applied as high on the arm as possible.

After sterile preparation of the hand and arm with povidone-iodine or Hibitane (ICI Pharmaceuticals, Macclesfield, UK) the tourniquet is draped out of the operative field with a sterile plastic U-drape. A sterile stockinette is applied. Further sterile, preferably paper, drapes are then applied.

74 Arthropathies

Operation

Incisions

1 & 2

The Boyd posterolateral approach to the elbow joint is utilized.

The skin incision begins two fingers'-breadth proximal to the lateral epicondyle, lateral to the triceps tendon and continues distally to the lateral side of the subcutaneous border of the ulna, four fingers'-breadth distal to the tip of the olecranon.

An incision is made through the fascia, lateral to the subcutaneous border of the ulna, leaving enough fascia attached to the ulna for later repair; this fascial incision continues proximally along the border of the triceps tendon. The anconeus is released subperiosteally from the proximal ulna and retracted. Enough of the supinator is reflected from the proximal radius to expose the joint capsule.

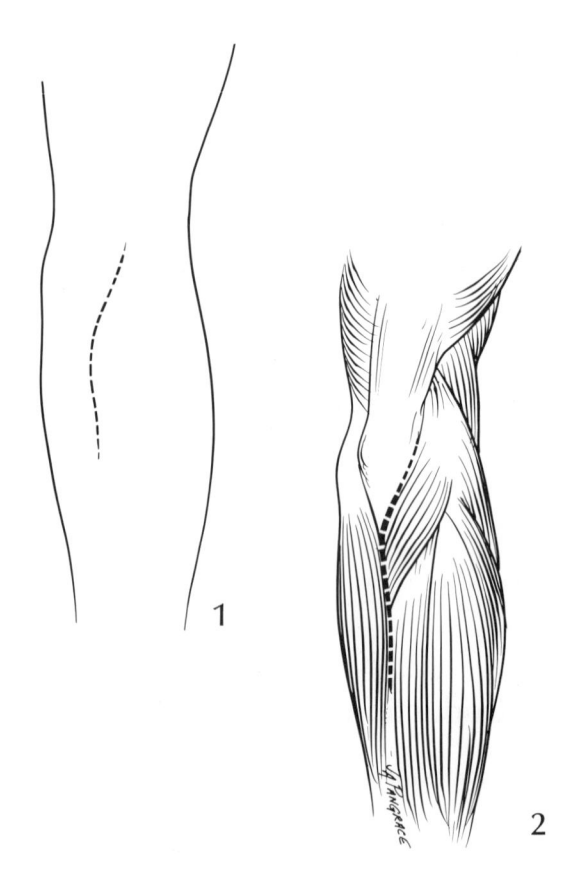

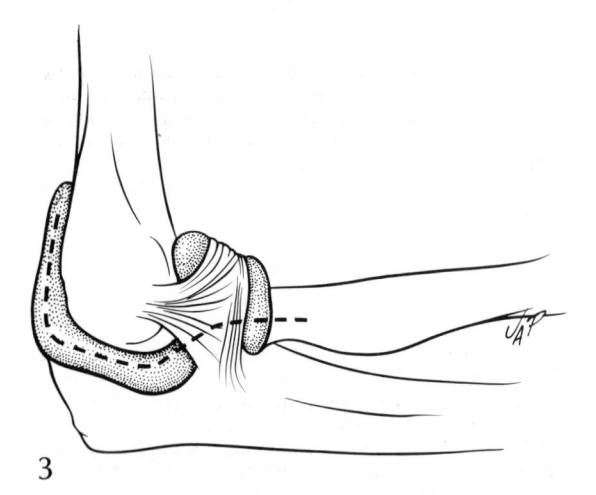

3

The capsule and annular ligament are incised longitudinally and the radial head and neck are exposed.

Resection

4

A small Bennett retractor is placed around the radial neck, and the anconeus and supinator are retracted. In the adult patient, the radial neck is osteotomized with a power saw or osteotome and the radial head is removed. The cut end of the radial neck is covered with bone wax to limit haemorrhage. Synovium from the anterior and posterior aspects of the elbow is removed with a rongeur. It is not necessary to replace the radial head with a Silastic (Dow Corning, UK) spacer, thus avoiding the potential complications of fracture of the Silastic radial head, subsequent silicone synovitis and bone destruction, and the 'squeak' that is noted at times with movement of the elbow in the presence of a Silastic radial head.

Closure

The wound is irrigated and the deep fascia is repaired with interrupted 2/0 sutures, the subcutaneous tissue with interrupted 3/0 sutures, and the skin with interrupted or continuous running 4/0 sutures. A suction drain is inserted with one catheter into the elbow joint and one into the subcutaneous space. A sterile dressing is applied over the wound. Sterile Dacron (El du Pont de Nemours and Comp, UK) is applied from the level of the metacarpophalangeal joints to the upper humerus and is compressed with the use of a compression flannel bandage.

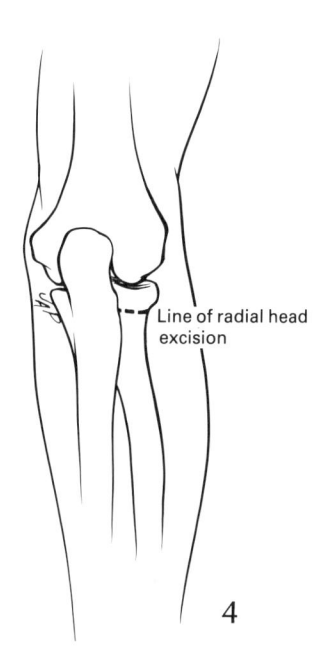

ULNAR NEURITIS

If there are accompanying symptoms of ulnar neuritis, the ulnar nerve should be decompressed rather than performing an anterior transposition of the ulnar nerve. Simple decompression gives least disturbance to the blood vessels of the nerve and produces minimal scar formation. There is also the lowest rate of sensory and motor nerve disturbances postoperatively.

5

To perform a decompression of the ulnar nerve as well as a synovectomy of the elbow, a posterior incision is made just off the midline of the elbow, lateral to the olecranon and along the subcutaneous border of the ulna. The medial skin flap is dissected in the plane between the superficial and deep fascia. The ulnar nerve is exposed four or five fingers'-breadth proximal to the ulnar notch. The dissection proceeds distally, carefully preserving the blood vessels to the nerve. The ligament forming the roof of the canal for the ulnar nerve over the medial epicondyle is released. The dissection continues to the flexor carpi ulnaris and any site of compression is released. At the completion of the dissection, the wound is irrigated and drained and closed as previously indicated.

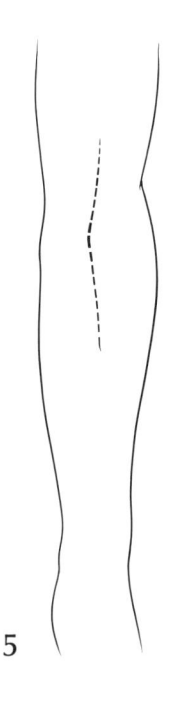

Postoperative management

Active flexion, extension, pronation and supination of the elbow are encouraged on the afternoon of surgery. Active range of movement exercises of the shoulder on the operative side are also employed to prevent stiffness of the shoulder. The suction catheter and compression dressing are removed on the second postoperative day. Active exercises of the elbow and shoulder are continued until maximum function has been obtained. Passive exercises should not be employed as this may result in permanent stiffness. The patient may use the operated arm in a normal fashion 6 weeks postoperatively.

Complications

Wound haematoma and haemarthroses are occasionally seen postoperatively. Usually it is not necessary to drain the wound unless the skin is so distended that skin necrosis is imminent, a complication which is very rare.

Instability of the elbow has been reported following synovectomy and radial head resection. This usually occurs when there is instability of the elbow preoperatively owing to an advanced degree of destruction of the elbow. Replacement of the elbow with an unconstrained prosthesis is a better choice in this situation than synovectomy. If synovectomy is performed in the presence of advanced changes in the elbow, then it is wiser not to resect the radial head. If significant disabling instability results following synovectomy and radial head resection, consideration should be given to an unconstrained elbow replacement.

Radial nerve palsy has also been reported following synovectomy. It is usually a traction injury and resolves spontaneously. Bracing should be used to provide wrist and finger extension until the nerve function returns. This complication is most unusual if a posterolateral exposure has been utilized.

Ulnar neuritis may occur following synovectomy if extensive dissection and mobilization of the ulnar nerve have been performed. If the blood supply of the ulnar nerve has been greatly disturbed, which is likely to occur in an anterior transposition, ulnar neuritis is common. Usually the paraesthesiae subside spontaneously in 6 to 12 months without further treatment, as does any disturbance of motor function of the nerve.

Wound infection is uncommon. Superficial wound infection should be treated by intravenous antibiotics. A deep wound infection requires re-incision, drainage of the wound and abscess, debridement, and preparation of cultures from the depths of the wound for investigation for aerobic and anaerobic bacilli, fungi and acid-fast bacilli. Intravenous antibiotics are given based on the sensitivities obtained. Treatment with intravenous antibiotics is required for 4 to 6 weeks.

Further reading

Brattstrom H, Al Khudairy A. Synovectomy of the elbow in rheumatoid arthritis. *Acta Orthop Scand* 1975; 46: 744–50.

Copeland SA, Taylor, JG. Synovectomy of the elbow in rheumatoid arthritis: place of excision of the head of the radius. *J Bone Joint Surg [Br]* 1979, 61-B: 69–73.

Porter BB, Richardson C, Vainio K. Rheumatoid arthritis of the elbow: the results of synovectomy. *J Bone Joint Surg [Br]* 1974; 56-B: 427–37.

Wilson DW, Arden GP, Ansell, BM. Synovectomy of the elbow in rheumatoid arthritis. *J Bone Joint Surg [Br]* 1973; 55-B: 106–111.

Illustrations by Philip Wilson and G. Bartlett

Surgical procedures in haemophilia

R. B. Duthie CBE, MA, ChM, FRCS
Nuffield Professor of Orthopaedic Surgery, University of Oxford, UK

I. W. Nelson MA, FRCS
Clinical Lecturer, Nuffield Department of Orthopaedic Surgery, University of Oxford, UK

Introduction

Deficiencies of blood clotting factors may be congenital or acquired. Classical haemophilia and Christmas disease are characterized by sex-linked congenital factor deficiencies which affect males almost exclusively. In the majority of cases a family history is present and in approximately 30 per cent of cases the condition arises as a result of a spontaneous mutation. Deficiences of other blood coagulation factors are exceptionally rare. The disorder is classified as follows.

Classical haemophilia (haemophilia A)

This is the commonest form of haemophilia and is characterized by a reduced level of active circulating Factor VIII (antihaemophilic globulin). The prevalence in the UK is approximately 16 per 100 000 of the male population. Factor VIII is a complex glycoprotein and the deficiency arises as a result of a genetic defect on the X chromosome; it therefore manifests itself in the male.

Christmas disease (haemophilia B)

This condition is characterized by a deficiency in the circulating level of active Factor IX. The genetic transmission is again sex-linked and recessive. Christmas disease is less common than classical haemophilia and the incidence is approximately 5 to 10 males per million of the population. The clinical manifestations of the disorder are identical to those of haemophilia.

Antibodies

Antibodies directed against Factor VIII arise in two classes of patient. The commonest are in the severely affected haemophiliac in whom the stimulation of antibody formation is the infused factor which is a protein and is antigenic. They are present in 6 per cent of patients with classical haemophilia, and the levels fluctuate in response to the amount of infused factor. The significance of their presence is the rapidity of inactivation of infused Factor VIII and elective surgery is therefore absolutely contraindicated in the presence of Factor VIII antibodies. In the second group, previously normal patients who often have evidence of autoimmune disease, antibodies to Factor VIII may develop resulting in so-called 'acquired haemophilia'.

Clinical manifestations

Severity of bleeding in haemophiliacs is related to the amount of Factor VIII present in the blood (Table 1). Severely affected patients are characterized by repeated haemorrhages into joints and muscles. Table 2 summarizes the incidence of bleeds in the period of 1981 to 1986 in patients requiring admission to hospital in Oxford.

Table 1 Severity of bleeding[1]

Plasma level of Factor VIII (iu/dl)	Bleeding manifestations
40	None
20–40	Tendency to bleed after major injury. Often not diagnosed
5–20	Bleeding after minor injury and surgery
1–5	Severe bleeding after minor injury. Occasional haemarthrosis and 'spontaneous' bleeding
<1	Severe haemophilia. Spontaneous haemarthrosis and muscle haematomas. Joint ankylosis and crippling

Table 2 Incidence of bleeds 1981–1986

Haemarthroses		Soft tissue	
Knee	103	Iliopsoas	34
Elbow	52	Thigh	29
Ankle	24	Calf	22
Shoulder	19	Buttock	21
Wrist	9	Forearm	13
Hip	9	Arm	7
Temporomandibular joint	1	Miscellaneous	16
Nerve palsies			
Femoral	14	Lateral popliteal	3
Median	7	Radial	2
Ulnar	4	Cutaneous, in leg	2
Sciatic	4		

Haemarthroses

Severe haemophiliacs bleed into joints more commonly than elsewhere. The frequency of haemarthroses in the knee, elbow and ankle is attributed to the large amount of synovium within the joints. The source of bleeding is thought in most cases to be from the vessels of the synovial membrane which may become trapped within the articulation of the joint. Repeated haemarthroses result in synovial thickening, joint contracture and eventually articular cartilage destruction. Clinically, chronic haemophilic arthropathy is characterized by joint contracture and stiffness and concomitant muscle wasting. Radiographically, there is evidence of metaphyseal widening, joint space narrowing and osteoporosis.

Muscle haematomas

In the severe haemophiliac these are often spontaneous and usually self-limiting. As a result of confinement of the fascial sheaths, anatomically-related structures such as the femoral nerve under the iliacus fascia may be compressed. However, the consequent neurapraxia usually resolves completely. The injured muscle may heal by fibrosis and contracture, obliterating the original site of the haemorrhage.

Haemophilic cysts and pseudotumours

These uncommon lesions present difficult management problems. The pathogenesis is still not understood but they may arise as simple cysts within a muscular fascial envelope and extend to the periosteum, giving cortical thinning; or, rarely, they may be the result of interosseous haemorrhage. They may also follow fractures.

Preoperative

The circulating levels for Factor VIII are quantified and it is essential to confirm the absence of factor antibodies.

HIV (human immunodeficiency virus)

It has been estimated that 70 per cent of severe haemophiliacs in the UK have evidence of being exposed to this virus. All haemophiliacs should be screened preoperatively. However, it is possible that seroconversion may be occurring and screening tests may be negative. It is routine at the Nuffield Orthopaedic Centre to treat all haemophiliacs for surgery as if they are positive. Rigorous precautions are essential: isolation of the operating team and patient within a vertical laminar-flow operating room, together with rigorous techniques of instrument cleaning postoperatively and of waste disposal are mandatory.

Hepatitis B

Hepatitis B occurs in about 3 per cent of all haemophiliacs per annum and serum should be screened before surgery. The presence of the Australia antigen requires special precautions to be taken to prevent risk to the operating team during surgery[2].

Principles of coagulation control[1]

Control of haemorrhage during and after surgery is achieved by factor replacement to maintain adequate levels so that haemostasis may be maintained until wound healing is complete. Before surgery is undertaken it is essential that the total factor requirement for the operative and postoperative period is calculated and banked.

For major surgery a preoperative transfusion of Factor VIII is given which must be sufficient to raise the patient's plasma level of the factor to 100 iu/dl. Assays are carried out immediately after the dose and 4–6 hours later, and further doses are given if the assays indicate these are required. Typically it is necessary to give factor replacement three times in the first 24 hours and 12-hourly thereafter to maintain the factor level above 40 iu/dl. As considerable variation occurs in patient response to Factor VIII infusion, the following formula gives a rough guide to dosage:

$$\text{Dose (i.u.)} = \frac{\text{weight(kg)} \times \text{desired increase (iu/dl)}}{2.0}$$

In the case of Factor IX concentrate, for 2.0 substitute 1.0. A unit of Factor VIII is defined as the Factor VIII activity contained in 1 ml of fresh citrated normal plasma.

The variety of materials available for the treatment of haemophilia are summarized in Table 3. In practice, lyophilized human Factor VIII or cryoprecipitate are generally used. The first dose is administered within 1 hour prior to surgery.

Antifibrinolytic agents

Epsilon aminocaproic acid and tranexamic acid are the two drugs which have been widely used. The latter is preferred as the side-effects of gastrointestinal upset are less. The antifibrinolytic agents, if tolerated by the patient, reduce the overall factor requirement of the patient during the postoperative period. The adult dose of tranexamic acid is 1 g three times a day and it is given until wound healing is well advanced, usually for 2–3 weeks after surgery.

Factor IX concentrate

There is relatively poor recovery of Factor IX in patients' blood following infusion with Factor IX. For major surgery to be carried out in patients with Christmas disease it is necessary to give continuous infusion of Factor IX concentrate, which has a half-life of only 30 hours in the patient's circulation. The Factor IX level must be kept above 25 per cent of normal.

Principles of surgical technique

The availability of Factor VIII and Factor IX concentrates has expanded the range and volume of reconstructive surgery. Standard surgical approaches and techniques are used and when possible a pneumatic tourniquet is applied to obtain a bloodless field. Meticulous attention to haemostasis is essential, and electrocautery is used for tissue dissection. Exposure is kept to a minimum, as is stripping of tissue planes as this will predispose to pocketing of haematoma. Wounds are closed by coaptation of tissue planes with continuous haemostatic polyglycolic acid sutures. The wounds are not drained but a firm compression bandage is applied and rigid immobilization is achieved with a plaster of Paris splint. Splintage discourages haematoma formation and is continued until wound healing is achieved.

Percutaneous and external fixation devices are avoided because of the potential complication of pin track

Table 3 Therapeutic materials available for the treatment of haemophilia

Source of Factor VIII	Level of Factor VIII which may be achieved in patient's blood (iu/dl)	Advantages	Disadvantages
Fresh whole blood	4–6	No preparation needed	Insufficient quantity of Factor VIII. Factor VIII unstable in stored blood
Fresh-frozen plasma	15–20	Cheap	May overload circulation. One hour to administer. Serum hepatitis in pooled plasma
Cryoprecipitate	60–80	One donor only: little risk of hepatitis	Cannot be assayed until the time of transfusion. Stored below −20°C
Lyophilized human AHG	60–80	Units of Factor VIII known	Hepatitis risk. HIV risk
Lyophilized animal AHG	150	Very potent source of Factor VIII	Antigenic

AHG, antihaemophilic globulin

bleeding and infection. In general, definitive operations with predictable good results are preferred to multiple or staged operations.

Implant surgery is carried out in isolation in a laminar-flow operating theatre and prophylactic antibiotics are administered preoperatively and until the wound has healed.

Postoperative management

Compression and rigid immobilization are continued until skin and soft tissues have healed. Isometric exercises are started as soon as the patient is comfortable. The factor replacement is used to cover removal of sutures and is maintained during early postoperative mobilization. Rehabilitation is commenced in the hydrotherapy pool and then subsequently with appropriate support on land. It is important to continue postoperative rehabilitation and to keep the patient in hospital as long as rehabilitation is required, as this allows easy administration of the factor and early detection of possible complications.

Operations

TOTAL HIP REPLACEMENT[3]

Indications

The hip, while a relatively infrequent site of haemarthroses, is particularly susceptible to the development of haemophilic arthropathy. This often presents in the young and middle-aged and is becoming an increasingly common problem. Clinically, there is increasing pain and restricted range of movement, often with fixed contractures. Radiographically, the changes of chronic haemophilic arthropathy are compounded by secondary degenerative changes.

Procedure

A standard approach and technique is used following the general principles of meticulous haemostasis (see chapter on 'Total hip replacement arthroplasty', pp. 943–964). Electrocautery is used for soft-tissue dissection. A cemented low-friction arthroplasty is employed and the greater trochanter is not osteotomized.

Coagulation control

The total dose of the factor required is calculated and banked. The dose of Factor VIII required immediately preoperatively is calculated from the patient's weight and the initial level of the serum Factor VIII. Factor replacement is given by intravenous infusion using a 21-gauge needle. Tranexamic acid, if tolerated by the patient, is also commenced preoperatively.

Postoperative management

A compression bandage is applied to the region of the hip and the patient is mobilized in a one-and-a-half hip spica incorporating the whole of the leg on the operated side. The immobilization reduces the amount of haematoma formation, allows primary healing of the soft tissues and reduces the Factor VIII required; it is continued for 3 weeks. Following removal of the cast and sutures under factor cover, mobilization is commenced in the hydrotherapy pool, and the patient graduates to walking with elbow crutches.

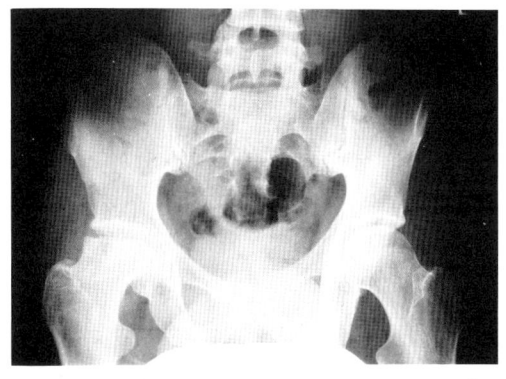

Case history

1a & b

A 32-year-old haemophiliac with 1 per cent of normal levels of circulating Factor VIII and no antibodies to Factor VIII had suffered repeated bilateral knee bleeds; haemophilic arthropathy was established in both of these joints. For the 18 months prior to admission he complained of increasing pain in the right hip. Examination of the right hip showed a range of flexion from 10° of fixed flexion to 70°, adduction fixed at 10° and lateral rotation limited to 10°. The patient walked with a marked antalgic gait. Radiographs showed superior segment collapse at the femoral head with joint space narrowing, subchondral sclerosis and a marginal osteophyte.

A standard Charnley total hip replacement was performed under full Factor VIII cover, with the initial dose being given 1 hour before surgery.

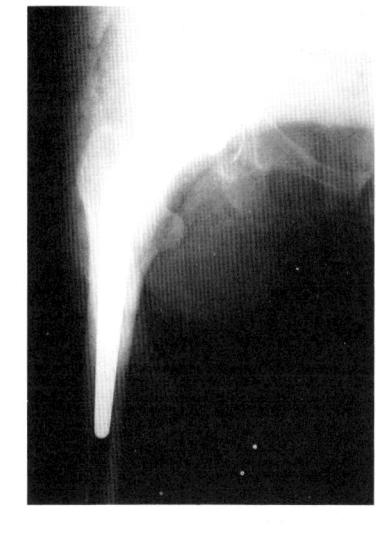

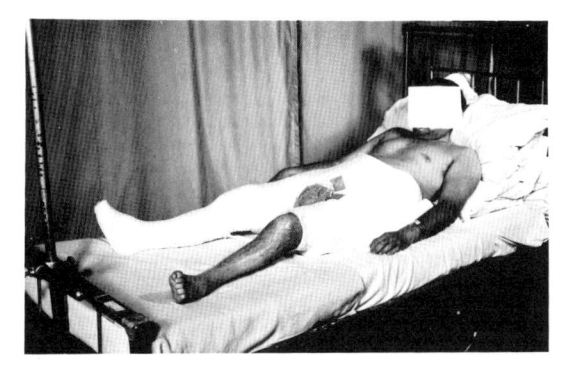

2

Postoperatively the patient was immobilized in a full leg-hip spica for 3 weeks. After removal of the spica and the sutures (with factor cover), mobilization was commenced in the hydrotherapy pool. Mobilization was continued with the help of elbow crutches and the patient was discharged 5 weeks after surgery with a well-healed wound and a range of movement of the hip showing flexion from 0° to 90°, abduction 20°, adduction 10° and a combined rotation 20°. The Factor VIII requirement and serum levels achieved are shown in *Figure 1*.

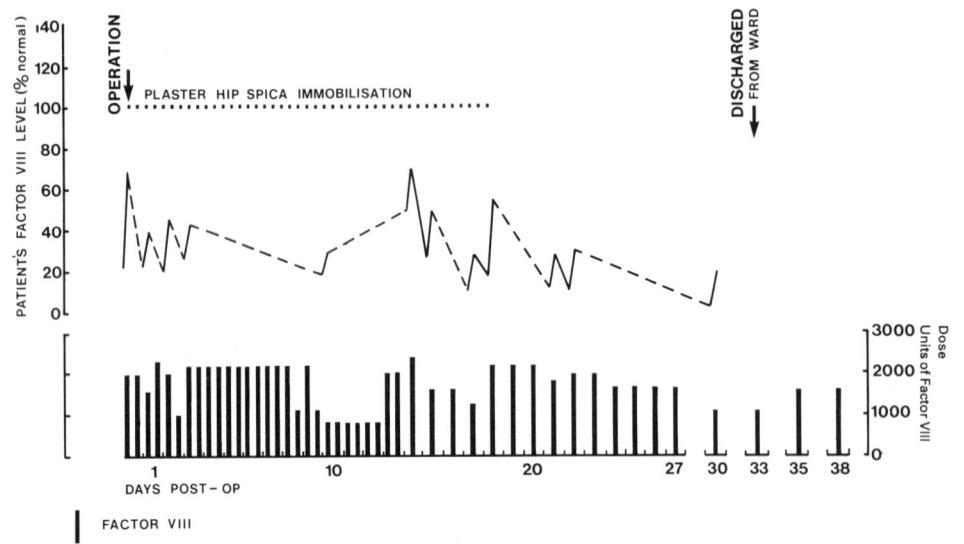

Figure 1 Factor VIII requirements of a patient undergoing total hip replacement.

SYNOVECTOMY OF THE KNEE[4]

Indications

Synovectomy is indicated when there are frequent repeated haemarthroses with evidence of considerable synovial thickening, which have failed to respond to conservative management by repeated compression, adequate factor infusion and strict bed-rest for a 3-week period. The patient should be near skeletal maturity with minimal fixed flexion deformity and a range of flexion to at least 90°. The objective of synovectomy is a reduction in the frequency of haemarthroses. There is no evidence that it alters the natural history of haemophilic arthropathy.

Procedure

An anterior two-thirds synovectomy is performed through a medial parapatellar incision. Meticulous haemostasis is maintained throughout. A firm compression bandage and a plaster of Paris backslab are applied to the leg.

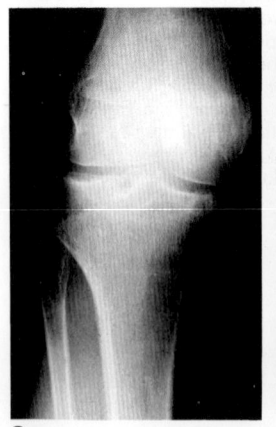

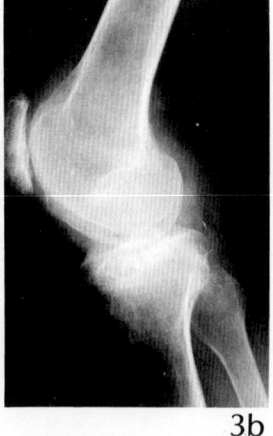

Postoperative management

Coagulation control is maintained following the principles outlined above. The limb remains immobilized in the compression bandage and plaster backslab until wound healing is complete. Isometric quadriceps exercises are commenced in the compression bandage. Two weeks after surgery the sutures are removed and physiotherapy is commenced with Factor VIII cover. Flexion of 90° should be regained after 2 weeks of physiotherapy, and weight-bearing is then permitted.

Case history

3a & b

A 24-year-old labourer with no circulating Factor VIII and no antibodies had had multiple haemarthroses, particularly in his knees. In the year before admission he had suffered recurrent haemorrhages into the right knee which failed to respond to two prolonged periods of rest and rigid immobilization with factor replacement. Prior to admission he was suffering from approximately two haemarthroses a week. Examination of the right knee showed considerable synovial thickening and a range of movement from 5° to 110° of flexion. Radiographs showed evidence of early haemophilic arthropathy.

Anterior two-thirds synovectomy of the right knee was carried out under an initial infusion of Factor VIII concentrate. Postoperatively a compression bandage and a plaster of Paris backslab were applied.

The wound healed by primary intention. Intensive physiotherapy was started 2 weeks after the operation and the patient was allowed to bear weight at 4 weeks. At this stage 80° of flexion were present in the joint. Following the operation he has had no further haemarthroses in the knee and has now gained 100° of flexion.

3a 3b

ARTHRODESIS OF THE KNEE[5]

Indications

Pain is the main indication for arthrodesis of the knee in haemophilia. This may be associated with flexion contracture, deformity, instability and recurrent haemarthroses, all of which are functionally disabling.

Procedure

4, 5 & 6

An exsanguinating tourniquet is applied to the lower limb. A medial parapatellar approach is made to the knee joint and the undersurface of the patella decorticated. The condylar surfaces of the femur are removed up to the level of the intercondylar notch, and the surface of the tibia is excised just below the subchondral bone layer. Fixation is achieved with crossed cancellous compression screws. The knee should be arthrodesed in from 10° to 30° flexion, depending on coexistent hip or ankle deformity.

Postoperative management

The arthrodesis is protected by external splintage with a compression bandage in a long-leg plaster of Paris cast. Two weeks after surgery the sutures are removed and the cast is changed under factor cover. It is important to raise the serum level of Factor VIII to 80–100 per cent during this procedure. Isometric quadriceps exercises are started in the cast and the patient is mobilized without weight-bearing. The arthrodesis is protected by external splintage until there is radiographic union at the site of the arthrodesis.

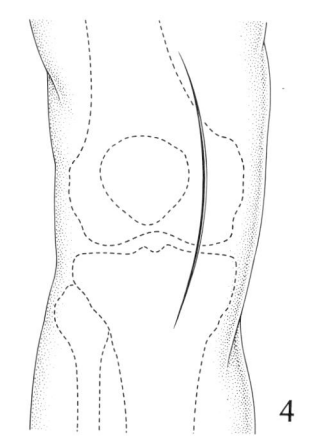

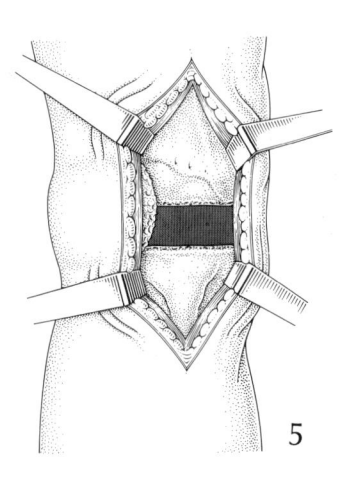

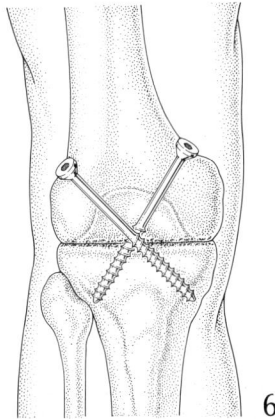

84 Arthropathies

Case history

7a & b

A 35-year-old man with severe haemophilia, and no Factor VIII or antibodies, had severe haemophilic arthropathy affecting both knees. He presented complaining of unremitting pain in the left knee and with a limited range of movement. On examination there was a fixed flexion deformity of 5° of the left knee with only 10° of further flexion available. Radiographically, he had evidence of severe haemophilic arthropathy.

Immediately before operation an infusion of Factor VIII concentrate was given. An arthrodesis of the left knee was carried out and crossed-screw fixation used to immobilize the arthrodesis. A full-leg plaster of Paris cast was applied.

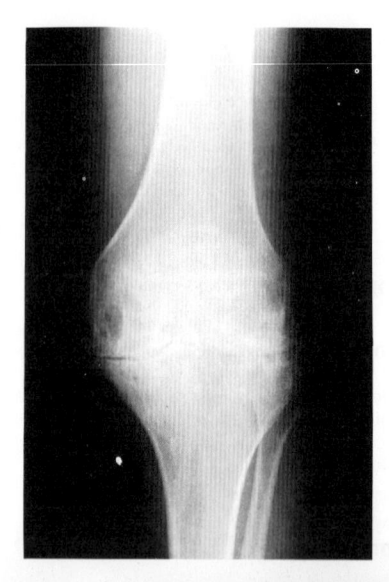

7a

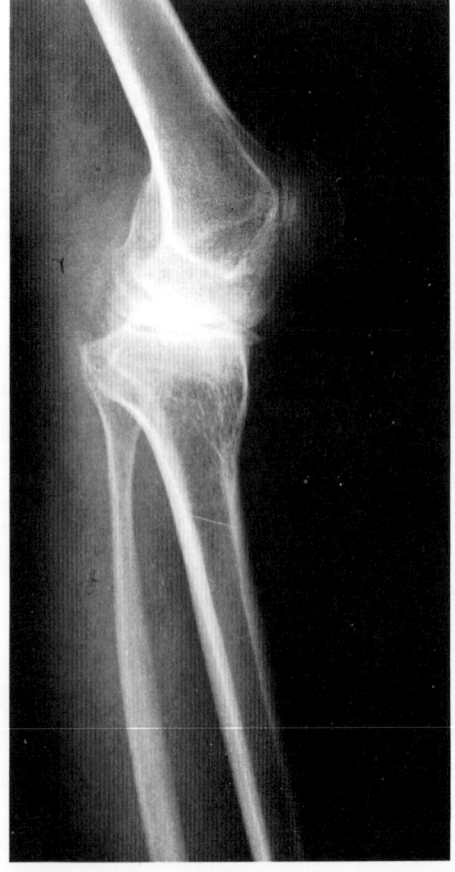

7b

8a & b

The wound healed by primary intention. The sutures were removed and plaster changed under factor cover 2 weeks after the operation. Sound arthrodesis was obtained after 4 months and as a result of the operation the patient had increased function in the limb and no pain from the knee. The factor requirements of a patient undergoing knee arthrodesis are shown in *Figure 2*.

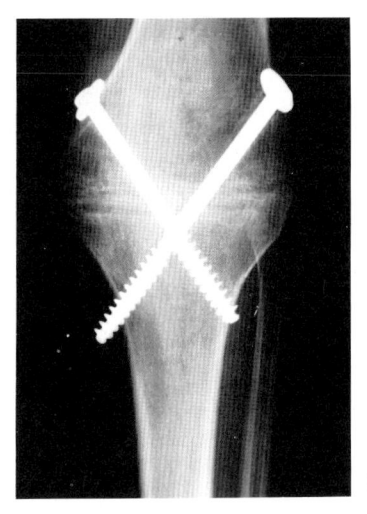

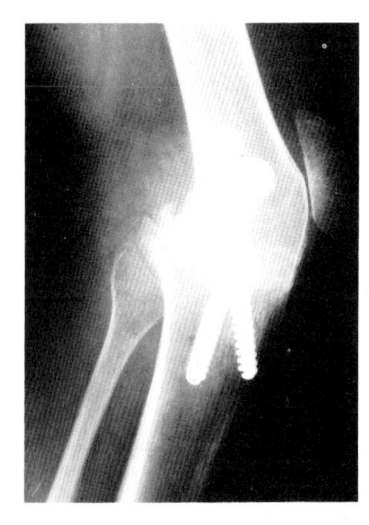

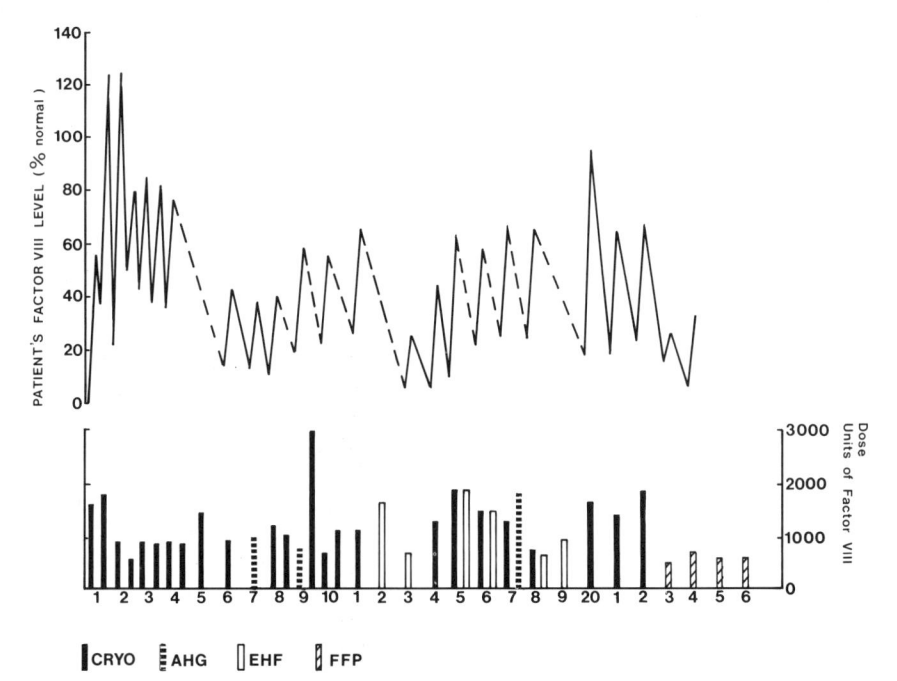

Figure 2 Factor VIII requirements of a patient undergoing knee arthrodesis. Cryo, Cryoprecipitate; AHG, Factor VIII concentrate (anti-haemophilic globulin); EHT, non-assayed AHG; FFP, fresh frozen plasma.

86 Arthropathies

9 & 10

REVERSED DYNAMIC SLINGS AND PRESSURE GARMENTS[6, 9]

Indications

Fixed flexion deformity of the knee (or elbow) secondary to intra-articular fibrosis, capsular adhesions and contraction, may cause considerable disability. Reversed dynamic slings, while effective with larger fixed flexion contractures, are less well-tolerated by the patient. Force *a* is converted to a downward pressure on the lower end of the femur via a canvas sling around the Thomas' splint. Longitudinal skin traction is applied to the leg (force *b*). Over a period of 10–14 days the knee flexion is approximated to the Thomas' splint, thus straightening the leg.

Pressured garments (e.g. Flowtron, Medicross Ltd, Eastleigh, UK) are better tolerated by patients but are only effectively able to correct smaller deformities. The garment is repeatedly inflated and deflated throughout the treatment. It is possible to continue isometric quadriceps exercises with the garment on. Factor VIII replacement is usually required during treatment.

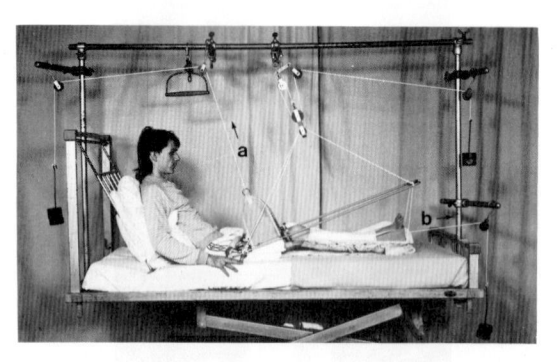

9

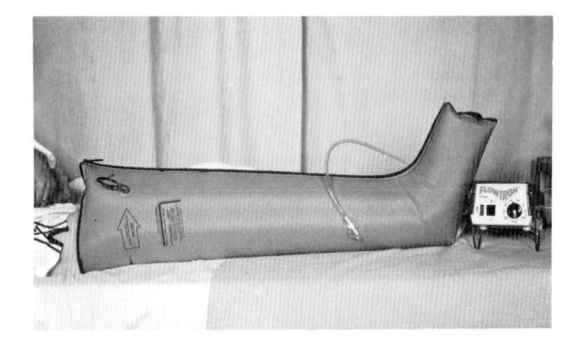

10

ARTHRODESIS OF THE ANKLE

Indications

The main indication for arthrodesis of the ankle is pain; in the majority of cases this is not associated with fixed deformity. In the absence of deformity, modification of the Pridie technique[7] is employed. Where there is significant deformity present requiring correction, the RAF technique is used[8].

Procedure

11, 12 & 13

The operation is carried out under tourniquet. A longitudinal incision is made over the medial or lateral malleolus. The medial malleolus and anterior and posterior joint capsule are exposed. Under image intensification, a guide wire is introduced through the medial malleolus, across the ankle joint and then through the lateral malleolus. Cannulated drills are used sequentially to remove a cylinder of bone including the joint space, lower tibia and upper talus, up to three-quarters of an inch in diameter. Drilling is continued into the fibula but should not broach the lateral fibular cortex. The bone chips removed are retained and mixed, if necessary, with graft from bank bone. The mixture is returned to the cylindrical defect and packed into place with a punch. Accurate haemostasis is maintained throughout surgery and a below-knee plaster applied.

Postoperative management

The arthrodesis remains immobilized in the below-knee plaster of Paris cast until the sutures are removed and the plaster changed at 2 weeks, during which factor cover is necessary. Weight-bearing is commenced after 6 weeks and the time to radiographic union is approximately 3–4 months.

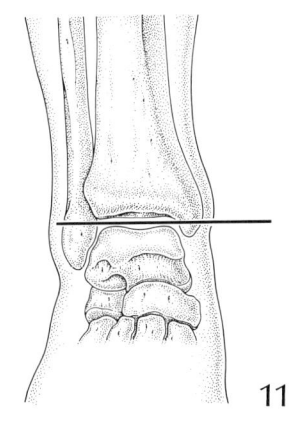

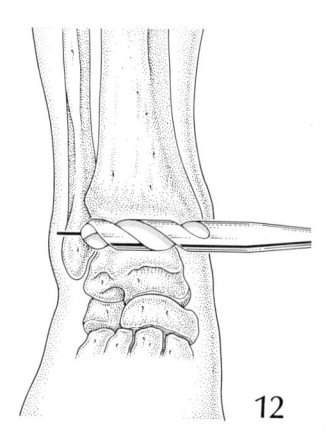

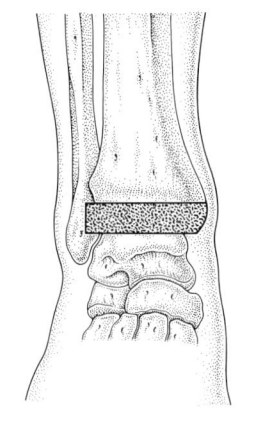

88 Arthropathies

Case history

A 35-year-old male haemophiliac, with no Factor VIII nor antibodies, had previously had multiple bleeds into both knees, both elbows, and both ankles. He gave a 6-month history of severe pain affecting the right ankle.

14a & b

On examination, the right ankle was in the neutral position with 5° of plantarflexion, available only with associated severe pain. Inversion and eversion were pain-free.

Operation was preceded by an initial infusion of Factor VIII concentrate. A cylinder of bone was removed through the medial malleolus as far as the lateral cortex of the lateral malleolus, including the ankle joint. The bone chips obtained were supplemented with bank bone and replaced into the defect.

15a & b

Postoperatively the limb was kept in a below-knee plaster cast. The patient had previously had a left knee arthrodesis and commenced partial weight-bearing 10 days after the operation. Full weight-bearing was commenced at 6 weeks and the plaster discarded at 3 months.

The Factor VIII requirements of a patient undergoing ankle arthrodesis are shown in *Figure 3*. The Factor VIII infused was kept to a minimum by the administration of ε-aminocaproic acid.

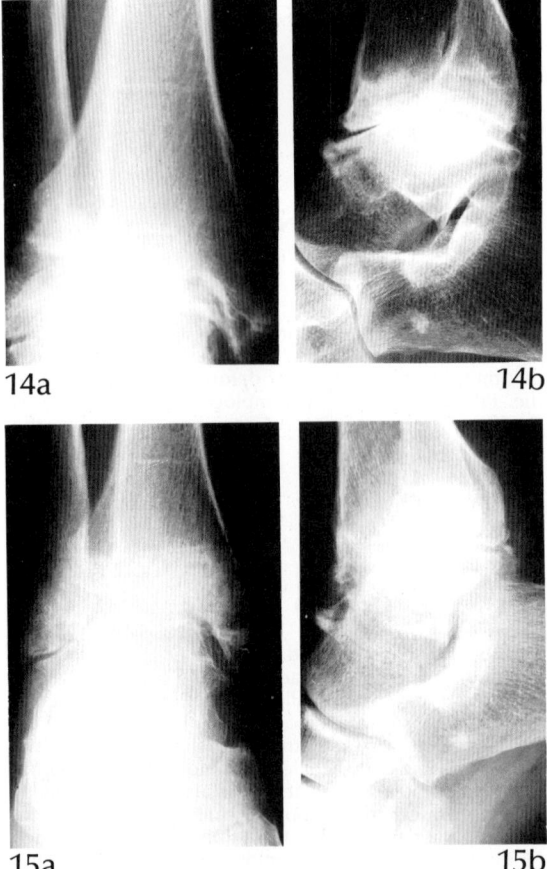

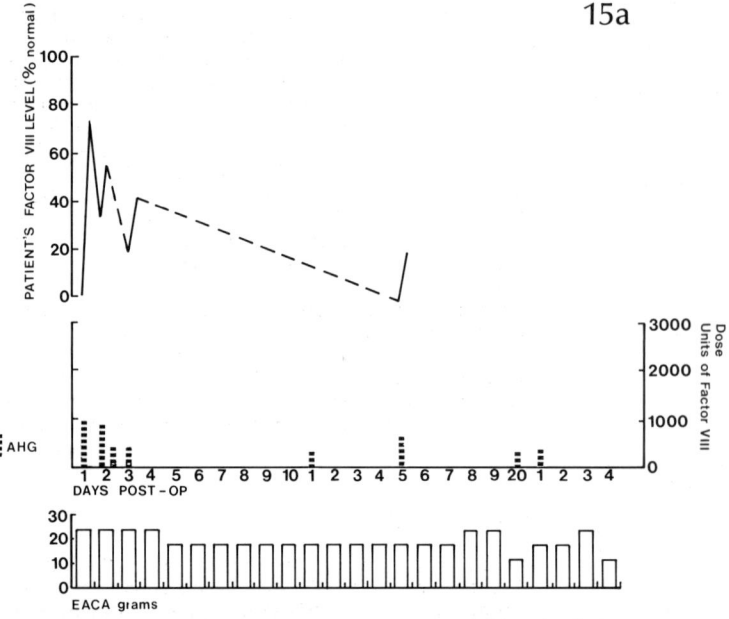

Figure 3 Factor VIII requirements of a patient undergoing ankle arthrodesis.

Management of fractures in haemophilia

Haemophiliacs do not have an increased incidence of fractures compared with the rest of the population. The principles of management of fractures in haemophiliacs are as follows.

Coagulation control

Serum factor level must be raised by intravenous infusion to 30–40 per cent of normal. The high level of Factor VIII must be maintained for approximately 4 days in the uncomplicated fracture, but may be continued for a further 2–3 weeks in a major fracture with displacement or in an open fracture. If surgical treatment is required or if the fracture is complicated, the Factor VIII levels should be raised 80–90 per cent in a similar manner to that of any other surgical procedure. With adequate serum levels of Factor VIII there is less haematoma formation and less soft-tissue destruction, and the fracture can be expected to unite and consolidate in the usual way.

Fracture treatment

The best method of immobilization of the fracture is that which adequately holds the reduction and has least chance of initiating further bleeding. Conservative measures of treatment are preferred unless the fracture is unstable or involves the joint surfaces. Skeletal traction with percutaneous pins as external fixation devices are avoided as the pin tracks are potential sites for repeated haemorrhage and infection. With stable fractures the limb is supported with a compression bandage until bleeding has ceased and a definitive plaster cast is then applied with minimal manipulation of the fracture.

Unstable fractures and intra-articular fractures, where there is incongruity of joint surfaces, are best treated by internal fixation.

Secondary manipulations and operations should be avoided, but if they are required Factor VIII replacement should be adequate. Factor VIII replacement is also needed when removing sutures, renewing or changing the plaster cast and during the early phase of mobilization.

Haemophilic cysts and pseudotumours

Severe haemophiliacs may suffer the rare complication of cyst or pseudotumour formation. This condition is becoming less frequent, probably owing to improved early management of haemorrhage. Cysts may develop in muscle, subperiosteally or in bone. The initial treatment is conservative using the following principles.

1. Immobilization of the affected part to reduce haematoma formation and potentiate healing.
2. Adequate Factor VIII replacement to achieve a serum level of 30–40 per cent of normal. This method of conservative management may need to be prolonged and is continued until there is little pain and the swelling is noted to subside. Radiographs may show that the resolution of the cyst is taking place.

Should conservative therapy fail and the complications of skin ulceration, infection or haemorrhage occur, surgical intervention may be required in the form of cyst excision. Excision of large pelvic cysts is a major undertaking with a high mortality, but may be the only option if vital structures such as ureters or an inferior vena cava are compromised. Excision is usually the method of treatment if the cyst lies in an extremity. Amputation is only required if the circulation is compromised with necrosis.

Complications of surgery in haemophilia[2]

The complications that have been encountered in 11 patients are summarized in Table 4. The commonest complication is haemorrhage, often associated with secondary infection. Rarely, antibodies develop in the postoperative period when high levels of antigenic Factor VIII are administered. This serious complication renders effective treatment difficult: rigid immobilization and compression, together wth animal Factor VIII, offer the best prospect of arrest from haemorrhage.

Conclusions

Many other orthopaedic operations have been reported as having been performed on patients with haemophilia. Where possible, standard surgical approaches and techniques are used, but great care must be taken to ensure and maintain haemostasis, both operatively, by attention to detail, and by adequate factor replacement both during surgical procedure and during the postoperative period. With the advancement of surgical technique, further operations will become available to the haemophiliac in the future. In particular, total knee replacement has been associated in haemophiliacs with raised incidence of infection and wound breakdown and is currently not practised in this unit.

The best results of orthopaedic surgery in haemophiliacs are achieved in centres where expertise has grown up over the years and where there is greater experience of both surgical and haematological complications and their treatment. It is recommended that elective surgery should be carried out in such centres in preference to those with less expertise.

Acknowledgements

We would like to thank the physicians of the Oxford Haemophilia Centre, Dr Charles Rizza and Dr James Matthews, for their assistance in the management of patients with haemophilia.

Table 4 Complications of surgery in 100 patients

Operation	Complication	Cause	Management
Knee arthrodesis	Delayed union for 7 months	–	Prolonged immobilization
Knee arthrodesis	Delayed union for 11 months	–	
Knee arthrodesis	Delayed union for 12 months	–	
Knee arthrodesis	Haematoma	Poor coagulation control (1968)	Aspiration under Factor VIII cover
Knee arthrodesis	Wound infection	Secondary to haematoma	Antibiotics: Factor VIII replacement
Ankle arthrodesis	Haematoma	Inadequate compression	Compression bandage and Factor VIII replacement
Ankle arthrodesis	Haematoma and wound dehiscence	Poor coagulation control (1967)	Factor replacement and daily dressings for 4 months
Total hip replacement	Died	Intraoperative collapse: cardiac arrest	
Total hip replacement	Dislocation on fifth day	Inadequate hip spica	Conversion to full hip spica
Femoral plate for fracture (at other hospital)	Infection and antibody development	Poor coagulation control, with haematoma	Multiple debridement under Factor VIII cover; died 18 months after fracture
Excision of pelvic pseudocyst	Died	Uncontrollable haemorrhage Day 3 after operation	Re-exploration failed to stop bleeding from aberrant arteriovenous blood vessels

References

1. Biggs R, Rizza CR, eds. *Human blood coagulation, haemostasis and thrombosis*, 3rd ed. Oxford: Blackwell, 1984.

2. Houghton GR, Duthie RB. Orthopaedic problems in haemophilia. *Clin Orthop* 1978; 138: 197–216.

3. Duthie RB. Reconstructive surgery in haemophilia. *Ann NY Acad Sci* 1975; 240: 295.

4. Storti E, Traldi A, Tasatti E, Davoli PG. Synovectomy, a new approach to haemophilic arthropathy. *Acta Haematol (Basel)* 1969; 41: 193.

5. Houghton GR, Dickson RA. Lower limb arthrodesis in haemophilia. *J Bone Joint Surg [Br]* 1978; 60-B: 143–4.

6. Stein H, Dickson RA. Reversed dynamic slings for knee flexion contractures in the hemophiliac. *J Bone Joint Surg [Am]* 1975; 57-A: 282–3.

7. O'Hara JN, Pearson JR. Arthrodesis of the ankle joint: a new technique. *J R Coll Surg Edinb* 1986; 31: 224–6.

8. Duthie RB, Matthews J, Rizza CR, Steel WM. *The management of musculo-skeletal problems in the haemophilias*. Oxford: Blackwell, 1972.

9. Nelson IW, Atkins PA, Allen A. Flowtron in haemophilic knee flexion contractures. *J Bone Joint Surg [Br]* 1989; 71-B: 327.

Illustrations by Laurel L. Cook

Techniques of bone biopsy

Mark C. Gebhardt MD
Assistant Professor of Orthopaedic Surgery, Harvard Medical School, Massachusetts General Hospital and The Children's Hospital, Boston, Massachusetts, USA

Henry J. Mankin MD
Edith M. Ashley Professor of Orthopaedic Surgery, Harvard Medical School; Chief, Orthopaedic Service, Massachusetts General Hospital, Boston, Massachusetts, USA

Introduction

In considering the technical details of performing a bone biopsy, it must be remembered that biopsy is but a final important step in the evaluation of a disease process or neoplasm. Although this chapter will focus on bone neoplasms, the techniques and principles are similar for infections and metabolic bone disease. Since a biopsy is relatively simple to perform, emphasis will be placed on the preliminary staging and decision-making process, and the choice of the biopsy site. It is a procedure which requires thoughtfulness and is not to be delegated to the most junior member of the surgical team, as improper biopsies may lead to misdiagnosis or loss of a limb.

Preoperative

Evaluation of a patient with a bone neoplasm is a complex process. There are a variety of benign and malignant neoplasms in a wide spectrum of tissues: bone, cartilage, fibrous tissue, marrow elements, vascular and neural tissues, and others[1]. The age and sex of a patient influences the incidence, as does the location. Multidisciplinary consultation is required to arrive at the correct diagnosis and treatment protocol.

Screening

The initial evaluation involves a screening history and physical examination, laboratory tests, plain radiographs or xeroradiograms of the lesion, radionuclide bone scans and a chest radiograph (Table 1). The goal is to arrive at a tentative decision as to whether the lesion is a benign or malignant primary bone tumour, a metastatic deposit or a round cell lesion.

Except in a very few instances, the history is non-specific. Most often the patient complains of *pain* which is first noted after minor trauma to the part, but many benign and an occasional malignant lesion are discovered incidentally on radiographs obtained for other purposes. The character of the pain is usually dull and aching. A notable exception is the osteoid osteoma where the pain is described as sharp and boring, often worse at night and characteristically relieved with aspirin[1]. On occasion a lump or pathological fracture may be the presenting problem.

On physical examination the findings may be minimal for benign lesions. An osteoid osteoma may show local *tenderness* and limitation of joint movement, or, in children, may present as a scoliosis, limp or growth disturbance. Malignant lesions are often associated with a palpable *soft tissue mass* which is tender to palpation. The mass should be assessed accurately for size, the distinctness of its margins, its consistency, mobility and location. Large lesions are more likely to be malignant, as are tumours that are tender to palpation. In some malignant tumours, heat, redness, oedema, venous distension and even lymphangitis may be present, at times making the differentiation from infection difficult. *Systemic findings* are usually lacking, except in patients with Ewing's sarcoma or lymphoma who may present with fever, chills, anorexia and weight loss consistent with a chronic or subacute infection process.

Laboratory tests include a complete *blood-cell count* and sedimentation rate which are helpful in excluding diseases such as myeloma, leukaemia and infection. *Calcium and phosphorus* determinations are useful to

Table 1 Protocol for staging of bone tumours

First order screen	History and physical examination
	Radiographs: plain, xero and chest
	Laboratory investigations: cell count, ESR; Ca, P and alkaline phosphatase; serum immunoelectrophoresis, SGOT; blood urea nitrogen and blood sugar
	Radionuclide bone scan

DIAGNOSTIC DECISION

Second order studies

Benign
Biopsy (open, incisional)

Primary malignant
Lung tomogram or CT
Arteriogram
Lesion: CT or MRI
Biopsy (culture, EM and immunohistochemistry)

Round cell
Lung tomogram or CT
Lymphangiogram
Liver/spleen scan
Gallium scan
Bone marrow biopsy
Lesion: CT or MRI
Biopsy (culture, EM surface markers and immunohistochemistry)

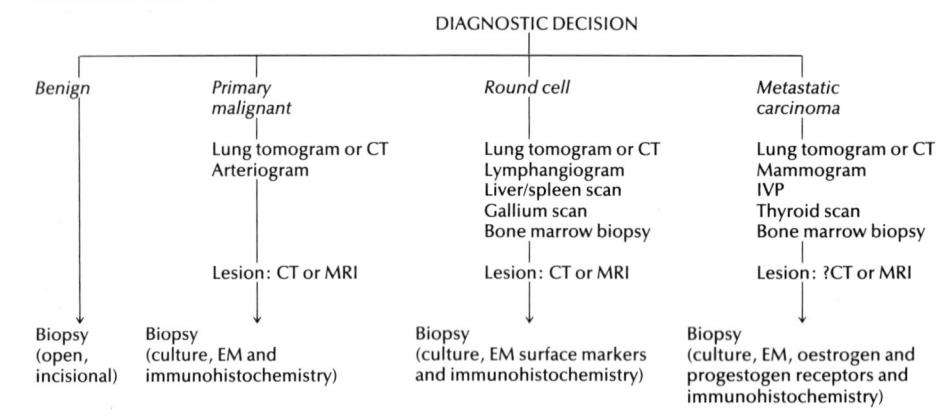

Metastatic carcinoma
Lung tomogram or CT
Mammogram
IVP
Thyroid scan
Bone marrow biopsy
Lesion: ?CT or MRI
Biopsy (culture, EM, oestrogen and progestogen receptors and immunohistochemistry)

detect metabolic bone disease, and for hypercalcaemia which can occur with metastatic bone disease; alkaline phosphatase level is useful in the assessment of metabolic disease, but may be significantly elevated in patients with osteosarcoma, lymphoma or Ewing's sarcoma. A serum *immunoelectrophoresis* is helpful in detecting multiple myeloma.

Plain radiographs of the lesion in two or more planes help in assessing location, size, cortical integrity, margination, and the presence or absence of a soft tissue mass. They may show *osseous, chondroid, fibrous or 'other' tissues* and some non-neoplastic disorders such as bone infarcts, infection or stress fractures can be excluded. The xeroradiogram is particularly helpful in delineating a soft tissue extension of the lesion. The radionuclide bone scan (usually ^{99m}Tc di- or poly-phosphonate) is useful in *assessing the activity* of the lesion relative to its bone production and blood flow, and shows any bony lesions at other sites. On occasion, lesions such as eosinophilic granuloma, unicameral bone cyst, and multiple myeloma may appear normal or actually decreased in activity on bone scan. A *chest radiograph* is obtained in any patient with a suspected malignant bone tumour to search for evidence of metastatic disease or a primary focus from which a metastasis may have arisen.

Diagnosis

After these preliminary studies, a decision is made. If the lesion is believed to be a primary benign bone tumour, one may observe it or proceed with biopsy for confirmation. If the lesion is thought to be a primary malignant tumour of bone, further 'second order' studies are required. These include a computed tomogram (CT) or magnetic resonance image (MRI) of the lesion, an arteriogram (in cases deemed to be resectable or to assess the extent of the soft tissue extension), and/or tomograms of the lesion. These tests are principally directed toward determining the *extent of the lesion* in the bone and in the adjacent soft tissues, especially the relationship to the neurovascular bundle. It is important to obtain these results before the biopsy because they may be affected by the haematoma associated with the biopsy[2]. Tomograms or CT scans of the lungs are obtained prior to general anaesthesia on all patients suspected of having malignant bone tumours to detect metastases.

In lesions thought to be metastatic, a preliminary work-up seeking the site of the primary tumour is required. In addition to the history and physical examination, the studies may include mammograms, urinalysis, intravenous pyelography or ultrasound of the kidneys, acid phosphatase determination, a thyroid scan, and lung tomograms or CT. On occasion it is not possible to locate the primary tumour, and the diagnosis will depend upon the histological interpretation of the bony lesions[3].

For tumours thought to be round cell lesions (Ewing's tumour, myeloma and lymphoma) further staging studies should include a gallium scan, abdominal CT and lymphangiography[4]. Myeloma patients require a serum electrophoresis, a skeletal survey and a bone marrow biopsy prior to biopsy of the bony lesion (this latter may obviate the need for a bone biopsy)[5].

Planning the biopsy

Once the staging process has been completed, attention is directed toward obtaining tissue for histological diagnosis, and careful consideration given to placement of the incision relative to limb-salvage planning. In addition, complete staging may lead to a tentative but likely diagnosis of the lesion which, if confirmed by frozen section analysis, allows for a definitive operation to be performed at the same session.

The biopsy may be accomplished by either an open or a closed (needle) technique. Open biopsies are classified as *incisional* when the lesion is entered and representative tissue is removed for pathological evaluation without removing the lesion. *Excisional* biopsies are those in which the entire lesion is removed ('shelled out'), usually through the pseudocapsule of the lesion, without obtaining prior diagnostic tissue.

Advantages of closed biopsy

Needle biopsies may be performed under local anaesthesia under CT control as an outpatient, or in the operating theatre under general anaesthesia, depending upon the location and size of the lesion. The small puncture wound can either be ignored or excised at the time of definitive resection. This technique lessens the chance of a large haematoma, reduces contamination of normal tissue and does not create large defects in bone which might result in pathological fracture. In addition, it is usually possible to obtain tissue from the centre of the lesion, rather than the periphery, which might be helpful in certain instances[6]. Needle biopsies, especially those controlled by CT, are most appropriate in the spine or pelvis, and when the suspected diagnosis is metastasis, infection, a round cell lesion or a local recurrence[7-11]. Their major drawback is failure to provide the pathologist with a satisfactory tissue sample for diagnosis. In 60 to 80 per cent of biopsies, this procedure obtains adequate tissue, the variation depending upon the diagnosis, the skill of the operator, and the expertise of the pathologist[6,12-15]: the accuracy is greater for infectious and metastatic lesions than it is for primary bone tumours.

Advantages of open biopsy

Open biopsy is considered to be a more reliable method and is often preferred in musculoskeletal tumours in order to ensure that sufficient tissue is obtained for accurate diagnosis and to avoid sampling error[2]. The technique, even when properly performed, has the disadvantages of creating a larger operative haematoma, violating tissue planes, increasing the possibility of infection or skin slough, and increasing the chance of subsequent pathological fracture if the cortex is violated.

Excisional biopsies are performed for small, obviously benign lesions such as osteochondromas, osteomas, and on occasion low-grade malignancies when the diagnosis is certain by the staging studies. Certain malignant or benign, aggressive lesions can be treated by excisional biopsy (marginal excision) when they are located in expendable bones such as the proximal fibula, clavicle and rib.

Incisional biopsies are appropriate when the diagnosis is still in doubt after staging, and the options of treatment vary considerably depending upon the proper diagnosis. In general, this applies to most benign aggressive lesions in weight-bearing bones (e.g. giant cell tumour, osteoblastoma, chondroblastoma) and primary malignant lesions (e.g. osteosarcoma, chondrosarcoma), metastases and round cell lesions (e.g. Ewing's sarcoma, lymphoma, myeloma), where the treatment varies greatly depending upon the diagnosis.

Operation

The technique of biopsy is crucial and should be performed by an experienced surgeon knowledgeable in musculoskeletal tumours. Whether closed or open, the incision must be placed in a location where it can be excised with the specimen at the time of definitive operation. Anaesthesia may be local, regional or general, but it is inadvisable to inject large amounts of local anaesthesia in the vicinity of a malignant mass because of the possibility of contaminating a larger area with tumour cells. The patient's involved part is prepared and draped in a sterile manner, and it is wise to localize a soft tissue mass, if present, by palpation and by review of the staging studies as an aid to planning the incision. When there is no soft tissue mass an image intensifier may help to ensure proper localization of the lesion.

NEEDLE BIOPSY

Needles

There are various types of needles commercially available. They are broadly classified into those for *trephine* biopsies[7-11] in which a core of tissue is removed and those for *aspiration* where a 'fine needle' technique is used to obtain tissue for cytology and frequently other studies[14-19].

It is more common in our institution to use one of two types of needles. The first is the 'Tru-cut' needle which is excellent for soft tissue masses (manufactured by Baxter Health Care Corp, Baxter Parkway, Deerfield, Illinois). It is a single use, sterile-packed needle which is inserted percutaneously to the pseudocapsule of the mass. A trocar is advanced into the lesion, and then a sharp, outer sleeve is advanced over it which cuts a core of tissue 1.6 × 20 mm for pathological evaluation. Several cores may be taken without much risk of haematoma, but it is important to limit the number of needle paths in order to make it possible to excise the tracks.

1

For bony lesions, or those where more diagnostic tissue is needed, a Craig needle system (distributed by Codman and Shurtleff Inc, Randolph, Massachusetts), or the similar Turkel needle is employed. This is particularly useful in the spine. In this case, a small incision is made, and a stylet (a) is advanced to the bone or pseudocapsule. An outer sleeve (b) is slid over this, and stabilized by the surgeon. A 3 mm core needle with either a corrugated (c) or smooth (d) cutting tip is advanced through the sleeve and twisted, with the aid of a T-handle (e), into the lesion. The length of penetration into the lesion is limited to 2.5 cm for safety, especially in the spine. Precise placement of this needle is mandatory, at times necessitating CT or image intensification for control[7-8, 20]. It is helpful to apply some negative pressure on the needle core prior to its removal with a syringe, or to use a 'pigtail' attachment to ensure that the tissue remains in the instrument as it is withdrawn. The stylet (f) is used to push the specimen out of the core needle.

OPEN BIOPSY

The technique of open incisional biopsy is simple, but hazardous. Since the technique will vary with each type and location of tumour, only general principles can be outlined. The most crucial decision is placement of the biopsy incision[2]. It should be planned with the definitive surgical procedure in mind. *In no instance should transverse incisions be made in the extremities.* Usually, the most direct route to the lesion is the best choice.

2

For malignant, matrix-producing lesions with a demonstrable soft tissue mass the incision is placed over the soft tissue mass as shown in this CT scan of the mid-thigh, where the preferred approach for this tumour is through the vastus medialis (white arrow). This approach avoids the femoral artery and vein deep to the sartorius (black arrow) without disrupting many soft tissue planes, and allows the surgeon to obtain tissue from the periphery of the mass. This location usually provides the most aggressive, immature tissue for diagnostic purposes, and because matrix-producing lesions are usually most heavily mineralized centrally, a peripheral specimen is easier to cut on frozen section.

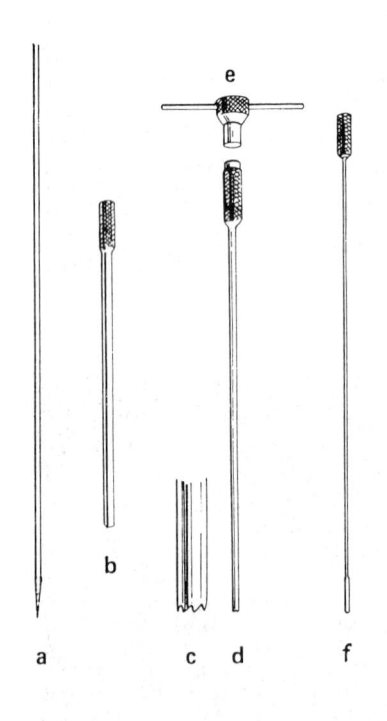

Modified from Operative Surgery: Orthopaedics *3rd edition, 1979, page 336, from a drawing by Miss A. McNeil.*

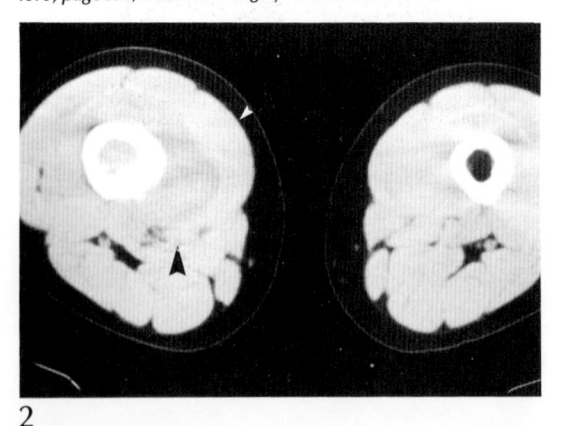

3a, b & c

For lesions without a soft tissue mass, such as the chondrosarcoma illustrated, the most lytic area on plain films (a) or tomograms (b) will usually reveal the most diagnostic tissue, when this is confirmed in the gross specimen (c).

In most instances the biopsy is performed without a tourniquet (based upon theoretical considerations of tumour biology), but this decision is largely the surgeon's preference. If used, the tourniquet must be deflated at the completion of the procedure to obtain adequate haemostasis. It is important to avoid exposing major neurovascular structures, because if contaminated by tumour cells they would have to be resected at the time of definitive operation. The one exception to this rule is the deltopectoral groove, which is employed for most shoulder region biopsies so as to avoid denervation of the anterior deltoid when the tract is excised. It should be possible to approach the lesion without entering more than one anatomical compartment, so that at closure the haematoma is contained.

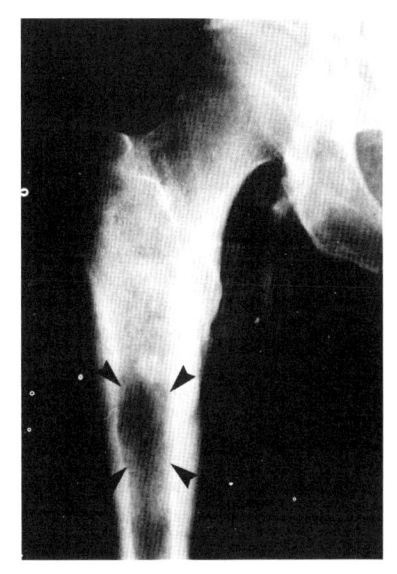

3a

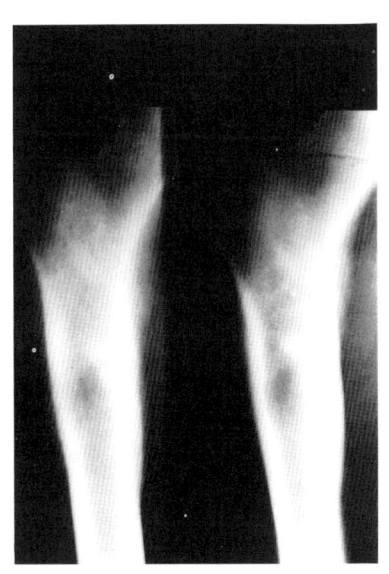

3b

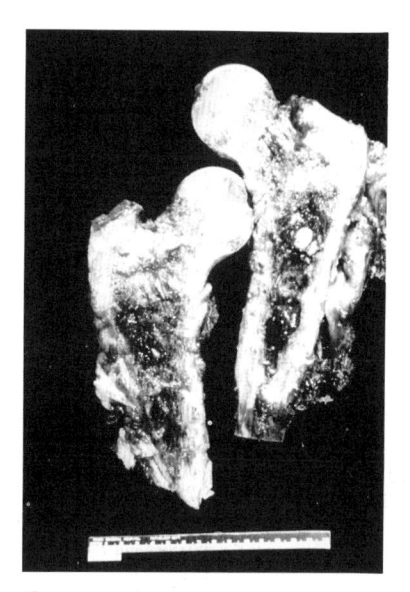

3c

4a, b, c & d

The incision is carried directly through the subcutaneous tissues to the deep fascia which is opened in line with the incision. The muscle is divided or spread directly to the pseudocapsule of the lesion while maintaining absolute haemostasis. It is imperative to avoid Bennet-type retractors, which, if placed around the bone, could pierce the tumour and thereby contaminate more than one compartment. A wedge of tissue is removed and sent for frozen section analysis. If there is no soft tissue mass, a small oval hole is made in the cortex of the bone and a curette is employed to obtain a sample for pathological examination[21].

A culture should always be obtained and a frozen section is usually examined to ensure that diagnostic tissue has been procured. It is not always possible to reach a definitive diagnosis at the time of biopsy, but it should be possible to establish a tentative diagnosis sufficient to allow for proper processing of the tissue. The pathologist should be aware of the clinical and radiographic information for correlation. For certain lesions, especially round cell lesions, Ewing's sarcoma and soft tissue sarcomas, tissue should be obtained for immunohistopathology and electron microscopy, the latter requiring fixation in glutaraldehyde. For metastatic lesions and lymphomas, the presence of certain surface markers, such as oestrogen and progesterone receptors, and T- and B-cell markers are essential to confirm the diagnosis.

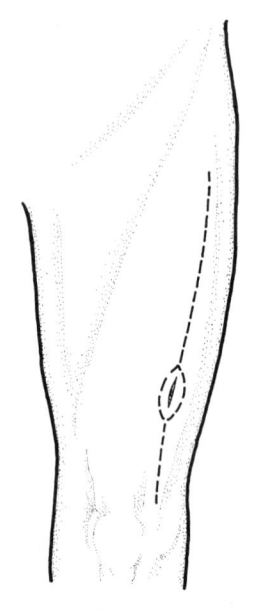

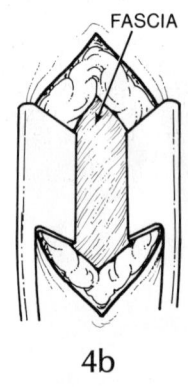

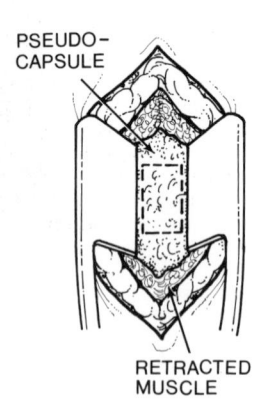

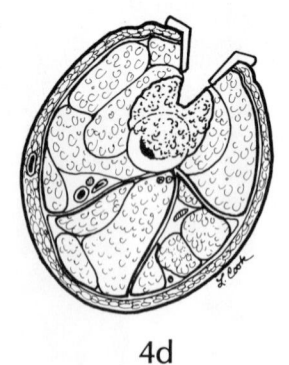

Haemostasis

Prior to closure, haemostasis must be achieved. For soft tissue lesions, compression and closure of the fascia with a running suture is usually sufficient, but in an extremely vascular lesion, packing with a haemostatic agent such as absorbable gelatin sponge or Avitene (Med Chem Products, Woburn, MA, USA) may be necessary. For malignant primary or metastatic bone tumours, plugging the cortical window with methylmethacrylate cement aids in achieving haemostasis, avoids propagation of the haematoma, and prevents pathological fracture. Caution should be used to avoid pressure packing, however, because one experimental study suggests that the use of cement packing increases the number of metastatic foci spreading to the lung[22].

The use of a drain is controversial. If it is employed in an extremely vascular lesion, it should either be brought out through the wound or immediately adjacent to it in line with the incision. Placement of drain wounds distant from the biopsy incision can make subsequent resective surgery difficult or impossible.

A theoretical concern in high-grade malignancies is that intravascular tumour spread during the biopsy manipulation might increase the possibility of metastatic spread. A tourniquet placed proximal to the biopsy site might prevent such an occurrence (avoid the use of an Esmarch bandage), especially if immediate amputation above the tourniquet is indicated and possible. One study, however, has failed to demonstrate a worse prognosis in those patients with osteosarcoma in whom a delay of up to 1 month had occurred between biopsy and definitive resection[23].

At the completion of the biopsy procedure it will be necessary to decide whether to proceed immediately to definitive resection or whether to wait for the final pathological interpretation based upon permanent sections. This will depend upon the clinical situation, the desires of the patient and his or her family, the experience of the pathologist and the certainty of the frozen section diagnosis. It is the authors' opinion that it is preferable to wait for a definitive permanent section diagnosis, rather than proceed on the basis of insecure frozen section diagnoses.

If the decision is made to proceed with the definitive operation the wound is closed, the site is prepared and draped again, the gowns and gloves of the surgical team are changed, and new instruments are employed. The biopsy tract is completely excised *en bloc* with the malignant lesions.

Postoperative management

The routine postoperative management is bed rest, elevation and protection in a splint for 24–48 hours to avoid spread of the haematoma. Lesions requiring wide excision of bone (especially lymphoma or Ewing's sarcoma which may be treated with radiation) will require a plaster of Paris cast, brace or crutches until the bony defect heals.

Complications

One should always be prepared for adverse situations, the most devastating of which is unexpected excessive haemorrhage. It is usually possible to control the bleeding with pressure, packing and patience, but it is wise to have blood available for lesions noted for their vascularity, such as renal cell carcinoma and aneurysmal bone cysts. In extreme situations, immediate amputation or embolization may be required. In patients with suspected renal cell carcinomas, or for lesions in the pelvis or spine (e.g. giant cell tumour, osteosarcoma) it may be wise to precede the biopsy (and the definitive procedure) with intra-arterial embolization.

Other complications that may be encountered from closed or open techniques are pathological fracture from making a large, rectangular, rather than an oval window in the cortex[21], peripheral nerve damage, paralysis and pneumothorax[6]. With proper planning and careful execution, aided in closed techniques with CT or image intensifier direction, most of these hazards should be avoidable.

98 Bone biopsy

5a, b, c & d

Perhaps the greatest complication that can arise from a biopsy is that of performing it improperly. The consequences of such an incident can be devastating, and range from failing to establish the correct diagnosis, obtaining a misdiagnosis which delays critical treatment (and which may be life-threatening), and misplacement of the biopsy incision which may lead to amputation in cases which were otherwise suitable for limb salvage.

An example is illustrated. Anteroposterior and lateral radiographs of this 11-year-old girl show a destructive osteosarcoma of the distal femur (*a, b*). The bone scan (*c*) shows the intraosseous extent of the lesions. A medially placed biopsy tract can be seen at the time of attempted resection of her distal femur (*d*, white arrow). There was a large haematoma in the adductor canal from extensive muscle mobilization during the biopsy (black arrow), and an amputation was required.

Failure to pay suffucent attention to the details of asepsis and incisions can lead to wound infections and skin sloughs, making amputation all but a certainty. In a survey of members of the Musculoskeletal Tumor Society, Mankin et al.[24] reported upon 329 biopsies performed at the referring institution (45 per cent) and the treating centres (55 per cent). There were 18.2 per cent major errors in diagnosis and 10.3 per cent non-representative or

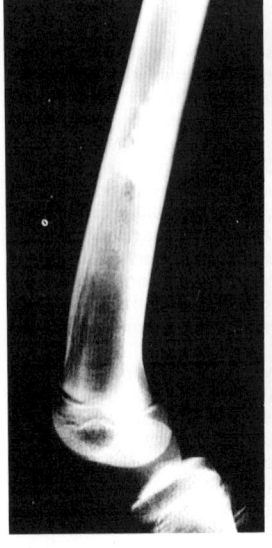

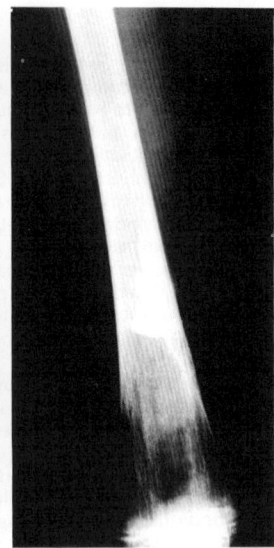

5a

5b

technically poor biopsies. Problems with skin, soft tissue or bone arose in 17.3 per cent of the biopsies. The optimal treatment plan was prevented in 18.2 per cent, an unnecessary amputation was required in 4.5 per cent, and in 8.5 per cent the prognosis and outcome were considered to have been adversely affected as a result of improper biopsy technique. Problems with the biopsy occurred more frequently when the biopsy was performed in the referring institution, indicating that surgeons and pathologists not familiar with musculoskeletal neoplasms or their treatment, should probably refer them to a tumour centre *prior* to biopsy.

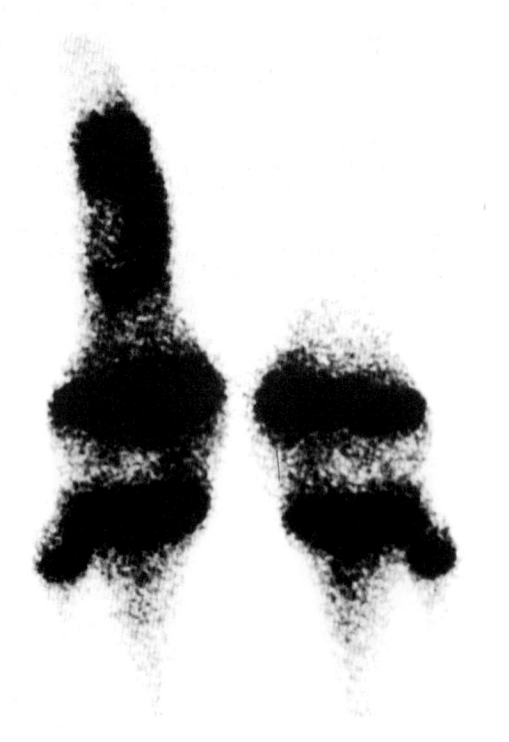

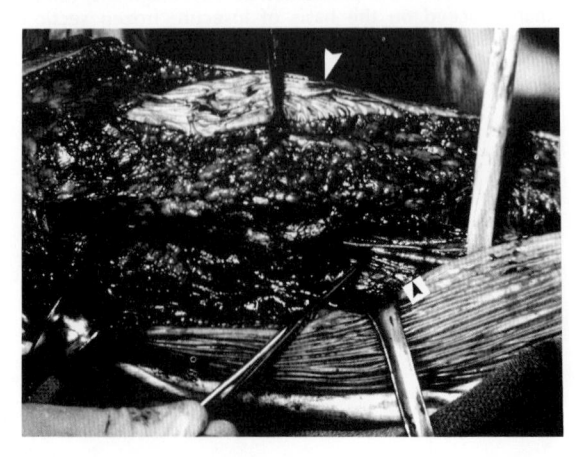

5c

5d

References

1. Spjut HA, Dorfman HD, Fechner RE, Ackerman LV. *Atlas of tumour pathology*, 2nd series Fascicle 5: Tumors of Bone and Cartilage. Washington: Armed Forces Institute of Pathology, 1971.
2. Simon MA. Biopsy of musculoskeletal tumours. *J Bone Joint Surg [Am]* 1982; 64-A: 1253–7.
3. Simon MA, Karluk MB. Skeletal metastases of unknown origin: diagnostic strategy for orthopaedic surgeons. *Clin Orthop* 1982; 166: 96–103.
4. Sweet DL, Mass, DP, Simon MA, Shapiro CM. Histiocytic lymphoma (reticulum-cell sarcoma) of bone: current strategy for orthopaedic surgeons. *J Bone Joint Surg [Am]* 1981; 63-A: 79–84.
5. Kyle RA. Multiple myeloma: review of 869 cases. *Mayo Clin Proc* 1975; 50: 29–40.
6. Moore TM, Meyers MH, Patzakis MJ, Terry R, Harvey JP Jr. Closed biopsy of musculoskeletal lesions. *J Bone Joint Surg [Am]* 1979; 61-A: 375–80.
7. Craig FS. Metastatic and primary lesions of bone. *Clin Orthop* 1970; 73: 33–8.
8. Craig FS. Vertebral body biopsy. *J Bone Joint Surg [Am]* 1956; 38-A: 93–102.
9. Evarts CM. Diagnostic techniques: closed biopsy of bone. *Clin Orthop* 1975; 107: 100–11.
10. Ottolenghi CE. Aspiration biopsy of the spine: technique for the thoracic spine and results of twenty-eight biopsies in this region and over-all results of 1050 biopsies of other spinal segments. *J Bone Joint Surg [Am]* 1969; 51-A: 1531–44.
11. Ottolenghi CE. Diagnosis of orthopaedic lesions by aspiration biopsy: results of 1,061 punctures. *J Bone Joint Surg [Am]* 1955; 37-A: 443–64.
12. den Heeten GJ, Oldhoff J, Oosterhuis JW, Schraffordt-Koops H. Biopsy of bone tumors. *J Surg Oncol* 1985; 28: 247–51.
13. Mink J. Percutaneous bone biopsy in the patient with known or suspected osseous metastases. *Radiology* 1986; 161: 191–4.
14. Schajowicz F, Derqui, JC. Puncture biopsy in lesions of the locomotor system: review of results in 4050 cases, including 941 vertebral punctures. *Cancer* 1968; 21: 531–48.
15. Schneider R. Percutaneous needle bone biopsy. *Orthop Rev* 1983; 12: 119–25.
16. Akerman M, Berg NO, Persson BM. Fine needle aspiration biopsy in the evaluation of tumor-like lesions of bone. *Acta Orthop Scand* 1976; 47: 129–36.
17. Palombini L, Marino D, Vetrani A, Fulciniti F. Fine-needle aspiration biopsy in primary malignant and metastatic bone tumors. *Appl Pathol* 1983; 1: 76–81.
18. Taylor SR, Nunez C. Fine-needle aspiration biopsy in a pediatric population: report of 64 consecutive cases. *Cancer* 1984; 54: 1449–53.
19. Thommesen P, Frederiksen P. Fine needle aspiration biopsy of bone lesions: clinical value. *Acta Orthop Scand* 1976; 47: 137–43.
20. Gatenby RA, Mulhern CB Jr, Moldofsky PJ. Computed tomography guided thin needle biopsy of small lytic bone lesions. *Skeletal Radiol* 1984; 11: 289–91.
21. Clark CR, Morgan C, Songstegard DA, Mathews LS. The effect of biopsy-hole shape and size on bone strength. *J Bone Joint Surg [Am]* 1977; 59-A: 213–7.
22. Robertson WW Jr, Janssen HF, Pugh JL. The spread of tumour-cell-sized particles after bone biopsy. *J Bone Joint Surg [Am]* 1984; 66-A: 1243–7.
23. Brostrom LA, Harris MA, Simon MA, Cooperman DR, Nilsonne U. The effect of biopsy on survival of patients with osteosarcoma. *J Bone Joint Surg [Br]* 1979; 61-B: 209–12.
24. Mankin HJ, Lange TA, Spanier SS. The hazards of biopsy in patients with malignant primary bone and soft-tissue tumours. *J Bone Joint Surg [Am]* 1982; 64-A: 1121–7.

Illustrations by Peter Cox

Principles of fracture management

C. E. Ackroyd MA, FRCS
Consultant Orthopaedic Surgeon, Southmead Hospital, Bristol, UK

Introduction

Fractures of the long bones have been treated by simple splintage for more than 5000 years. The ancient Egyptians used simple wooden splints that were bandaged onto the injured limb to give support and maintain alignment. In the eighteenth and nineteenth centuries numerous bracing devices were designed and with them the simple principles of modern functional treatment evolved. In 1852 Mathijsen[1] described the application of a plaster of Paris bandage which still forms the foundation of the present treatment of most fractures.

Many of the great surgeons of the past had a clear vision of the aims of fracture treatment. Sir Robert Jones[2] stated in 1913, 'the object of treatment is the restoration of complete function with the least risk or inconvenience to the patient and the least anxiety to the surgeon'. This aim remains true today. Since that time there has been a great increase in our knowledge of both the biological and mechanical factors concerned with fracture healing. This biomechanical understanding, coupled with technical advances in material science and equipment design, has led to great improvements in the methods of both operative and non-operative treatment. There is much discussion about the place of the different methods of management for particular fractures. The principles of fracture management remain the same. It is only the application of the principles in the light of modern methods that poses the dilemma for management. For most surgeons there are two questions. Which method of treatment is most suited to this particular fracture, with the special requirements of this particular patient? Does he have the surgical skill, knowledge and means to effect the method satisfactorily?

In the pages that follow the established principles of management will be described and the different methods of management discussed.

Aims of treatment

Restoration of normal function after fracture implies union of the bone in good alignment, perfect restoration of the joint surfaces and good movement of surrounding joints. The loss of function of the soft tissue envelope due to scarring and secondary joint stiffness can be prevented only by early mobilization. Modern fracture treatment therefore emphasizes the importance of proper management of the soft tissues, with early movement of muscles and joints. Treatment of the bone is a secondary consideration. When the skeleton is unstable the application of the specialized techniques of traction and bracing is difficult. The aim is therefore to give rigid fixation which will provide the fracture with sufficient strength to resist the forces of muscle activity and gravity. When properly performed this operative technique holds out the best chance of restoring to perfect function the most severely injured limbs.

Many surgeons in the past have recognized the importance of early functional treatment, but there has been considerable disagreement as to how this should be achieved. Non-operative treatment inevitably involves a period of rest, either in a plaster splint or after a period of skeletal traction. It takes several weeks for the inflammatory response to settle and during this time marked wasting of muscles can occur and stiffness of the soft tissues develops. Provided function starts rapidly within 3–4 weeks, recovery of the soft tissue envelope generally occurs satisfactorily without too much delay. It does, however, involve considerable determination on the part of the patient and great help from the physiotherapist to restore movement to the joints. By contrast, the attractions of primary stable internal fixation of the fracture are evident. The potential for the inflammatory response to cause swelling and soft tissue oedema is considerably reduced. Muscle function and joint movement can resume at any earlier stage. Internal fixation is, however, a potentially dangerous treatment and in each case the benefits and risks should be carefully assessed before deciding on the definitive method of management.

Principles of fracture management 101

Bone healing and union

The process of fracture healing of an unsplinted long bone has been known for many years but a full understanding of the mechanisms initiating and controlling it has yet to be achieved. There are four main biological processes which may be evoked in the healing of a fracture; these have different characteristics and may be modified by the physical environment[3].

1 & 2

Primary callus response and *external bridging callus* can occur in the presence of movement in the fracture ends although under some conditions the external bridging fails and delayed or non-union of the fracture may occur. Danis[4] observed that under conditions of rigid internal fixation fracture healing took place with minimal callus formation.

3

Schenk and Willineger[5] demonstrated that this was due to *cortical haversian remodelling*, and in areas of bone contact primary bony union could occur. In the areas of gap between the fracture ends, the space is filled by woven bone probably derived from the medullary callus. This then undergoes remodelling by new haversian systems. The effectiveness of this form of union depends on the vascularity of the bone ends; if there is a considerable length of necrotic bone, the remodelling process may take many months or even years to reach completion. In the presence of minor degrees of movement, this process is inhibited, the mechanical environment being critical.

The fourth biological response is that of *medullary callus* forming from the endosteal surface. This develops slowly over a period of weeks and months and is probably independent of the mechanical environment. Kenwright and Goodship[6] have made a major contribution to the understanding of the callus response and the influence of the mechanical environment. Much remains to be elucidated, including its direct application to fracture treatment.

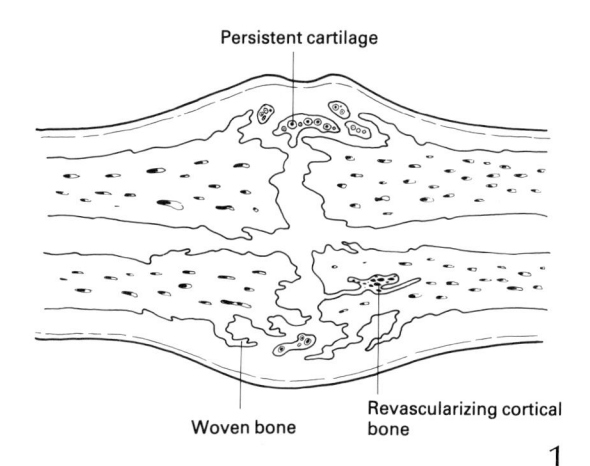

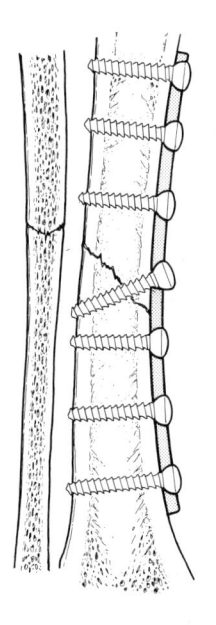

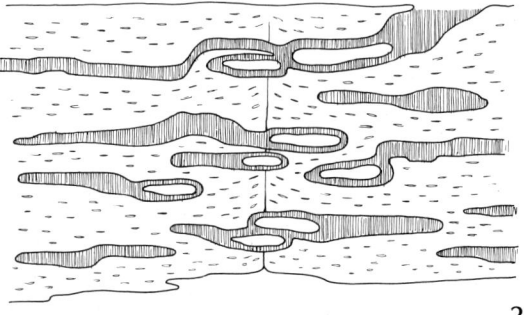

History and mechanism of injury

A careful clinical history invariably produces a clear understanding of the mechanism of injury and it is often possible to predict accurately the type of fracture most likely to be involved. The method of management will depend on the characteristics of the fracture and the condition and aspirations of the patient, and on the degree of damage to the soft tissue envelope.

The principal mechanical function of bone is to act as a supporting structure and to transmit load. The loads to which a bone may be subjected are those of compression, tension, bending and torsion. Bone is strongest in compression and weakest in tension.

4 & 5

Bone is a viscoelastic material and fractures are therefore related not only to the force but to the rate of application of force. Bone is better able to withstand a rapid application of a large force. The energy is stored within the bone and when failure occurs the energy is released. If high energy levels are present, fracturing will produce comminution of bone. If low levels of energy are present a simpler fracture pattern results.

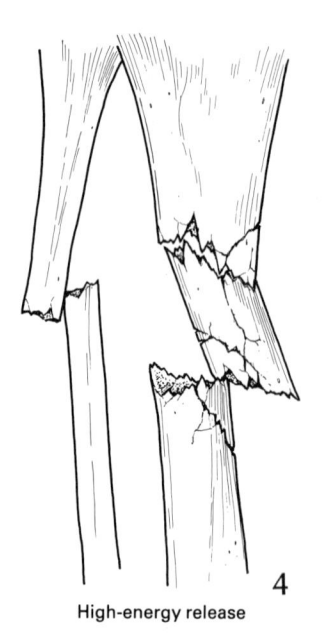

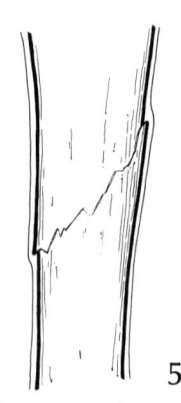

4 High-energy release

5 Low-energy release

6

The immature bone of the child or adolescent has a lower modulus of elasticity and a lower bending strength than the adult. It therefore deflects and absorbs more energy before breaking. The typical greenstick fracture surface of the child's bone requires more energy for its production than the relatively smooth surface of the adult fracture. Children's bones are also capable of considerable plastic deformation without fracturing.

Throughout adult life mechanical properties of bone do not change significantly. In old age energy absorption of bone decreases, partially caused by an increase in mineralization. The porosity of bone also increases with corresponding overall decrease in strength. The extent of plastic deformation decreases as the bones become more brittle; and the process of crack propagation requires less energy and thus fracturing in the elderly becomes more frequent. The three most common fractures of the elderly are the Colles' fracture of the wrist, femoral neck fracture and vertebral compression fractures.

A combination of different forces and methods of application results in the different patterns of fracture.

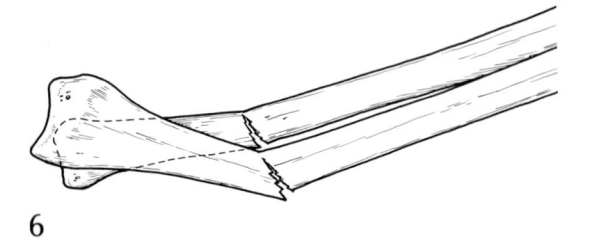

Principles of fracture management 103

7a & b

Pure compression fractures occur mainly in the cancellous areas such as the vertebral bodies and os calcis and there is often an element of compression in the metaphyseal fracture.

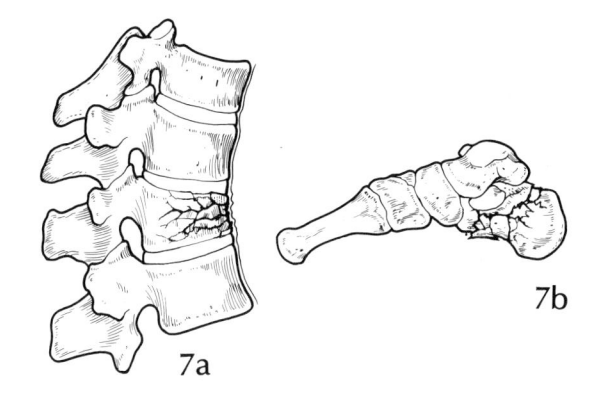

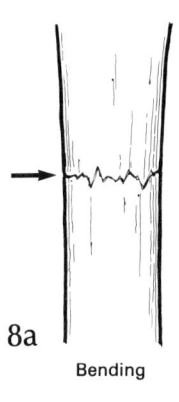

7a

7b

8a
Bending

8b
Bending and compression

8c
Torsion

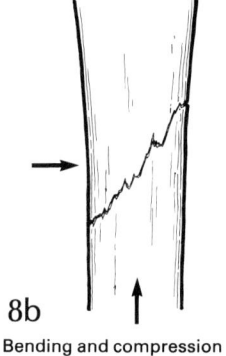

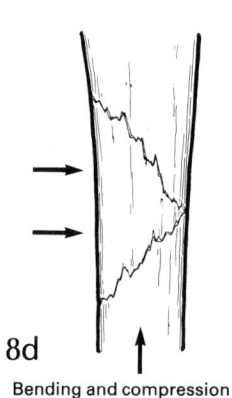

8d
Bending and compression

8a–d

Transverse, oblique and spiral fractures with and without butterfly fragments result from a combination of pure bending, torsion or a combination of these forces with axial compression loading.

It is also easy to distinguish the low-velocity injuries resulting in little soft tissue damage from the high-velocity injuries which produce comminuted fractures with considerable soft tissue damage.

104　Fracture treatment

Diagnosis

Radiological investigations

Standard anteroposterior and lateral radiographs are the first requirement. Oblique radiographs are often helpful to show the fracture lines and degree of displacement, particularly where there are complex bone shadows in the joints of the upper and lower limbs.

9

Simple strain radiographs can be performed in the accident department to assess joint stability but it is often necessary to perform this under general anaesthesia.
　　The more complex injuries of joints and of the spine require more detailed investigation with the use of tomography or computed axial tomography.

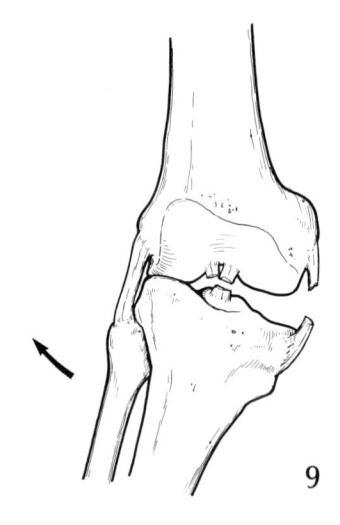

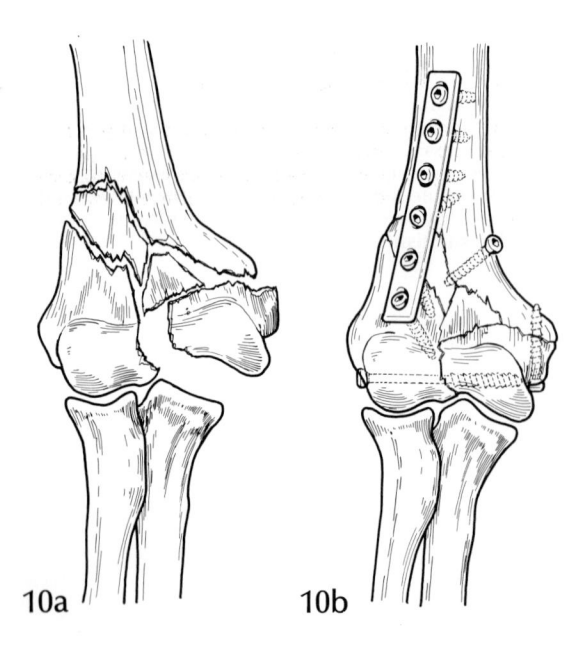

10a & b

It is essential that an accurate diagnosis of the fracture is made prior to treatment, and it is often helpful to draw out the fracture on celluloid or tracing paper particularly prior to operative reduction.

Diagnostic manipulation

11

Manipulation has a valuable diagnostic role. Initial manipulative reduction of a displaced fracture may be successful only to result in the fracture becoming displaced within the next few days. It is necessary to have a clear understanding of the stability of the fracture after it has been reduced in order to plan the most appropriate method to hold it in the reduced position. The stability depends on the shape and number of fragments, obliquity of the fracture line, and integrity of the soft tissues.

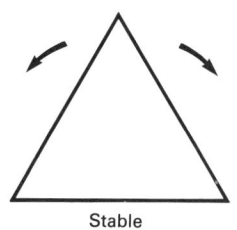

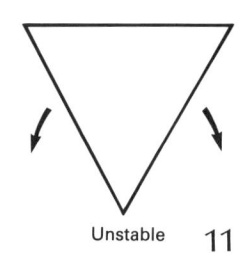

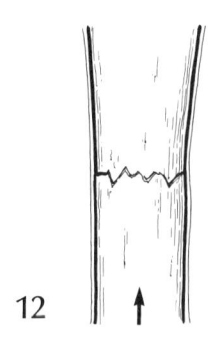

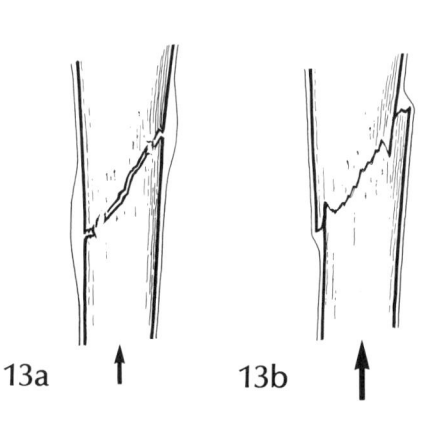

12, 13a & b

Once the fracture has been reduced to the best possible position it is then tested in different ways. First the part is subject to longitudinal compression. A transverse fracture or one that is short, oblique and impacted will not shorten.

14

The greater the area of contact the less the ease with which the fragments can be rocked. If the rocking movement is carried out in two directions at right angles it is possible to identify the direction in which the deformity needs to be further reduced.

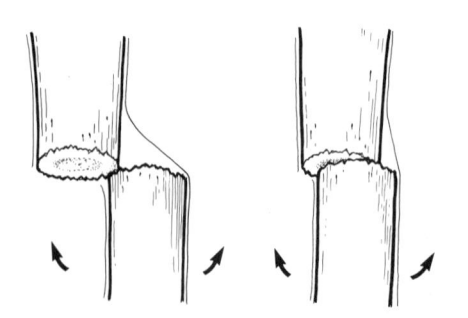

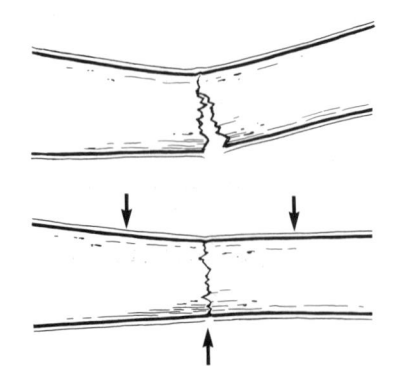

15

If there is a soft tissue hinge it is easy to determine its position by this rocking technique. It is essential to show its position prior to the application of plaster in order to apply three-point fixation.

16

When a fracture is oblique, spiral or comminuted, stressing in compression shows not only how easily but how far it can be displaced. The soft tissues impose a restraint on fracture movement and the stability can be felt and visualized under image intensification.

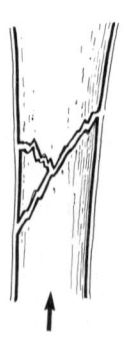

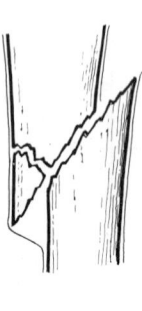

17a, b, c & d

Special circumstances apply when a transverse fracture is overlapped. The soft tissue hinge (*h*) often prevents reduction by longitudinal traction. This problem can usually be solved by bending the fracture as much as 70° and then using the thumb on the distal fragment to slide it distally on the proximal fragment until it is clear (with *b* equivalent to *b'*) and it is then able to reduce into line. An area of end-to-end contact is then established by pushing and rocking the fragments.

This situation often occurs with children's forearm fractures and can be particularly difficult to reduce when only one bone is broken. The technique is more difficult when there is marked swelling of the limb and the neurovascular structures must be protected.

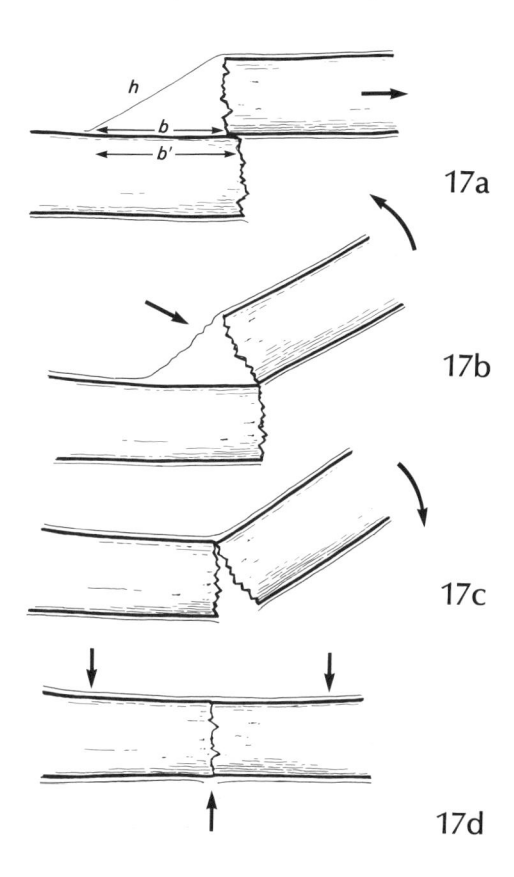

Fracture reduction

Reduction of most fractures can be satisfactorily achieved by closed means when the mechanism of injury is understood[7]. There are, however, some circumstances where interposition of muscle, tendon, periosteum or other soft tissue structures makes it impossible to achieve adequate bony contact. In other circumstances gross displacement of bony fragments, often with rotation, may make it impossible to reduce the fracture by closed means. This is particularly true with intra-articular fractures. Sometimes imbalanced muscle activity may prevent an adequate reduction or make maintenance of the position difficult. When there has been a significant delay in treatment, reduction becomes increasingly difficult and closed methods may not be successful after the first week, particularly in children when healing can occur very rapidly.

Successful manipulation requires an understanding of the fracture mechanism and type and an appreciation of what it can be expected to achieve. The advent of the image intensifier has helped with visualization of the fracture fragments. It may, however, lead to a loss of the traditional diagnostic and manipulative skills.

Once successful manipulation of the fracture has been achieved it must now be held in the reduced position until healing occurs. Maintenance of the position in unstable or partially stable fractures may be difficult or impossible. This is particularly true for intra-articular fractures where the criteria for adequacy of reduction are much more exact.

Methods of holding fractures

SELF-STABILIZING FRACTURES

18a & b

Undisplaced fractures generally have an intact soft tissue envelope including the periosteum. The tendency to displacement will vary with the length of the lever arm, the direction of the fracture line and the magnitude of the applied force. For example, an oblique undisplaced fracture of the lateral malleolus can be treated as satisfactorily with adhesive strapping as with plaster of Paris provided care is taken not to overload the ankle. Similarly, the fracture of the base of the fifth metatarsal can be treated with strapping provided pain can be controlled satisfactorily and there is minimal soft tissue damage. Other examples apply to the neck of the humerus, the clavicle and the metacarpals and phalanges of the hand.

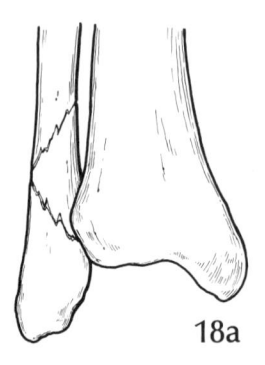

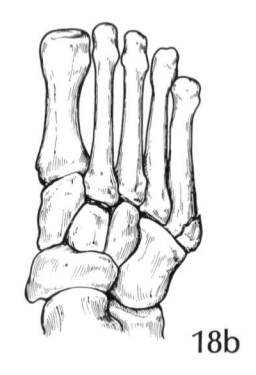

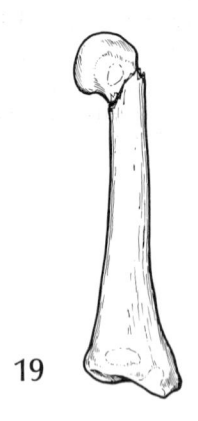

19

Some fractures may be driven into a stable position. Fractures of the neck of the fifth metacarpal, even if considerably displaced, may be treated with wool and bandaging and early mobilization.

Principles of fracture management 109

PLASTER OF PARIS

Plaster of Paris is a considerable encumbrance to the patient but is extremely effective in protecting the injured part from external forces: it immediately reduces the movement at the fracture of both the bone and the soft tissues, and helps to relieve pain. A plaster cast does not totally immobilize a fracture but merely provides a comfortable splinted environment for healing to occur. Indeed some micro-movement at the fracture is desirable to stimulate the callus response. The role of most plaster casts is to prevent bending and twisting and to rest the soft tissues.

There are three ways in which a plaster cast can be applied apart from a simple cylinder in order to improve the mechanical effect of immobilization.

Joint position

Immobilization of the joint above and below the fracture will to some extent reduce the deforming forces acting at the fracture site, and it can be used to maintain satisfactory alignment and rotation. However, once muscle activity recovers such casts can actually increase movement at the fracture site and predispose to non-union. Such casts should be applied for as short a time as possible, generally until soft tissue swelling has settled, anything from 2 to 4 weeks. Thereafter casts using bracing principles should be applied.

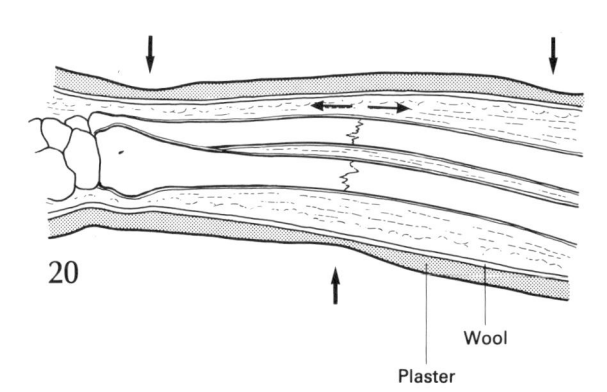

Three-point fixation

20

The use of a soft tissue hinge is of great advantage in maintaining fracture immobilization. Such hinges are common in the greenstick fractures of childhood and can be identified during the diagnostic manipulation procedures. This technique employs the simple application of pressure at strategic points to create tension and compression forces in the soft tissue envelope of a long bone and so maintain fracture stability.

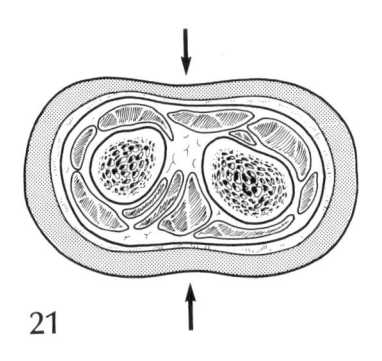

20
Wool
Plaster

Moulding

21

An additional technique involves moulding of the plaster in such a way as to take advantage of other soft tissue pressures. Such moulding can be used between the forearm bones, at the wrist and ankle and as an integral part of the bracing techniques.

21

110 Fracture treatment

FRACTURE BRACING

Braces have been available for fracture treatment for well over 200 years. Recently, Sarmiento developed the techniques for use with modern materials[8].

22a & b

The tibial fracture is ideally suited for this technique because of the relatively long levers and the fact that it has one subcutaneous surface enhancing the grip of the cast. Similar factors operate for the ulna. The essential requirement is that the soft tissue swelling should have settled completely and a nearly skin-tight cast is applied and moulded to grip upper and lower ends of the fractured bones. The upper end of the tibia is triangular and with the bellies of the gastrocnemius muscles forms a heart-shaped cross-section which provides good rotational stability. A hinge can be applied at the ankle to control alignment of the lower fragment.

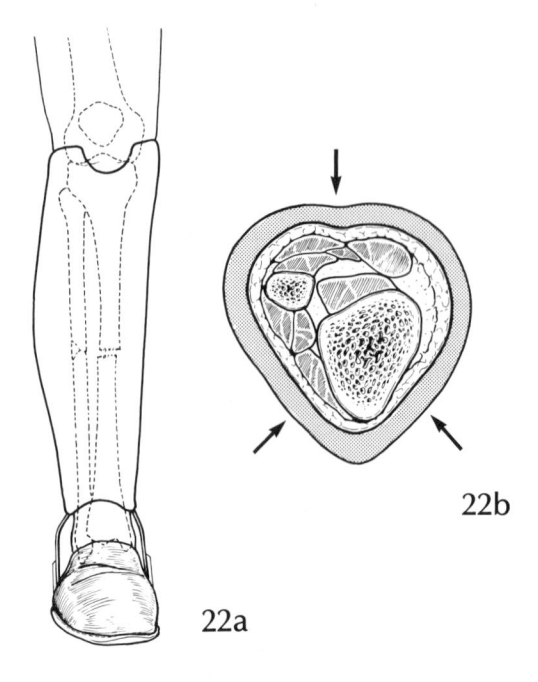

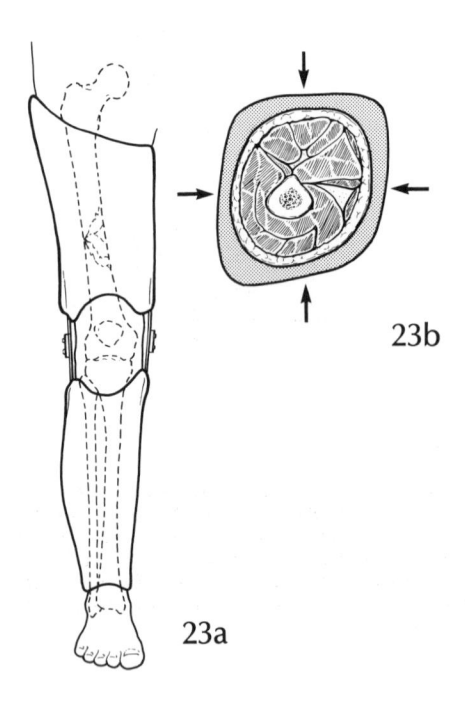

23a & b

Similar techniques can be applied to the humerus and femur using the quadrilateral socket principle; the soft tissues are shaped into a quadrilateral and, on weight-bearing, fracture shortening, angulation and rotation are resisted.

TRACTION

Traction can be applied either through the skin or through a skeletal pin or screw.

Skin traction

24a, b, c & d

Adhesive strips are applied to the skin after application of benzoin tincture (Tinct. Benz) and then closely bandaged to the limb. As an alternative, corrugated foam strips can be bandaged to the limb for temporary traction. The malleoli should be protected either by passing the traction cords around the side bars of the Thomas' splint or by application of plaster felt around the malleoli. The skin must be inspected daily to ensure that no damage is occurring, particularly in the elderly who may have frail, poor quality skin. The maximum weight that can be applied safely to a single limb is 2.7 kg (6 lb).

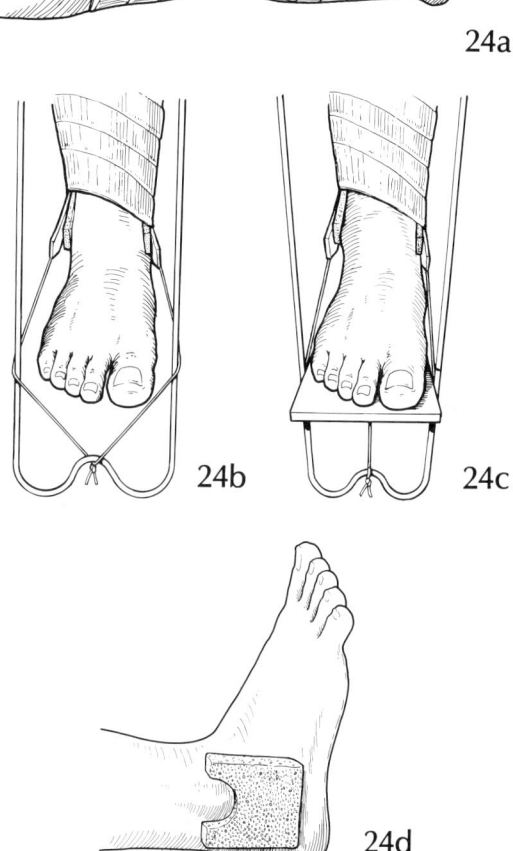

Skeletal traction

Skeletal traction should be used on adults when more than 2.7 kg is applied or when traction is likely to last several weeks. The need for traditional skeletal traction for long-bone fractures has been considerably reduced with the advent of external skeletal fixation of fractures when there is an increasing tendency to use fully-threaded half pins.

25

A Denham pin is most satisfactory, particularly when going through cortical bone, as it reduces the incidence of a loosening and subsequent pin-track infection.

26a

The upper tibial pin site is 2.5 cm below and 2.5 cm behind the tibial tuberosity. The lower end of the tibia can also be used and occasionally a pin can be inserted in the os calcis.

Skeletal traction can also be applied to the upper limb through the olecranon for humeral and supracondylar fractures. It is also occasionally applied to the lower end of the femur and to the greater trochanter.

26b

Pin insertion can be done under local anaesthesia, though more often manipulation of the fracture is required at the same time and general anaesthesia is necessary. The upper tibial pins should be inserted from the lateral side through a small puncture incision. The pin should be inserted by hand at right angles to the line of the tibia in both sagittal and coronal planes.

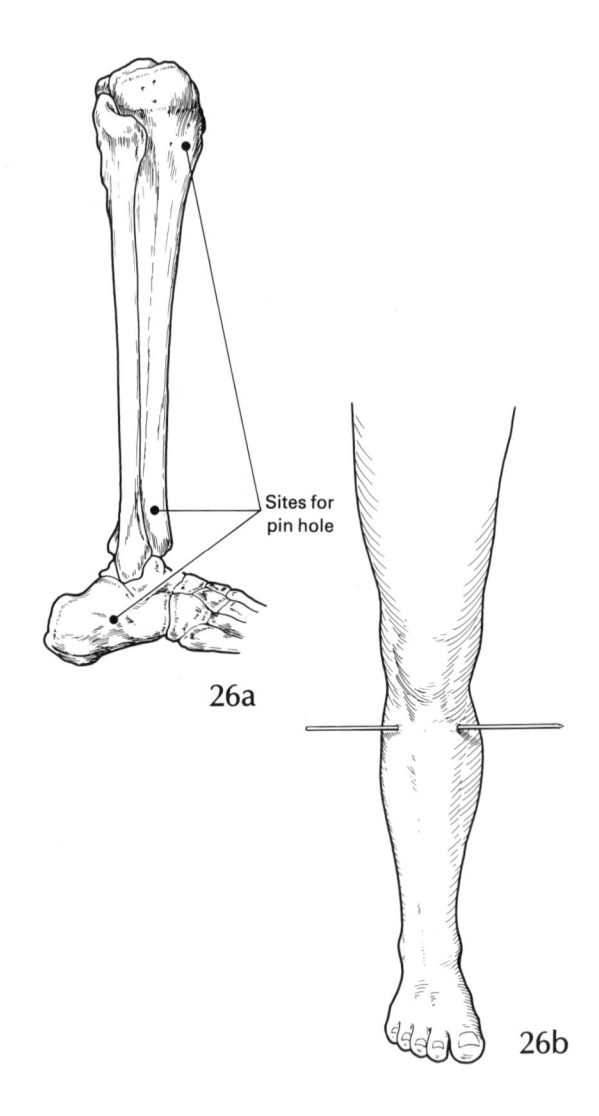

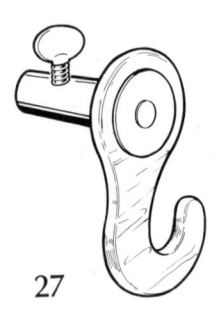

27

Traditional stirrups and swivel hooks are unsatisfactory as they invariably bind with the pin and promote loosening. The Simionis swivel traction hook is a very satisfactory alternative.

EXTERNAL SKELETAL FIXATION

28

External skeletal fixation has been available as a method of management of fractures for more than 80 years. There are now many systems available to produce versatile and satisfactory stabilization of the skeleton whilst allowing access to any related wound. Skeletal stabilization allows the injured limb to be managed with much greater ease and there is good evidence that this reduces the incidence of wound infection in open fractures. Wound management involving simple excision and packing or complex plastic surgical treatment can be performed easily.

The key to satisfactory external fixation is the integrity of the pin–bone interface. Suitably sized pins should be chosen for the particular bone. When inserting pins into cortical bone the holes should be predrilled and the soft tissue protected with guides.

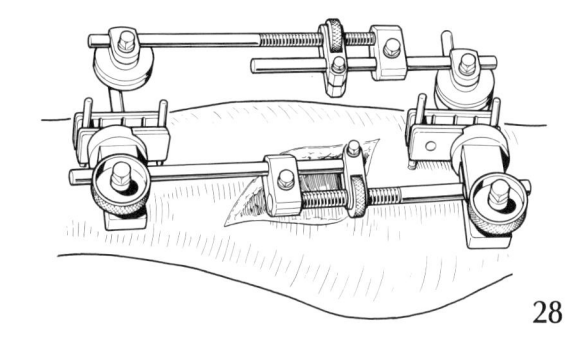

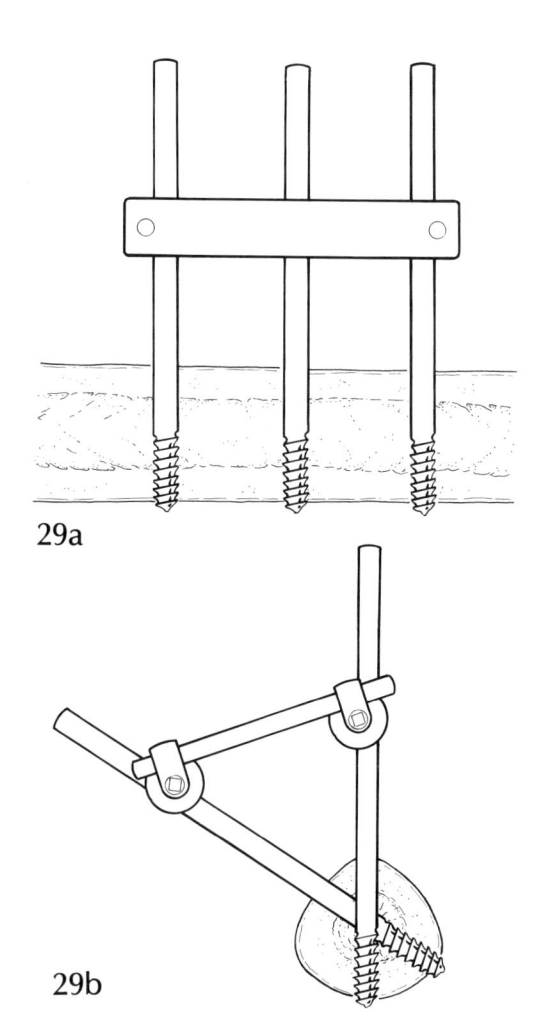

29a & b

A firm grip of the bone fragment can be obtained by the use of up to three pins in one plane and if necessary one or two of these pins can be introduced in separate anatomical planes at an angle of greater than 60°. Transfixion pins should be avoided when they cross muscle and fascial compartments.

The clamps will vary with the different systems, the best allowing versatile geometry. The geometrical arrangement of the clamps and bars may give a frame which is unilateral, bilateral, triangular or quadrilateral. The arrangement chosen will depend on the mechanical conditions of stability required and the position of the soft tissue wounds.

External skeletal fixation allows the surgeon to alter the mechanical environment at will and create conditions favourable to reducing infection and stimulating fracture healing. Detailed text should be consulted before attempting to apply this technique for anything other than the simplest fracture[9].

INTERNAL FIXATION

Indications

There are a wide range of indications for internal fixation. The basic principle, however, must remain that the method of treatment chosen for any fracture should be as simple and non-invasive as possible provided the criteria of acceptable anatomical alignment, rapid fracture healing and early functional treatment can be satisfied.

Absolute indications

Failure of reduction Any fracture which cannot be reduced satisfactorily by closed means must be opened to restore anatomical alignment. There are circumstances when soft tissue interposition can prevent fracture reduction. In other circumstances, particularly with joint injuries, closed reduction is not possible.

Loss of position When the fracture position has been lost after initial non-operative treatment, further manipulation is seldom successful and an open reduction becomes necessary.

The presence of multiple injuries The primary stabilization of certain fractures can considerably simplify management of multiple injuries and reduce the risks of adult respiratory distress syndrome.

Relative indications

There are many relative indications when primary fixation, or delayed primary fixation as a planned procedure can simplify the post-injury period, assuring an anatomical position of the fracture and speeding up the rehabilitation, often with greater convenience to the patient.

Optional indications

There are circumstances when both surgeon and patient will decide that internal fixation is a more convenient method though the risks and benefits must be carefully assessed.

Whenever open operation is performed it is essential to consider very carefully the risks of the procedure and weigh them against the benefits. This discussion must involve careful consultation with the patient to ensure that he fully understands the nature of the procedure. Considerable skill, care and attention to detail is required in performing and managing such cases. Ill-advised or improperly performed internal fixation can end in complete disaster.

Screw fixation

30

Screws can be used either to hold plates onto the bones or to produce interfragmentary compression between two fragments of bone. The bone should always be predrilled and tapped prior to screw insertion and the drill should be irrigated to prevent overheating.

Whenever an interfragmentary technique is used the proximal piece of bone should be free to slide and be compressed against the distal piece of bone. This can be achieved either by overdrilling the proximal fragment so that it slides over the screw threads or by using a screw with a smooth shank. In shaft fractures it is invariably necessary to supplement single screw fixation with a neutralization plate.

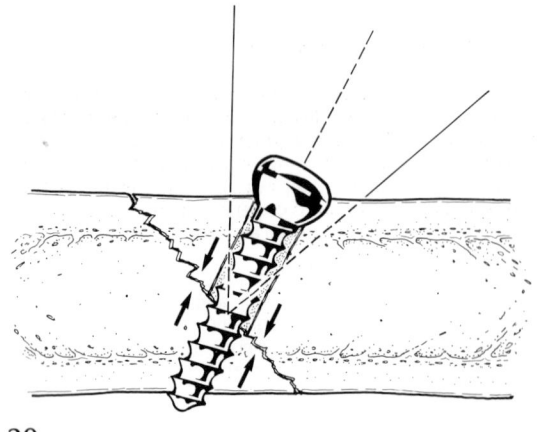

30

Principles of fracture management 115

31a, b & c

Screws engaging cancellous bone should be larger and have coarse threads. A large variety of screw sizes are available from 1.5 mm up to 6.5 mm. These are available in the various fracture fixation sets.

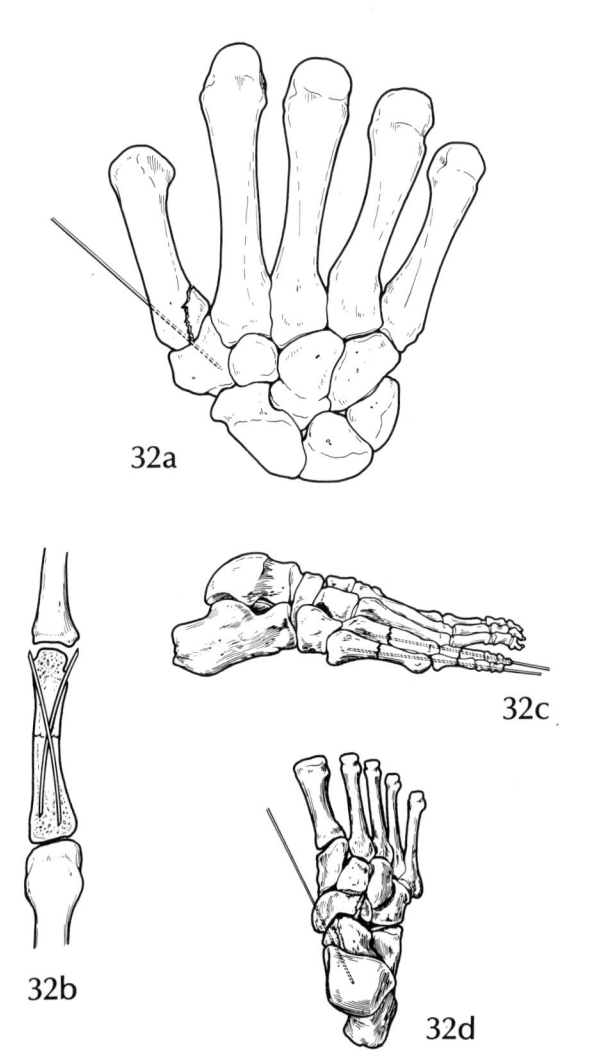

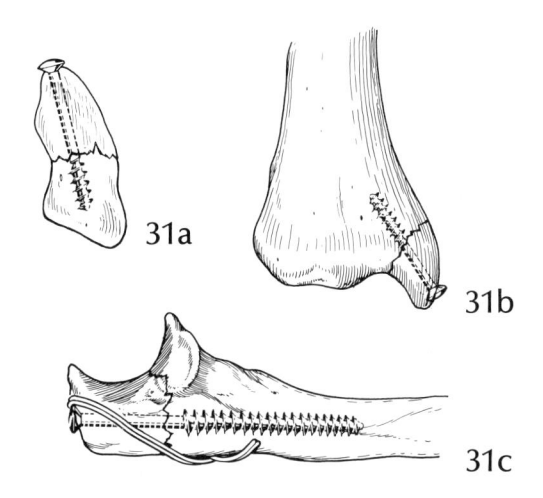

31a

31b

31c

Wire fixation

32a, b, c & d

Kirschner wires are a very satisfactory method of producing skeletal stabilization. This technique is particularly useful with small fragments of bone such as in fractures of the fingers, metacarpals and metatarsals. Temporary Kirschner wire fixation is an essential part of the reconstruction of more complex fractures of the larger joints.

32a

32b

32c

32d

33a, b, c & d

Various special techniques of Kirschner wire fixation are available using the addition of tension-band wiring and this is most appropriate for the patella, olecranon, greater trochanter and medial malleolus.

For detailed description of the tension-band technique for patellar fractures *see* the chapter on 'Fractures of the patella' (pp. 252–255) and for olecranon fractures *see* the chapter on 'Fractures of the elbow in adults' (pp. 165–174).

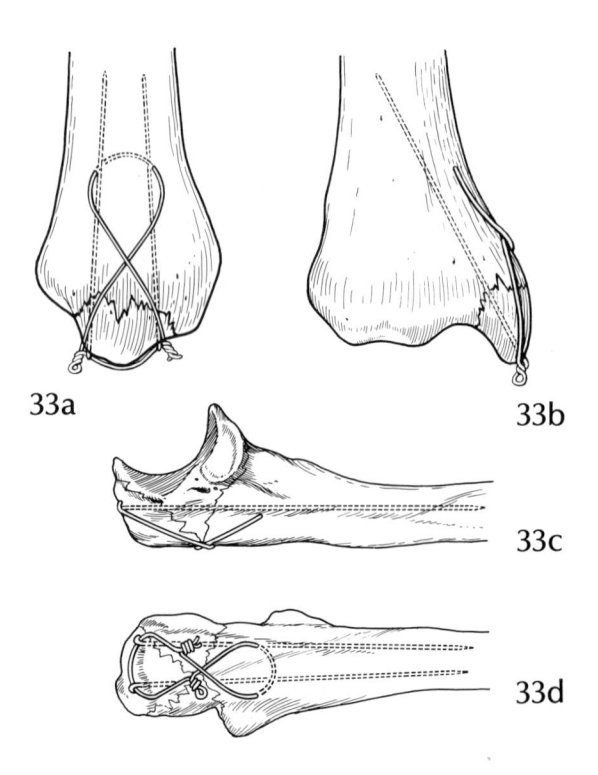

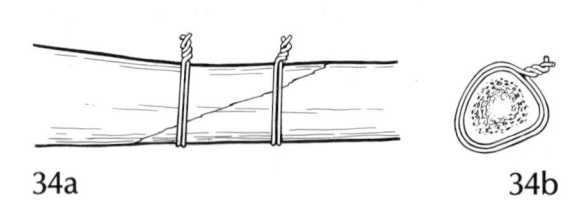

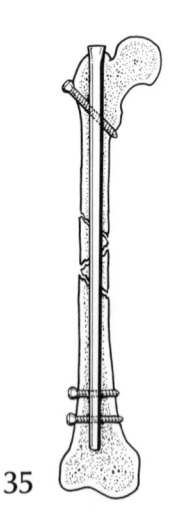

33a

33b

33c

33d

34a & b

Circlage wiring can also be used as a means of holding bone temporarily in place while screws or plates are inserted or as an adjunct to intramedullary fixation in long oblique and spiral fractures.

Intramedullary nailing

35

Traditionally, intramedullary nailing has required an approach to the fracture site. Recently, techniques have been developed using thin guide rods and the image intensifier which allow a closed reduction to be performed. Reaming is carried out over the rod with closed introduction of the nail. The nails can also be locked with one or two crossed screws and this has considerably increased the indications for the intramedullary techniques.

Great success can be achieved with the tibia and the femur and techniques are being developed for the humerus and some of the other long bones. A detailed description of the technique is described in the chapter on 'Kuntscher's closed intramedullary nailing technique for the treatment of femoral shaft fractures' (*see* pp. 223–241).

Plate fixation

Fixation of fractures by the use of plate and screws was pioneered by Lane and Hey Groves in the early part of this century. Until the mid-1960s this form of fixation was not rigid in nature and additional plaster of Paris splintage was required. The results were generally poor with infection, non-union and joint stiffness being amongst the complications.

In the early 1960s the Swiss AO group developed techniques of plate fixation which result in compression of the fracture surfaces, thus increasing the mechanical stability of the unit to provide a very rigid environment. This rigidity modifies the fracture healing process, much reducing callus formation from the periosteum. Fracture healing relies on primary haversian remodelling or secondary medullary bone ingrowth from the endosteal surface. The strength of the fixation is generally sufficient to allow unsupported use of the limb. Provided the bone ends are viable, fracture union takes place within a reasonable period and superb functional results can be obtained. If, however, the blood supply of the fracture surfaces is compromised, the remodelling process can be delayed by many months; and if excessive loading of the fixation occurs, the screws and plate can loosen or the plate can fatigue and break. There are therefore great advantages to be obtained if the healing processes are satisfactory, but there are potential drawbacks which must be recognized and action may have to be taken to prevent complications occurring.

A detailed description of the techniques is to be found in the *Manual of internal fixation* published by the AO group[10]. The techniques are demanding and careful attention to detail is essential to obtain the best results.

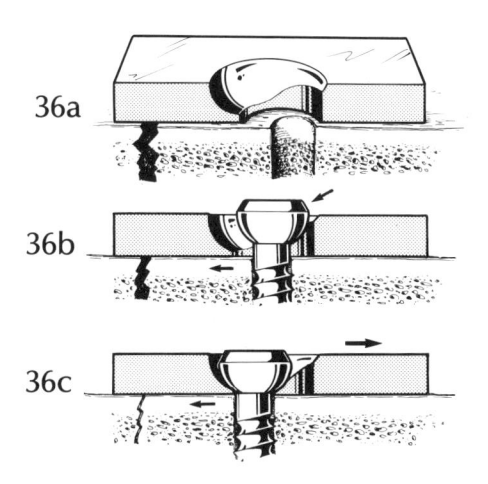

36a–c

The plate in most common use today is called the 'dynamic compression plate'. It has oval holes for screws which are designed to create compression at the fracture site and tension in the plate as the screws are tightened. The plates vary in size and strength depending on the size of the bone to be fixed.

118 Fracture treatment

37

Plates may be used in different mechanical ways. A tension-band plate is applied to the convex surface of the bone, resisting the tension forces; however, there must be an intact opposite compression cortex or the fixation will fail.

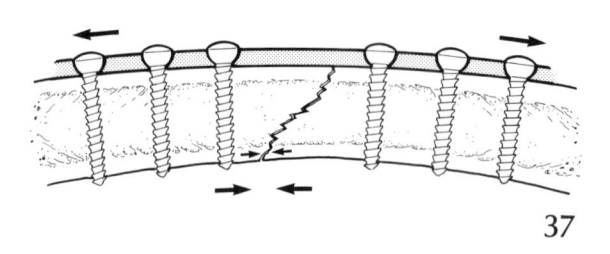

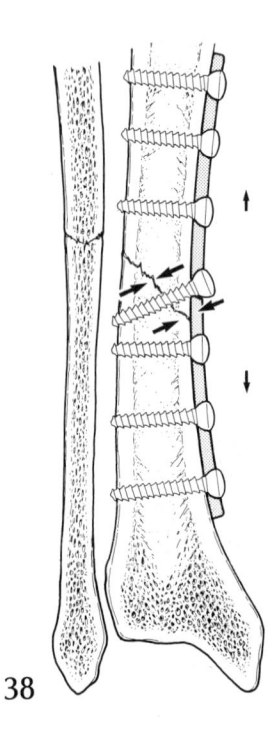

38

The plate may also be used to neutralize the external deforming forces in a situation where interfragmentary screw fixation has compressed the fracture surfaces together. This use of the plate is essential to maintain the integrity of the fixation in order to allow functional treatment.

Plates may also be used to buttress concave surfaces such as at the lower end of the radius and at the tibial plateau.

39a & b

There are also several specialized plates for use in the spine, the dynamic hip screw and plate for femoral neck fractures and the dynamic condylar screw for supracondylar fractures of the femur. Detailed descriptions may be found in the relevant chapters.

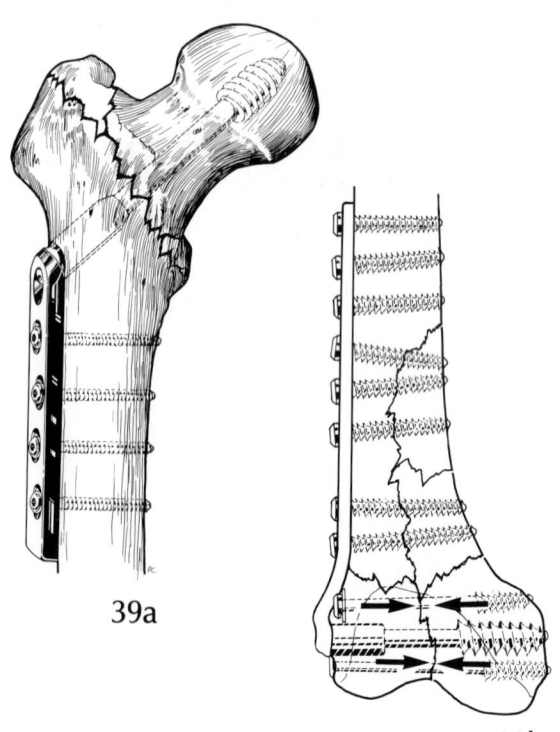

Bone grafting

40

The use of autogenous bone graft is an important additional technique in the management of fractures. When open reduction and internal fixation with plate and screws is being performed, fracture comminution with fracture gaps is an important cause of fixation failure. It is essential that in all circumstances fracture fragments that cannot be fully incorporated into the fixation are either replaced with autogenous cancellous bone graft or bone graft is applied under the periosteal sleeve.

Bone grafting should also be carried out whenever there is significant bone loss such as occurs in major open fractures.

Grade II and Grade III open fractures[11,12] are often associated with significant soft tissue damage and damage to the blood supply of the bone. Delayed primary or secondary bone grafting is often necessary in order to stimulate callus formation. This should be carried out early to ensure that healing occurs within a reasonable time period of 4–6 months. Thus bone grafting of fracture gaps should take place within 4–6 weeks of the initial injury provided the soft tissue conditions are satisfactory. If there is no evidence of good callus formation within 6–12 weeks then bone grafting should definitely be carried out.

When a fracture has failed to unite within 6 months the healing potential for union should be assessed. Bone grafting is often required in the management of delayed union or non-union and it is essential in the atrophic case.

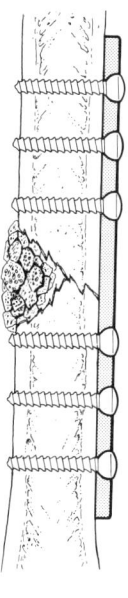

Implant removal

It is generally recommended that large implants should be removed from the long bones of adult and middle-aged patients. This is to allow the bone structure to return to normal and prevent the possibility of stress-protection osteoporosis weakening the bone which may predispose to a subsequent refracture. It now seems unlikely that this is an important consideration. As the years pass, the bone remodels around the implant and there are seldom any significant adverse effects.

A recent study of plate removal from the forearm demonstrated a high complication rate. Only 20 per cent of patients requested plate removal as a result of significant symptoms[13]. In general, therefore, whereas plates and screws should be removed from the weight-bearing bones of the tibia and femur after at least 2 years have elapsed, in the upper limb and in the ankle, plates should be removed only if clinical symptoms dictate. Intramedullary rods often produce irritation at the upper end and should be removed when radiographs show adequate callus formation, usually some 18 months after injury.

Isolated screws seldom require removal. Tension-band wiring, particularly in subcutaneous areas such as the patella and olecranon, often produces prominent tender nodules; these implants therefore require removal once sound fracture healing has occurred.

Complications of injury

Open fractures

Open fractures should be graded according to the classification of Gustilo and Anderson[11,12]. The Grade I fracture, which is no more than a puncture wound, can be treated as if it was a closed injury. Grade II and Grade III fractures are more serious with significant damage to skin, soft tissue and bone. The Grade III fractures have been further classified into three subdivisions depending on the severity of the skin and neurovascular lesions.

Successful management of open fractures depends entirely on correct primary treatment and most wounds should be healed within 4 weeks of injury. Initial management should include a polaroid clinical photograph of the wound, a culture swab should be taken and a dressing soaked in povidone-iodine applied. It is not disturbed until the patient is anaesthetized in the operating theatre. Broad spectrum, high dose, intravenous antibiotics should be given for up to 5 days to help prevent infection.

The management of open fractures naturally falls into two parts: wound treatment and fracture management.

Wound treatment

The primary traumatic wound should be extended so that full exploration of the extent of the injury can be determined, dirt and debris should be irrigated out of the wound and damaged soft tissues excised. The wounds should then be packed with an antiseptic and left open for subsequent inspection at 48 hours. It may be permissible to close the surgical wound but under no circumstances should the traumatic wound be closed unless it is completely clean and there is no tension on the soft tissues.

The skin should be closed by delayed primary closure or skin grafting. If there is a large skin defect then plastic surgical procedures involving tissue transfers will be necessary and should be carried out at an early stage.

Fracture management

After the bone ends have been cleaned and irrigated the fracture should be reduced and stabilized. In Grade II and III open fractures it is generally best to use external skeletal fixation carefully planned to allow satisfactory access to the wound, minimal interference with joint function and a frame geometry that will confer satisfactory stability to the fracture and a relatively rigid environment for the first few days.

If rigid fixation is maintained for more than a few days fracture union is inevitably delayed and it is therefore important to reduce the fracture stiffness within a week or apply techniques of loading with intermittent compression or, if conditions allow, early weight-bearing.

Delayed union and non-union

The definition of these conditions depends on the attitude of the surgeon and the patient and the nature of the fracture. In practice, delayed union is what makes a surgeon think he is going to have to operate on a fracture whereas non-union is what persuades him that he must. The time scale of delayed union is subject to interpretation whereas non-union is the state where the fracture is unlikely to unite spontaneously.

41a

Non-union is divided into three basic types. The hypertrophic type is where there is abundant callus formation but bridging of the fracture gap has not occurred. Both bone ends are fully viable and the failure is generally due to the mechanical environment. If such fractures are held rigidly, either by internal fixation or by external fixation, mineralization of the fracture gap and bridging callus usually occurs within a few weeks.

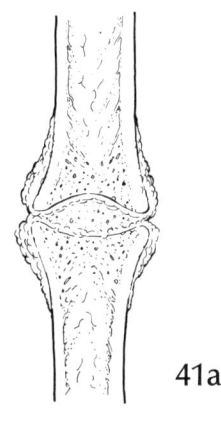

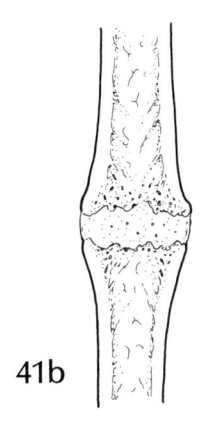

41b

Oligotrophic fractures have some callus response but there is often biological and mechanical inadequacy. Bone grafting and rigid fixation is generally necessary for successful union.

41c

The third pattern is the atrophic response. There is no callus formation and the bone ends have a poor or absent blood supply. In these circumstances it is essential to carry out generous cancellous bone grafting which responds well to a rigid mechanical environment that can be provided either by various types of rigid internal fixation or rigid external fixation.

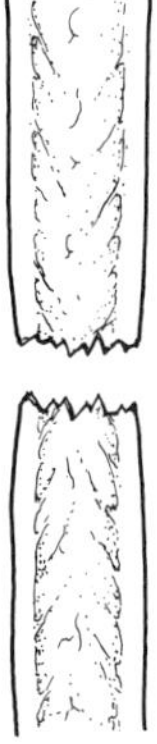

Malunion

Malunion of fractures should be prevented before it occurs. The wedging of long bone fractures in a plaster of Paris cast is a simple but effective technique. Provided there is no significant translation of the fracture fragments, angulation can be corrected quite easily within the first 2–4 weeks.

When callus formation is developing, the only way of altering fracture alignment is by applying external skeletal fixation. It is possible to distract the callus and correct alignment up to the time of fracture union. Thereafter it is necessary to break the callus in order to correct alignment, in which case it may be more satisfactory to allow full remodelling and then carry out a definitive corrective osteotomy.

Infection

The best treatment for infection of fractures is prevention. Correct management of open fractures, paying attention to both the soft tissues and the bone, can reduce the infection rate very considerably. Infection after open reduction and internal fixation is an ever-present hazard and the surgeon undertaking such treatment should be fully conversant with the techniques necessary to overcome such problems.

Primary infection occurs within a few weeks of operation or injury and should be treated along conventional lines by draining haematomas and abscesses, by high-dose intravenous antibiotics and by maintaining fracture stability.

Once infection becomes established it is necessary to remove all dead tissue, including bone that may be of structural importance. The sooner this is done, the sooner will the infection be overcome. If medullary or plate fixation is sound then the fixation should be left *in situ*. If the implants are loose they should be removed immediately at the same time as the sequestrectomy, and the limb stabilized with rigid external skeletal fixation.

When the wound is fully vascularized, reconstruction should be performed with either open cancellous bone grafting techniques or free vascularized tissue transfers. Treatment of bone infection is a complex problem and detailed texts should be consulted[14,15].

Acknowledgement

Illustrations 17, 24 and 26 were drawn by Peter Cox after G. Lyth.

References

1. Mathijsen A. Nouveau mode d'application du bandage au platre dans les fractures. *Archives belges de médecine Militaire*, 1852.

2. Jones R. An orthopaedic view of the treatment of fractures. *Am J Orthop Surg* 1913; 11: 314–35.

3. McKibbin B. The biology of fracture healing in long bones. *J Bone Joint Surg [Br]* 1978; 60-B: 150–62.

4. Danis R. *Theorie et pratique de l'osteosynthese*. Paris: Masson, 1949.

5. Schenk R, Willenegger H. Morphological findings in primary fracture healing. *Symposia Biologica Hungarica* 1967; 875: 75–86.

6. Kenwright J, Goodship AE. Controlled mechanical stimulation in the treatment of tibial fractures. *Clin Orthop* 1989; 241: 36–47.

7. Charnley J. *The closed treatment of common fractures*. 3rd ed. Edinburgh and London: Livingstone, 1970.

8. Sarmiento A, Latta L. *Closed functional treatment of fractures*. Berlin: Springer-Verlag, 1981.

9. Ackroyd CE, O'Conner BT, de Bruyn PF. *The severely injured limb*. London: Churchill Livingstone, 1983.

10. Müller ME, Allgöwer M, Schneider R, Willenegger H. *Manual of internal fixation*. 2nd ed. Berlin: Springer-Verlag, 1979.

11. Gustilo RB, Anderson JT. Prevention of infection in the treatment of one thousand and twenty five open fractures of long bones. *J Bone Joint Surg [Am]* 1976; 58-A: 453–8.

12. Gustilo RB, Mendoza RM, Williams DN. Problems in the management of type III (severe) open fractures: a new classification of type III open fractures. *J Trauma* 1984; 24: 742–6.

13. Langkamer VG, Ackroyd CE. Removal of forearm plates: a review of the complications. *J Bone Joint Surg [Br]* 1990; 72-B: 601–4.

14. Burri C. *Post-traumatic osteomyelitis*. Berne: Huber, 1975.

15. Weber BG, Cech O. *Pseudarthrosis: pathophysiology, biomechanics, therapy and results*. Berne: Huber, 1976.

Illustrations by Peter Cox after J. M. P. Booth

Traction treatment of fractures

John D. M. Stewart MA, FRCS
Consultant Orthopaedic Surgeon, Chichester District Health Authority, West Sussex, UK

Introduction

The correct management of a fracture entails reduction of the fracture, maintenance of that reduction and exercises, so that union of the fracture occurs in the best functional position as rapidly as possible, the development of joint stiffness is prevented or minimized and as much muscle power as possible is retained. In addition, demineralization of the skeleton is kept to a minimum, and the risk of pneumonia, venous thrombosis and renal calculi is decreased. Traction is often used to achieve these aims.

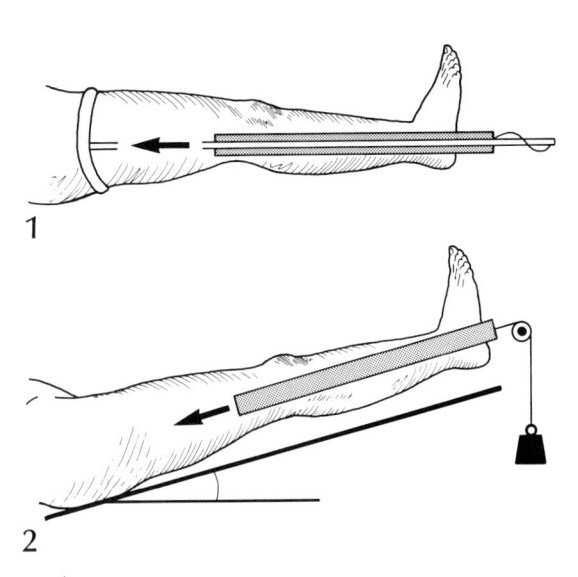

TRACTION

Traction helps to counteract the deforming forces acting upon a fracture and to control the amount and direction of movement which can occur at a fracture site, thus aiding the healing of bone and soft tissues.

To apply traction a satisfactory hold must be obtained on the affected part of the body. The traction force may be applied, in the case of a limb, through the skin – *skin traction* – or direct to the skeleton – *skeletal traction*.

1 & 2

When traction is applied, counter-traction, acting in the opposite direction, must be applied also to prevent the body from being pulled in the direction of the traction force. When counter-traction acts through an appliance which obtains purchase on a part of the body, the arrangement is called *fixed traction*. When the weight of all or part of the body, acting under the influence of gravity, is used to provide counter-traction, the arrangement is called *sliding traction*.

Fixed traction can maintain, but not obtain, the reduction of a fracture. Sliding traction can be used for both purposes, but as the initial traction weight required to obtain reduction of the fracture, in a sliding traction arrangement, is greater than that required to maintain the reduction, great care must be taken to avoid distraction of the fracture by keeping maintenance traction to a minimum.

124 Fracture treatment

SKIN TRACTION

Skin traction is used in preference to skeletal traction in the treatment of lower limb fractures in children, in adults when the traction force required is not great, and occasionally in the management of fractures of the upper limb.

To spread the load, the traction force is applied over a large area of skin distal to the fracture site, by using either adhesive or non-adhesive strapping. Skin traction frequently may need to be reapplied, especially if non-adhesive strapping is used.

Prepared Elastoplast skin traction kits for use in children or adults are available, or the necessary apparatus can be assembled. For patients who are allergic to adhesive strapping containing zinc oxide, other adhesive preparations can be used – Orthotrac, Seton Skin Traction Kit, Skin-Trac, or Tractac. Non-adhesive skin traction preparations are Notac Traction, Specialist Foam Traction, and Ventfoam Skin Traction Bandage. (For manufacturers' details see p. 144.)

Contraindications to skin traction

Contraindications to skin traction are abrasions or lacerations of the skin over the area to which the traction is to be applied; impairment of circulation – varicose ulcers, impending gangrene, or stasis dermatitis; and where there is marked overriding of the bony fragments which might indicate that the required traction force might need to be greater than can be applied through the skin.

Application of adhesive skin traction

3a–d

(a) The area of skin to which the strapping is to be applied is shaved (shaving is not required with Orthotrac, Skin-Trac or Tractac).
(b) The malleoli (or ulnar head and radial styloid process) are protected with a strip of felt, foam rubber or a few turns of bandage under the strapping.
(c) Starting at the ankle (or wrist) but leaving a loop projecting 5–15 cm (2–6 inches) beyond the distal end of the limb, the widest possible strapping is applied to both sides of the limb. For the lower limb it is placed parallel to a line between the lateral malleolus and the greater trochanter. On the lateral aspect, the strapping must lie slightly behind, and on the medial aspect slightly in front of, this line to encourage medial rotation of the limb. To ensure that it lies flat, there should not be any wrinkles or creases in the strapping; any that there are should be nicked. Bony prominences, such as the malleoli, tibial crest, patella, ulnar head, radial styloid process and humeral condyles, should be avoided.
(d) A crêpe or elasticated bandage is applied over the strapping, again starting at the ankle (or wrist). A spreader bar and cord are attached to the distal end of the strapping and the required traction weight added.

The maximum traction weight that can be used with adhesive skin traction is 6.7 kg (15 lb).

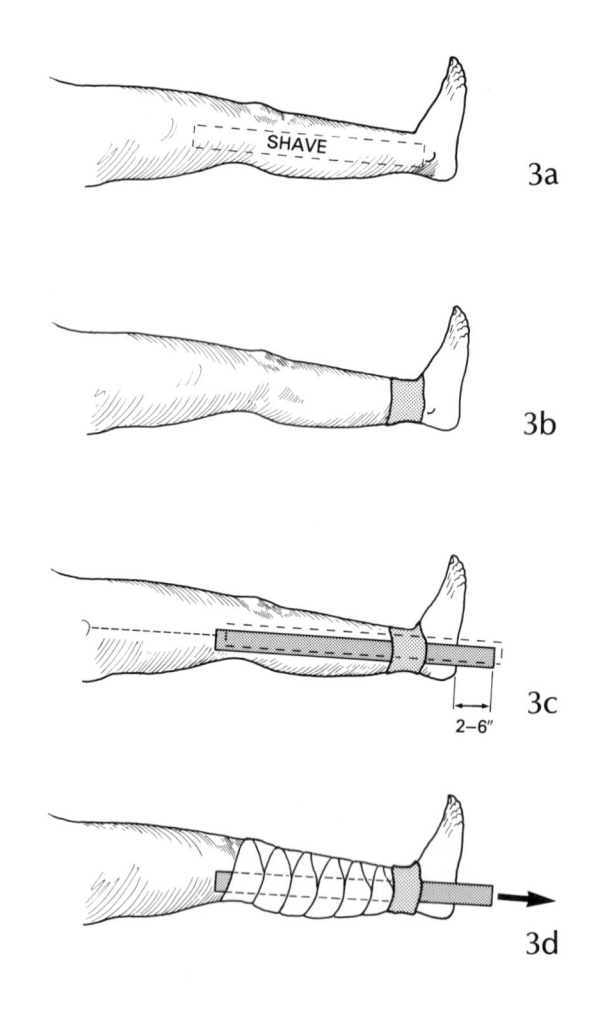

Application of non-adhesive skin traction

Non-adhesive skin traction is applied basically as described above. Shaving is not required. As the grip is less secure than that of adhesive strapping more frequent reapplication is likely to be necessary. The traction weight should not exceed 4.5 kg (10 lb).

Complications of skin traction

The complications of skin traction are allergic reaction to the adhesive; excoriation of the skin from wrinkling or slipping of the adhesive strapping; pressure sores over bony prominences and over the tendo Achillis; and palsy of the common peroneal nerve. This palsy may result from pressure on the nerve either by the strapping and encircling bandage if these are allowed to slide downwards until they are halted at the head of the fibula, or by the slings on which the limb rests, when lateral rotation of the lower limb is not prevented.

SKELETAL TRACTION

Skeletal traction is used chiefly in adults in the management of dislocation of the hip, certain fractures of the femur and tibia, in fractures and fracture-dislocations of the cervical spine (skull traction), and occasionally in fractures of the upper limb. Generally its use is avoided in children and when skin traction would be adequate.

In skeletal traction the traction force is applied directly to the skeleton. For a limb, a metal pin (Steinmann or Denham) or a wire (Kirschner) is driven through the bone.

Steinmann pin

4a & b

Steinmann pins[1] are rigid stainless steel pins of varying length, 4–6 mm in diameter. After insertion, either a special stirrup[2] (Böhler) or hooks with swivelling connections (Simonis) are attached, to allow the direction of pull to be varied without turning the pin in the bone.

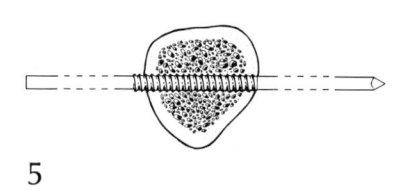

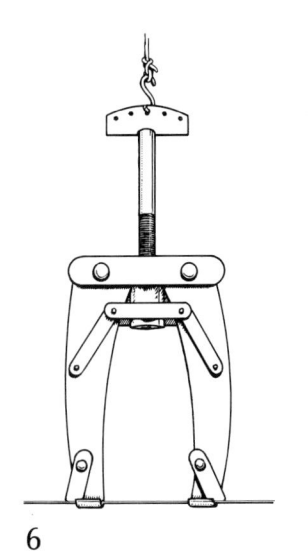

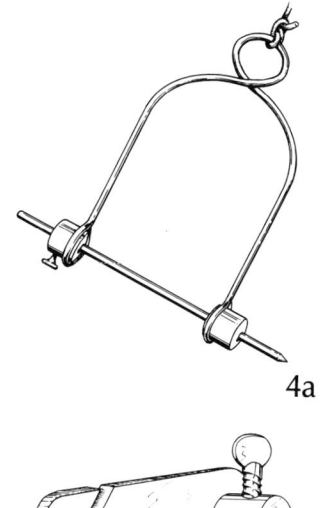

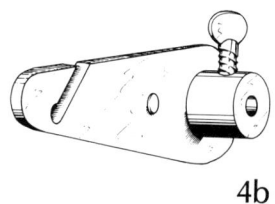

Denham pin

5

The Denham pin is identical to the Steinmann pin except for a short threaded length, situated towards the end held in the introducer, which engages the bony cortex and thus reduces the risk of the pin sliding in the bone. It is particularly suitable for use in the calcaneum or in osteoporotic bone.

Kirschner wire and special stirrup or strainer

6

A Kirschner wire[3] is of small diameter and is insufficiently rigid until pulled taut in a special stirrup[4]. The wire cuts easily out of bone if a heavy traction weight is applied, and rotation of the wire occurs with rotation of the stirrup. It can be used in the lower limb but is used more often in the upper limb.

Common sites for application of skeletal traction

Upper end of femur

7

At 2.5 cm (1 inch) below the most prominent part of the greater trochanter on the lateral surface of the femur, midway between the anterior and posterior surfaces.

Lower end of femur

8

Just proximal to the most superior bony protrusion of the lateral femoral condyle. Alternatively, a line is drawn from before backwards at the level of the upper pole of the patella and a second line is drawn from below upwards anterior to the head of the fibula; where these two lines intersect is the point of insertion. Care must be taken to avoid entering the knee joint.

To minimize knee stiffness, the metal pin at the lower end of the femur should be removed after 2–3 weeks and replaced by one through the upper end of the tibia.

Upper end of tibia

At 2 cm (¾ inch) behind the crest, just below the level of the tubercle of the tibia.

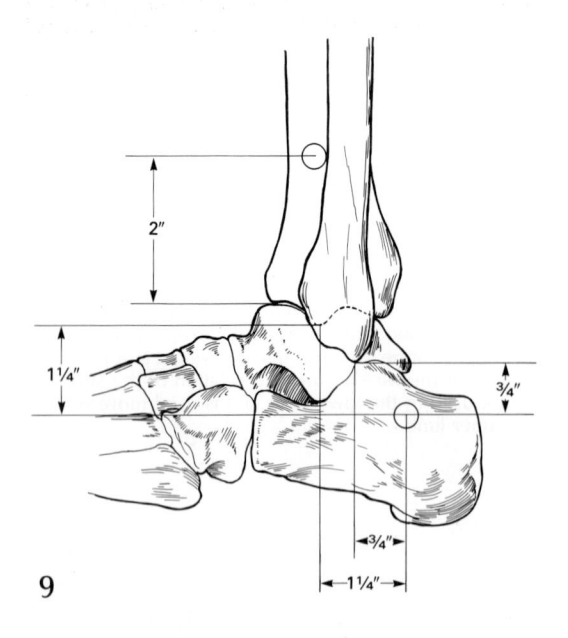

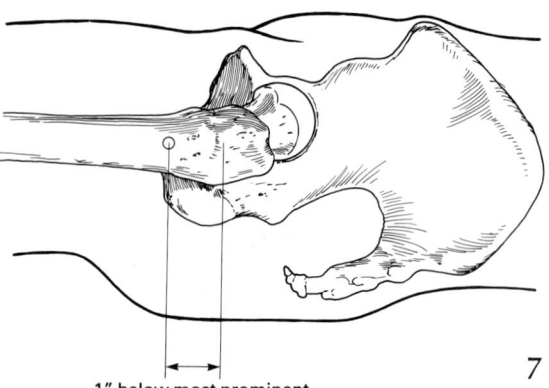

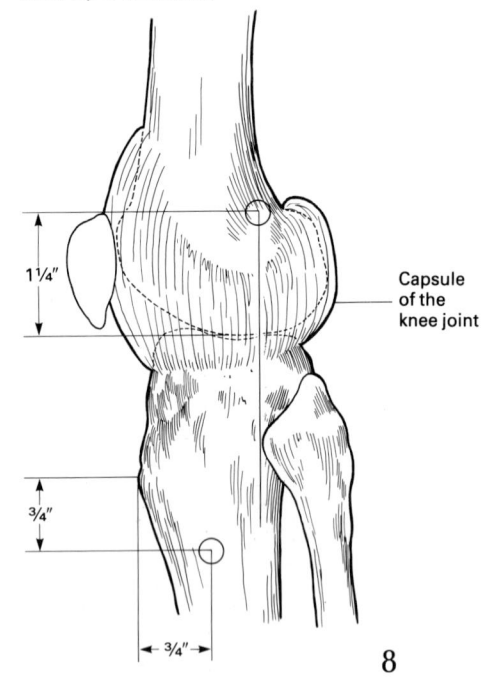

Lower end of tibia

9

At 5 cm (2 inches) above the level of the ankle joint, midway between the anterior and posterior borders of the tibia.

Calcaneum

At 2 cm (¾ inch) below and behind the lateral malleolus. This corresponds with a point 3 cm (1¼ inches) below and behind the medial malleolus.

Traction treatment of fractures 127

Olecranon

10

At 3 cm (1¼ inches) distal to the tip of the olecranon just deep to the subcutaneous border of the ulna. The Kirschner wire should be inserted from medial to lateral to avoid the ulnar nerve.

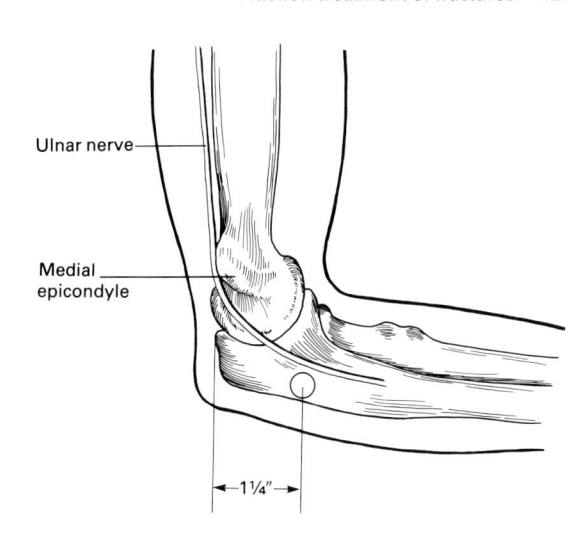

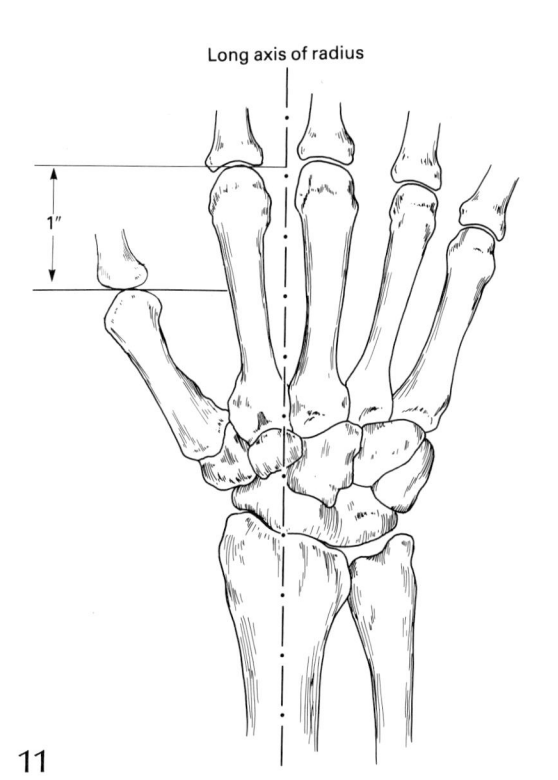

Second and third metacarpals

11

At 2.5 cm (1 inch) proximal to the distal end of the second metacarpal. The Kirschner wire passes through the second and third metacarpals at right angles to the longitudinal axis of the radius.

Insertion of a Steinmann pin in the lower limb

General or local anaesthesia is used; with the latter the skin and periosteum must be infiltrated. The skin is shaved locally and, using full aseptic precautions, is painted with iodine. Skin towels are draped under and around the limb.

12a

An assistant holds the limb in the same degree of lateral rotation as the normal limb, and with the ankle at a right angle. The correct rotational position is very important to avoid one end of the pin from impinging on the bed or splint and thus causing malrotation at the fracture site, or movement of the pin in the bone, and hence infection.

12b

The pin is mounted in the introducer and the site of insertion identified. The pin, held horizontally and at right angles to the long axis of the limb, is driven from lateral to medial, through the skin and the bone with a gentle twisting movement of the forearm, while keeping the elbow flexed against the side of the body. The surgeon must take care not to place his hand over the exit point of the pin. He should also ensure that the skin is not too tight around the pin.

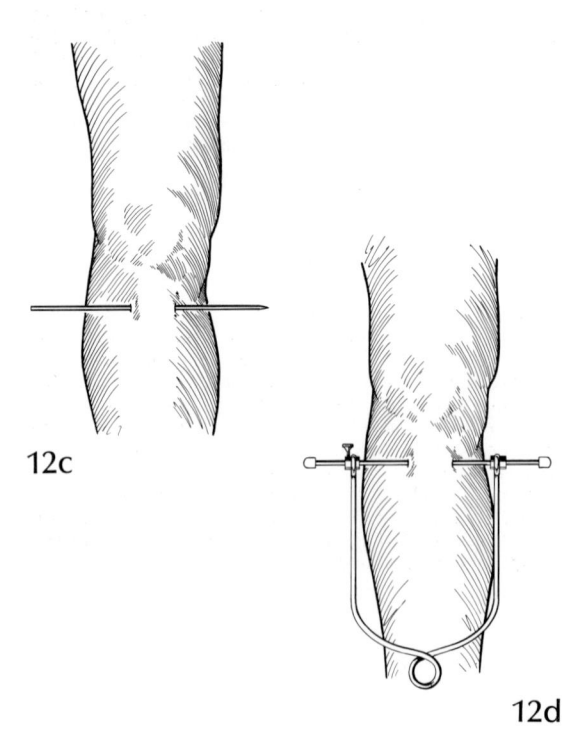

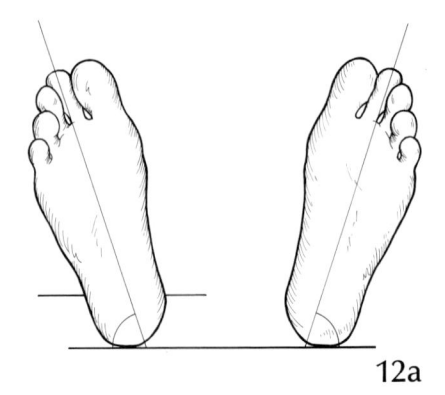

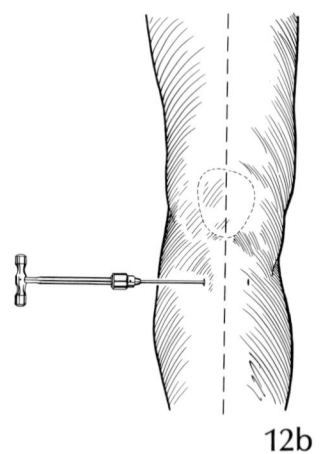

12c

A small cotton wool pad, soaked in benzoin tincture, is applied around the pin on each side to seal the wounds. Two separate pads should always be used. A strip of gauze wound back and forth across the shin and around the pins may cause a pressure sore.

12d

The Böhler stirrup is fitted and guards are applied over the ends of the pin.

Complications of skeletal traction

Infection

Unless full aseptic precautions are taken, infection can be introduced into the bone when the metal pin or wire is either inserted or removed. Infection can extend also along the pin tract from the skin wound. This is likely to occur if the skin does not encircle the pin closely or if the pin rotates or moves in and out of the bone.

Splintering or loosening

The bone may be splintered during the insertion of the pin. Rarely, the pin or wire may cut out of the bone. This is more likely to occur when the bone is porotic or a Kirschner wire is used.

Laxity or stiffness

Prolonged traction through a joint may cause ligamentous laxity. Stiffness of neighbouring joints can result either from the joint being entered during incorrect placing of the pin, or by the promotion of fibrosis in the muscles moving the joint.

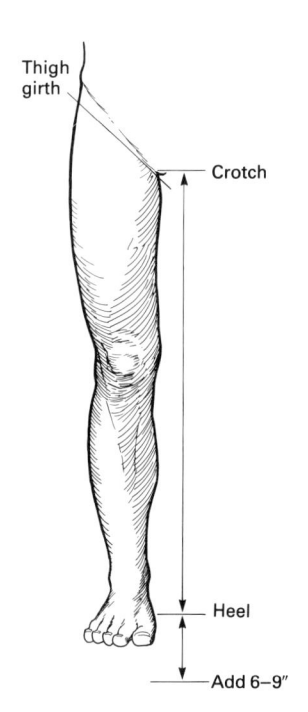

Damage to growth-plates

Damage may occur to epiphyseal growth-plates when skeletal traction is used in children. The late development of genu recurvatum can follow the treatment of a fracture of the femoral shaft with traction through the upper end of the tibia[5,6].

Delayed union

As a much greater traction force can be applied with skeletal traction, it is possible to distract the fracture, causing delay in union. It is better to allow 1.25 cm (½ inch) of overlap than to risk distraction.

SPLINTS

The Thomas' splint[7] is made in different sizes. It consists of a padded, leather-covered metal ring to which are attached two side-bars. These bars bisect the oval ring, are of unequal length so that the ring is set at an angle of 12° to the inner side-bar, and are joined together distally in the form of a W. The outer side-bar may be angled 5 cm (2 inches) below the ring, to clear a prominent greater trochanter.

How to choose a Thomas' splint

13

To obtain the *internal* circumference of the padded ring, the oblique circumference of the thigh is measured immediately below the gluteal fold and ischial tuberosity, in line with the inclination of the ring of the splint. This measurement must be accurate if fixed traction is intended. Accuracy is not so important with sliding traction. (This measurement can be taken from the uninjured limb to avoid causing pain, but one must remember to allow for swelling of the injured thigh.)

The distance from the crotch to the heel is measured and 15–23 cm (6–9 inches) is added to determine the length of the inner side-bar.

FISK SPLINT

14

In the Fisk splint[8], the groin ring, the front half of which is a padded strap and buckle, is attached by swivel joints to the side-bars, so that the same splint can be used for either limb. The distal ends of the side-bars are connected, just beyond the knee, by a squared-off frame which has a small eyelet at each upper corner. The knee-flexion piece is fixed to the side-bars, just proximal to the squared-off frame, through offset double-cog hinges. The side-bars of the thigh and knee-flexion parts of the splint are adjustable telescopically to allow all lengths of lower limb to be accommodated.

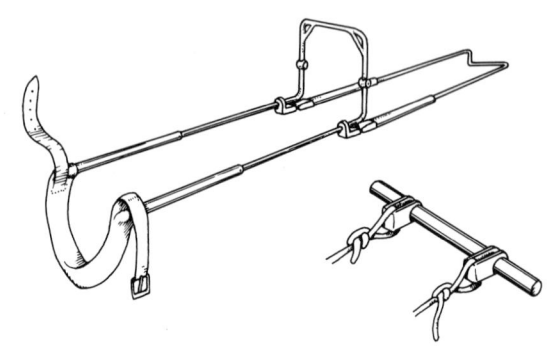

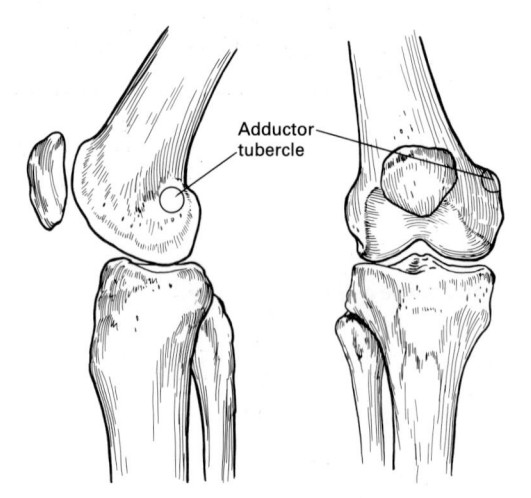

Knee hinge

15

When a knee-flexion piece in conjunction with a Thomas' splint or a Fisk splint is used, the hinge must lie level with the adductor tubercle of the femur, to coincide with the axis of movement of the knee joint.

Traction treatment of fractures 131

How to prepare a splint

16a

Slings are fashioned between the side-bars by taking several lengths of 15 cm (6 inches) wide Domette bandage and passing each around the inner side-bar, then passing the two ends over the outer side-bar and fastening to the lax sling so formed with two large safety pins. The slings must be lax initially: the tension can be adjusted easily to assist in the management of the fracture, but care must be taken to avoid excessive pressure on the skin and soft tissues, especially in the region of the neck of the fibula and tendo Achillis.

To prevent the slings sliding distally on the side-bars, they can be pinned to each other, or zinc oxide strapping can be applied around the side-bars under the slings. The distal sling must end at least 6 cm (2½ inches) above the back of the heel to avoid pressure sores developing over the tendo Achillis.

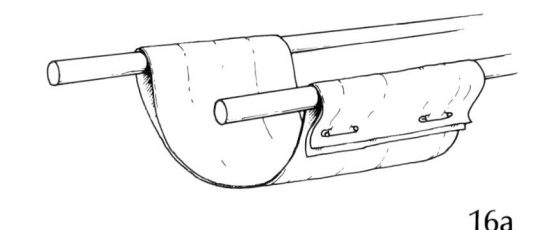

16b

The slings are lined with Gamgee tissue. One large pad, 15 × 23 cm (6 × 9 inches) and about 5 cm (2 inches) thick when compressed, is fashioned from Gamgee tissue and placed under the lower thigh to maintain the normal anterior bowing of the femoral shaft.

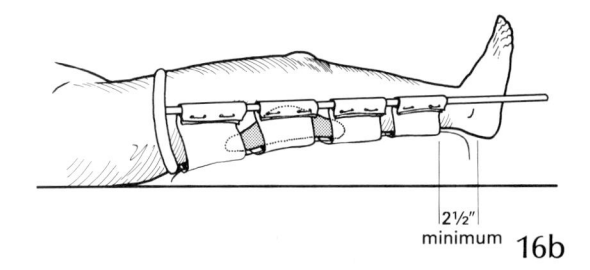

16c

To avoid leaving a triangular area of thigh unsupported proximally, the length of Domette bandage is passed around the ring of the splint and the side-bars. (Tubigrip, placed over the end of the splint, instead of individual slings, can be used to support that part of the limb which is not fractured.)

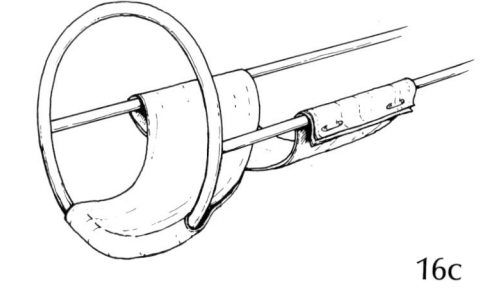

Prevention of equinus deformity at the ankle

When a lower limb is in traction there is a risk of an equinus deformity of the ankle developing unless active dorsiflexion of the ankle is carried out regularly. This risk can be reduced by clamping a footplate to the side-bars of a Thomas' splint; using a traction unit or Tulloch Brown traction; or using lengths of stockinette or elastic which pass around the sole of the foot.

132 Fracture treatment

Suspension of splints

Splints are suspended from an overhead frame by cords, running over pulleys, attached to weights. This increases the mobility of the patient, eases nursing and reduces the dangers of immobility – pressure sores, thrombosis and embolism, muscle wasting, joint stiffness, decalcification, pneumonia, renal stones and urinary infection.

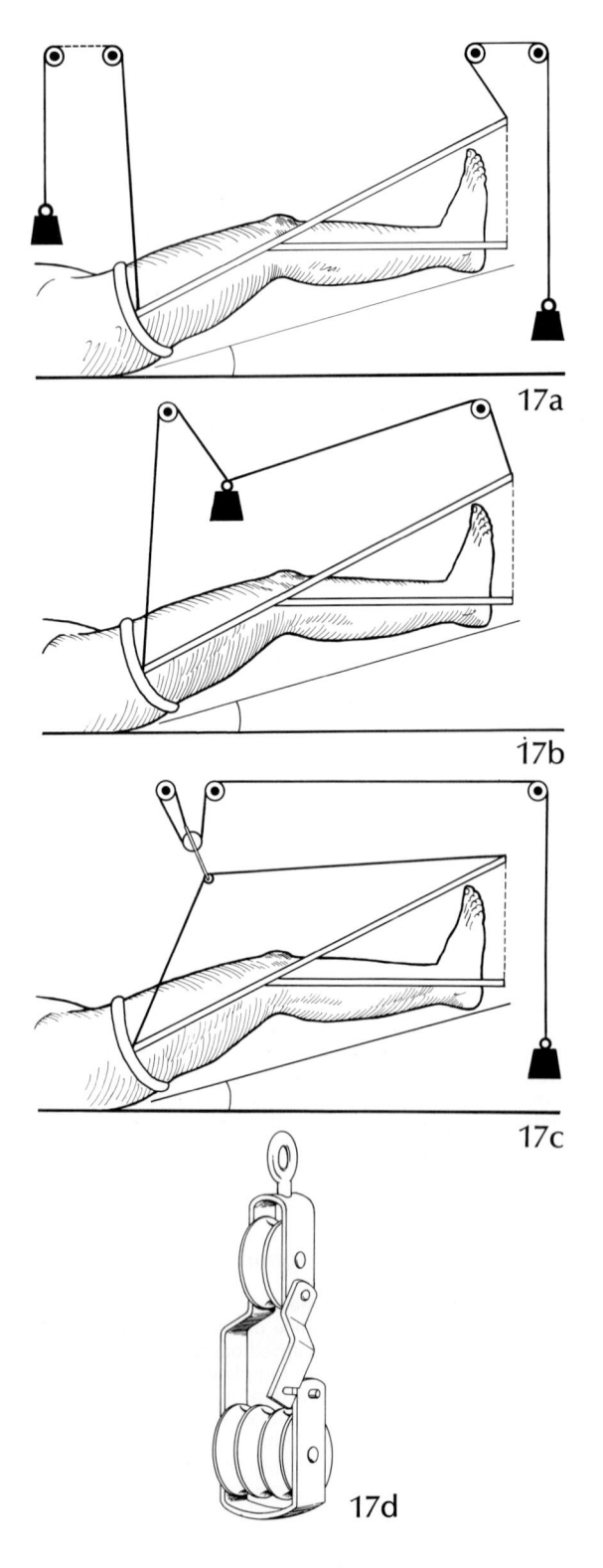

Methods of suspending a Thomas' splint

Method 1

17a

A small loop of cord is formed between the side-bars at each end of the splint and a suspension cord is tied to the centre of each loop. These pass up and cranially to two pulleys. From these pulleys the cords are passed over another two pulleys, situated at the foot or the head of the bed, and are then attached to weights.

Rotation of the splint is controlled by moving the point of attachment of the suspension cords to the proximal and distal loops on each end of the splint.

Method 2

17b

Two lengths of cord are tied, one on each side, to each end of the splint. Each cord is passed over two pulleys. A single suspension weight is attached firmly to both cords at a point nearer the pelvis, thus linking the two cords together.

Rotation of the splint is controlled by adjusting the length of one cord relative to the other.

Method 3

17c & d

Two lengths of cord, one on each side, are tied to each end of the splint. Both cords pass over the smaller wheels of a compound pulley block placed over the patient's thigh.

A further cord passes up from the ring on the compound pulley block, over a pulley on the overhead frame, down around the larger wheel of the pulley block then up around a second pulley on the overhead frame, before passing over a pulley at the foot of the bed to a weight.

Rotation of the splint is controlled by adjusting the length of one cord relative to that on the other side of the splint.

Suspension of a Fisk splint

18

The ends of a long loop of cord are tied to the eyelets at the corners of the squared-off frame. The loop is passed upwards and cranially over a pulley situated over the patient's abdomen so that when the hip is flexed to 45°, the cord is at right angles to the long axis of the femur. A single suspension weight of 1.8–3.6 kg (4–8 lb) is attached to the loop by a slip knot. This loop of cord must be long enough so that the suspension weight hangs within easy reach of the patient.

The distal end of the knee-flexion piece is suspended by a length of cord looped over the overhead frame. The length of this cord is such that when the hip is flexed 45°, the leg is horizontal.

After suspending the splint, the traction cord is checked to ensure that it is in line with the shaft of the femur when the hip is flexed 45°.

Rotation is controlled by varying the length of the cord attached to the knee-flexion piece and by varying the length of each arm of the loop attached to the squared-off frame.

In the Fisk splint the patient, as soon as possible, flexes his hip and at the same time flexes his knee and dorsiflexes his ankle, assisting the movement by pulling downwards on the suspension weight. He then actively extends his hip and knee and plantarflexes his ankle while gradually releasing the pull on the suspension weight. Passive movements are not encouraged.

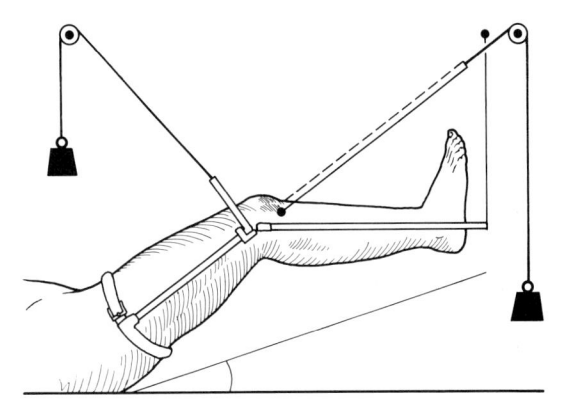

18

Traction weights

The exact traction weight required to reduce or hold the reduction of a fracture is determined by trial and observing the behaviour of the fracture, since it depends upon the site of the fracture, the age and weight of the patient, the power of his muscles, the amount of muscle damage, the degree of friction in the traction system and whether the traction weight is being used to reduce the fracture or only to maintain a reduction. For fractures of the femoral shaft an initial traction weight of 4.5–9.1 kg (10–20 lb) is usually sufficient for an average adult, and 1.0–4.5 kg (2–10 lb) for an average child. Proportionally lesser weights are used for fractures of the tibia. The heavier the traction weight used, the higher the foot of the bed must be raised to provide counter-traction.

TRACTION SYSTEMS FOR THE LOWER LIMB

BUCK'S TRACTION

Buck's traction[9] is used in the temporary management of fractures of the femoral neck in adults and of the femoral shaft in older and larger children. Lateral rotation of the limb is not controlled by this method.

Application of Buck's traction

19

Below-knee skin traction is applied. The leg is supported on a soft pillow to keep the heel clear of the bed. The cord is passed from the spreader over a pulley attached to the foot of the bed, and a weight of 2.4–3.2 kg (5–7 lb) is attached to the cord. The foot of the bed is elevated.

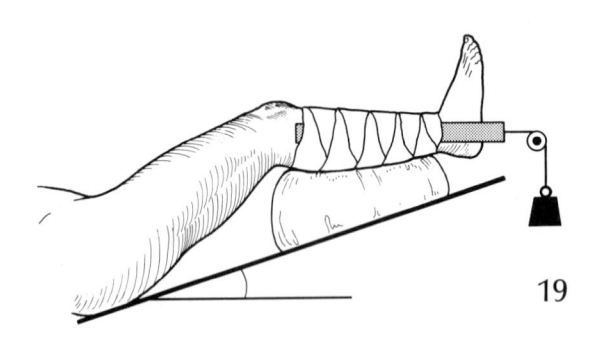

PERKINS' TRACTION

Perkins' traction[10] is used in the management of fractures of the tibia and of the femur from the subtrochanteric region distally in all age groups and of trochanteric fractures of the femur in patients under 45 years of age.

A Denham pin is inserted through the upper tibia for fractures of the femur, the mid-tibia or a point at least 2.5 cm (1 inch) below the lower limit of the associated haematoma for fractures of the condyles of the tibia, and the calcaneum for other fractures of the tibia. Early movement of the injured limb is encouraged.

A Hadfield split bed, in which the distal one third of the mattress and the base of the bed can be removed, is required in the management of a fracture of the femur, so that knee flexion can occur. An ordinary standard bed can be used for fractures of the tibia.

Application of Perkins' traction

A Denham pin is inserted at the selected site and a Simonis low-friction swivel attached to each end. Two traction cords are connected, one to each swivel. With the cords parallel they are passed over two separate pulleys fixed to the foot of the bed, where a weight is attached to each cord. For the average adult, two weights of 4.6 kg (10 lb) are required for fractures of the femur, and two of 2.3 kg (5 lb) for fractures of the tibia. For fractures of the femur, pillows are placed under the thigh to maintain the normal anterior bowing of the femur. The foot of the bed is elevated.

Anteroposterior and lateral radiographs are taken. Rotation of the limb is controlled by adjusting the height of one pulley.

For femoral fractures, active quadriceps exercises are started as soon as possible. After about one week, active knee flexion against resistance is commenced under the supervision of a physiotherapist, the injured limb being supported while the bed is split. For fractures of the tibia, ankle movements are started immediately and flexion of the knee as soon as possible.

Traction treatment of fractures 135

HAMILTON RUSSELL TRACTION

Hamilton Russell traction[11] can be used in the management of fractures of the shaft and trochanteric regions of the femur and after arthroplasty operations on the hip.

Application of Hamilton Russell traction

20

Below-knee skin traction is applied, with a pulley attached to the spreader. A soft broad canvas sling is *placed under the knee* NOT under the thigh. The limb is supported on two soft pillows, one above and the other below the knee, with the knee slightly flexed and the heel clear of the bed.

A length of cord is tied to the knee sling, and is then passed over pulley A, which is placed well *distal* (not proximal) to the knee, around one of the pulleys B, around pulley C, and then around the other pulley B before being attached to a weight. The pulleys B must be at the same level as the foot when the leg is lying horizontally on a pillow. The weight attached to the cord is generally of 3.6 kg (8 lb) for adults and 0.28–1.8 kg (0.5–4 lb) for children.

Theoretically the two pulley blocks B double the pull on the limb, but in practice the pull is modified by the friction present in the system. The resultant of the two forces acting along all the cords produces a pull in the line of the femoral shaft. In an alternative arrangement, two cords can be used, each cord passing over pulleys to separate weights.

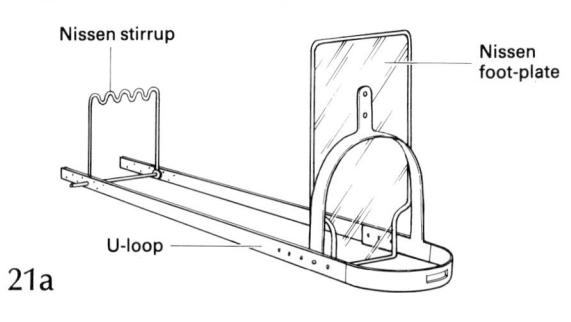

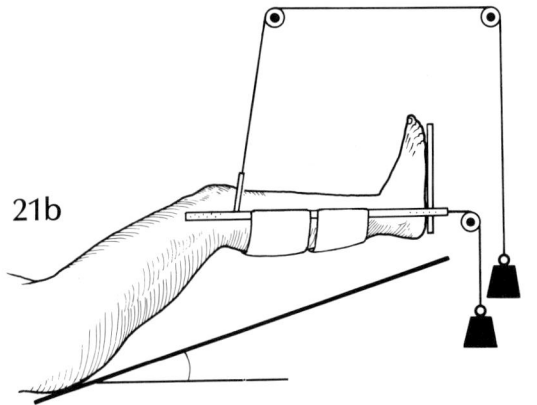

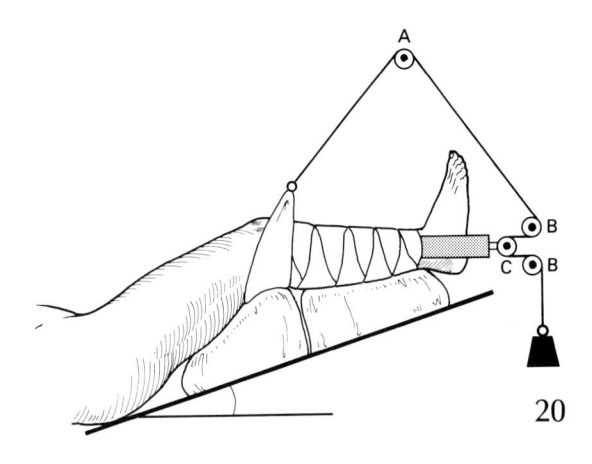

TULLOCH BROWN TRACTION

21a

Tulloch Brown traction, with a U-loop tibial pin and a Nissen foot-plate and stirrup, is used in the management of a fracture or fracture-dislocation of the hip, fracture of the shaft of the femur or after an arthroplasty or pseudarthrosis operation on the hip. It is not used in children.

Application of Tulloch Brown traction

21b

A Steinmann or Denham pin is inserted through the upper end of the tibia. The U-loop is slipped over the ends of the Steinmann pin, ensuring that it lies evenly on each side of the leg which is supported on slings from the U-loop. The slings, which are lined with Gamgee tissue, should not be tight as this leads to compression of the tissues of the calf.

The Nissen stirrup is hooked around collars attached to the Steinmann pin. The detachable Persplex foot-plate is mounted on the U-loop to support the foot. Two pulleys and cords with weights, or the Hamilton Russell system, are used for traction and suspension. The foot of the bed is elevated.

The correct rotation of the limb is obtained by varying the attachment of the cord to the Nissen stirrup.

NINETY-NINETY TRACTION

Ninety-ninety traction[12], in which the hip and knee joints are both flexed to 90°, is used in the management of compound fractures of the femur with wounds on the posterior aspect of the thigh, and in fractures of the proximal third of the shaft of the femur which cannot be controlled in a Thomas' splint. It can be used in the management of fractures in children as well as adults.

Skeletal traction is applied through the lower femur or upper tibia. In children, skin traction applied to the thigh can be used; if skeletal traction is used in children, great care must be taken to avoid injury to the epiphyseal growth-plates. Humberger and Eyring[13] reported on the use of 90/90 traction in the treatment of fractures of the shaft of the femur in children, with skeletal traction through the upper tibia. There was no evidence of injury to or growth disturbance of the proximal tibial epiphysis, nor of limitation of movement or instability of the knee, or cases of ischaemic contracture. However, children over 10 years of age or those who weighed over 45 kg (99 lb) did tend to develop pain in the knee after about 4 weeks in traction, and therefore its use is not recommended in such children.

Support of the leg in 90/90 traction

22a, b & c

There are three methods of supporting the leg in 90/90 traction: (a) Tulloch Brown U-loop with Nissen foot-plate; (b) a second Steinmann pin through the lower end of the tibia fitted with a Böhler stirrup; (c) a below-knee plaster cast which is well padded over the tendo Achillis and back of the heel and around the malleoli, and which incorporates the upper tibial Steinmann pin, if used.

A cord is attached to the end of the U-loop, Böhler stirrup or lower part of the cast, and passed vertically upwards over a pulley before being attached to a weight. The weight must be enough to keep the leg suspended with the knee flexed to 90°.

Application of 90/90 traction

The knee is flexed to 90° to allow the soft tissues to move into the position in which they will lie when the limb is in traction. Then, in adults, a Steinmann or Denham pin is inserted through the lower end of the femur, or alternatively in the upper tibia. In children, skin traction is applied to the thigh; if skeletal traction is required, a Kirschner wire can be inserted through the upper tibia, great care being taken to avoid injury to the epiphyseal growth-plate.

A Böhler stirrup is attached to the Steinmann pin, and the leg is supported with the hip and knee joints both flexed to 90°. From the stirrup a cord passes vertically upwards and over a pulley situated over the hip, and thence to a weight of 4.6–9.2 kg (10–20 lb) for the average adult. When unilateral 90/90 traction is used, the traction weight must not be so great as to lift the buttock on that side of the bed, otherwise valgus angulation can occur at the fracture site[14].

Rotation is controlled by the knee being flexed and by ensuring that the leg and thigh are in line when the patient is viewed from the foot of the bed.

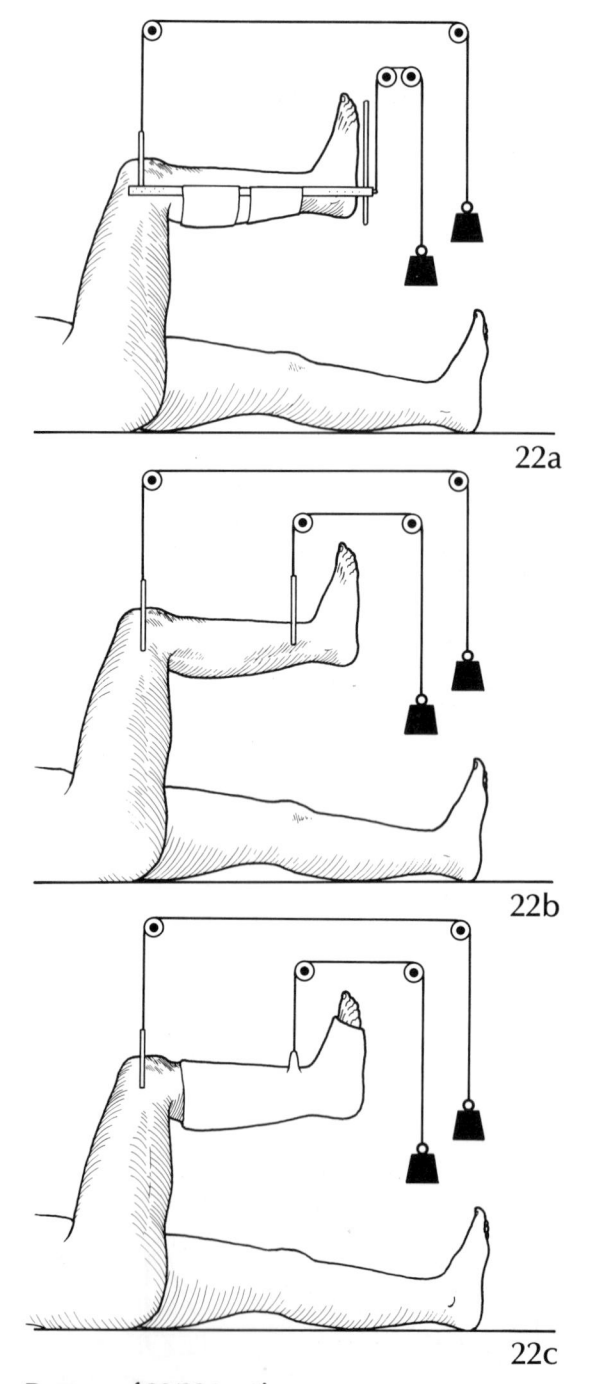

22a

22b

22c

Dangers of 90/90 traction

The dangers of 90/90 traction are those of skeletal traction (see p. 129): stiffness of and loss of extension of the knee, flexion contracture of the hip, neurovascular damage, and injury to epiphyseal growth-plates in children.

REDUCTION OF A FEMORAL SHAFT FRACTURE

Fixed traction in a Thomas' splint

Skin traction is used for children, and skeletal traction with an upper tibial Steinmann pin (Denham pin for the elderly) with a Böhler stirrup for adults.

The prepared splint is passed under the limb. The dorsalis pedis and posterior tibial pulses are palpated. The radiographs are studied to determine the type of fracture, and thus the subsequent procedure.

Transverse fractures

An assistant holds the Böhler stirrup and exerts traction in the long axis of the limb, simultaneously forcing the ring of the splint against the ischial tuberosity. The surgeon stands at the side of the limb, grips the limb above and below the fracture site and manipulates the fracture, reducing the distal fragment to the proximal fragment. Maintaining careful traction, he carefully lowers the limb onto the prepared splint, with the large pad under the lower part of the thigh, and then arranges the tension in the other slings to allow 15°–20° of flexion at the knee. Traction cords are attached to each end of the Steinmann pin and tied to the lower end of the splint. The pull on the Böhler stirrup is released.

Anteroposterior and lateral radiographs are taken to check the reduction of the fracture. If necessary the fracture is remanipulated. The pulses are palpated and if they are absent, the traction force is reduced. If the pulses do not return, the fracture should be remanipulated very gently. If the pulses are still absent arteriography and open exploration are required. If the pulses are present and the reduction is satisfactory, the Böhler stirrup is removed and the thigh is bandaged into the splint.

The splint is suspended and a 2.3 kg (5 lb) traction weight is attached to the end to reduce partly the pressure of the padded ring of the splint around the root of the limb.

Oblique, spiral or comminuted fractures

Formal manipulation of these fractures is not required. Traction is applied in the long axis of the limb until the fractured femur is restored to its correct length, and traction is maintained until the traction cords are tied to the lower end of the splint. Placement of the pad, radiography, palpation of peripheral pulses and suspension of the Thomas' splint are as described above.

Sliding traction with a Thomas' splint and Pearson knee-flexion piece

This method is often used to obtain and then maintain the reduction of a spiral, oblique or comminuted fracture of the shaft of the femur. Knee flexion controls rotation, prevents the development of laxity of the posterior capsule and cruciate ligaments of the knee, and allows variation in the direction of pull when an upper tibial Steinmann pin is used.

Application of sliding traction with a Thomas' splint and Pearson knee-flexion piece

23

The correct size of splint is chosen, and the splint and the knee-flexion piece are prepared. An upper tibial Steinmann pin is inserted. The prepared splint is passed under the limb, and the limb is rested on the slings. The large pad is placed under the lower part of the thigh.

The position of the hinge of the knee-flexion piece is checked to see that it is placed correctly opposite the adductor tubercle. The distal end of the knee-flexion piece is suspended from the distal end of the splint, by two cords, one on each side, so that the knee is flexed 20°–30°.

The splint is then suspended by the chosen method (p. 132). The position of the thigh pad and the tension in the sling supporting the pad are adjusted to obtain the normal anterior bowing of the femoral shaft. The thigh is bandaged into the splint.

A Böhler stirrup and cord are attached to the Steinmann pin. The cord is passed over a pulley at the foot of the bed so that the line of the cord is in line with the shaft of the femur. A weight is attached to the cord. The foot of the bed is elevated to provide counter-traction.

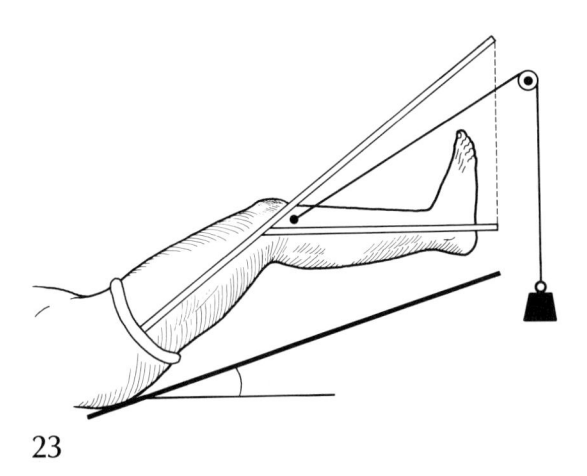

138 Fracture treatment

GALLOWS (BRYANT'S) TRACTION

24

Gallows or Bryant's traction[15] is convenient and reasonably safe for the treatment of fractures of the shaft of the femur in children up to the age of 2 years. Vascular complications may occur in either the injured or the normal limb. These are more likely to occur between the ages of 2 and 4 years[16, 17], but their occurrence is less likely if posterior gutter splints are applied to keep the knees in slight flexion. *Over the age of 4 years the use of gallows traction is absolutely contraindicated.* The cause of vascular complications is the reduction in the blood pressure in the lower limbs which occurs with elevation[18].

Application of gallows traction

Adhesive skin traction is applied to *both* lower limbs. The traction cords are tied to an overhead beam and are tightened sufficiently to raise the child's buttocks just clear of the mattress.

The state of the circulation in the limbs should be checked frequently because of the dangers of vascular complications. Observe the colour and temperature of *both feet*. Dorsiflex *both ankles* passively. *Dorsiflexion should be full and painless*. If dorsiflexion is limited or painful, muscle ischaemia may be present; the limbs should therefore be lowered and all bandages and adhesive strapping removed immediately.

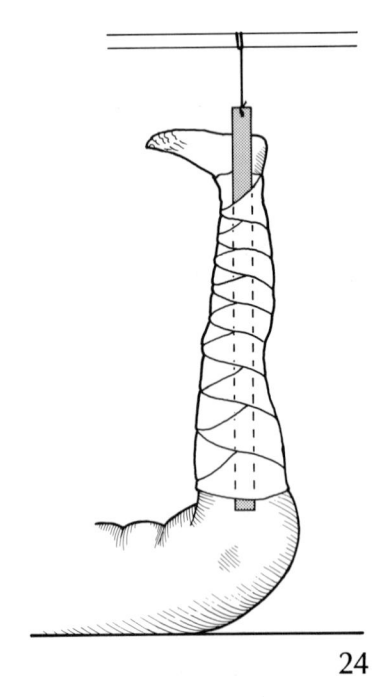

24

SLIDING TRACTION WITH A BÖHLER–BRAUN FRAME

Sliding traction with a Böhler–Braun frame can be used for the management of unstable fractures of the tibia. Skeletal traction is commonly used.

Application of sliding traction with a Böhler–Braun frame

25

Slings are fashioned between the sides of the frame to support the thigh and leg. The slings are covered with Gamgee tissue.

A Steinmann or Denham pin is inserted where necessary. Frequently an above-knee, well-padded plaster cast is applied, incorporating the pin when a tibial fracture is being treated. A Böhler stirrup is attached to the pin.

The limb is placed on the slings. A cord is attached to the stirrup, passed over the required pulley, and a 3.2–4.5 kg (7–10 lb) weight is attached. The foot of the bed is then elevated.

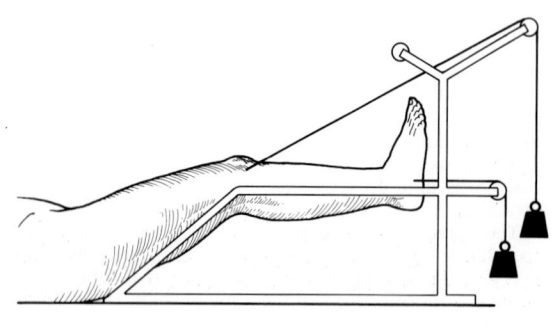

25

LATERAL TRACTION THROUGH UPPER END OF FEMUR

26a

In central fracture-dislocations of the hip, skeletal traction in the long axis of the femur (Tulloch Brown traction) may be coupled with lateral traction through the upper end of the femur to restore the relationship between the dome of the acetabulum and the weight-bearing portion of the femoral head.

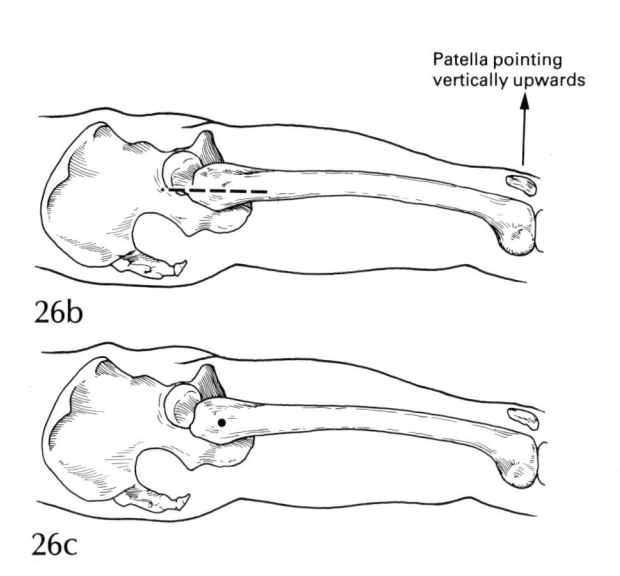

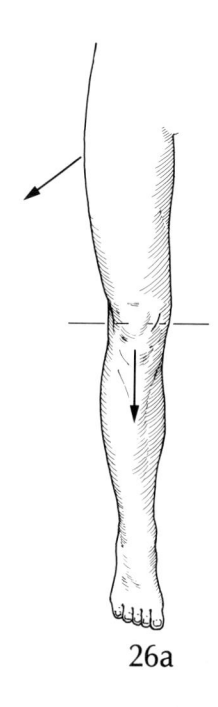

Application of lateral traction

26b & c

A small longitudinal incision is made, centred just below the most prominent part of the greater trochanter on the affected side, and is then deepened down to bone. The point on the lateral surface of the femur 2.5 cm (1 inch) below the most prominent part of the greater trochanter, mid-way between the anterior and posterior surfaces of the femur, is identified.

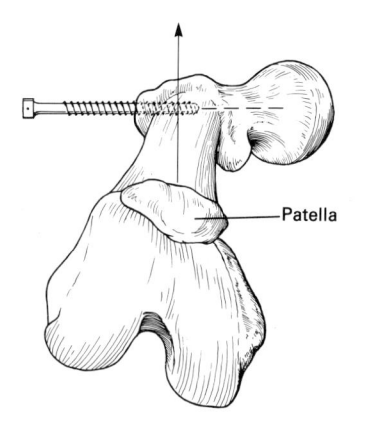

26d

An assistant is asked to rotate the lower limb medially so that the patella points vertically upwards. This eliminates the normal forward angulation (anteversion) of the femoral neck and ensures that the femoral neck is lying horizontally.

26e

A hole is drilled in the lateral cortex of the femur, using the correct size of drill for the coarse-threaded screw or bolt.

A finger is placed on the femoral artery at the groin (this point lies over the head of the femur).

The drill is held horizontally and directed cranially and medially towards the finger on the femoral artery. The drill will thus be directed up the neck of the femur. A hole 3.75–5 cm (1½–2 inches) deep is then drilled, the drill removed and the coarse-threaded screw or bolt, 7.5–10 cm (3–4 inches) long, is inserted.

26f

A length of stainless steel wire is attached to the end of the screw or bolt, and brought out through the wound, which is then sutured. A cord is attached to the stainless steel wire and passed over a pulley at the side of the bed to a traction weight of 3.6–6.7 kg (3–15 lb).

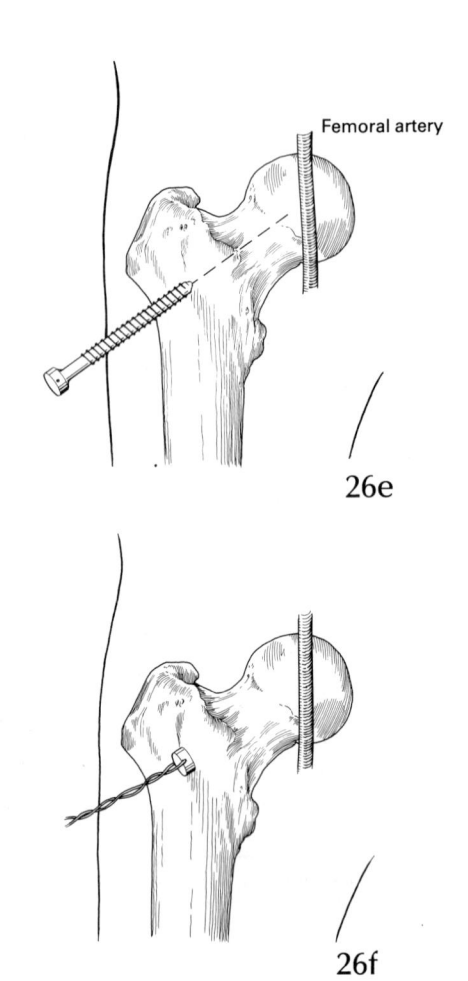

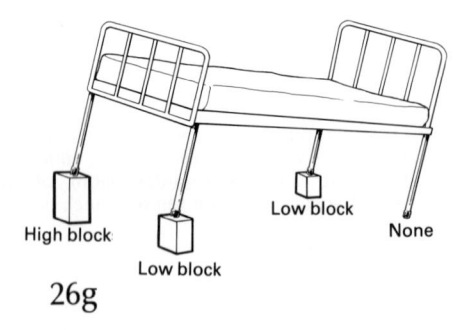

26g

The patient's bed is arranged to tilt in two planes, the foot of the bed being highest on the affected side and the head of the bed being lowest on the unaffected side. This is achieved by using three wooden blocks of two different heights.

Lateral traction is continued for 3–4 weeks and Tulloch Brown traction for a total of 8–10 weeks. Active movement of the hip and knee is encouraged.

As an alternative to a screw or bolt, a Denham pin can be inserted through the greater trochanter in an anteroposterior direction with some lateral inclination. The disadvantages of this method are that infection of the pin tract is likely to occur, and the posterior end of the pin sticks into the mattress, making it uncomfortable for the patient.

TRACTION SYSTEMS FOR THE UPPER LIMB

DUNLOP TRACTION

Dunlop traction[19] is used in the management of supracondylar and transcondylar fractures of the humerus in children, and gives the best results when the distal fragment is displaced posterolaterally[20]. It is especially useful if flexion of the elbow causes loss of the radial pulse.

Application of Dunlop traction

27

With the patient supine, skin traction is applied to the forearm. The shoulder is abducted 45°, and with the elbow flexed also about 45°, the traction cord is passed over a pulley. A padded sling is passed over the upper arm.

Weights are attached both to the padded sling and the traction cord, and the upper arm must be just clear of the bed. The weights required will depend upon the size of the child but often 0.5–1.0 kg (1–2 lb) will be enough initially. The side of the bed on the affected side is elevated.

The weights are increased daily under radiographic control until a satisfactory reduction is obtained.

Check on the circulation

The circulation in the limb is checked *hourly* during the first 12 hours and then twice daily while the traction weight is being increased.

It is *more* important to check that full painless active and passive extension of the fingers is present and that sensation in the fingers is normal than whether the radial pulse is present. Ischaemia of the forearm muscles can occur even in the presence of a radial pulse. If ischaemia is present, active extension of the fingers will be absent and passive extension will be painful.

When ischaemia is suspected, traction should be discontinued. It is better to risk malunion of the fracture rather than Volkmann's ischaemic contracture of the forearm. If circulatory embarrassment is not relieved by discontinuing traction, the fracture should be gently manipulated before exploring the brachial artery or carrying out a fasciotomy of the forearm.

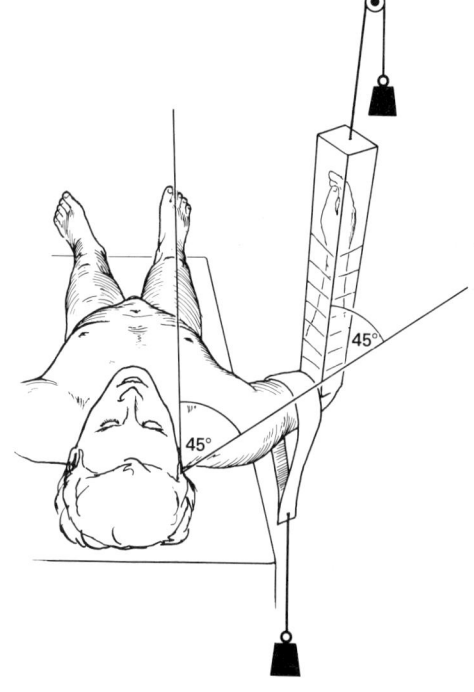

142 Fracture treatment

OLECRANON TRACTION

Olecranon traction is used in the management of supracondylar and comminuted fractures of the lower end of the humerus, and unstable fractures of the shaft of the humerus in adults.

Application of olecranon traction

28a

With the forearm supported across the patient's chest, the upper arm elevated and the elbow flexed to 90°, a Kirschner wire is inserted deep to the subcutaneous border of the upper end of the ulna, 3.0 cm (1¼ inches) distal to the tip of the olecranon, in a medial to lateral direction, taking care to avoid the ulnar nerve. A Kirschner wire strainer and traction cord are attached.

With the shoulder abducted a few degrees, and the upper arm lying horizontally the traction cord is passed distally to a pulley at the foot of the bed. A weight of 1.3–1.8 kg (3–4 lb) is attached.

Two cords, tied one to each end of the Kirschner wire, are passed vertically upwards over two pulleys placed above the elbow on an overhead frame, and attached to weights of 0.5–1.0 kg (1–2 lb). Soft loops are fashioned between these cords to support the forearm.

The weights are adjusted until satisfactory alignment of the fracture is obtained. The patient must exercise his fingers and wrist fully every hour. A daily check must be kept on the circulation, sensation and movement of the fingers.

Rotation at the fracture site is controlled by moving the pulleys over which the cords from each end of the Kirschner wire pass. Medial rotation is obtained by moving the pulleys towards the patient and lateral rotation by moving them away from the patient.

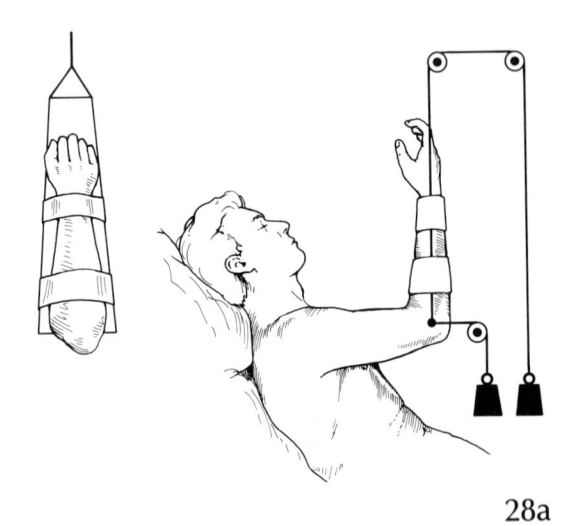

28a

28b

A screw eye can be used instead of a Kirschner wire, but support of the forearm requires the application of skin traction. Through a 1.25 cm (½ inch) incision over the subcutaneous surface of the olecranon placed at 3.0 cm (1¼ inch) distal to the tip of the olecranon, a 3.0 mm (⅛ inch) hole is drilled into which the screw eye is inserted.

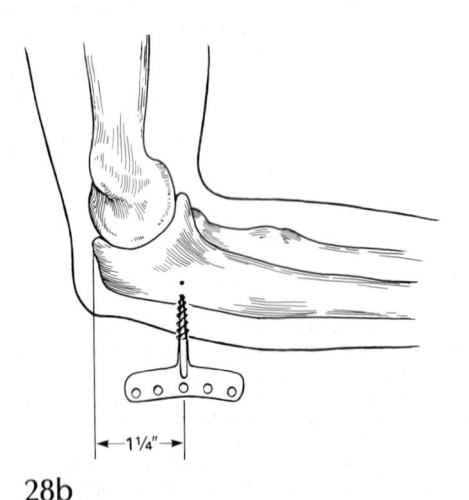

28b

METACARPAL PIN TRACTION

Traction through the second and third metacarpal bones is used in the management of comminuted fractures of the bones of the forearm, especially those of the lower end of the radius.

Application of metacarpal pin traction

29a & b

The hand is squeezed to increase the transverse metacarpal arch. This exposes the distal ends of the second and third metacarpals, as the fourth and fifth metacarpals are relatively more mobile.

A Kirschner wire is inserted from the radial to the ulnar side through the distal ends of the second and third metacarpals 1.25 cm (1 inch) proximal to the end of the second metacarpal, at right angles to the long axis of the radius. The metacarpophalangeal joints must be avoided. A Kirschner wire strainer and traction cord are attached.

The cord passes vertically upwards over a pulley and is tied to a weight. An initial weight of 1.3–1.8 kg (3–4 lb) is used. The weights are adjusted until a satisfactory reduction is obtained. A sling, to which a weight can be attached, is passed over the upper arm to provide counter-traction.

Although movement of the fingers is difficult, the patient must exercise his fingers regularly as much as possible. Once a satisfactory reduction has been obtained, the Kirschner wire can be incorporated in an above-elbow plaster cast. To reduce the risk of permanent stiffness of the fingers from fibrosis in the interosseous muscles, the Kirschner wire must be removed as soon as the fracture is stable.

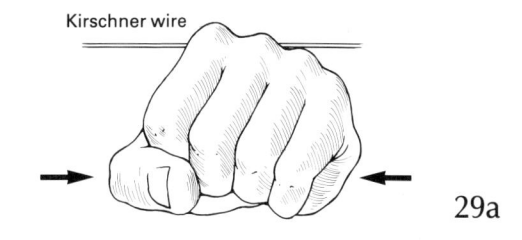

Management of patients in traction

Patients in traction and traction-suspension systems do not look after themselves. Successful management depends upon the continuing interest and care of medical, nursing, physiotherapy and other paramedical staff[21]. Everyone must be aware of potential problems and complications to ensure that none develop.

The patient generally, as well as the injured limb and the traction-suspension system, must be examined morning and evening, and after each period of physiotherapy and radiographic examination.

Injured limb

Pain may arise from pressure sores on the sacrum, groin, ankle, or under strapping, or from infection of the pin tract or compound fracture.
Paraesthesiae result from impairment of normal nerve function, from ischaemia, pressure or excessive traction.
Swelling may be due to lack of exercise, a bandage which is too tight or deep vein thrombosis.
Skin irritation may arise from allergy to adhesive strapping.
Weakness may result from impaired nerve function, from disuse or muscular atrophy.
Painful limitation of joint movement results from ischaemia of muscles, or if not painful, from lack of exercise or joint contractures.

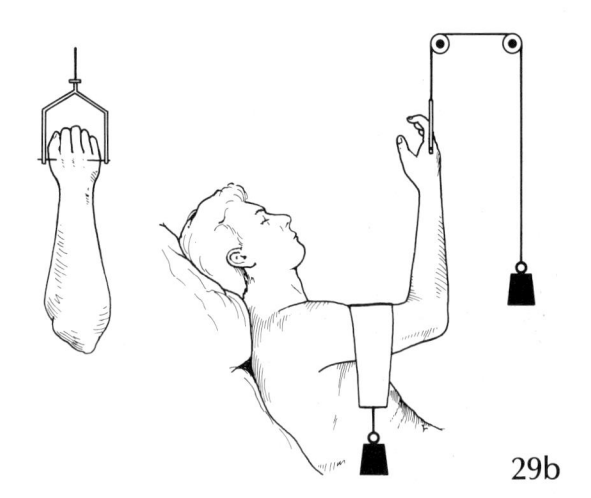

It is better to lose the position of the fracture than to allow serious complications to develop.

Traction-suspension system

The following must be checked:

1. Overhead frame securely fastened to the bed.
2. Bed elevated as necessary to provide counter-traction.
3. Splint, sling or pad correctly sited.
4. Skin traction not wrinkled or sliding down the limb.
5. Pin immobile in bone and infection absent.
6. Stirrup moving freely on its pin.
7. Cords not frayed and running freely on pulleys.
8. Weights hanging freely and not directly over the patient.

Radiographic examination

Radiography is generally advisable two or three times in the first week while adjustments are being made to the traction, then weekly for the next three weeks, followed by monthly examinations until union occurs. A radiograph should also be taken after each manipulation of the fracture or change in the traction weight.

Removal of traction

Traction is continued until either the fracture is stable (that is until any deformity which can be provoked at the fracture site disappears when the deforming force is removed) or an alternative method of supporting the fracture is substituted until union occurs.

For adults, a rough guide on the duration of fraction is shown in Table 1.

Table 1 Duration of traction

Fracture	Traction
Elbow fracture with olecranon pin	3 weeks
Tibial fracture with calcaneal pin	3–6 weeks
Trochanteric fracture of femur	6 weeks
Femoral shaft fracture	12 weeks

Table 2 Proprietary products

Proprietary products	Manufacturer
Domette Bandage Gamgee Tissue*	Robert Bailey & Son Ltd, Great Moor, Cheshire, UK
Elastoplast	Smith & Nephew, Welwyn Garden City, UK
Notac Traction Seton Skin Traction Kit	Seton Products Ltd, Oldham, Lancashire, UK
Orthotrac	Biomet Ltd, Bridgend, South Glamorgan, UK
Skin-Trac	Zimmer Inc, Warsaw, Indiana, USA
Specialist Foam Traction Tractac	Johnson & Johnson Ltd, Slough, Berkshire, UK
Tubigrip	Seton Products Ltd, Oldham, UK
Ventfoam Skin Traction Bandage	The Scholl Manufacturing Co Ltd, London, UK

(* Sampson Gamgee: British Surgeon 1828–1886. A surgical dressing consisting of a thick layer of absorbent cotton between two layers of absorbent gauze).

References

1. Steinmann F. Die Nagelextension. *Ergeb Chir Orthop* 1916; 9: 520–60.
2. Böhler L. *The treatment of fractures,* English translation by Steinberg ME. Vienna: Maudrich, 1929: 38, 39, Fig. 56.
3. Kirschner M von. Ueber Nagelextension. *Beitr Klin Chir* 1909; 64: 266–79.
4. Kirschner M von. Verebesserungen Der Drahtextension. *Arch Klin Chir* 1927; 148: 651–8.
5. Bjerkreim I, Benum P. Genu recurvatum: a late complication of tibial wire traction in fractures of the femur in children. *Acta Orthop Scand* 1975; 46: 1012–9.
6. Van Meter JW, Branick RI. Bilateral genu recurvatum after skeletal traction: a case report. *J Bone Joint Surg [Am]* 1980; 62-A: 837–9.
7. Thomas HO. *Diseases of the hip, knee and ankle joints, with their deformities, treated by a new and efficient method,* 2nd ed. Liverpool: Dobb, 1876: 98, Plate 13, Fig. 4.
8. Fisk GR. The fractured femoral shaft: new approach to the problem. *Lancet* 1944; i: 659–61.
9. Buck G. An improved method of treating fractures of the thigh illustrated by cases and a drawing. *Trans NY Acad Med* 1861; 2: 232–50.
10. Perkins G. *The ruminations of an orthopaedic surgeon.* London: Butterworth, 1970.
11. Russell RH. Fracture of the femur: a clinical study. *Br J Surg* 1924; 11: 491–502.
12. Obletz BE. Vertical traction in the early management of certain compound fractures of the femur. *J Bone Joint Surg* 1946; 24: 113–6.
13. Humberger FW, Eyring EJ. Proximal tibial 90–90 traction in treatment of children with femoral shaft fractures. *J Bone Joint Surg [Am]* 1969; 51-A: 499–504.
14. Brooker AF, Schmeisser G. *Orthopaedic traction manual.* Baltimore: Williams & Wilkins, 1980.
15. Bryant T. On the value of parallelism of the lower extremities in the treatment of hip disease and hip injuries, with the best means of obtaining it. *Lancet* 1880; i: 159–60.
16. Thomson SA, Mahoney LJ. Volkmann's ischaemic contracture and its relationship to fractures of the femur. *J Bone Joint Surg [Br]* 1951; 33-B: 336–47.
17. Miller DS, Markin L, Grossman E. Ischaemic fibrosis of lower extremity in children. *Am J Surg* 1952; 84: 317–22.
18. Nicholson JT, Foster RM, Heath RD. Bryant's traction: a provocative cause of circulatory complications. *JAMA* 1955; 157: 415–8.
19. Dunlop J. Transcondylar fractures of the humerus in childhood. *J Bone Joint Surg* 1939; 21: 59–73.
20. Prietto CA. Supracondylar fractures of the humerus: a comparative study of Dunlop's traction versus percutaneous pinning. *J Bone Joint Surg [Am]* 1979; 61-A: 425–8.
21. Stewart JDM, Hallett JP. *Traction and orthopaedic appliances.* 2nd ed. Edinburgh: Churchill Livingstone, 1983: 105–17.

Illustrations by Gillian Oliver

External skeletal fixation

J. Kenwright FRCS
Consultant Orthopaedic Surgeon, The Nuffield Orthopaedic Centre, Oxford, UK

Introduction

There have been major increases in the frequency of use of external skeletal fixation over the last ten years for several reasons.

Advances in soft tissue plastic reconstructive surgery have led to a need for stabilization of the skeleton in a manner which can only be supplied by external fixation. Similar advances in bone reconstructive surgery for infected non–union and for traumatic bone loss require prolonged stabilization of the skeleton, and external skeletal fixation has been found to be most effective for this purpose.

Fracture instability treated by internal fixation is associated with a significant incidence of wound and fracture infection; the use of external skeletal fixation instead of internal fixation reduces the incidence of such problems. Frame and screw technology has improved so that most fractures can now be stabilized with external skeletal fixation even if they are very comminuted or juxta–articular; fixation of pelvic fractures and small bone fractures is also possible. The incidence of serious screw–tract complications has been reduced.

Indications

The main indications are as follows.

1. Diaphyseal fractures with associated soft tissue injury (Grade 2 or 3).
2. Unstable diaphyseal fractures with overlying contused skin, making internal fixation risky.
3. Multiple trauma: stabilization of multiple fractures of the limbs reduces the risk of acute respiratory distress syndrome; this situation is a very strong indication for the use of external skeletal fixation in the early hours after injury. Such stabilization also allows early function of adjacent joints.
4. Stabilization of diaphyseal fractures after decompression of compartment syndrome, or after repair of neurovascular structures.
5. Acute bone loss in diaphyseal fractures.
6. Infected non-union after uncompromising excision of dead bone: external fixation is strongly indicated here, whichever method of bone reconstruction – cortico-cancellous bone graft, free vascularized graft, or bone transport.

Other specialized uses of external skeletal fixation include arthrodesis, leg lengthening and spinal stabilization.

Choice of frame

There are many types of frame available and most will allow stabilization of diaphyseal fractures of the tibia. Specialized frames are needed for the treatment of pelvic fractures, juxta-articular fractures, fractures of the forearm, and short bone fractures within the foot or hand.

In planning treatment it is important to assess the mechanical demands to be placed upon the fixation system in order to know whether the frame available can deal with the given situation with improvisation or whether a special frame is needed.

Application of external skeletal fixation

The same principles of meticulous application apply to external skeletal fixation as to internal fixation of fractures.

It is important to pre-plan screw insertion so that a screw does not tent the skin edge at the site of the incision. The screw should be close to the centre of the bone so as to achieve sound mechanical fixation and must pass completely through both cortices.

Neurological and vascular injuries are common and the anatomical structures adjacent to the screw hole need to be considered at every screw entry and the safe corridor chosen[1,2]; frequently it is safest to make an open exposure to protect nerves and this applies particularly in the arm.

Sufficient screws need to be inserted to give stability; from the mechanical viewpoint, greater stability is gained if the screws are widely spread and the frame-to-bone distance is minimized. However, the frame should be attached to allow for the considerable oedema which very often follows open fractures.

Frames should be applied so that secondary wound surgery and dressings are not obstructed. If there is an open wound associated with the fracture, maximum effort should be made at the initial surgery to achieve fracture reduction through the wound.

Postoperative management

Stability of the fracture is not usually a problem with modern frames and appropriate application technique. The frame should be checked for stability and tightness of the clamps at every clinic visit.

Screw-tract problems are very common. The screw holes should be inspected to see there is no skin tenting for different positions of function; if tenting is seen, a small incision should be made under local anaesthetic to allow freedom. Erythema around screw holes frequently settles with rest alone. If there are other physical signs of infection, rest is needed, together with antibiotic therapy. If there are persistent signs of infection and the screw is frankly loose, it should be replaced at a distance of at least 2 cm. Osteomyelitis after screw removal is rare; if infection persists after removal, the tract should be curetted thoroughly.

Post-fixation fracture through screw holes is a risk but the incidence is low. Screw breakage is seen rarely with modern equipment.

Rehabilitation programme

Firm rehabilitation is usually needed whilst the frame is on to avoid the risk of development of joint deformity and to re-educate muscle function. Equinus deformity of the foot can develop in an insidious manner: if the patient is unable to dorsiflex the foot, a temporary splint should be used immediately.

Removal of the frame

As a general principle, frames should be removed as soon as possible and when the soft tissues are stable. There is controversy concerning the time of removal for tibial diaphyseal fractures, and many surgeons advocate retaining the frame until fracture healing occurs if there are no serious screw-tract problems. If this method is chosen it is important that functional loading of the fracture is increased progressively, either by decreasing the rigidity of the frame or by increasing the loading by the patient.

Failure of fracture consolidation

The fracture may not consolidate and a bone graft may be needed for serious diaphyseal fractures, performed with the frame *in situ*. Alternatively, the method of stabilization may be changed to internal fixation with a supplementary bone graft. It is safest to treat the patient in a cast for 1 month after removal of the frame before proceeding with the internal fixation. This reduces the risk of infection from screw tracts.

Surgical technique

TIBIAL DIAPHYSEAL FRACTURES

Indications

These are as detailed in the introduction.

Frame selection

Unilateral frames are satisfactory for nearly all tibial diaphyseal fractures; and all frame types are designed to embrace treatment of this type of injury.

Occasionally more complex frames are needed for very comminuted fractures, or fractures with a juxta- or intra-articular component.

In the present description a unilateral frame, the Dynabrace Oxford Fixation system (Richards, UK), is described for the treatment of tibial diaphyseal fractures but the same principles apply to all frames.

Procedure

1

Pre-planning of the screw position is important. Medial placement of the screws prevents inhibition of muscle function by avoiding penetration of the anterior compartment; medially inserted screws pass through little soft tissue and fewer screw-tract problems are seen. Screws should be kept away from mobile skin, such as that seen over the anterior aspect of the ankle and close to the patellar tendon.

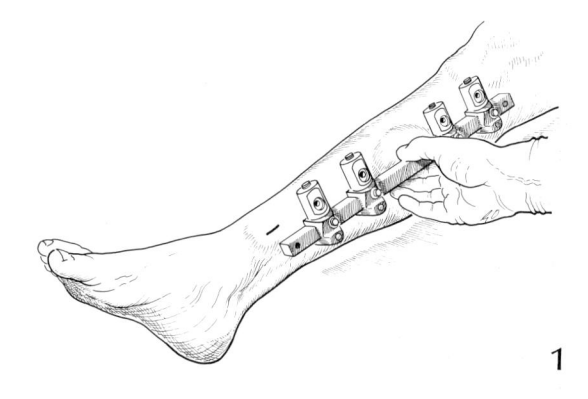

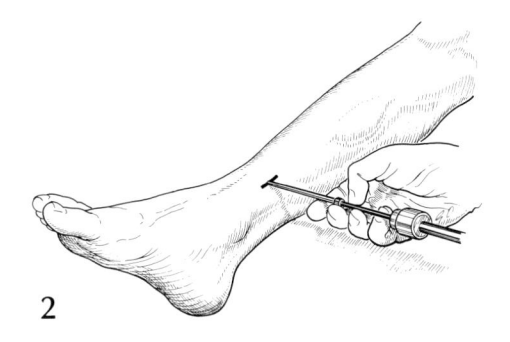

2

A longitudinal 1 cm incision is made in the skin. Pre-drilling is performed, protecting the skin with a trocar. Care is taken to ensure the drill hole is in the centre of the skin incision to prevent tenting of the screw on the skin edges. The pre-drilled hole should be through the centre of the bone.

148 Fracture treatment

3

Pre-drilling is made so that deep penetration of the anterior compartment does not occur; the anterior tibial vessels and deep peroneal nerve are very close to the lateral tibial surface, at the level between one and two hands'-breadth above the medial malleolus.

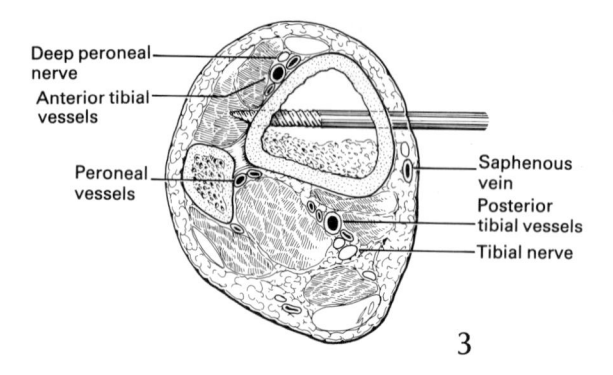

4

The screw is inserted by hand, this being a self-tapping screw; the distal cortex should be penetrated fully. Power insertion regularly leads to over-penetration.

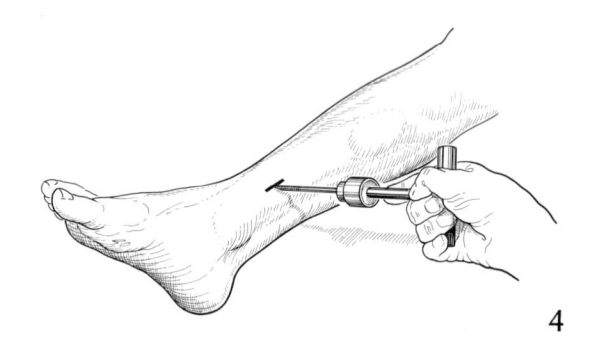

5

Further screws are inserted in a similar manner after reduction of the fracture. The frame is positioned to allow for postoperative oedema. Check radiographs are taken with standard X–ray cassettes, and fracture position is assessed in both planes; complete screw penetration of both cortices of the tibia is confirmed. The foot and knee are moved through their range of movement to ensure that tenting of screws on the skin does not occur in different positions.

Postoperative management

Screw holes are dressed each day; if moist, small dry dressings are applied; if dry, no dressings are needed. Scabs should be removed if proliferative to prevent accumulation of discharge within the screw holes.

External skeletal fixation 149

DISTAL FOREARM FRACTURES

Indications

This technique is used for unstable fractures in the distal radius with serious comminution; and for fractures with major wounds overlying them.

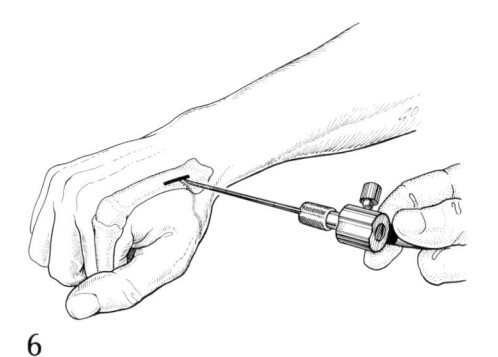

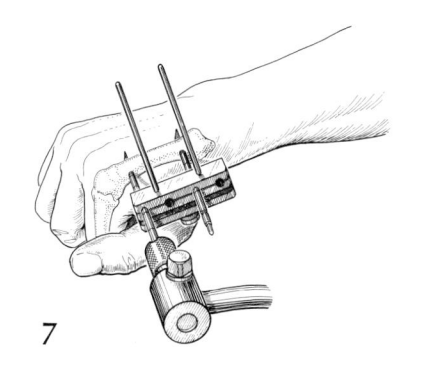

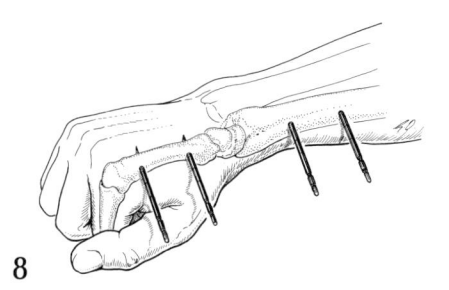

Frame selection

The most appropriate type of frame for these injuries is the Hoffmann frame with small series C-components. Other frames can be used with improvisation.

Procedure

6

The arm is placed extended on a board, and the fracture reduced into approximate alignment. The wounds are debrided.

The first pin is inserted into the proximal base of the second metacarpal with the index finger flexed, so that the finger will have full movement postoperatively. A 1 cm longitudinal mid-lateral incision is made and the bone exposed by direct dissection, so as to avoid nerve injury. A 3 mm diameter, 80 mm long, half-pin with continuous thread is inserted manually, parallel to the palm of the hand. The screw is inserted through both cortices.

7

The second pin is inserted in a similar manner using the pre-drill guide as a template. The screw is inserted distally in the second metacarpal, using the first and third holes in the guide.

8

The third and fourth screws are inserted into the distal third of the radial shaft. Direct exposure of the bone should be made through a 1.5 cm skin incision, taking care to avoid injury to the terminal branches of the radial nerve and to the radial artery; screws should not be over-inserted.

150 Fracture treatment

9

The frame is attached using small four-hole universal ball-joints with straight smooth rods between them; final reduction is achieved. The ball-joints are tightened and check radiographs taken. There needs to be sufficient offset to allow for oedema.

Postoperative management

Mobilization of the hand is started immediately. Screw holes are dressed as previously described (p. 148)

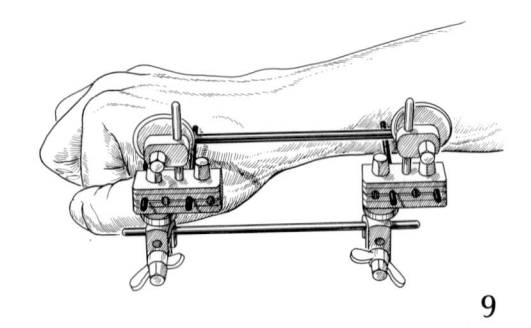

PELVIC FRACTURES

Indications

This technique is indicated for emergency treatment of unstable pelvic fractures with associated major blood loss or visceral damage, or in patients with multiple leg fractures. The pelvis is stabilized with a simple anterior frame in the receiving room of the accident department.

It is also the definitive treatment of pelvic fracture dislocations with anterior instability. Each injury needs careful assessment for pattern and stability to assess the type of stabilization required, which varies considerably.

Anterior frames alone will not stabilize serious injuries to the sacroiliac complex, and particularly will not stabilize vertical shear dislocations. Additional fixation is needed for the definitive treatment of these complex injuries.

Frame selection

It is possible to improvise with many of the types of unilateral frame but a most appropriate frame for pelvic fractures is constructed from the Hoffmann system; the method for anterior stabilization is described here.

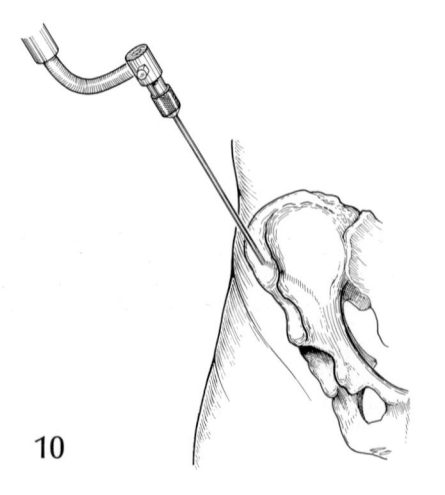

Procedure

10

To ensure correct placement of the screws in the pelvic brim, the anterior iliac crest is exposed through a 7 cm incision by direct dissection. Bone levers are inserted on the inside and outside of the iliac crest, so as to locate the position and angle of the ilium. A 4 mm diameter, 180 mm long, Hoffmann pin with continuous thread is inserted on the hand drill 2 cm behind the anterior superior iliac spine. Pins should be inserted so that all the thread is within the bone. Care is taken to ensure the screw remains within the walls of the ilium.

External skeletal fixation 151

11

The half-pin guide is placed over the first pin, and then the posterior pin is inserted as far posteriorly as possible – at least hole 5. Then the third pin is inserted.

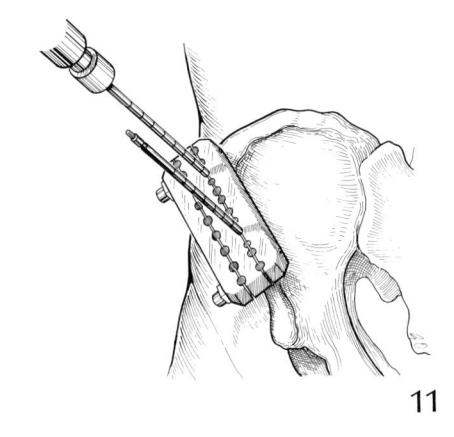

12

A clamp is attached to the three inserted pins well away from the bone. The procedure is repeated on the opposite side of the pelvis.

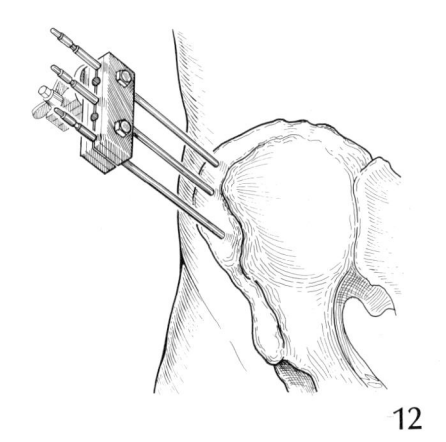

13

The frame is attached in a trapezoid manner and at 70° to the angle of the body. The wings of the locking nuts on the articulation couplings should face away from the patient, so as to allow easy adjustment and tightening.

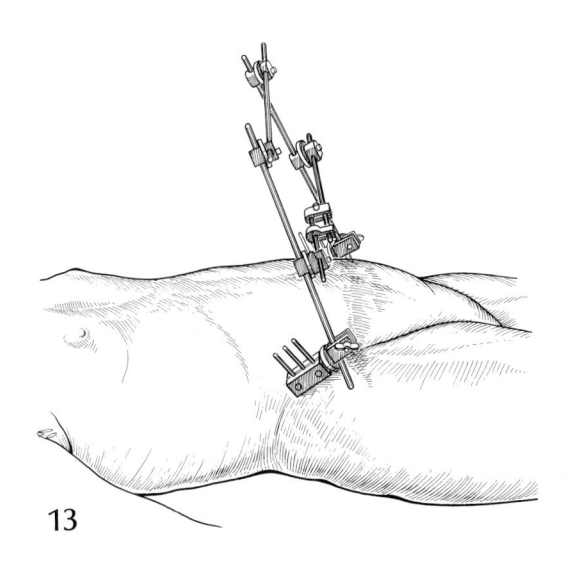

14

Connecting rods are attached and the fracture reduced manually. The couplings on the distal rod are tightened. A radiograph is then taken to check that reduction is adequate.

Further lateral compression can be applied by tightening the wheel to shorten the central connecting rods.

It is important that allowance is made for oedema and abdominal distension, which may be very considerable; the frame position should allow the patient to sit comfortably.

The wounds are closed around the screw holes.

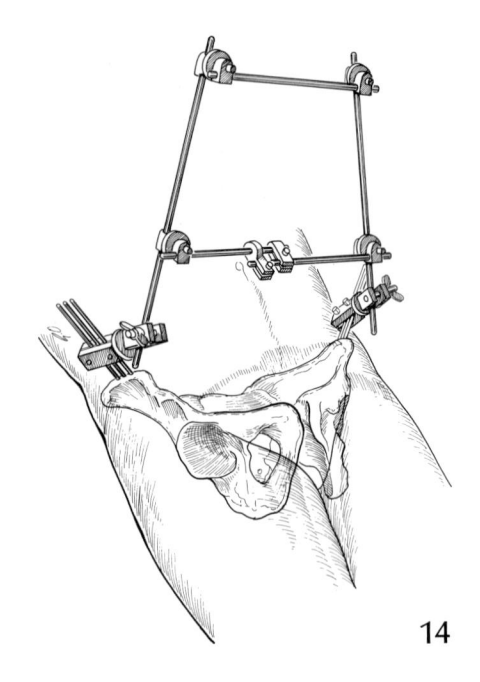

Postoperative management

Screw-hole care is the same as for all external skeletal fixation (p. 148)

Frames are maintained until sufficient stability is achieved, which is usually a period of at least 6 weeks; but each frame needs to be reviewed as there are individual variations in the pattern of injury. Similar caution is needed before weight-bearing is prescribed for more severe injuries, especially if there is posterior pelvic instability. Frames can be removed without anaesthesia.

References

1. Behrens F, Searles K. External fixation of the tibia: basic concepts and prospective evaluation. *J Bone Joint Surg [Br]* 1986; 68–B: 246–54.

2. Green SA. *Complications of external skeletal fixation: causes, prevention and treatment.* Springfield, Illinois: Thomas, 1981.

Illustrations by Mark Iley

Fractures of the long bones of the upper limb

Paul T. Calvert MA, FRCS
Consultant Orthopaedic Surgeon, St George's Hospital, London, UK

FRACTURES OF THE PROXIMAL HUMERUS

Indications for operation

An understanding of the classification of proximal humeral fractures described by Neer[1] is the most important prerequisite for determining which of these fractures require operation. All undisplaced and minimally displaced fractures can be treated conservatively; this constitutes the majority (80 per cent). There are four displaced fractures for which surgical treatment is indicated.

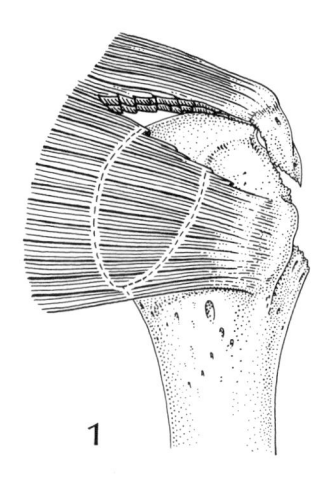

1

1. Fractures of the greater tuberosity with wide separation (greater than 1 cm) of the tuberosity fragment; the supraspinatus and infraspinatus muscles are attached to this fragment, and retract it superiorly and posteriorly; there is an associated longitudinal tear of the rotator cuff.
2. Fracture of the surgical neck if the shaft fragment is widely displaced and cannot be reduced by manipulation. The proximal end of the shaft may be lying in the deltoid muscle with soft tissue interposition which prevents reduction.

154　Upper limb fractures

2a–d

3. Displaced three-part fractures in younger patients; these require open reduction and internal fixation.
4. Displaced four-part fractures and both three- and four-part fracture-dislocations; these are best treated by hemiarthroplasty in most patients[2].

Techniques

All the operations described require the patient to be supine or semi-seated on the operating table with the shoulder close to the edge of the table and a sandbag between the scapulae. The shoulder and arm are draped so that the whole arm can be manoeuvred freely during the operation.

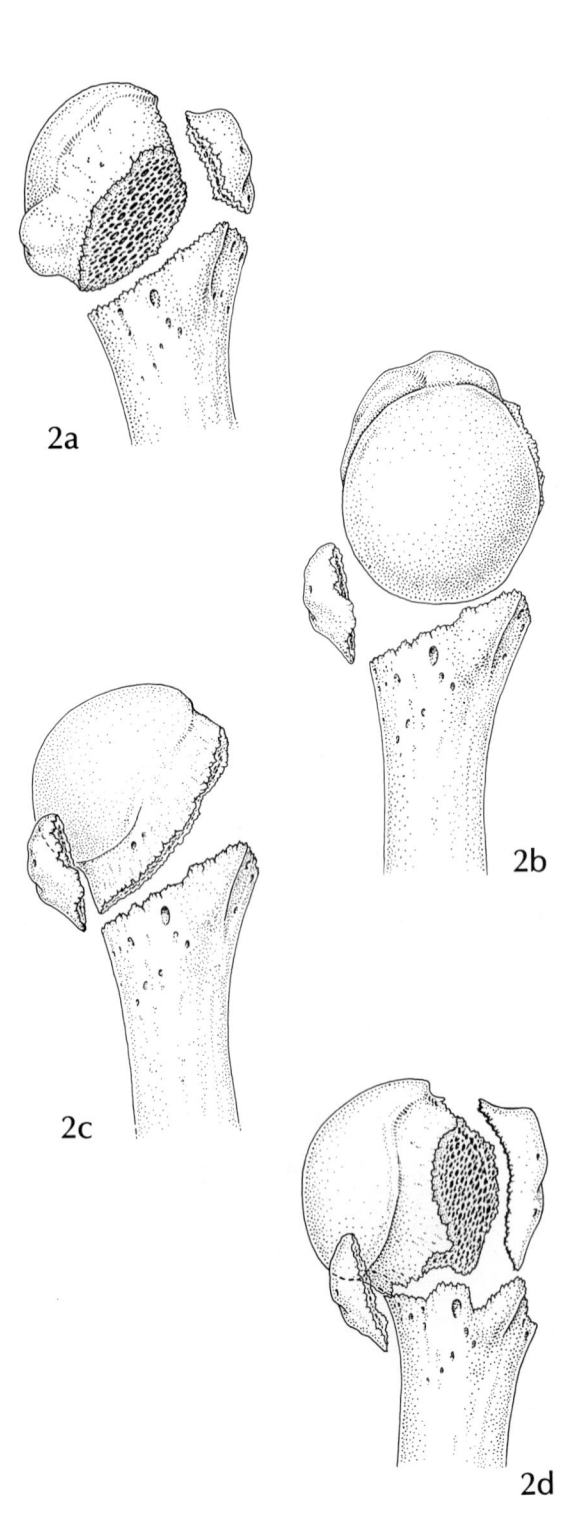

DISPLACED FRACTURE OF THE GREATER TUBEROSITY (displacement more than 1 cm)

3a, b & c

A 7 cm deltoid splitting incision is made starting at the most lateral edge of the acromion. The deltoid muscle is not detached from the acromion. The deltoid is split in the line of the incision to expose the subacromial bursa in the proximal part of the wound and the greater tuberosity distally. The axillary nerve lies approximately 5 cm distal to the acromion. If the tuberosity has retracted with the rotator cuff muscles under the acromion, the incision can be extended into a transacromial approach[3], taking care to preserve the continuity of the trapezius and deltoid as an osteoperiosteal flap across their acromial insertion. The tuberosity is exposed, reduced and fixed with a figure-of-eight heavy non-absorbable suture or, occasionally, two 4 mm cancellous screws. The wound is closed over a suction drain.

Postoperative management

The patient returns from the operating theatre with the shoulder supported in some abduction on a wedge support. Passive mobilization in the range 90°–180° is commenced by the physiotherapist on the first postoperative day. The arm can be brought down to the side at 5 days, but a full passive range of movement must be maintained. Assisted active elevation can begin at 3 weeks, but unassisted active elevation in the entire range should not be permitted for 6 weeks.

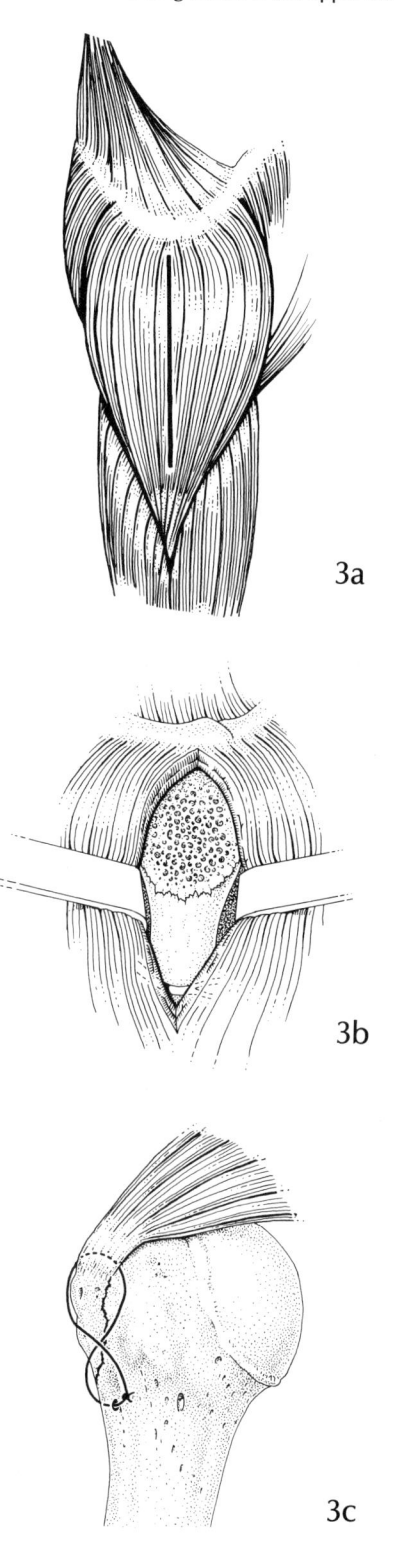

NEER HEMIARTHROPLASTY

4a–e

An anterior deltopectoral approach preserving the cephalic vein is made. The deltoid is not detached from either its clavicular or acromial origins. If additional exposure is required the deltoid origin is reflected distally and this will allow easier retraction of the muscle. The coracoacromial ligament and clavipectoral fascia are divided. The long head of biceps and its tendon are identified – this is the essential landmark which locates the interval between the tuberosities – and this interval is developed. The shaft fragment is usually easy to find. By retracting the lesser tuberosity medially and the greater tuberosity laterally, the head fragment can be found and removed. To increase exposure it may be necessary to extend the split in the rotator cuff along the junction of the supraspinatus and subscapularis; this must be repaired at the end of the operation.

The humeral shaft is reamed with the appropriate reamers and the correct sized trial humeral component is selected. There are two head sizes (15 mm and 22 mm) and three stem diameters (6.3 mm, 9.5 mm and 12.7 mm). It is important that the head diameter is correct so that the rotator cuff muscles are reconstructed at their original length and tension. The humeral shaft may need trimming but this will depend on the level of the fracture. The trial component is inserted in approximately 35° of retroversion and the tuberosities are checked to ensure that they come together over the fin of the prosthesis. The humeral component is cemented into place (in some patients cement may not be required) and the tuberosities reconstructed as shown using heavy (No. 5) non-absorbable braided sutures. The wound is closed over a suction drain.

Postoperative management

The postoperative rehabilitation is as important as the operation. The arm is placed in a sling and bandaged to the side for 5 days. Passive medial and lateral rotation, and elevation in flexion are commenced at 5 days. These are continued for 6 weeks, at which stage the tuberosities should be united to themselves and to the shaft. Thereafter the patient can progress to assisted active movements and active (unassisted) movements.

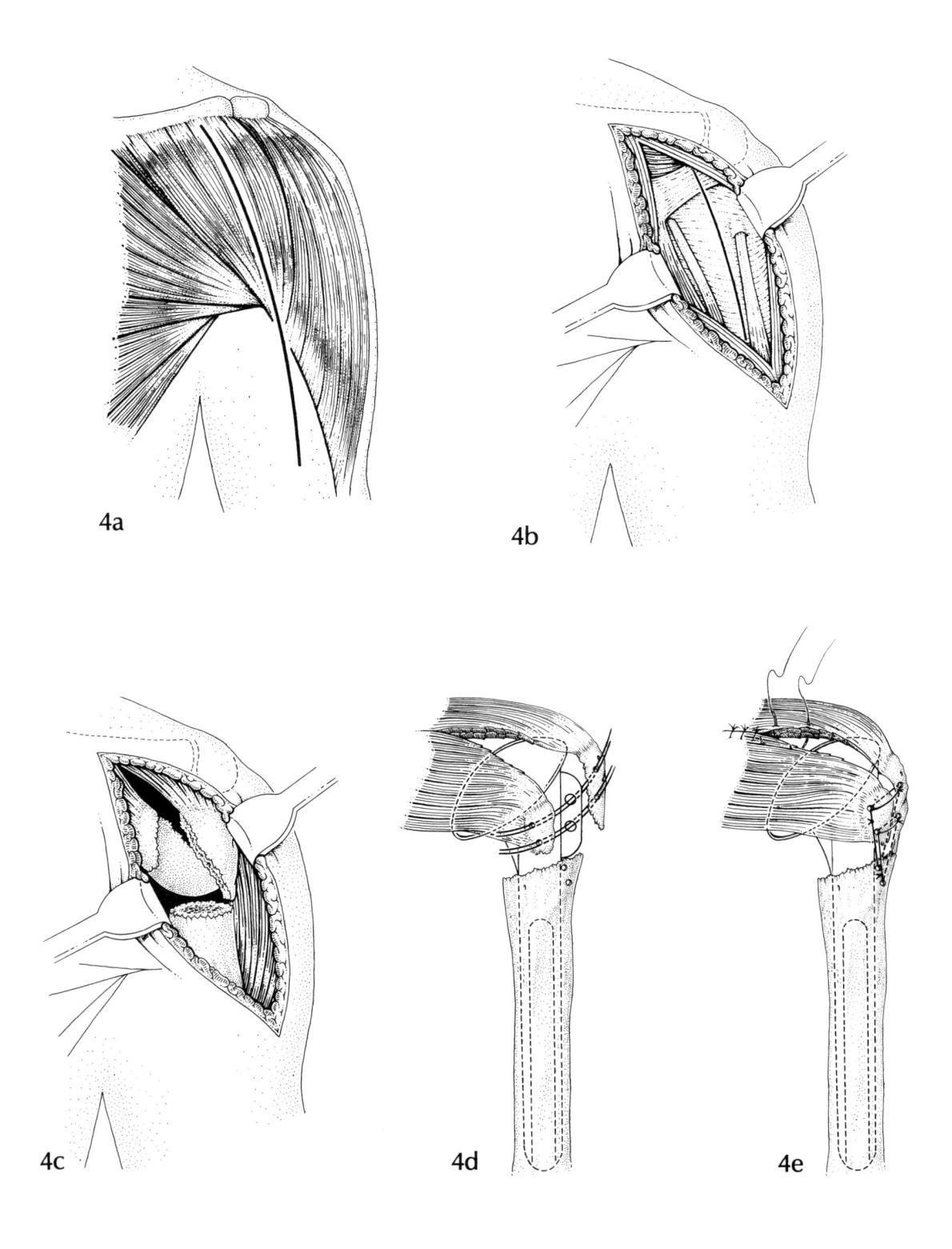

Fractures of the long bones of the upper limb 157

4a

4b

4c

4d

4e

OPEN REDUCTION OF DISPLACED TWO- AND THREE-PART FRACTURES

5a, b & c

The same anterior deltopectoral approach for the Neer hemiarthroplasty is used. Available fixation methods are illustrated. The T-plate is satisfactory in younger patients with good quality bone, but in older patients tends not to grip the proximal fragment and should be avoided.

Postoperative management

Mobilization should be individualized according to the stability of the fixation. Pendulum exercises and passive mobilization should be commenced as soon as they are judged to be safe.

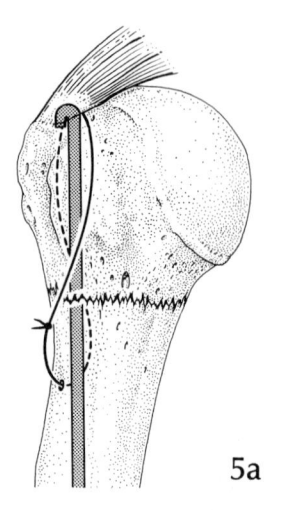

5a

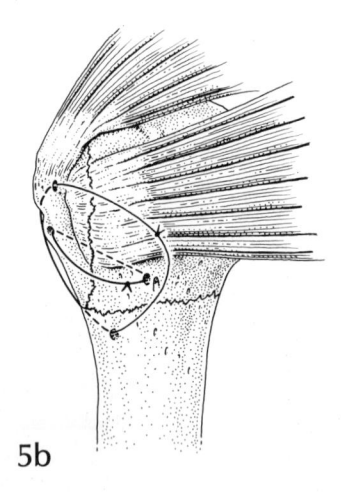

5b

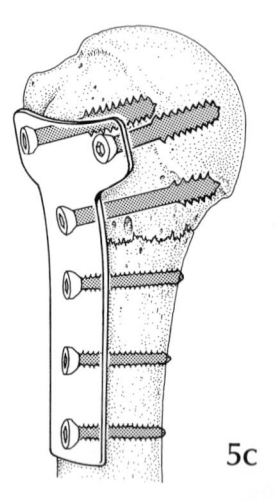

5c

FRACTURES OF THE HUMERAL SHAFT

Indications

Most fractures of the shaft of the humerus heal satisfactorily with conservative management and are best treated by a collar and cuff, hanging cast or functional brace[4,5].

The indications for operative treatment are limited but may be listed.

1. Patients with multiple injuries, severe head injuries or spinal cord injury for whom conservative management is very difficult[6,7].
2. When there is an associated ipsilateral forearm or elbow fracture[8].
3. Associated vascular injury in the same limb[9].
4. Pathological fractures.
5. Secondary radial nerve palsy. The majority of primary radial nerve palsies resolve with conservative treatment.

Technique

Plating is the most generally applicable technique and can be used for most humeral shaft fractures which require internal fixation. Intramedullary nailing by the closed technique may be used for the transverse or short oblique midshaft fracture but is most useful for pathological fractures.

Fractures of the long bones of the upper limb 159

PLATING

6a–d

An anterior exposure of the humerus is used. A longitudinal incision of approximately 12–15 cm is made along the lateral border of the biceps muscle. At the proximal end of the wound, the cephalic vein, which lies in the deltopectoral groove, is identified, ligated and divided. The interval between the pectoralis major and the deltoid is developed to expose the deltoid insertion into the humerus. In the middle and distal parts of the wound, the dissection is continued down along the lateral border of the biceps muscle, which is retracted medially, exposing the brachialis muscle which lies on the anterior surface of the humerus. To expose the proximal humeral shaft, the deltoid insertion is reflected laterally, the brachialis muscle distal to this is split in the midline, reflected and the humerus exposed subperiosteally. Care should be taken not to retract too vigorously with bone levers on the lateral aspect of the humerus because this can damage the radial nerve.

A broad 4.5 mm dynamic compression plate (DCP) is applied to the exposed humerus using the technique described in the chapter on 'Principles of fracture management' (see pp. 100–122). It is important to use a plate of sufficient length so that there are at least three screws gripping both cortices on either side of the fracture. If there is considerable comminution of the fracture or if the plating is being performed because of non-union, then a cancellous bone graft should be used in addition to the plate, taking bone from the ipsilateral iliac crest.

The wound is closed over a suction drain and a well-padded dressing is applied.

Postoperative management

The arm is supported in a triangular sling giving support to the elbow. Active shoulder and elbow movements are started as soon as the drain is removed. Unrestricted use of the arm should not be permitted until the fracture has united and this will take at least 6–12 weeks. If it is decided to remove the plate this should not be done until at least 1 year has elapsed.

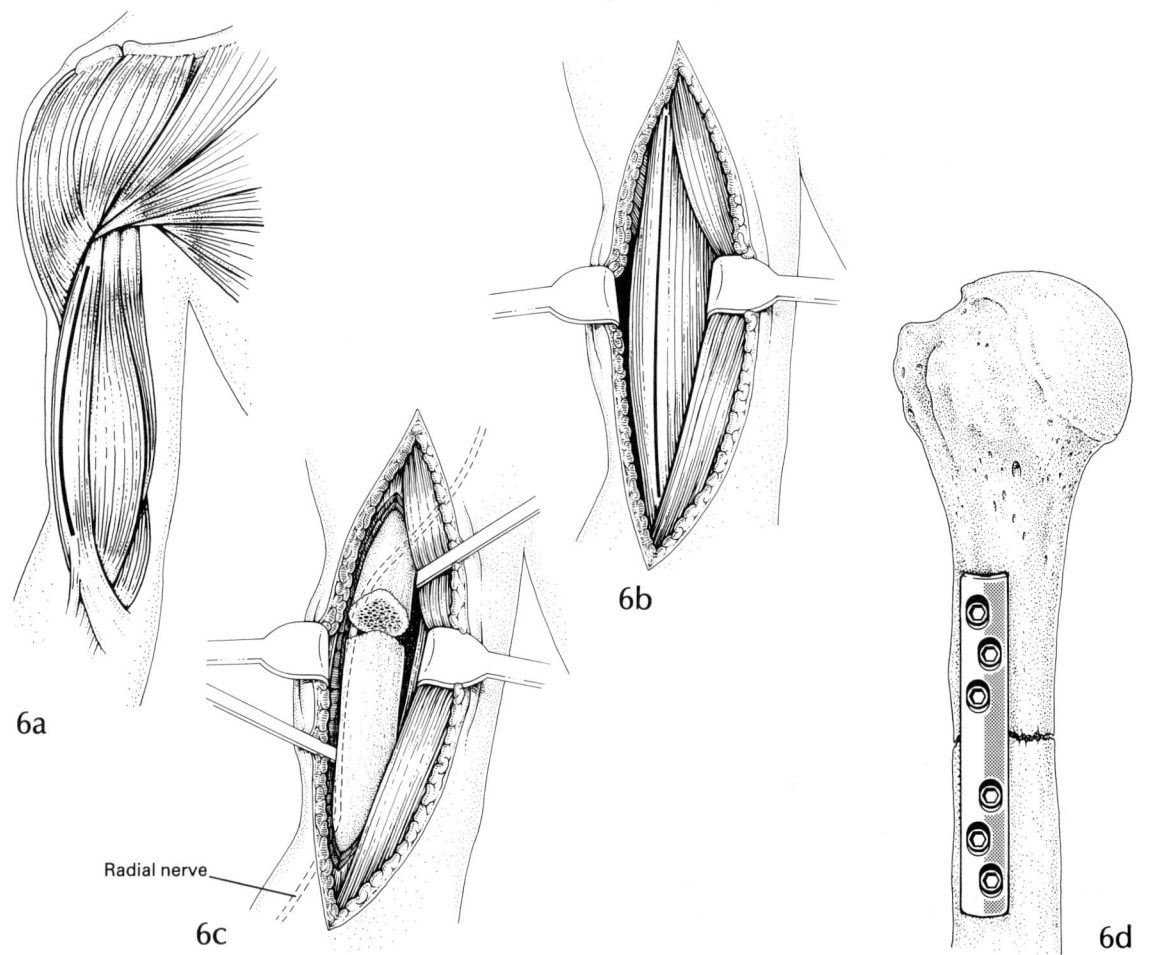

6a

6b

Radial nerve
6c

6d

CLOSED INTRAMEDULLARY NAILING

7

The patient is positioned in a lateral position with the affected arm uppermost, supported on an arm rest; it is important that the elbow can be flexed to more than 90°. An image intensifier is positioned as shown so that views of the humerus can be obtained in two planes at right angles.

A 6 cm longitudinal incision is made in the midline posteriorly over the distal humerus and olecranon. The triceps aponeurosis is reflected as a distally based triangular flap to expose the olecranon fossa which is cleared of all soft tissue. The elbow is flexed beyond a right angle, and a bone awl or drill used to make a hole in the cortex at the apex of the olecranon fossa into the medullary cavity. It is important to enlarge this hole with bone nibblers to allow good access to the medulla because otherwise there is a danger of producing a fracture. A hand reamer is passed into the medulla and across the fracture site under image intensifier control; an experienced assistant is required to manipulate the fracture. The medulla is reamed until the cortex is just felt to 'bite' onto the reamer. The length of nail is chosen so that it will pass into the humeral head proximally and its distal end will be just buried in the medulla. An intramedullary nail is passed across the fracture under radiographic control and is hammered into position. A 3.5 mm cortical screw is placed transversely across the distal humerus so that it just traverses the apex of the olecranon fossa; this prevents the nail from backing out. The wound is closed in layers. Flexible nails can be used as an alternative to a Küntscher nail, and the patient can be positioned supine with overhead traction; this is useful for the patient with multiple injuries[6].

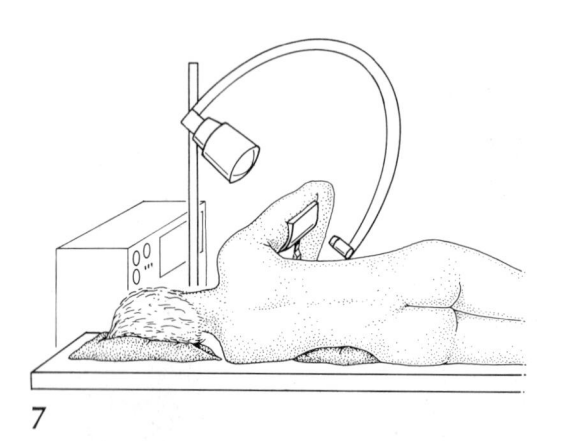

7

Postoperative management

This is the same as for plating except that more vigorous use of the arm can be permitted at an earlier stage.

FRACTURES OF THE SHAFTS OF THE RADIUS AND ULNA

Indications

The indications for open reduction and internal fixation are:

1. Displaced fractures of both bones of the forearm in adults[10].
2. Monteggia and Galeazzi fracture-dislocations in adults[11,12].
3. Isolated fractures of the ulna which are displaced more than 100 per cent.
4. Displaced fractures of both bones of the forearm in older children and adolescents in which an acceptable reduction cannot be achieved or maintained. The older the child the more important it is to obtain a good reduction. (The reader is referred to the excellent study by Fuller[13] for guidance about the degree of acceptable deformity.)
5. Monteggia fracture-dislocations in children which can usually be treated by closed means, but if a satisfactory reduction cannot be maintained, then open reduction and internal fixation of the ulna is required.

Techniques

Most authors agree that the best results are obtained by rigid plate fixation. In adults it is essential to use the 3.5 mm DCP plates and to employ a plate of sufficient length so that at least six cortices are held by the screws on either side of the fracture. This requires a minimum of a six-hole plate. Semitubular and one-third tubular plates are inadequate and should not be used except in children. For all these fractures the radius and ulna should be approached through separate incisions. The ulna can be approached throughout its length along the subcutaneous border. The radius is approached by either an anterior Henry approach or a dorsal approach over its extensor aspect; the anterior approach will be described here because it is applicable to the whole length of the radius and the volar surface presents a flatter surface more suitable for plate application. All or part of the exposure described is used, depending on the site of the fracture and the length of plate required.

A high-arm pneumatic tourniquet is used.

RIGID PLATE FIXATION

Exposure of the radius

8a–d

A 10 cm longitudinal incision is made on the volar aspect of the forearm, centred on the radial fracture. The deep fascia is incised in the line of the wound. The biceps tendon is at the most proximal end, and the lateral side of this is dissected. The recurrent leash of radial vessels, beneath which lies the bicipital bursa and supinator muscle, is ligated and divided. Distal to the biceps, the interval between the brachioradialis and the flexor carpi radialis is developed. The radial nerve, which lies on the medial surface of the brachioradialis, is retracted carefully with the muscle in a radial direction; the artery is retracted towards the ulnar side. At the proximal end of the wound, the insertion of the supinator muscle is exposed; the insertion of the pronator teres is more distal, and then, in order, are the origins of flexor pollicis longus, flexor digitorum superficialis and pronator quadratus; directly beneath these lies the radius. To gain exposure of the proximal radius, the insertion of the supinator is incised along the medial side of the radius, and the supinator muscle is reflected laterally by subperiosteal dissection; this protects the posterior interosseous nerve as it lies within the muscle. To expose the more distal part of the radius, the forearm is pronated and the muscle insertions along the lateral border of the radius incised and reflected subperiosteally in an ulnar direction.

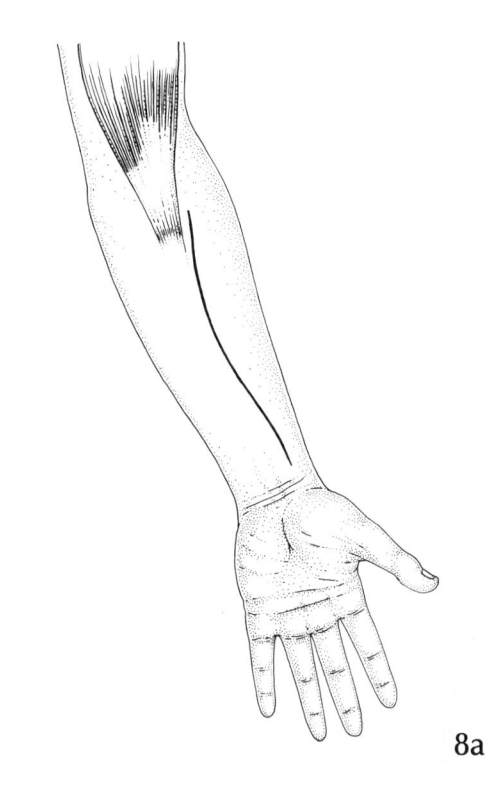

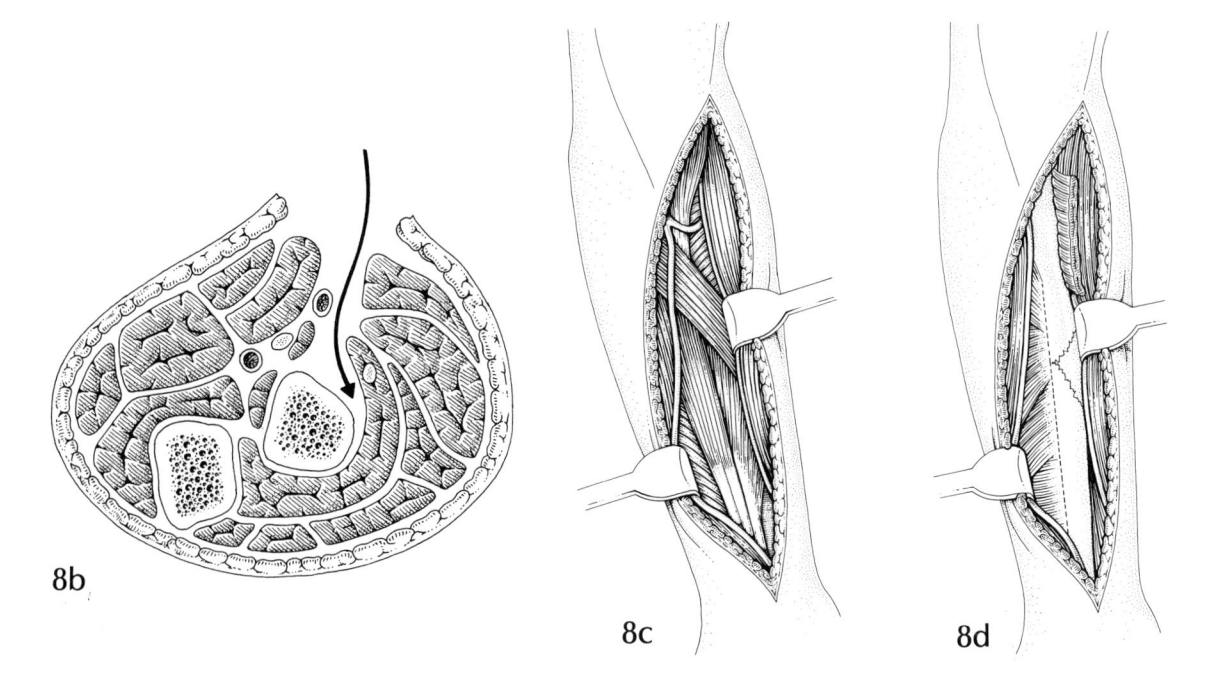

Exposure of the ulna

A 10 cm longitudinal skin incision is made along the subcutaneous border of the ulna. This incision is continued directly down onto the bone which is exposed subperiosteally. The fracture is reduced and fixed with a 3.5 mm DCP plate.

Plating of the fracture

9a–d

Adequate exposure of bone should be obtained so that a plate of suitable length can be inserted without excessive soft tissue retraction. It is as important to handle the soft tissues gently as it is to fix the fracture adequately. The fracture ends should be cleaned, the two ends are grasped with small bone-holding forceps and the fracture reduced. A 3.5 mm DCP plate of sufficient length is chosen and contoured so that it fits the surface of the bone accurately. The plate is held in position with bone-holding forceps. Before the plate is screwed into position on either bone, the other fracture is exposed to ensure that it can be reduced; sometimes it is necessary to release one to reduce the other.

Using the neutral guide, a 2.5 mm hole is drilled through one of the holes in the plate adjacent to the fracture; the length of screw required is measured with the depth gauge; the hole is tapped with the 3.5 mm tap and the screw inserted. This procedure is repeated in the adjacent hole on the same side of the fracture. Using the compression guide with its arrow directed towards the fracture, the hole which is adjacent to the fracture on the other fragment is drilled into eccentrically; a screw is inserted after measuring and tapping. As this screw is tightened the fracture will be seen to compress. The fixation is completed by inserting screws in the same manner into the remaining holes, using the neutral drill guide.

If there is a separate butterfly fragment this must be fixed with lag screws. If the fracture is oblique, a lag screw may also be used and the configuration of the fracture determines to which fragment the plate is first fixed (see *Illustrations 9c and d*).

Closure

The wounds are closed with subcutaneous and skin sutures only; the deep fascia is not closed. Suction drains should be inserted in both wounds, and a well-padded bandage is applied.

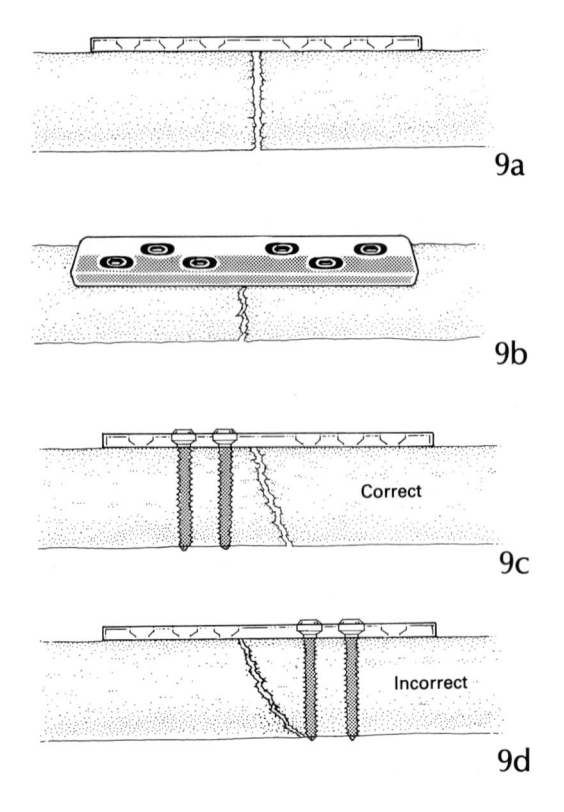

Postoperative management

The arm should be elevated in a suitable support such as a roller towel for 24 to 48 hours, at which time the drains should be removed. If the fixation is good and the patient reliable then no external splintage is necessary and early active mobilization can be allowed. A triangular sling should be used for 6 weeks. If there is any doubt about the adequacy of fixation or the cooperation of the patient, then an above-elbow plaster of Paris cast should be applied either immediately or at about 5 days when the wound is satisfactory.

Progress towards union and consolidation should be monitored radiographically. In young people it may be necessary to remove the plates. This should be done not less than 1 year after the original plating to avoid the complication rate associated with plate removal[14].

MONTEGGIA FRACTURE

The ulna is plated as described. The reduction of the radial head must be checked by a radiograph in the operating theatre. The position of maximum stability should be determined and an above-elbow plaster of Paris cast must be applied in this position and retained for 6 weeks. Radiographs are obtained at 2 and 4 weeks to ensure that the radial head remains reduced.

If, at the time of operation, the radial head is not reduced, then a small incision is made over the lateral aspect of the radial head, the annular ligament is identified and incised to allow the radial head to return to its anatomical position. The ligament is repaired with fine absorbable sutures.

GALEAZZI FRACTURE

The radius is plated as described. The reduction of the inferior radioulna joint is checked with a radiograph in the operating theatre. It is usually satisfactory, but occasionally the tendon of extensor carpi ulnaris becomes interposed and the joint must be opened to restore its correct anatomical position. An above-elbow plaster of Paris cast is worn for 6 weeks.

FRACTURES OF THE DISTAL RADIUS

Indications

The vast majority of fractures of the distal radius with dorsal displacement (Colles' type) are best treated by closed methods. In younger patients in whom an acceptable reduction cannot be maintained, there is an occasional indication for the use of an external fixator. The main indication for open reduction and internal fixation of a fracture of the distal radius is where there is volar displacement (Smith's type).

Technique

10a–e

An anterior longitudinal incision is made over the flexor carpi radialis, starting at the distal flexor wrist crease and extending 6–8 cm proximally. The fascia is divided in the line of the incision. The flexor carpi radialis and median nerve are retracted to the ulnar side, and the flexor pollicis longus and the radial artery are retracted to the radial side. The pronator quadratus is divided at its radial insertion to expose the fracture.

The wrist is extended over a kidney dish and this manoeuvre usually reduces the fracture. Either an Ellis plate[15] or a small fragment AO buttress plate is fixed to the proximal fragment. This is usually sufficient to hold the fracture but it may sometimes be necessary to insert a screw through the volar fragment. The wound is closed over a small suction drain.

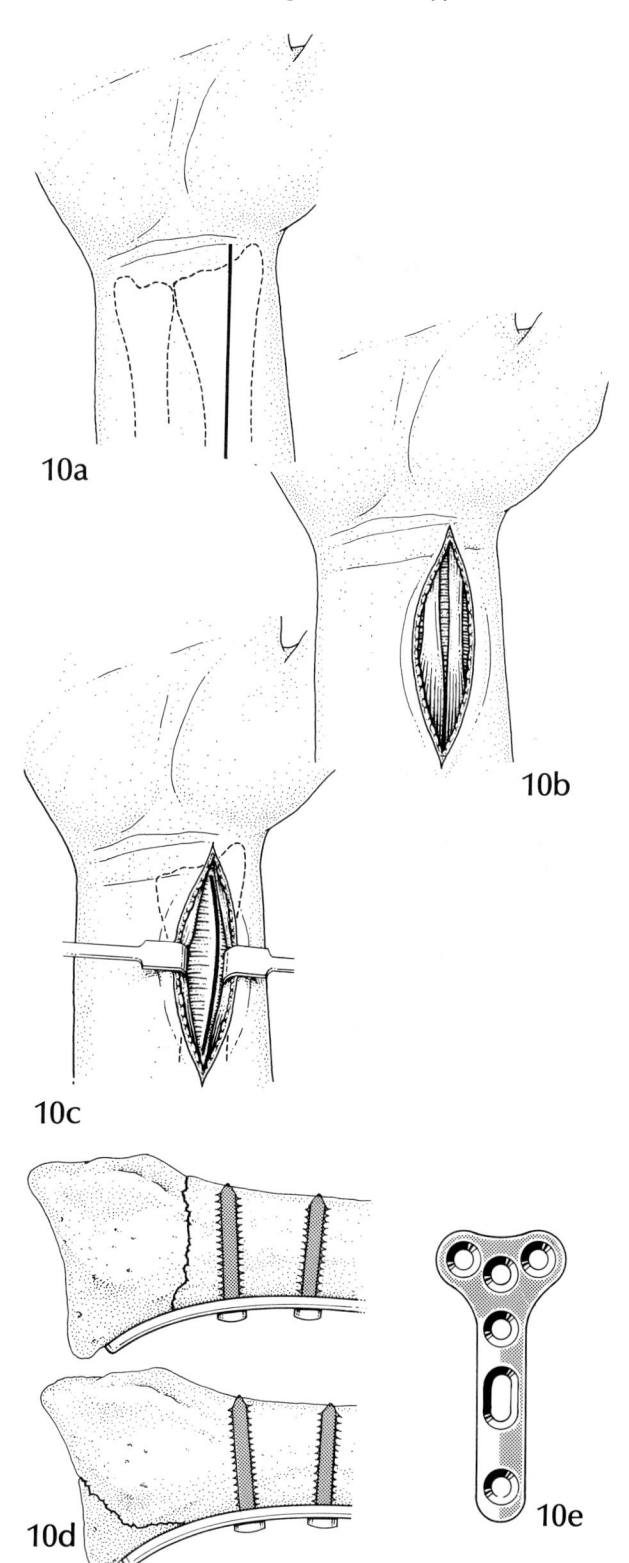

Postoperative management

A backslab is applied and the arm is elevated. If the fixation is adequate, the wrist can be mobilized under supervision on the third postoperative day. If there is any doubt about the strength of the fixation, then a forearm cast is applied as soon as swelling permits and is retained for 4 weeks, when the wrist is mobilized.

References

1. Neer CS II. Displaced proximal humeral fractures. Part I Classification and evaluation. *J Bone Joint Surg [Am]* 1970; 52-A; 1077–89.

2. Stableforth PG. Four-part fractures of the neck of the humerus. *J Bone Joint Surg [Br]* 1984; 66-B: 104–8.

3. Kessel L, Watson M. The painful arc syndrome: clinical classification as a guide to management. *J Bone Joint Surg [Br]* 1977; 59-B: 166–72.

4. Epps C Jr. Fractures of the shaft of the humerus. In: Rockwood CA, Green DP, eds. *Fractures in adults*. 2nd ed. Philadelphia: J. B. Lippincott, 1984: 653–74.

5. Sarmiento A, Kinman PB, Calvin EG, Schmitt RH, Phillips JG. Functional bracing of fractures of the shaft of the humerus. *J Bone Joint Surg [Am]* 1977; 59-A: 596–601.

6. Bell MJ, Beauchamp CG, Kellem JK, McMurty RY. The results of plating humeral shaft fractures in patients with multiple injuries. *J Bone Joint Surg [Br]* 1985; 67-B: 293–6.

7. Brumback RJ, Bosse MJ, Poka A, Burgess AR. Intramedullary stabilization of humeral shaft fractures in patients with multiple trauma. *J Bone Joint Surg [Am]* 1986; 68-A: 960–70.

8. Rogers JF, Bennett JB, Tullos HS. Management of concomitant ipsilateral fractures of the humerus and forearm. *J Bone Joint Surg [Am]* 1984; 66-A: 552–6.

9. Rich NM, Baugh JH, Hughes CW. Acute arterial injuries in Vietnam, 1000 cases. *J Trauma* 1970; 10: 359–69.

10. Hadden WA, Reschauer R, Seggl W. Results of AO plate fixation of forearm shaft fractures in adults. *Injury* 1983; 15: 44–52.

11. Krause B, Horne G. Galeazzi fractures. *J Trauma* 1985; 25: 1093–5.

12. Hughston JC. Fracture of the distal radial shaft: mistakes in management. *J Bone Joint Surg [Am]* 1957; 39-A: 249–64.

13. Fuller DJ, McCullogh CJ. Malunited fractures of the forearm in children. *J Bone Joint Surg [Br]* 1982; 64-B: 364–7.

14. Hidaka S, Gustilo RB. Refracture of bones of the forearm after plate removal. *J. Bone Joint Surg [Am]* 1984; 66-A: 1241–3.

15. Fuller DJ. The Ellis plate operation for Smith's fracture. *J Bone Joint Surg [Br]* 1973; 55-B: 173–8.

Further reading

Müller ME, Allgöwer M, Schneider R, Willenegger H. *Manual of internal fixation*. 2nd ed. Berlin: Springer-Verlag, 1979.

Illustrations by Paul Richardson

Fractures at the elbow in adults

G. S. E. Dowd MD, MChOrth, FRCS
Consultant Orthopaedic Surgeon, St Bartholomew's and Homerton Hospitals, London, UK

Introduction

Fractures around the elbow frequently occur as a result of a fall onto the outstretched hand. The force is transmitted along the radius from the wrist resulting, in some cases, in fractures of the radial head as it impacts against the capitellum. If the force is transmitted across to the ulna, then this may result in a condylar fracture or a T–Y fracture of the distal humerus. Resistance to extension of the elbow by contraction of the triceps muscle during a fall onto the outstretched hand may result in an avulsion fracture of the olecranon.

Diagnosis of an elbow fracture may be obvious on clinical examination, but radiographic confirmation is essential. In cases of doubt, in adolescents for example, where epiphyseal lines can be mistaken for a fracture, comparative radiographs of the opposite elbow are very useful. In certain difficult fractures, oblique radiographs may elucidate the true extent of the bony injury.

In all elbow injuries a careful examination for neurological and vascular complications is essential. Depending on the type of fracture, any one of the three major nerves to the forearm and hand may be damaged. In closed fractures, the majority of nerve injuries are in continuity and recovery can be expected in 3–6 weeks. Vascular complications classically occur after displaced supracondylar fractures, when the brachial artery may be torn or caught over a spike of bone. If the circulation to the forearm does not return rapidly on reduction of the fracture, surgical exploration is mandatory, together with a fasciotomy of the forearm and fixation of the fracture.

In the majority of displaced fractures around the elbow, open reduction and internal fixation is required to restore the joint surface and to allow early movement. Undisplaced fractures may be treated conservatively provided careful follow-up is arranged and serial radiographs show no deterioration in position.

Perhaps the commonest complication of elbow fractures is reduced elbow movement. Occasionally, despite expert care, this complication occurs and the patient should be warned, at the outset, of this potential problem and warned against over-vigorous mobilization.

FRACTURES OF THE HEAD OF THE RADIUS

The majority of radial head fractures are relatively minor injuries in which the fragments are small and minimally displaced. This type of fracture may be treated by aspirating the fracture haematoma and resting the elbow in a sling for a few days until the pain has settled, and then mobilizing it out of the sling with active flexion and extension exercises. An almost full range of movement is to be expected. A severely comminuted displaced fracture with incongruity of the joint surface may require operative treatment to remove the fragments of the head. This should only be performed in adults because of the risk of proximal migration of the radius in children during growth. There is still dispute concerning the early or late removal of the fragmented radial head. The advantage of early removal of the head is that the elbow can be mobilized early rather than waiting several weeks before undergoing an operative procedure, by which time the elbow may be stiff. Occasionally the head may be split into two main fragments and their reconstitution should then be performed where possible to prevent late inferior radio-ulnar joint problems.

EXCISION OF THE HEAD OF THE RADIUS

Position of patient

1

The patient lies supine on the operating table with a well-padded pneumatic tourniquet applied to the upper arm. The skin is prepared and the arm draped, leaving adequate access to the elbow joint. The elbow is flexed and fully pronated and supported on an arm board.

Incision

2

The lateral epicondyle is identified by palpation with the radial head lying distally, and a skin incision is made from above the epicondyle, over the radiohumeral joint and across the radial head. The incision must not pass distal to the neck of the radius (2.5 cm distal to the joint) since the posterior interosseous nerve may be inadvertently divided as it passes round the proximal radius into the extensor compartment of the forearm.

Exposure

3

The incision is deepened to identify the extensor muscle mass inserted into the lateral epicondyle. A longitudinal split is made between fibres of anconeus posteriorly and the extensor muscle mass anteriorly. A retractor is placed between the two edges of muscle to reveal the capsule which is divided. Bone levers should not be used since heavy traction may injure the posterior interosseous nerve which lies between the two parts of the supinator muscle a little distal to the wound. Proximally lies the lateral epicondyle and the capitellum, with the radial head distal. The fragments of the radial head are removed and the separate pieces reconstituted on a green towel to ensure that all the fragments have been retrieved: a check radiograph should be made to confirm this. The radial neck should then be examined and any sharp edges removed with bone nibblers. Pronation and supination of the forearm will bring the whole circumference of the neck into the wound.

Closure

The wound is irrigated with saline. The two edges of the extensor mass and anconeus are gently apposed with interrupted absorbable sutures. The skin is closed with interrupted nylon sutures. A dressing is applied to the wound and the elbow is covered with wool and a crêpe bandage. The elbow is rested in a broad arm sling in 90° of flexion.

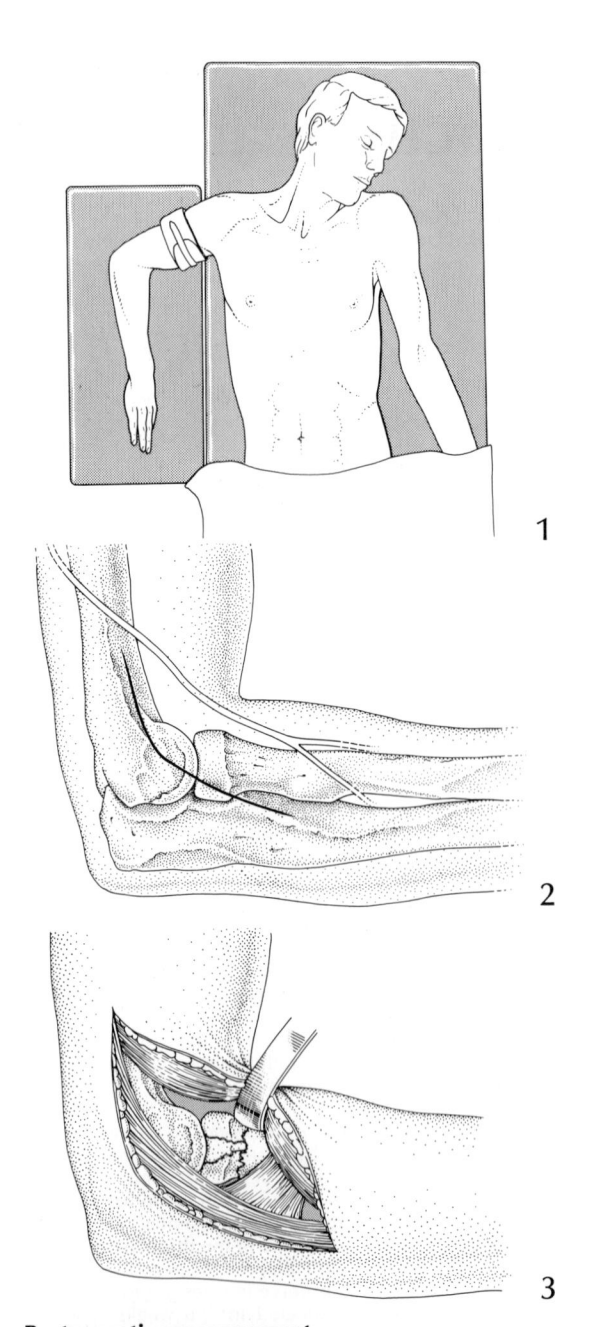

Postoperative management

Gentle active flexion and extension exercises should begin 24–48 hours after operation, together with pronation and supination exercises of the forearm. Sutures should be removed at 10 days. The elbow should be supported in a sling for 14–21 days when exercises are not being carried out. The elbow should not be forcefully extended since this may result in permanent stiffness of the elbow.

RECONSTRUCTION OF A SPLIT RADIAL HEAD

The position of the arm and the exposure is the same as for excision of the radial head.

Procedure

4a, b & c

The two fragments of the radial head are identified. The fracture surface is carefully cleaned of clot and an accurate reduction is performed, ensuring the articular surface of the radial head is reduced. The fracture can be held temporarily with a fine Kirschner wire. A stable fixation can be obtained by fixing the two fragments with either a 4 mm cancellous AO screw or two 2.7 mm lag screws. The heads should be countersunk to avoid irritation of the overlying annular ligament.

Postoperative management

This is similar to the management described for excision of the radial head.

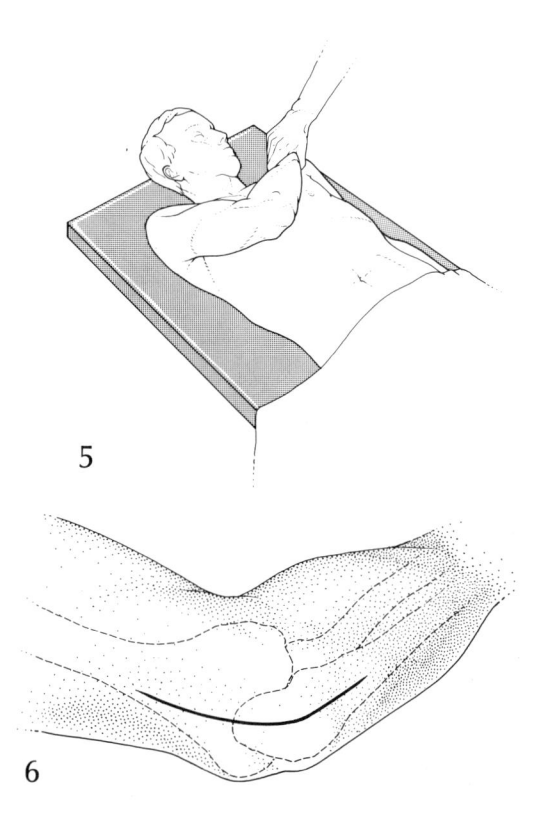

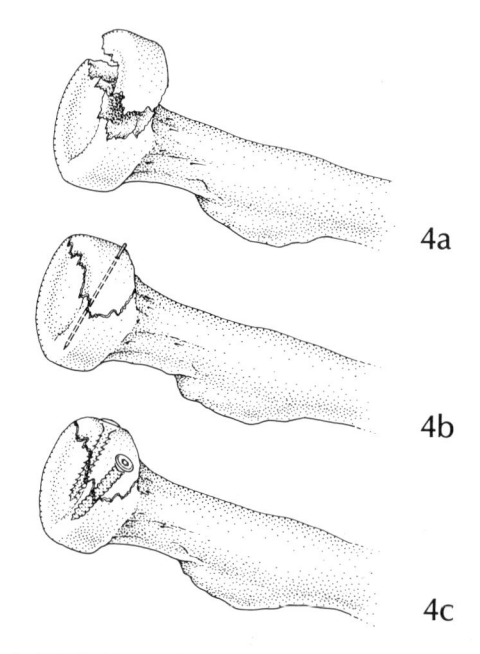

FRACTURE OF THE OLECRANON

There are several methods of fixing an olecranon fracture including the use of cancellous lag screws and tension-band wiring. The aim common to any method of fixation is to obtain a perfect reduction of the articular surface of the olecranon and to hold the position until union has occurred. This is sometimes difficult using a lag screw. The technique favoured by the author is tension-band wiring.

5

Position of the elbow

The patient is placed supine on the operating table with a tourniquet placed high on the upper arm. The elbow is prepared and draped to leave access to the joint. The arm is brought over the patient's chest and held by an assistant.

Incision

6

A posterior longitudinal incision is made from the midpoint of the triceps muscle, approximately 5 cm proximal to the tip of the olecranon, and is continued distally slightly to the radial side of the subcutaneous border of the ulna in order to protect the ulnar nerve passing round the medial epicondyle.

168 Upper limb fractures

Procedure

7a, b, & c

The fracture gap will be immediately identified beneath the skin incision and will be filled with haematoma. It is not usually necessary to dissect out the ulnar nerve, but if there is doubt about its position it should be dissected free and protected with a tape, carefully avoiding traction. The fracture ends should be carefully cleaned by removal of haematoma and any soft tissue interposition. Any small fragments of bone should be removed. The fracture gap should be thoroughly irrigated with saline. A 2 mm hole should be drilled in a transverse direction across the subcutaneous border of the ulna, about 4 cm distal to the fracture. The fracture can be accurately reduced by extending the elbow until the cortices of the two fragments are accurately apposed. The reduced fracture is held with a towel clip gripping the two fragments, and the elbow is flexed to facilitate transfixation of the fracture by two 2 mm Kirschner wires.

The Kirschner wires are drilled across the fracture in the longitudinal plane of the ulna, parallel to each other, and inserted about 1 cm proximal to the subcutaneous border of the ulna with the elbow flexed. They should cross the fracture line by at least 3 cm and be left to protrude out of the bone. A 26-gauge wire is then passed through the hole drilled across the subcutaneous border of the ulna, leaving a length on either side. A small eye is made in one length of the wire approximately 2 cm from the drill hole. The other length of wire is bent round the two Kirschner wires protruding from the ulna and twisted onto the end of the other wire. The eye and loose ends of the wires are tightened simultaneously to apply equal compression on both sides of the fracture. The wire loops are cut short and buried in soft tissue. The ends of the Kirschner wires are bent beyond a right angle, cut short and knocked further into the ulna.

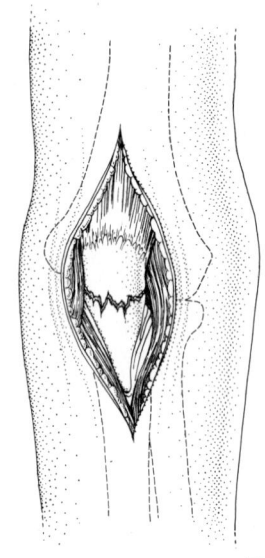

Closure

After checking that there are no sharp ends protruding from the wires, and that full extension and flexion of the elbow can be obtained without opening of the fracture line, the subcutaneous tissue is closed with interrupted absorbable sutures and the skin with interrupted non-absorbable sutures. A dressing is applied to the wound, covered with firm wool, and a crêpe bandage applied to the elbow.

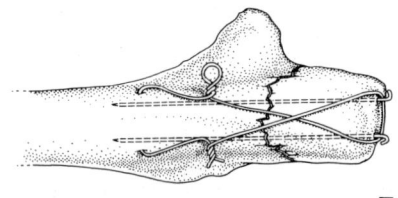

Postoperative management

The elbow is rested in a broad arm sling in 90° of flexion. At 7–10 days, gentle active flexion and extension excercises are started, providing the wound is satisfactory. Sutures are removed between 10 and 14 days and the broad arm sling discarded at about 3 weeks.

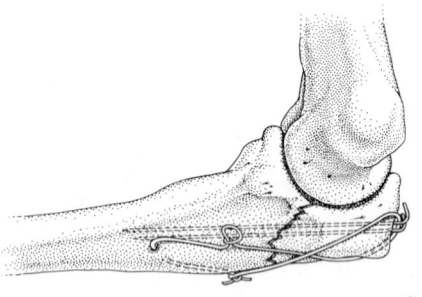

7a

7b

7c

MONTEGGIA FRACTURES

INTERNAL FIXATION

A Monteggia fracture is one in which the proximal ulna is fractured and angulates, levering out the radial head from its normal position within the confines of the annular ligament. The aim of treatment is to restore the length and reduce the angulation of the ulna, allowing the radial head to return to its anatomical position. In most cases, accurate reduction of the ulna results in spontaneous reduction of the radial head. If this does not occur, the radial head must be explored and any block to reduction, especially by interposition of the annular ligament, must be cleared.

Incision

8

The subcutaneous border of the ulna proximal and distal to the fracture is identified and a longitudinal skin incision approximately 15 cm in length is made. The bony border lies between the extensor and flexor carpi ulnaris muscles.

Procedure

9

The periosteum over the ends of the fracture is divided longitudinally to allow exposure of the bone. The fracture ends are thoroughly cleaned of haematoma and periosteum. The fracture is accurately reduced by manipulation, ensuring that the irregular surfaces interdigitate as perfectly as possible. A six-hole AO dynamic compression plate is recommended for fracture fixation, although other types of plate may be used. If the forearm can be fully pronated and supinated following fixation of the ulna, then reduction of the radial head is likely. However, anteroposterior and lateral radiographs of the fracture and radial head should be obtained on the operating table to ensure that the radial head has been reduced.

Closure

If possible, the periosteum should be sutured over the plate with absorbable sutures. The subcutaneous tissue is closed with absorbable sutures and the skin is closed with interrupted nylon sutures.

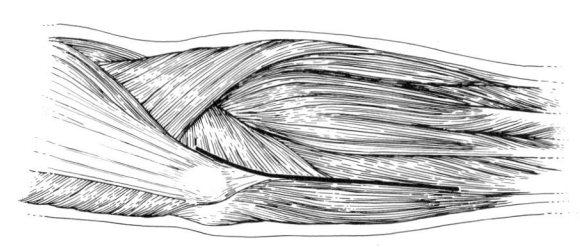

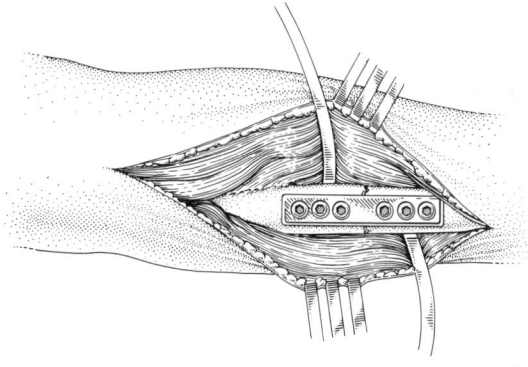

Postoperative management

The limb is placed in a plaster cast from the metacarpal heads to above the elbow, with the forearm in neutral rotation and the elbow flexed between 90° and 110°. It is maintained for approximately 4 weeks to allow soft tissue healing to stabilize the radial head. The plaster is removed and gentle flexion and extension exercises of the elbow commenced. Pronation and supination exercises are also started with the arm resting in a broad arm sling for about 2 weeks until a good range of movement is obtained.

OPEN REDUCTION OF THE RADIAL HEAD

Incision

10

A longitudinal incision is made over the lateral aspect of the elbow, based on the lateral epicondyle, and extending two fingers'-breadth above and two fingers'-breadth below. The skin is retracted and the space between the anconeus and the extensor mass is identified and split longitudinally to reveal the capsule, which is then divided. Care must be taken at the distal end of the wound where the posterior interosseous nerve passes round the proximal end of the radius.

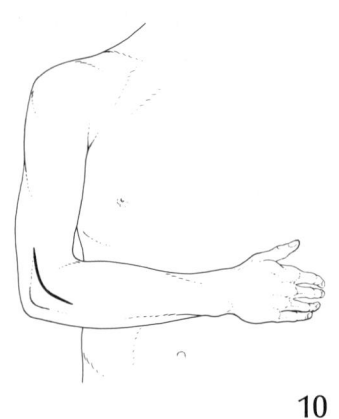

Procedure

11

Frequently, the radial head will be found lying over the flattened annular ligament. In younger patients, the head may have been levered out of an intact annular ligament, in others the ligament will have been ruptured. The ligament should be gently cleared to allow the radial head to return to its normal position, articulating with the capitellum. If possible, the edges of the annular ligament should be sutured over the neck of the radius. If instability remains, a Kirschner wire may be inserted across the radial head into the capitellum where it should remain for about 3 weeks until the soft tissues have healed. In this instance the elbow must be prevented from moving postoperatively by a plaster cast.

Postoperative management

This is the same as for closed reduction of the radial head.

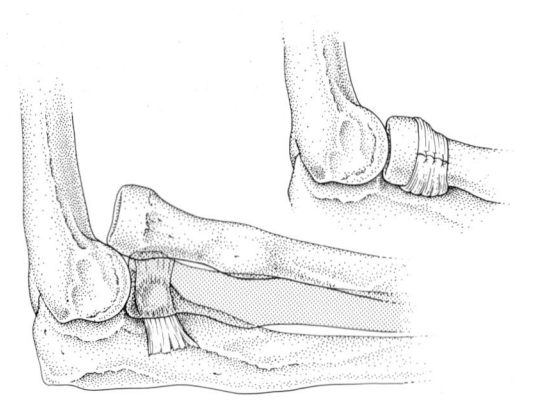

T–Y FRACTURES OF THE DISTAL HUMERUS

T–Y fractures of the distal humerus are frequently caused by a fall on the outstretched hand, with the force transmitted through the coronoid area of the ulna, splitting the two halves of the trochlea. The split in the trochlea passes to the two weak areas of the lower humerus in the supracondylar region and produces a three-part fracture. In some cases, comminution is severe and operative treatment cannot possibly accurately reconstitute the elbow. A reasonable closed reduction followed by skeletal traction through the distal ulna and early mobilization is an alternative approach to a very difficult operative procedure, especially in the elderly osteoporotic patient. Where the three main articular fragments can accurately be reduced and fixed, then operative treatment is advised to allow early movement and reduce the risk of elbow stiffness.

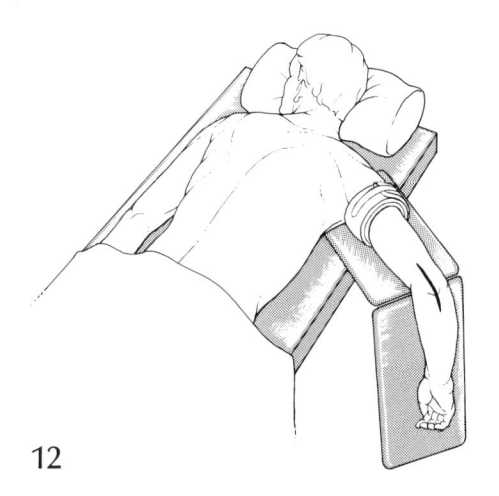

INTERNAL FIXATION

Position of patient

12

The patient lies prone with the shoulder abducted and medially rotated to bring the posterior aspect of the elbow into a convenient operating position. The elbow is allowed to hang over the edge of an arm board. A tourniquet is applied to the upper arm well above the elbow. The elbow is prepared and draped to allow access to the joint.

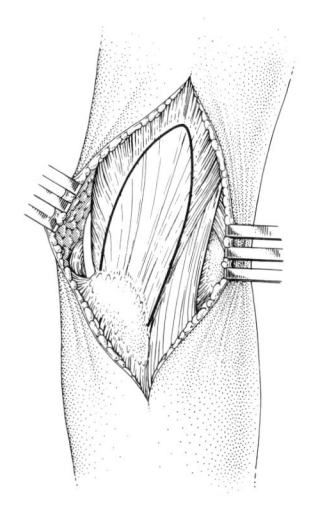

Incision

13

The posterior incision begins approximately 5 cm above the elbow joint and is continued over the tip of the olecranon and distally to the radial side of the subcutaneous border of the ulna for a distance of approximately 3 cm.

Exposure

14

Although the exposure can be performed without identifying the ulnar nerve, it is advisable to locate it on the medial side of the incision and to protect it with a moist tape. A triangular tendinous tongue of the triceps aponeurosis is fashioned, based on its insertion at the tip of the olecranon (see *Illustration 13*). The fracture will be identified beneath the aponeurosis after dividing the remaining muscle fibres in the midline, together with periosteum and capsule. Wider exposure can be obtained by stripping the periosteum on each side of the midline, releasing the muscular and capsular attachments. An alternative, less satisfactory, approach is to osteotomize the olecranon and to retract the proximal fragment of bone and the insertion of triceps to reveal the whole of the distal end of the humeral articular surface.

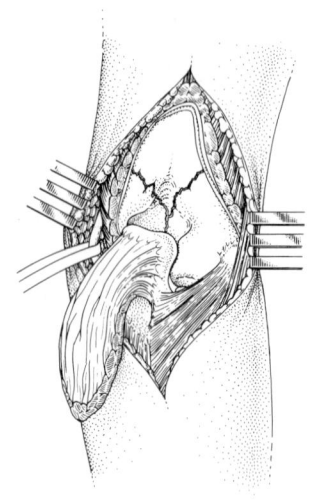

Procedure

15

The two main fragments forming the distal articular surface of the humerus are identified and the surfaces cleaned of haematoma and interposed periosteum.

A 3.2 mm drill hole is made through the fracture surface of the lateral fragment to the lateral epicondyle. The two articular fragments are reduced as accurately as possible and held with a towel clip. The drill is passed through the first drill hole from the lateral epicondyle, across the fracture site into the medial fragment towards the medial epicondyle. A depth gauge is used to measure the length of the AO malleolar screw required. The appropriate malleolar screw is inserted across the two distal articular fragments from the lateral side and the fracture is compressed. The screwed distal fragments are then fixed onto the humeral shaft using two semitubular plates placed over the supracondylar ridges, ensuring that the olecranon fossa remains clear to allow full extension of the elbow.

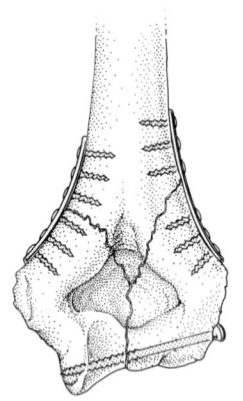

Closure

The wound is irrigated with saline. The aponeurotic tongue of triceps is sutured back into position with interrupted absorbable sutures and the skin with non-absorbable sutures. If an osteotomy of the olecranon has been performed, it should be fixed into position using the tension-band wiring technique or screw fixation. The wound is dressed and the elbow rested in a broad arm sling with the elbow flexed 90°–100°.

Postoperative management

Providing a strong and stable fixation of the fracture has been secured by operation, the elbow can be released from the sling at 7 days and gentle active assisted exercises, supervised by the physiotherapist, are carried out. Passive stretching of the elbow is forbidden since this may result in severe permanent stiffness of the elbow. Once the patient is relatively free of pain and has a reasonable range of movements, the sling can be discarded but no heavy activities are allowed until the fracture has united.

FRACTURE OF THE CAPITELLUM AND LATERAL CONDYLE

Fractures of the capitellum may vary from small cartilage-capped fragments of bone to a fragment containing the complete capitellum and the lateral half of the trochlea. The detached fragment may have little or no soft-tissue attachments. If the fragments are undisplaced, a conservative approach to treatment is advisable, especially in the elderly. Small displaced fragments should be removed since they may cause symptoms of a loose body, including locking and pain. In displaced fractures, open reduction and fixation of large fragments is essential for elbow stability and a good range of movements. Lateral condylar fragments, when displaced, also require open reduction and screw fixation.

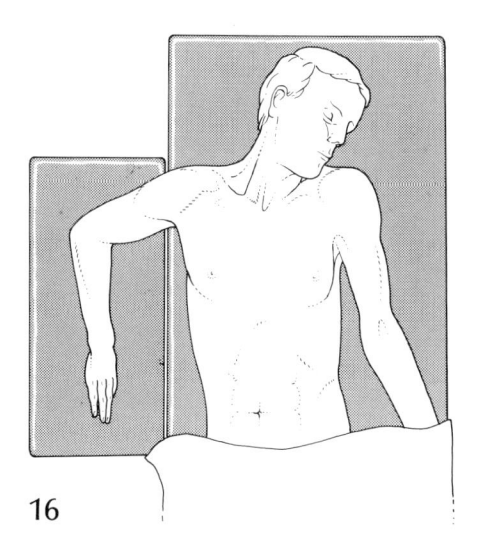

Position of patient

16

The patient is placed supine on the operating table with the elbow resting on an arm board.

After application of a padded pneumatic tourniquet to the upper arm, the elbow should be prepared and draped to allow a clear exposure of the joint. The elbow is abducted and medially rotated and placed on an arm rest.

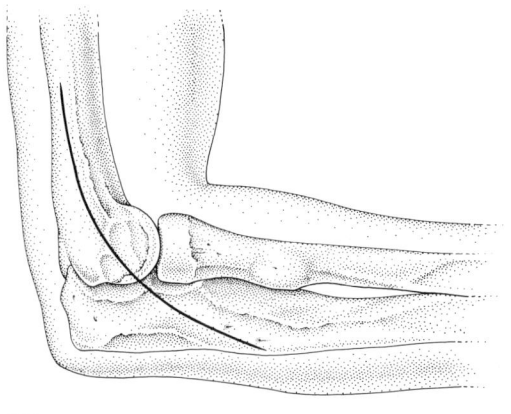

Incision

17

The skin incision is centred on the lateral epicondyle, extending three fingers'-breadth above it, but only two fingers'-breadth below the head of the radius to protect the posterior interosseous nerve.

Exposure

18

The incision is deepened to expose the attachment of the common extensor origin into the lateral epicondyle. The space between the anconeus muscle and the common extensor origin is identified and the latter is dissected forwards off the epicondyle. If a greater exposure is required, the radial extensors and brachioradialis are also stripped off the bone at the lateral supracondylar ridge. The radial nerve lies deep to these muscles and should be protected during exposure of the elbow joint. The capsule of the joint is divided vertically to expose the capitellum and the radial head.

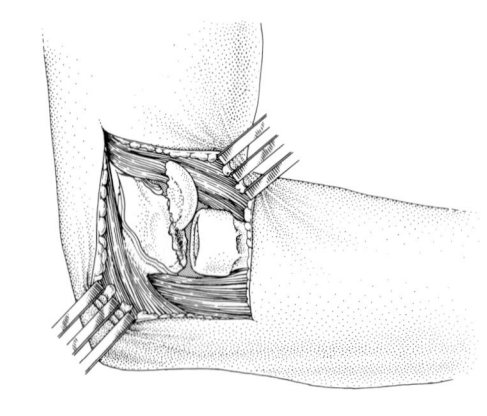

Procedure

19a & b

Small osteochondral fragments may be removed and discarded, but large fragments of the capitellum and those including the trochlea must be accurately reduced and fixed into position. After careful cleaning of the cancellous fracture ends, the fragments are accurately reduced. In many cases, accurate placement of two Kirschner wires provides a satisfactory fixation of the fracture. The ends of the wire should be bent to a right angle and excess wire broken off with wire cutters and buried in soft tissue. A very large lateral condylar fragment may be fixed with a cortical screw, using the lag screw principle.

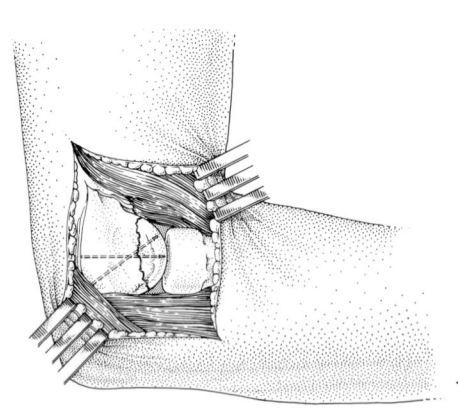

Closure

The wound is irrigated. Muscle is closed with interrupted absorbable sutures and the skin with interrupted non-absorbable sutures. A dressing is applied to the wound, and wool and a crêpe dressing applied to the elbow.

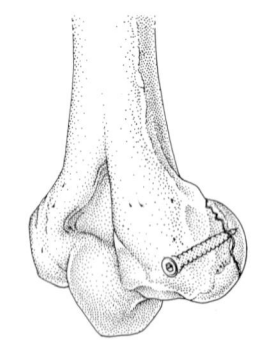

Postoperative management

Postoperative care is similar to that described for T–Y fractures.

Further reading

Colton CL. Fractures of the olecranon in adults: classification and management. *Injury* 1973; 5: 121–9.

Jupiter JB, Neff U, Holzach P, Allgower M. Intercondylar fracture of the humerus: an operative approach. *J Bone Joint Surg [Am]* 1985; 67-A: 226–39.

Reckling FW. Unstable fracture dislocations of the forearm (Monteggia and Galeazzi lesions). *J Bone Joint Surg [Am]* 1982; 64-A: 855–63.

Strachan JCH, Ellis BW. Vulnerability of the posterior interosseous nerve during radial head resection. *J Bone Joint Surg [Br]* 1971; 53-B: 320–3.

Illustrations by Geoff Lyth and Peter Cox

Operative treatment of fractures of the hand

N. J. Barton FRCS
Consultant Hand Surgeon, Nottingham University Hospital and Harlow Wood Orthopaedic Hospital, Mansfield, Nottinghamshire, UK

Introduction

Badly done internal fixation of fractures of bones of the hand gains nothing and often leads to complications such as stiffness or even non-union, which could have been avoided by simple conservative treatment. In order to achieve effective internal fixation that will allow immediate mobilization of joints and tendons, the correct equipment is essential and the surgeon must be familiar with its use[1]. The techniques are more difficult than those for large bones and there is very little margin for error. They should never be attempted in the Accident and Emergency Department.

Indications

1, 2a, b & 3

Operative treatment is indicated only in a small minority of fractures of the hand, perhaps 5 per cent. The indications were defined 30 years ago by Robins[2] as follows.

1. Fractures of the shafts of the phalanges, especially the proximal phalanx, in which it has proved impossible to obtain or maintain anatomical reduction by conservative means.
2. Fractures involving joints, with either:
   (a) a large displaced fragment of bone covered with articular cartilage; or
   (b) subluxation or dislocation of the joint.
3. Severe hand injuries with multiple fractures of the metacarpals and/or phalanges.

These indications remain valid, despite improvements in equipment and techniques, and will be discussed in turn. To them can now be added a fourth.

4. During reattachment of amputated digits. Here, since the distal part is completely detached, special considerations apply. The reader is referred to the chapter by Matiko and Lister[3].

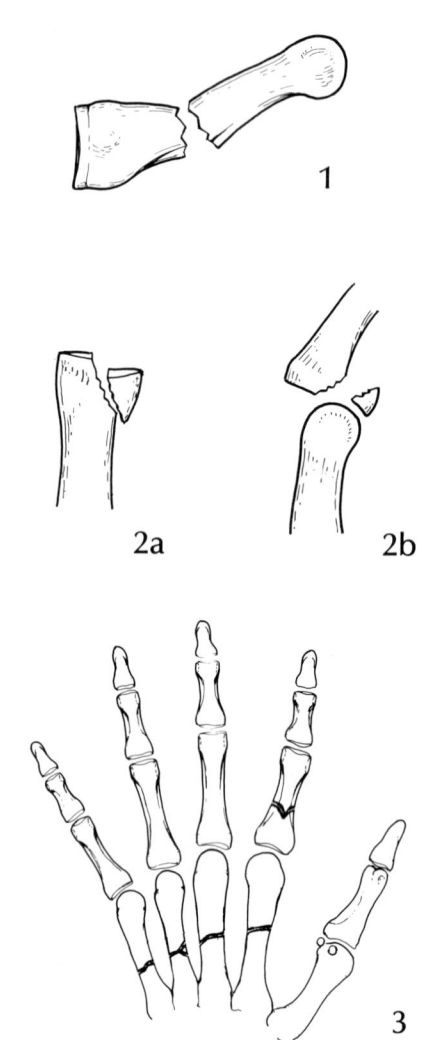

Equipment

Kirschner wires are difficult to insert obliquely by hand as they tend to go in too transverse a direction or else skid off and run longitudinally along the outside of the bone. It is helpful to have a power tool that can be held and controlled in one hand, leaving the surgeon's other hand free to control the fracture. The mini-driver made by the 3M Company (Loughborough, UK) is particularly suitable as the length of the wire projecting can be adjusted very quickly by a grip-release control.

Dental screws and plates can be used but the AO (ASIF) mini and small fragment sets, especially designed for use on hands and feet, are better. These sets include various types and sizes of screws, drills, taps and handles to hold them: the surgeon must be familiar with these and with the principles which will enable him to use them correctly[1].

A tourniquet should always be used (except for percutaneous wiring) to ensure a bloodless field and a clear view of the fracture.

Fracture of shaft of proximal phalanx

These fractures can often be reduced by closed manipulation and held by external splintage, and this should always be the first line of treatment. It is, however, necessary to obtain anatomical reduction, as the front of the phalanx is the floor of the tunnel in which the flexor tendon must glide up and down. If perfect reduction cannot be achieved by conservative means, then open reduction and internal fixation are indicated, provided the fracture is not comminuted.

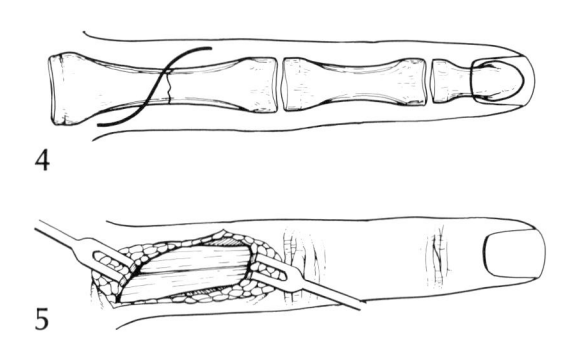

INTERNAL FIXATION BY CROSSED K-WIRES

Incision

4 & 5

An oblique, slightly sinuous incision is made along the back of the proximal phalanx and the extensor tendon split in its midline[4].

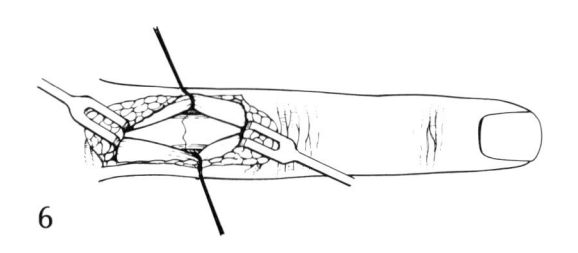

Exposure of the fracture

6

With small blunt hooks, the two halves of the extensor tendon are retracted to each side to expose the fracture, which is almost always angulated with its apex anterior. Its angulation must now be reversed to expose the broken ends of bone.

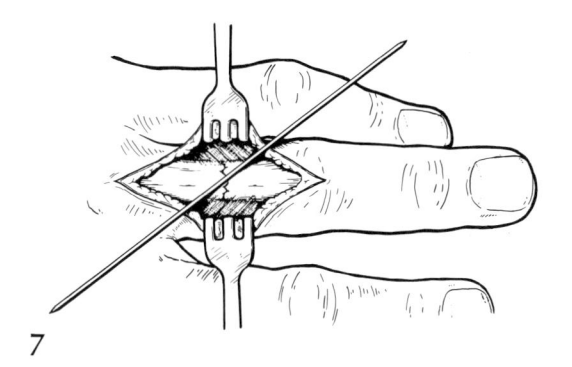

'Preview pin'

7

A Kirschner wire is laid across the dorsum of the reduced fracture to help plan the direction and angle of entry of the wires which will be used for fixation[5].

178 Upper limb fractures

Insertion of K-wires

8, 9 & 10

A Kirschner wire about 10 cm long and 1 mm wide and pointed at *both* ends is fitted into the chuck of a power tool, with about 2.5 cm of wire projecting. The point of the wire is inserted into the fracture surface of the distal fragment, in the midline but close to the dorsal cortex. The wire is then angulated in the coronal plane so that it is pointing half-laterally at an angle of 45° to the axis of the phalanx, and advanced through the cancellous bone and cortex (it is impossible to do this at the correct angle by hand: a power tool is essential).

The wire is further advanced so that it comes out through the skin in the midlateral line of the finger with at least 2 cm projecting. The power tool is then removed from the proximal end of the wire, and the distal end of the wire grasped in a small hand-held introducer and slowly and carefully withdrawn with a twisting motion, until the proximal end of the wire is flush with the fracture surface.

A second wire is inserted into the distal fragment but anterior to the first wire and passing obliquely to the other side of the bone. It is then advanced in a similar manner until its proximal end is flush with the fracture surface.

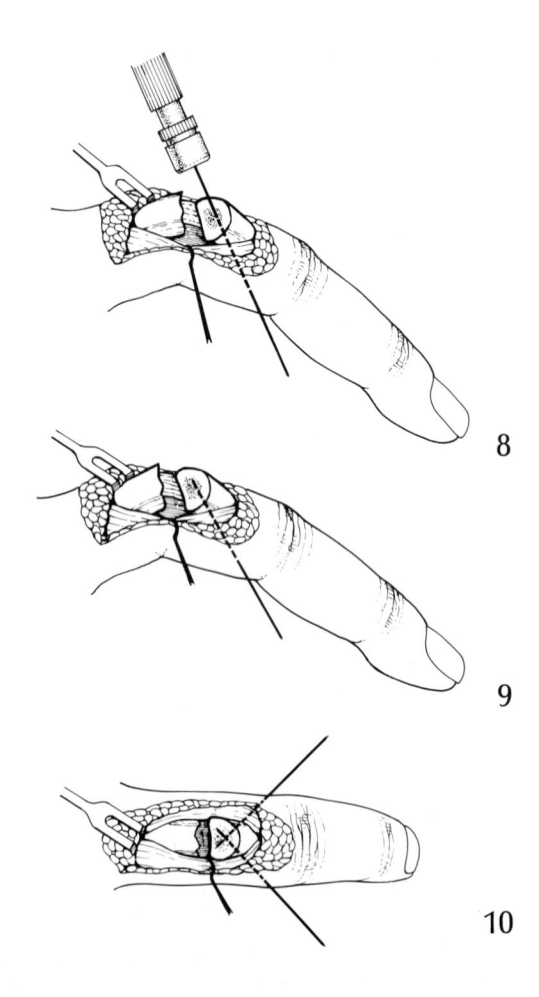

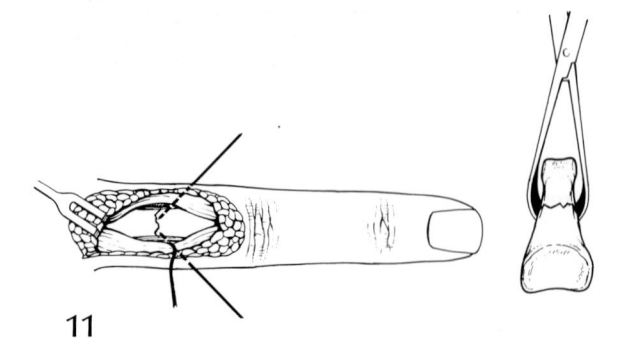

Reduction of the fracture

11

This is the most critical stage of the procedure. Keeping the other fingers flexed out of the way, the fracture is reduced under direct vision into an anatomical position and held from side to side with an instrument such as an Allis tissue forceps or, if the fracture line is slightly oblique, a towel clip (which may be inserted percutaneously if this is easier).

Retrograde insertion of first wire into proximal fragment

12 & 13

The distal end of either K-wire is now grasped in the power tool and the wire driven proximally (in the opposite direction to before), into the proximal fragment. As it reaches the cortex, the fracture will tend to displace and in particular to distract, so accurate reduction and compression must be maintained until the point of the wire is through the cortex and can be palpated through the skin. This end of the wire should not pierce or displace the skin.

The fracture is now loosely held but it is not stabilized against rotational forces. The distal part of the finger must be grasped and pushed proximally to compress the fracture surfaces together in the reduced position. While this reduction and compression are maintained, the other Kirschner wire is similarly driven into the proximal phalanx until it has just crossed the cortex.

If the fracture surfaces are allowed to part while this is being done, the second wire will keep them apart and delay or prevent union.

Any retractors are now removed from the dorsal wound and the fixation is tested by flexing the finger. It should be possible to move it through a fairly full range without movement occurring at the fracture site.

The distal ends of the wires should be cut off as short as possible, so that they are buried subcutaneously.

Closure

The extensor tendon is sutured with interrupted 4/0 nylon sutures, taking only the edge of the tendon to avoid bunching it up. The skin is carefully sutured and the tourniquet released.

The wound is dressed with tulle gras (or one of its variants), as bleeding from the wound makes ordinary dressings become hard and adherent. The finger is encircled with plaster wool 2.5 cm wide and then wrapped in a crêpe bandage of the same width (it is often necessary to cut these from wider rolls) to provide a firm supporting cylinder. However, this must not be so tight as to impair the circulation to the finger tip, which should therefore be left exposed for inspection.

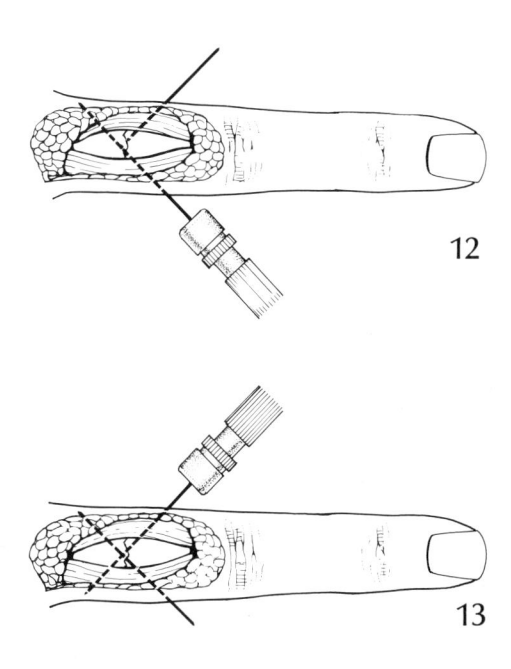

Postoperative management

The patient should remain in hospital with the hand elevated for at least 24 hours. Next day, the surgeon removes the dressings, replaces them by a small elastic adhesive plaster and instructs the patient in active finger flexion exercises to be performed every hour: this is the most important part of the treatment and it is the surgeon's responsibility to explain it to the patient and ensure that he is doing it satisfactorily before he is allowed home. The movements are needed not only for the joints but to prevent the extensor tendon getting stuck down. The physiotherapist reinforces this and continues supervision after the patient is discharged. Resisted exercises such as squeezing of putty or a rubber ball are forbidden, as they might cause redisplacement of the fracture.

The Kirschner wires should not be removed in less than 6 weeks and, if they are causing no trouble, need never be removed.

180 Upper limb fractures

OTHER METHODS

Longitudinal Kirschner wires

These are not recommended. They provide no resistance to rotation and little stability against angulation, and they usually cross a joint, unnecessarily increasing the risk of stiffness.

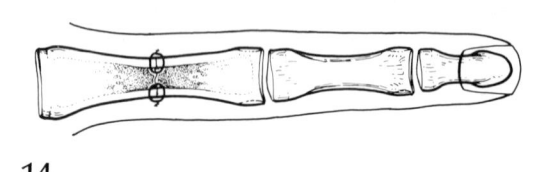

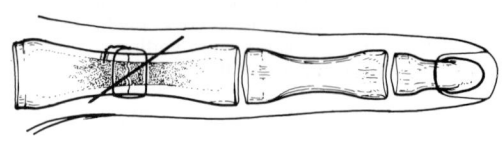

Parallel oblique Kirschner wires

This technique is particularly suited to oblique fractures. The method reduces the risk of distraction with crossed wires but retains the control of rotation.

Semicircular wiring

14

Small holes are drilled in each fragment close to each side of the fracture line on both sides of the finger and two small loops or circles of malleable wire (24 or 26 s.w.g.) are passed through the holes, one loop on each side of the phalanx. After reduction of the fracture, the wires are carefully tightened to hold the cortices together. Just twisting the wire usually breaks it at the base of the twist: the correct technique is to put on a preliminary slack twist, tighten by traction and twist only to take up the slack, repeating until the desired tension is achieved.

14

Lister's intraosseous wiring[6]

15

One short stout oblique Kirschner wire is combined with a single larger loop of flexible 24 or 26 s.w.g. wire which passes through both cortices on each side of the fracture. When the loop is tightened, the fracture surfaces are compressed together along the Kirschner wire. The redundant K-wire is cut off and the twisted ends of the flexible wire buried in a separate adjacent hole in the cortex. This method gives strong fixation but is tricky to perform, and should be practised on a dry bone first.

Both the above methods require exposure of both sides of the phalanx and should be done through two midlateral incisions.

There is no place for the use of plates on phalanges, as their application needs a larger exposure and the tendons become adherent, causing a stiff finger.

15

Oblique fracture of head of proximal phalanx

These fractures are uncommon, but their obliquity means that they usually displace, and this always results in a stiff, painful and deformed finger if open reduction and internal fixation are not done.

SCREW FIXATION

Exposure of fracture

16

A midlateral incision is made along the distal half of the proximal phalanx on the side of the displaced condyle. The extensor tendon is retracted dorsally and the neurovascular bundle anteriorly, using blunt hooks. This exposes the fracture on the side of the phalanx. The origin of the collateral ligament will be seen on the distal fragment.

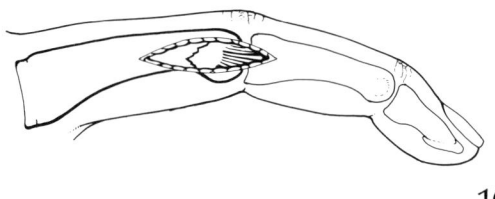

Reduction of fracture

A small instrument, such as a Watson Cheyne dissector or a dental probe, is inserted into the fracture to disimpact the surfaces. The distal part of the finger is then angulated away from the operator while the condylar fragment is guided with the instrument into a position of perfect reduction. It is not necessary, and is indeed undesirable, to open the proximal interphalangeal joint: if the proximal half of the fracture-line, including its dorsal aspect, which can be seen by retracting the extensor tendon, is *perfectly* reduced, then the distal (intra-articular) part, which cannot be seen, will also be reduced.

Reduction is held by a towel clip with one point in the most distal part of the distal fragment (leaving the middle of the fragment clear) and the other point penetrating the skin on the far side of the finger to enter the far side of the phalanx (the AO small fragment set contains a special reduction forceps with one flat end which may be used instead of the towel clip).

Drilling and tapping

17

With a 1.1 mm drill bit held in a small hand-tool, which can be operated with one hand, a hole is very carefully drilled in the cortex of the centre of the distal fragment (it may be necessary to make a small longitudinal incision in the origin of the collateral ligament to expose the bone, and then retract the ligamentous fibres on each side with skin hooks). The drill bit is very fine and fragile, and will break if bent or treated roughly.

Reduction is checked as perfect and kept firmly held with the towel clip. With counterpressure on the far side of the finger, drilling is continued in a transverse direction, across the fracture line and through the far cortex, until the drill can be felt beneath the skin. Using the depth gauge, the hole is measured to determine the required length of screw.

The 1.5 mm tap is then used to cut a thread in the walls of the hole.

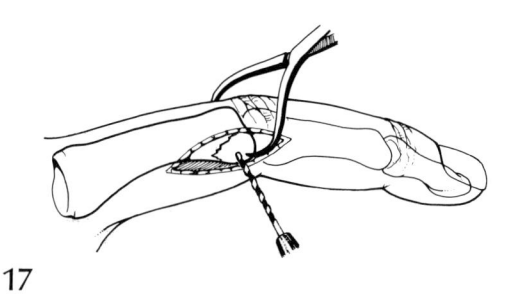

182 Upper limb fractures

Overdrilling the near fragment

18a–d

After checking the reduction again, the hole in the near cortex (i.e. on the distal fragment) is enlarged with a 1.5 mm drill, to allow the threaded part of the screw to slide in this fragment so that compression may be achieved *(a, b)*. If overdrilling is not done, a gap remains at the fracture site *(c, d)*. There is no need to overdrill the soft cancellous bone.

Insertion of screw

19

A screw of the chosen length and of 1.5 mm diameter is inserted across the fracture from the near to the far cortex and then tightened to compress the two fragments together. The 1.5 mm screws go up to 16 mm in length which is usually enough. (Alternatively, a 2.0 mm screw can be employed, though this has a rather large head: in this case the 1.5 mm drill is used first, then the 2.0 mm tap and the 2.0 mm drill to make the gliding hole in the nearest cortex.)

The towel clip is removed and fixation tested by gently flexing the proximal interphalangeal joint to 90°. There should be no movement at the fracture site. A check radiograph may be taken at this stage.

Closure and postoperative care

The skin is sutured with 5/0 nylon, the wound covered with a patch of tulle gras and a small supporting cylindrical dressing of wool and bandage applied as described above. Next morning the dressings are removed, or reduced to a minimum which will not restrict flexion, and active and passive movements begun.

In younger patients it is probably wise to remove the screw after about 3 months. This can be done under local anaesthesia, but the head of the screw may be difficult to find in the collateral ligament.

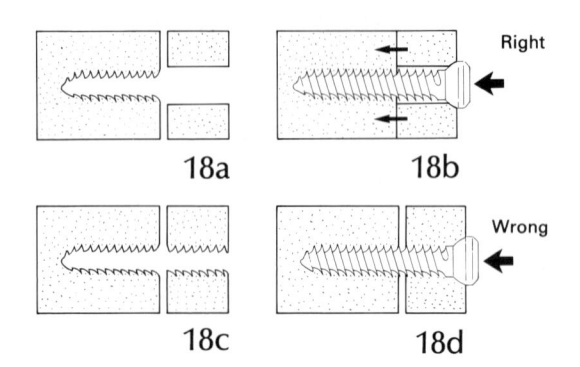

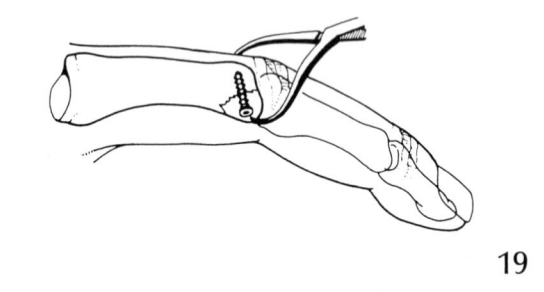

OTHER METHODS

Satisfactory fixation, though without compression, can be achieved by a transverse Kirschner wire, using the same approach and method described above. A 0.8 mm wire should be used: a larger one may split the distal fragment. Two parallel Kirschner wires give better fixation but increase the risk of shattering the distal fragment and losing all fixation.

Fracture-subluxation with a small bony fragment

In a fracture-subluxation it is essential to restore a normal relationship between the main joint surfaces, i.e. to reduce the subluxation. If this is done, the fracture will look after itself; if the subluxation is not corrected, then the joint cannot be expected to work normally.

PERCUTANEOUS KIRSCHNER WIRE FIXATION OF BENNETT'S FRACTURE-SUBLUXATION

The method described is that of Wagner[7]. Since no skin incision is made, a tourniquet is not necessary for this procedure.

Reduction of fracture

20

The base of the first metacarpal, which is subluxated laterally, is pushed medially towards the other metacarpals by the thumb of the surgeon's non-dominant hand while the index finger pulls the head of the first metacarpal laterally to extend (or radially abduct) it. The subluxation reduces easily and palpably.

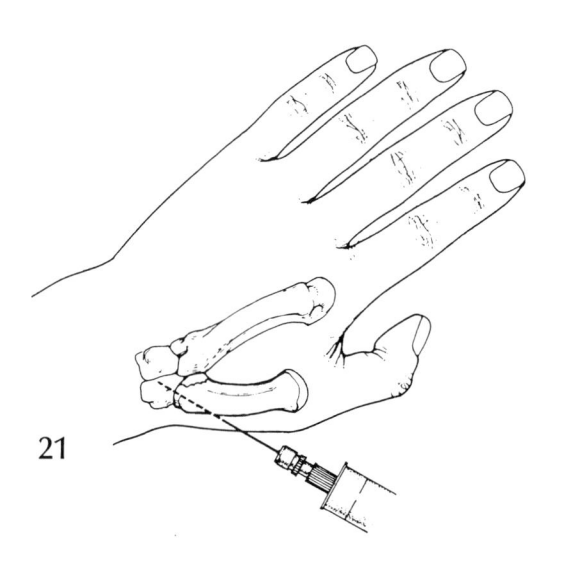

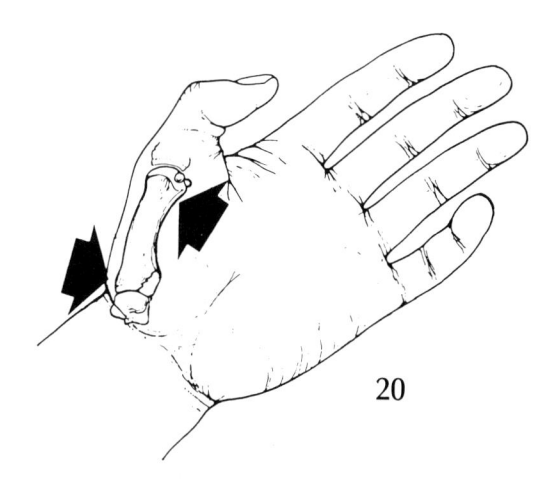

Insertion of K-wire

Reduction is maintained by the surgeon's non-dominant hand, or by the hands of a trusted and trusting assistant. A stout (e.g. 1mm) Kirschner wire of measured length, mounted on a power tool, is inserted into the dorsoradial aspect of the shaft of the first metacarpal near the junction of its proximal and middle thirds. Once the point of the wire has engaged the cortex, the wire is angled so that it lies almost parallel to the shaft of the metacarpal and is then driven proximally, aiming towards the centre of the trapeziometacarpal (saddle) joint. No attempt is made to transfix the small bony fragment.

Transfixion of joint in reduced position

21

After checking that reduction is still maintained, the wire is driven further proximally until it crosses the joint and enters the trapezium. The position can be checked by radiography (an image intensifier saves much time), but this is not essential; if it is no longer possible to subluxate the joint, then the aim has been achieved, wherever the wire is. In practice, it sometimes goes into the second metacarpal but this does not matter.

Optional introduction of second wire

Salgeback et al.[8] recommend using a second wire, which enters the medial or ulnar side of the first metacarpal and crosses the first wire obliquely.

Application of below-elbow cast

The part of the wire still outside the patient is bent to a right angle just above the skin and cut off, leaving the bent end sticking out but covered with a small dressing. A padded below-elbow cast of plaster of Paris is applied, immobilizing the carpometacarpal and metacarpophalangeal joints of the thumb but leaving the interphalangeal joint of the thumb and all the finger joints free. The cast is well moulded over the lateral side of the base of the first metacarpal.

Removal of cast and wires

The cast and wire(s) are removed after 6 weeks and there is usually little difficulty in regaining movement of the joint. It is a mistake to remove the wire(s) too soon as the subluxation may recur.

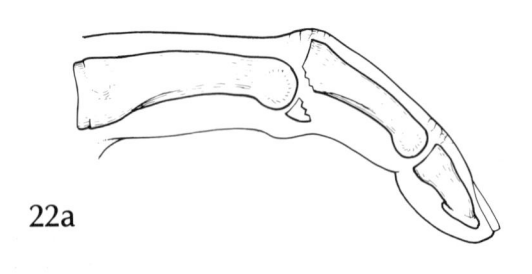

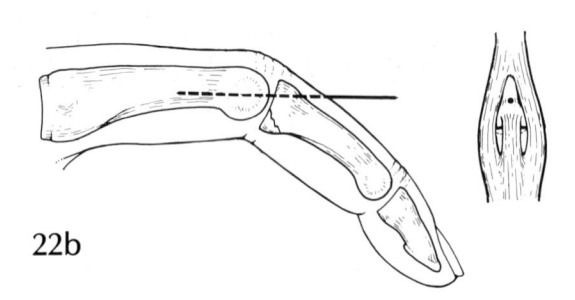

22a & b

PERCUTANEOUS K-WIRE FIXATION OF FRACTURE-SUBLUXATION OF PROXIMAL INTERPHALANGEAL JOINT

A similar method may be used for fracture-subluxation of the proximal interphalangeal joint with a small anterior fragment and dorsal displacement of the middle phalanx. The wire is introduced through the triangular bare area of bone on the dorsum of the base of the middle phalanx, just distal to the insertion of the central slip and in between the lateral bands of the extensor mechanism. It should be removed after 3 weeks, when an extension block splint[9] is applied and the permitted range of extension is gradually increased over another 3 weeks.

Fractured shafts of metacarpals

When only one metacarpal is broken, angulation is limited by its intact neighbours and fixation is not necessary.

SCREW FIXATION

Long spiral fractures may be fixed by one or two transverse screws, inserted to produce interfragmentary compression, as described above for intra-articular fractures with a large fragment, though in the metacarpal the bigger 3.5 mm or 2.7 mm screws can be used.

PLATING

Plating may be indicated for transverse or short oblique fractures of two or more metacarpals[10].

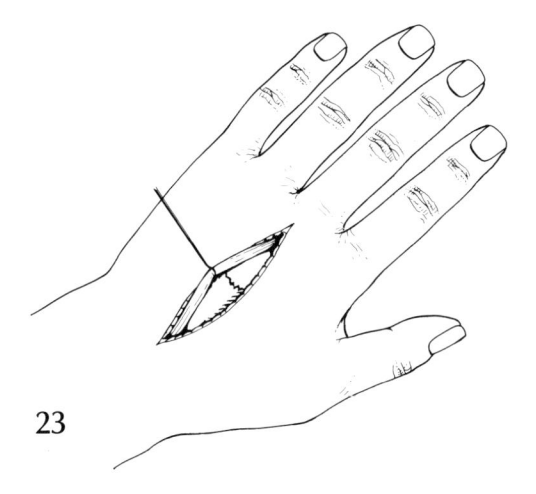

Exposure

23

Two adjacent metacarpals can be exposed through one dorsal longitudinal incision over the intermetacarpal space, about 6 cm long and centred over the fractures. If three or four metacarpals are to be plated, a second incision is needed: the incisions should be parallel and not too close together. The first fracture to be dealt with is exposed by retracting the overlying extensor tendon to one or other side with a blunt hook.

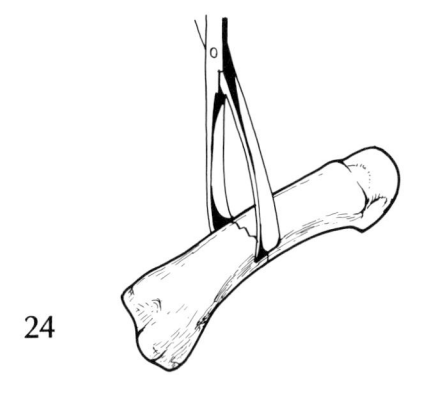

Reduction

24

The fracture is anatomically reduced and held with a suitable instrument.

186 Upper limb fractures

Selection of plate

25a & b

A plate is chosen from the AO small fragment set. It must have a minimum of two holes on each side of the fracture, i.e. at least a four-hole plate (a). If the fracture is near one end of the metacarpal, a T-shaped plate may be preferred (b).

The plate is laid over the fracture and held in position with its midpoint over the fracture line.

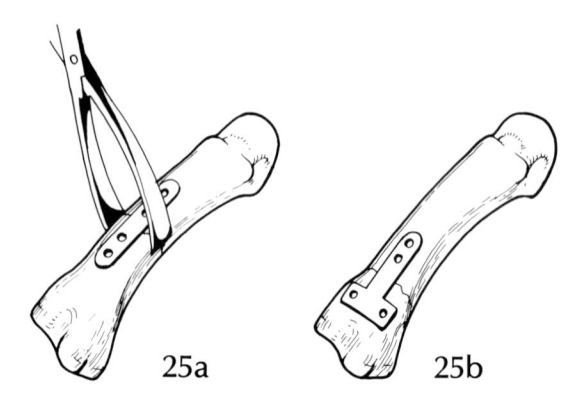

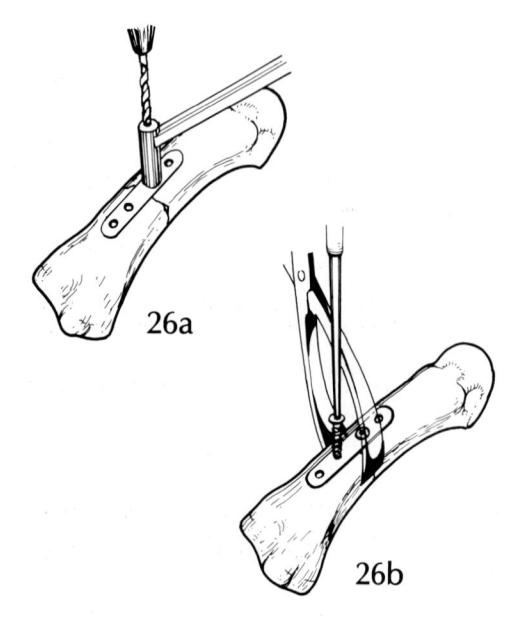

Drilling, tapping and insertion of first screw

26a & b

Using a 2.5 mm drill through the corresponding drill guide seated in the hole of the plate which is just distal to the fracture, a hole is drilled across the distal fragment until it has passed through both cortices. The length of the hole is measured with the depth gauge and the appropriate length of screw chosen. A 3.5 mm tap is then used to cut a thread in the bone surrounding this hole and a cortical screw of the same diameter inserted to its full length but not finally tightened at this stage. If the bones are very small, the 2.7 mm tap and screw may be used instead.

Insertion of second screw

27

The reduction must now be checked or, if it has been lost during the foregoing procedures, restored. This is a critical stage, and the plate must be held firmly onto both fragments, with the fracture perfectly reduced, while the second screw is inserted.

This should be into the plate hole in the proximal fragment nearest the fracture, and the drill should be introduced in the most proximal part of the hole in the plate, rather than its centre. Once the plate is seen to be lying correctly along the bone, the first screw is tightened. Then the second screw is tightened in the eccentric drill hole, so that its head comes up against the lip of the hole and is forced to slide distally, carrying the proximal bony fragment with it, thus compressing the fracture surfaces together.

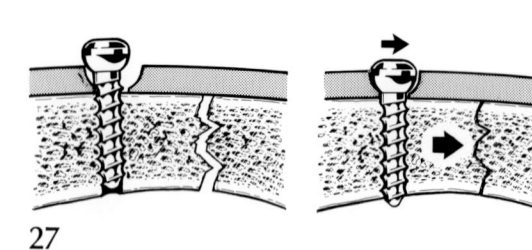

Insertion of remaining screws

28

Once fixation has been achieved, the remaining holes are drilled in the centre of their plate holes. They are measured and tapped, and the third and fourth screws inserted to complete fixation.

Closure

If possible, very fine sutures are used to appose periosteum or areolar tissue over the plate to separate it from the extensor tendon, to prevent adherence of the tendon which would limit flexion of the fingers.

The skin is sutured and a firm supportive dressing of wool and bandages applied.

Postoperative management

The hand is elevated in hospital for 48 hours. The dressings are then reduced to a minimum, and active flexion and extension exercises started under the guidance of the physiotherapist. Only when these are being achieved satisfactorily may the patient go home, continuing the exercises as an outpatient.

In a young patient, the plate and screws should probably be removed after the bone is fully united and full function has been regained, which usually takes 3 or 4 months.

Acknowledgement

I am grateful to my colleague Mr C. L. Colton, FRCS FRCS(Orth)Ed for his advice on the details of screw fixation.

References

1. Heim U, Pfeiffer KM. *Internal fixation of small fractures. Technique recommended by the AO-ASIF group*. 3rd ed. Berlin: Springer-Verlag, 1988.

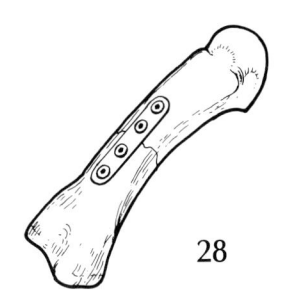

2. Robins RHC. *Injuries and infections of the hand*. London: Edward Arnold, 1961.

3. Matiko J, Lister G. Fixation of fractures in reattachment of amputated parts. In: Barton NJ, ed. *Fractures of the hand and wrist*. Edinburgh: Churchill Livingstone, 1988: 191–206.

4. Pratt DR. Exposing fractures of the proximal phalanx of the finger longitudinally through the dorsal extensor apparatus. *Clin Orthop* 1959; 15: 22–6.

5. Edwards GS, O'Brien ET, Heckman MM. Retrograde cross-pinning of transverse metacarpal and phalangeal fractures. *Hand* 1982; 14: 141–8.

6. Lister G. Intraosseous wiring of the digital skeleton. *J Hand Surg* 1978; 3: 427–35.

7. Wagner CJ. Method of treatment of Bennett's fracture dislocation. *Am J Surg* 1950; 80: 230–1.

8. Salgeback S, Eiken O, Carstam N, Ohlsson NM. A study of Bennett's fracture – special reference to fixation by percutaneous pinning. *Scand J Plast Reconstr Surg* 1971; 5: 142–8.

9. Strong ML. A new method of extension-block splinting for the proximal interphalangeal joint: a preliminary report. *J Hand Surg* 1980; 5: 606–7.

10. Ford DJ, El-Hadidi S, Lunn PG, Burke FD. Fractures of the metacarpals: treatment by AO screw and plate fixation. *J Hand Surg* 1987; 12-B: 34–7.

Illustrations by Department of Medical Illustration, Western Infirmary, Glasgow

Primary treatment of the acutely injured hand

Campbell Semple FRCS
Consultant Hand Surgeon, Western Infirmary, Glasgow, UK

Introduction

Aetiology

The patient can always describe how or by what the injury was caused – *this is important*. It makes a tremendous difference to diagnosis, treatment and prognosis of a wound if it has been caused by a broken bottle, a football boot or the roller of a printing press – each mechanism will produce very different types and degrees of tissue damage. Any surgeon dealing with a steady flow of hand injuries should be familiar with the industries and machinery common in the locality. Quite apart from the knowledge gained about the injury itself, the circumstances of the injury may well be of medicolegal significance – the time to note these down is *now*, at the first meeting with the patient.

1

It is preferable to have a simple clinical examination form relating to hand injuries, with some of the more important structures noted on it, so that the staff, particularly the junior staff, in an accident department or emergency room, do not miss important aspects of examination and diagnosis of injured hands.

Types of injury to the hand

Blunt injury

2a & b

Blunt injury to the hand generally produces bone or joint injury only. A *direct* blow to the finger or hand usually causes a transverse fracture, and if a particularly localized force is involved, a compound skin wound may be present.

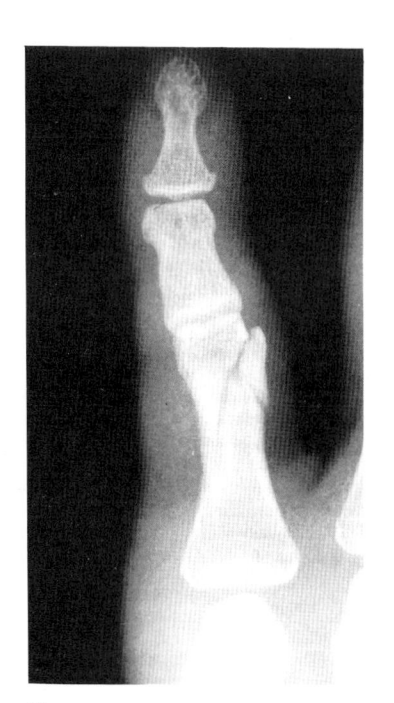

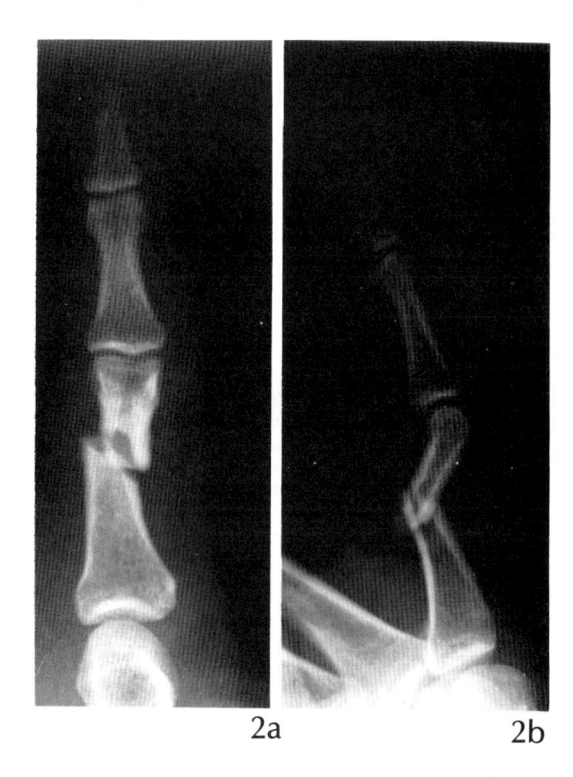

3

An *indirect* force, such as the twisting injury when a finger is caught in an opponent's shirt, is more likely to produce a spiral or oblique fracture of the proximal phalanx, or a tear of a joint, for example the metacarpophalangeal joint ligament injury which follows falls while skiing. The subsequent displacement of these bone and joint injuries usually bears little relation to the original force, but is caused by the pull and imbalance of local tendons and muscles.

Sharp injuries

4

When a hand or finger is damaged by a knife, broken glass or other sharp edge, tendons and nerves are usually damaged. The diagnosis may not be obvious, but tendon and nerve damage *must* be suspected in any hand that has been cut by a sharp object. It must be remembered that the force behind a fall on to a broken bottle or through a window is considerable, and the glass will penetrate the hand until stopped, that is until it strikes bone. There is much vulnerable anatomy between the skin and the skeleton on the palmar aspect of the hand and fingers, and all these tendons, nerves and muscles are very liable to injury. While the entry wound itself may be relatively small, a great deal of damage may have been caused which, if not recognized and repaired promptly, can result in sensory loss and weakness distally in the fingers.

High-pressure injuries

Any injury in the hand involving high pressure must be treated most carefully as there is generally much more damage present than is initially apparent. Widespread damage to the whole thickness of the hand, including the intrinsic muscles and deep fascial compartments, may lead to swelling and oedema over the following few days, often producing secondary necrotic changes in these deep compartments and permanent contractures of the hand and fingers. Emergency fasciotomy of the forearm, wrist and hand should be considered in an attempt to avoid these secondary contractures.

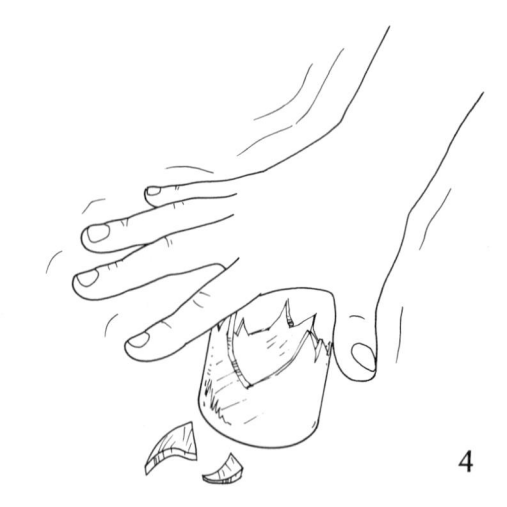

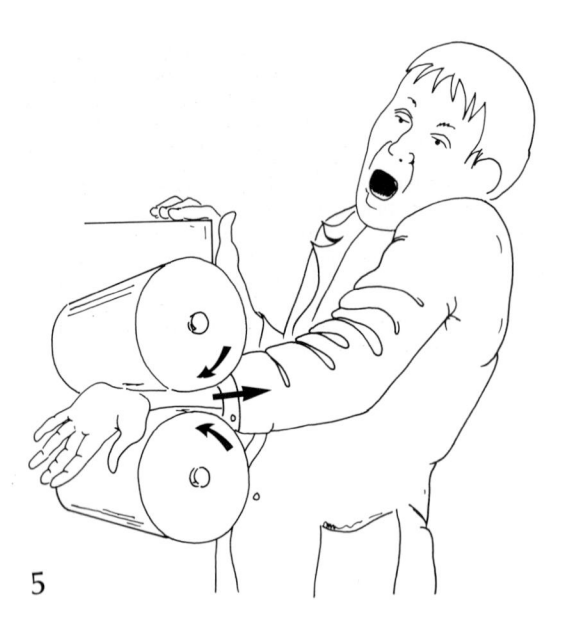

5

Roller injuries High-pressure rollers are used in many industries, such as printing, textiles and paper works, as well as in the home. Apart from the high-pressure injuries described above, there may be a degloving injury caused by the patient's attempt to withdraw the hand from the rollers. The flaps are generally distally based and have a poor prognosis because of the impaired venous return. While in a partially degloved finger it may be possible to carry out microvascular anastomosis and preserve the skin of the finger, with a completely degloved finger a primary amputation is generally necessary. Degloved skin on the palm of the hand generally requires excision of at least part of the flap – the more proximal portion – and application of a thick split-skin graft either primarily or a few days later.

6

High-pressure injection injuries These are caused by industrial implements, such as oil or grease guns, paint sprays or hydraulic or diesel-injection pipes. The entry wound is often tiny, and the patient may hardly be aware of the specific injury. Whether the injected material is oil, grease, paint, paint solvent, hydraulic or diesel oil it will produce a chemical irritation of the tissues – especially paint, light oils or thinners/solvents. Because the fluid is injected at high pressure it is generally distributed throughout a considerable volume of tissue and is often impossible to remove by excision or washing. The serious implications of these injuries must be appreciated, however, and the hand or finger promptly explored in an operating theatre. Thicker more viscous materials, like grease, may well be removable, but if there is evidence of widespread thinner, organic fluid, formal primary amputation of the digit may be necessary (*see* chapter on 'High pressure injection injuries', *The Hand* pp. 85–92).

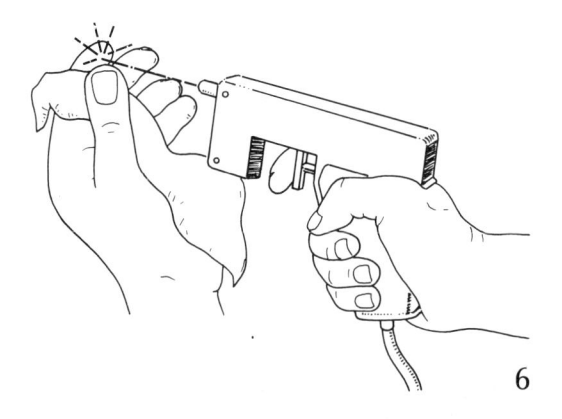

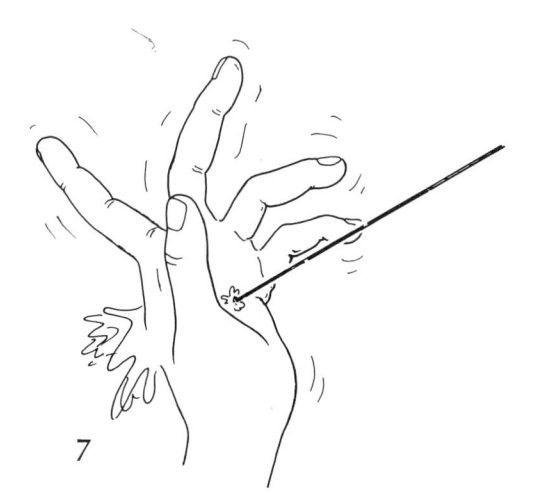

7

Gunshot wounds Injuries caused by low-velocity projectiles, such as airgun and shotgun pellets at more than a few yards range, may be treated as simple wounds with a contained foreign body. Removal of the pellets need not be carried out on the day of injury: it is generally better to leave them where they are until later, more formal exploration being easier when the oedema and inflammation of the initial injury have settled.

High-velocity gunshot wounds are an entirely different problem. If the hand or forearm has been struck by a bullet from a modern rifle, particularly a military rifle, then very much more damage will have occurred than is immediately apparent (*see* chapter on 'Blast injuries of the hand', *The Hand* pp. 82–84).

192 Upper limb fractures

Primary management of the injured hand

8a & b

The patient must initially be reassured, as he must be relaxed and in a cooperative mood before proper examination of the hand, and particularly of the distal nerve function, can be carried out.

It must be stressed that there is nothing to be gained by trying to look *into* the wound of the hand. For example, in a transverse cut on the front of the wrist there is nothing to be seen in the wound apart from a bit of blood and perhaps some tendon ends: it is impossible to identify these tendons or achieve anything worth while by poking about in the wound, and indeed you may do a considerable amount of harm and you will certainly alarm and hurt the patient (a).

A brief look *at* the wound (*b*), noting its approximate extent coupled with awareness of the cause of the injury, should suffice, and the wound can then be covered by a simple temporary moist dressing.

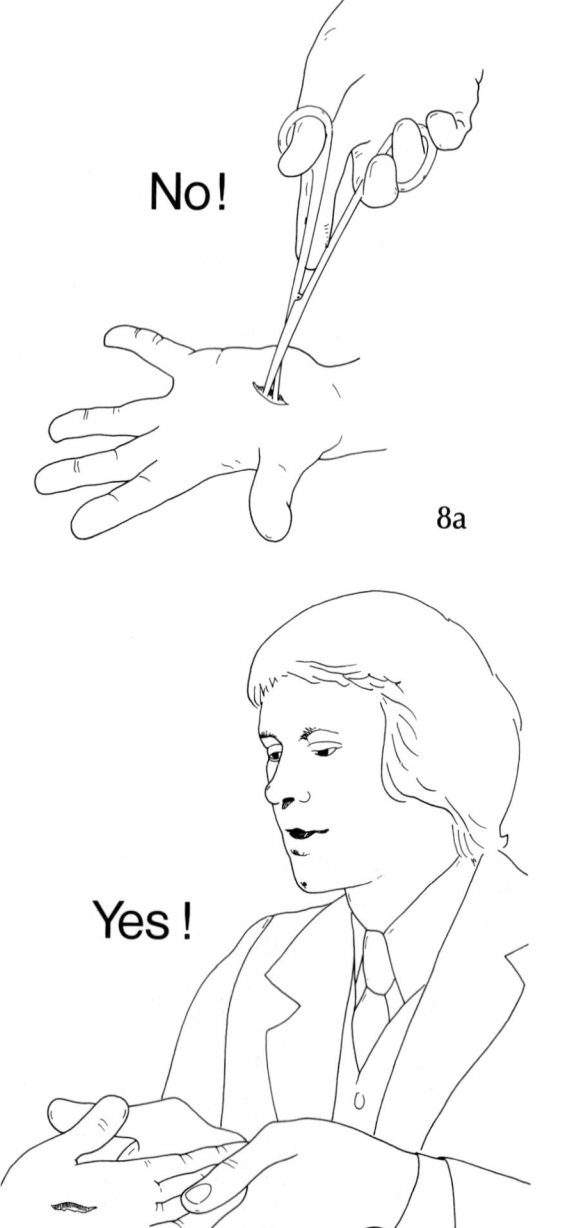

No!

8a

Yes!

8b

9

Attention should then be turned to the function of the hand distal to the wound: careful examination of the movement and sensation in the fingers and thumb should establish an effective diagnosis regarding divided or damaged structures. For example, the patient may have altered sensation in the median nerve territory, and be unable to flex the index and middle fingers; this implies that the patient has cut at least the median nerve and the flexor tendons to the index and middle fingers. Further damage may become apparent when the wrist is formally explored in the operating room.

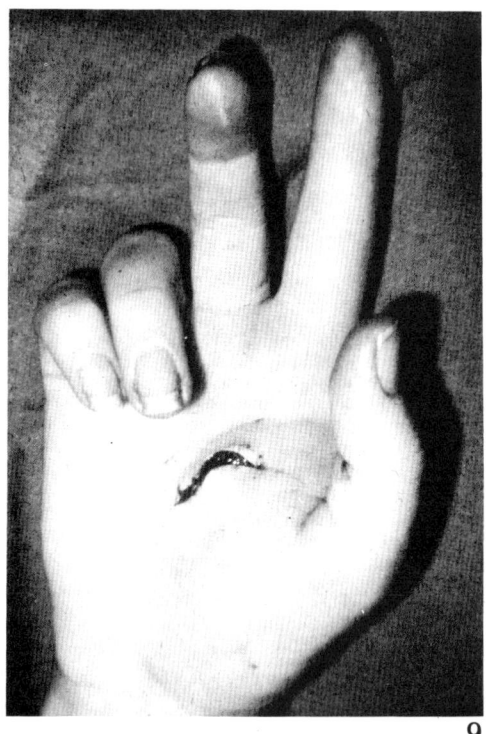

10

When a single digit has been badly damaged, it may be better for the hand and the patient to advise primary amputation of the digit rather than to embark on a long and complicated series of operations and reconstructive work to salvage a poor-quality digit. It is generally preferable to amputate fingers which have been caught in machinery and badly mangled, the aim being to achieve primary healing of good skin over the amputation stump.

Replantation of a finger or fingers is possible in selected cases when the following conditions are met: there is a clean-cut amputation of the digit; the digit itself is of significant value to the hand, for example the thumb, and the patient is young and robust enough to undergo the rather lengthy surgery and long-term rehabilitation that will be necessary. It is also assumed that there is a surgical team available who are skilled in this type of work. The primary treatment in such a case should be to (1) reassure and resuscitate the patient; (2) place the amputated part in a clean plastic bag which is then put inside another bag containing ice; and (3) telephone the appropriate microsurgical unit for advice.

In assessing skeletal injury, routine radiographs of an injured hand should be carried out in three planes: anteroposterior, lateral and oblique. With fractures in the regions of the proximal interphalangeal joint it is often worth obtaining further films, magnified if possible, and carefully centred on the actual fracture site, before planning specific treatment.

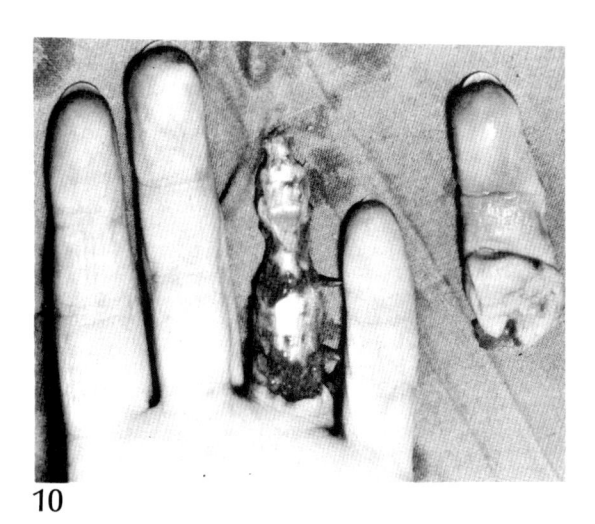

11

All bleeding from the hand should stop following simple elevation and a pressure dressing. There is no case for inserting clamps or haemostats into a wound of the hand in an attempt to arrest bleeding. This type of treatment will only cause further trouble by clamping or otherwise damaging peripheral nerves and tendons. Formal identification and treatment of the various structures in the hand requires proper operating theatre facilities.

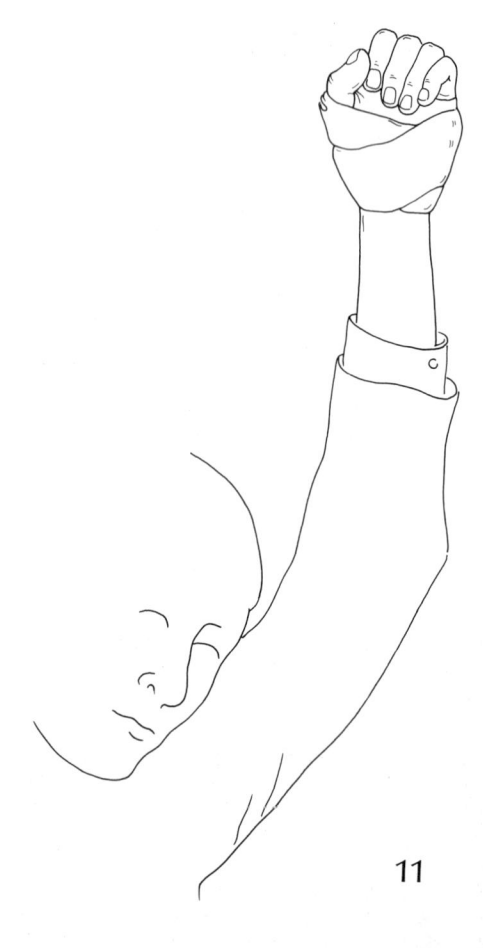

11

Anaesthesia

Adequate anaesthesia of the hand must be achieved before proper treatment can be carried out. A general anaesthetic will certainly produce this, but an anaesthetist is not always available. There are certain advantages in carrying out good regional anaesthesia, particularly if one of the longer acting anaesthetic agents, such as bupivacaine (Marcain, Astra, UK), is used. An axillary or supraclavicular brachial block can produce excellent anaesthesia for the arm, and any surgeon carrying out a considerable amount of hand surgery is well advised to learn these techniques.

For simple manipulations and very short operations intravenous regional anaesthesia (Bier block) may well be appropriate, although it is not easy to carry out careful dissection techniques on the hand under this type of anaesthetic block. One must be aware of the possible fatal result of using bupivacaine in a Bier block and allowing a large amount of bupivacaine to enter the general circulation. For injuries or surgical treatment in the distal half of the finger, a digital or metacarpal nerve block may be used, but this type of anaesthesia is rarely adequate for working on the proximal interphalangeal joint or the proximal phalanx (for further information, *see* chapter on 'Anaesthesia for hand injury', *The Hand* pp. 12–19).

Operative treatment

Once the patient is in the operating theatre and adequate anaesthesia has been achieved, the decision must be taken as to whether to use a tourniquet or not. Most wounds in the front of the hand or wrist will require a bloodless field. A tourniquet with efficient pneumatic control, keeping the pressure at approximately 300 mmHg, will allow proper identification of divided structures, nerves etc. in the wound. Once the various structures have been identified it is advisable to release the tourniquet and achieve haemostasis in order to avoid postoperative haematomas and complications of wound healing. Some surgeons prefer to keep the tourniquet in place until all the wound dressings and bandaging are completed, but this requires skill and experience in judging the pressure to apply in the various dressings.

The wound

12

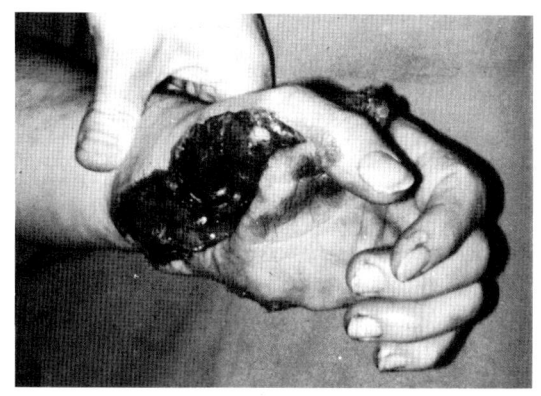

Palmar degloving injury following a roller press accident, which would be most unsuitable for primary closure as skin necrosis would be very likely to develop

12

With the majority of clean incised wounds of the hand, wound edge excision is not necessary. This precaution is only really necessary in wounds which have been caused by very dirty or potentially infected mechanisms, such as agricultural machinery, or where there is a crushing element involved in the skin edges of the wound, as in a hand that has been caught in gear machinery. With all wounds, however, thorough cleaning of the skin edges is necessary and this requires copious amounts of saline and a mild detergent. Surgical preparation of the skin prior to surgery is best carried out with a solution of chlorhexidine (Hibitane, ICI Pharmaceuticals, UK); a solution of chlorhexidine in alcohol is appropriate when there is no skin wound, but if there is a significant wound of the skin then chlorhexidine and water is safer.

Once the various damaged structures in the hand have been identified the question of repairing them primarily or leaving them until later arises. The majority of civil and industrial injuries are reasonably clean wounds, there is no significant contamination, and it is very much better to repair all divided structures at the initial operation. Both flexor tendons and digital and wrist nerves should be repaired on the day of injury. This assumes of course that the damage has been *diagnosed*, and that an *adequately skilled surgeon is available*. Suture of nerves and tendons is not easy, and requires experience and skill – in general, most surgeons should be capable of handling 6/0 nylon easily. If he is uncertain of his ability with tendons or nerves he should contact a more experienced surgeon promptly.

There are three exceptions to this general rule of primary repair.

1. Gunshot wounds, especially high-velocity missile wounds. These are very difficult and deceptive wounds to manage.
2. Infected, or potentially infected, wounds with considerable contamination, particularly by Gram-negative or anaerobic organisms. The surgeon should beware especially of wounds caused by human or animal teeth, as these are highly contaminated by such organisms and wound infection invariably follows primary skin closure.
3. Wounds caused by high-pressure machines, where a considerable amount of deep hidden damage is likely to be present.

Foreign bodies

Foreign bodies in the hand, such as pieces of glass, bits of wood or metal objects, i.e. needles or portions of gunshot, should only be removed if they are perfectly obvious and require little in the way of dissection or surgery. It is generally a mistake to go looking for foreign bodies, particularly if the entry wound is small, as a great deal of harm can be done by such dissection. It is generally best to wait until the wound is fully healed, and if the foreign body is then causing symptoms it will be easy to identify and remove it at formal elective surgery.

Fractures and dislocations

13

It should be possible to reduce all skeletal deformities on the day of injury. Some fractures, such as those in the metacarpal region and in the region of the distal phalanx, may not require accurate reduction or significant fixation. It is important, however, to concentrate on fractures and dislocations lying between the head of the metacarpal and the base of the middle phalanx, i.e. injuries involving the metacarpophalangeal joint, the proximal phalanx and the proximal interphalangeal joint. This problem zone gives rise to considerable morbidity if these injuries are not accurately reduced, and later reconstruction can be almost impossible.

It is not easy to reduce and maintain the reduction in a displaced fracture in this problem zone, and some form of internal fixation is generally required, for example a Kirschner wire or a small screw. In a straightforward transverse fracture of a proximal phalanx a longitudinal Kirschner wire will provide simple but adequate fixation of the fracture for the week or two required for initial healing. In multiple fractures, particularly when compound, Kirschner wires are the only safe method of dealing with the problem. More complex methods using screws or plates or intraosseous wiring involve considerable dissection and are likely to lead to infection and other postoperative complications. The reader is referred to the appropriate fracture chapters for further details on fracture management.

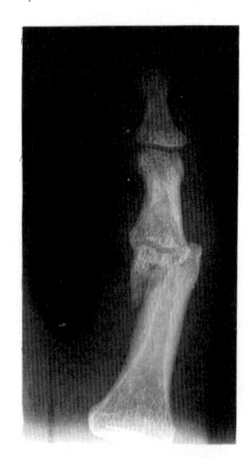

14

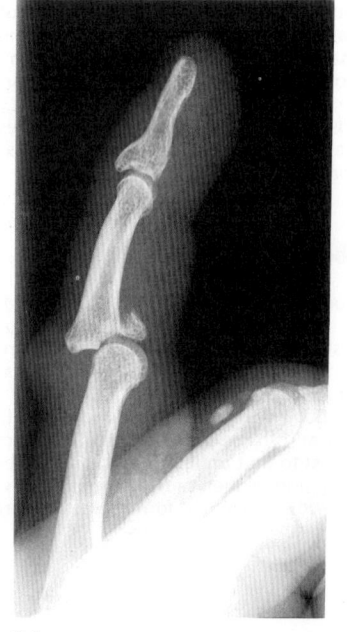

Simple dislocations of the proximal interphalangeal joint such as often occur on the football field are often reduced at the time of injury and give rise to few further problems. One should beware, however, of dislocation or subluxation of the joint which is associated with a fracture of the base of the middle phalanx. These can be extremely difficult injuries to deal with and often result in considerable stiffness of the proximal interphalangeal joint, with significant loss of function. It is vitally important that the subluxation or dislocation is fully reduced and held reduced, without doing too much damage to the joint itself. The simplest method of doing this is to reduce the dislocation and hold it with a longitudinal Kirschner wire; opening the joint and replacing the fracture fragment at the base of the middle phalanx should only be attempted if the surgeon is fully confident of his ability to operate in this small and difficult zone.

15 & 16

Most fractures and dislocations of the hand can be treated, after reduction if necessary, in a simple volar plaster cast, as illustrated. The aim of the splint is to rest the hand in a comfortable yet natural position for a week or so to allow the swelling and pain to settle, so that the patient can then begin to move the fingers. There is no difficulty in fracture healing in the hand, but a careful eye should be kept on the fractures to make sure that they do not displace during this period.

It should not be imagined that a plaster cast can hold any fractures of the hand in a particular position or reduction and thereby regain normal anatomical alignment.

If this type of reduction is required, for example in fractures in the problem zone, then some form of internal fixation is required. The use of sharp Kirschner wires, inserted by means of a small modern power drill, makes this type of fixation relatively simple, and the majority of difficult fracture-dislocations, such as Bennett's fractures and fractures of the proximal interphalangeal joint, can be simply and effectively treated by this method. All fracture-dislocations, and most fractures, require the Kirschner wire to be inserted across at least one joint, but a thin sharp Kirschner wire inserted across a joint does no harm for 2 or 3 weeks, by which time the fracture will have gained enough stability for the wire to be removed and gentle mobilization commenced.

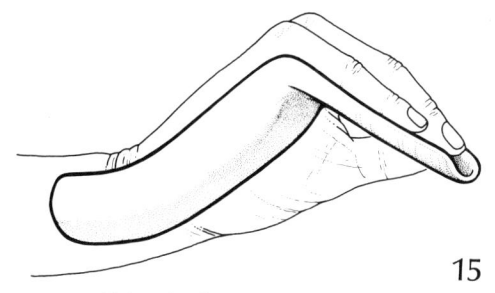

Volar splint for phalangeal fractures 15

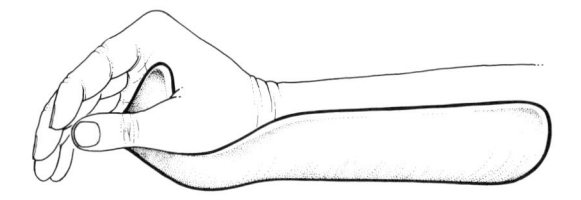

Volar splint for metacarpal fractures 16

Skin closure

The skin does not *have* to be closed at primary treatment. Indeed, much damage can be caused by excessive attempts to pull tight skin edges or flaps together. If skin will not come easily together with neat interrupted 5/0 nylon sutures, it should probably be left open or other methods found to close the wound. Covering any defects with split skin grafts is easily done, but again there is no compelling need to carry out these on the day of injury – delayed skin grafting, say at 5 or 6 days, has much to commend it, and the wounds should then be clean and fresh, and should provide a suitable bed.

At the end of primary treatment the hand should look and feel comfortable, and should be comfortable in its natural resting position. It should be remembered that after any trauma, and certainly after a significant crushing injury, the hand and fingers are going to swell considerably. After a few hours it will be impossible to manipulate the digits into a natural position, and all effort must be made to achieve and hold this position at the primary treatment. Even if the hand does end up somewhat stiff, a stiff hand in the position of function is infinitely more useful than one which has been allowed to stiffen in an extended or clawed position.

Hand injuries in children

Children are likely to injure their hands in domestic situations, involving burning, or crushing injuries from doors and falling stones, but they also can receive nasty lacerations from broken glass or sharp knives. Establishing a diagnosis following a cut in the hand can be quite difficult because a child is generally very apprehensive and uncooperative and the surgeon may have to advise formal exploration of a wound under general anaesthesia before he can properly establish what structures have been divided. Primary repair of all divided structures is probably advisable in most cases with children, although it must be fully explained to the parents that a considerable period of physiotherapy and rehabilitation will be required after damage to tendons or nerves, and it may require a lot of patience on the part of physiotherapists and others working in this field to achieve cooperation and worthwhile results in small children. On the other hand, the ability of the various tissues of the hand to heal rapidly and well is very much better in small children, and one often achieves very gratifying results following wounds that might have caused considerable problems in an adult hand.

Postoperative management

All patients with an open wound should be protected against the possibility of tetanus infection; it is rarely possible to establish a patient's tetanus-immune status on the day of injury, and standard practice is to cover the patient with an injection of active antitetanus serum, and 1 mega-unit of long-acting procaine penicillin. Anaerobic infection by tetanus or gas gangrene bacilli is much more likely in wounds that have been severely contaminated by earth or farmyard material. In these circumstances a thorough removal of all tissue of doubtful viability is required, together with careful vigilance and a high dose of penicillin in the postoperative phase.

It should be possible to make a reasonable guess at the likely infecting organisms if there is concern about postoperative infection. Most such infections are caused by *Staphylococcus aureus* and a prophylactic antibiotic regimen should therefore include a penicillinase-resistant penicillin, such as cloxacillin, or a cephalosporin.

Where Gram-negative infection is a possibility, a broader spectrum antibiotic will be indicated.

The overall aim of primary treatment should be to repair all structures that have been divided by sharp injury, and to reduce fractures and dislocations, particularly those in the danger zone, into satisfactory alignment. At the end of the primary treatment the patient's hand should lie in a natural comfortable position and should not be unduly painful. Elevation of the hand is essential to prevent swelling following severe injuries in the first 24 hours. Any patient who has a painful hand, in particular if they have poor feeling in their fingers, more than 24 hours after primary surgery, should have the dressing taken down, and if necessary the hand re-explored to find the cause. Considerable damage can be caused to the hand by excess pressure and tension inside the hand due to haematoma formation, over-tight bandaging or infection.

Most wounds of the hand should be well on their way to healing within a day or two, and at the end of a week the patient should be able to move his fingers, perhaps through a small range of movement only but certainly comfortably. Multiple wounds of the hand and those involving tendons will require careful supervision by a physiotherapist for a number of weeks after the injury.

Illustrations by Peter Cox

Intracapsular fractures of the neck of the femur

C. E. Ackroyd MA, FRCS
Consultant Orthopaedic Surgeon, Southmead Hospital, Bristol, UK

G. C. Bannister MChOrth, FRCS
Consultant Senior Lecturer, Southmead Hospital, Bristol, UK

V. G. Langkamer FRCS
Orthopaedic Registrar, Southmead Hospital, Bristol, UK

Introduction

Proximal femoral fracture is predominantly a disease of the elderly. The geriatric population has not only increased in size, but the fracture rate has increased. It is estimated that there are over 40000 new cases per year and half of these fractures are intracapsular[1]. Fractures in the elderly are associated with weak, osteoporotic bone, whereas in the small number of young patients who sustain this injury it occurs only after considerable violence.

Classification

1a–d

The fracture has been classified by Garden according to the degree of displacement. As the displacement increases, so the integrity of the blood supply to the head of the femur is compromised. This may lead to delayed union or non-union of the fracture or to the late complication of avascular necrosis. Complete and undisplaced fractures (Garden Stages I and II) unite in 99.5 per cent of cases, compared with 65 per cent of displaced fractures (Garden Stages III and IV). Fracture union declines with age and immobility[2].

Avascular necrosis occurs at between 18 months and 3 years after injury in approximately 20 per cent of patients, of whom one-quarter complain of significant symptoms[2]. Stability of the fracture after closed reduction and internal fixation is essential for a successful result. Comminution of the posterior cortex of the femoral neck is often present and this increases the difficulty in maintaining an anatomical reduction.

Stage I

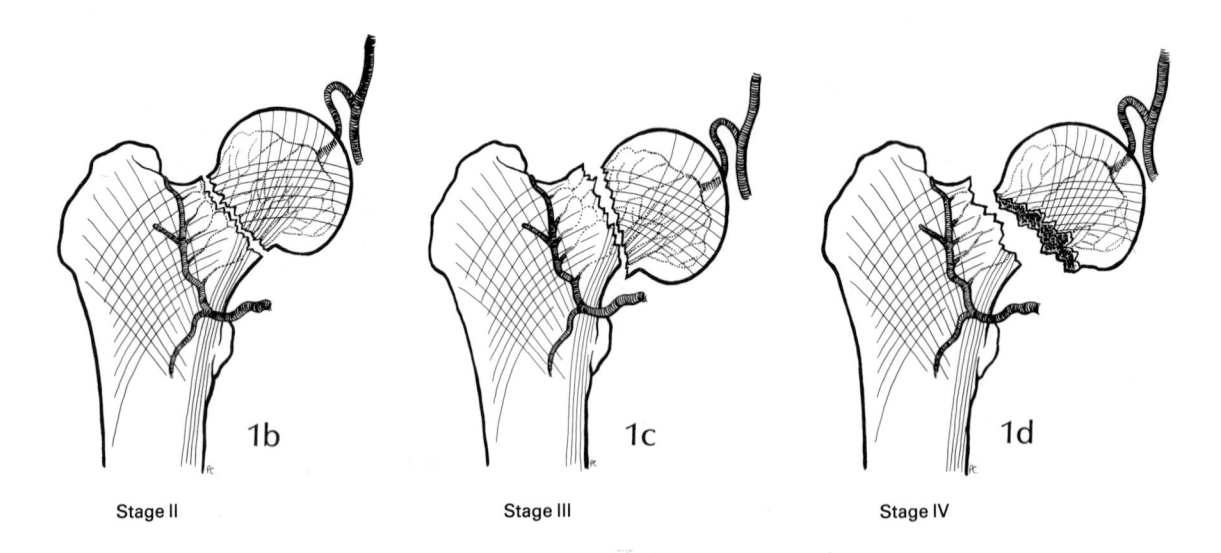

Stage II

Stage III

Stage IV

Indications for internal fixation

If undisplaced fractures are managed without fixation, 12 per cent displace and are therefore less likely to unite[3]. The trabecular bone is already impacted and fixation with two screws is sufficient to maintain stability.

British and Danish controlled trials suggest that in patients over 70 years of age with displaced fractures, primary prosthetic replacement results in lower morbidity, fewer reoperations and comparable mortality over 6 months[4,5] when compared with internal fixation. However, femoral head replacement results in progressive acetabular erosion and after 5 years 20 per cent of survivors have undergone total hip replacement[6].

Internal fixation may reasonably be offered to mentally alert, independent and fully mobile patients, whose life expectancy is likely to exceed 5 years provided that the fracture can be accurately reduced. In patients under 60 years of age every effort must be made to preserve the femoral head. Prosthetic replacement will inevitably fail with the passage of time.

Fixation devices

The profusion of fixation devices is testimony to the poor union rate of intracapsular fractures and the endeavours to improve this by more secure fixation. The literature is confused by reports quoting wide differences in results between individual authors and from different institutions but when randomized prospective controlled trials have been carried out by some authors, results[4,5,7] are all very similar.

The evidence suggests that displaced subcapital fractures unite better with adequate internal fixation[8]. Two implants are better than one[9], and a screw can be inserted with less trauma than a nail and is less likely to disturb the reduction[2].

2 & 3

The concept of controlled collapse and transient or continuous compression has been studied for almost four decades, yet clinical superiority of fixation devices possessing these properties remains to be clearly demonstrated[10,11]. Christie et al.[12] have shown that a single sliding screw has a higher rate of non-union compared to divergent Garden screws.

Two sturdy implants, such as Garden screws, offer fixation as good as any and the opportunity to perform the operation percutaneously. If a sliding hip screw is used, a further cancellous screw should be inserted above it to control rotation and shear.

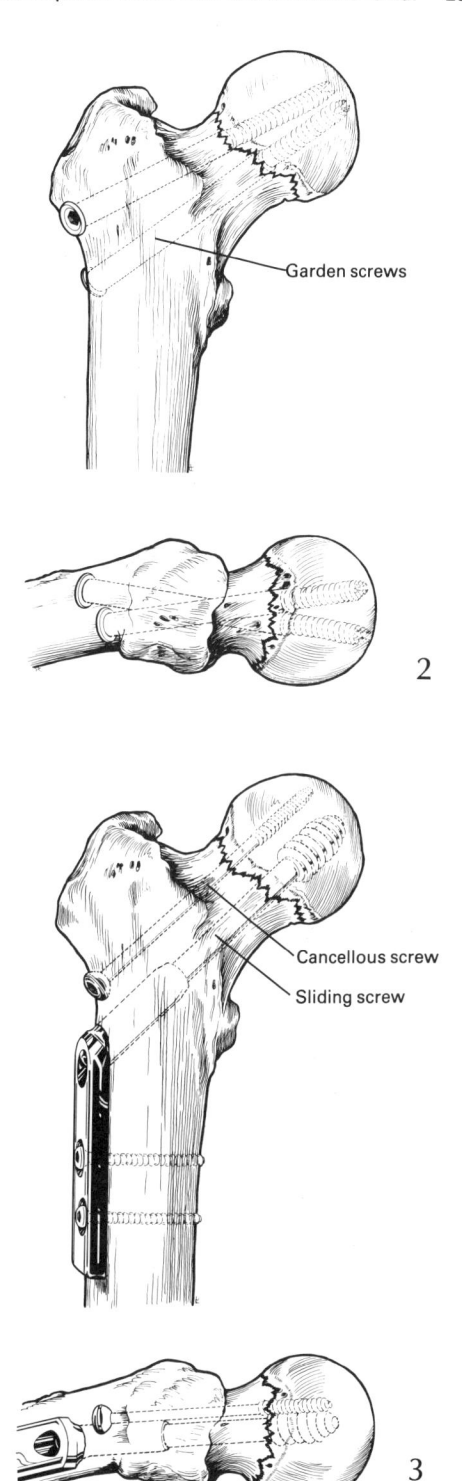

Preoperative preparation

If the fracture is unstable, the patient should be made comfortable with Pugh's skin traction and 2.72 kg (6 lb) weight. Prophylactic antibiotics are of proven value in reducing infection in femoral neck fracture fixation[13].

Timing of surgery

Mortality rises if surgery is delayed more than 4 days from the fracture, but union rate declines only after 1 week[2].

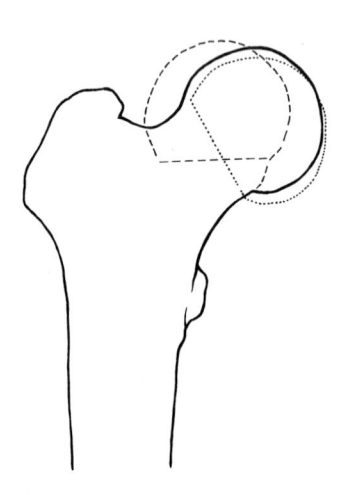

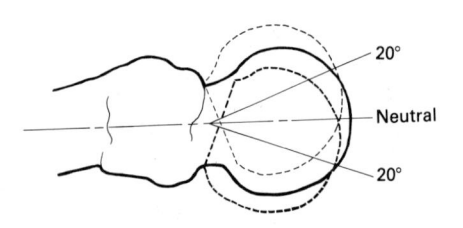

Anaesthesia

Spinal anaesthesia maintains higher perioperative arterial oxygen levels and has a lower initial mortality than general anaesthesia. After 2 weeks, however, mortality from local and general anaesthesia are similar[14].

Operation

Aim of the operation

The operation in the elderly involves closed reduction and internal fixation. Without accurate reduction, the fixation is doomed. If this cannot be achieved by closed means, open methods must be employed if the femoral head is to be retained. There is no place for fracture fixation in an unsatisfactory position.

Criteria for satisfactory reduction

4

The normal angle between the long axis of the shaft of the femur and the vertical trabeculae of the femoral neck is 160° on the anteroposterior radiograph and 180° on the lateral radiograph. The acceptable standard of reduction is 5° of varus to 20° of valgus on the anteroposterior view and 20° of displacement on either side of the neutral 180° line on the lateral view[2].

Use of the fracture table and image intensifier

The fracture table is prepared before operation. The perineal pole against which traction takes place must be radiolucent (wood or plastic) and padded. The sacral rests must be placed centrally on the fractured side or the pelvis will sag and obscure the lateral projection of the radiographic image. The unaffected leg should be abducted to 45° or flexed to the 90/90 position to allow access for the radiographic equipment. Preliminary screening should be performed to ensure an adequate radiograph and to check the reduction.

CLOSED REDUCTION[15]

The capsule of the hip joint is tight in extension and medial rotation and relaxed in flexion and lateral rotation. Reduction should be a gentle manoeuvre and is aided by muscle relaxation.

5a, b & c

The surgeon should stand beside the injured limb just below the knee facing the head. The upper hand is placed over the front of the thigh to grip the medial side, the lower hand grips the limb at the level of the knee with the calf supported against the body. The thigh is flexed to 30° in lateral rotation, the limb is manipulated by slight abduction, and gradually increasing traction is exerted along the line of the neck of the femur. The thigh is then gradually rotated medially and extended, allowing the capsule to tighten and maintain the reduction. The hips should now be positioned in medial rotation of some 15° and abduction of 20°, and the foot secured. Tension in the limb is adjusted so that it is just possible to flex the knee.

Screening of the hip with an image intensifier while gently rotating the limb will aid visualization of the fracture. Care should be taken to ensure correct interpretation of the radiograph; a metal marker placed on the anterior skin surface may help orientation. The neck of the femur should be positioned horizontally in the lateral view. This facilitates placement of the guide wires. More than 90 per cent of fractures can be reduced in this way[16].

The skin is now prepared with two applications of a suitable antiseptic and the patient draped with sterile towels or one of the all-in-one adhesive transparent sheets.

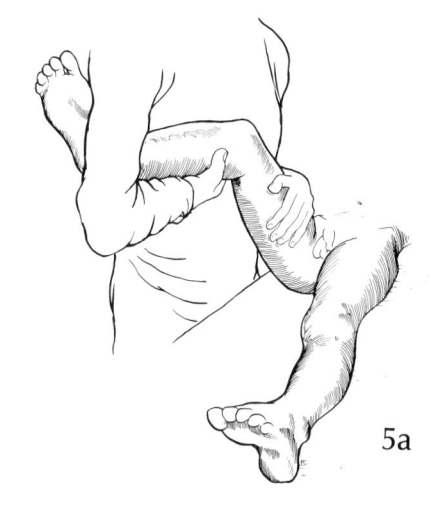

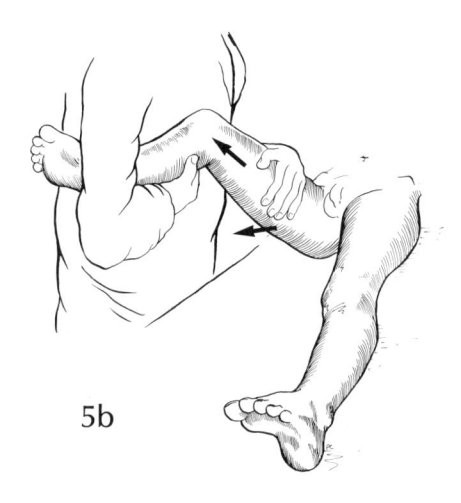

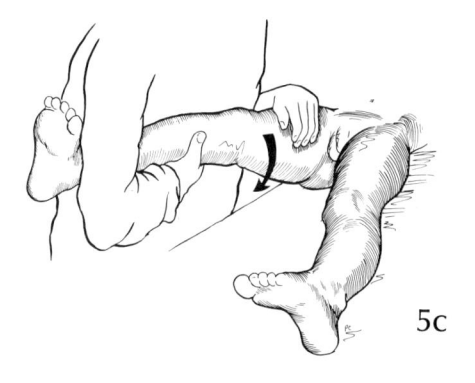

OPEN REDUCTION

6

If closed reduction cannot be achieved, the fracture should be exposed by one of the anterolateral approaches to the hip. Most convenient is a slightly modified Watson-Jones approach. This consists of a straight incision running obliquely over the lateral part of the thigh. It commences 5 cm behind the anterior superior iliac spine, runs to the midpoint of the greater trochanter, proceeding distally down the thigh to run slightly behind the line of the shaft of the femur.

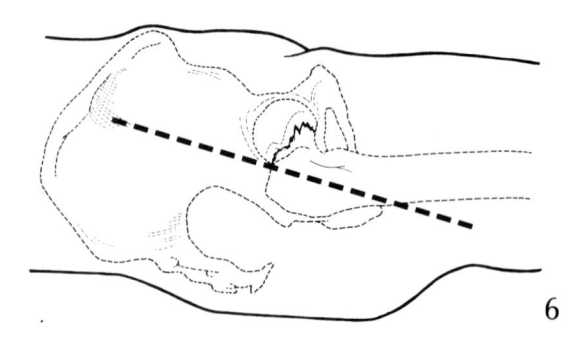

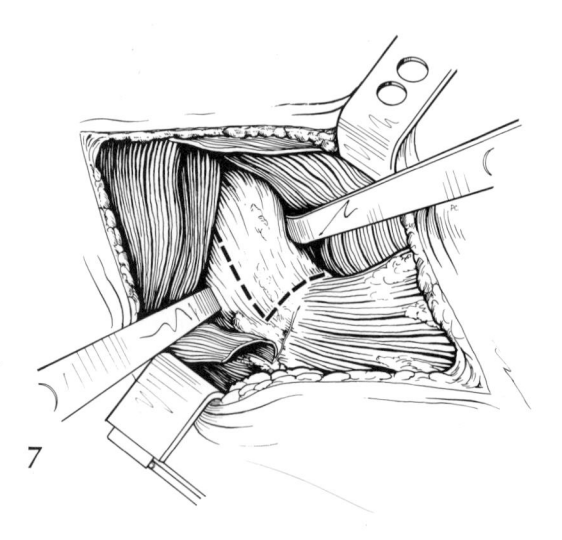

7

The deep fascia is split in line with the incision and the anterior flap reflected forwards. The anterior margin of gluteus medius is identified, retracted upwards and stripped off the undersurface of the fascia lata to develop the space between gluteus medius and tensor fasciae latae. Branches of the superior gluteal artery are coagulated and the inferior branch of the superior gluteal nerve running to tensor fasciae latae is preserved. The anterior one-third of the insertion of gluteus medius is divided and a lever inserted into the trochanteric fossa. The extracapsular fat and reflected head of rectus femoris are elevated to expose the capsule of the hip joint. The capsule is incised in line with the femoral neck and extended to an L at its distal end to facilitate exposure of the fracture.

8

The fracture is then reduced under direct vision and held with two stout guide wires running along the neck of the femur and crossing the hip joint to enter the pelvis.

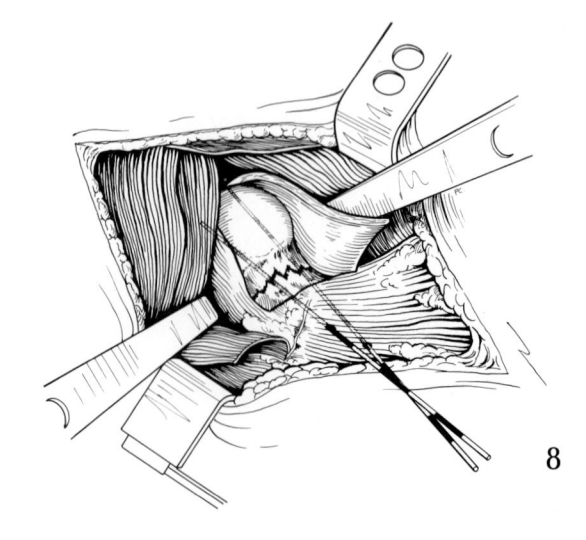

FRACTURE FIXATION

Cannulated screw fixation

If an accurate closed reduction has been obtained under image intensification control it is then possible to carry out percutaneous fixation with cannulated screws. Two divergent Garden screws provide satisfactory stability.

9

Orientation of the guide wires in the two planes can be considerably simplified by the use of a reference guide wire (wire 1A) placed on the skin parallel to the femoral neck in the lateral plane. If possible this wire should also correspond to the correct angle for the first screw in the anteroposterior plane. This wire gives immediate reference for the anteversion plane and allows the surgeon to concentrate on getting correct alignment in the anteroposterior plane. The wire is adjusted so that its tip is at a point midway between the anterior superior iliac spine and the pubic tubercle and running to a point 3 cm distal to the trochanteric ridge. The position is checked on the image intensifier. This wire indicates the position for the skin incision.

A 2 cm incision is made over the lateral aspect of the femoral shaft and the vastus lateralis is split down to the femur. A 3.2 mm drill with drill guide is inserted through the incision and the lateral cortex of the femur penetrated at a point slightly posterior to the midpoint of the shaft.

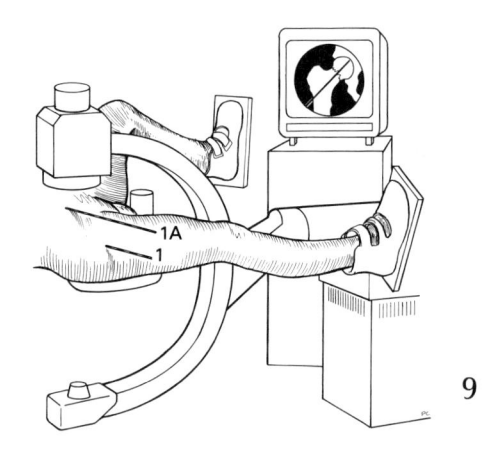

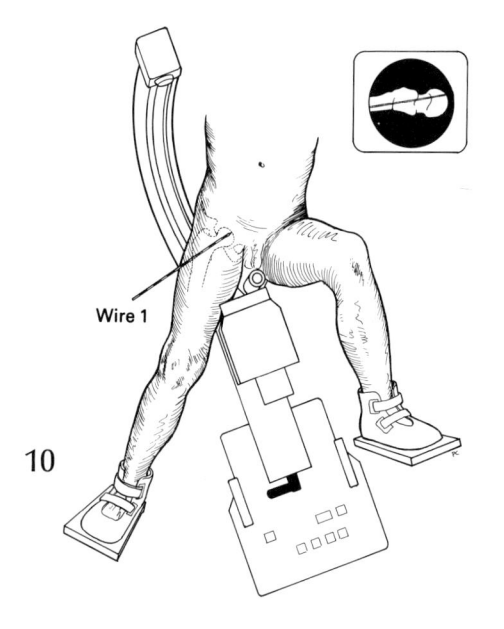

10

The drill is then moved in line with the reference guide wire. A stout guide wire (wire 1) is then mounted in the power drill and placed in the pilot hole in the femur. The guide wire is inserted parallel to the reference wire in each plane. In the lateral plane the guide wire should be aimed very slightly anteriorly so that it enters the anterior part of the femoral head and runs as far as the subchondral bone. The guide wire is then measured and an appropriate screw chosen so that its tip is at least 1 cm short of the subchondral bone. The entry hole is then prepared with a reamer or tap depending on the type of screw to be inserted.

206 Lower limb fractures

11

The second guide wire (wire 2) is now positioned commencing with a placement wire on the skin so that in the anteroposterior plane it is running slightly more horizontally from 1 cm below the vastus lateralis ridge, along the femoral neck to the inferior part of the femoral head. The drill hole in the lateral cortex should be placed slightly anterior to the midpoint of the femoral shaft and when the guide wire is inserted it should be aimed slightly posteriorly so that its tip lies in the posterior-inferior part of the femoral head. This screw will support the comminuted posterior cortex.

Once the second guide wire has been satisfactorily positioned the lateral cortex of the femur is enlarged with a power reamer to the correct diameter of the screw and the two screws are then inserted. Radiographic screening is carried out in the anteroposterior and lateral views at strategic points during the procedure.

In very unstable fractures it is often desirable to drive the guide wires across the joint surfaces to control the fracture while the screws are being inserted. The skin wounds are closed with nylon sutures.

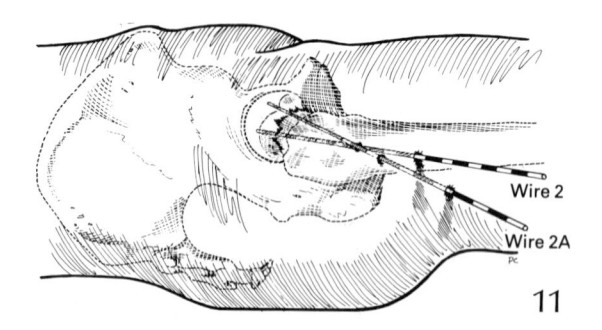

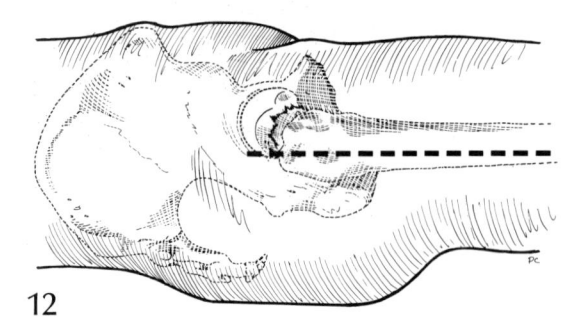

Compression screw and plate

12

Extensive exposure of the lateral surface of the femur is necessary to insert this device and the approach is identical to that required for trochanteric fractures (see chapter on 'Trochanteric fractures of the femur' pp. 209–215). The skin is incised vertically from the level of the greater trochanter, proceeding 12 cm down the thigh in line with the shaft of the femur.

13 & 14

The fascia lata is incised to expose vastus lateralis. This should be detached from the vastus lateralis ridge, and the vastus fascia incised for 8 cm along its posterior attachment to the linea aspera. The posterior attachment of vastus lateralis should then be elevated from the femur leaving a thin cuff for reattachment. The perforating branches of the profunda femoris are isolated and coagulated. The periosteum can then be incised down to bone and, with sweeping movements from distal to proximal using a periosteal elevator, the vastus lateralis is displaced forwards.

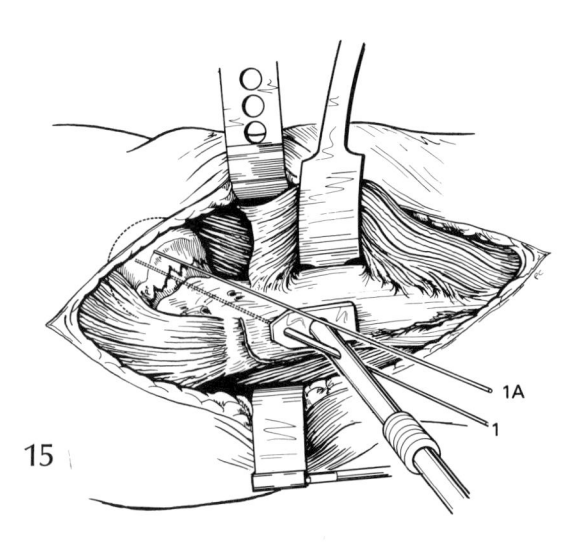

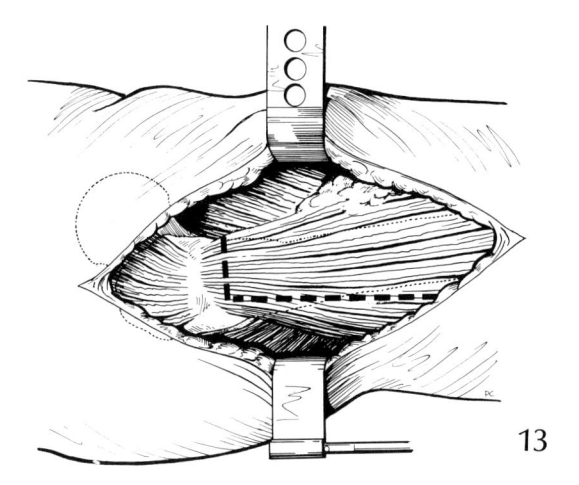

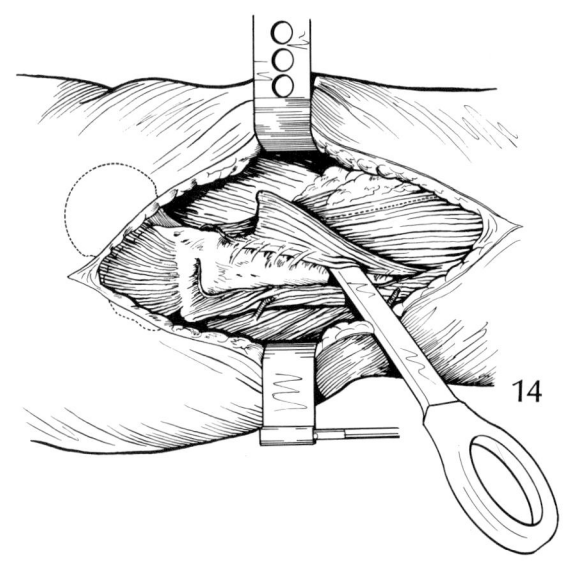

15

Accurate placement of wires is easier with the femur exposed. The anteversion reference wire (wire 1A) is easily inserted along the anterior border of the femoral neck and impacted into the head. The guide wire (wire 1) for the screw should be inserted centrally along the neck of the femur to enter the centre of the head.

The guide wire protractor with an angle of 45° to the shaft is positioned to determine the site of entry of the guide wire, and a 3.2 mm drill hole made at the midpoint of the shaft. The guide wire is then inserted at the correct angle using the reference wire 1A to align the lateral plane and the protractor, and checked with the image intensifier in both the lateral and anteroposterior planes.

After measurement using the reverse calibrated depth gauge, a screw 10 mm shorter than the depth is selected and the lateral cortex is reamed with the triple reamer in preparation for tapping and insertion of the screw. At least one further guide wire is necessary to maintain provisional reduction of the fracture; in young hard bone several guide wires are required to avoid displacement. After insertion of the screw a two-hole plate is applied and the compression screw tightened. Fixation should be supplemented by a cancellous screw positioned superiorly in the femoral neck to prevent rotation of the fracture. Tapping of the screw threads should always be carried out in the younger patient.

The wound is now closed over one or two suction drains, vastus lateralis being folded over the plate and resutured to its site of origin. The deep fascia is closed with absorbable sutures. The subcutaneous sutures, incorporating the superficial layer of the deep fascia (Sherman's fascia), take tension off the skin wound which can then be closed with continuous nylon sutures.

Postoperative management

The patient should be nursed in bed until the suction drains are removed at 48 hours after operation. Movements of the hip, knee and ankle are encouraged immediately and antithrombogenic stockings may be worn. There is a slightly higher union rate if patients do not bear weight and this should be encouraged in young patients. The elderly have usually fallen as a result of poor balance and non- or partial weight-bearing is impracticable. Routine anticoagulation of patients with femoral neck fractures has been shown to reduce the incidence of thromboembolic complications[17]. However, the risks of this therapy in elderly patients may be considerable and there is an increased risk of wound haematoma. The surgeon should therefore balance the advantages and disadvantages of such a policy in each individual case.

References

1. Boyce J, Grimley-Evans J. Incidence and outcome of fractured proximal femur. *J Bone Joint Surg [Br]* 1986; 68-B: 156.

2. Barnes R, Brown JT, Garden RS, Nicoll EA. Subcapital fractures of the femur: a prospective review. *J Bone Joint Surg [Br]* 1976; 58-B: 2–24.

3. Bentley G. Impacted fractures of the neck of the femur. *J Bone Joint Surg [Br]* 1968; 50-B: 551–61.

4. Sikorski JM, Barrington R. Internal fixation versus hemiarthroplasty for the displaced subcapital fracture of the femur: a prospective randomised study. *J Bone Joint Surg [Br]* 1981; 63-B: 357–61.

5. Söreide O, Molster A, Raugstad TS. Internal fixation versus primary prosthetic replacement in acute femoral neck fractures: a prospective randomised clinical study. *Br J Surg* 1979; 66: 56–60.

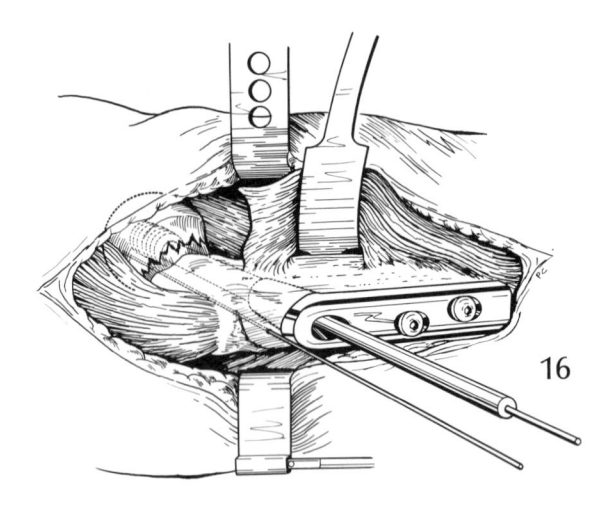

6. Maxted MJ, Denham RA. Failure of hemiarthroplasty for fractures of the neck of the femur. *Injury* 1984; 15: 224–6.

7. Riley TBH. Knobs or screws? A prospective trial of prosthetic replacement against internal fixation of subcapital fractures. *J Bone Joint Surg [Br]* 1978; 60-B: 136.

8. Smith-Petersen MN, Cave EF, Van gorder GW. Intracapsular fractures of the neck of the femur: treatment by internal fixation. *Arch Surg* 1931; 23: 715–59.

9. McQuillan WM, Abernethy PJ, Guy JG. Subcapital fractures of the neck of the femur treated by double divergent fixation. *Br J Surg* 1973; 60: 859–66.

10. Clawson DK. Trochanteric fractures treated by the sliding screw plate fixation method. *J Trauma* 1964; 4: 737–52.

11. Charnley J, Blockey NJ, Purser DW. The treatment of displaced fractures of the neck of the femur by compression: a preliminary report. *J Bone Joint Surg [Br]* 1957; 39-B: 45–65.

12. Christie J, Howie CR, Armour PC. Fixation of displaced subcapital femoral fractures: compression screw fixaton versus double divergent pins. *J Bone Joint Surg [Br]* 1988; 70-B: 199–201.

13. Ericson L, Lidgren L, Lindberg L. Cloxacillin in prophylaxis of postoperative infection of the hip. *J Bone Joint Surg [Am]* 1973; 55-A: 808–13.

14. McKenzie PJ, Wishart HY, Dewart KMS, Grey I, Smith G. Comparison of the effects of spinal anaesthesia and general anaesthesia on postoperative oxygenation and perioperative mortality. *Br J Anaesth* 1980; 52: 49–54.

15. Flynn M. A new method of reduction of fractures of the neck of the femur based on anatomical studies of the hip joint. *Injury* 1974; 5:309–17.

16. Compton EH. Accuracy of reduction of femoral subcapital fractures. *Injury* 1977–78; 9: 71–3.

17. Sevitt S, Gallagher NG. Prevention of venous thrombosis and pulmonary embolism in injured patients: a trial of anticoagulant prophylaxis with phenindione in middle-aged and elderly patients with fractured neck of femur. *Lancet* 1959; ii: 981–9.

Illustrations by Peter Cox

Trochanteric fractures of the femur

G. C. Bannister MChOrth, FRCS
Consultant Senior Lecturer, Southmead Hospital, Bristol, UK

C. E. Ackroyd MA, FRCS
Consultant Orthopaedic Surgeon, Southmead Hospital, Bristol, UK

V. G. Langkamer FRCS
Orthopaedic Registrar, Southmead Hospital, Bristol, UK

Introduction

Fifty per cent of proximal femoral fractures involve the trochanteric region. In contrast to the intracapsular fractures, union occurs in 99 per cent of cases and avascular necrosis of the femoral head is unlikely to occur.

Classification

1a & b

Trochanteric fractures are classified as stable or unstable. This classification is relative. The stable type often have minimal displacement and when reduced there is good apposition of the medial cortex of the calcar femoralis. The unstable type are comminuted with three or four main fragments, often with considerable displacement.

The stable two-part fractures displace and collapse but to a lesser extent than the unstable three- or four-part fractures.

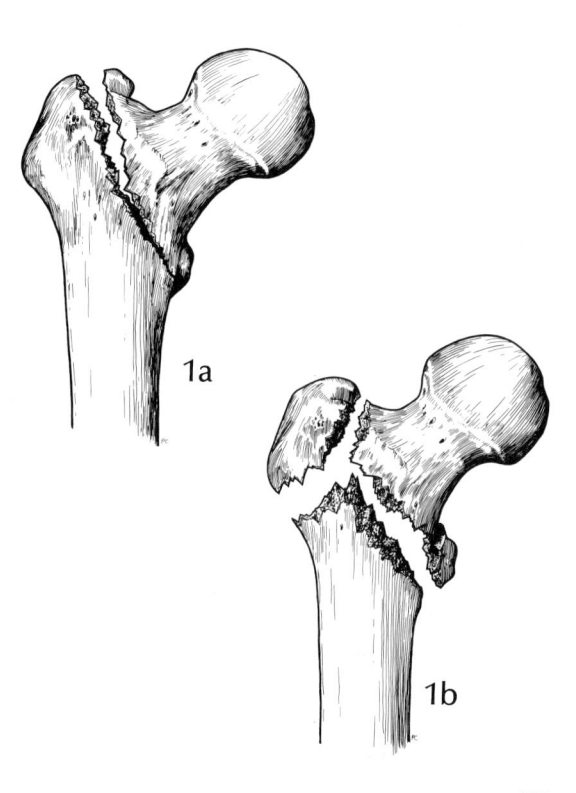

Indications for internal fixation

Unstable trochanteric fractures can be treated by traction in bed, provided nursing care is excellent, or by internal fixation; the mortality is comparable. The fracture usually unites satisfactorily in traction in 8–12 weeks in the elderly; however, there may be difficulty in maintaining satisfactory alignment. In young patients with stable fractures reduction and traction is the method of choice since union occurs within 3–4 weeks. After internal fixation, patients can start walking within a few days and leave hospital earlier. The more comminuted fractures may be painful for several weeks, delaying mobilization.

Techniques of fixation

There are three types of device available for fixation of these fractures: the fixed-angle, fixed length, nail–plate, intramedullary rods, and the sliding screw with fixed plate.

2 & 3

In the 1930s the fixed length nail–plates evolved as side plates were added to Smith-Petersen trifin nails (e.g. the Jewett nail–plate). In the 1950s sliding screws were designed to allow impaction of subcapital fractures but were found to be more effective in the trochanteric region.

More recently, intramedullary nailing techniques have been pioneered but found to be disappointing in unstable fractures[1]. In stable fractures all techniques are comparable.

In unstable fractures sliding-screw fixation appears to be superior to fixed-length devices[2–4]. Efforts to restore medial bone contact in three-part fractures have included a valgus[5] and a medial[6] displacement osteotomy. Both these osteotomies are difficult to perform and do not show clear advantage over fixation of the fracture *in situ* using a sliding-screw device[7,8].

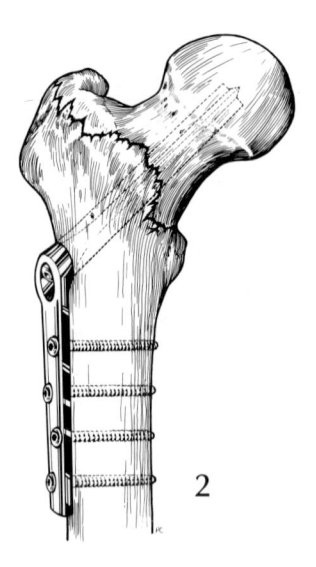

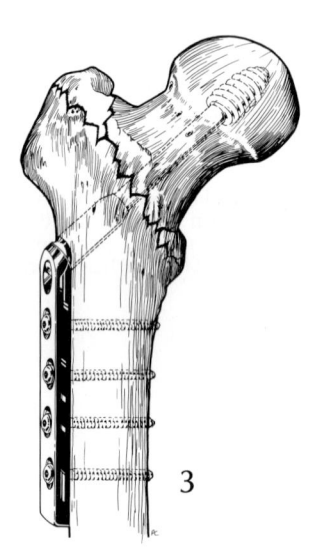

Preoperative

Preparation of patient

Patients should be made comfortable with temporary skin traction. Two units of blood are usually required and prophylactic antibiotics are of proven value in reducing infection. The operation should be carried out as soon as the patient is considered fit after adequate screening for medical conditions. The simplest and most reliable operation is closed reduction of the fracture and internal fixation with a sliding hip screw.

Preparation of fracture table

4 & 5

The fracture table is prepared with a radiolucent perineal pole (wood or plastic) and the sacral support placed centrally or on the affected side. The screws on the traction device which control distraction, adduction and abduction should be loose. The distraction ratchet adjacent to the foot should be prepared so that traction can be applied to the limb. The perineum is placed firmly against the traction pole and the unaffected limb abducted and flexed to allow adequate views of the affected hip to be obtained from the image intensifier. The correct position of the guide wires is shown.

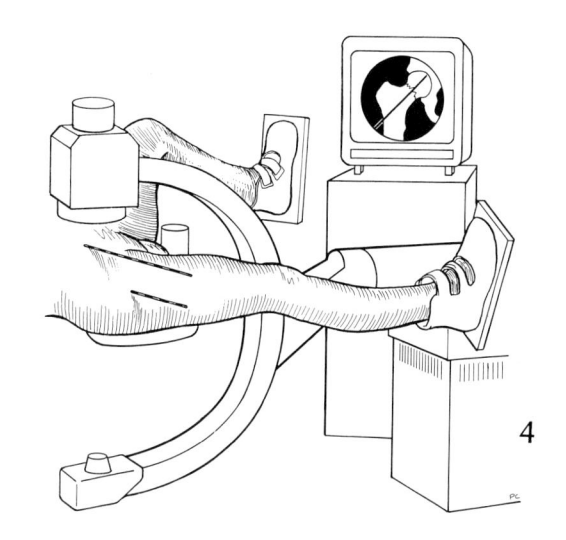

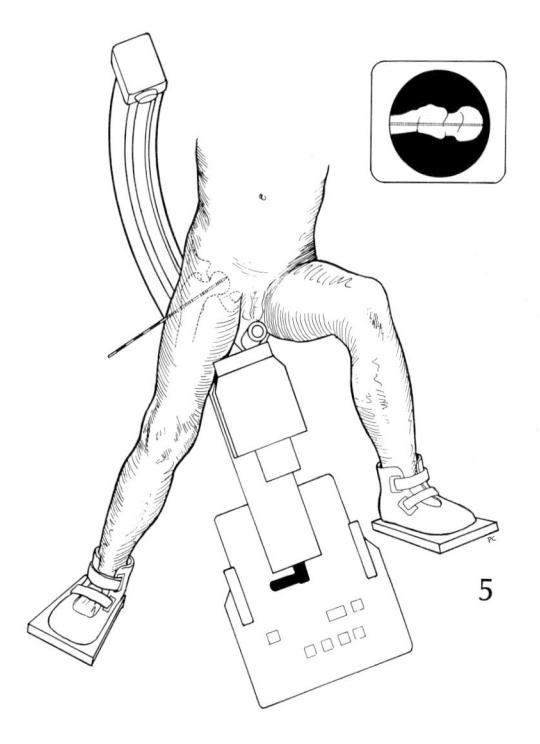

Operation

Reduction

6 & 7

The reduction is best carried out under image intensifier control. The optimum position of rotation and traction can then be assessed. Two- and three-part fractures are best reduced in neutral or 15°–20° of medial rotation. Four-part unstable fractures are best reduced in neutral in 75 per cent of cases and lateral rotation in 25 per cent of cases. Excessive medial rotation should be avoided as this may cause malunion with an inturned foot and produces a significant handicap.

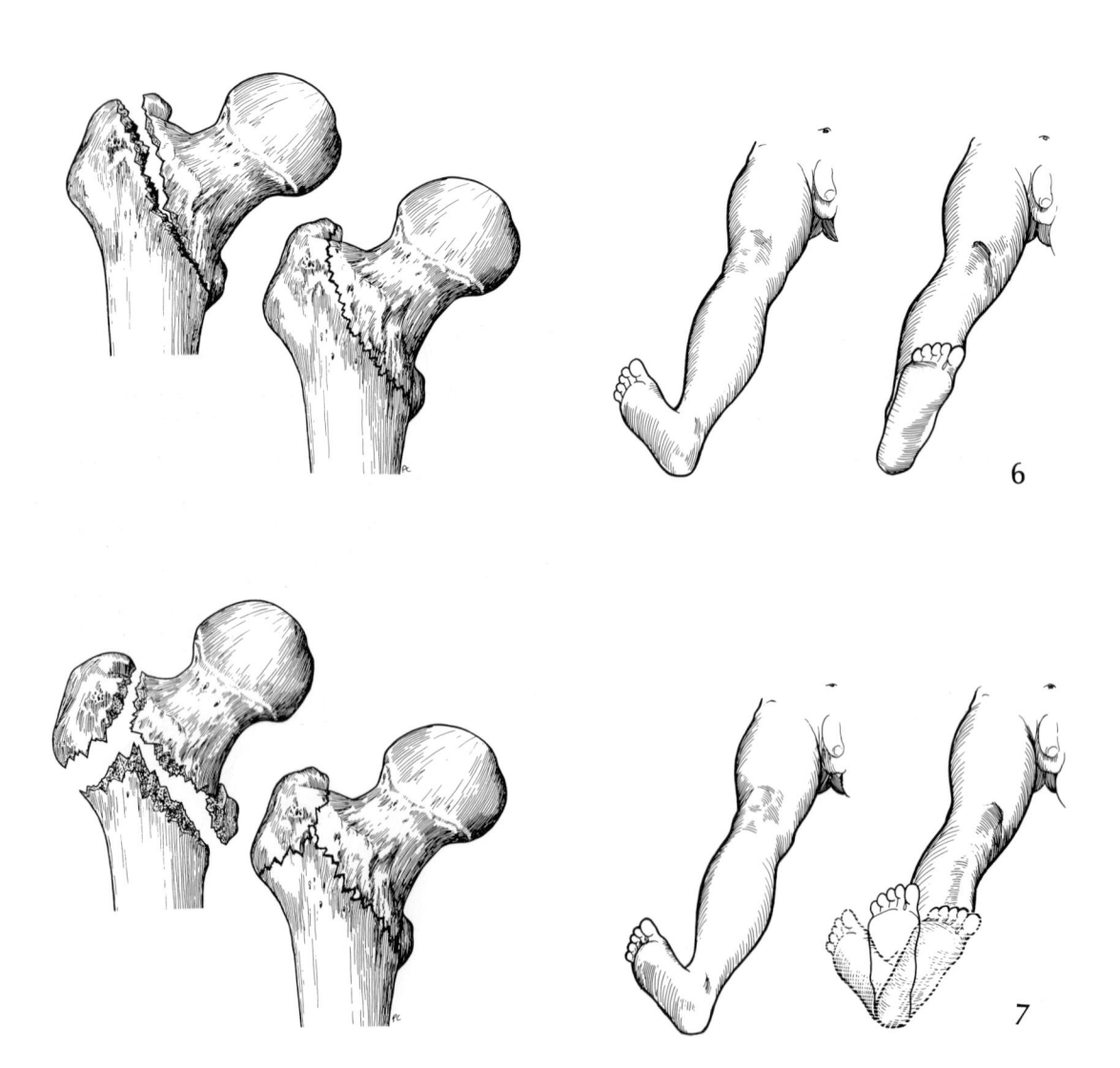

Trochanteric fractures of the femur 213

Internal fixation

8

The limb is prepared and draped with sterile towels or an all-in-one disposable transparent adhesive drape. The incision starts 1 cm proximal to the midpoint of the vastus lateralis ridge and extends distally for 12 cm.

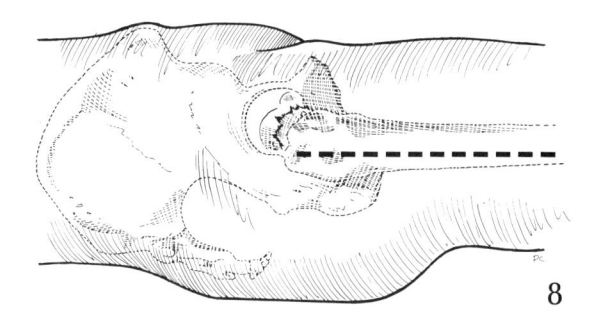

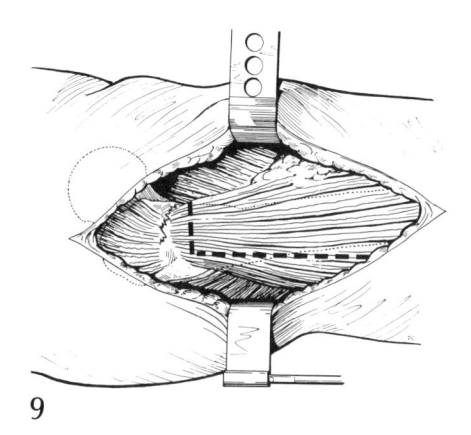

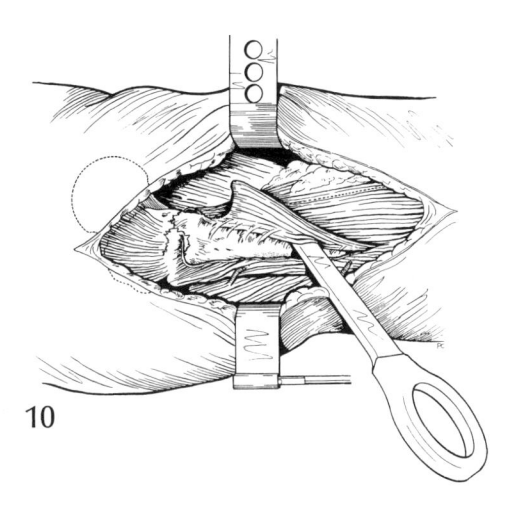

9 & 10

The fascia lata is split and vastus lateralis exposed. The origin of vastus lateralis is divided at the vastus lateralis ridge of the femur, a small cuff of muscle being left for resuture. The vastus lateralis fascia is incised longitudinally near its posterior border where it originates from the linea aspera. The lateral intermuscular septum curves medially to attach to the femur, and just superficial to the periosteum lie the perforating vessels of the profunda femoris artery. These should be identified and coagulated. The periosteum and muscle can then be mobilized using a periosteal elevator and swept forwards by passing the instrument from distal to proximal against the line of the muscle fibres as they arise from the femur. The muscle is then pushed forwards medially to expose the lateral side of the femur. Bone levers are then inserted on the medial side of femur to hold the muscle forwards.

11

The first guide wire (1A) is then placed manually along the anterior border of the femoral neck to show the lateral plane and to correspond with the 135° angle that the screw will make with the shaft in the anteroposterior plane. This guide wire is tapped into the side of the femoral head and its position checked on the lateral radiograph. When accurately placed this guide wire provides the reference line for the lateral plane of the femoral neck.

The entry point on the lateral cortex of the femur is 2.5 cm below the vastus lateralis ridge at the midpoint of the shaft. A 3.2 mm drill hole is made and the guide wire can then be inserted with a power drill using the 135° guide resting against the lateral surface of the femur. This wire (wire 1) is maintained parallel to the anterior guide wire (wire 1A) in the lateral plane which facilitates correct insertion. Anteroposterior and lateral radiographs are taken to ensure the correct position of the guide wire which should be placed centrally in the femoral head and neck. The guide wire is now measured with the reverse calibrated gauge and a correct screw is selected which is 10 mm shorter.

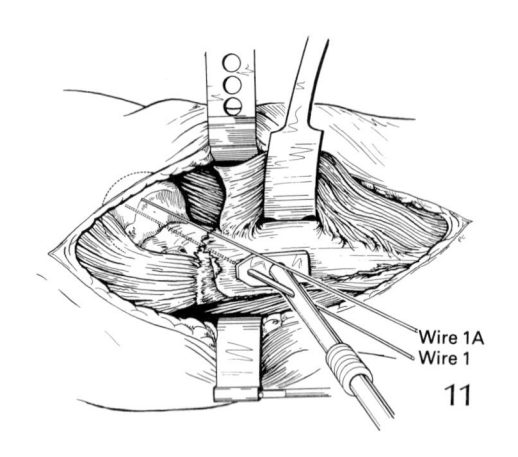

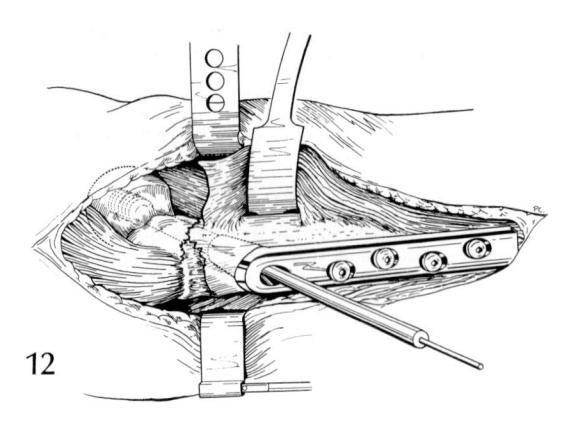

12

The lateral cortex is then reamed using the triple drill-guide adjusted to the length of the screw. In young patients or those with hard bone it may be necessary to tap into the cancellous bone of the femoral head. In elderly osteoporotic patients this is not necessary. The selected screw with its assembly is inserted along the guide wire and screwed into position within 10 mm of the subchondral bone surface.

A four- or six-hole plate is then inserted onto the screw assembly and secured to the femur. After removal of the screw assembly and guide wire a compression screw can be inserted. As compaction of the fracture occurs any compression effect of the screw is quickly lost.

The flap of vastus lateralis is now returned to its correct position to cover the plate and sutured to the periosteum of the greater trochanter and along the linea aspera. The fascia lata is closed over a suction drain with absorbable sutures. Subcutaneous fat is closed with absorbable sutures incorporating the superficial layer of the deep fascia and the skin closed with nylon.

Variations of the technique

If a sliding screw is not available a fixed-length device can be used with equal success in stable fractures. The failure rate of these implants in unstable fractures rises to 30 per cent[3].

If an unstable fracture is being internally fixed with a fixed-length device there will be a much lower incidence of penetration into the joint if the blade is placed proximal to the junction of Ward's triangle.

The Jewett nail–plate has a keel at the junction of the trifin nail and the plate. It is necessary to nibble away a small piece of bone distally at the inferior aspect of the penetrating hole in the lateral cortex to avoid fracturing the shaft when this nail is inserted.

Postoperative management

The patient is nursed in bed with an air-ring under the sacrum and pillows to support the leg, maintaining some flexion of the hip and knee. Active movement of the limb is encouraged. The suction drains are removed at 48 hours.

Check radiographs should be obtained to confirm a satisfactory position of the fracture and implant. The patient may then be permitted to walk with a frame or crutches within the limits of pain.

When using the sliding screw a certain amount of pain may occur as the fracture settles into its position of stability. There is no evidence that non-weight-bearing has any effect on union, although in unstable fractures when a fixed-length device has been used, it may reduce the tendency for the nail to penetrate into the hip joint. Some shortening of the limb inevitably results in the comminuted unstable fractures but its functional significance is minimal. A shoe-raise can be used if necessary.

Provided placement of the screw is satisfactory the mechanical failure rate of the sliding screw is less than 5 per cent[3]. It is seldom necessary to remove the implant unless there is discomfort over the lateral aspect of the thigh or loosening of the screw in the femoral neck. A large implant of this type produces significant stress-protection osteoporosis and great care should be taken with weight-bearing in the months following removal.

References

1. Marsh CH. Use of Ender's nails in unstable trochanteric femoral fractures. *J R Soc Med* 1983; 76: 550–4.

2. Jensen JS. Trochanteric fractures: an epidemiological clinical and biochemical study. Thesis. *Acta Orthop Scand* 1981; 52 (Suppl. 188): 1–100.

3. Bannister GC, Gibson AGF. Jewett nail-plate or AO dynamic hip screw for trochanteric fractures?: a randomised prospective controlled trial. *J Bone Joint Surg [Br]* 1983; 65-B: 218.

4. Esser MP, Kassab JY, Jones DHA (1986) Trochanteric fractures of the femur: a randomised prospective trial comparing Jewett nail–plate with the dynamic hip screw. *J Bone Joint Surg [Br]* 1986; 68-B: 557–60.

5. Sarmiento A, Williams EM. The unstable intertrochanteric fracture: treatment with a valgus osteotomy and I-beam nail–plate. A preliminary report of one hundred cases. *J Bone Joint Surg [Am]* 1970; 52-A: 1309–18.

6. Dimon JH, Hughston JC. Unstable intertrochanteric fractures of the hip. *J Bone Joint Surg [Am]* 1967; 49-A: 440–50.

7. Hubbard MJS, Burke, FD, Houghton GR, Bracey DJ. A prospective controlled study of valgus osteotomy in the fixation of unstable pertrochanteric fractures of the femur. *Injury* 1980; 11: 228–32.

8. Hunter G, Krajbich I. Results of medial displacement osteotomy for unstable intertrochanteric fractures of the femur. *J Bone Joint Surg [Br]* 1979; 61-B: 248.

Illustrations by Paul Richardson

Subtrochanteric fractures of the femur: Zickel nail fixation

Robert E. Zickel MD
Clinical Professor of Orthopedic Surgery, Columbia University, New York, USA

Introduction

The Zickel subtrochanteric nail was designed in 1964 and first used in January 1966. This appliance was developed to provide intramedullary fixation to the subtrochanteric area.

Prior to this, standard nail–plates used for intertrochanteric fractures were extended and used for the subtrochanteric area, with a significant rate of failure. The design concept was to provide an intramedullary nail that could be securely anchored to the head and neck of the femur, to provide secure intramedullary fixation for subtrochanteric fractures.

A preliminary report on the use of the appliance was first published in 1967[1], and subsequent articles have appeared since[2-3]; 9 years' experience was reported in 1976[4]. Its use in non-pathological and pathological fractures of the femur has subsequently been reported by several institutions.

Indications

Those fractures of the femur located in the proximal one-third of the femoral shaft, often referred to as the subtrochanteric region, are ideally suited for this device. Non-pathological fractures caused by trauma, or pathological fractures secondary to metastatic carcinoma, are included. Subtrochanteric fractures that extend into the intertrochanteric region may also be fixed with this appliance.

Contraindications

Fractures that are predominantly intertrochanteric with a small subtrochanteric component are usually better treated with sliding nail–plates or screw–plate devices. Unusual deformities of the femur secondary to previous fracture or bone disease may also be contraindications to the use of the Zickel nail. (For example: a severely bowed femur with Paget's disease with an obliterated medullary canal would be unsuitable.)

Classification

1 & 2

Seinsheimer[5] and Zickel have classified types of subtrochanteric fractures as demonstrated in the illustrations; Type I (not illustrated) comprises non-displaced fractures. All of the fractures Types II–V are suitable for Zickel nail fixation. Type V, in the Seinsheimer classification, with a significant intertrochanteric fracture, might present technical problems during insertion of the device.

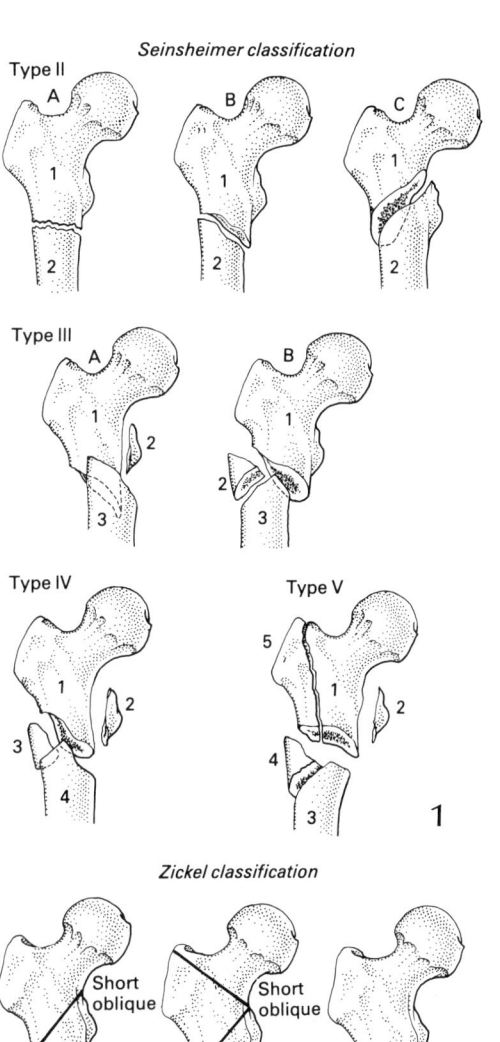

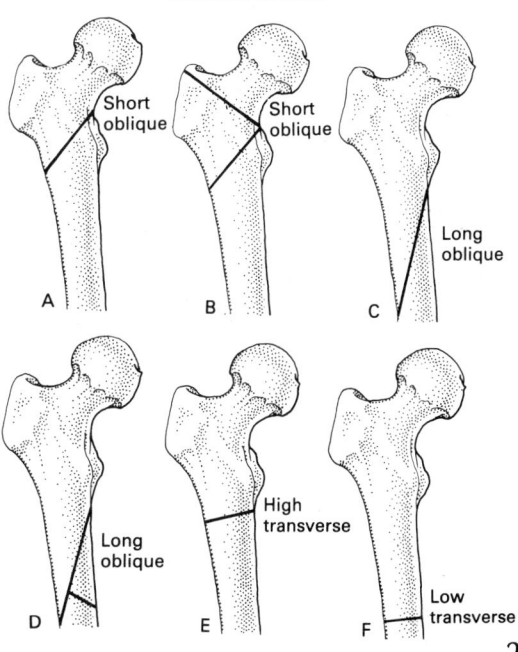

218 Lower limb fractures

Preoperative

Anaesthesia

General or spinal anaesthesia are acceptable.

Position of patient

3

The patient is placed semi-supine on a standard operating table with a roll under the flank to elevate the operated hip. Alternatively a lateral decubitus may be used if the surgeon is comfortable with the orientation of the femur in that position, or a fracture table may be used if the surgical team can control abduction, adduction and rotation of the leg intraoperatively.

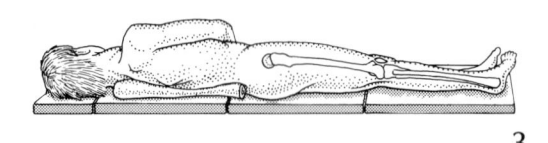

3

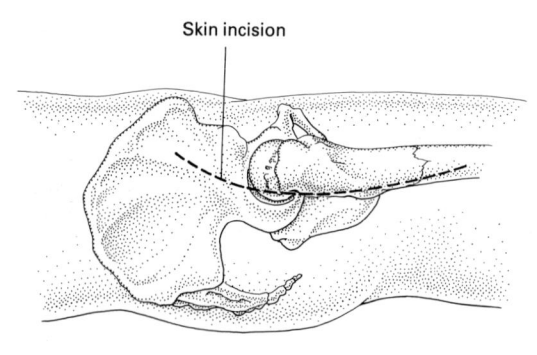

Operation

Draping is done in a manner that permits manipulation of the leg during the procedure.

4

The skin incision is curvilinear along the posterior border of the trochanter, extending four fingers'-breadths superior to the greater trochanter.

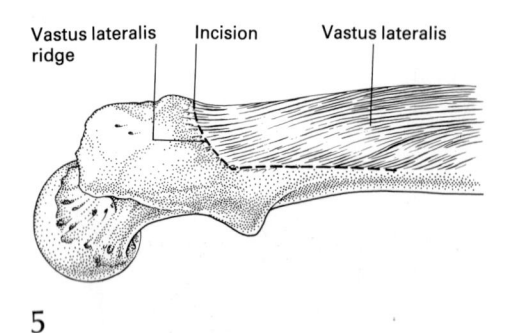

4

5

The fracture is exposed by detaching the vastus lateralis muscle and periosteum just lateral to the linea aspera.

5

Subtrochanteric fractures of the femur: Zickel nail fixation 219

6

After reaming the distal medullary canal, the rod is tested for size in the distal shaft where it should fit snugly. It is then extracted. Each rod is marked to indicate the stem diameter and side (right or left) into which it is to be inserted.

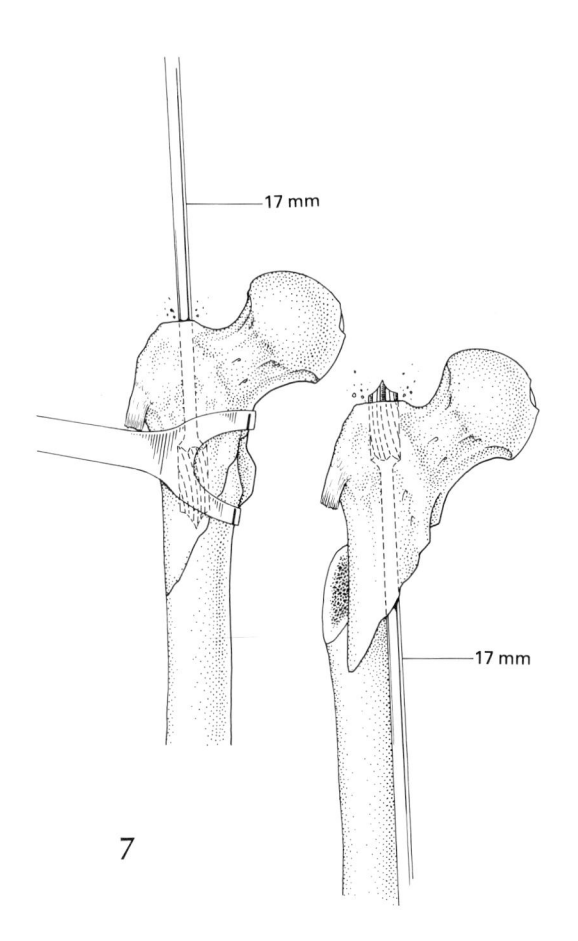

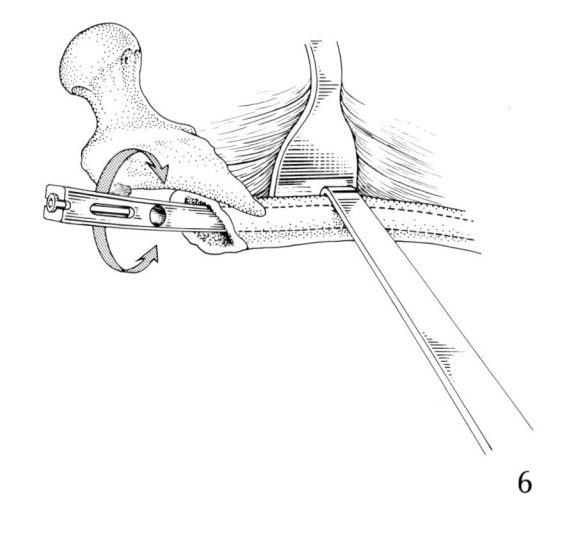

7

The trochanteric medullary canal is next prepared. This may be done by retrograde or anterograde reaming. Prior to reaming the small tip of the greater trochanter, it should be excised with a 12 mm osteotome to ensure proper placement of the medullary reamer. This is performed through a small gluteal muscle-splitting incision.

8

The intramedullary rod of the appropriate size and side is assembled with the tunnel locator and driver. A guide pin inserted through the tunnel locator should pass through the centre of the tunnel in the rod indicating proper orientation. The guide pin is now removed.

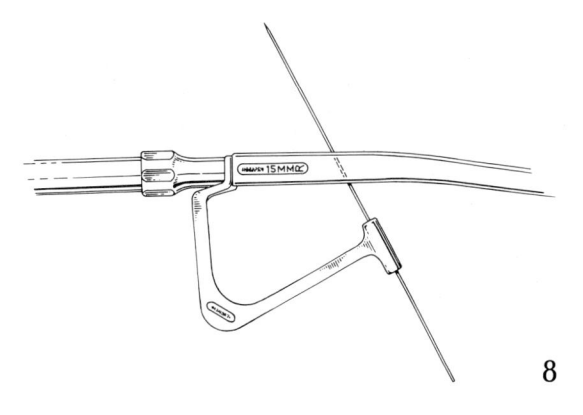

220 Lower limb fractures

9

With the fracture anatomically reduced, the leg is adducted and the assembled rod introduced through the tip of the trochanter.

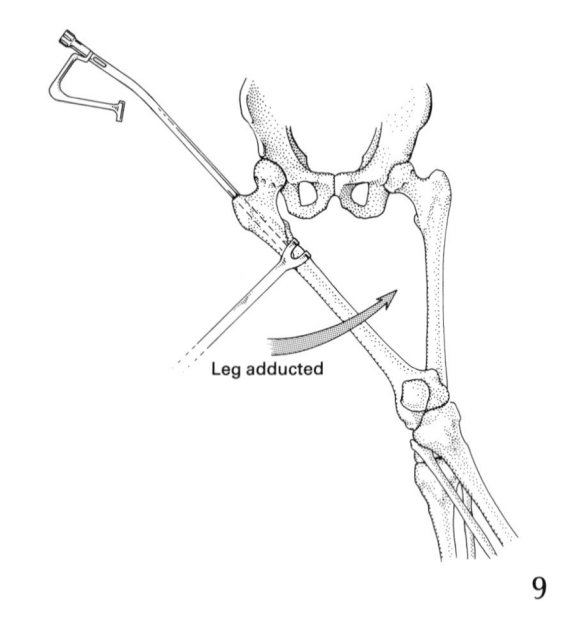

10

The correct orientation of the rod is controlled by the tunnel locator which serves as a handle during insertion of the appliance. This version should be determined immediately after the tip of the rod crosses the fracture site. With the leg in the neutral position, slight anteversion (approximately 15°) is the position of choice. Neutral position of the leg is determined by placing the leg with the patella pointing directly towards the ceiling as the surgeon steps back from the operating table and determines the version of the tunnel-locating gauge.

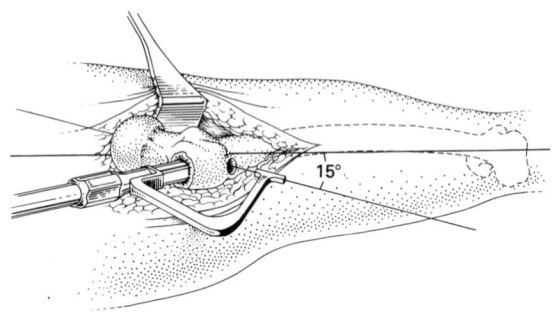

11

The rod is impacted until the tunnel locator is 2.5 cm below the vastus lateralis ridge. The guide pin is drilled through the arm of the locator into the neck and head of the femur, and radiographs are taken in two planes to determine the correct position.

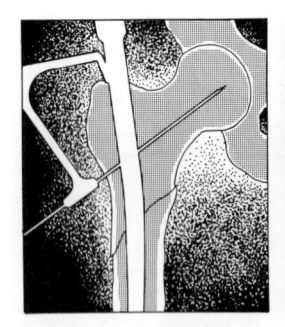

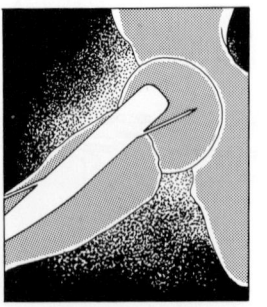

12

With the guide pin accurately positioned, the tunnel locator is removed. A 12 mm cortical reamer is passed over the guide pin and a cortical hole is drilled in the lateral cortex. The tunnel in the rod should now be visible and the wire is next extracted.

The hole in the bone may be enlarged with a curette so that a triflanged nail will pass easily through the tunnel in the rod. Difficulty encountered in this step is due to failure to remove sufficient cortical bone. The appropriate triflanged nail is driven through the tunnel in the rod to the correct depth in the femoral head. The grooves in the nail must face superiorly.

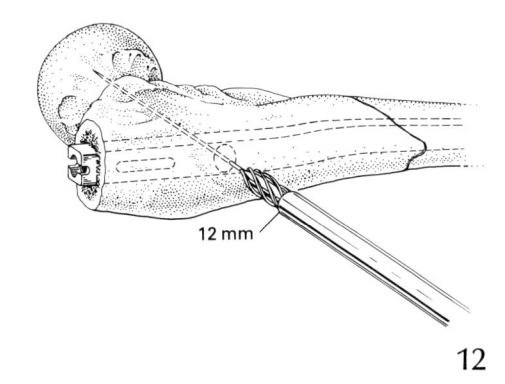

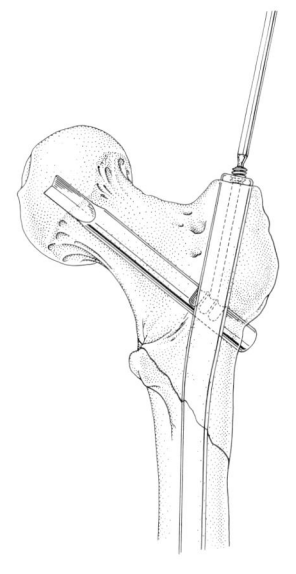

13

The set screw is inserted in the top of the rod with a hexagonal-head screw driver. When the blunt end of the screw has engaged a groove in the triflanged nail, the top of the screw will be level with the top of the rod. If more than one thread of the set screw is exposed it should be loosened and the nail driven or extracted slightly as the screw is being tightened. It should then engage the nail properly.

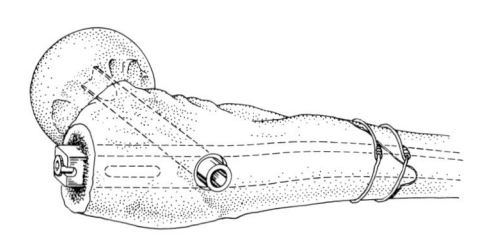

14

Accessory fixation, usually cerclage wires, is used when necessary.

The wound is closed in layers, as in other hip fractures.

Postoperative management

The patient may be mobilized with crutches as soon as comfortable. Full weight-bearing is not permitted until there is adequate radiographic evidence of fracture healing.

Complications

If the fracture is reduced correctly and the nail inserted accurately the success rate is very high. Most complications are due to faulty surgical technique and the failure to adhere to the surgical steps outlined.

References

1. Zickel RE. A new fixation device for subtrochanteric fractures of the femur: a preliminary report. *Clin Orthop* 1967; 54: 115–23.

2. Zickel RE. Subtrochanteric femoral fractures. *Orthop Clin N Am* 1980: 11(3): 555–68.

3. Zickel RE, Mouradian WH. Intramedullary fixation of pathological fractures and lesions of the subtrochanteric region of the femur. *J Bone Joint Surg [Am]* 1976; 58-A: 1061–6.

4. Zickel RE. An intramedullar fixation device for the proximal part of the femur: nine years' experience. *J Bone Joint Surg [Am]* 1976; 58-A: 866–72.

5. Seinsheimer F. Subtrochanteric fracture of the femur. *J Bone Joint Surg [Am]* 1978; 60-A: 300–6.

Illustrations by D. Howat, T. King and Paul Richardson

Küntscher's closed intramedullary nailing technique for the treatment of femoral shaft fractures

Kevin F. King FRCS, FRACS
Director, Department of Orthopaedic Surgery, The Royal Melbourne Hospital, Victoria, Australia

Introduction

Küntscher first described his closed femoral nailing operation in 1940 and over the next 30 years gradually improved the technique, particularly by the introduction of flexible intramedullary reaming over guide wires and by the use of the image intensifier radiographic unit in the late 1950s. Using this technique, a femoral shaft fracture can be fixed rigidly through a single small incision over the lateral aspect of the buttock. The procedure can be carried out with minimal trauma, with little interference to the fracture haematoma, and without further disruption to the periosteal blood supply of the femoral shaft. Over the last 10 years a further modification has been developed in the form of 'cross-pinning' to stabilize fractures otherwise unsuitable for closed nailing.

Preoperative

Indications

The prime indication for the closed nailing operation is a traumatic fracture of the midshaft of the femur. It is also suitable for use in some subtrochanteric fractures in the proximal one-third, and, with modifications (e.g. cross-bolts), it can be used to fix fractures of the lower third of the shaft internally. It is also readily applicable to the treatment of pathological fractures, particularly those due to osteoporosis and secondary neoplastic deposits where the patients are often frail, and minimal operative trauma is even more desirable than usual.

224 Lower limb fractures

Technical requirements

The following items of equipment are required.

Mobile image intensifier radiographic unit and a television screen

1

With sophisticated radiographic equipment it is possible to reduce the fracture, pass guide wires and to perform intramedullary reaming under direct radiographic screening.

A desirable extra piece of equipment is a video storage unit which allows radiographic images to be recorded, stored and recalled at will. This attachment not only makes the operative technique easier, but it also greatly diminishes the radiation to the patient and the theatre staff.

Orthopaedic operating table

This must be of a modern design with low-slung horizontal leg extension pieces which allow access for the image intensifier unit to be swung around the thigh through an arc of at least 110° from vertical to horizontal screening positions. It must have various types of perineal support bars, both of the horizontal and vertical variety, allowing the patient to be positioned either on the side or supine.

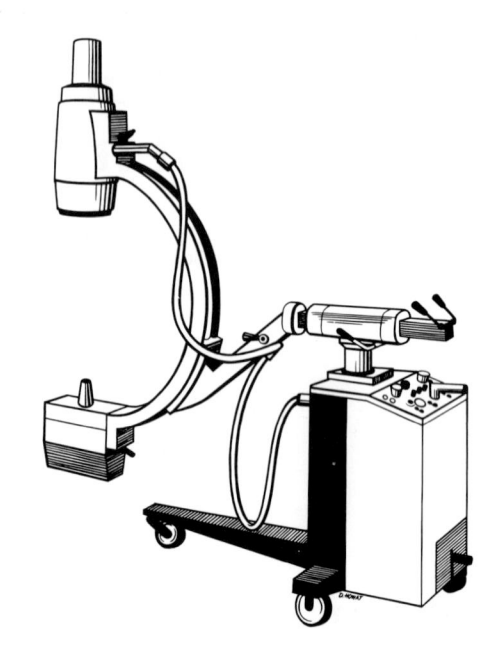

Complete set of Küntscher's instruments

2

A slow speed (up to 400 rev/min) right-angled air-powered drill with a cannulated chuck allowing the reaming bit to operate along a guide wire is required.

A full set of flexible cannulated intramedullary reamers increasing in diameter from 9 to 18 mm in 0.5 mm increments is also used.

A ball-tipped guide wire (3 mm in diameter, length 950 mm), over which the cannulated flexible intramedullary reamers are threaded, is used. In the event of reamer breakage, the ball tip allows for easy removal of the broken bits by withdrawal of the guide wire with the attached fragments.

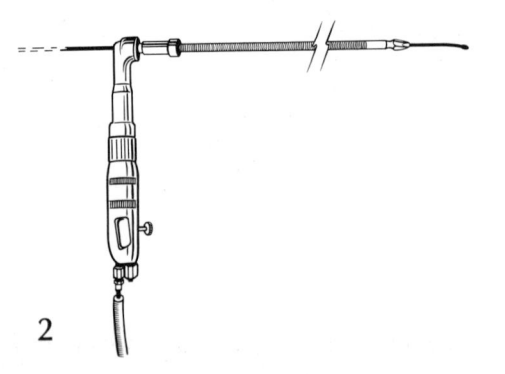

3

Medullary tube This is a plastic tube used for changing from reaming rod to inserting rod.

4

An inserting rod (4 mm in diameter, length 950 mm), over which the Küntscher's nail is inserted, is required.

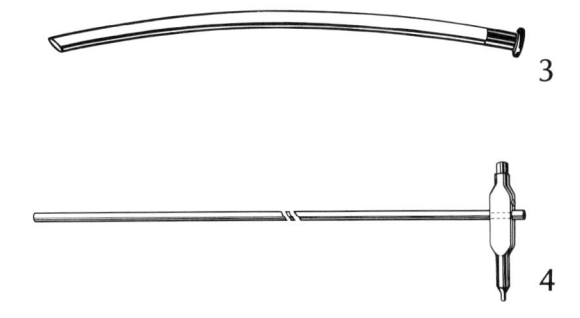

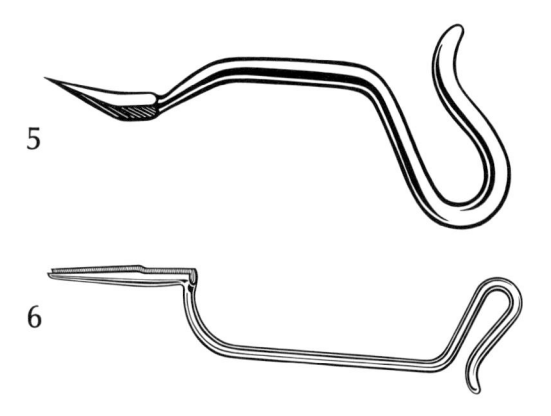

5 & 6

Awls A pointed awl is used to perforate the tip of the greater trochanter. The cannulated enlarging awl is used to enlarge and to straighten the initial hole in the greater trochanter and also gives some control over the proximal fragment of femur.

7

A *soft tissue guard* is used to protect the skin of the thigh at the upper margin of the incision.

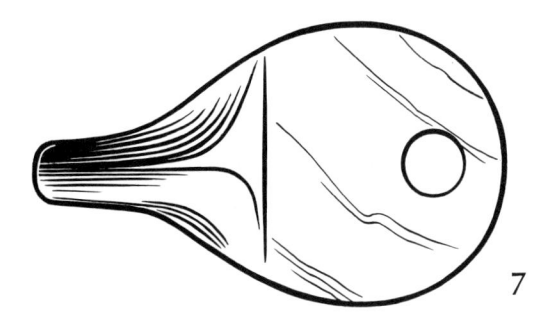

8

A *cannulated punch* and *split hammer* are used for the insertion of the nail over the guide wire.

A full set of Küntscher's nails is required. The minimum requirements are a set of nails varying in diameter from 10 to 18 mm and in length from 36 to 46 cm.

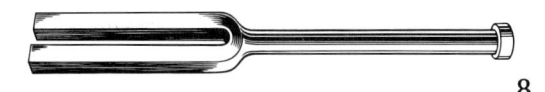

Supracondylar skeletal traction

9

A Steinmann pin should be inserted through the femoral condyles at the beginning of the operation. By means of a long stirrup connected to the footpiece of the orthopaedic table, routine traction forces of 24–74 kg (50–150 lb) can be applied to the lower femoral fragment, all traction through the knee itself being avoided. It is essential to the success of this operation that distraction of the bone ends should be achieved to permit reduction at the fracture site.

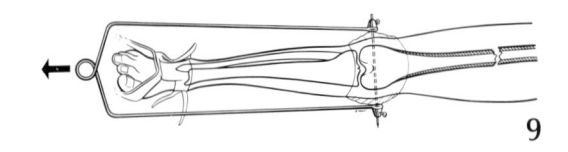

External correcting devices

These are designed to apply two-point pressure to the proximal and distal fragments, in a line at right angles to the line of the shaft, and are designed to be applied when the fracture site has been distracted by supracondylar traction.

10

Küntscher used a crutch and strap technique which was effective but which can be clumsy to use.

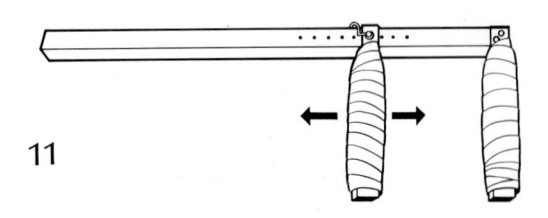

11

An alternative apparatus preferred by the author is made of square-section aluminium tubing which is radiotranslucent. It has padded jaws, the distance between which can be adjusted to fit varying thicknesses of thigh. With this instrument it is possible to apply corrective pressure and, possessing a long handle, it keeps the manipulator clear of the radiographic beam.

Protective lead-impregnated wrap-around aprons should be worn by all members of the surgical team working in the operating theatre. Thyroid shields should also be worn.

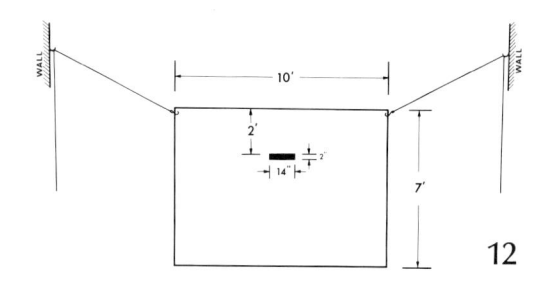

Special draping

12, 13 & 14

A large vertically-hung sheet with an operating slit 36 cm × 5 cm (14 × 2 inches) which fits over the lateral part of the buttock and upper thigh allows the surgeon access to the trochanteric region. It also leaves free access to the patient for the radiographer and anaesthetist. The sheet is suspended by its upper corners from opposite walls of the theatre and the upper free margin of the sheet lies over the midline of the patient. The surface of the sheet thus flows downwards and towards the surgeon over the curve of the buttock, allowing room for the use of reaming drills and other instruments. The long skirt of this sheet allows the image intensifier to swing up to the horizontal position without disturbing the sterile fields. The margins of the operating sheet are sutured to the lateral aspect of the upper thigh and buttock, and further secured with a Steridrape (Johnson & Johnson) to seal off the margins.

A Küntscher's nail extractor should always be available in case of need.

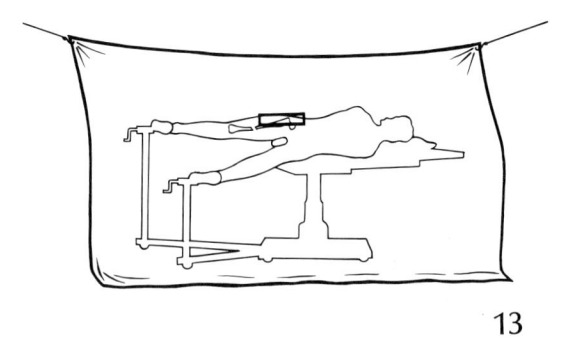

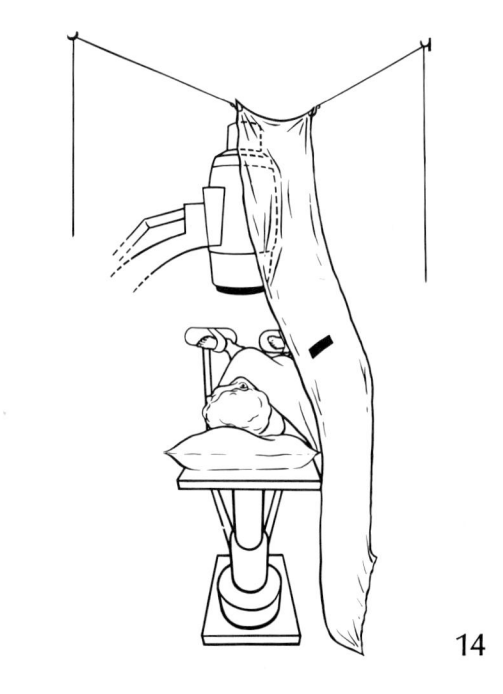

228 Lower limb fractures

Operation

Position of patient

The patient is anaesthetized on the anaesthetic trolley. The subsequent transfer to the orthopaedic table requires the cooperation of at least four people directed by the surgeon. The anaesthetist controls the head and shoulders, two assistants on opposite sides of the trolley and table lift the trunk, using a narrow lifting sheet under the buttocks, and a third assistant holds the feet and legs. The first stage is to transfer the patient onto the top of the orthopaedic table in a supine position, the perineal support having first been removed. At this stage the third assistant supports the weight of both legs. The next coordinated step is to switch the patient from a supine to a lateral position with the injured leg uppermost and the buttocks facing where the surgeon will stand.

15

The L-shaped perineal support is then attached to the orthopaedic table and its padded horizontal component is positioned in the perineum, separating the thighs. Both feet are now strapped to the footplates, the lower limb is fully extended at knee and hip, and the top limb is fully extended at the knee but flexed 30° at the hip. This flexion of the injured limb at the hip allows radiological screening in vertical and horizontal planes. The mobile image intensifier unit is now positioned with the plane on the C-arm at right angles to the line of the upper thigh. The beam is first centred in the vertical screening position, and once a satisfactory image has been obtained on the television screen, the C-arm is swung to the horizontal position and the height adjusted until a satisfactory image is obtained in this plane as well.

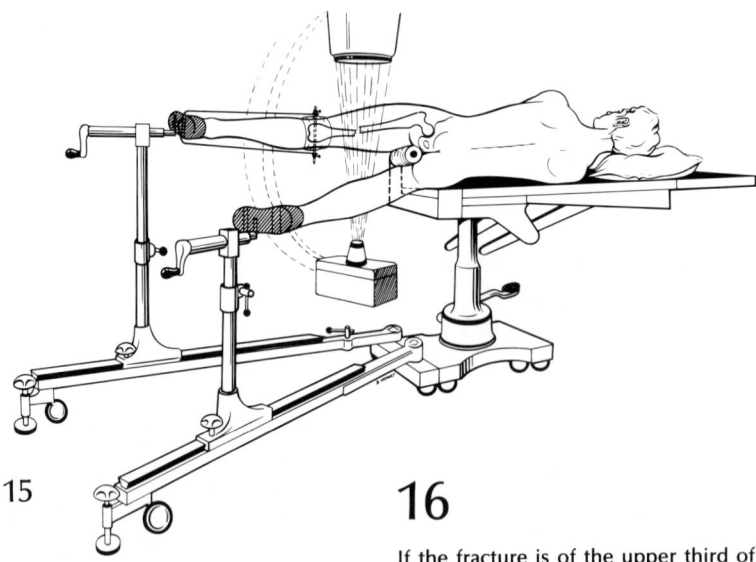

15

16

If the fracture is of the upper third of the femur, purely vertical screening may result in superimposition of the two thighs with a poor image. Therefore, in upper third fractures, the C-arm is swung 30° beyond the vertical to clear the lower thigh.

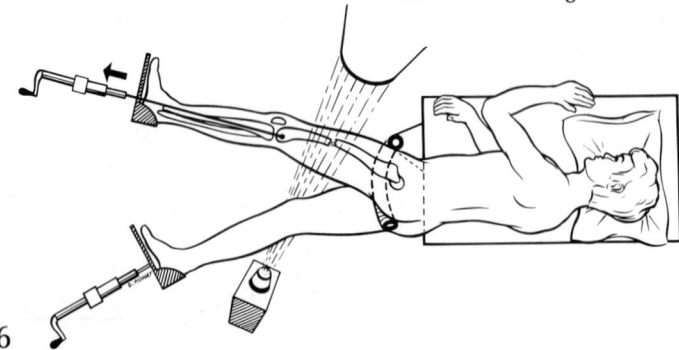

16

17

The above position is optimal for standard closed nailing. Another position is with the patient supine, the uninjured leg widely abducted and the image intensifier positioned between the legs. This arrangement is used when closed nailing of the femoral shaft is combined with fixation of a fracture of the neck of the femur in the same limb using Knowles' pins. An alternative lateral position is with the upper injured limb flexed 30° at the hip as described above, but the lower limb flexed as far as possible at both hip and knee with the subcutaneous surface of the tibia resting on a padded gutter support. This is an awkward position if there are other injuries affecting the opposite limb or if the patient has any stiffness at all of the knee and hip in the opposite limb.

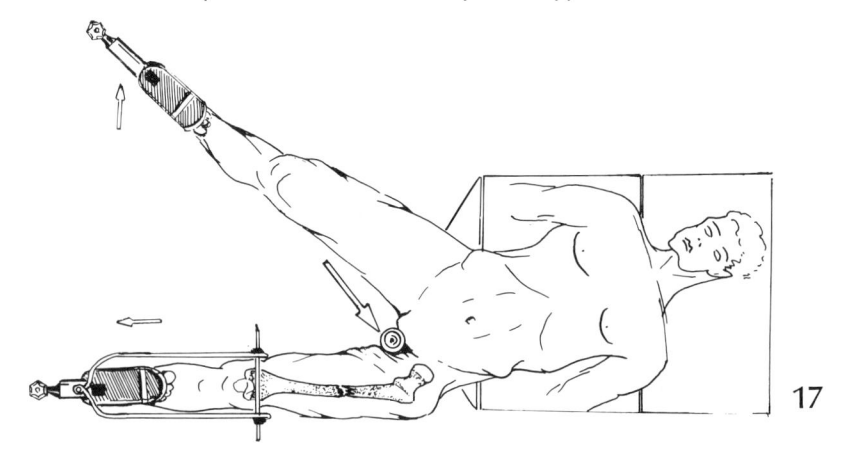

Insertion of supracondylar Steinmann pin and application of external correcting force

18

The outline of the femoral condyles is marked on the skin with a felt pen, the skin is prepared with iodine and a threaded Steinmann pin is drilled through the posterior halves of the lateral and medial femoral condyles, the placement avoiding the risk of the Küntscher's nail impacting on the Steinmann pin later in the operation. The long Steinmann pin stirrup is then attached and hooked around the footplate; through it, longitudinal traction may be applied without any strain being placed on the knee joint. Heavy traction forces of between 24 and 74 kg (50 and 150 lb) (as can' be measured on a spring balance) are then applied, and distraction of the bone ends is demonstrated on the radiographic screen. Once distraction is achieved, the external correcting device is applied and the bone ends are reduced under radiographic screening. The operation does not proceed unless preliminary reduction can be demonstrated on the image intensifier television screen. When reduction is achieved, the traction is partly released and the area of the greater trochanter is prepared and draped.

Heavy traction should be used for short periods only, initially to demonstrate reduction, then during the insertion of the guide wires, during reaming and then during the insertion of the nail. It should be relaxed in between these procedures to avoid any danger of pressure effects in the perineum.

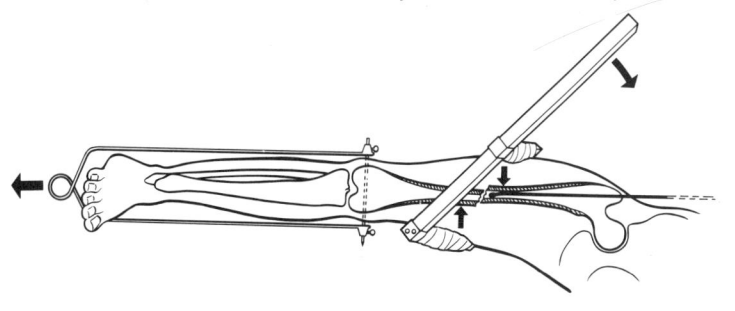

230　Lower limb fractures

Incision

19 & 20

A small 5 cm incision is made proximally from the tip of the greater trochanter in the line of the femoral shaft. The tip of the trochanter is palpated with a double-gloved finger, the conjoined fibres of the gluteus maximus and tensor fasciae latae are split in the line of their fibres, as are the distal fibres of gluteus medius. The upper border of the greater trochanter can then be palpated and seen; it is perforated with an awl midway between the anterior and posterior margins, and as far medially as is possible without actually passing over into the piriform fossa and onto the top of the femoral neck. Before making this awl hole it is essential to check once more the alignment of the proximal fragment of femur by placing a guide wire over the outer aspect of the thigh and screening both vertically and horizontally. If the awl hole is not made in the line of the medullary canal, a false passage may result and great difficulty can then be experienced in passing the guide wire down the femoral shaft. This initial awl hole is then enlarged with the enlarging awl, which also gives the operator some control over the proximal fragment. Through it, the ball-tipped guide wire is passed into the proximal shaft of the femur and heavy skeletal traction is reapplied. The external correcting device is used to reduce the bone ends and, under radiographic screening, the guide wire is passed into the distal fragment and advanced until it reaches the level of the femoral condyles. If the distal 2.5 cm of the guide wire is curved slightly this greatly assists its manipulation into the medullary canal of the distal fragment.

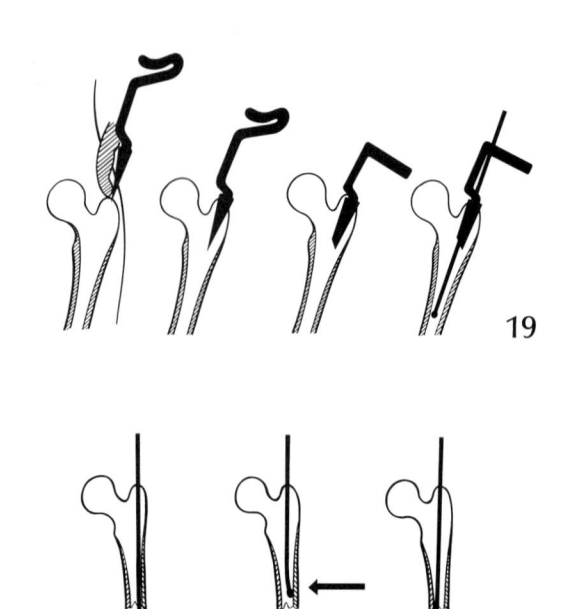

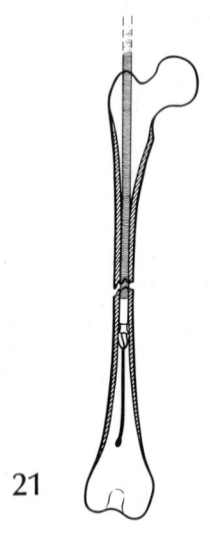

Flexible intramedullary reaming

21

The proximal and distal medullary canals are reamed in 0.5 mm increments, using the flexible intramedullary reamers over the ball-ended guide wire and starting at a diameter of 9 mm. In the average-sized adult, routine reaming up to 14 or 15 mm in diameter is used, the general principle being that the size of the reamer is increased until it can be felt to bite solidly on both proximal and distal medullary canals. When this occurs it is then advisable to ream at least several sizes above this. The larger the diameter of nail used the stronger and more rigid is the fixation.

Insertion of the nail

The length of the nail is gauged either by preliminary measurement of the opposite femur from the tip of the trochanter to the upper border of the patella (plus 1 cm) or, alternatively, by means of the intramedullary guide wire. The diameter of the nail must be 1 mm less than that of the largest reamer used to avoid any possibility of jamming. An inserting rod without a ball-tip is then substituted for the reaming guide wire, this manoeuvre being facilitated by the use of a plastic medullary tube which is temporarily passed down through the medullary canal while the exchange is being made.

The appropriate Küntscher's nail is then slowly tapped into the femur over the inserting rod, using the cannulated punch and split hammer.

22

As the tapered tip of the nail crosses the fracture site, it corrects the last few millimetres of lateral displacement and this stage must be closely observed under radiographic screening to ensure that the tip of the nail does not impact onto the distal fragment.

Traction is then released, and the rest of the nail is hammered into place, leaving 1 cm of nail exposed proximally above the tip of the greater trochanter to facilitate later removal.

Wound closure

The wound over the trochanter is now sutured and the Steinmann pin is removed from the supracondylar region of the femur.

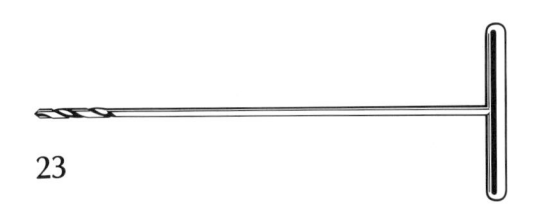

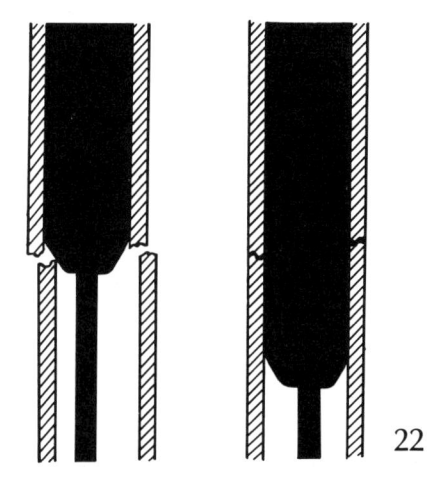

Complications and their management

Failure to reduce the bone ends preoperatively

If reduction cannot be demonstrated with supracondylar traction and external correcting force, the closed procedure should be abandoned.

Failure to pass the guide wire into the proximal medullary canal of the femur

23

This occurs if the awl hole in the tip of the trochanter is not made in the right direction at the correct point of entry. The direction in which the awl is inserted must be carefully checked by screening in two planes before the hole is made. If the guide wire does not glide easily into the medullary canal of the proximal fragment, the initial track is best made with a 9 mm diameter solid hand reamer.

232 Lower limb fractures

Jamming and breaking of reamers

If the full set of graduated reamers is used with a proper reaming drill and matching guide wires, this complication is rare. If, however, breakage or jamming does occur, then the remnants of the remaining drill can be removed by pulling out the guide wire. The ball on the end of the guide wire usually ensures that no fragments are left behind. Small broken metallic fragments lying loose in the medullary canal can be removed with sigmoidoscopy biopsy forceps, using the image intensifier for radiographic control.

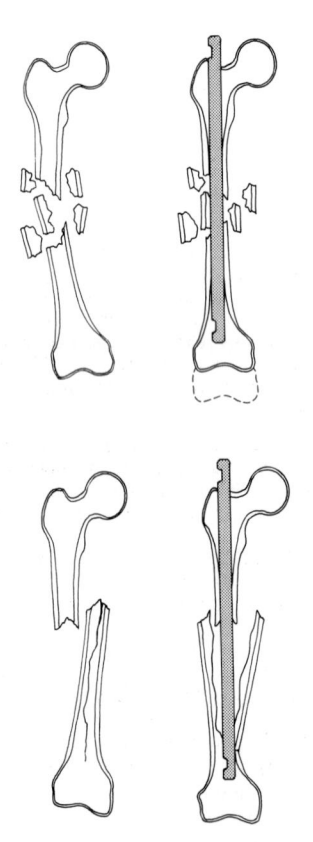

Impaction of the drill or nail on the edge of the distal cortex at the fracture site

This is avoided by reaming and inserting the nail under radiographic control in two planes and by screening continuously as the tip of the nail passes the fracture site.

Stuck nail

This should not happen if the femoral shaft in normal bones has been adequately reamed and if the diameter of the nail is 1 mm less than that of the largest reamer. In the case of Paget's disease affecting the femoral shaft, jamming may occur readily if the nail is not prebent to the shape of the bowed shaft.

Special indications

Interlocking nails

24

Comminuted fractures of the midshaft and fractures of the lower third of the femoral shaft are unsuitable for closed femoral nailing alone, as the nail will not grip on the distal fragment and thus will not control rotation or, in the case of comminution, shortening.

24

25

Over the last 10 years, various types of 'interlocking' or 'cross-pin' nails have been developed to overcome the stability problem. All rely upon operative techniques which allow threaded screws or pins to be inserted through the eyes in the proximal and distal ends of the intramedullary nail. In the case of the distal cross-pins, the nails are inserted by means of a closed, percutaneous technique using radiological control and require only a very small skin incision, approximately 0.5 cm in length.

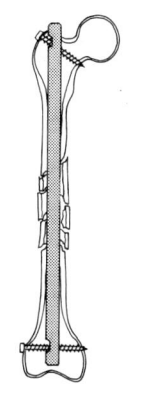

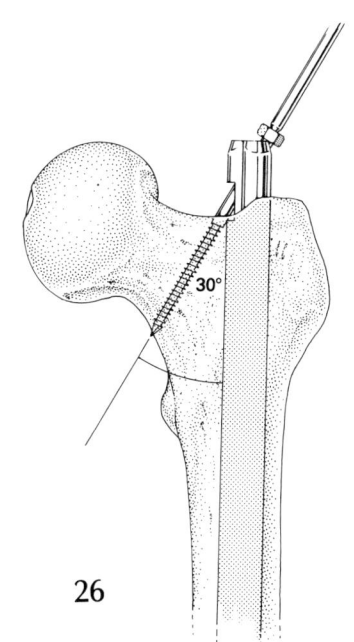

26

Insertion of the proximal cross-pin is not difficult as it can be performed either by a simple jigging system (as supplied with most types of interlocking nail) or under direct vision at the time of insertion of the nail through the proximal incision over the tip of the trochanter.

All techniques encounter major problems when endeavouring to insert the distal cross-pin. The methods used include:

1. An external jigging system attached to the image intensifier. This is generally regarded as being unsatisfactory as the aiming system is attached to an unstable platform, namely the C-arm of the image intensifier rather than to the patient's leg.
2. An external jigging system attached to the proximal end of the nail itself. This is theoretically effective but it has the disadvantage that intramedullary nails, like all hollow rods, will bend and twist if, over a length of 40–46 cm, they are exposed to the deforming forces which inevitably occur during the insertion of the nail down the intramedullary canal of a femur.
3. Hand-held external aiming devices. These do not supply a fixed or stable aiming platform and expose the operating surgeon to unnecessary radiation.

234   Lower limb fractures

MELBOURNE CROSS-PINNING TECHNIQUE

27

The technique routinely used by the author and his colleagues since 1976 involves making a mark on the skin over the outer side of the patient's lower thigh and knee, using this as the aiming point, and therefore as the jigging device, in conjunction with the image intensifier, for the insertion of the distal cross-pin. This has proved to be a simple, reliable, effective and cheap method of obtaining interlocking fixation and requires no extra specialized equipment.

For this method we have routinely used Howmedica vitallium double-ended Küntscher nails with eyes in both proximal and distal ends. It should be noted that these nails have an eye which measures 9 × 4 mm and, when viewed from the side, there is a distinct notch in the nail which can be visualized radiographically.

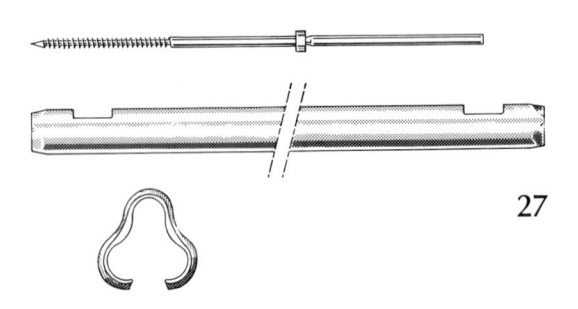

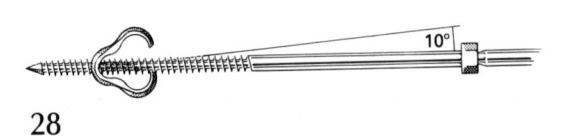

28

As cross-pins we have routinely used vitallium Knowles' pins threaded in the distal part of the shaft. These have proved to be suitable because they fit through the eye in the nail but will also allow approximately 10° of rock in the transverse plane of the femur, giving a margin of error during closed insertion. *It is essential, during insertion of the intramedullary nail, that the eye in the lower end of the nail should face exactly medially in the femoral shaft and that the longitudinal slit in the nail should face exactly laterally.* Careful control of this alignment must be observed during insertion of the nail as this accurate positioning is essential to the subsequent insertion of the distal cross-pin.

Position of patient

29

The patient remains on the orthopaedic table in the same lateral position used in the initial part of the operation for the insertion of the intramedullary nail. It must be emphasized once again that this nail must have been inserted with the longitudinal slit facing exactly laterally in the shaft and therefore directly up towards the roof of the operating theatre. If intraoperative supracondylar traction has been used, this is now removed.

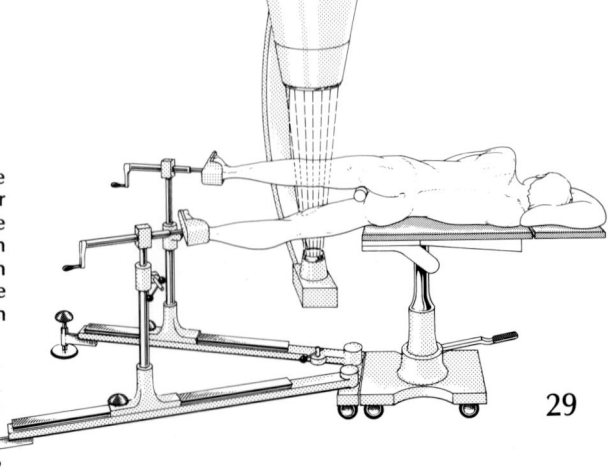

Küntscher's closed intramedullary nailing technique 235

30

The image intensifier is now positioned with the beam centred vertically over the lower end of the femur. If the intramedullary nail has been inserted as described, screening will now produce an image showing the 'eye' in the nail midway between anterior and posterior margins.

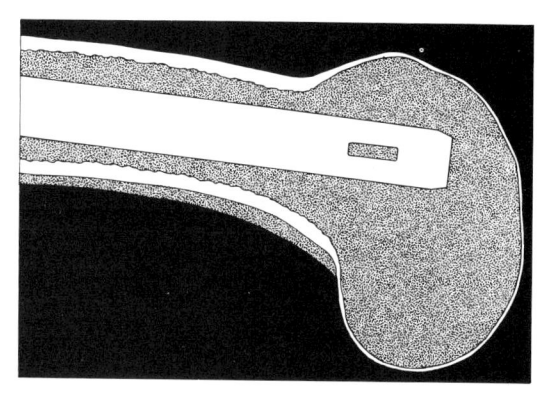

31

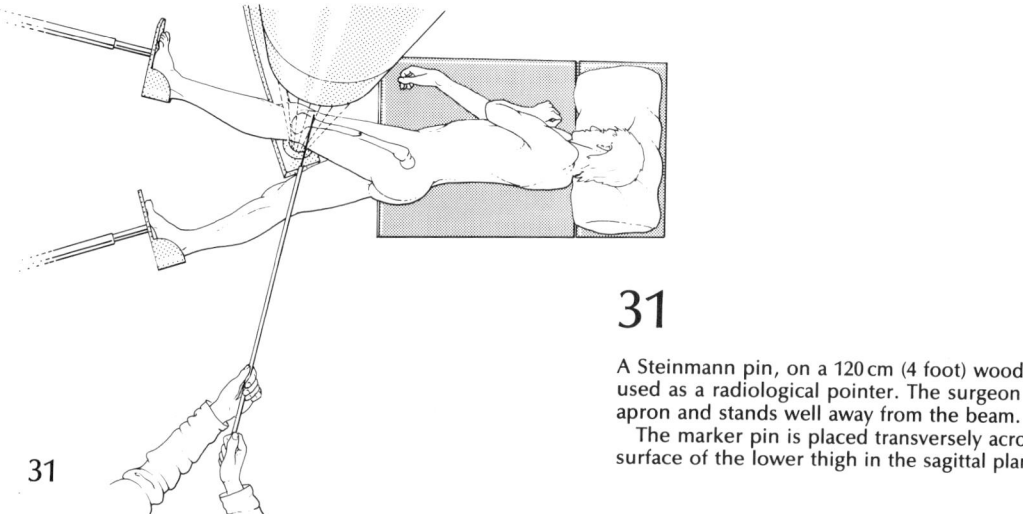

A Steinmann pin, on a 120 cm (4 foot) wooden handle, is used as a radiological pointer. The surgeon wears a lead apron and stands well away from the beam.

The marker pin is placed transversely across the upper surface of the lower thigh in the sagittal plane.

32

The pointer is then rolled up and down the thigh until, on intermittent screening, it is seen to cover the upper half of the eye.

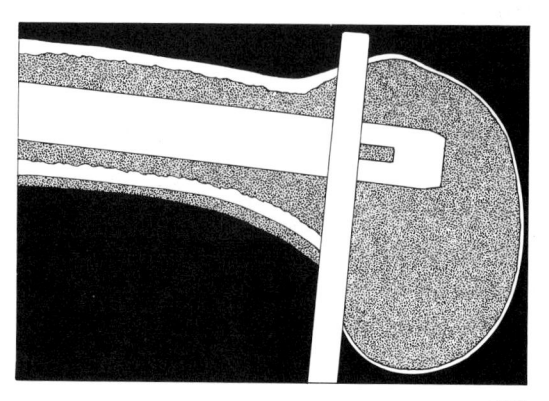

236 Lower limb fractures

33, 34 & 35

A transverse line is then drawn on the skin with a felt pen. Further oblique lines, 45° upwards and 45° downwards, are drawn on the skin using the same radiological screening technique. The surgeon now knows that, below this point, at a depth of approximately 3 cm, lies the lower eye in the intramedullary nail.

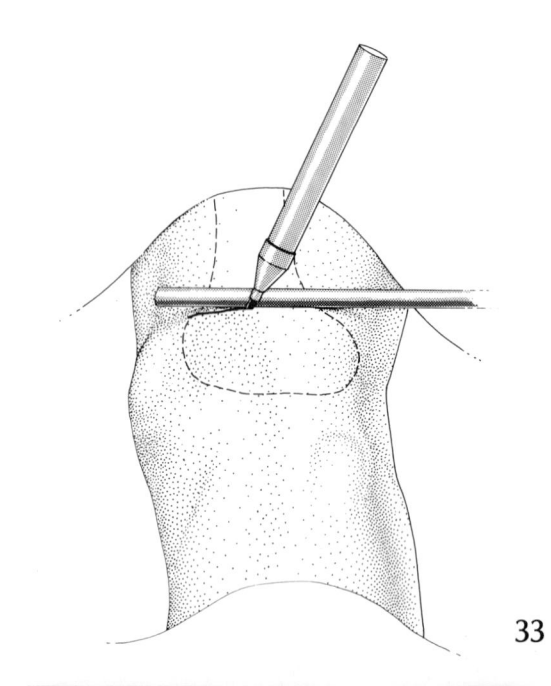

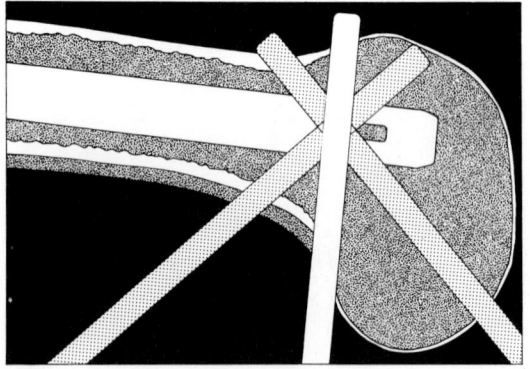

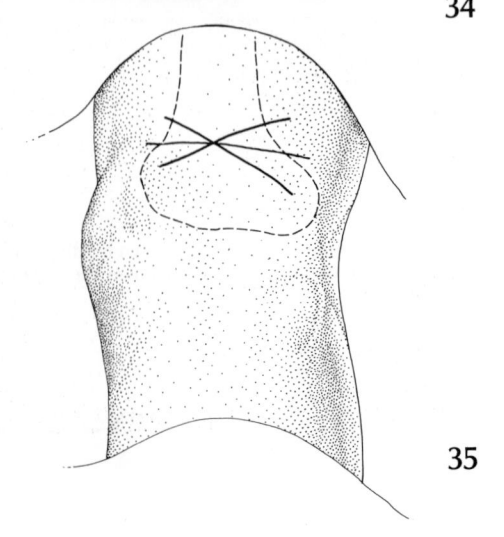

33

34

35

Küntscher's closed intramedullary nailing technique 237

36

A Knowles' pin of suitable length, as gauged by pre-operative radiography, is fitted into the chuck of the hand-drill. A small stab incision is made at the 'aiming point' at the junction of the three lines on the skin, and the Knowles' pin is drilled vertically downwards into the underlying lateral condyle of the femur to a depth of approximately 2–3 cm. The vertical alignment is controlled by the surgeon's eye.

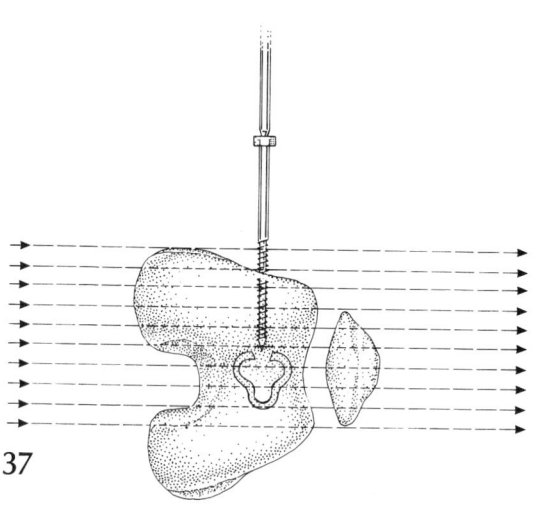

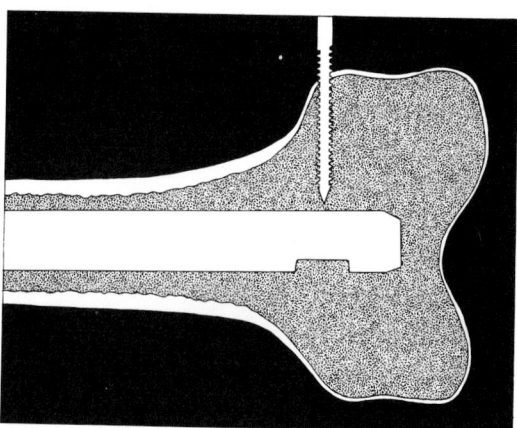

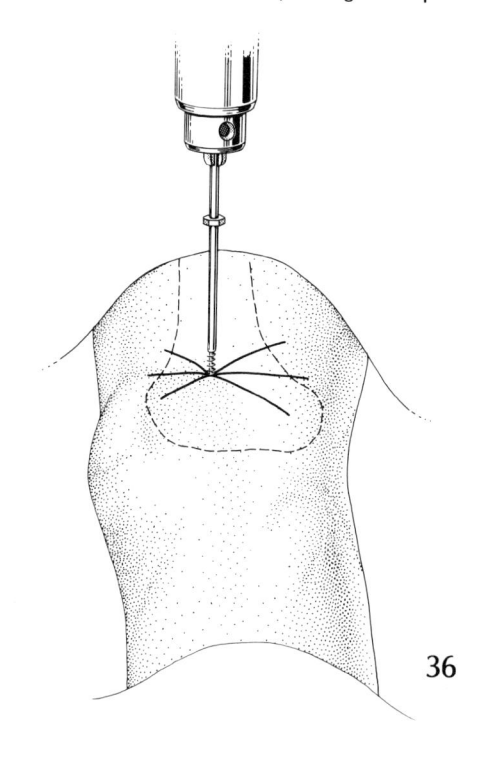

37 & 38

Radiological screening is then carried out in the horizontal plane to check that the Knowles' pin has been inserted at a suitable level in relation to the lower eye.

238 Lower limb fractures

39

The image intensifier is then used to screen vertically or, as close to the vertical plane as is required, to align the beam along the line of the Knowles' pin as it sits in its partially inserted position. The hand-drill is removed from the Knowles' pin before screening.

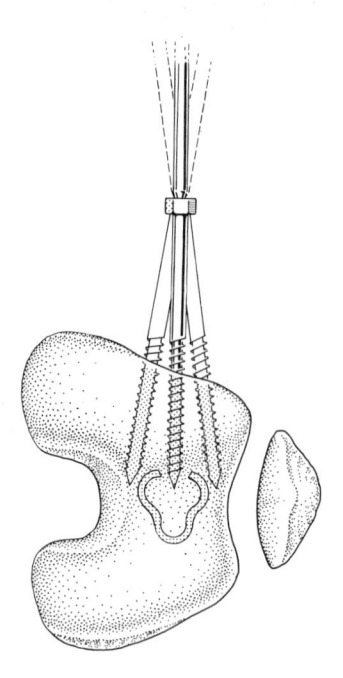

40

Ideally, the tip of the Knowles' pin should pass through the distal eye at the first attempt, but more frequently several passes are required.

41

If the Knowles' pin lies anteriorly or posteriorly, vertical screening along the line of the Knowles' pin will reveal this, the appearance being known as the 'sunrise' effect with the tip of the Knowles' pin appearing anterior or posterior to the lower margins of the nail.

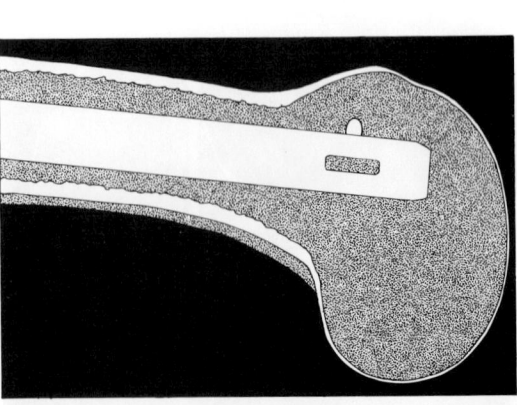

42

The Knowles' pin is then withdrawn 1 cm, swivelled on the lateral cortex and reinserted. After no more than several partial withdrawals and reinsertions, the Knowles' pin will pass through the eye. On vertical screening, the 'bull's eye' effect is seen with the tip of the Knowles' pin exactly filling the eye in the lower end of the nail. Each time the Knowles' pin is adjusted, the beam of the image intensifier must also be adjusted so that it is parallel to the Knowles' pin.

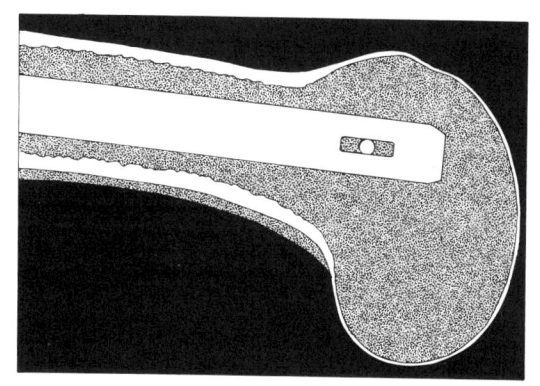

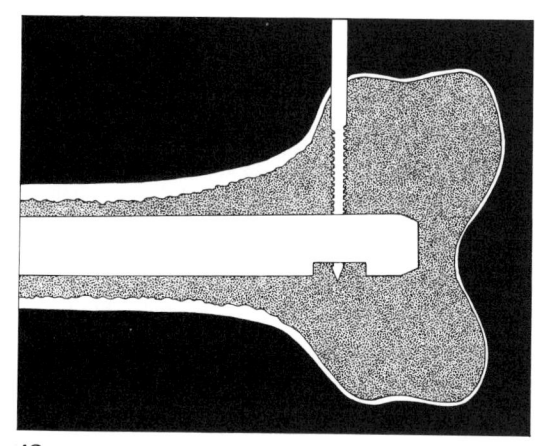

43

Accurate alignment is then confirmed by horizontal screening, the tip of the Knowles' pin being seen to appear just below the nail. The operator now knows that the Knowles' pin is lying within and the tip just through the eye.

44

The Knowles' pin is then drilled in to engage the opposite cortex. It is desirable to leave approximately 0.5 cm of the proximal shaft of the Knowles' pin protruding to allow easy removal at a later date.

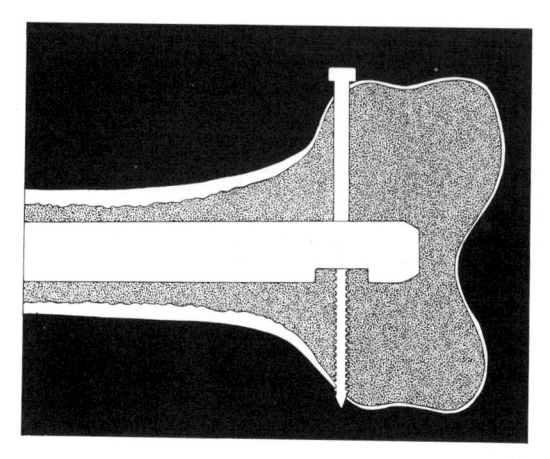

ADAPTION OF CROSS-PINNING TECHNIQUE TO VARIOUS FORMS OF COMMERCIALLY AVAILABLE INTERLOCKING NAIL SYSTEMS

This operative technique for cross-pinning is easily applied to the newer forms of cross-bolting device including the AO Universal, the Grosse and Kempf and the Russell–Taylor interlocking nail systems. The only minor changes that have to be applied to the technique are as follows.

1. In order to cross-bolt the proximal end of the nail the standard proximal jig, from any of the assorted sets, would be used.
2. For distal cross-bolting the standard 4.2 mm diameter AO type drill bit is used, in place of the Knowles' pin (without a proximal self-locking cuff), the soft tissue being protected by a 4.2 mm soft tissue protecting sleeve from the standard AO instruments. In all other respects, particularly for protection of the surgeon from unnecessary radiation when screening, the technique is exactly the same. Once this 4.2 mm drill bit has been seen to pass through the lateral cortex, through the two eyes in the lower end of the nail and on through the lateral cortex of the lateral femoral condyle, it is a simple matter to substitute the appropriate threaded cross-bolt.

Virtually any form of standard intramedullary nail, commercially available, can be modified for the cross-pinning technique by asking any hospital workshop to drill suitable holes through the distal end and, if necessary, the proximal end of the nail as well. Attention must be given, in these circumstances, to compatibility of the metals used in the nails and screws.

Postoperative management

Postoperative management for routine intramedullary nailing is to rest the limb in a sling or Thomas' splint for 1–2 days until pain and swelling have subsided. Full weight-bearing is started within several days of the operation.

In the average patient with an uncomplicated fracture of the middle third of the femoral shaft, where a firm grip has been obtained on both proximal and distal fragments, the patient can be discharged home within 10–14 days, fully weight-bearing. Quadriceps exercises and knee-bending are started within 24 hours.

In a case where cross-pinning has been used and the femoral shaft is comminuted, or the lower third of the shaft is involved, only partial weight-bearing is permitted from the second or third day onwards, up to a maximum of 9–14 kg (20–30 lb). This partial weight-bearing is maintained for 6 weeks. At the end of this time the distal cross-pin is usually removed as the patient often complains of some discomfort from the protruding head of the pin.

Appendix

Availability of equipment

The most complete and technically the most satisfactory set of instruments is that designed by the AO group, which is manufactured by Synthes. They have copied and improved Küntscher's original instruments, the only item missing being the enlarging trochanteric awl. The solid hand reamers in the AO set can be used as a substitute.

Zimmer produce a basic set of instruments, including the trochanteric enlarging awl and a right-angled air drill designed for reaming. This is neither as complete nor as technically satisfactory as the AO set but is significantly cheaper.

Howmedica supply a good set of flexible cannulated reamers produced by Ortopedia, a German subsidiary, but supporting instruments are limited.

In his last years, Küntscher himself had his instruments and implants supplied by an American company, the Orthopaedic Equipment Company. The author has had no experience with this particular set but assumes that they are satisfactory, having been designed to Küntscher's specifications.

In regard to 'cross-pinning', various types of interlocking nail have been produced over the last few years. Technically, the most satisfactory of these are the Grosse and Kempf system and the new AO interlocking system.

The instruments for the Grosse and Kempf system are complicated, and the external jigging system for insertion of the distal interlocking pin is associated with technical problems. In addition, different shaped nails are used for right and left femoral shafts.

The AO interlocking nail system is similar, but has the advantage of being completely compatible with the AO intramedullary reaming instruments. One shape of nail will fit both right and left sides but it has the problem of not supplying an entirely satisfactory aiming system for insertion of the distal interlocking pin.

Other types of interlocking pin available in recent years are the Huckstep intramedullary compression nail system (not really a closed system), the Biomet winged nail and the Russell–Taylor interlocking nail system (Richards). The author has had no personal experience of these systems.

Klemm and Boerner devised a cross-pinning technique based upon an idea of Küntscher and this was the first effective interlocking system. The instruments are manufactured by Ortopedia. The system used for inserting the distal cross-pin is similar to that produced much later by the AO school.

The long traction stirrups for supracondylar traction can be inexpensively made to order by any surgical supply firm or hospital splint shop. An aluminium external correcting device was designed and made in his own workshop by Mr E. Talkish, a radiographer at the Western General Hospital, Melbourne. The design is simple and the instrument can be easily reproduced by any hospital engineer or splintmaker.

There are various designs of mobile image intensifier unit available. The C-arm must rotate through an arc of at least 110°. Video storage units are expensive and are not essential. However, they are valuable, not only because they reduce radiation but also because they make the operation technically easier.

Protective lead aprons are used by all personnel in the operating theatre, are of standard design and readily available. The long pointer can be simply made from a suitable broomstick with a Steinmann pin fitted into one end. This device enables the operator to stand well away from the radiation beam while screening during the preliminary aiming process for cross-pinning.

Further reading

Decoulx J, Kempf I, Jenny G, Schvingt E, Petit P, Vives P. Enclouage à foyer fermé avec alésage du fémur selon Küntscher: technique, indications et résultats à propos de 399 cas. *Rev Chir Orthop* 1975; 61: 464–86.

Kempf I, Grosse A, Beck G. Closed locked intramedullary nailing: its application to comminuted fractures of the femur. *J Bone Joint Surg [Am]* 1985; 67-A: 709–20.

Klemm KW, Boerner M. Interlocking nailing of complex fractures of the femur and tibia. *Clin Orthop* 1986; 212: 89–100

Kootstra G. *Femoral shaft fractures in adults: a study of 329 consecutive cases with a statistical analysis of different methods of treatment.* Assen, The Netherlands: Royal Van Gorcum, 1973.

Küntscher G. *Practice of intramedullary nailing.* Springfield: Charles C. Thomas, 1967.

Illustrations by Peter Cox

Supracondylar fractures of the femur

C. E. Ackroyd MA, FRCS
Consultant Orthopaedic Surgeon, Southmead Hospital, Bristol, UK

Introduction

General considerations

Fractures of the supracondylar and intracondylar region of the femur are difficult to treat satisfactorily and require careful management to obtain good cosmetic and functional results. The main problem is obtaining and maintaining an adequate reduction of both shaft and articular fragments while allowing function of the knee to be regained at an early stage. There are powerful muscles which act across the knee, tending to maintain deformity of the fracture fragments. It is difficult to counterbalance these forces by closed methods, and if open reduction and internal fixation is performed the implants can be subjected to considerable loading.

Closed methods of treatment have traditionally been used for these injuries, using tibial traction or occasionally the two-pin skeletal traction technique described by Modlin[1]. The reports of Stewart et al.[2] and Neer et al.[3] of 25 years ago confirmed the place of non-operative treatment by the standards of those times. Improved results have been obtained by emphasis on earlier function using Perkins' technique of joint movement in traction and the application of cast-bracing to allow earlier mobilization of the patient[4].

In recent years great advances have been made in the understanding and techniques of internal fixation. Considerable skill is necessary to obtain anatomical reduction of the more complex fractures, and fixation is only an advantage if this can be sufficiently rigid to allow early function of the knee joint. Good results of open reduction and internal fixation have been reported[5-7].

In 1974 Shatzker et al.[8] published the results of 71 supracondylar fractures. They applied stricter criteria for the results and showed that those patients whose fractures had been treated according to the AO principles obtained 75 per cent good or excellent results, contrasting with 32 per cent good or excellent results in those patients who were treated non-operatively. A further study in 1979 on 35 patients treated by open reduction and internal fixation reinforced the importance of surgical technique[9]: 71 per cent of the 17 patients who were treated according to the AO principle achieved a good or excellent result. Only 21 per cent of 18 patients achieved a good or excellent result when the operation failed to achieve anatomical reduction and stable internal fixation. It is clear that properly performed operations can produce excellent results that are generally superior to non-operative treatment. However, non-operative treatment is better than operation improperly carried out or performed in less than ideal circumstances.

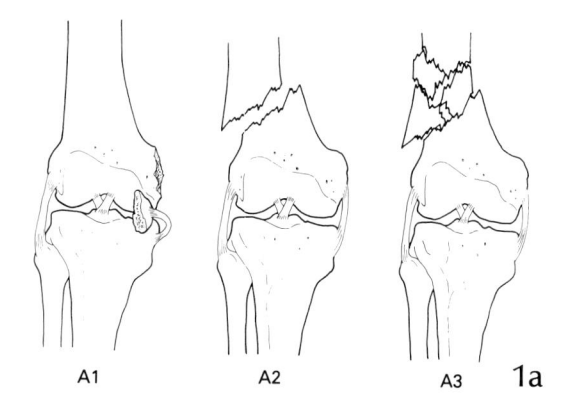

Classification

It is important to define the 'personality' of this fracture and take into account the various factors before deciding on open operation. High-velocity injuries, fracture comminution, and osteoporosis make the fracture much more difficult to treat. Supracondylar fractures may be undisplaced, impacted, displaced or comminuted.

1a, b & c

A useful classification has been designed by the AO group[5]. Type A fractures are extra-articular and vary in complexity from ligamentous avulsion through to severe comminution of the shaft in the supracondylar region. Type B fractures involve only one condyle and vary in the fracture fragment size and in the fracture plane. Type C fractures include the typical T and Y-shaped intra-articular and supracondylar types with varying degrees of comminution.

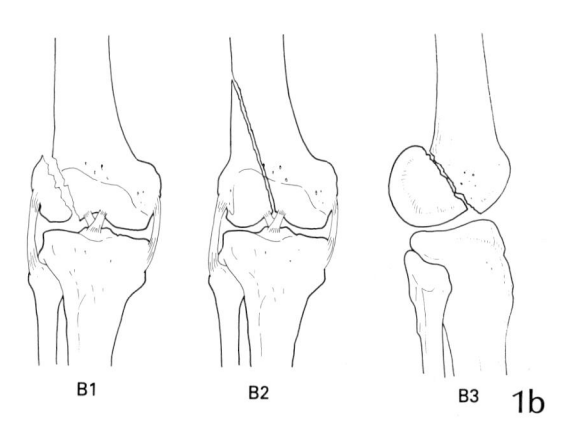

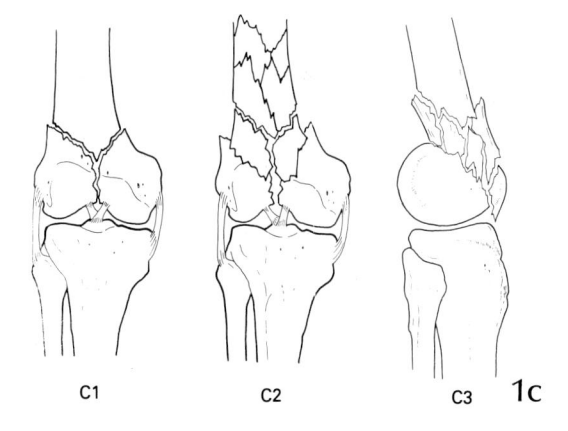

Indications for operation

Open reduction and internal fixation should only be carried out if the surgeon is sure that he can achieve the goals of anatomical reduction, rigid internal fixation and early return to full function. The surgeon must consider carefully his own personal results of internal fixation, and in each case consider the factors which may lead to an unsatisfactory result. These operations take several hours and they should not be performed late at night, when the surgeon is tired or when the theatre equipment or surgical team is less than optimal. Many fractures can be treated reasonably satisfactorily by the technique of skeletal traction with early active joint movement, followed by a functional brace.

Absolute indications

Extra-articular fractures Where adequate alignment of the fracture cannot be obtained or maintained by traction (Type A), internal fixation is indicated. It is quite reasonable to carry out delayed primary fixation if it proves impossible to maintain a satisfactory position within 1–2 weeks of injury. Fixation at a later stage is feasible but it is likely to produce a less satisfactory result.

Unicondylar fractures These can seldom be reduced satisfactorily by non-operative means (Type B). Redisplacement of a reduced fracture often occurs and joint mobilization cannot occur to any significant degree for several weeks.

Fractures in the coronal plane These cannot be reduced by closed means though failure to get a perfect reduction at open operation or damage to the soft tissue attachments of the fragment may compromise the final result.

T or Y bicondylar fractures Where there is rotation of the condyles, or when traction has not produced a satisfactory reduction (Type C), open reduction is indicated. Separation of the condyles by more than 2–3 mm, varus or valgus displacement or malrotation always suggests surgical treatment. Operation should be carried out within 1 week as significant delay will make the operation much more difficult. Extensive dissection may be required to reduce the fragments and the fracture surfaces in the cancellous areas tend to round off rapidly.

Open fractures Prevention of sepsis is the most important goal in these injuries. Clinical and experimental work suggests that stabilization of bone fragments is an important adjunct to the management of the traumatic wound.

Pathological fractures These injuries are an important indication for internal fixation as fracture healing is likely to be slow and early stabilization will help management of the tumour whether by radiotherapy or chemotherapy.

Other indications There are a variety of other circumstances where internal fixation is desirable. These include multiple injuries, fractures associated with neurovascular injury and cases where there are other major bony injuries to the same limb.

Relative indications

Experienced surgeons working in good conditions can achieve excellent results in the majority of cases. This fact should not encourage operative treatment by the less experienced. Open operation can be extremely difficult and the full armamentarium of instruments and techniques may be necessary to achieve satisfactory fixation.

Fixation of the articular fragments alone can be considered and the supracondylar component can be treated by skeletal traction and early active joint movement.

Preoperative

Adequate radiographs should be performed so that a precise diagnosis of the fracture type and severity of injury can be diagnosed. Anteroposterior, lateral and oblique views of the injured side are obtained as well as anteroposterior and lateral views of the uninjured side to aid the preoperative planning. Tomography can help to identify the fracture fragments and CT scanning may be useful in certain complex injuries.

Operative treatment is best carried out within 12 hours, before significant swelling and soft tissue oedema have developed. The fracture should be splinted in the accident department and light traction applied to the leg on a Thomas' splint to reduce pain and blood loss.

If circumstances are not satisfactory for an immediate operation then provisional reduction should be carried out under general anaesthesia with application of skeletal traction and a Thomas' splint with the knee flexed. The Denham pin should be inserted well below the tibial tubercle to avoid contamination of the skin incision. It is best to wait 5–7 days before operation, until the swelling has decreased. If the operation is delayed more than 2 weeks it becomes much more difficult. At 6–8 weeks the operation can be considered equivalent to treating a case of delayed union or non-union.

Preoperative planning

2a & b

Time spent planning the operation can reduce considerably the time of the surgical procedure. Celluloid sheets and felt tip pens should be available in theatre so that the fracture lines can be drawn on a tracing of the normal femur or on a plastic femur, which will help considerably in planning the surgical approach.

The position of the window for the seating chisel in the lateral femoral condyle is marked at the centre of the anterior half of the condyle (A–B). The lag screws used to secure fixation of the condyles are then marked and additional interfragmentary screws are considered. Threaded or gliding holes may need to be drilled prior to fracture reduction and these can be marked on the drawing.

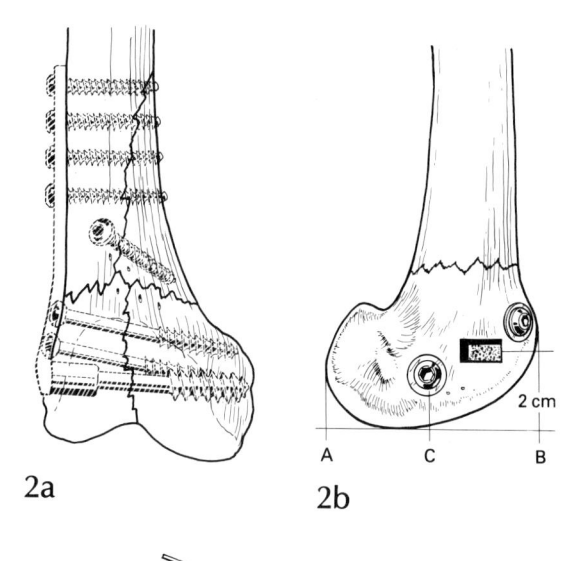

2c

It is important to note that the end of the femoral condyles form a quadrilateral shape, being higher on the lateral side. This is shown by the anterior Kirschner wire. The blade of the blade–plate or screw should be parallel to this wire and the correct length of implant should be measured. Transparent templates of the plates are available and this will enable judgement to be made about the length of the blade–plate. The experienced planner will be able to consider the order in which the screws are to be inserted.

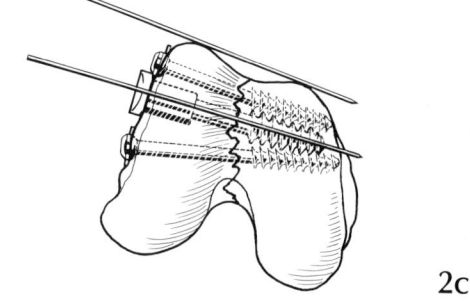

Positioning of patient

The operation is carried out under general anaesthesia. A tourniquet can be applied to the limb and used for periods of 2 hours to reduce the blood loss. Some surgeons prefer to operate without a tourniquet. The limb should be exsanguinated by elevation alone and the tourniquet inflated with the knee in the flexed position to prevent tightening of the quadriceps muscle. The pneumatic tourniquet is inflated to double the systolic blood pressure, though in large limbs a higher pressure may be required.

The patient should be positioned supine on the operating table with a sandbag under the ipsilateral buttock to facilitate exposure of the greater trochanter and iliac crest for bone grafting.

It is necessary to flex the knee during the operation and it is most convenient to be able to break the operating table at the level of the knee joint. The surgeon can be seated beside the fractured limb and it is important to ensure a long waterproof gown.

The skin of the entire limb, from the umbilicus above to the entire foot below, is cleansed with several applications of a suitable antiseptic. It is helpful if most of the limb is exposed, but using a glove or plastic sheet to cover the foot. This facilitates visualization of leg alignment. The towelling is prepared to allow good access to the bone-graft sites.

Operation

Incision

3

The approach to the supracondylar region of the femur should be from the lateral side. The skin is incised in the mid-lateral position just in front of the iliotibial tract. The incision starts some 15 cm above the lateral joint line and runs to the midpoint of the lateral condyle. It then curves forwards medially to a point just distal to the tibial tubercle. The length of the incision will depend on the type of fracture. Supracondylar fractures require exposure to the level of the joint line. Intra-articular and complex fractures require an extensive exposure, often with osteotomy of the tibial tubercle.

The deep fascia is divided along the line of the incision to expose the vastus lateralis and the quadriceps expansion. The latter is divided along the line of the incision and in the more complex fractures extended to the tibial tubercle.

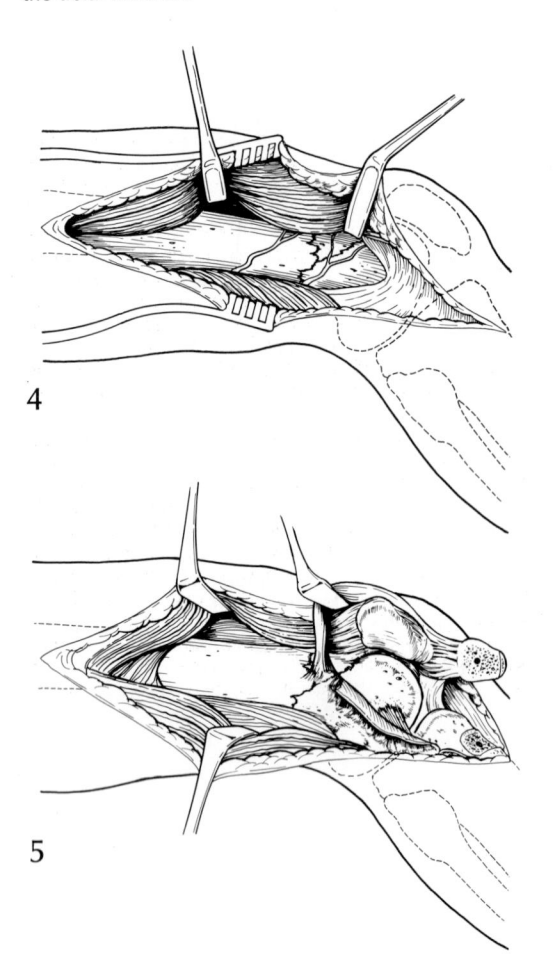

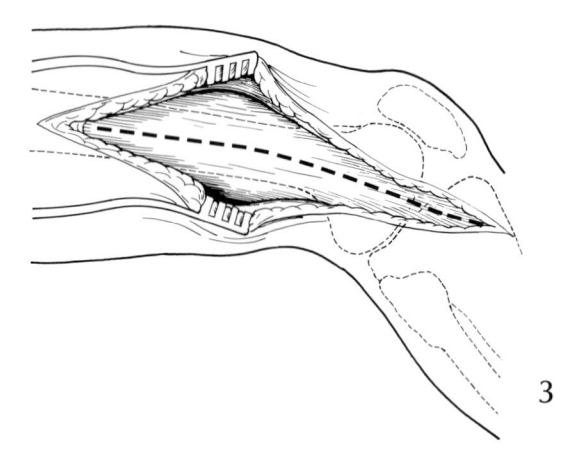

Exposure of fracture

4

Vastus lateralis is lifted forwards from the lateral intermuscular septum and separated from its attachment to the linea aspera. As in the approach to the femoral shaft, the perforating branches of the profunda femoris artery are divided and ligated. The line of dissection is continued downwards and the quadriceps expansion and the capsule of the knee joint are reflected forwards to expose the lateral femoral condyle. In the purely extra-articular fractures it may not be necessary to open the knee joint other than to obtain correct placement of the guide wires. In the more complex fractures the synovium is opened to expose the whole of the lateral aspect of the knee joint. In these cases the tibial tubercle is pre-drilled and tapped with two small or one large cancellous screw before the osteotomy so that the entire quadriceps mechanism can then be detached and reflected upwards and medially to expose the whole joint and the medial side of the shaft of the femur. It is important to preserve and carefully identify the tissue layers so that they can be closed satisfactorily at the end of the operation.

5

The fracture fragments are gently separated using a small bone hook and the fracture edges carefully cleaned, care being taken to maintain soft tissue attachments. Careful inspection of the fracture should be carried out at this stage in order to confirm the preoperative planning and define precisely the number of fragments present and the orientation of the fracture lines. Copious irrigation should be carried out with Ringer's solution to remove blood clot and keep the wound moist.

Supracondylar fractures of the femur 247

Reduction of the intercondylar fracture

In most cases the next stage in the operation is reduction of the articular surfaces. Flexion of the operating table at this stage often helps to get the fracture fragments reduced and particularly to correct rotational deformity.

In comminuted fractures the fracture jigsaw is assembled step by step and held with stout Kirschner wires. When there are two main fragments these are generally easily reduced and also held with stout Kirschner wires.

Care should be taken with placement of the interfragmentary screws, securing the condyles to ensure they do not interfere with placement of the blade–plate. Marking of the lateral condyle should be carried out at this stage to show where the plate will lie. The condylar fracture is fixed with two 6.5 mm cancellous screws one of which is inserted anterior to the plate and the second posteriorly. The 3.2 mm drill holes are made in the lateral femoral condyle and the screws are inserted after preliminary tapping of the proximal cortex. It is often necessary to use a washer on each screw.

It is now possible to reduce the simpler supracondylar components and the fracture is once again held with stout crossed Kirschner wires. More often the supracondylar component is comminuted and it is not possible to reduce the condyles onto the shaft until the blade or dynamic condylar screw has been inserted.

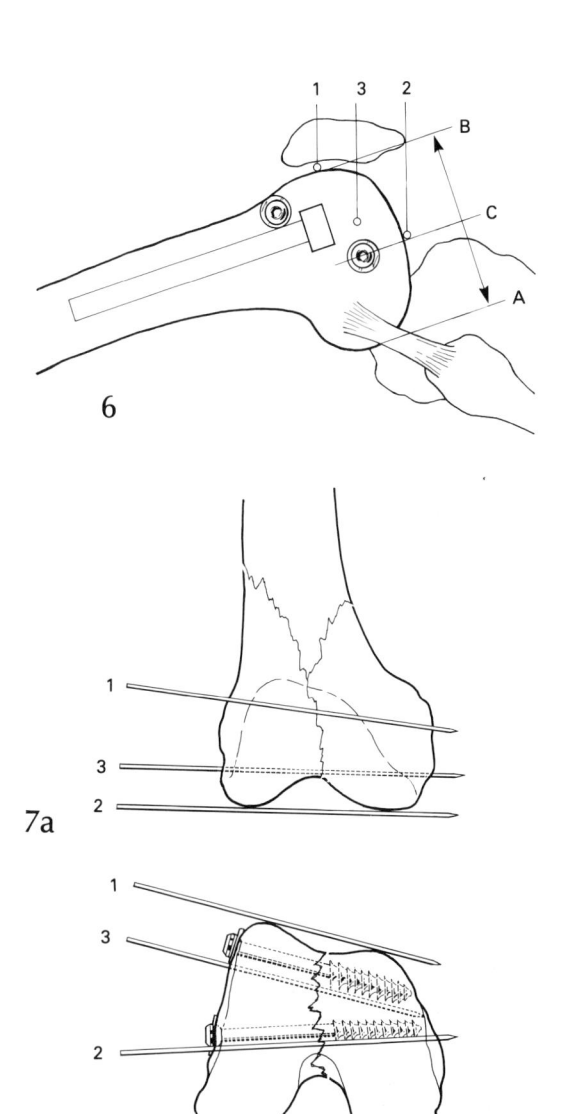

Placement of the lateral condylar window

6, 7a & b

The lateral profile of the femoral condyle is approximately twice the width of the femoral shaft which is in line with the anterior half of the condyle. Placement of the blade or condylar screw must be in the anterior half of the femoral condyles so that the plate will lie correctly along the femoral shaft. The anteroposterior width of the lateral femoral condyle should be measured (A–B) and the midpoint marked on the side of the femur with methylene blue (C). The anterior half is then bisected and the position for the window marked in the middle of the anterior half. The window is positioned 2 cm from the articular surface. This position is also marked with methylene blue.

Two guide wires are now placed across the joint to mark the surface alignment. Wire number 1 is placed parallel to the patellar surface of the femur and secured in the medial soft tissues. Wire number 2 is inserted transversely through the knee joint parallel to the surfaces of the femoral condyles. A third wire is now inserted on the power drill and passed through the middle of the femoral condyle, just above the articular surface. This wire is inserted parallel to guide wire 1 in the horizontal plane and parallel to wire 2 in the vertical plane. This then serves as a guide for the blade or condylar screw and its position should be checked with an anteroposterior radiograph.

8

If a 95° AO condylar blade–plate is to be used, the window in the lateral femoral condyle is now prepared. This should be 16 mm long and 8 mm wide with a bevelled proximal edge. This can be prepared easily with the 16 mm osteotome which is supplied in the blade–plate set. Alternatively, the triple-drill guide can be used to create three 4.5 mm screw holes in the outer cortex. These are then expanded using the router and the window is trimmed with the osteotome. A central hole is made with the 3.2 mm drill through the medial cortex for measurement of the blade–plate length. It is important to realize that the medial surface of the femoral condyle slopes at an angle of approximately 25° and care must be taken to choose a blade of the correct length. This cannot be judged from the radiograph because the posterior surface of the condyle is considerably wider than the anterior surface. If the blade protrudes on the medial side it will cause irritation within the knee joint and may damage the medial collateral ligament.

Considerable difficulties are encountered with the insertion of the condylar plate because the plate must be aligned with the femoral shaft. Comminuted fractures cannot be reduced and held until the blade has been inserted and it is necessary to judge the rotation of the condyles very carefully. Breaking the table will allow flexion of the knee which will rotate the condyles and aid positioning during insertion of the seating chisel. The degree of rotation of the condyles can be judged by observing the anterior patellar surface of the lateral femoral condyle which should be parallel with the femoral shaft.

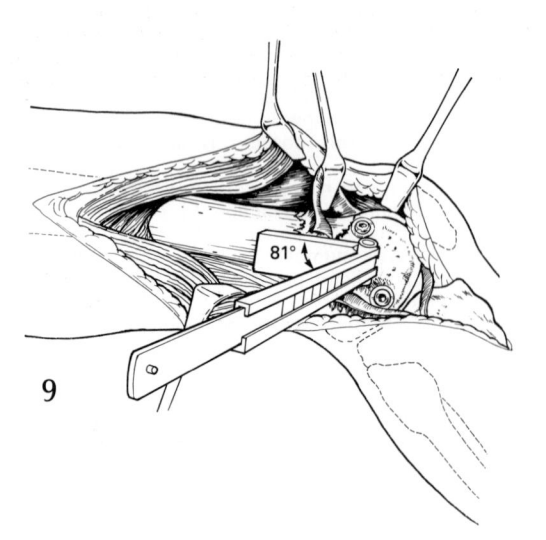

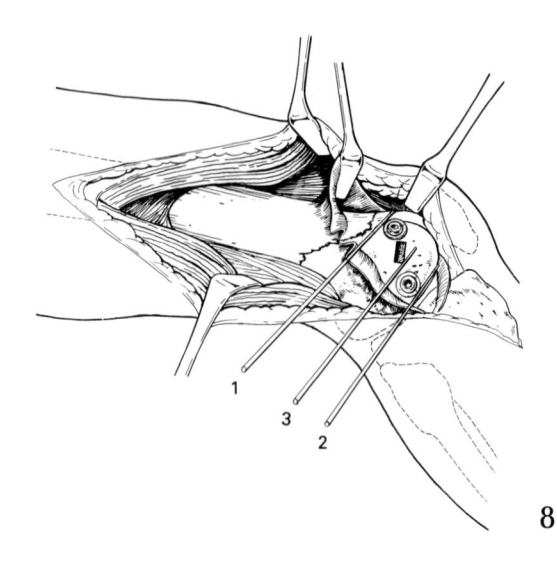

Insertion of the seating chisel or condylar screw

9

Now that the window in the lateral cortex has been prepared and the condyles have been aligned with the shaft, the seating chisel can be inserted. The flap of the guide is set at 81°, the angle necessary to ensure correct alignment of the blade in the condyles. The flap should be aligned with the femoral shaft.

The chisel is gently inserted using the slotted hammer to control its rotation, while the medial side of the condyle is supported by an assistant. Great care is necessary to prevent disruption of the intercondylar fracture. If the bone is hard or the chisel meets an obstruction, the track can be prepared with 3.2 mm drill holes to facilitate insertion. Once the chisel is inserted to the correct depth there is good control of the distal fragment and the position can be checked with radiographs.

Supracondylar fractures of the femur 249

10

The dynamic condylar screw has been developed as an alternative to the blade-plate to simplify insertion of the condylar component. The design is identical to the dynamic hip screw for the proximal femur. The reaming guide-wire is inserted in the centre of the area where the window for the seating chisel would have been cut and parallel to guide wire numbers 1 and 3. The reverse depth gauge is used to measure the length of the screw.

The track for the dynamic condylar screw and plate combination is then precut with the triple reamer. The track is 10 cm less than the width of the condyle and an appropriately sized screw is inserted. In hard bone it is necessary to tap the threads. This device has greatly simplified the insertion of this implant. An additional advantage is that rotation of the condyles in the sagittal plane is not critical. Adjustment can easily be made by removing the plate and turning the screw the desired amount to correct the malalignment.

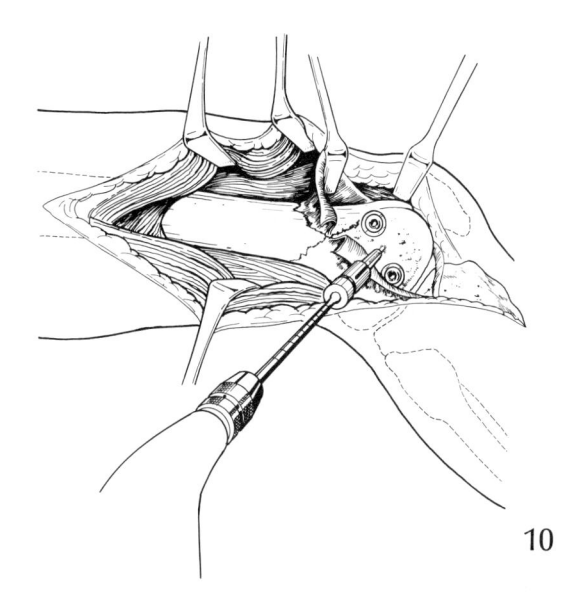

Insertion of the condylar blade–plate and reduction of the shaft

The seating chisel is removed and a suitably sized 95° blade–plate inserted along the groove prepared in the femoral condyles. The blade is impacted into the condyles and secured with one or two cancellous screws which may allow additional interfragmentary fixation of the intercondylar fracture.

11

When using the dynamic condylar screw a suitably sized plate is inserted over the screw and secured with a compression screw which increases the interfragmentary fixation of the intercondylar fracture.

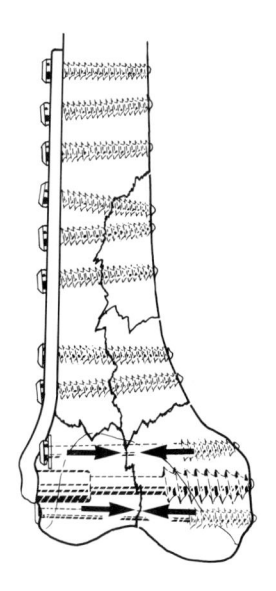

12

In comminuted fractures the femoral distractor can be used to restore length and alignment. One of the bolts of the distractor is inserted into the proximal shaft above the plate. The second is inserted through the first or second screw-hole of the condylar plate into the distal fragment. Slight over-distraction can be used to reduce comminuted fragments which can then be secured with interfragmentary screws. The plate is secured to the shaft with a single screw and the overall alignment checked with anteroposterior and lateral radiographs. The distraction is then eased off, the other fragments are fixed and the remaining screws inserted.

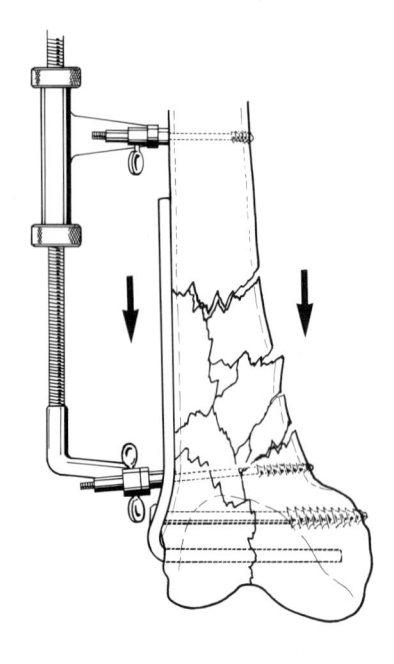

13

An alternative method is to use the compression distraction device attached to the proximal end of the plate. This will allow distraction of comminuted fragments or compression of fracture lines that are still separated. Fracture lines that are anatomically reduced can be compressed using the load guide and screws in the dynamic compression screw holes. The precise order of screw insertion will depend entirely on the type of fracture and the ease with which reduction can be obtained. Some screws may need to be lagged when they cross a fracture line. Schatzker[10] has described in detail the technical problems which can occur with the different types of supracondylar fracture.

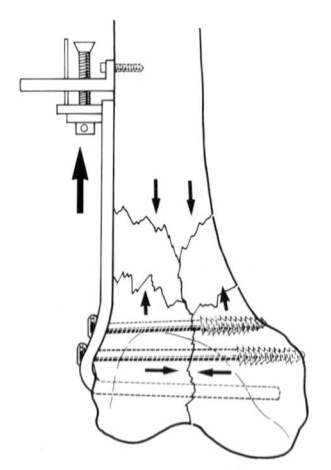

Bone grafting

Comminution and impaction of cancellous bone often occurs in these fractures. Restoration of normal length may leave an area of fracture gap. A comminuted fracture may have poor apposition of the medial cortex. In these circumstances it is essential to fill the gaps with cancellous bone graft. Excellent quality cancellous bone can be obtained from the ipsilateral greater trochanter. This graft can be packed into the cavities and can also be used to support comminuted fragments of articular surface. Larger defects in the shaft can be supplemented with corticocancellous strips from the iliac crest.

Closure

Prior to wound closure thorough irrigation is carried out with Ringer's solution. The wound is closed in layers using an absorbable type of suture, care being taken to ensure that the correct layers are apposed. Suction drainage helps to prevent haematoma formation. The vastus lateralis provides good soft-tissue cover of the plate and is held in position after resuture of the fascia lata. The skin can be sutured with interrupted or continuous polypropylene sutures and a wool and crêpe bandage dressing applied.

When operating on a pathological fracture it may not be possible to fill the defect with bone graft. An alternative is the use of methylmethacrylate which can be injected into the medullary cavity to fill the bone defect prior to the placement of the central screws. In cases of severe osteoporosis it may not be possible to get a good grip with the screws. In these circumstances the use of methylmethacrylate injected into the screw hole prior to screw insertion will greatly enhance the grip of the screws.

Postoperative management

14

At the end of the operation the surgeon must make an assessment of the quality of his fixation. If a good quality and rigid fixation has been obtained it will be desirable to start early joint movement. The advent of continuous passive motion machines has greatly improved the postoperative rehabilitation in these cases. The range of movement should initially be 0°–40° and it is better to position the leg on the machine immediately after the operation. The range can be rapidly increased to 90° over the following 3–4 days. The treatment should continue for approximately 7 days by which time the patient should have good active flexion and have satisfactory control of the quadriceps muscles.

Where a continuous passive motion machine is not available a good alternative is the 90°/90° position. The knee, hip and ankle are all immobilized at 90° and the limb is straightened daily for 30 minutes in order to do quadriceps exercises. The knee is kept in this position for 3–4 days after surgery. This reduces the risk of postoperative adhesions and improves the arc of movement.

The use of anti-inflammatory analgesics helps to reduce postoperative pain and inflammation and considerably eases the rehabilitation.

The suction drains are removed at 48 hours. During the second week the patient should concentrate on developing full control of extension. The sutures are removed at the 10th to 14th day. When wound healing is satisfactory and there is good quadriceps control the patient may be allowed out of bed to commence walking with crutches but not weight-bearing. The programme of active exercises should be continued under supervision of the physiotherapist together with the use of hydrotherapy if this is available.

When rigid fixation has not been obtained it may be necessary to keep the patient in bed for several weeks and the limb may be supported on a Thomas' splint, in Hamilton Russell traction or on a continuous passive motion machine. Once wound healing is complete and the swelling reduced a protective cast–brace can be applied.

Partial weight-bearing may be introduced at between 4 and 6 weeks after operation depending on the stability of the fixation and the cooperation of the patient. The use of a cast–brace may give added confidence and support and allow safer and earlier weight-bearing while maintaining knee flexion.

Removal of the implants can be considered at 18 months to 2 years after injury. It is no longer considered essential to remove the plates in the middle-aged and elderly, though in younger patients it is probably desirable so that full remodelling of the underlying bone can occur. Care should be taken after plate removal to avoid excessive activity and particularly twisting because of the risks of refracture through a screw hole.

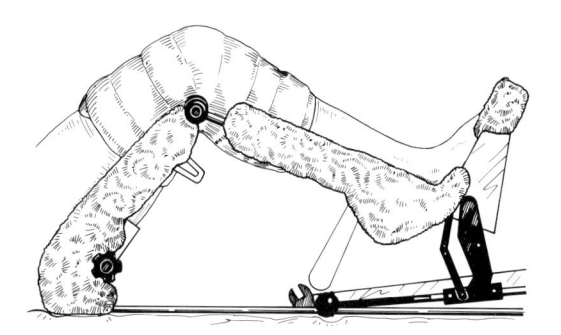

References

1. Modlin J. Double skeletal traction in battle fractures of the lower femur. *Bull US Army Med Dept* 1945; 4: 119–20.

2. Stewart MJ, Sisk TD, Wallace SL. Fractures of the distal third of the femur: a comparison of methods of treatment. *J Bone Joint Surg [Am]* 1966; 48-A: 784–807.

3. Neer CS, Grantham SA, Shelton ML. Supracondylar fracture of the adult femur: a study of one hundred and ten cases. *J Bone Joint Surg [Am]* 1967; 49-A: 591–613.

4. Mooney V, Nickel VL, Harvey JP, Snelson R. Cast-brace treatment for fractures of the distal part of the femur: a prospective controlled study of 150 patients. *J Bone Joint Surg [Am]* 1970; 52-A: 1563–78.

5. Müller ME, Allgöwer M, Willenegger H. *Manual of internal fixation.* Berlin: Springer-Verlag, 1970.

6. Olerud S. Operative treatment of supracondylar-condylar fractures of the femur: technique and results in 15 cases. *J Bone Joint Surg [Am]* 1972; 54-A: 1015–32.

7. Mize RD, Bucholz RW, Grogan DP. Surgical treatment of displaced comminuted fractures of the distal end of the femur: an extensile approach. *J Bone Joint Surg [Am]* 1982; 64-A: 871–9.

8. Schatzker J, Home G, Waddell J. The Toronto experience with the supracondylar fracture of the femur 1966–1972. *Injury* 1974; 6: 113–28.

9. Schatzker J, Lambert DC. Supracondylar fractures of the femur. *Clin Orthop* 1979; 138: 77–83.

10. Schatzker J. Supracondylar fractures of the femur. In: Schatzker J, Tile M, eds. *The rationale of operative fracture care.* Berlin: Springer-Verlag, 1987: 255–73.

Illustrations by Peter Cox

Fractures of the patella

V. G. Langkamer FRCS
Orthopaedic Registrar, Southmead Hospital, Bristol, UK

C. E. Ackroyd MA, FRCS
Consultant Orthopaedic Surgeon, Southmead Hospital, Bristol, UK

Introduction

Fractures of the patella are caused by direct or indirect violence. This results in varying degrees of displacement of the fragments and interrupts the quadriceps mechanism. Accurate reconstruction of the articular surface is important in safeguarding the long-term health of the joint.

Indications for operation

Loss of active extension of the knee, with fragment separation of more than 2 mm, and a step in the articular surface of more than 2 mm are indications for operation[1]. In older patients a more conservative approach can be adopted if there is gross continuity of the quadriceps mechanism.

In children, small avulsion fractures, of either pole, may be difficult to see on the radiographs and may consist of a considerable portion of the articular surface[2]. If displacement is more than 2 mm, operation should be carried out.

Restoration of normal anatomy is recommended for transverse fractures and for comminuted fractures when the articular surface is not severely damaged and can easily be reduced. Where there is a small fragment of the upper or lower pole, bony reconstruction to restore the quadriceps mechanism is preferable to excision of the fragment and reinsertion of the tendon. In severely comminuted fractures, reconstruction of the bone may be impossible and excision of the patella should be carried out, with repair of the quadriceps expansion[3]. Anatomical reconstruction and tension-band wiring gives the best result and should be attempted. Partial excision of the patella gives good results providing that three-fifths of the patella can be preserved[4].

The decision whether or not to attempt reconstruction depends upon the integrity of the articular surface of the patella and may thus only be carried out at the time of operation. Significant fissuring or fibrillation of the articular cartilage, except in the young patient, or evidence of osteoarthritis will favour patellectomy. The patella should be preserved if at all possible, as excision may result in considerable residual disability[5,6].

Preoperative

Operation should be performed as soon as possible after injury unless there is local skin infection, extensive abrasions, or more serious injuries that demand priority. The skin in the operative area is lightly shaved and a suitable antiseptic applied. While awaiting operation, the patient's leg should be rested in a foam gutter splint.

Anaesthesia

The operation should be carried out under general anaesthesia. The limb should be elevated and a pneumatic tourniquet applied high up on the thigh, over a layer of wool. The tourniquet should be inflated to 350–400 mmHg and may be left in position for up to 2 hours.

Position of patient

The patient is placed supine with the knees straight. The operative area is prepared with at least two applications of antiseptic and the whole limb draped in sterile towelling. The skin around the site of the incision may be protected by adhesive plastic.

Operation

Incision

1

A transverse incision 10 cm long is made on the anterior aspect of the knee. It is extended proximally on the medial side and distally on the lateral side to form a superior and inferior skin flap. The incision should be centred over the lower half of the patella with the knee extended. During flexion and extension of the knee, the skin on the anterior aspect slides in relation to the aponeurosis with the intervening pre-patellar bursa. Scar adherence between these layers may lead to long-term discomfort. The loose areolar tissue is usually infiltrated with haematoma, and identification of the deep fascia may be difficult.

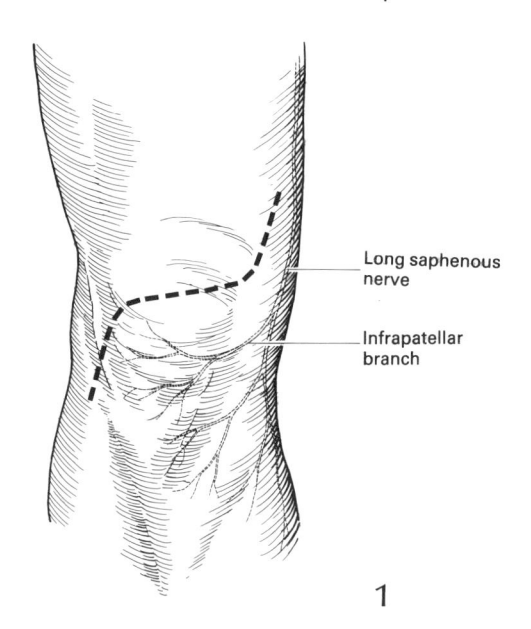

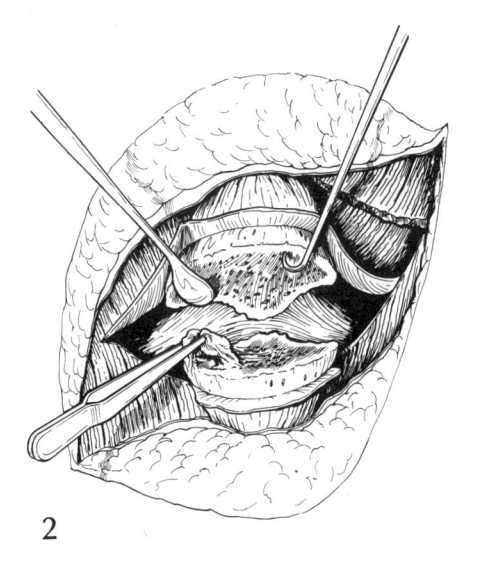

Exposure of the fracture

2

The deep fascia is divided and the skin flaps are elevated and retracted using sharp dissection. The fractured patella and torn patellar retinacula are now exposed. The blood clot is removed from both the fracture surfaces using a dissector or small curette. A sucker with lavage is useful to remove the adherent clot and debris. A small bone hook is used to elevate proximal and distal fragments so that the articular surface of the patella can be inspected and the knee joint cleaned and irrigated with Ringer's solution. The periosteum and retinacular fibres are scraped back from the edge of the fracture some 2–3 mm, using a small periosteal elevator so that reduction is not obstructed.

254 Lower limb fractures

Reduction of the fracture

3

The bone fragments are now reduced. It is important that there should be perfect apposition of the articular surface. Difficulty with reduction may be due to small bone fragments or soft tissue which have not been removed from the fracture surface. The reduction is maintained with reduction clamps or temporary Kirschner wires, inserted with the power drill. It may be desirable to obtain a radiograph to ensure that the articular surface is well apposed.

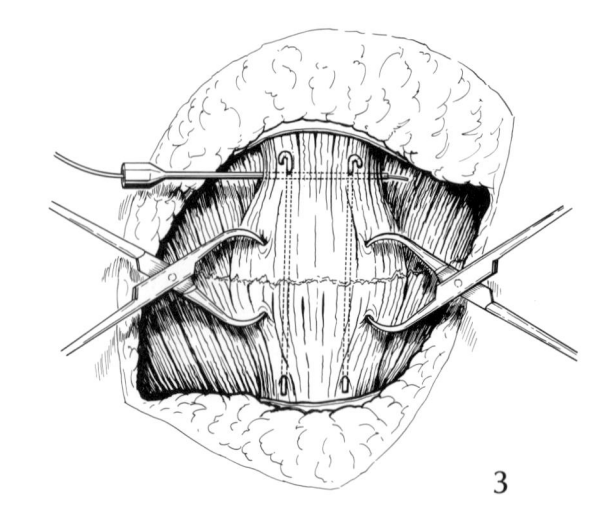

Rigid internal fixation

4

The tension-band wire technique provides excellent fixation. The fracture is held with two longitudinal wide-gauge Kirschner wires. A loop of 18-gauge circlage wire is then passed through the introducer deep to the quadriceps tendon. The passage of the wire under the tendon can be facilitated by using a slightly curved large-bore needle and by passing it through the tendon close to the bone at exactly the desired location. The wire is then pushed into the lumen of the needle and the needle and wire are then withdrawn together. The wire is passed distally on either side of the patella, and deep to the patellar tendon, and positioned so that the tightened knot lies to the side of the patella. A further tightening loop on the other side provides two-point tension and gives a better tightening effect. The Kirschner wires are now bent over the circumferential wire to provide an anchorage point[7].

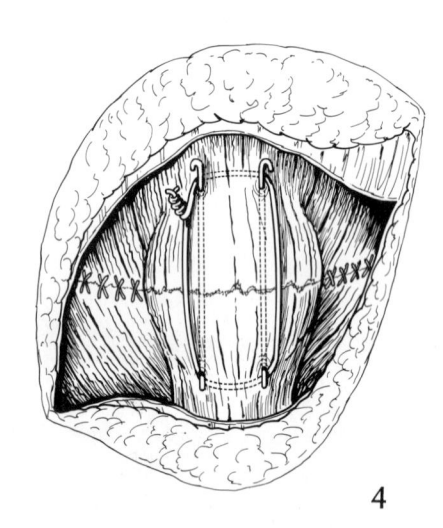

5

This method, when tested on cadaveric transverse fractures using apparatus to measure fracture separation and muscle strength, gives a very favourable result compared to simple circumferential wiring or a double tension wire[8]. When the wires are tightened, slight overcorrection at the fracture occurs. On flexing the knee or contraction of the quadriceps, the fracture surfaces are squeezed together under compression. In T-fractures or other more comminuted types, Kirschner wires, or interfragmentary screws may be used to create two main fragments which are then suitable for the tension-band wiring technique.

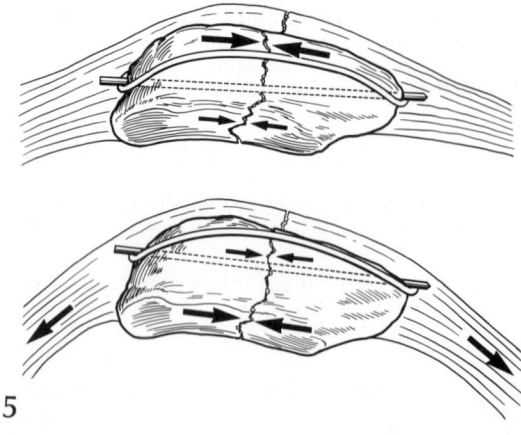

6

Distal pole fractures are best treated by a combination of cancellous screw fixation with a ligament washer and crossed circlage wiring. After all the patellar fixation has been completed, it is essential to repair any defects in the retinaculum and the quadriceps mechanism.

A suction drain is inserted and the deep fascia is closed with sutures of polyglycolic acid or polyglactin 910, ensuring good soft tissue cover of the wires. The skin is closed with subcuticular 2/0 polypropylene sutures.

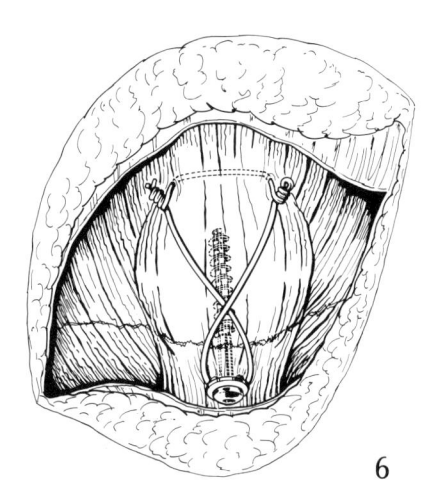

6

Postoperative management

A sterile dressing is placed on the wound and a generous layer of plaster wool applied to the entire limb. The limb is then immobilized in a plaster of Paris cylinder. The tourniquet is removed and the surgeon awaits return of the circulation to the foot. The limb should be elevated on pillows or a frame at 45° for 3–5 days and quadriceps activity encouraged within the plaster cylinder. The patient should commence straight-leg raising exercises immediately after the operation. When this is achieved and the leg is comfortable, mobilization with crutches, with partial weight-bearing, may commence. The patient may be discharged when he is walking satisfactorily.

The plaster cylinder is bivalved at between 7 and 14 days; provided wound healing is satisfactory, knee flexion may be commenced together with static quadriceps exercises. The sutures are removed at 14 days and a removable plaster of Paris back-splint may be used with advantage during weight-bearing for a further 2 weeks; it is essential if there is inadequate control of the quadriceps muscle.

Alternatively, wool and crêpe dressing can be used after the operation, with no plaster support. As this is often very painful, the plaster cylinder applied for 1–2 weeks may be preferred, as it assists comfort.

Experimental studies have confirmed that, with secure tension-band fixation, early active movement throughout the 90° range and weight-bearing may safely be allowed without loss of reduction[8]. If there is any doubt about the fixation, the plaster cylinder may be maintained for 4–6 weeks[7].

The institution of early active movement seldom results in postoperative stiffness, and a full range of movement should be achieved within 8–10 weeks. However, if stiffness persists, manipulation should not be carried out until at least 2 months or when radiological union has been demonstrated. Removal of the metal is often necessary as it may cause some discomfort under the skin. This should be carried out after 6–9 months, when clear radiological union of the fracture has taken place.

References

1. Boström A. Fractures of the patella: a study of 422 patellar fractures. *Acta Orthop Scand* 1972; suppl 143: 1–80.

2. Houghton GR, Ackroyd CE. Sleeve fractures of the patella in children: a report of three cases. *J Bone Joint Surg [Br]* 1979; 61–B: 165–8.

3. Hohl M. Fractures of the patella. In: Rockwood CA, Green D P, eds. *Fractures*. Philadelphia: Lippincott, 1984.

4. Böstman O, Kiviluoto O, Nirhamo J. Comminuted displaced fractures of the patella. *Injury* 1981; 13: 196–202.

5. Scott JC. (1949) Fractures of the patella. *J Bone Joint Surg [Br]* 1949; 31–B: 76–81.

6. Levack B, Flannagan JP, Hobbs S. Results of surgical treatment of patellar fractures. *J Bone Joint Surg [Br]* 1985; 67–B: 416–9.

7. Müller ME, Allgöwer M, Schneider R, Willenegger H. *Manual of internal fixation*. Berlin, Heidelberg, New York: Springer-Verlag, 1979.

8. Weber MJ, Janecki CJ, McLeod P, Nelson, CL, Thompson JA. Efficacy of various forms of fixation of transverse fractures of the patella. *J Bone Joint Surg [Am]* 1980; 62–A: 215–20.

Illustrations by Gillian Oliver

Tibial plateau fractures

J. K. Webb FRCS
Consultant Orthopaedic Surgeon, University Hospital, Queen's Medical Centre, Nottingham, UK

Introduction

1a & b

Tibial plateau fractures are intra-articular, occurring as a result of vertical loading as well as a bending movement which occurs in the classical 'bumper' injury. Axial malalignment may occur and as a result the weight-bearing axis is shifted and the overload may result in osteoarthrosis.

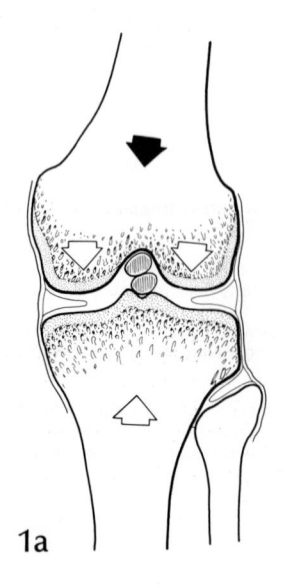

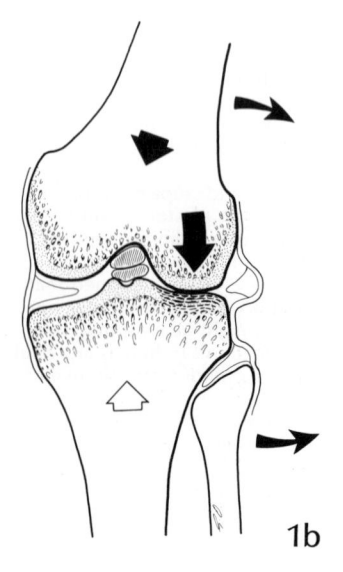

1a

1b

2

No classification of tibial plateau fractures can encompass all the variables seen in orthopaedic practice, and as a result various classifications have been proposed.

The classification of Schatzker et al.[1] into six types is recommended because it has certain merits; in particular, it alerts the clinician to the associated soft tissue injuries. It appreciates pathoanatomical factors, aetiological factors, and directs the surgeon to appropriate operative techniques. A more detailed classification has been proposed by the AO group (Arbeitgemeinschaft fur Osteosynthesefragen), and the Schatzker types can be incorporated into it.

AO classification

A. Tibia proximal, extra-articular fracture

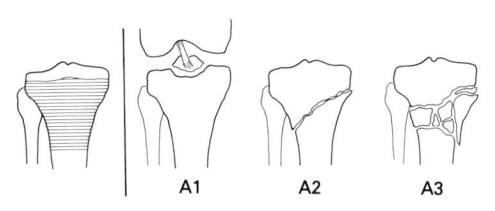

A1 A2 A3

B. Tibia proximal, partial articular fracture

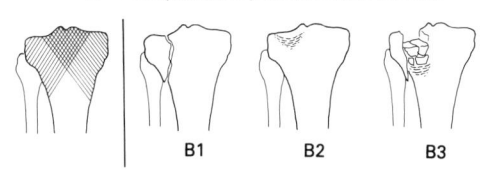

B1 B2 B3

C. Tibia proximal, complete articular fracture

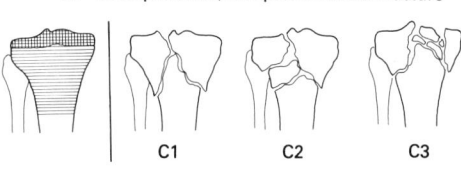

C1 C2 C3

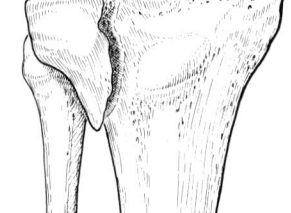

Type 1 – pure cleavage fracture (B1)

3

This is a wedge-shaped non-comminuted fragment which has become detached and displaced laterally and downwards. This fracture usually occurs in young patients without osteoporotic bone.

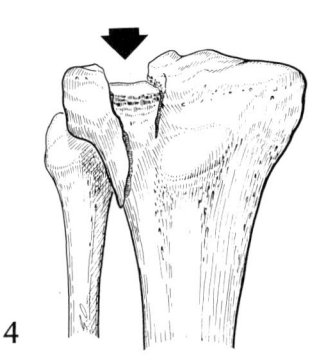

Type 2 – cleavage combined with depression (B3)

4

A lateral wedge is separated from the plateau but in addition there is an associated depression of the articular surface. This fracture is more common in older patients. A depression of more than 5–6 mm should be treated with open reduction, elevation of the depressed plateau, and a bone graft. Fixation of the fracture is performed with cancellous screws and a buttress plate should be applied to the lateral cortex.

Type 3 – pure central depression (B2)

5

The articular surface of the lateral plateau is depressed and driven into the tibial condyle. The lateral cortex is intact. This fracture tends to occur in osteoporotic bone. If the depression is severe or instability is demonstrated on stress radiographs, the articular fragment should be elevated and the defect beneath the elevation grafted. The lateral cortex should be supported with a buttress plate.

Type 4 – fractures of the medial condyle (B1)

6

The medial condyle is split. There are two types.

1. A wedge fragment is split off from the tibial plateau. This type occurs in younger people.
2. There is depression and comminution of the medial plateau. This occurs in older patients.

The treatment should be similar to that described for the lateral condylar fracture.

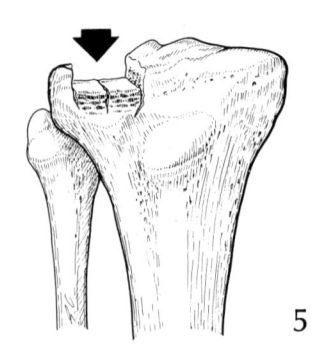

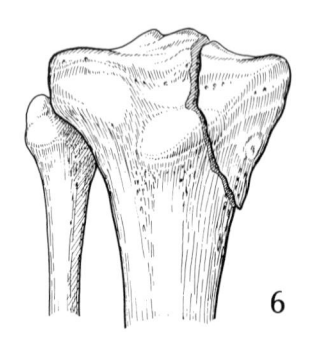

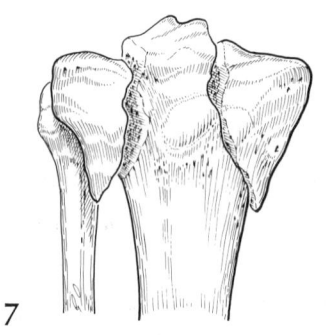

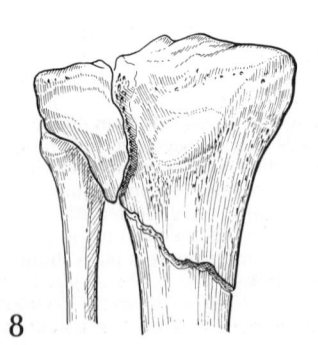

Type 5 – bicondylar fractures (C1)

7

Both tibial plateaux are disrupted, but there is no disruption of the metaphysis. Both condyles should be reduced and held with buttress plates and cancellous screws.

Type 6 – tibial plateau fracture with associated fracture of the tibial metaphysis and diaphysis (C2)

8

The essential feature of this fracture is a transverse or oblique fracture of the proximal tibia, which results in the interassociation of the metaphysis and the diaphysis. There are varying degrees of comminution in one or both tibial condyles as well as damage to the articular surface. The tibial plateau fracture is treated by appropriate methods of elevation, bone grafting and buttress plate. The fixation should extend across the more distal fracture.

Preoperative

Clinical symptoms and signs

The knee is painful, swollen and haemarthrosis is present, although if the capsule is torn then fluid may extrude into the soft tissues. Tenderness is present over the knee and especially at the fracture site. Movement is exceedingly painful. Stress testing may reveal some instability but it may well be too painful to be contemplated.

The objectives of the treatment are union of the fracture with:

1. Full extension, and flexion greater than 120°
2. Prevention of instability
3. Prevention of angular deformity.

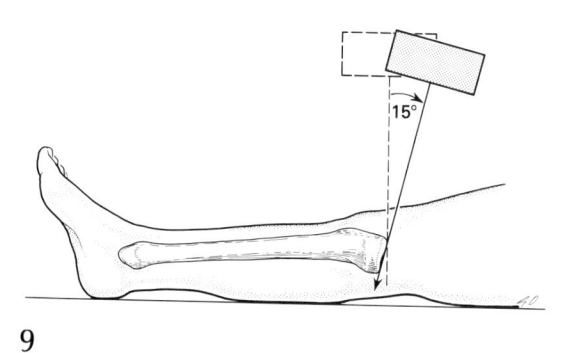

Assessment

9

Radiographic assessment is essential to classify the tibial plateau fracture. Standard radiographs in most cases are inadequate and should be supplemented with oblique films. The tibial plateau slopes posteroinferiorly 5°–10° from the horizontal, and the best correlation of the radiographic measurement with the actual depression of the central or posterior portion of the lateral plateau is obtained with the X-ray tube tilted 15°.

Anterior and posterior tomograms are recommended to assess articular damage and are necessary to aid reconstruction of the articular surface.

Stress views are recommended with the knee in full extension and 15° of flexion with radiographic documentation. CT scans, particularly three-dimensional reconstructions, are the ideal investigation for severe tibial plateau fractures.

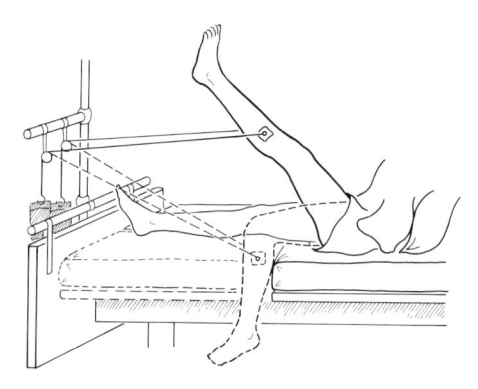

Treatment of undisplaced fractures

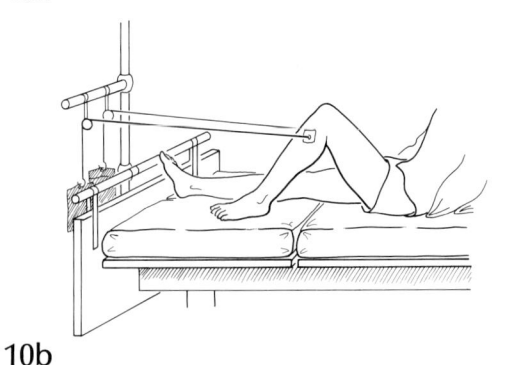

10a & b

If haemarthrosis is present, aspiration is performed. The knee must be stable in extension, especially to varus and valgus strain. Skeletal traction is applied to the leg.

(a) A pin is placed through the distal tibia and 20 kg of longitudinal traction is applied.
(b) Active knee flexion is encouraged.

At 4 weeks a cast-brace is applied with a hinge to protect the knee against varus and valgus forces. The cast-brace is worn for a period of 10 weeks, after which further physiotherapy is prescribed to strengthen the quadriceps and hamstring muscles. In the more elderly osteoporotic patient, if the deformity is minimal and the knee stable, then a light-weight long leg cast is applied. It is converted to a cast-brace at 6 weeks and worn for a further 4 weeks.

Operative approach

The approach to the tibial plateau is dictated by the pattern of injury. Hence the importance of accurate assessment of the bone and soft tissue injuries.

260 Lower limb fractures

LATERAL PLATEAU INJURIES

A lateral parapatellar approach is utilized.

Technique

11

The patient is anaesthetized, the leg exsanguinated and the tourniquet inflated. The knee is flexed 50°–60° over a roll and the whole of the leg, including the foot, is draped so that the knee can be easily manipulated during the operative procedure.

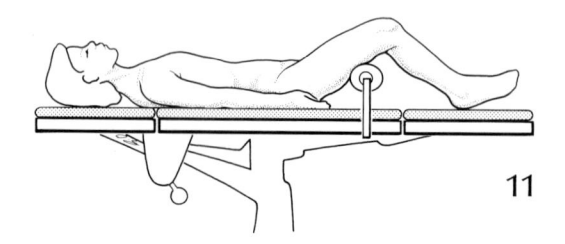

12

With the leg extended, the incision starts over the vastus lateralis, 2.5 cm lateral to the superior pole of the patella. The incision is carried lateral to the patella and for a few centimetres below and lateral to the tibial tuberosity.

13

The fascia, skin and subcutaneous tissue are then reflected laterally to expose the neck of the fibula. Care is taken to identify and protect the peroneal nerve. A portion of the soft tissues is detached from the upper lateral border of the tibia. A transverse incision is made in the capsule and the lateral meniscus is identified. Care must be taken that this is not damaged.

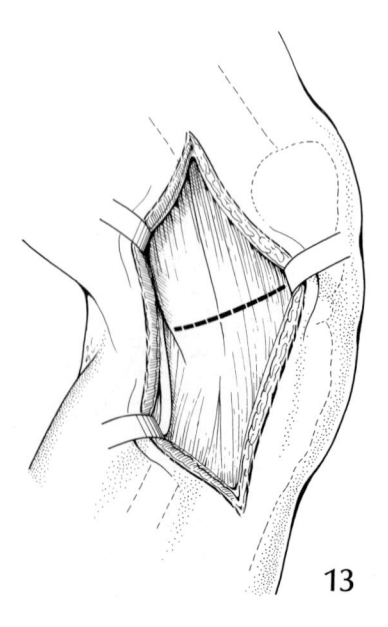

14

The meniscus is elevated cranially so that a clear view of the damaged plateau is obtained. The meniscus must be preserved at all costs and must not be removed.

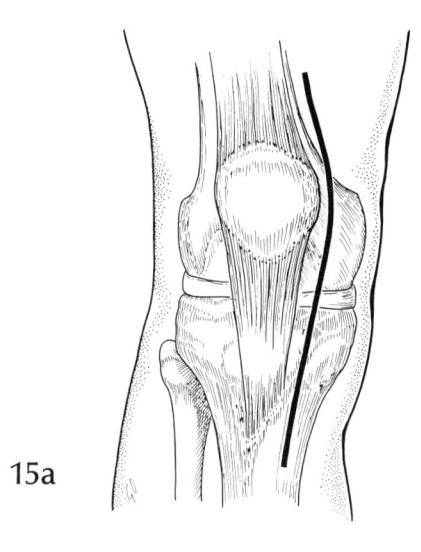

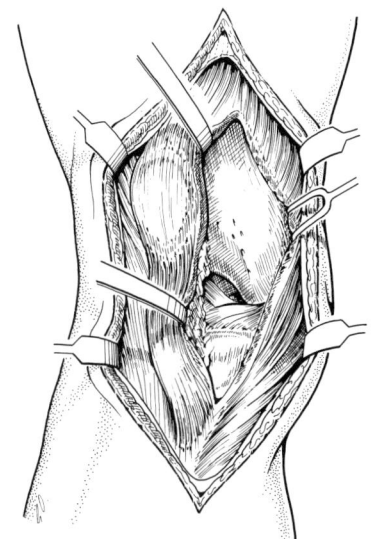

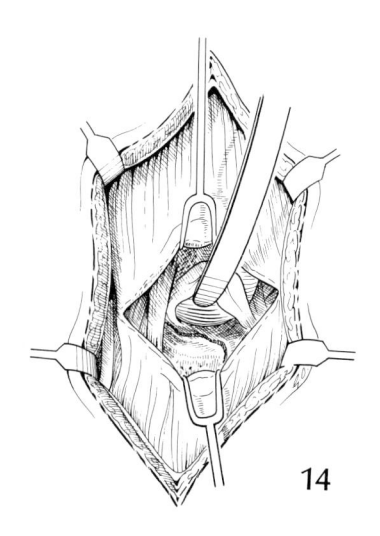

MEDIAL PLATEAU

15a & b

The skin and subcutaneous tissue are reflected medially and the upper portion of the tibia exposed. The tibiocollateral ligament is preserved. It may be necessary to reflect part of the pes anserinus complex to allow a plate to be applied to the medial aspect of the tibia.

APPROACH TO BOTH TIBIAL PLATEAUX

16a & b

A midline longitudinal incision is performed. This incision must be at least 10–12 cm so that tension is not applied to the skin edges when retraction is performed. The skin and subcutaneous tissue and fascia are reflected medially and laterally so that the whole of the patella and patellar tendon is clearly exposed. Parapatellar incisions are made on each side of the patella, extending to each side of the patella and then extending to each side of the ligamentum patellae beyond the tibial tuberosity.

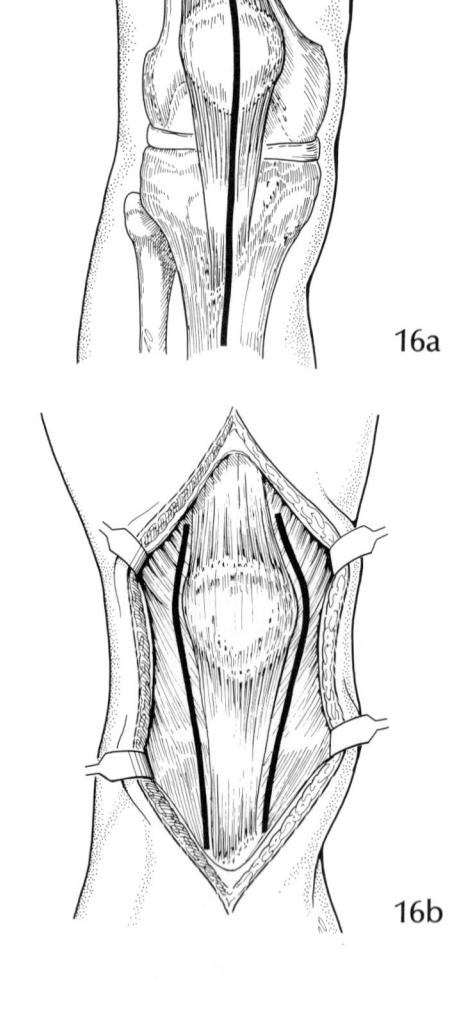

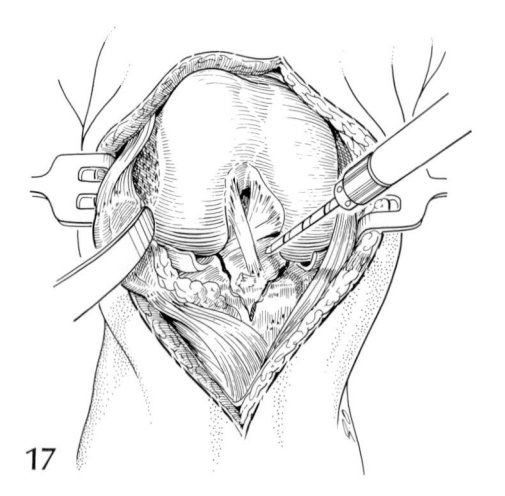

16a

16b

17

A 3.2 mm drill hole is made through the tibial tubercle and the posterior cortex of the tubercle is also drilled. Care should be taken when penetrating the opposite cortex to avoid potential damage to the posterior tibial vessels. The depth of the hole is measured and then tapped with a 4.5 mm tap.

Tibial plateau fractures 263

18

Four drill holes are made, two on each side of the tibial tuberosity, and are then linked with a sharp osteotome.

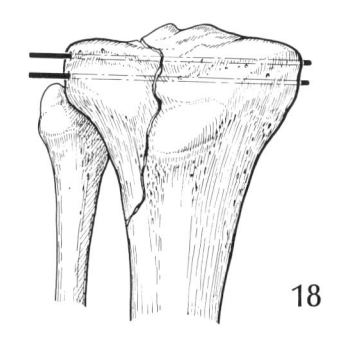

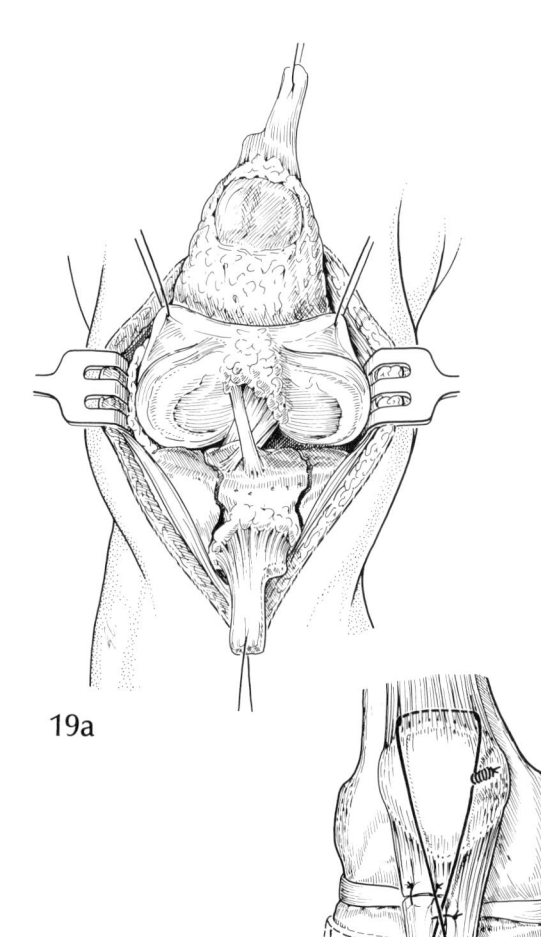

19a & b

The tibial tuberosity is elevated and then, with its ligamentum patellae lifted cranially, the soft tissues are dissected on each side of the patella (a). Alternatively, the ligamentum patellae can be split with a Z-plasty and later closed with repair and the use of a tension-band wire (b). This exposure allows both tibial plateaux and intercondylar areas to be clearly visualized, and allows anatomical reconstruction of the joint.

264 Lower limb fractures

Reconstruction and fixation

CLEAVAGE FRACTURES

20

In wedge fractures, which are pure cleavage injuries in young patients, with good quality bone, the fractures can be anatomically reduced and held with cancellous lag screws.

The articular surface is reduced and held in place with two parallel Kirschner wires (see *Illustration 18*). Radiographs are taken to ensure perfect anatomical reduction.

21

Beneath the subchondral bone a 3.2 mm drill is used to penetrate the opposite cortex.

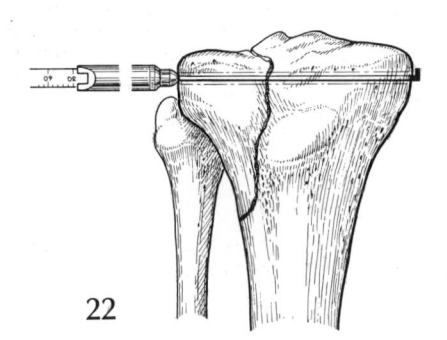

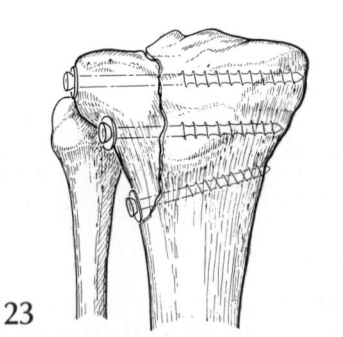

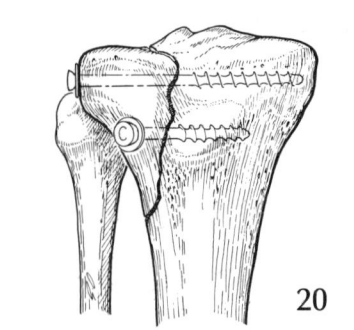

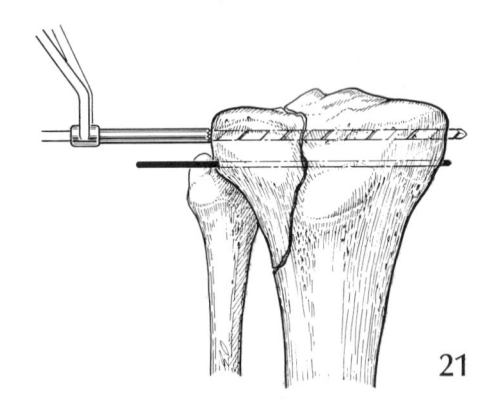

22

The depth is measured, only the proximal cortex is tapped and the appropriate length cancellous screw is inserted. It is imperative that the thread does not cross the fracture site (see *Illustration 20*).

23

A further screw is placed parallel to the articular surface in a similar way. A third screw can be placed at the caudal end of the fragment when large fragments are present – this acts as a buttress.

DEPRESSED PLATEAU FRACTURES

Elevation is essential.

24

A small flap is lifted in the bone 3–4 cm below the articular surface using an osteotome.

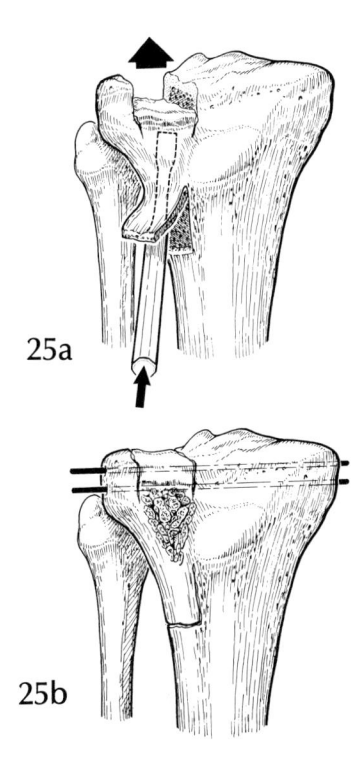

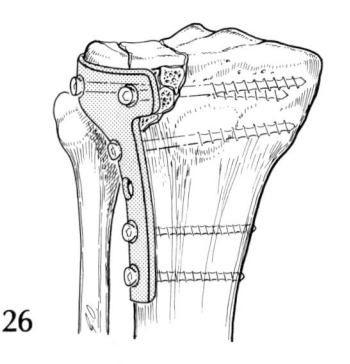

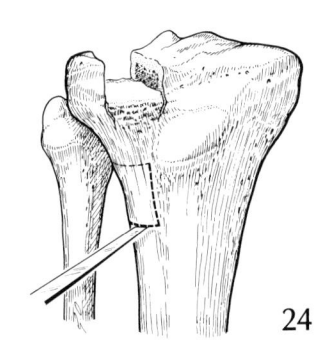

25a

A punch is then inserted through the elevated flap beneath the depressed articular surface and with great care the surface is elevated. The articular surface is visualized throughout this procedure and, once the surface has been anatomically reduced, it is held with Kirschner wires which are placed parallel to the articular surface.

Radiographs are then taken to ensure that anatomical reconstruction is satisfactory.

An iliac bone graft is required. The bone should be cancellous and this is packed into the defect which has been left beneath the elevated articular surface. It is essential that this whole area is packed as tightly as possible with cancellous bone. The elevated flap of bone is replaced.

25b

Initially two K-wires are placed parallel to the articular surface beneath the subchondral bone.

26

A buttress plate is then applied to the condyle of the tibia and cancellous screws are inserted in the manner described above. The remaining holes are filled with cortical screws applied using:

1. A 3.2 mm drill
2. A depth gauge
3. A 4.5 mm tap
4. An appropriate cortical screw.

The wound is closed in layers and a vacuum drain applied to subcuticular sutures of the skin.

266 Lower limb fractures

SEVERE BICONDYLAR FRACTURES

The more severe fractures are treated in a similar manner to unicondylar fractures. Good exposure is necessary; the skin should not be damaged before making a vertical incision.

27a & b

Too large buttress plates should be avoided as they compromise the blood supply to the bone.

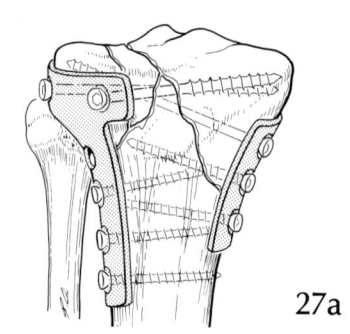

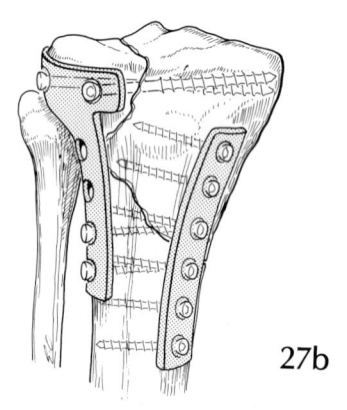

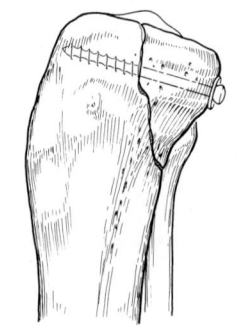

27a

27b

Posterior fragment

28

The fracture is reduced through a posterior approach and is held in place with a K-wire. Radiographs are used to confirm an anatomical reduction, and the fragment is held in place with a 6.5 mm cancellous screw.

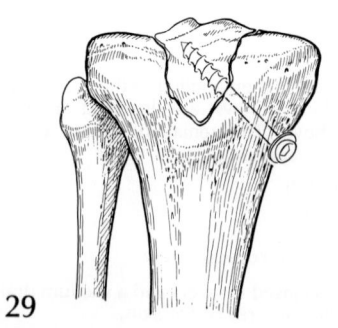

28

Intercondylar fragment

29

The fragment is reduced by direct vision and is then held with screws using the lag-screw principle.

29

Aid to reduction

30a & b

Severely comminuted fractures are difficult to reduce; the use of a distractor will help to realign the fragments.

Postoperative management

The wound is closed in layers and subcuticular sutures are applied to the skin. A vacuum drain is placed beneath the skin to prevent the formation of haematoma.

The leg is placed on a continuous passive motion machine. The drains are removed after 48 hours. Once 90° of knee movement is obtained, the patient may be allowed home. Weight-bearing is not allowed for 10 weeks. If the patient is unreliable, then a cast-brace should be applied for this period of time.

Reference

1. Schatzker J, McBroom R, Bruce D. The tibial plateau fracture: the Toronto experience. *Clin Orthop* 1979; 138: 94–104.

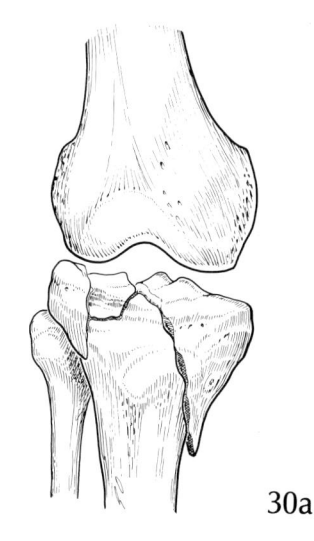

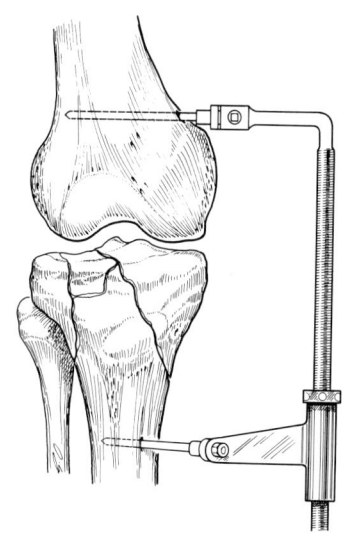

30a

30b

Illustrations by Peter Cox

Management of tibial shaft fractures

J. K. Webb FRCS
Consultant Orthopaedic Surgeon, University Hospital, Queen's Medical Centre, Nottingham, UK

R. J. Langstaff MA, FRCS(Ed)
Honorary Senior Registrar, University Hospital, Queen's Medical Centre, Nottingham, UK;
Senior Specialist (Orthopaedics), Royal Air Force Medical Services

Introduction

Soft tissues

The assessment of soft tissues is the essential element to the management of limb fractures; early soft tissue healing with wound cover is paramount, wound cover being obtained within 4–7 days. Treatment should be regarded in terms of the potential mechanical stability of bone and the extent of the soft tissue injury. The surgeon must grade closed injuries and be alert to the possibility of a compartment syndrome. Injudicious surgical incisions may lead to skin edge necrosis, wound breakdown and potential sepsis. Bone and soft tissue damage reflect the dissipation of energy, and classification of injuries to the limbs should allocate the severity into low- or high-energy injuries; this differentiation is of great importance in decision-making and all current classifications appreciate this concept.

Classification of open wounds

The commonest classification of open wounds was presented by Gustilo and Anderson[1].

Grade I fracture

1

This is a simple fracture where the puncture wound is less than 1 cm long with minimal muscle contusion and no crushing injury.

Grade II fracture

2

This is a simple fracture where the laceration is more than 1 cm, without extensive soft tissue damage, flaps or avulsions. There is minimal to moderate crushing injury.

Grade III fracture

3

This is a multifragmentary fracture. There is extensive soft tissue damage, including skin muscle and neurovascular structures. This arises from a high-energy injury with severe crushing components.
  This group includes all segmental fractures, all fractures with bone loss, gunshot wounds, traumatic amputations, and farm injuries with soil contamination.

Grade IIIA has adequate soft tissue coverage of the bone despite extensive soft tissue laceration or flaps. The infection rate is 4 per cent but amputation rate 0 per cent.

Grade IIIB has extensive soft tissue injury with periosteal stripping and bone exposure. There is major wound contamination, an infection rate of 52 per cent and an amputation rate of 16 per cent.

Grade IIIC is an open fracture associated with an arterial injury requiring repair. The infection rate is 42 per cent and the amputation rate is 42 per cent.

Bacterial considerations

Antibiotics are usually advocated in open wounds with a single dose in Grade I injuries, and 24–36 hours of cephalosporins and an aminoglycoside in Grades II and III injuries.

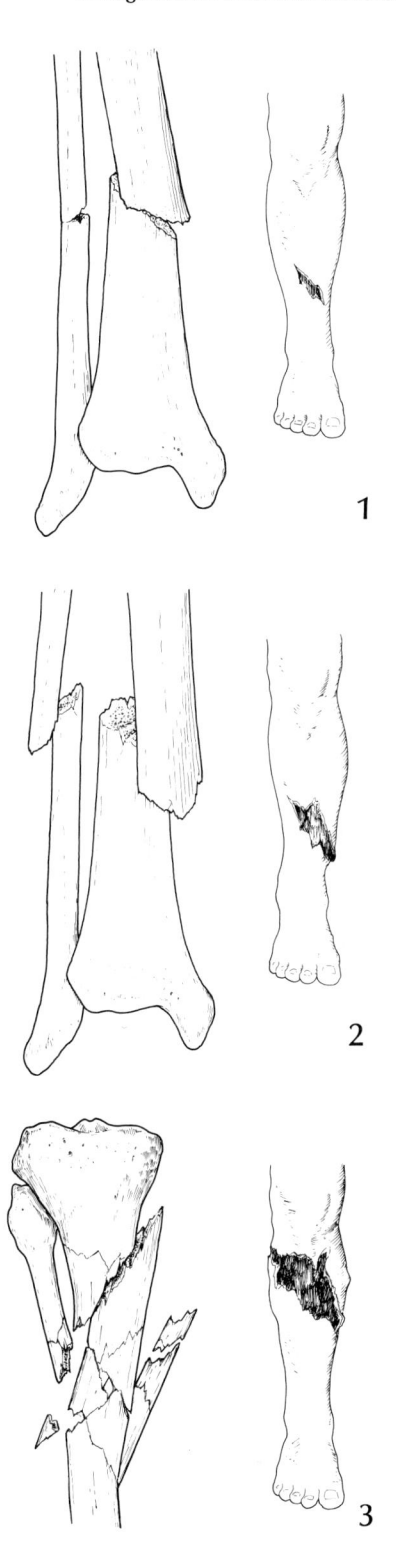

Non-operative management

Indications

Non-operative management is indicated for closed wounds and for injuries of Grade I; where there is minimal fragmentation; where shortening of less than 1 cm is anticipated; and where there is minimal soft tissue injury.

Contraindications

Conservative treatment is contraindicated in severe soft tissue injuries of Grades II and III; in segmental fractures; in multifragmentary fractures; and where there is an associated articular fracture.

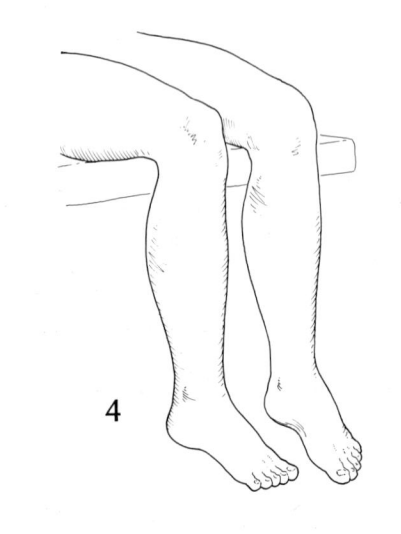

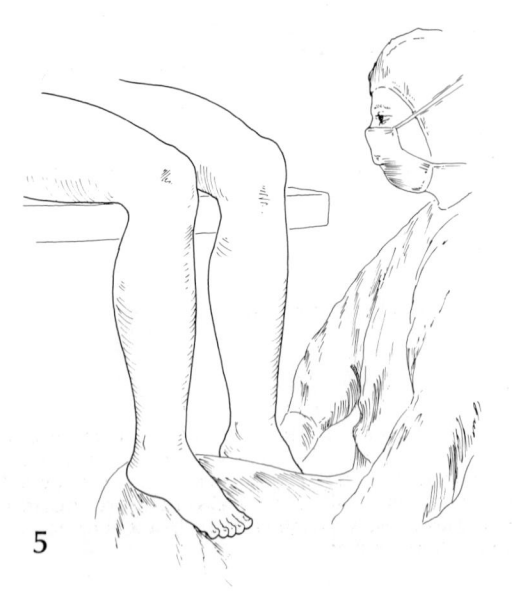

Timing of non-operative treatment

If treatment by means of manipulation and plaster is to be undertaken, several points must be considered if an ideal result is to be achieved. The injury tends to become swollen over the first day, and the distended tissue tends to cause shortening. Reduction is best performed as soon as possible. Once the limb is swollen and shortened, efforts at manipulation will prove both arduous and unrewarding.

The levels of stability achieved by means of plaster are generally not high enough to provide satisfactory defence against infection. The treatment of wounds greater than Grade I by plaster is not recommended.

Application of plaster for tibial fractures

General anaesthesia is usually required, where more than angulatory correction is necessary.

4 & 5

The patient should be supine with the leg dependent over the end of the operating table, avoiding pressure on the popliteal fossa. The surgeon sits on a low stool at the foot of the table having adjusted the height until the toes of the injured leg, with the ankle in relaxed equinus, touch the surgeon's knee.

6

The tibia is reduced by traction and gentle manipulation to produce a slightly varus position with rotation similar to the dependent uninjured limb. Plaster wool and wet plaster is applied below the knee by the surgeon. Once the plaster has set, the fracture position is checked by means of radiographs before completion of the cast to an above-knee cast.

7 & 8

With more difficult fractures, strong manipulation and careful reduction is required. When the patient is supine, a block is placed behind the supracondylar region of the thigh, avoiding pressure on the popliteal vessels. The surgeon's assistant stands at the foot of the table holding the leg. If an adequate reduction cannot be achieved, traditionally os calcis skeletal traction may be applied to aid reduction.

However, if reduction is that difficult, there are more satisfactory methods of treatment such as external fixation or internal fixation. If the surgeon encounters difficulty in maintaining the reduction, it is likely that displacement will occur later, and an alternative approach should be considered.

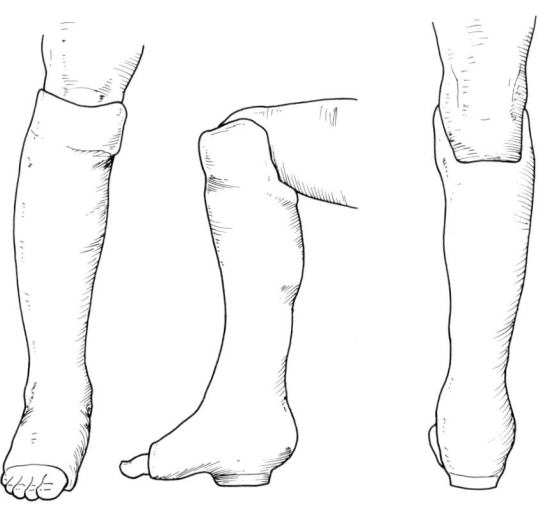

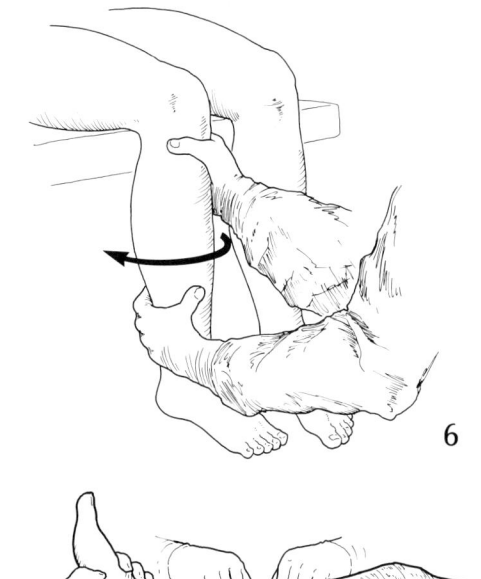

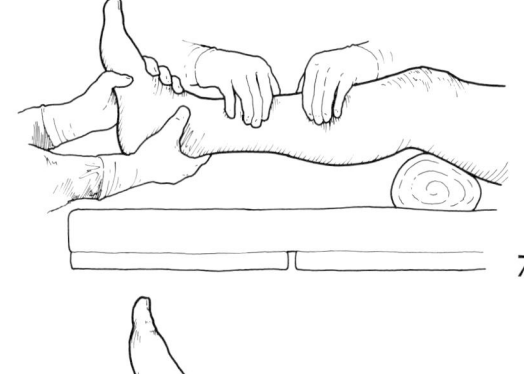

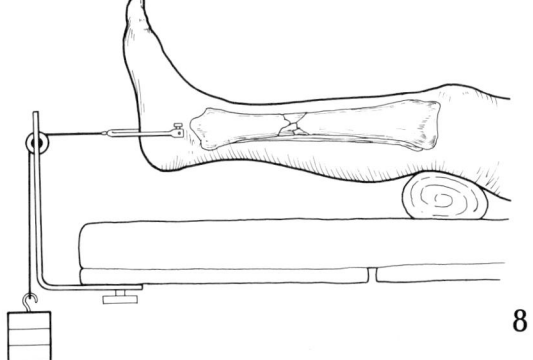

Functional fracture orthosis

9

A tibial fracture is managed in a long-leg cast for 3 weeks, and then placed into a functional cast, although a complex multifragmentary fracture may require a longer period until the fracture is stiff, and 6 weeks in a long-leg cast may be required. Early weight-bearing is essential to encourage bone healing.

272 Lower limb fractures

Operative treatment

EXTERNAL FIXATION

The application of an external fixator allows ready access to the soft tissue.

10

The external fixation as a unilateral frame is sufficient in the vast majority of tibial fractures.

Application of external fixator

The correct insertion of pins is important to prevent complications, in particular loosening and infection. The weak link in a fixator is the bone–pin interface. Aseptic technique is essential.

11a & b

The fracture should be reduced and the limb aligned before insertion of the pins.

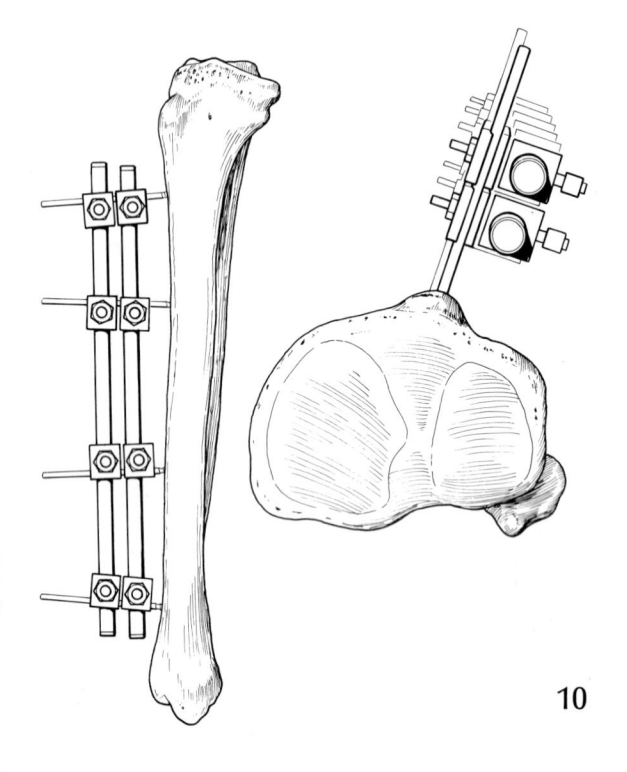

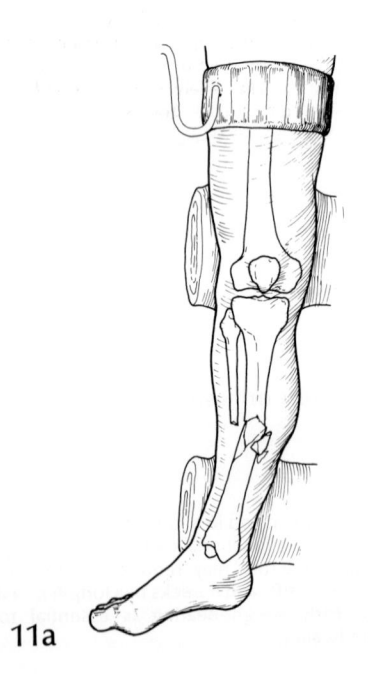

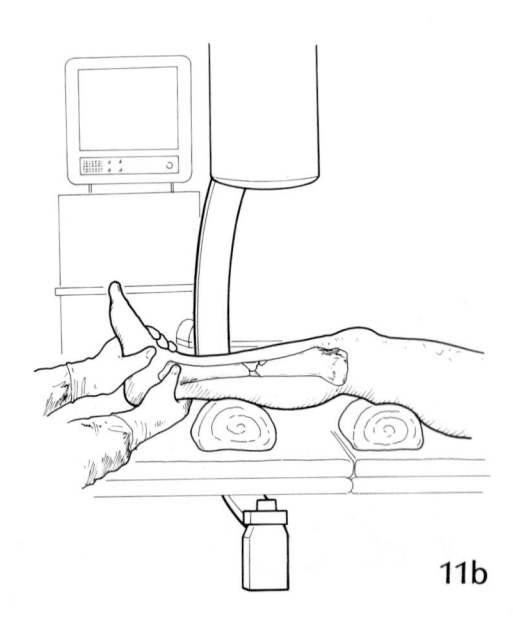

12

For pin insertion, longitudinal skin incisions are made down to the bone.

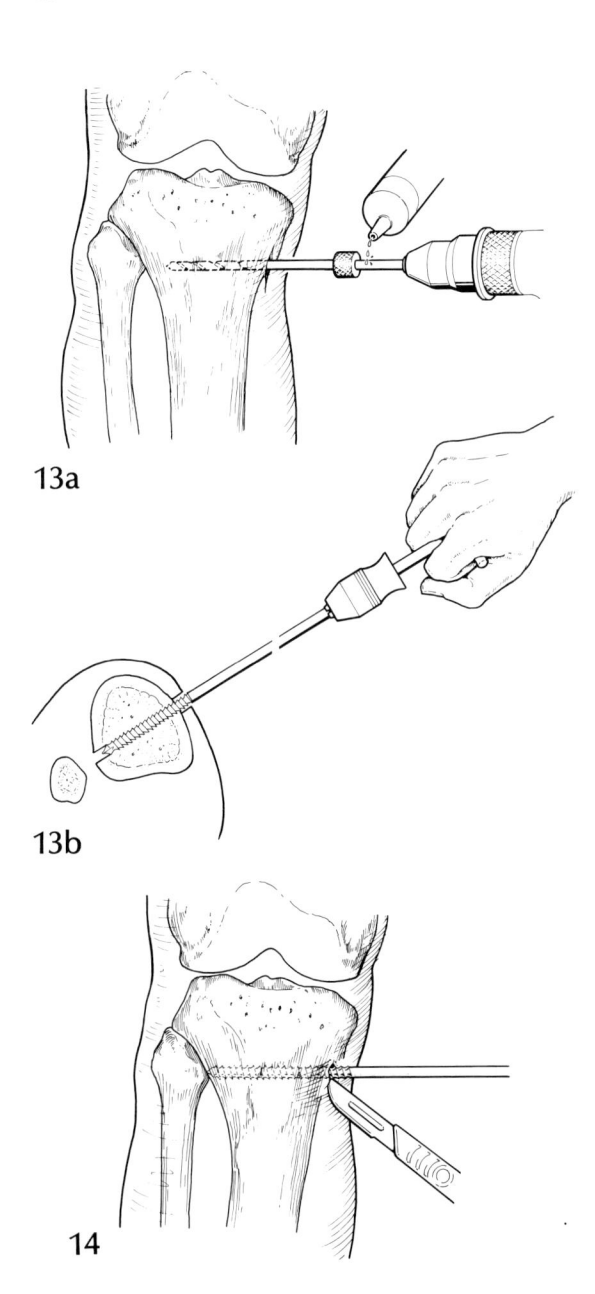

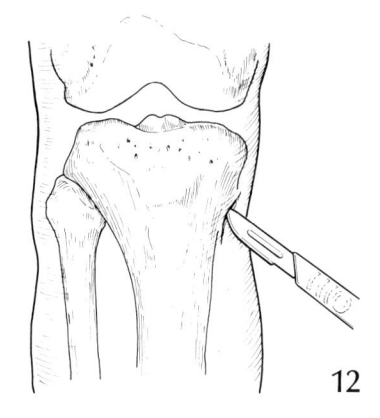

12

13a, b & 14

Pin tracks in the bone are first made with a slow-speed drill, using a guard, which is well irrigated to reduce thermal injury. The pins must then be inserted by hand. Tenting of the skin should be released with a scalpel. Light dressings are applied to the pin tracks.

13a

13b

14

274 Lower limb fractures

15 & 16

The fixator is applied and can be used to elevate the limb. Dependent oedema of the calf is prevented by firm pressure dressings. It is essential to prevent equinus deformity by the use of an anti-foot drop orthosis.

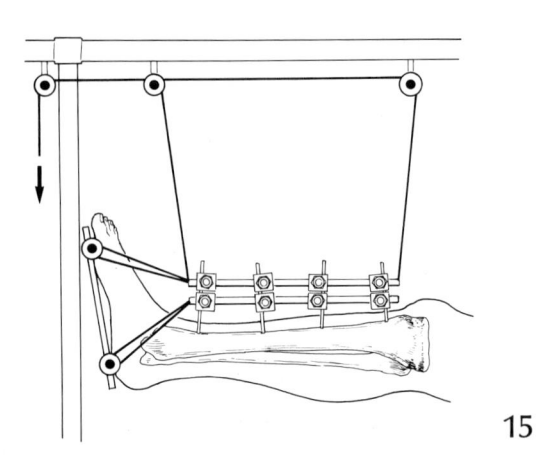

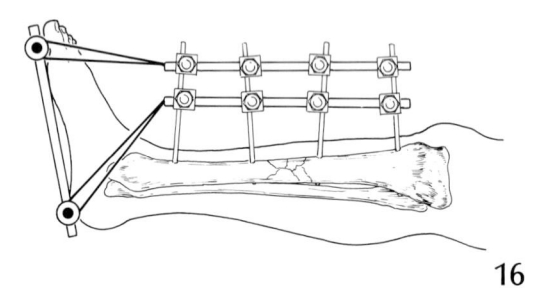

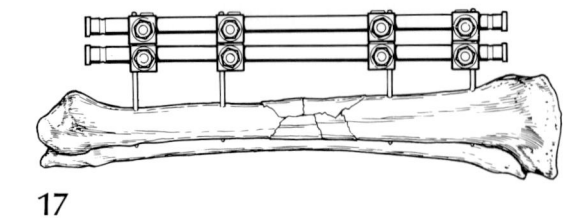

15

16

Number of pins

17

The use of six pins instead of four leads to a 30 per cent increase in stiffness, and this allows early weight-bearing and callus generation. Where four uniaxial pins are used, the pins should be as widely separated as possible.

17

Dynamization

Initially, an external fixator should be stiff, but then, as the soft tissue healing occurs, the rigidity should be reduced progressively to stimulate callus formation.

Timing of dynamization

Dynamization should occur as early as possible, preferably within 14 days of bone fragment apposition being present.

Complications of external fixation

Complications include refracture, compartment syndrome, delayed union, pin track infection, and neurovascular damage.

INTERNAL FIXATION BY TIBIAL PLATING

Internal fixation by means of lag screws and a neutralization plate is a method of fracture care. Like any surgery, plating of tibial fractures is not for the inexperienced.

Principles of internal fixation

Anatomical reduction, stable fixation and early movement of adjacent joints underlies this form of management.

Indications

The ideal indication for plating is a Grade I or II open fracture at the junction of the diaphysis and metaphysis; or a tibial fracture associated with an articular fracture of the knee or ankle.

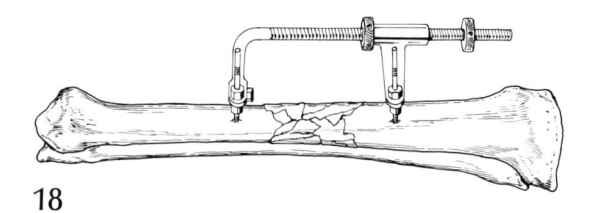

18

The complex fracture should not be pieced together with multiple interfragmentary screws, destroying the blood supply, but reduced by traction with the aid of a femoral distractor and then held by a plate.

18

Technique

19 & 20

Minimal dissection should be undertaken to protect the vascular supply of soft tissue and bone. The incision should be placed 1 cm lateral to the anterior tibial crest, extending distally to follow the line of tibialis anterior tendon towards the medial malleolus. The incision should pass directly to fascia without undermining of the skin edges. The plate is placed on the subcutaneous border of the tibia superficial to the periosteum.

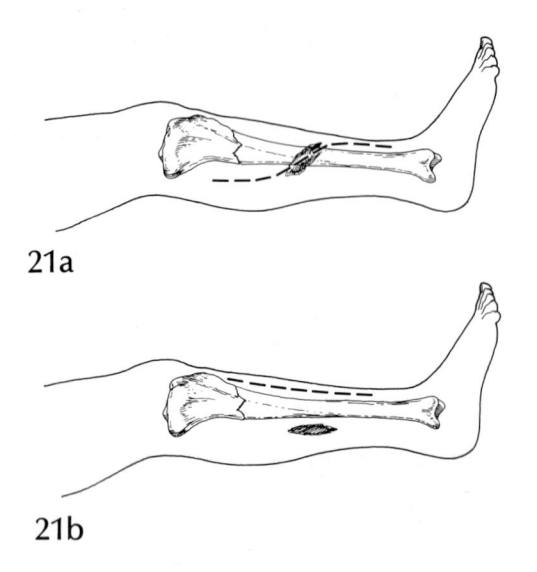

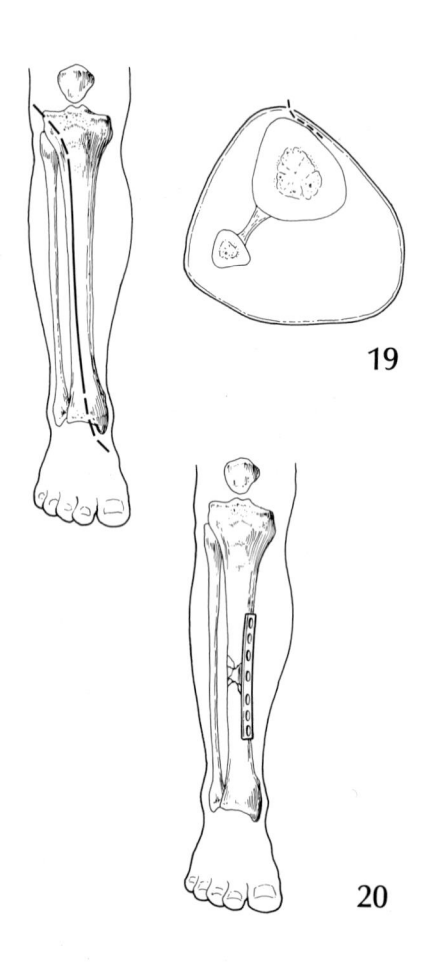

21a & b

If a wound is present on the subcutaneous border, it may be incorporated into the incision, although the wound must be left open at the end of the procedure. Where doubt exists regarding the health of the skin, then surgery should either be delayed or alternative methods of management undertaken.

Plate fixation

The fracture is exposed preserving the periosteum, and the ends of the fracture are cleaned; haematoma and soft tissue interposition are removed.

Anatomical reduction is essential; interfragmentary fixation must be achieved with a lag screw, and then a plate is applied using it in the neutralization mode. Six cortices (i.e three screws through both sides of the intact bone) above and below the fractures must be held with the inserted screws.

Uses

22–26

Internal fixation by screws or plate may be used for:

1. Reduction of a fracture (*Illustration 22*).
2. Stabilization of a fracture with lag screws (*Illustration 23*).
3. Contouring of a plate, initially using a malleable plate (*Illustration 24*).
4. Application of a plate using 3.5 mm screws (*Illustration 25*).
5. Placing a lag screw through the plate and across the fracture, if the configuration of the fracture allows (*Illustration 26a, b & c*).

When the plate is applied, it is essential that six cortices be held above and below the fracture by the screws.

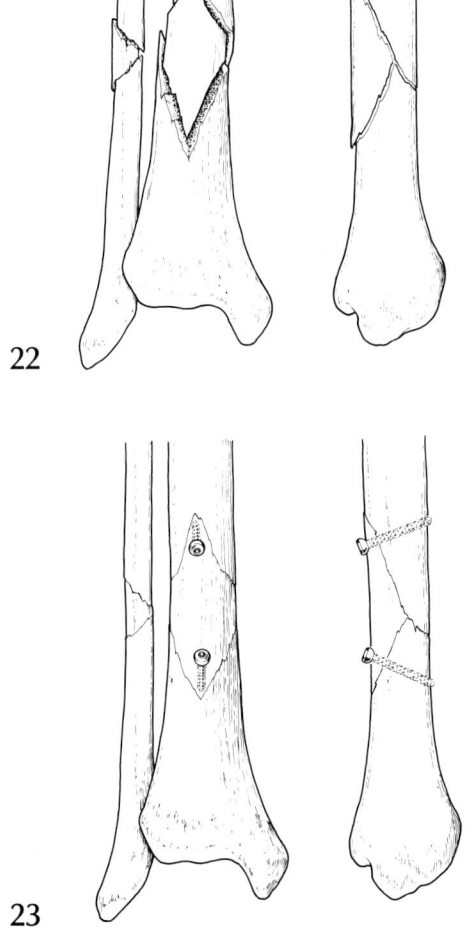

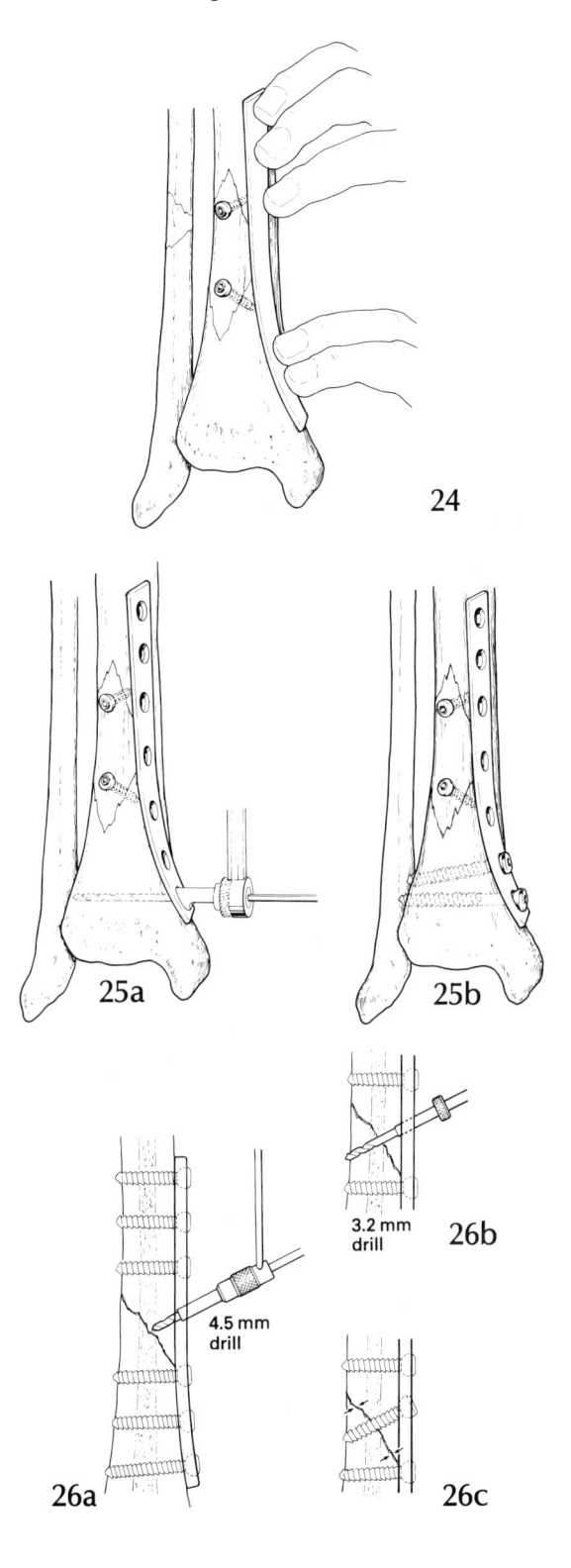

24

22

25a 25b

23

26a 26b 3.2 mm drill

4.5 mm drill

26c

Postoperative management

27

The purpose of internal fixation is to obtain a stable fixation which allows early movement of the limb, facilitating good functional recovery. The immediate postoperative management is elevation, prevention of haematoma with a suction drain, and prevention of equinus deformity with a plaster backslab; 10 kg weight-bearing is allowed.

In patients with stable fixation, the recommended regimen consists of 10 kg weight-bearing for 6 weeks; if at that stage the radiographs are satisfactory, with no increase in the fracture line, or irritation callus is not present, then increased weight-bearing is permitted until full weight-bearing is reached at 10–12 weeks.

The unreliable patient should be managed by keeping the patient in hospital for 5–7 days, preferably on a continuous passive motion machine until swelling has resolved and a good range of ankle joint movement has returned, and then and only then apply a cast.

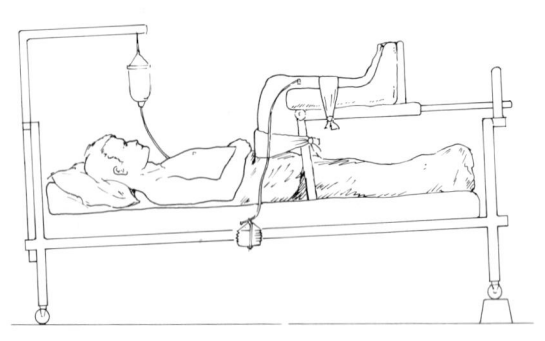

INTERNAL FIXATION BY INTRAMEDULLARY NAILING

Indications

Intramedullary nailing is indicated for (a) transverse fractures which are closed, or open fractures of Grade I or II; and (b) multifragmentary diaphyseal fractures, either closed or open Grades I or II.

Position of patient

28

The position of the patient on the table is crucial for the successful performance of this operation.

The patient is positioned supine on the table, with the knee flexed over a support bar to give 90° of flexion. The other leg is extended at the knee and extended at the hip, and adducted to bring the two legs close together. This allows the X-ray C-arm to swing into the anteroposterior and lateral direction. The surgeon should confirm that adequate anteroposterior and lateral views of the proximal and distal end of the tibia, and of the fracture site, can be obtained before preparing and draping the patient.

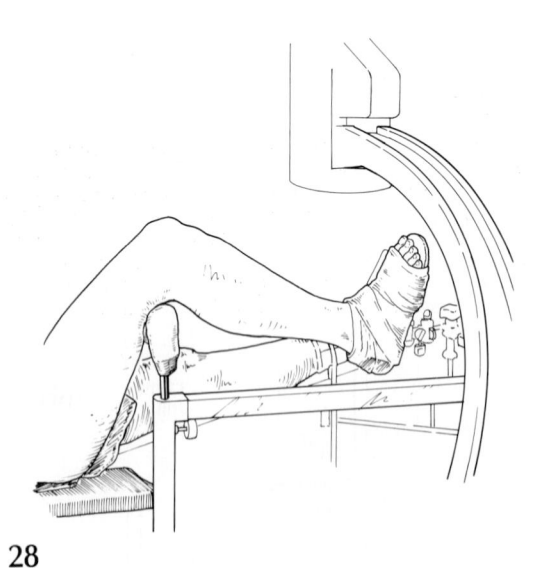

Management of tibial shaft fractures 279

29

In the position shown, the fractures can be reduced using the traction table, with the foot secured to the foot piece using sticking plaster. It is only usually necessary to use a calcaneal wire for skeletal traction if there is considerable shortening at the fracture site, or delay in surgery. If the fracture cannot be adequately reduced, closed nailing is inappropriate.

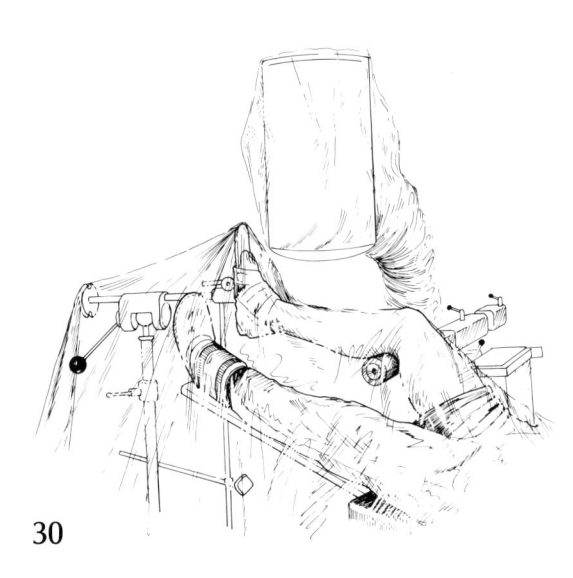

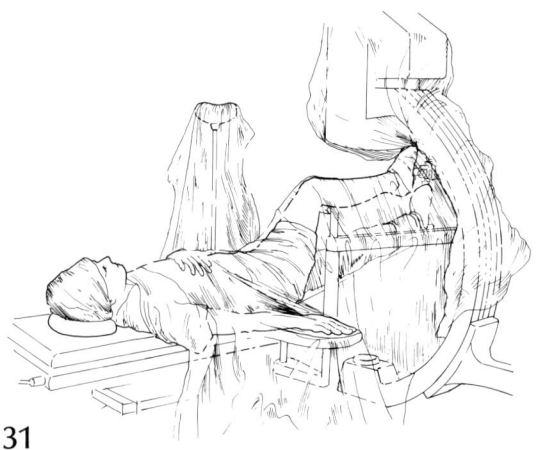

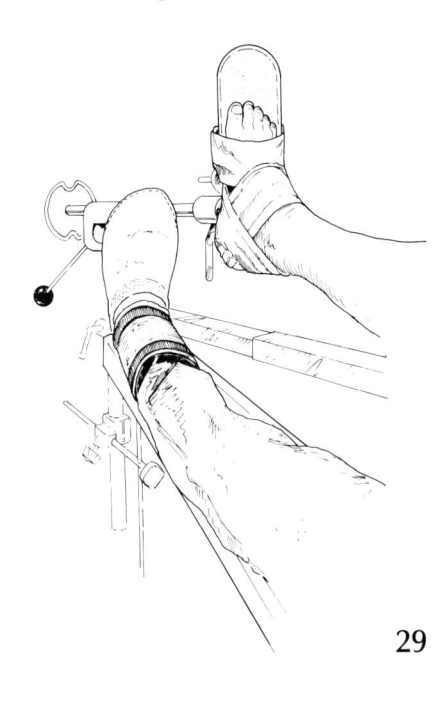

Draping

30 & 31

The skin is prepared in the usual way, and draped with a large polythene drape, incorporating an iodine-impregnated adhesive area, which is the most suitable way of draping a patient for this procedure. In order to allow the C-arm to swing through into the lateral position, a sterile bag is incorporated into the drapes over a dripstand. This allows adequate radiographic views to be taken while maintaining sterility at all stages of the procedure.

280 Lower limb fractures

Incision

32

A longitudinal incision is used. It is made slightly medial to the midline, about 8 cm long. The patellar tendon can be retracted out of the way.

Nail insertion

33

The insertion point is just medial to the tibial tubercle. The cortex is broached using the small and large awl, care being taken not to damage the edge of the tibial plateau. Hand-reamers are used to enlarge the initial insertion hole; then, under radiographic control, the bent guide-wire is passed into the hole. A small, straight nail slid over the wire into the enlarged insertion hole gives excellent control over the proximal fragment, and aids manipulative reduction of the fracture in order to achieve easy passage of the wire. A cannulated chuck inserted over the wire, about half-way down, guides rotation, and this, together with the nail, makes passage of the wire down the tibia a relatively easy exercise.

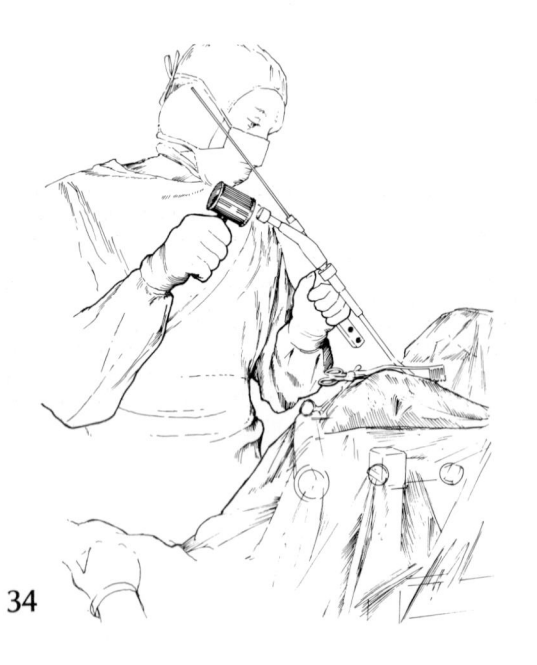

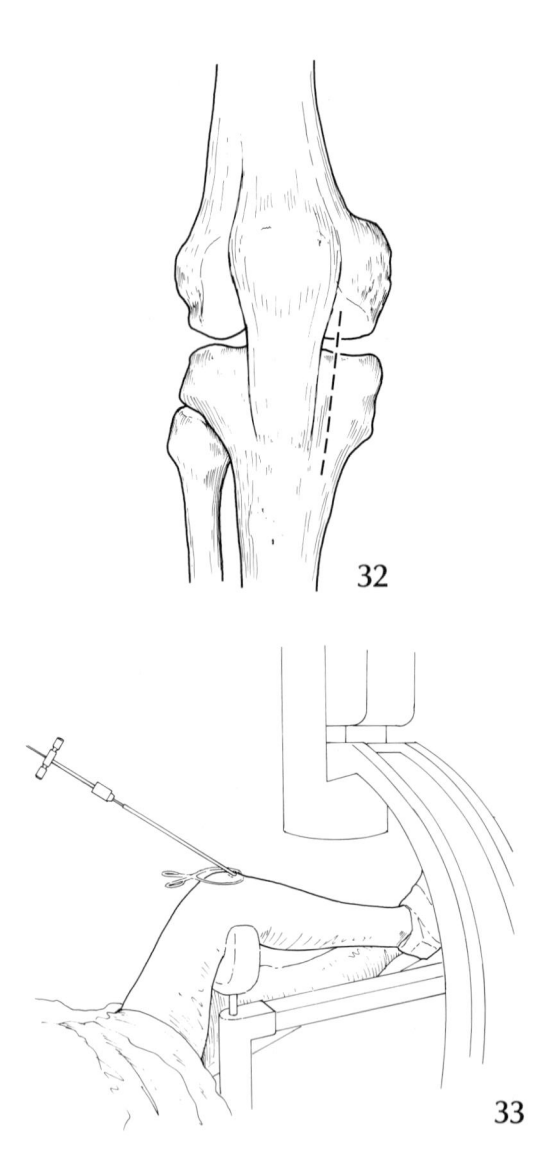

34

Once the wire is passed, it is advanced to the end of the tibia, and its position checked on the X-ray screen. The tibia is then reamed in the usual fashion commencing with the end-cutting reamers and advancing in 0.5 mm increments with the side cutters. Once reaming is completed, the plastic guide-tube is inserted over the wire, and the reaming guide-wire exchanged for the nail-insertion wire. The length is measured and a nail of appropriate size inserted. It should advance easily with each blow of the hammer; if it does not, over-reaming by 0.5 mm may be appropriate. Its passage across the fracture site should be checked with the image intensifier.

The proximal locking screw jig is used as a handle to control rotation of the nail during insertion.

Management of tibial shaft fractures 281

Locking

35

The decision as to whether or not to lock a tibial nail in the static or dynamic manner is based on assessment of the fracture stability. Static locking is recommended in multifragmentary fractures; dynamic-mode locking can be used with good bone contact and inherent stability. Insertion of the locking screws is straightforward.

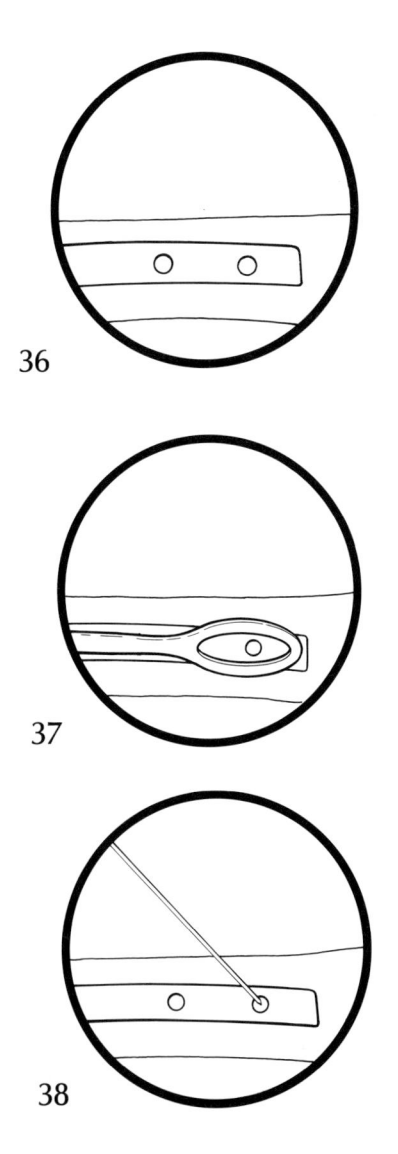

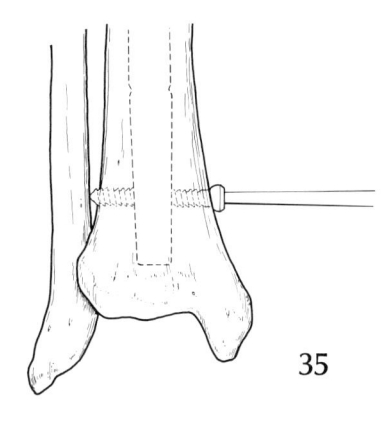

35

36

The distal screws should be inserted first, and can be the more difficult. We have modified the original AO technique and now perform this part of the operation without the use of the cutting device. The image intensifier is positioned in the lateral plane so that the distal holes are visible as perfect circles in the middle of the screen. In order to ensure this, the nail must not have rotated within the medullary cavity, and it may be necessary to adjust the position of the nail before the screws are inserted.

36

37 & 38

To insert the distal locking screws, a pair of Lane's tissue forceps are positioned over the skin on the medial side of the tibia, so that on the X-ray screen, the perfectly circular hole in the nail is surrounded by the bars of the Lane's forceps. This indicates the correct position for the skin incision. Having made the skin incision, the Lane's forceps are moved away and the tip of a 3 mm Kirschner wire, mounted on an AO universal drill is positioned on the cortex so that, on the X-ray screen the tip of the K-wire is seen as a sharp point in the middle of the distal hole in the nail.

37

38

282 Lower limb fractures

39

Having achieved this position, the K-wire is then swung into the coronal plane at 90° to the long axis of the tibia, the X-ray equipment swung into the anteroposterior plane, the position checked, and the wire drilled across the tibia and through the locking holes of the nail. The locking screws, which are of a self-tapping variety, can be inserted down the track left by a 3 mm K-wire with little trouble. Once the first screw has been positioned, the operation is then repeated for the second hole. The position of the screws is then checked finally with the image intensifier in the anteroposterior and lateral plane.

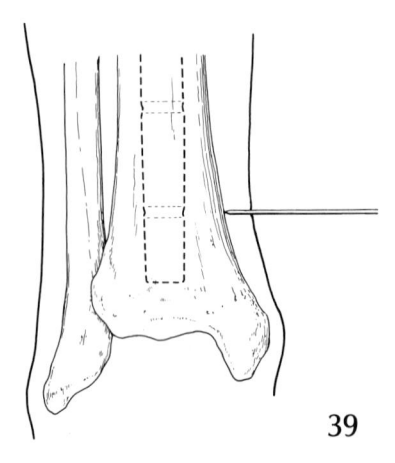

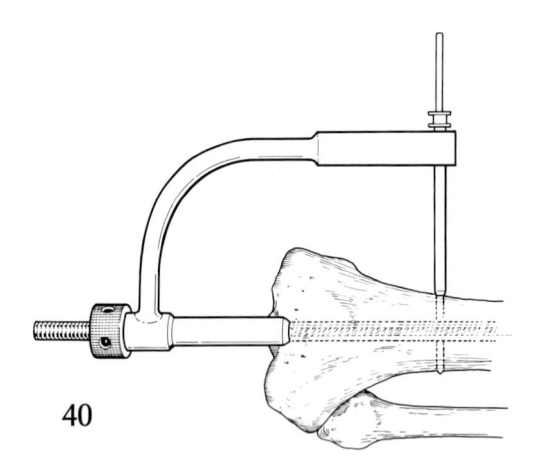

40

For the proximal holes, a jig is provided on the nail, making insertion simple. Problems arise only if the locking lugs between the nail and the jig have become loose, and the handle has been allowed to rotate.

Closure

We use a proximal drain; this should not be inserted directly into the medullary cavity, as this may result in heavy blood loss and intense pain. The wound is then closed in the usual fashion. A wool and crêpe dressing is applied.

Postoperative management

Compartment syndrome has in the past been considered a risk of closed tibial nailing. In practice, this does not seem to be a significant problem, although it must be watched.

Check radiographs are taken before the patient is mobilized. If these are satisfactory, the patient may be mobilized allowing touch weight-bearing, once the drain has been removed. Routine antibiotic prophylaxis should be used, with a cephalosporin in a three-dose regime.

Follow-up

Healing of the fracture should be monitored with radiographs at 6 weeks and 3 months.

References

1. Gustilo RB, Anderson JP. Prevention of infection in the treatment of 1025 open fractures of long bones. *J Bone Joint Surg [Am]* 1976; 58-A: 453–8.

Illustrations by Peter Cox

Fractures of the ankle

C. L. Colton FRCS, FRCS (Ed)
Consultant Orthopaedic Surgeon, University Hospital, Queen's Medical Centre, Nottingham, UK

C. E. Ackroyd MA, FRCS
Consultant Orthopaedic Surgeon, Southmead Hospital, Bristol, UK

Introduction

Classification

Fractures of the ankle occur as a result of a variety of injury mechanisms, each deforming force producing its characteristic sequence of anatomical disruptions, leading, if unchecked, to a pattern of fracture-dislocation typical of that force. It is therefore possible, by studying the fracture pattern, to deduce the direction of the injuring force and the associated ligamentous ruptures[1,2]. This concept has been especially helpful in understanding the mechanism of injury, establishing an accurate anatomical diagnosis and thereby assisting closed reduction in conservative management. In the field of surgical management, such an understanding leads to more confident prediction of those joint fractures that will be difficult to maintain in a position of perfect reduction throughout the healing period.

Danis[3] classified ankle injuries using the level of the fibular fracture as an indicator of integrity of the inferior tibiofibular syndesmosis, a most crucial structure in the maintenance of the intimate relationship of the talus with the ankle mortise. This classification, modified by Weber[4], forms the basis of this widely used, working classification of three basic types of injury.

Type A injuries

1a

In Type A injuries, the fibula fractures at or below the level of the horizontal portion of tibial articular surface (the tibial plafond), so that, apart from a few of the lower fibres of the anterior tibiofibular ligament, the syndesmosis is intact. This injury is usually the result of a force which causes the talus to adduct in the mortise, producing a tensile force on the lateral structures and a compressive force on the medial malleolus, the latter being all the greater if axial loading of the limb is taking place as the angulation occurs. The lateral tension results in any of the following.

1. A *pull-off* fracture of the whole lateral malleolus
2. A mixed osseo-ligamentous disruption with only the malleolar tip avulsed
3. A disruption of the lateral ligament complex without fibular fracture.

If the deforming force then continues, a compression fracture of the medial malleolus, with a vertical fracture plane and often an associated crushing of the *medial corner*, will supervene.

A much less common mechanism of injury, which can produce a fibular fracture at the level of the tibial plafond, is where the talar body is forcibly abducted in the mortise, producing a comminuted, compression fracture of the fibular malleolus and a traction fracture of the medial malleolus.

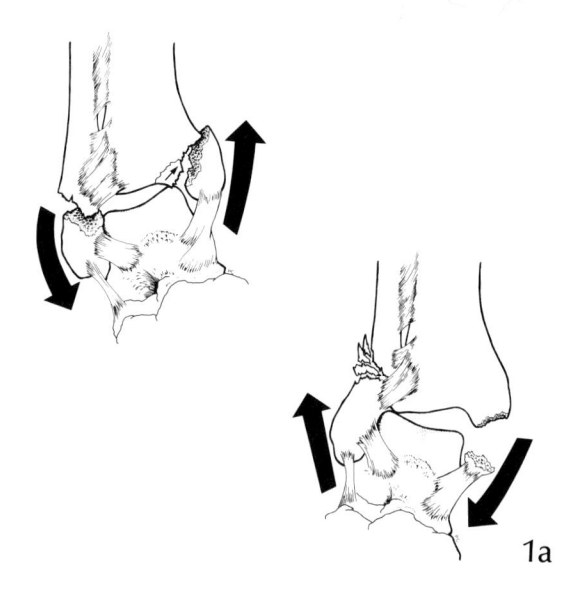

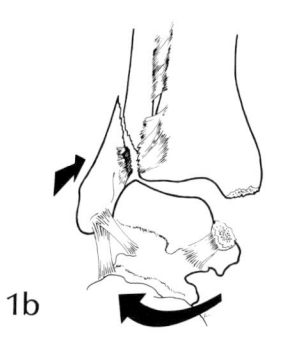

Type B injuries

1b

In the Type B injury, the fibular fracture runs obliquely downwards and forwards to the level of the tibial plafond and is caused by lateral rotation of the talus in the mortise. Such a displacement of the talus first pushes the lateral malleolus backwards, rupturing the anterior tibiofibular ligament and causing the oblique fibular fracture. If the force then continues to impart lateral rotation to the talus, the posterior lip of the tibial plafond is often pushed off as a 'posterior malleolar fracture' (Volkmann's triangle) and the talus, as it exits the back of the ankle joint, pulls off the medial malleolus (or ruptures the deltoid ligament).

Type C injuries

1c

The Type C injury also results from the lateral rotation of the talar body in the mortise, but (for reasons determined by the position of the subtalar joint at the time of the injury) in this instance, the medial structures are first to fail – in tension – either by a pull-off fracture of the medial malleolus or as a deltoid ligament rupture. The talus then swings forwards as it rotates and opens up the syndesmosis by sequentially tearing the anterior tibiofibular ligament, the interosseous ligament and then finally the posterior tibiofibular ligament. The fibula, now free of its syndesmotic tether to the tibia, separates from it (*diastasis*, meaning spreading) and the fibular shaft then breaks somewhere above the upper level of the syndesmosis. It is to be noted that the anterior syndesmotic failure may be represented by an avulsion of the origin of the anterior tibiofibular ligament at the anterior tibial tubercle (Tillaux fracture).

1c

Indications for internal fixation

The ankle joint has a number of characteristics which render it very liable to degenerative change if its biomechanical configuration is even slightly disturbed[5-7]. This, in combination with our modern knowledge of the capacity of articular cartilage in animals to heal where there is anatomical reduction plus stability plus early joint movement[8,9], suggests that, where possible, unstable and displaced joint fractures of the ankle should be treated by rigid internal fixation and early joint mobilization. Only stable, totally undisplaced fractures into the ankle joint, such as the isolated, oblique crack fracture of the lateral malleolus (Type B), are likely, regularly and predictably, to do well with cast immobilization. Conversely, it is extremely difficult, even in the most skilled hands, to achieve an excellent result from the conservative treatment of a grossly unstable, bimalleolar or trimalleolar ankle joint injury: in between these two extremes there is a spectrum of relative indications for internal fixation of ankle joint injuries, the final decision being determined by the skills of the surgeon, the facilities at his disposal, degree of osteoporosis and comminution of the fracture, as well as the general health of the patient.

What is indefensible, in the context of our modern understanding of the ankle as a biomechanical unit, is to operate upon the ankle, incompletely stabilizing the injury complex and then to immobilize the joint in a cast for several weeks immediately after surgery.

Preoperative

The limb should be immobilized in a temporary splint as soon as possible after immediate reduction of obvious deformity. Open injuries should be covered with an antiseptic-soaked dressing, which must remain undisturbed until the wound is uncovered under full aseptic conditions in the operating theatre at the earliest opportunity.

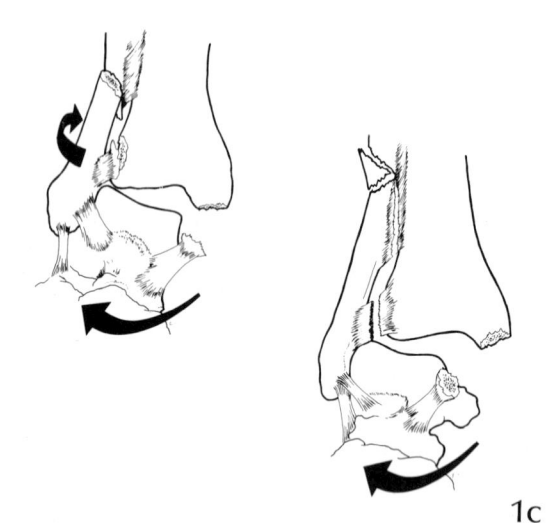

The timing of operation for closed injuries is also vitally important. Unless surgery can be undertaken in the first 24 hours and before there is blistering, marked swelling and/or *peau d'orange* (indicative of intradermal oedema), then operation should be delayed to permit rest in elevation for several days to reduce local oedema: in this context, the tell-tale sign of the appearance of 'wrinkling' of the skin is the clinical feature to be awaited.

Complete radiological assessment of the injury is essential prior to operation, and oblique views may be helpful.

Anaesthesia

Where possible, surgery should be performed under general anaesthesia. The use of a pneumatic tourniquet, after exsanguination by elevation, inflated to double the systolic blood pressure for up to 2 hours is safe in patients with normal vasculature. The tourniquet may then be deflated for 20 minutes and reinflated for a further 1 hour for long procedures.

Position of patient

The patient is positioned supine on the operating table, with a sandbag under the buttock, usually on the side of the injury. The skin should be prepared with more than one application of an antiseptic solution and the limb draped with sterile towelling, the foot being covered with a sterile rubber glove. The skin of the operating area may be covered with adhesive plastic draping material.

Operation

LATERAL COMPLEX

Incision

2

The approach to each fracture should be carefully planned in advance, based on the anatomy of the injury as revealed by the preoperative evaluation. It is prudent to confirm reduction of both the medial and lateral components of the injury prior to the final commitment to a particular fixation method; most surgeons will start with the reduction of the lateral side to bring the fibula out to length and to correct any rotation. A posterolateral, or anterolateral, slightly J-shaped incision is used, exercising care to avoid damage to the sural nerve. As the incision is deepened through the subcutaneous tissues, small superficial veins are divided and secured. When the deep fascia over the fibula is reached, the skin flaps are elevated, using sharp dissection, and gently retracted. Incisions should be generous in length as forcible retraction and 'folding' of the skin flaps can greatly prejudice viability.

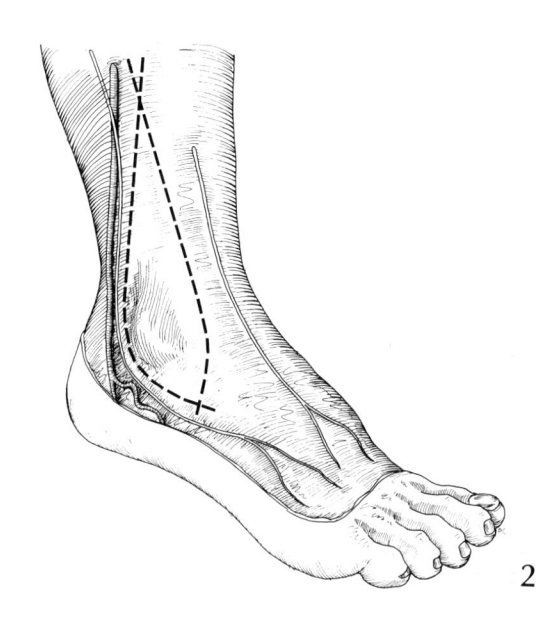

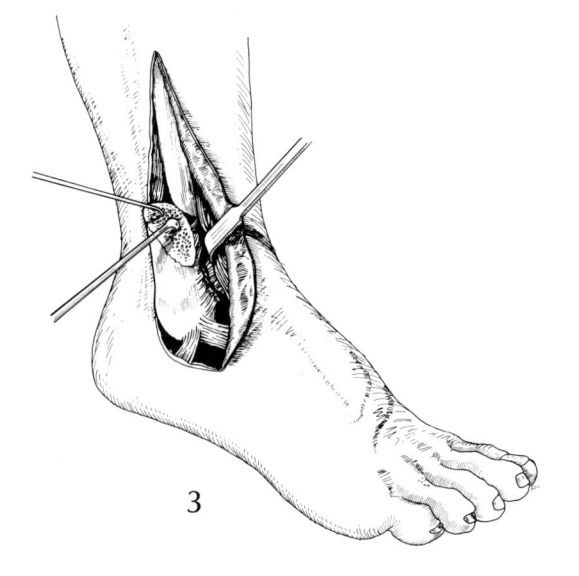

Exposure of the fracture

3

The deep fascia is divided to expose the fracture. Often the injury itself will have stripped some of the fascia and the exposure of the fracture site, certainly in the subcutaneous zone of the distal fibula, is rarely a problem. The fracture ends are separated gently using a small bone hook and any blood clot or small loose bone fragments removed with a fine curette. The periosteum at the fracture edge is scraped back for 1–2 mm so that it will not impede perfect reduction.

Reduction of the fracture

4a

The fracture is now reduced using pointed reduction forceps, with the assistant manipulating the foot in the opposite direction to the original deforming force. Difficulty of reduction may be due to the following.

1. Entrapment of bony fragments between the fibular bone ends, such as a small Tillaux fragment with the attached anterior tibiofibular ligament
2. Soft tissue interposition medially – either an inverted torn deltoid ligament, or occasionally the tibialis posterior tendon. For this reason, the medial side should be opened before the lateral fixation is begun.

The fibular reduction is then held with a pointed reduction forceps, whilst the closure of the medial joint space and reduction of the medial malleolus is undertaken, whereafter an intraoperative radiograph should be taken to confirm anatomical reposition before fixation is performed.

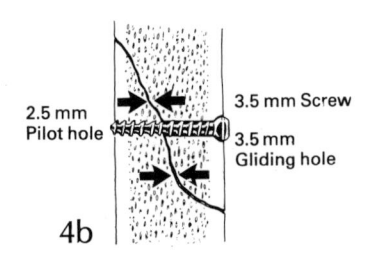

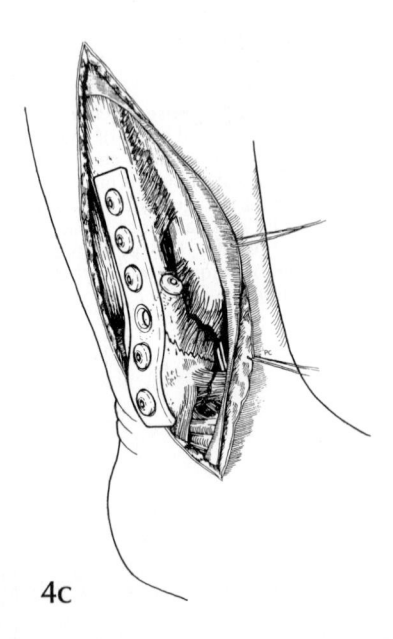

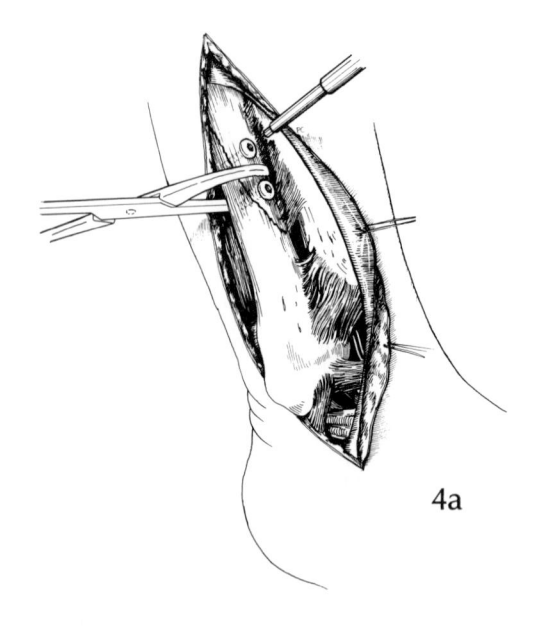

4b

The choice of fixation technique for the fibular fracture depends upon the fracture characteristics, but, in general, oblique fractures will be fixed by an interfragmentary lag screw technique, protected by a plate fulfilling a neutralization function. For the lag screwing, a 3.5 mm cortical screw is chosen. The near (usually anterior) cortex is drilled with a 3.5 mm drill bit to provide a gliding hole, and then through a 3.5–2.7 mm insert sleeve passed into this gliding hole, the opposite cortex is pierced with a 2.5 mm drill bit. After countersinking the near cortex and measuring the depth of the hole to give the required screw length, the far cortex is threaded using a 3.5 mm cortical tap. The screw is then inserted and as it is tightened, compression of the fracture surfaces is noted. In long oblique fractures, two such lag screws may be inserted. A five- or six-hole, one-third-tubular plate is then contoured, as necessary, to the precise shape of the fibular surface and fixed with 3.5 mm screws to span the fracture line and protect the lag screw fixation.

4c

The oblique Type B fractures are fixed in this way. The anterior inferior tibiofibular ligament is approximated with stout sutures.

5a & b

For transverse fractures of the fibular shaft in the Type C injury, a one-third-tubular plate with three holes on each side of the fracture is chosen, and light axial compression is applied by drilling an eccentric screw hole (on the side of the plate away from the fracture) through one of the shaft fragments after fixing the plate to the other shaft fragment. This technique must never be used in combination with direct lag screwing of a fracture – a neutralization (or protection) plate should not be loaded to produce axial compression at the fracture.

Transverse fractures of the lateral malleolus (adduction Type A) should also be fixed using a one-third-tubular plate, accurately contoured. This is fixed to the malleolar fragment using small 3.5 mm cancellous screws, and to the shaft using similarly sized cortical screws, the first of which, after fixing the plate to the malleolus, may be inserted eccentrically to produce slight tension in the plate, thereby causing a little compression at the fracture surface. Tension-band wiring[10] is an alternative technique for this type of fracture.

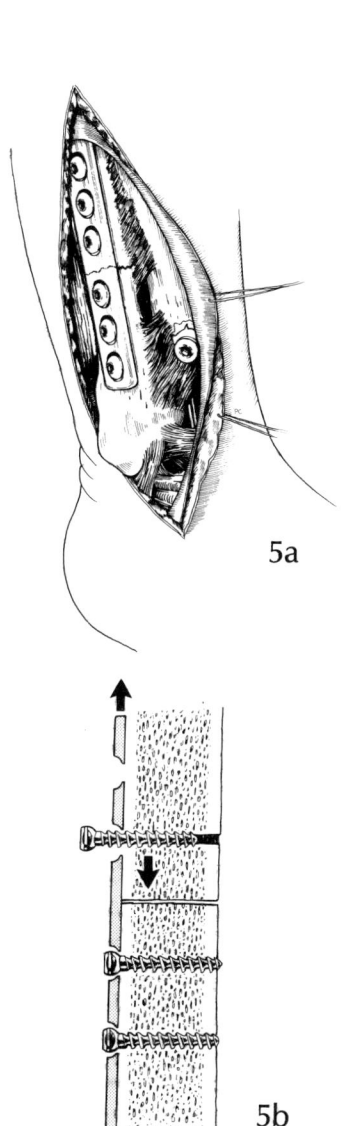

Tibiofibular syndesmosis

Once the fibular fracture has been fixed and, where appropriate, the medial side stabilized, it is necessary to test the stability of the inferior tibiofibular joint. In Type B fractures, the interosseous ligament may, or may not, be intact and the integrity of the posterior tibiofibular ligament complex will depend on whether there is a Volkmann's fracture posteriorly. In Type C fractures, the whole syndesmosis is ruptured, but after fixation of the fibular fracture, the syndesmotic stability will be restored if either a posterior malleolar fracture has been rigidly fixed, or a Tillaux fracture has been fixed thereby reconstituting the function of the anterior tibiofibular ligament.

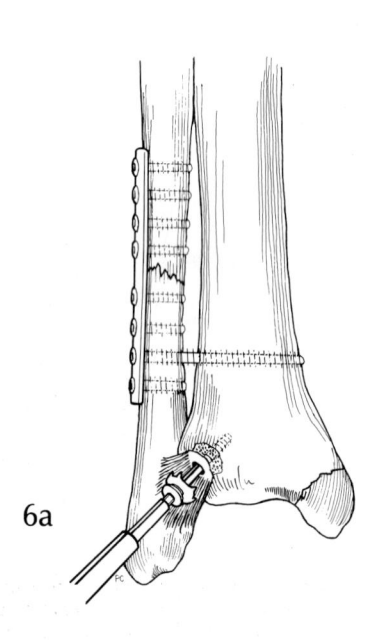

6a

In any case, at the conclusion of the operation, a small bone hook is passed around the fibula and gentle traction is applied in a lateral direction in an attempt to draw the fibular away from the tibia. If any diastasis persists, then a stabilizing fibulotibial screw is inserted. It has to be fully appreciated that this screw is *not* a compression screw – it is inserted to maintain the fibula in its correct position in the incisura fibularis. The steps in its insertion are as follows.

1. With the ankle dorsiflexed, so that the wide part of the talar body is in the mortise, accurate relocation of the fibula in relation to the tibia is secured
2. At a site above the syndesmosis, either through a plate hole or separately, a 2.5 mm hole is drilled through the fibula and into both tibial cortices and its length measured
3. With the location of the fibula carefully maintained, this hole is tapped with the 3.5 mm cortical tap
4. The appropriate 3.5 mm cortical screw is inserted.

The reason for engaging both tibial cortices is to ensure that the screw protects against any tendency for the fibula to shift proximally. This diastasis screw will have fulfilled its role as soon as the syndesmotic ligaments have healed, and as normal ankle function requires that the fibula moves in relation to the tibia, the screw should be removed at 6–8 weeks after insertion, prior to unprotected weight-bearing.

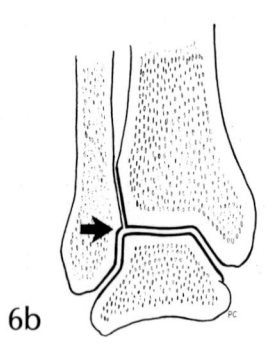

6b

At the conclusion of the operative procedure, a lateral radiograph is taken, and also an anteroposterior view with the limb in 20° of medial rotation; these will show the quality of the reduction and fixation. On the anteroposterior film, the correct relationship of the fibula to the tibia will be confirmed by noting that the small beak of bone, which projects from the medial surface of the fibula at the level of the junction of the articular with the non-articular portions of the lateral malleolus, forms a continuous curve with the subchondral bone of the tibial plafond[11] – the 'Shenton's line' of the ankle.

Posterior malleolus

If a posterior tibial lip fracture (Volkmann's fracture) has been produced as the talus exits from the back of the ankle mortise (usually in the Type B injury), it may bear a radiologically visible portion of the articular surface, in which case it should be reduced and fixed with one or two cancellous lag screws. As such a fragment will bear the tibial origin of the posterior tibiofibular ligament, its stabilization will contribute to the restoration of the integrity of the inferior tibiofibular syndesmosis. A non-articular Volkmann's fragment need not normally be internally fixed.

On the preoperative radiographs, it is often possible to assess whether the posterior fragment is predominantly posterolateral or posteromedial. This will then determine the choice of surgical approach. If posterolateral, then the incision for the fibular approach will have been curved a little more posteriorly (always having regard to the path of the sural nerve), and can be deepened behind the fibula, between flexor hallucis longus and the peroneal tendons, which can be retracted forwards after partial release, if necessary, of the peroneal retinaculum. Alternatively, a predominantly posteromedial fragment can be exposed behind the medial border of the tibia.

7a

The reduction of the fragment is secured using a sharp bone hook and held using a stout Kirschner wire passed forwards through the thickest portion of the fragment and at right angles to the fracture plane. This wire is gently advanced until it is felt to pierce the anterior tibial cortex. A small stab wound over the tip of this wire in the front of the ankle region allows the wire to be driven on to protrude about 1 cm through the skin. Using an appropriate 'triple-barrelled' drill guide slipped over the protruding end of the wire, a 2 mm hole is drilled anteroposteriorly into the centre of the Volkmann's fragment. A 4 mm cancellous lag screw, fitted with a washer, is then inserted from in front after tapping the cortex at the point of entry, producing interfragmentary compression. A second such screw may be inserted if the posterior fragment is of sufficient size.

Care must be taken to ensure that the whole threaded portion of the screw lies entirely within the posterior fragment, in order that interfragmentary compression be achieved. If the length of screw indicated by the depth gauge has a threaded portion of such a length that it would cross, and not pass fully beyond, the fracture line, then a slightly longer screw is chosen and its threaded portion trimmed to the appropriate length with wire-cutters or bolt-cutters prior to insertion.

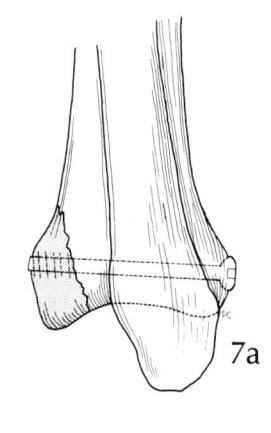

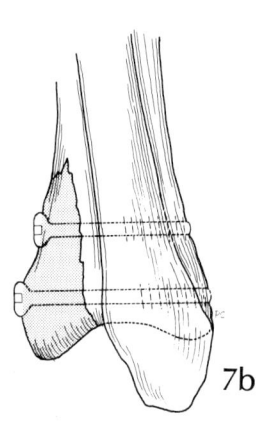

7b

An alternative approach, using the standard posterolateral or anterolateral incisions, exposes the Volkmann fragment through the disrupted syndesmosis. Once the ankle is exposed, the foot is displaced into lateral rotation subluxing the talus, which carries with it the distal fibular fragment. The ankle joint cavity itself can be inspected and the Volkmann fragment cleaned and reduced using a sucker, curette and small bone hook. A stab incision is made over the anterior part of the tibia and a stout Kirschner wire passed backwards through the lower tibia into the fragment, so providing temporary stabilization. The triple-barrelled drill guide is then used to drill an appropriately placed 2 mm drill hole into the thickest most-lateral part of the Volkmann fragment and a cancellous lag screw inserted as above. Care must be taken to ensure that the Kirschner wire is placed eccentrically to allow optimum positioning of the screw. Continuity of the posterior inferior tibiofibular ligament has now been restored, the talus and the fibular fracture can now be reduced and the anterior tibiofibular ligament reconstructed.

MEDIAL COMPLEX

Incision

8

The ipsilateral sandbag under the buttock may be removed for ease of access medially. Slightly curved longitudinal or horizontal incisions may be used, depending upon the area to be exposed, as judged by the preoperative evaluation. Care should be taken to avoid division of the saphenous nerve, especially if the long saphenous vein has to be ligated.

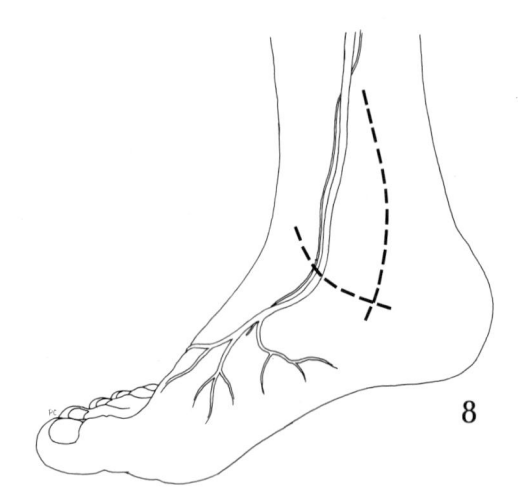

Exposure of the fracture

9

The incision is deepened through the fascia to expose the periosteum of the medial malleolus and the fracture site. There may be a sizeable flap of periosteum tucked between the fracture surfaces, which will need to be lifted out. The fracture edges are cleared for 1–2 mm so that the accuracy of reduction can be checked. Before reduction, however, the malleolar fragment is pulled down so that the interior of the joint can be irrigated, using Ringer's or Hartmann's solution, any loose chondral fragments removed and the state of the articular surfaces assessed. The fracture surfaces are then cleaned free of blood clot and tiny free bony fragments carefully removed before the malleolus can be restored to its correct position.

Reduction and fixation of the fracture

10a

The fracture has now to be reduced anatomically and temporary fixation obtained with a Kirschner wire and pointed reduction forceps. The usual fixation chosen is a small cancellous lag screw with a washer. The screw must be inserted perpendicular to the fracture surface in both planes, and its thread should be totally beyond the fracture so that interfragmentary compression is achieved. The soft tissues are cleared from the chosen site of entry of the screw and a 2 mm drill hole made across the fracture. Excessive length of the screw is no advantage as the densest cancellous bone of the distal tibia is immediately above the subchondral bone of the tibial plafond. For injuries of Types B and C a screw 30 mm long is usually ideal. In Type A injuries, where the fracture line is vertical, the screws will be lying virtually horizontal in the dense spongy bone.

After drilling, the depth of the hole is checked. The malleolar fragment *only* is then threaded with a small cancellous tap (to assist passage of the screw through the fragment without splitting or twisting it), prior to insertion of the chosen screw and washer. In a larger fragment, a second screw, parallel to the first, may be inserted in a similar manner to provide rotational stability. In a smaller fragment, the Kirschner wire may be left in, cut short and the end bent over.

An alternative technique in Type B or C (but not the adduction Type A) fractures, especially for small malleolar fragments, is to use the Weber–Vasey tension-band wiring technique (see chapter on 'Fractures of the Patella', pp. 252–256).

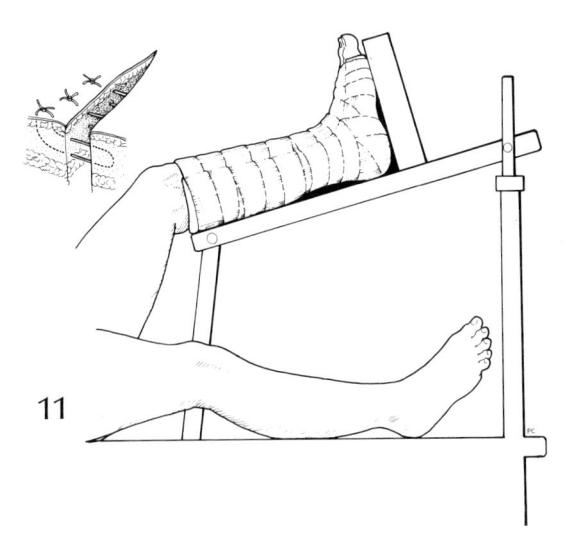

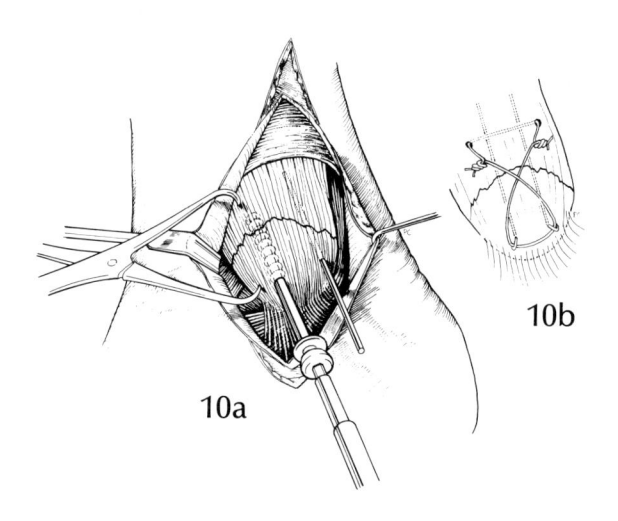

Wound closure

11

The wounds are closed using fine interrupted absorbable sutures in the subcutaneous tissue and interrupted 3/0 or 4/0 monofilament nylon sutures for the skin. A suction drain to the subcutaneous space of each wound is mandatory. Care is taken that there is no tension in the wound edges and the use of the Donati–Allgöwer skin suture technique[10] protects the vascularity of the delicate skin edges. Where there is marked swelling, it is better to leave a portion of the wound open rather than suture it under tension, so long as the implants are not exposed. In open fractures, the original wound must, of course, be left open. A sterile dressing is applied, followed by 'plaster wool' and then a firm, evenly wound crêpe bandage. In order to prevent the foot from dropping into an equinus posture, a strong plaster of Paris backslab is applied after tourniquet release. The limb is elevated on a frame at 45°.

Postoperative management

Elevation of the limb is maintained for several days until all swelling has resolved. The suction drains are removed at 48 hours and the dressings reduced to simple gauze.

At 48 hours, under the supervision of a physiotherapist, active ankle movements within the comfortable range are encouraged several times daily, but the backslab is reapplied in the intervals between treatments, at least until comfortable active dorsiflexion above the right angle is easily performed. At that stage, the backslab can be used only as a night splint. The use of an ankle continuous passive motion (CPM) machine, if available, is preferable.

Once wound healing is assured and progress is observed in regaining joint movement, the patient may begin walking, using crutches but without bearing weight. The skin sutures are removed 10–12 days postoperatively in most cases and, provided the fixation is regarded as satisfactory, touch weight-bearing is safe from about 15–20 days after surgery. Where there is any doubt about the patient's compliance, a protective walking cast should be applied before discharge from hospital.

Unprotected weight-bearing is delayed until 6–8 weeks from operation, and where a diastasis screw has been used, this should first be removed (see above). The introduction of weight-bearing will vary from patient to patient, and will depend on the quality of the surgical fixation, local tissue factors and radiological control of the progress to bony union. Any appearance of additional swelling, local warmth or redness would indicate the need to adopt a more cautious programme of rehabilitation.

In general, implants should be removed between 6 and 12 months from insertion; trouble-free, single metaphyseal screws may be left *in situ*.

References

1. Lauge-Hansen N. Fractures of the ankle: combined experimental-surgical and experimental-roentgenologic investigations. *Arch Surg* 1950; 60: 957–85.

2. Colton CL. Injuries of the ankle. In: Wilson JN, ed. *Watson-Jones fractures and joint injuries*, 6th ed. Edinburgh: Churchill Livingstone, 1982: 1104–51.

3. Danis R. *Théorie et pratique de l'ostéosynthèse*. Paris: Masson et Cie, 1949.

4. Weber BG. *Die Verletzargen des oberen Sprunggelenkes: Aktuelle Probleme in der Chirurgie*. Bern: Huber, 1966.

5. Riede UN, Schenk RK, Willeneger H. Gelenkmechanische Untersuchungen zum Problem der posttraumatischen Arthrosen im oberen Sprungselenk: I Die intraartikuläre Modellfraktur. *Langenbecks Arch Chir* 1971; 328: 258–71.

6. Simon WH, Friedenburg S, Richardson S. Joint congruence: a correlation of joint congruence and thickness of articular cartilage in dogs. *J Bone Joint Surg [Am]* 1973; 55-A: 1614–20.

7. Tillmann B, Bartz B, Schleicher A. Stress in the human ankle joint: a brief review. *Arch Orthop Trauma Surg* 1985; 103: 385–91.

8. Salter RB. Regeneration of articular cartilage through continuous passive motion: past, present and future. In: Straub R, Wilson PD, eds. *Clinical trends in orthopaedics*. New York: Grune and Stratton, 1982, Chap. 12.

9. Mitchell N, Sheperd N. Healing of articular cartilage in intra-articular fractures in rabbits. *J Bone Joint Surg [Am]* 1980; 62-A: 628–34.

10. Müller ME, Allgöwer M, Schneider R, Willenegger H. *Manual of internal fixation*. Berlin: Springer-Verlag, 1979: 46.

11. Weber BG, Simpson LA. Corrective lengthening osteotomy of the fibula. *Clin Orthop* 1985; 199: 61–7.

Illustrations by Donn Johnson

Recognition and treatment of compartment compression syndromes

Thomas E. Whitesides Jr MD
Professor of Orthopaedics, Department of Orthopaedic Surgery, Emory University School of Medicine, Atlanta, Georgia, USA

Michael H. Heckman MD
Consultant Orthopaedic Surgeon, South Texas Sports Medicine and Orthopaedics, Corpus Christi, Texas; Department of Orthopaedic Surgery, University of Texas Health Science Center, San Antonio, Texas, USA

Introduction

The late complications of ischaemic contracture of the upper and lower extremities has been classically documented by Seddon[1,2] and Owen et al.[3] Retrospectively, they advised the necessity of early recognition of ischaemia and recommended therapy, including fasciotomy, of affected limbs. They noted that the classical signs of pain, pallor, paralysis, and pulselessness associated with ischaemic changes could not be relied upon entirely in evaluation of suspected patients, and their description of the catastrophic results of an unrecognized compartment syndrome are well known.

In the last 15 years further investigations by Whitesides et al.[4] have established the histology and biochemical changes associated with tissue ischaemia in acute injuries and research has clarified the parameters of timing and necessity for fasciotomy. Compartment syndromes[5] have occurred following arterial injury[6], burns[7], crush injuries[8], arterial injections[9], osteotomy[10], embolectomy, snake bite[11], drug overdose[12], acute and chronic exertional states[13], gunshot wounds[14] and both open[15] and closed[16,17] fractures. Patients sustaining these injuries require critical evaluation for elevated tissue pressure and ischaemia, which may lead to a compartment syndrome.

Pathogenesis

Compartment syndromes generally result from a muscle injury that leads to swelling, which is proportional to the tissue damage. In those patients sustaining fractures, the coincident formation of a fracture haematoma adds to the problem of increased pressure as it has the effect of increasing the volume within a closed space. Because the extremities are anatomically arranged in unyielding fascial compartments, as tissue pressures rise there is ultimately circulatory embarrassment, ischaemia, and compartment syndrome.

In cases of arterial injury the tissues are deprived of their blood supply, resulting in ischaemia. Re-anastomosis or re-establishment of circulation produces swelling within the tissues and elevation of tissue pressures.

In those injuries that produce complete ischaemia, skeletal muscle will remain electrically responsive for up to 3 hours, and will survive up to 4 hours without irreversible damage. Eight hours of total ischaemia produces completely irreversible changes[4].

Nerve tissue can conduct impulses 1 hour after the onset of total ischaemia and may survive 4 hours with only neurapraxic damage. Axonotmesis is usual after 8 hours of total ischaemia, with irreversible changes in the nerve.

Evaluation of the patient

Pain, pulselessness, pallor, and paralysis or paraesthesia have been described as the clinical hallmarks of a compartment syndrome[4].

Pain is the most important feature of a compartment syndrome, and pain aggravated by passive stretching of the compartment in question is the most reliable physical finding in making the diagnosis. In a normotensive patient with a diastolic blood pressure of 70 mmHg, an increase in tissue pressure from the normal resting pressure of 0–4 mmHg to 30–40 mmHg will result in significant discomfort, with passive stretching of the affected tissues. Paraesthesia, paralysis, and sensory changes are noted only after ischaemia has been present for a long time. Lack of distal pulses, pallor, and diminution of capillary refill will rarely occur unless there is an arterial injury, or the artery passing through an affected compartment is subjected to tissue pressures approaching the patient's systolic blood pressure.

In unconscious patients a close evaluation to rule out a compartment syndrome is warranted, and tissue pressure measurements should be performed in any suspicious case to exclude ischaemia. In those patients in shock or in a hypotensive state there is a decreased ability to perfuse the tissues, related to the low blood pressure, and only a slightly elevated tissue pressure may indicate an impending compartment syndrome.

Tissue pressure

A number of methods for the measurement of tissue pressures have been described and are currently in use. These methods include the infusion technique (Whitesides[18]), the Wick catheter (Hargens[19]), the Howmedica slit catheter (Rorabeck[20]), and the Stryker STIC device (Stryker–Whitesides[16]). Properly used, all of these methods are accurate and measure the same phenomena.

The critical tissue pressure at which ischaemia occurs is debated but currently it is believed that ischaemia is directly related to the perfusion gradient of the tissue in question. This gradient is directly related to the patient's blood pressure – more specifically, the diastolic or mean arterial pressure. Tissue perfusion within a compartment diminishes as these pressures are approached; ischaemia generally occurs at 10 mmHg below the diastolic pressure and 30 mmHg below the mean arterial pressure[40].

Indications for fasciotomy

We recommend that fasciotomy be performed at 20–30 mmHg below diastolic pressure in any patient with a worsening clinical condition, a documented rising tissue pressure, or a history of 6 hours of total ischaemia of an extremity.

Understanding pressure measurements

Tissue pressures need to be measured throughout an extremity to document that the area of the greatest tissue damage and highest pressure has been recorded.

In recent studies of patients sustaining lower extremity injuries, differences in pressure over a distance as small as 5 cm were found to be significant in making the diagnosis.

In those patients in whom tissue pressures are approaching the critical level for fasciotomy, careful follow-up is required in the form of repeat pressure readings every 1–2 hours, and monitoring of all the signs and symptoms associated with a compartment syndrome. Tissue pressures may remain elevated for as long as 48–72 hours after injury[21] and readings should be continued until a decrease or stabilization in pressure is noted or until an increase is noted to the point when fasciotomy is needed.

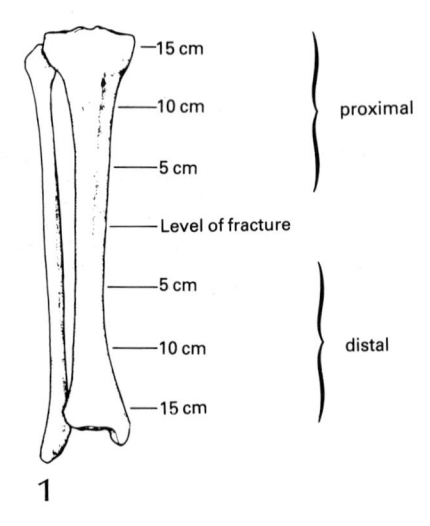

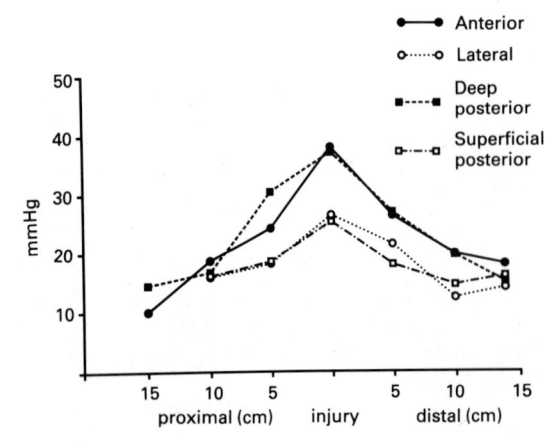

Figure 1 Mean pressure change with distance from the fracture

Measurement techniques

Utilizing the Whitesides or infusion technique, the equipment for tissue pressure measurements is inexpensive and should readily be available in hospitals, emergency rooms, and doctors' surgeries. The equipment needed is listed as follows: (1) a mercury manometer; (2) two plastic intravenous extension tubes; (3) two 18-gauge needles; (4) one 20 ml syringe; (5) one three-way stopcock; and (6) one vial of bacteriostatic normal saline.

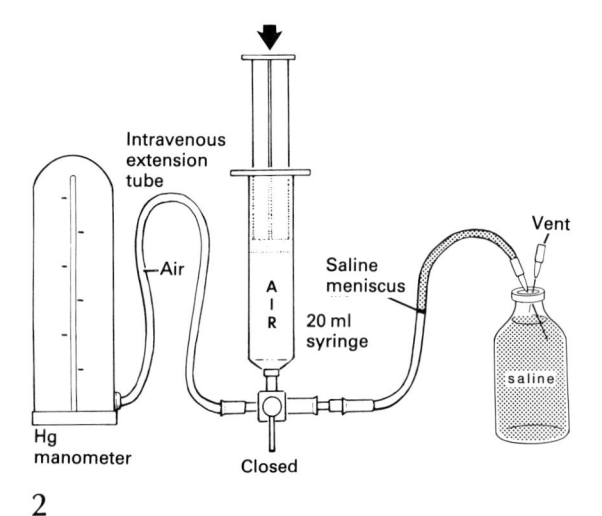

Steps in technique

2

1. The extremity to be evaluated is cleaned and prepared so that pressure measurements may be performed both proximal and distal to the level of injury, e.g. the level of fracture.
2. The vacuum in a sterile bottle of saline is broken with a sterile 18-gauge needle so that fluid may be easily withdrawn.
3. The 20 ml syringe is assembled with the three-way stopcock and one of the intravenous extension tubes (right of illustration). The second 18-gauge needle is placed at the end of the extension tubing. The third unused port of the three-way stopcock is closed off.
4. The 18-gauge needle at the end of the extension tubing is inserted into the bottle of saline and the saline aspirated without bubbles into approximately one-half the length of the extension tubing. The first 18-gauge needle should act as a vent to keep a vacuum from forming during aspiration. The three-way stopcock is turned to close off the extension tubing so that saline is not lost during the transfer of the needle from the saline to the patient.
5. The second extension tubing (left in illustration) is connected to the three-way stopcock at its remaining open port. The other end of this tubing should then be connected to the hose from the mercury manometer thus completing construction of the apparatus.

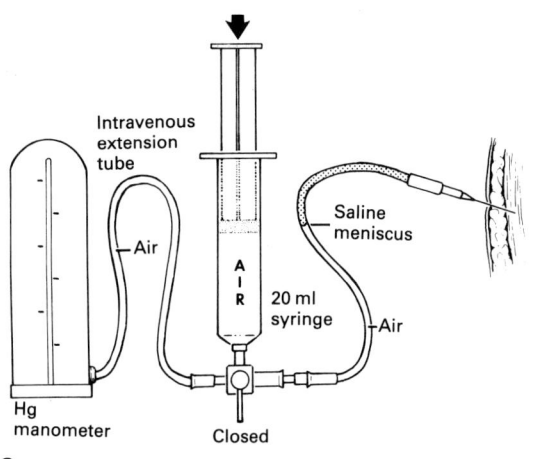

3

6. With the stopcock still closed to the extension tubing containing the saline, the syringe is removed from the apparatus and approximately 15 ml of air is aspirated. The syringe is reconnected to the three-way stopcock. The saline needle is now transferred to the patient and inserted through the skin and fascia, into the muscle at the site to be measured.
7. The stopcock is now turned so that the syringe is open to both extension tubes forming a 'T'-connection and an open system from the muscle to the mercury manometer. This creates a system that allows air from the syringe to flow into both extension tubes as pressure within the system is increased.

4

8. Taking care that the extension tubings and the site being measured are at the same level, so as not to create a fluid column that would artificially elevate the pressure being measured, a minute amount of fluid is injected to clear the system of any soft tissue. The column of saline in the tubing, by capillary attraction, normally forms a convex meniscus away from the patient. By slowly depressing the syringe the air column pressure is gradually raised, increasing the pressure in the system. The saline meniscus will be seen to flatten when the air pressure in the system equals the interstitial pressure of the tissue. If the air pressure is raised higher than the interstitial pressure of the tissue, the saline meniscus will form in the direction of the patient. While carefully watching the column of saline, an assistant monitors the pressure on the mercury manometer. The measurement should be recorded when the meniscus flattens. It is helpful in performing measurements to place the meniscus against a white background for better visualization. Care should be taken not to read the pressure as the saline is beginning to inject into the muscle as this will result in an erroneously high reading.

9. Once the pressure has been recorded the system is equilibrated by withdrawing on the syringe until pressure on the manometer reads 0 mmHg. This prevents saline from being lost from the system as the needle is withdrawn from the leg. Subsequent measurements may now be performed utilizing the same apparatus.

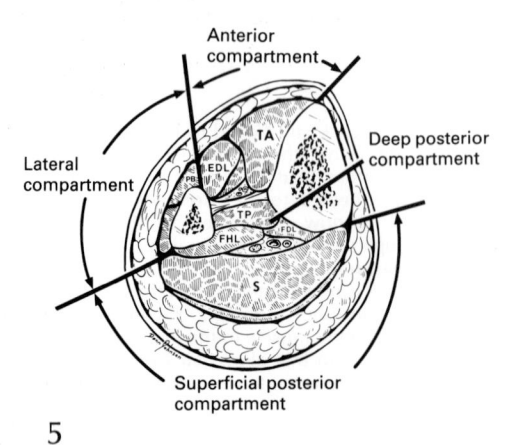

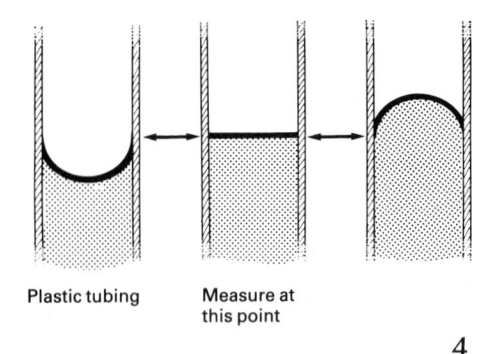

Plastic tubing   Measure at this point

4

Evaluation and treatment

When a compartment syndrome or increased tissue pressures are diagnosed, a set of guidelines needs to be observed. All circumferential dressings need to be split or removed immediately and the affected extremity raised to the level of the heart to maximize perfusion without compromising venous drainage. The cast padding must be split as well as the plaster. If resolution of the signs of ischaemia does not occur and the tissue pressures remain elevated, a surgical decompression is advised.

THE LEG

5

The leg is divided into four compartments, the anterior, the lateral, the superficial posterior and the deep posterior. The anterior compartment contains the tibialis anterior (TA), the extensor hallucis longus (EHL), the extensor digitorum longus (EDL), and the peroneus tertius muscles with the anterior tibial artery and the deep peroneal nerve. The lateral compartment contains the peroneal longus (PL) and brevis (PB) muscles with their nerve supply the superficial peroneal nerve. The deep posterior contains the tibialis posterior (TP), flexor hallucis longus (FHL), and the flexor digitorum longus (FDL) muscles and the posterior tibial artery and nerve. The superficial posterior compartment contains the gastrocnemius, the plantaris and the soleus (S) muscles and receives its nerve and blood supply from the posterior tibial nerve and artery. Tissue pressures need to be measured at multiple sites in each of these four compartments in evaluating any patient with a suspected compartment syndrome.

The anterior compartment is easily palpable on the anterolateral side of the tibia, offering easy access for pressure measurements. This is also true for the lateral compartment overlying the fibula and the superficial posterior compartment which is composed of the palpable gastrocnemius–soleus complex. The deep posterior compartment, on the other hand, is difficult to measure because of its location behind and adhering to the tibia, and must be approached posteromedially to the tibia if pressures are to be measured.

5

6

The needle placement in each of the four compartments is illustrated.

Perifibular fasciotomy

Fasciotomy of the leg may be performed through a lateral perifibular approach[22,23], a lateral approach with fibulectomy[4,24], or through a two-incision mediolateral approach[25,26]. Any of these, if carried out correctly, will result in decompression of all four compartments of the leg. A subcutaneous fasciotomy[27] through limited skin incisions is not recommended because the blind dissection of this technique endangers veins and sensory nerves; and without a complete release of the skin, a circumferential compressive force is still being applied to the underlying tissues, increasing their interstitial pressure.

The perifibular approach using a single lateral incision provides adequate exposure of all four compartments. A second medial incision is not needed to decompress the superficial posterior or deep posterior compartments.

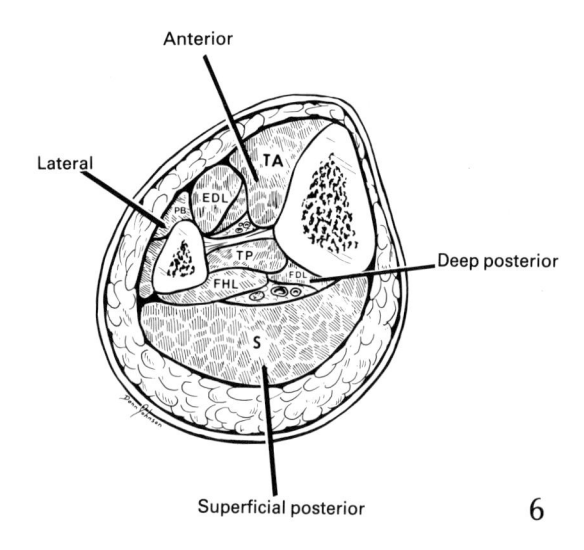

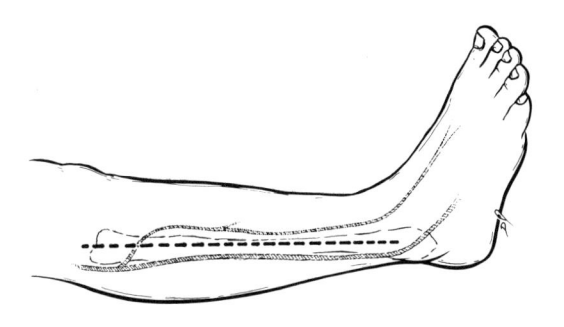

7

The perifibular fasciotomy is carried out through a straight lateral incision just posterior to the fibula, from the level of the fibular head to a point 5–6 cm above the tip of the lateral malleolus. At the level of the fibular head the common peroneal nerve passes subcutaneously around the fibular neck; it should be exposed and protected.

8

After the nerve has been mobilized and protected, the incision is deepened to incise the fascia overlying the lateral compartment for the length of the wound. This decompresses the compartment and allows inspection of the peroneal muscles. The anterior edge of the incision is then retracted to expose the anterior compartment and a second long fascial incision is made to decompress the extensors. Care is taken to avoid the superficial peroneal nerve as it exits the fascia of the lateral compartment and runs anterior in the distal third of the leg. The posterior edge of the wound is then retracted to expose the superficial posterior compartment, and the gastrocnemius–soleus complex is decompressed through a full-length fascial incision. Finally, the plane between the peroneus longus and the soleus is identified. This plane in many patients may be identified by a longitudinal fat strip that when dissected through will provide a true internervous dissection between the superficial peroneal nerve (serving the peroneus longus) and tibial nerve (to the soleus).

With deep dissection the periosteum of the fibula will then be exposed. The fibula should then be stripped of the soleus posteriorly. As the fibres of the soleus originate from the fibula, running distally toward the foot, elevation of the muscle should be carried out in a distal to proximal direction. The soleus can then be retracted posteriorly to visualize the deep posterior compartment. The fascia encasing the flexors of the foot and tibialis posterior can then be incised and, if necessary, epimysiotomy of any severely involved muscles in any of the compartments may be carried out.

Postoperative management

The wound is left open and a large, non-restrictive bulky dressing is applied. Usually there is a significant amount of drainage and the large dressing will help to contain this. At 3–4 days a delayed primary closure may be attempted or a split-thickness skin graft may be placed for muscle coverage.

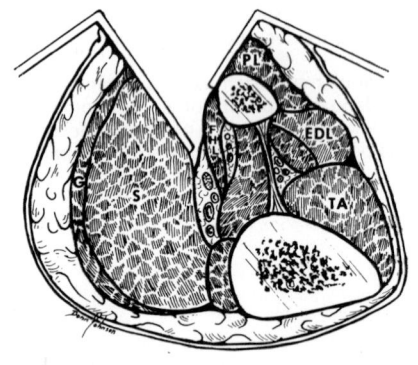

8

THE THIGH

9

Though the thigh is recognized as a site of rare involvement of compartment syndromes, the possibility exists for the development of the condition. The thigh contains three definite fascial compartments: anterior, medial, and posterior. The anterior compartment contains the quadriceps femoris (RF, VL, VM, VI), sartorius (S), iliacus, psoas, and pectineus muscles; the femoral artery and vein; and the femoral and lateral femoral cutaneous nerves. The medial compartment contains the adductor longus (AL), adductor magnus (AM), adductor brevis, gracilis (G), and the obturator externus muscles; the profundus femoris and obturator arteries and veins; and the obturator nerve. The posterior compartment contains the biceps femoris (B), a portion of the adductor magnus, semitendinosus (ST) and semimembranosus (SM) muscles; the perforating branches of the profundis femoris artery; and the sciatic and posterior femoral cutaneous nerves. Each of the three compartments is divided from the others by intermuscular septa originating from the femur.

Pressure measurements and fasciotomy technique

All three compartments of the thigh are easily accessible for pressure measurements, which should be taken in the quadriceps, the adductors, and the hamstring group. Again, multiple measurements should be performed to rule out a localized increase in tissue pressure.

Fasciotomy is performed through an incision parallel to the lateral shaft of the femur, from the level of the lesser trochanter to the proximal edge of the lateral epicondyle. The anterior compartment is decompressed by incising the underlying fascia lata for the whole length of the wound. The vastus lateralis is then retracted anteromedially to expose the lateral intermuscular septum and the underlying posterior compartment. The septum is then opened for the length of the incision, decompressing the posterior compartment.

After the anterior and posterior compartments have been decompressed, tissue pressure measurements should then be performed again on the medial compartment. If pressures remain elevated a second incision parallel to the gracilis should be made through the skin and subcutaneous tissues to the underlying adductor group. The underlying fascia may then be incised, thus providing decompression and access for evaluation of the medial compartment.

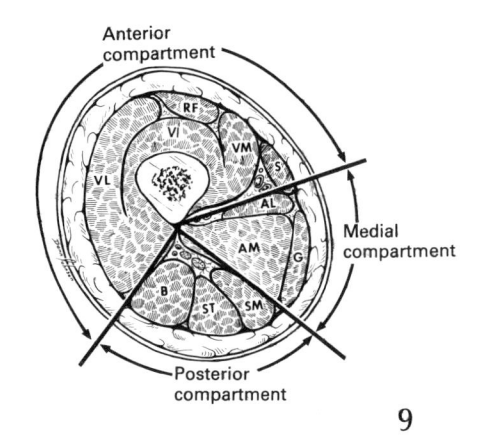

THE FOOT

10

Compartment syndromes of the foot do occur[28] and evaluation of the foot should be carried out in any patient with a more proximal ischaemic event, such as a crush injury, or tarsal or metatarsal fractures or dislocations[29]. The foot is divided into four compartments: the medial, the central, the lateral, and the interosseous[28]. The medial compartment contains the abductor hallucis (Abd H) and flexor hallucis brevis muscles (FHB); the central compartment contains the adductor hallucis (Add H), quadratus plantae (QP), flexor digitorum brevis (FDB), and the tendons of the flexor digitorum longus and flexor hallucis longus; the lateral compartment contains the flexor digiti minimi (FDM) and the abductor digiti minimi (AD) muscles; and the interosseous compartment contains the interossei of the foot (INT) and the plantar arterial arches and digital nerves.

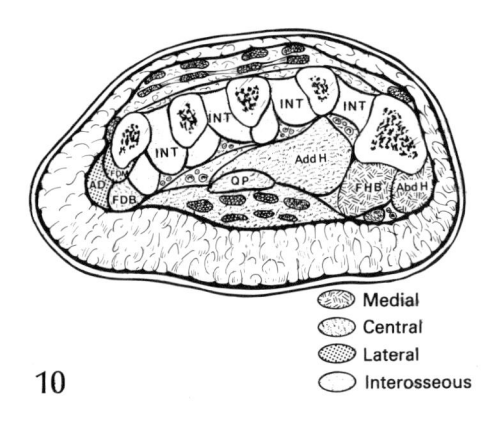

11

In the foot, tissue pressures should be recorded plantarly in the medial, lateral, and central compartments and dorsally in each of the interossei. The needle placements are illustrated.

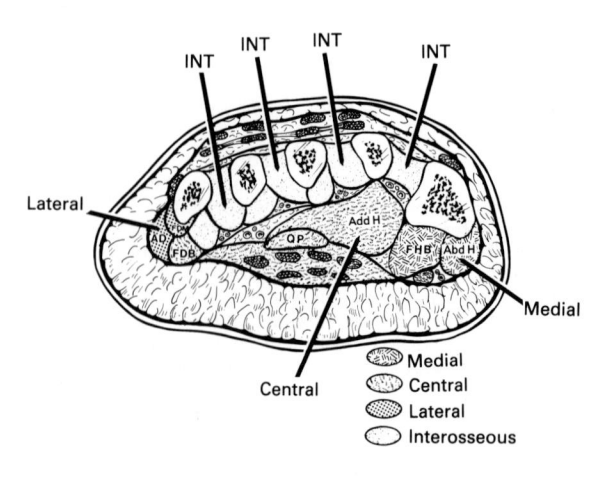

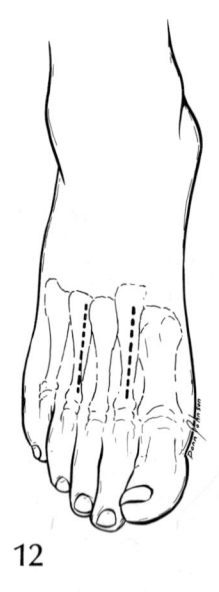

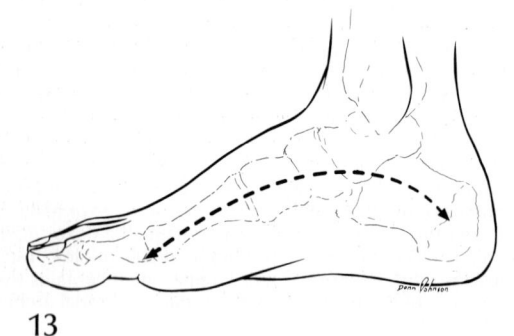

12 & 13

Decompression of the foot may be carried out through three separate incisions: two dorsally with each incision releasing two of the interossei, and a single medial incision utilizing Henry's[30] approach to the plantar structures of the foot.

14

Henry divides the muscles of the foot into four distinct layers. Through a medial incision overlying the first metatarsal and navicular tuberosity, the skin and subcutaneous tissues are divided. The abductor hallucis (Abd H) is then identified and dissected plantarly from the first metatarsal, navicular, and underlying fibres of the flexor hallucis brevis. The knot of Henry is then exposed and incised, taking care to locate the medial and lateral plantar neurovascular bundles. With the release of the knot, the first, second and third layers of the foot may be retracted plantarly sufficiently to trace the paths of the medial and lateral plantar nerves and arteries on the dorsal side of the first layer. With plantar retraction of the third layer, the plantar fascia of the interossei may be visualized and decompressed. We have found that decompression of the interossei may be performed more simply through two dorsal incisions on the foot, allowing for direct visualization and decompression of each of the four muscles.

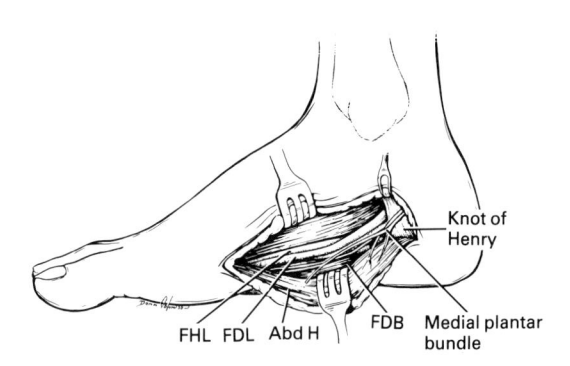

14

THE FOREARM

There are many conditions that produce compartment syndromes of the forearm. A high index of suspicion is warranted after fractures of the radius and ulna, supracondylar fractures of the humerus, and crush and arterial injuries[31].

15

The forearm is divided into three compartments: the dorsal, the volar, and the mobile wad[32]. The mobile wad consists of three muscles: the brachioradialis (B), the extensor carpi radialis longus (ECRL), and the extensor carpi radialis brevis (ECRB). The dorsal compartment contains all those muscles responsible for extension of the wrist and fingers: extensor pollicis brevis (EPB), extensor carpi ulnaris (ECU), extensor digitorum (ED) and extensor digitorum communis (EDC). These muscles are innervated by the posterior interosseous nerve and receive their blood supply from the posterior interosseous artery and perforators from the anterior interosseous artery. The volar compartment constitutes those muscles responsible for flexion and pronation/supination of the wrist, hand, and fingers: flexor pollicis longus (FPL), flexor carpi radialis (FCR), flexor carpi ulnaris (FCU), flexor digitorum superficialis (FDS), flexor digitorum profundus (FDP), and palmaris longus (PL). These muscles are innervated by the median and ulnar nerves and receive their blood supply from the radial, ulnar, and anterior interosseous arteries.

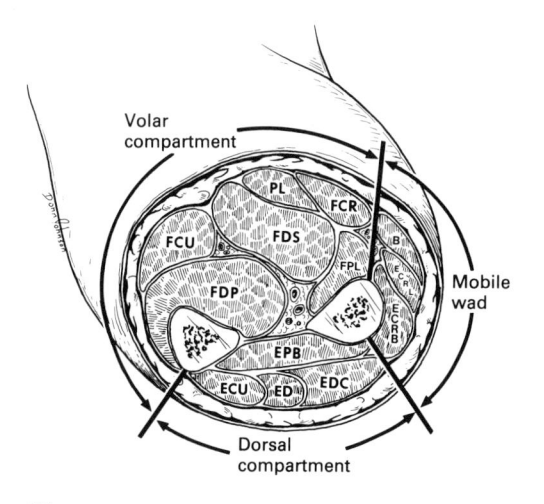

15

In evaluating any patient for a suspected compartment syndrome of the forearm, all three compartments should be measured both preoperatively and intraoperatively should a fasciotomy be necessary. Fasciotomy is carried out utilizing first volar then dorsal incisions on the forearm.

The volar (volar-ulnar) incision begins above the elbow laterally and is extended transversely across the antecubital fossa to the proximal-ulnar forearm. It is then continued distally, staying on the ulnar side of the forearm to the level of the wrist where it is then curved radially across the flexor crease of the wrist and is extended into the palm parallel to the thenar crease. The fascia of the forearm is opened under direct visualization for the full length of the incision, from above the elbow to the mid-palm, and an epimysiotomy is carried out of any enveloped muscles. The lacertus fibrosus is routinely released at the level of the elbow; in cases with median nerve involvement, the nerve should be explored for the full length of the forearm. The pronator teres and flexor digitorum superficialis may need to be released distally to complete decompression of the nerve in certain cases. A carpal tunnel release is routinely done in all cases.

After completion of the volar decompression, tissue pressure measurements should be performed again in all compartments. In some cases tissue pressures in the dorsal compartment and mobile wad will decrease significantly after volar release, making a dorsal fasciotomy unnecessary. In those cases in which pressures remain elevated, a dorsal incision is made in line with the lateral epicondyle of the humerus and the distal radio-ulnar joint. The incision should include at least the proximal two-thirds of the forearm but should not disrupt the extensor retinaculum of the wrist. The underlying dorsal fascia is then incised in line with the skin incision, decompressing the dorsal compartment.

Tissue pressures at this point should again be performed in the dorsal compartment and the mobile wad. Rarely, if decompression has still not been achieved in the mobile wad after the volar and dorsal incisions, and if tissue pressures remain elevated, a third incision parallel to the brachioradalis may be necessary to complete decompression of the forearm.

An alternative approach for decompression of the forearm is McConnell's combined exposure of the median and ulnar nerves as described in Henry's *Extensile exposure*[30]. The advantage of the volar-ulnar approach we have described over this approach is that the flexor tendons and median nerve are left with soft tissue coverage in the distal forearm. Either of the approaches if completed correctly will result in adequate decompression of the affected extremity. In no case should a subcutaneous fasciotomy be performed: without direct visualization of the fascia, superficial nerves and veins will be injured up and down the forearm.

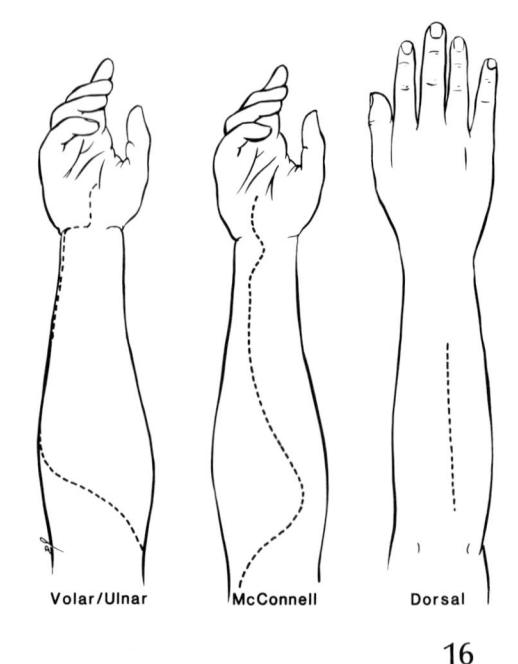

Postoperative management

Postoperatively the arm is immobilized in a bulky non-compressive dressing, with plaster splints to give stability if a fracture has been sustained. Delayed skin closure or split-thickness skin grafting of the forearm should take place at 48–72 hours after decompression has taken place, to provide soft tissue coverage of exposed muscles and tendons.

THE HAND

Compartment syndromes of the hand should be suspected in all patients presenting with documented ischaemia of the forearm. A high index of suspicion for development of the condition is warranted in any patient sustaining a crush, burn, arterial, injection, snake bite, or limb compression injury to the upper extremity[33].

17

Anatomically the hand is divided into four dorsal interosseous compartments (with no interconnections between one compartment and the next), three volar interosseous compartments, the adductor pollicis compartment, the thenar compartment, and the hypothenar compartment[34]. Each of the fingers and the thumb are enveloped in tight investing fascia attached to tough palmar skin and are compartmentalized by this fascia and skin at each of the flexor creases[33].

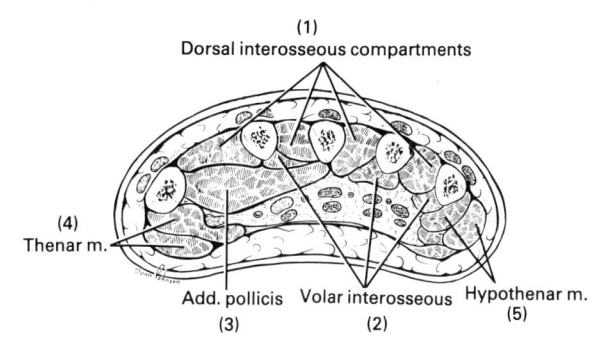

18

Tissue pressure measurements may be easily performed in the thenar and hypothenar compartments but care must be taken to measure pressures in each of the interosseous compartments. Fasciotomy of the hand, if necessary, may be performed through four separate incisions. The dorsal and volar interosseous muscle compartments and the adductor pollicis muscle compartment are released through two dorsal longitudinal incisions overlying the second and fourth metacarpals.

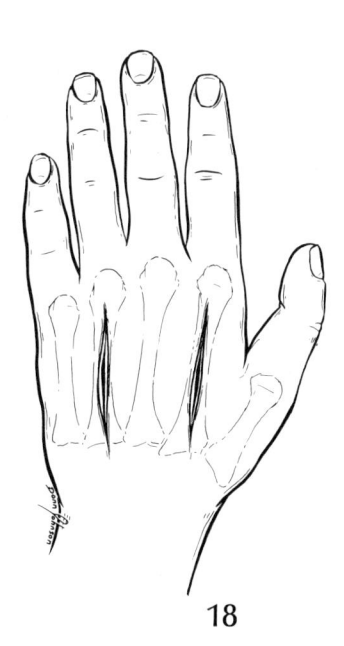

19

After incising the skin, the underlying fascia is opened along both sides of the metacarpals decompressing the dorsal interossei. The first dorsal interosseous muscle should be decompressed by incision radial to the second metacarpal. The first volar interosseous compartment and the adductor pollicis compartment are exposed by deep dissection next to the ulnar side of the second metacarpal. The second and third volar interosseous compartments may be decompressed by deep dissection along the radial sides of the fourth and fifth metacarpals.

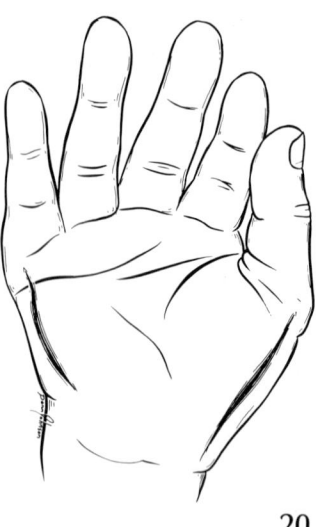

20

The thenar and hypothenar muscle compartments are decompressed through longitudinal incisions parallel to the radial aspect of the first metacarpal and the ulnar aspect of the fifth metacarpal[33].

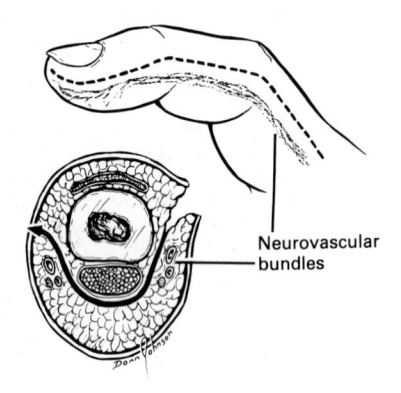

20

21

Excessive swelling in the fingers may cause tissue loss secondary to the tissue's inability to yield with increased interstitial pressure. If swelling is so severe that skin loss is imminent, a decompression of each of the fingers may be carried out utilizing mid-axial incisions. In most patients, depending upon their vocation, decompression should be done on the ulnar sides of the index, middle and ring fingers, and on the radial sides of the little finger and thumb[33].

Postoperative management

Postoperatively the hand is splinted with the forearm, and a bulky dressing is applied while the joints are in a safe position. The wrist should be dorsiflexed, the metacarpophalangeal joints should be in flexion, and the thumb should be placed in palmar abduction. The extremity should be elevated to the level of the heart and postoperative evaluation of neurovascular status continued. Delayed skin closure or split-thickness skin grafting of the hand should be carried out at 48–72 hours to provide soft tissue coverage.

21

Late complications: Volkmann's ischaemic contracture

THE LEG

In the lower extremity Volkmann's contracture has been reported after closed tibial shaft fractures in 1–10 per cent of cases[16,35], but potentially it may occur in any injury resulting in ischaemic damage to the tissues. Clinically affected patients complain of burning pain and anaesthesia of the extremity and may present with ulcerations of the skin and difficulty in walking[2].

How the extremity is affected is dependent upon the compartment involved in the ischaemic event. In those cases involving the deep posterior compartment there are findings ranging from simple clawing of the toes to more extensive deformity with severe injuries, including cavus of the foot, dorsiflexion of the talus, equinus and adduction of the forefoot, and a tendency for varus of the heel. If the posterior tibial nerve is affected, sensory changes will be reflected in an insensitive sole of the foot and plantar aspect of the toes[36].

If the anterior compartment is affected the initial result will be a foot drop, but as contracture of the muscles increases this will diminish. If the deep peroneal nerve is damaged this will result in loss of sensation to the first web space on the dorsum of the foot[25].

Involvement of the superficial posterior compartment results in an equinovarus deformity at the ankle, with contracture of the soleus and gastrocnemius muscles. If the sural nerve is affected, loss of sensation to the lateral side of the foot will result.

Involvement of the lateral compartment results in no apparent clinical deformity but contracture of the peronei[2]. Damage to the superficial peroneal nerve results in loss of sensation to the dorsum of the foot.

Treatment of Volkmann's contracture of the leg is conservative in the acute setting: it relies on splinting or bracing of the leg and foot with daily passive stretching. If foot deformities are present, the patient may require special shoes to allow for greater mobility[37].

If after three months[25] reconstruction is deemed necessary to improve function, surgical exploration will be required. Exploration of the involved compartments is carried out and areas of necrotic or fibrosed muscle are excised as necessary. Tendon lengthenings, if needed, may be performed and neurolysis may be carried out for diagnostic purposes or for release of any extrinsic compression of the nerve. Arthrodeses, tendon transfers, and in some cases amputation may be necessary to improve the functional status of the patient[2,10].

THE UPPER EXTREMITY

Classically, Volkmann's contracture of the forearm results from an ischaemic injury after a supracondylar fracture of the humerus[17,31]. The deep flexor muscles of the forearm are most frequently involved, with the flexor digitorum profundus being the most common and severely affected. As the condition progresses with time, the contractures become more fixed and severe with flexion at the elbow, forearm pronation, wrist flexion, thumb adduction and clawing of the fingers.

Treatment of the condition in the upper extremity depends upon the severity of the contractures, the neurological and functional status of the hand, and the time elapsed from the time of injury. Mild contractures are usually secondary to localized infarcts of the flexor digitorum profundus in patients with normal hand sensation and strength. Early treatment should consist of dynamic and passive splinting to maintain metacarpophalangeal joint flexion, interphalangeal and wrist joint extension and width of the first web space[38]. Late treatment consists of excision of the localized infarct in those cases refractory to conservative measures.

Moderate and severe contractures usually result from involvement of the flexor digitorum profundus, flexor pollicis longus, and often partial involvement of the flexor digitorum superficialis, wrist flexors, and extensors. Treatment initially involves release of any compression of the median, ulnar and radial nerves, followed by release or treatment of the forearm contractures through infarct excision, flexor tendon lengthening, and a flexor-pronator slide when necessary. Tendon transfers for substitution and reinforcement, if available, are delayed till adequate time for nerve recovery has elapsed[39]. In severe cases, proximal row carpectomy, radius and ulna shortening, and wrist or digital joint fusion may be necessary to release or control contractures and to improve function.

References

1. Seddon HJ. Volkmann's contracture: treatment by excision of the infarct. *J Bone Joint Surg [Br]* 1956; 38-B: 152–74.

2. Seddon HJ. Volkmann's ischaemia in the lower limb. *J Bone Joint Surg [Br]* 1966; 48-B: 627–36.

3. Owen R, Tsimboukis B. Ischaemia complicating closed tibial and fibular shaft fractures. *J Bone Joint Surg [Br]* 1967; 49-B: 268–75.

4. Whitesides TE Jr, Harada H, Morimoto K. Compartment syndromes and the role of fasciotomy, its parameters and techniques. *Am Acad Orthop Surg Instr Course Lect* 1977; 26: 179–96.

5. Von Volkmann R. Verletzungen und Krankheiten der Bewegungsorgane. *Handbuch der allgemeinen und speciellen Chirugie* 1882; 2 pt 2 section A: 234–920.

6. Hughes CW. Vascular injuries in the orthopaedic patient. *J Bone Joint Surg [Am]* 1958; 40-A: 1271–80.

7. Kingsley NW, Stein JM, Levenson SM. Measuring tissue pressure to assess the severity of burn-induced ischemia. *Plast Reconstr Surg* 1979; 63: 404–8.

8. Adams JP, Fowler FD. Wringer injuries of the upper extremity; a clinical pathological and experimental study. *South Med J* 1959; 52: 798–804.

9. Hawkins LG, Lischer CG. The main line accidental intra-arterial drug injection. *Clin Orthop* 1973; 94: 268–74.

10. Kikuchi S, Hasue M, Watanabe M. Ischemic contracture in the lower limb, *Clin Orthop* 1978; 134: 185–92.

11. Clement JF, Pietrukso RG. Pit viper snakebite in the United States. *J Fam Pract* 1978; 6: 269–79.

12. Schreiber SN, Liebowitz MR, Bernstein LH. Limb compression and renal impairment (crush injury) following narcotic and sedative overdose. *J Bone Joint Surg [Am]* 1972; 54-A: 1683–92.

13. Detmer DE, Sharpe K, Sufit RL, Girdley FM. Chronic compartment syndrome: diagnosis, management, and outcome. *Am J Sports Med* 1985; 13: 162–70.

14. Chandler JG, Knapp RW. Early definitive treatment of vascular injuries in the Vietnam conflict. *JAMA* 1967; 202: 960–6.

15. Delee JC, Stiehl JB. Open tibia fracture with compartment syndrome. *Clin Orthop* 1981; 160: 175–84.

16. Heckman MM, Whitesides TE, Grewe SR. Spatial relationships of compartment syndromes in lower extremity trauma. *Orthop Trans* 1987; 11: 537.

17. Lipscomb PR, Burleson RJ. Vascular and neural complications in supracondylar fractures of the humerus in children. *J Bone Joint Surg [Am]* 1955; 37-A: 487–92.

18. Whitesides TE Jr, Hanley TC, Morimoto K, Harada H. Tissue pressure measurements as a determinant for the need of fasciotomy. *Clin Orthop* 1975; 113: 43–51.

19. Mubarak SJ, Hargens AR, Owen CA, Garretto LP, Akeson WH. The wick catheter technique for measurement of intramuscular pressure. *J Bone Joint Surg [Am]* 1976; 58-A: 1016–20.

20. Rorabeck CH, Castle, GS, Hardie R, Logan J. Compartmental pressure measurements: an experimental investigation using the slit catheter. *J Trauma* 1981; 21: 446–9.

21. Halpern AA, Nagel DA. Anterior compartment pressures in patients with tibial fractures. *J Trauma* 1980; 20: 786–90.

22. Matsen FA, Winquist RA, Krugmire RB. Diagnosis and management of compartmental syndromes. *J Bone Joint Surg [Am]* 1980; 62-A: 286–91.

23. Nghiem DD, Boland, JP. Four compartment fasciotomy of the lower extremity without fibulectomy: a new approach. *Am Surg* 1980; 46: 414–7.

24. Ernst CB, Kaufer H. Fibulectomy – fasciotomy: an important adjunct in the management of lower extremity arterial trauma. *J Trauma* 1971; 11: 365–80.

25. Mubarak SJ, Hargens AR. *Compartment syndromes and Volkmann's contracture,* Philadelphia: Saunders, 1981.

26. Mubarak SJ, Owen CA. Double incision fasciotomy of the leg for decompression in compartment syndromes. *J Bone Joint Surg [Am]* 1977; 59-A: 184–7.

27. Bate JT. A subcutaneous fasciotome: an instrument for relief of compressions in anterior, lateral, and posterior compartments of the leg from trauma and other causes. *Clin Orthop* 1972; 83: 235–6.

28. Bonutti PM, Bell GR. Compartment syndrome of the foot: a case report. *J Bone Joint Surg [Am]* 1986; 68-A: 1449–51.

29. Jahss MH. *Disorders of the foot.* Philadelphia: Saunders, 1982: 1201.

30. Henry AK. *Extensile exposure,* 2nd ed, New York: Churchill Livingstone, 1973.

31. Eaton RG, Green WT. Volkmann's ischemia – a volar compartment syndrome of the forearm. *Clin Orthop* 1975; 113: 58–64.

32. Gelberman RH, Zakaib GS, Mubarak SJ, Hargens AR, Akeson WH. Decompression of forearm compartment syndromes. *Clin Orthop* 1978; 134: 225–9.

33. Rowland SA. Fasciotomy. In: Green DP, ed. *Operative hand surgery*. New York: Churchill Livingstone, 1982: 565–81.

34. Halpern AA, Mochizuki RM. Compartment syndrome of the interosseous muscles of the hand: a clinical and anatomic review. *Orthop Rev* 1980; 9 (3): 121–127.

35. Ellis H. Disabilities after tibial shaft fractures with special reference to Volkmann's ischaemic contracture. *J Bone Joint Surg [Br]* 1958; 40-B: 190–7.

36. Matsen FA, Clawson DK. The deep posterior compartmental syndrome of the leg. *J Bone Joint Surg [Am]* 1975; 57-A: 34–9.

37. Von Volkmann R. Die ischaemischen Muskellamungen and Kontraktunen. *Zentralbl Chir* 1881; 81: 801–3.

38. Goldner JL. In: Flynn JE, ed. *Hand surgery*. Baltimore: Williams and Wilkins, 1975.

39. Zancolli E. Tendon transfers after ischemic contracture of the forearm: classification in relation to intrinsic muscle disorders. *Am J Surg* 1965; 109: 356–60.

40. Heppenstall RB, Sapega AA, Scott R, et al. The compartment syndrome: an experimental and clinical study of muscular energy metabolism using phosphorus nuclear magnetic resonance spectroscopy. *Clin Orthop* 1988; 226: 138–55.

Illustrations by F. Price

Fractures and dislocations in the foot

P. S. London *MBE*, FRCS, MFOM, FACEM(Hon)
Formerly Surgeon, Birmingham Accident Hospital, Birmingham, UK

Introduction

In practice three main groups of injuries require prompt operation: (1) fractures and dislocations of the talus and calcaneum; (2) disruptive injuries of the tarsometatarsal region; and (3) crush injuries of the toes.

In general, it may be proposed that, as far as it is possible to do so, the uninjured joints of an injured foot should be kept in motion from the beginning. If this is accepted, it follows that external splintage should be avoided whenever internal fixation can be carried out. A further proposition is that if a foot is to be stiffened by the effects of injury it should be as nearly as possible of normal shape. If, on the other hand, deformity is inevitable it is particularly important to preserve as much movement as possible.

Surgical approaches in the foot

1, 2 & 3

A useful general purpose incision follows a line from in front of the lateral malleolus to the cleft between the first two toes.

It can, if necessary, be extended upwards to give access to the ankle (*see* Emergency operations on the ankle, *Accident Surgery*, page 645, incision 1 in *Illustration 1*). It allows thorough decompression of the dorsum of the foot and, if there has been disruption in the metatarsus, it permits the plantar haematoma to be removed. It allows both the medial and lateral sides of the foot to be seen and although it may not provide enough room for Kirschner wires to be inserted through the incision, there is no objection to driving these through the skin while they are directed by eye through the appropriate bones and joints. The extensors of the toes can be retracted *en masse* or separately in either direction and there is no objection to dividing one or both extensor retinacula in order to displace the long tendons more effectually.

In other cases, shorter incisions over one or two injured joints will suffice, but it may then be necessary to confirm with radiographs that the parts have been correctly restored. Such incisions should generally be longitudinal.

Other incisions for special purposes will be described in the relevant sections.

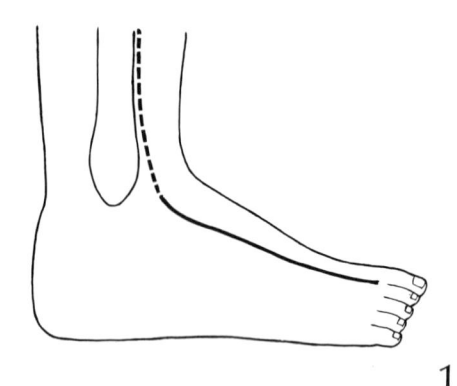

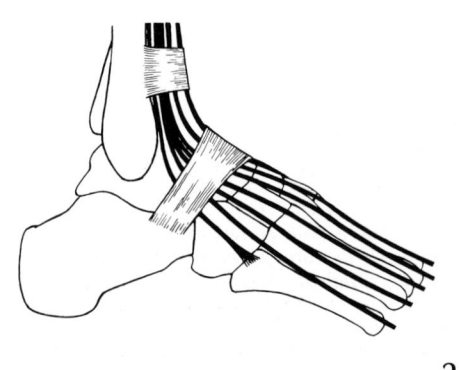

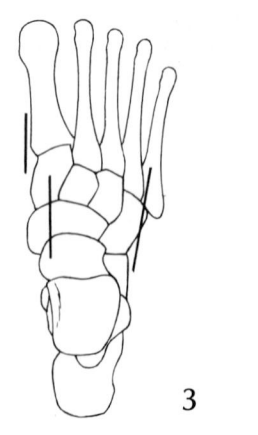

INJURIES OF THE TALUS

FRACTURE OF THE NECK OF THE TALUS

4, 5 & 6

If there is more than a crack through the neck or the body of the bone, it is preferable to fix it with a Kirschner wire rather than putting the foot in plaster.

If fluoroscopy is not available it is easiest to expose the bone and see where to insert the wires. There is in many cases no need to remove the wires and so, for the sake of comfort and convenience, their ends should be within the skin. There are two simple ways of doing this. One is to measure the length of wire required and mark this with a notch made by rotating the wire within the lightly closed jaws of a wire cutter. The wire is inserted at the chosen place, driven in until the notch is level with the bone and then snapped off. Alternatively, an unnotched wire can be driven in nearly as far as is necessary, cut off flush with the skin and then driven home by means of a punch with a slightly cupped end that is fine enough to follow the wire through the skin.

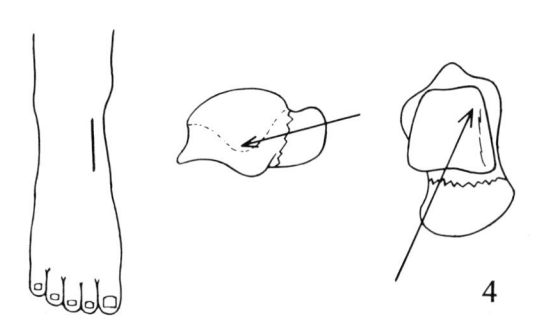

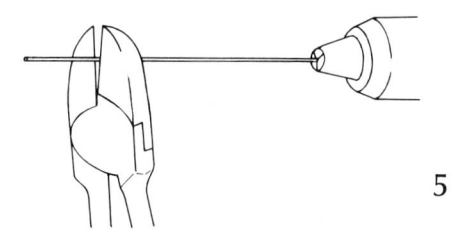

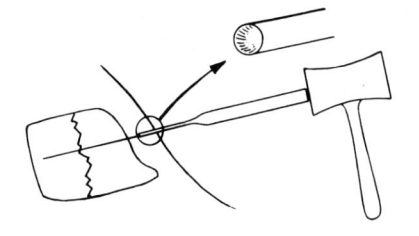

312 Lower limb fractures

FRACTURE-DISLOCATION OF THE TALUS

7 & 8

The experienced eye can usually identify the main features of a confusing jumble of shadows in the X-ray appearances of this injury, in which the body of the bone is expelled from its normal resting place along a curved and twisting course to the inner side of the heel, where it lies under tightly stretched skin that needs early relief from pressure. Although it may be possible to replace the displaced bone by pulling the heel downwards (by skeletal traction if necessary) so as to open the tibiocalcanean gap and then pushing the body upwards, forwards and inwards, it is undesirable to persist in such efforts and the further damage that they may inflict upon the skin that is already, and literally, hard-pressed. (Note that the wire through the heel is fairly far back.)

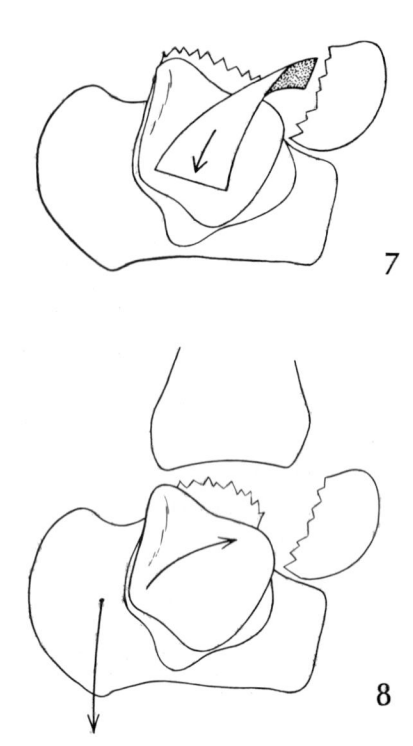

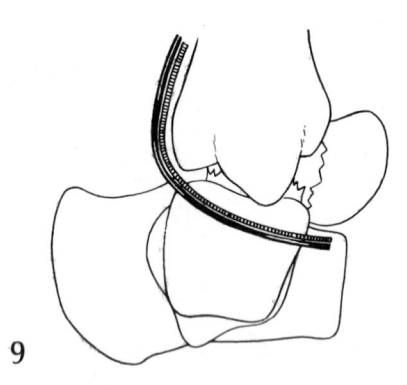

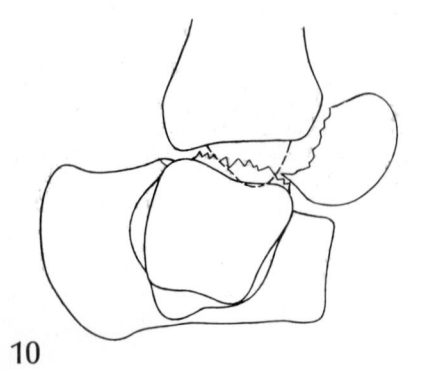

9 & 10

If closed manipulation fails the bone should be exposed by a gently curved cut across the prominence it causes, but this must be done with great care because the posterior tibial nerve and vessels lie between the much thinned skin and the bone immediately beneath it. A bone hook, rather than a Kirschner wire through the bone, can be used to pull the calcaneum away from the tibia and it may then be quite easy to push the displaced body into place. This may, however, be prevented by tendons or capsule and sometimes by a spike of bone that sticks up from the neck. Although the medial malleolus may hide this cause of obstruction, if the soft tissues are carefully retracted it can be seen and the spike can then be tilted downwards and out of the way. It should be mentioned that it is rarely necessary to divide any soft tissues other than the skin; retraction is usually possible and effective in the absence of the bony obstruction just described. Once the body has been accurately replaced it should be fixed to the head by one or two Kirschner wires.

Fractures and dislocations in the foot 313

TOTAL DISLOCATION OF THE TALUS

11 & 12

This is the result of violent inversion of the foot that causes the talus to be thrust right out of its socket to lie on the outer side of the foot, with its upper surface tightly stretching the skin below the lateral malleolus. In some cases the skin splits so that the bone falls out and may be lost.

If the talus can be returned to its socket without having to cut the skin, it is probably wise to do so in order to avoid adding surgically to the damage that the skin has already suffered, but it must be understood that the bone has no blood supply and that there is in consequence a strong likelihood that it will have to be operated on later.

If, on the other hand, the skin has already given way, the bone should not be replaced and if conditions are favourable primary tibiocalcanean fusion can be carried out by cutting the bones to fit in a position of 10° or so of equinus and then clamping or screwing them together. Note that the navicular bone should stand clear of the tibia. With the heel of the shoe raised 1 cm or so this operation gives a useful foot and the generous trimming of crushed and torn skin allowed by the loss of bone favours uneventful healing of the wound.

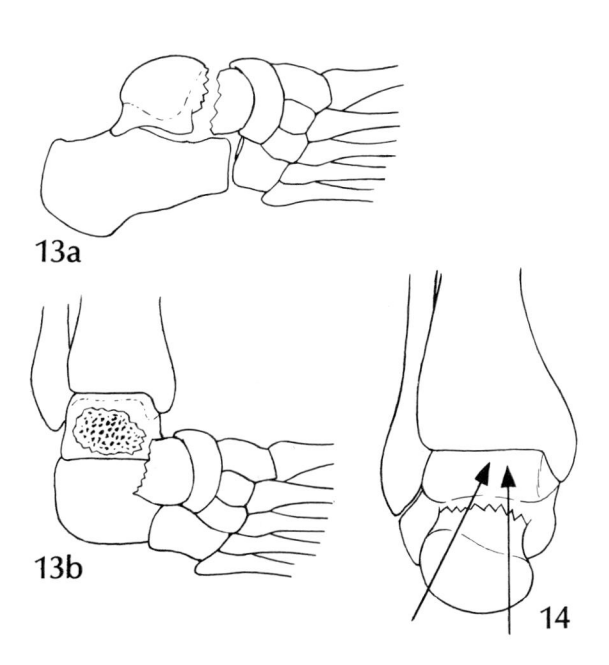

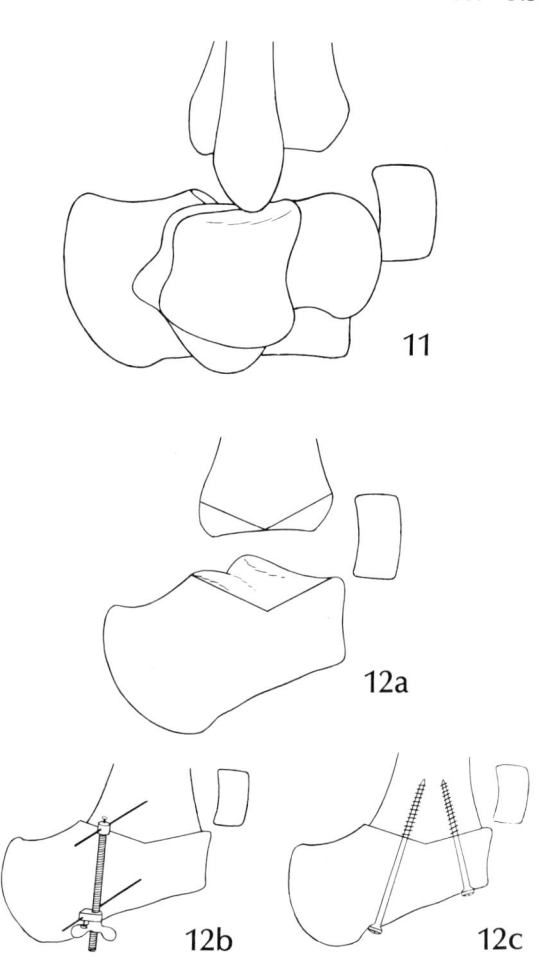

INVERSION FRACTURE OF THE TALUS

13 & 14

As well as the injuries that have already been described, fracture of the talus can occur as a result of supination or inversion, with the sharp, broken edge of the body of the talus blanching the skin in front of the ankle. The deformity is often easily corrected but it is best maintained by one or two Kirschner wires.

314   Lower limb fractures

FRACTURE OF THE LATERAL PROCESS OF THE TALUS

15 & 16

This injury is included not because it constitutes an emergency or because it occurs frequently but because it is often unrecognized and can give rise to disability that could have been prevented by timely operation. The patient is thought to have sprained the ankle and X-ray examination may support that diagnosis. Even if the films are examined with particular care the fracture may not be recognized in the ordinary anteroposterior and lateral views. The condition should be suspected when there is acute tenderness just below the tip of the lateral malleolus with an effusion into the ankle joint. The fracture is most easily seen in an anteroposterior view made with the foot at a right angle to the leg and rotated medially by 10°–20°.

Large fragments should be fixed in place with a Kirschner wire and if the fracture is comminuted the fragments should be removed and the soft tissues repaired snugly.

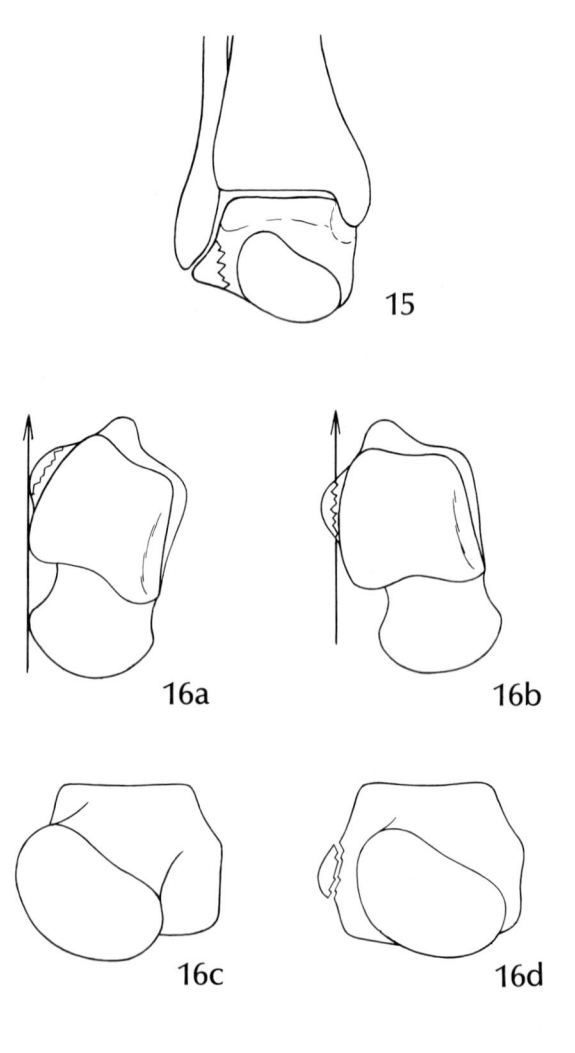

INJURIES OF THE CALCANEUM

Fractures for which early operation may be advantageous are the posterior avulsion ('beak') fractures and the crush fractures that affect particularly the posterior part of the talocalcanean joint.

BEAK FRACTURES

17 & 18

Although the smooth surface for a bursa extends quite a long way down the back of the calcaneum these are in fact avulsion fractures and the principal reason for operating on them promptly is that the sharp edge of the displaced fragment is liable to blanch the skin over it.

The incision should be vertical and on the medial side of the tendo Achillis so as to avoid the pressure that is applied by a shoe to the lateral side of the heel. A coarsely threaded screw passed downwards has the advantage over a staple in that it is not liable to come out.

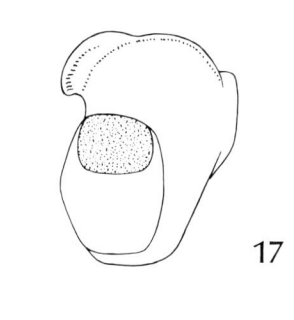

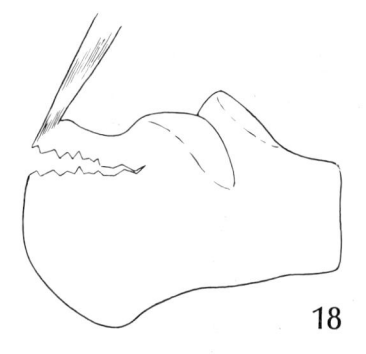

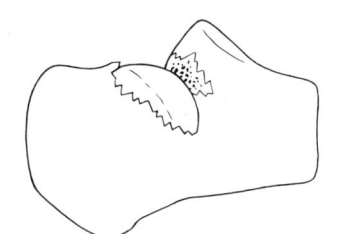

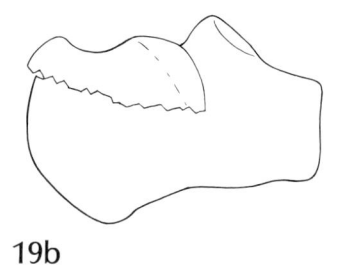

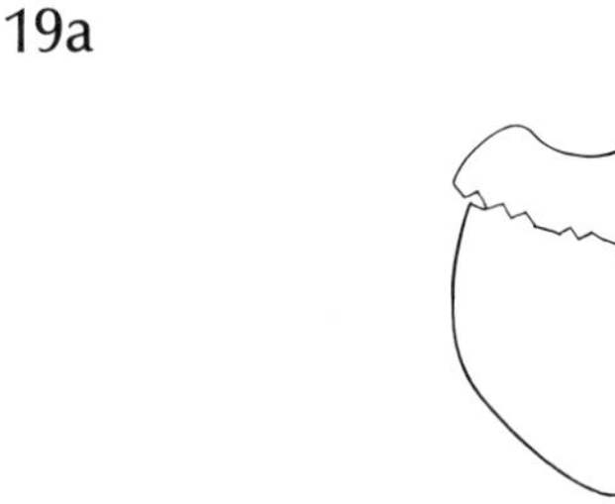

CRUSH FRACTURES

There is still much argument about the best way to treat these fractures. It is a matter of common experience that a useful foot with no more than tolerable discomfort can coexist with severe deformation of the heel. Success depends upon immediate, determined and continuing efforts to reduce swelling and to restore movement. On the other hand, there is marked deformation of the shoe and there may be discomfort caused by pressure between the lateral malleolus and the outward bulge of the subjacent calcaneum. Each surgeon must decide for himself whether to operate on these fractures and, if so, by what method.

19a & b

The fractures fall into two groups, according to whether or not the fragment carrying the posterior articular facet for the talus has a backward extension to the tendo Achillis.

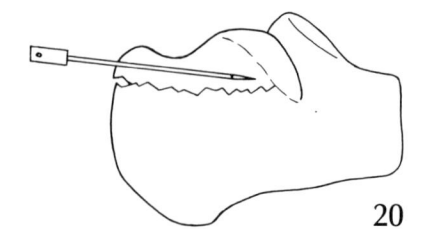

Correction of deformity by indirect methods

20–23

If there is a backward extension, this can be used as a handle for the articular surface by driving a spike into it from behind. With the patient prone, the flexed knee is raised from the table by one hand under the spike and the other placed as close to the front of the ankle as possible. The weight of the limb causes the fragment to return to its correct position and by removing it from the body of the bone it makes it possible to correct the broadening of the heel that is an essential part of the injury. This can be done quite easily by squeezing the heel firmly between two hands; it is not necessary to use a powerful clamp. The corrected position is maintained by a plaster cast that includes the spike but leaves both the ankle and the talocalcanean joints free to be exercised.

This method can be very successful in restoring the shape of the foot and maintaining some movement at the talocalcanean joint in persons under 50 years of age but more or less displacement can recur and there is the risk of infection.

Direct methods of correcting deformity

These methods have to be used when the depressed articular facet has no backward extension and they can be used when it has.

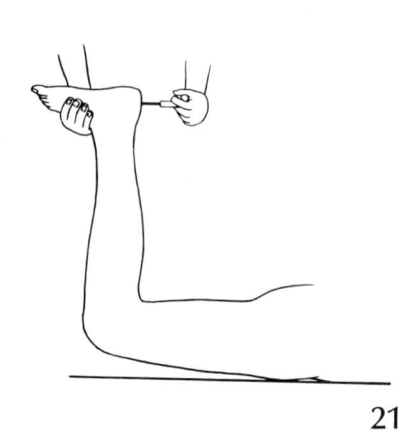

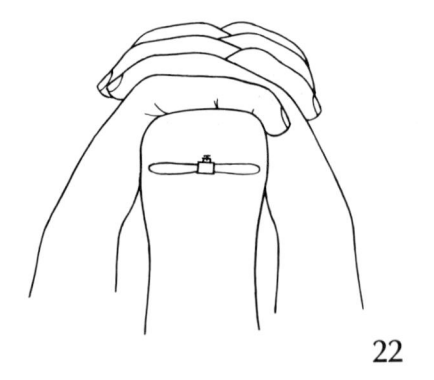

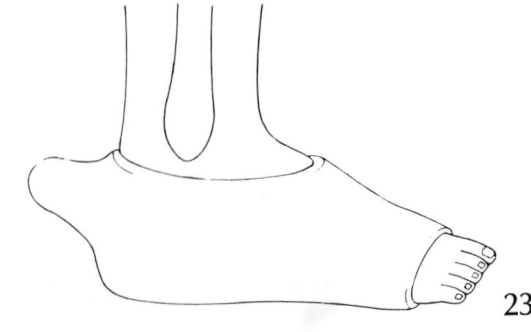

Lateral approach

24, 25 & 26

The skin is cut just below the lateral malleolus; it should expose the calcaneofibular ligament but it should not be necessary to divide it. The peroneal tendons may be pulled downwards if necessary.

The depressed facet is partly buried in the body of the bone and while it remains there it maintains the outward bulge. It is put back in place by levering up its anterolateral edge, which causes it to swing and twist up to fit accurately against the talus. The broadening of the heel can then be corrected easily by hand.

The depressed fragment can be propped up by a strong spike driven up from behind and below or by Kirschner wires that fix it to the talus. Transfixing the talocalcanean joint adds negligibly to the damage that has already been done. Once the depressed fragment has been fixed in place the other fragments may not require any fixation, but there need be no hesitation about using other wires, screws or staples to prevent them from displacing. Although bone grafts have been recommended for the purpose of filling the gap caused by crushing of cancellous bone they are not essential.

If a strong spike is used a plaster slipper should be applied but it is convenient rather than necessary if Kirschner wires have been used, with or without supplementary fixation. The wires transfixing the talocalcanean joint can be removed after 4–6 weeks.

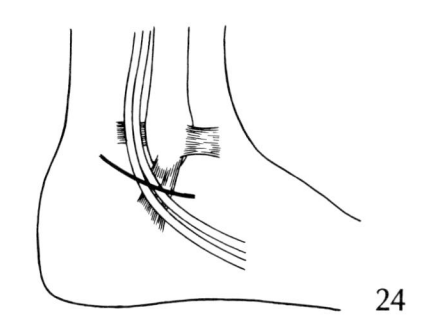

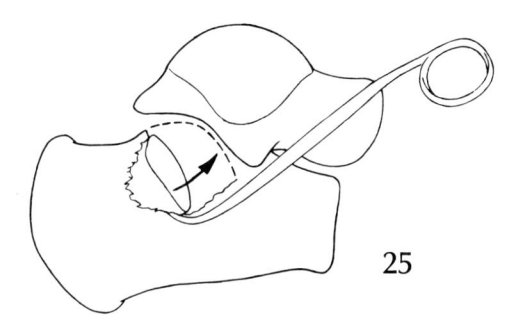

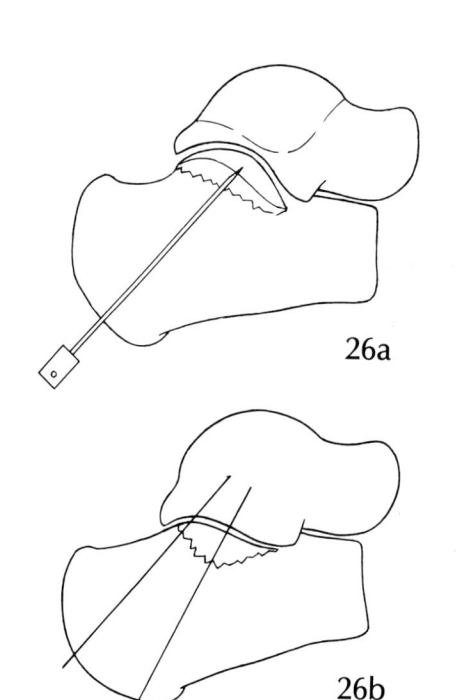

318　Lower limb fractures

Removing the calcaneum

27 & 28

This is a successful way of dealing with a fracture that is too comminuted for internal fixation and particularly if the fracture is also open. The patient should be prone and the heel is opened by a straight, longitudinal ('cloven hoof') incision after which the bone should be removed piecemeal from the surrounding soft tissues. The tendo Achillis should be stitched to the plantar fascia, with the foot in 20° or 30° of equinus. It is advisable to use suction drainage. The deformity is less than might be supposed and the patient walks with a normal heel-and-toe gait, though lacking spring. It is advisable to pad the heel of the shoe.

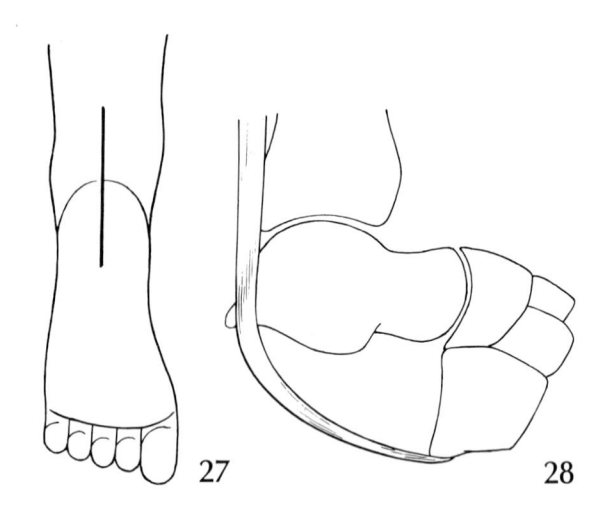

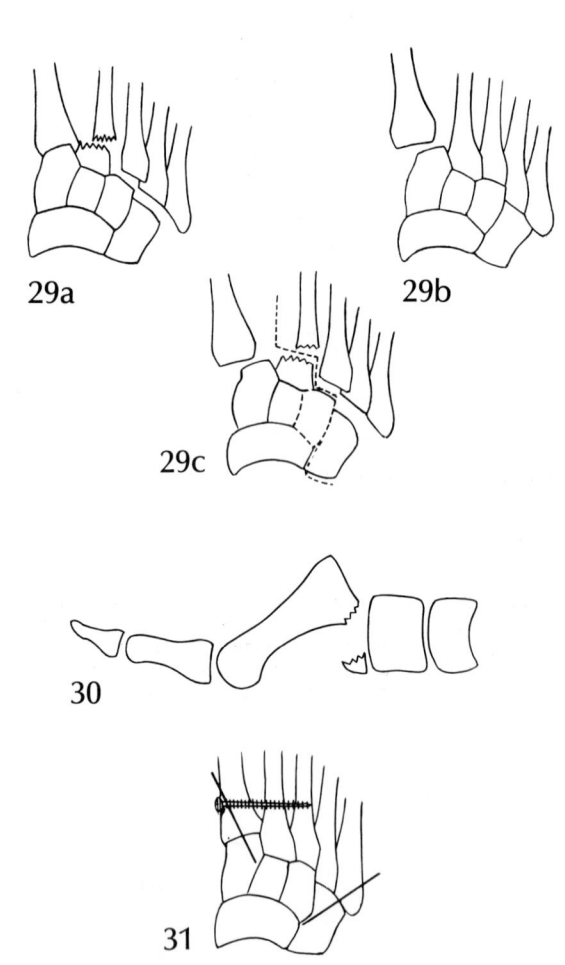

MAJOR DISRUPTIVE LESIONS OF THE FOOT

Although the X-ray appearances may be very confusing, these injuries fall into a few fairly well-defined patterns, albeit with variations in detail. The first requirement is to recognize that serious injury has occurred – failure of diagnosis is not all that rare. It is necessary to understand these patterns in order to treat the injuries successfully, which in most cases is best done by internal fixation. If fluoroscopy is available it may not be necessary to open some of these injuries but there need be no hesitation to open the foot for reasons that have already been stated.

TARSOMETATARSAL DISRUPTION

29, 30 & 31

The four, or fewer, lateral metatarsals may be displaced laterally and the first may be displaced medially either as a separate injury or in combination with the foregoing. The lateral line of disruption often follows the line of tarsometatarsal joints but it may follow an irregular course through the tarsus.

Occasionally, there is an isolated dorsal fracture-dislocation of the base of the first metatarsal bone, which is accompanied by hyperextension of the metatarso-phalangeal joint.

Fixation can usually be achieved with the aid of Kirschner wires and sometimes by screws, which it is not always necessary to remove.

Fractures and dislocations in the foot 319

DISRUPTION OF THE TARSUS

Talonavicular fracture-subluxation

32 & 33

This injury occurs when the forepart of the foot is swung inwards with simultaneous longitudinal compression. It is usually sufficient to transfix the talonavicular joint with a wire or a screw but if there are also fractures of metatarsals it may be advisable to fix them as well.

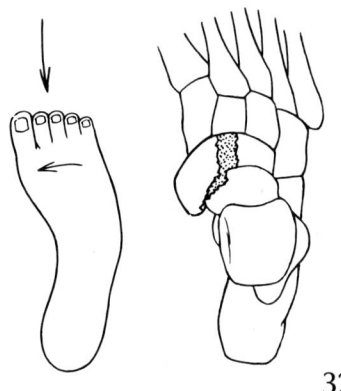

32

33

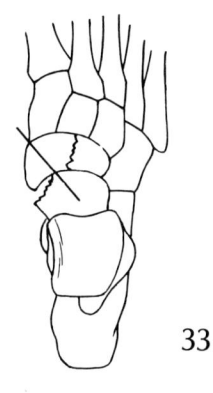

Talonavicular dislocation

34

Violent pronation may displace the navicular bone towards the sole. It is not usually necessary to operate on this injury but sometimes correction of the deformity is prevented by soft tissues – the figure shows how the tendon of tibialis anterior may act in this way.

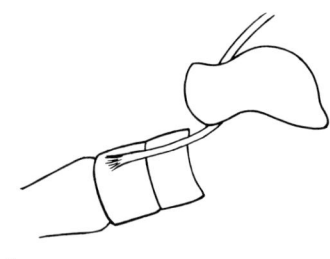

34

CRUSH INJURIES OF THE TOES

SUBUNGUAL HAEMATOMA

35

The pain can be alleviated by perforating the nail with a red-hot paper clip.
  The operation is painless. A dressing should be worn until the haematoma is dry.

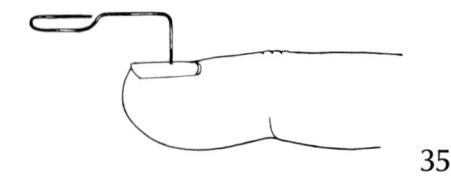

OPEN FRACTURES

Careful toilet and closure will often be followed by healing by first intention but too often the toes are treated much more casually than the fingers and the results are consequently poor. An advantage with injured toes is that there need be less reluctance to sacrifice parts of them than parts of fingers in order to be sure of prompt healing.

36a & b

For the sake of comfort in shoes, it may be desirable to fix fractures of toes and metatarsals so that they will heal in good position. Kirschner wires are particularly useful for this purpose and can safely be driven across joints. Whenever possible, wires should first be driven distally from fractures (a) because this is so much easier than trying to drive them proximally from the tip of a toe (b).
  Wires that are going to have to stay in place for several weeks should, whenever possible, not be left sticking out through the skin to provide portals of bacterial entry.

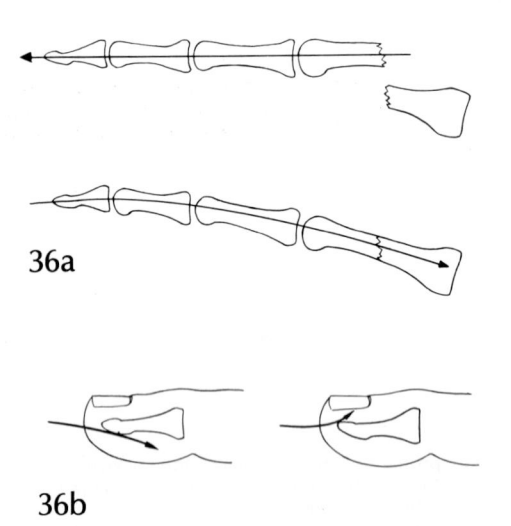

y Peter Cox after F. Price

Display, correction and fixation of stove-in hip joints

E. Letournel MD
Professor of Orthopaedic Surgery and Traumatology, Centre Medico-Chirurgical de la Porte de Choisy, Paris, France

Introduction

A stove-in hip is associated with different types of acetabular fracture.

To give the hip its original appearance and arrangement, the central dislocation of the head has first to be corrected and then to be prevented by reconstructing the acetabulum. Restoring perfect articular congruency and stability gives the patient the best chance of avoiding post-traumatic osteoarthritis.

322 Pelvis and acetabulum

Preoperative

1a, b & c

In order to gain a clear understanding of the fracture lines disrupting the iliac bone, four radiographic views are essential:

1. The anteroposterior view of the whole pelvis in case there are fractures on both sides.
2. The standard anteroposterior radiograph of the injured hip.
3. The obturator oblique view, with the patient supine but rolled 45° away from the side of the injury.
4. The iliac wing oblique view with the patient supine but rolled 45° towards the affected site.

The typical landmarks are studied carefully in each view.
A CT scan is advisable. This must involve the whole height of the pelvis and the cuts of the scan should be a maximum of 5 mm thick at the level of the joint. The scan should never be read alone, but conjointly with the standard views.

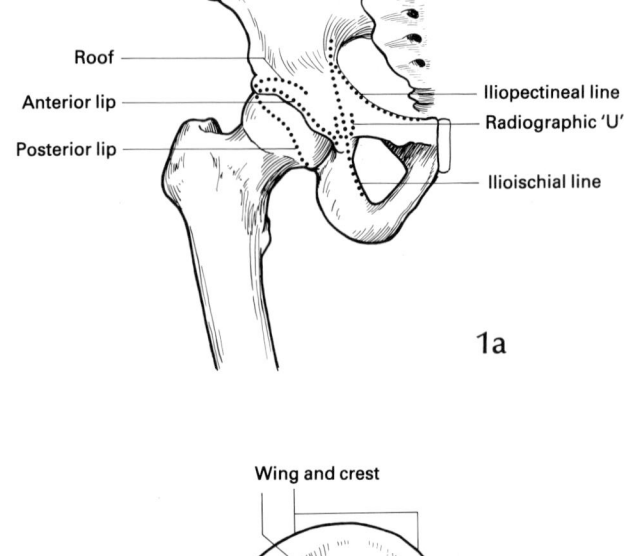

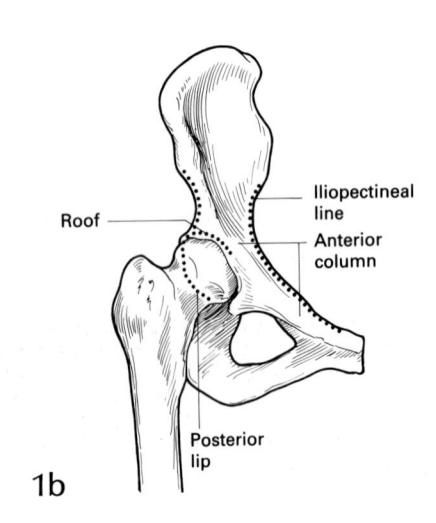

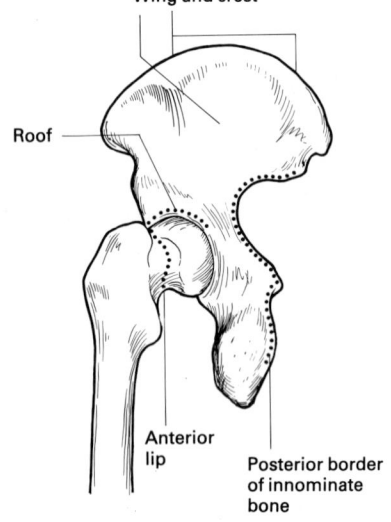

Indications

All displaced fractures of the innominate bone resulting in a stove-in hip should be treated surgically. This applies whether the incongruity is shown by three, two or only one radiographic view and confirmed by the CT scan. Even if the head can be reduced under a remaining part of the roof, surgical fixation offers the only possibility of restoring complete articular congruency.

One exception can be made. In some of the most complex fractures, the different parts of the articular crescent are shown, by all three radiographic views and the CT, to be congruent with the centrally displaced head. In these cases bed rest and active exercises may lead to a good result, but the hip is never perfect and it remains centrally displaced. Thus, if there is no contraindication, operation is advised in order to restore a congruent hip to its normal place. The choice must depend on the surgeon, who must be confident of restoring an accurately fitting and correctly placed hip.

Time of operation

Operation for stove-in hip joint is never an emergency, and the operation is perhaps easier when performed after 3–6 days when bleeding from pelvic veins disrupted at the time of injury has stopped.

Approach

This depends on the type of acetabular fracture associated with the stove-in hip.

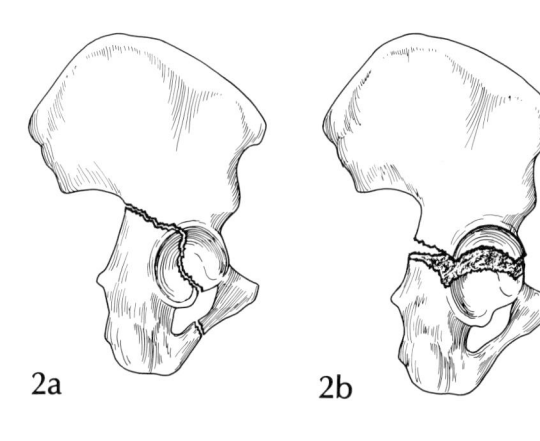

2a, b, c & d

1. If the centrally dislocated head is associated with (a) a posterior column fracture, (b) a transverse fracture not involving the roof; or (c) a T-shaped fracture; or (d) an associated transverse and posterior fracture of which the transverse fracture component spares the roof, good access is gained through a posterior or Kocher–Langenbeck type of incision.

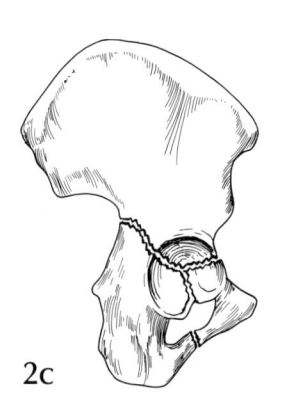

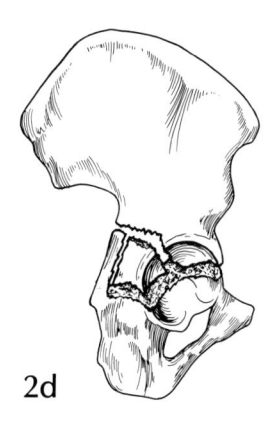

3a, b & c

2. If the associated fracture is either (a) an anterior wall; or (b) an anterior column fracture; or (c) a combination of anterior and transverse fractures, the ilioinguinal anterior approach has to be used.

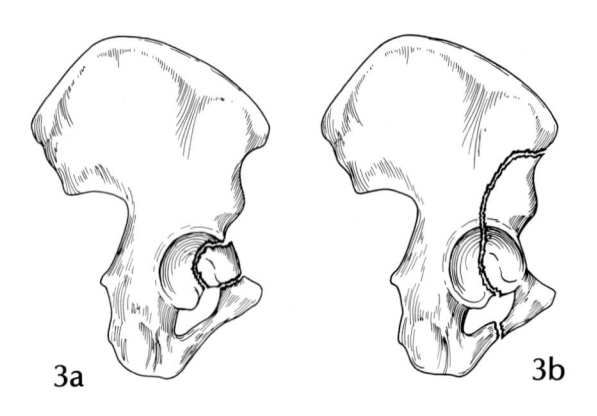

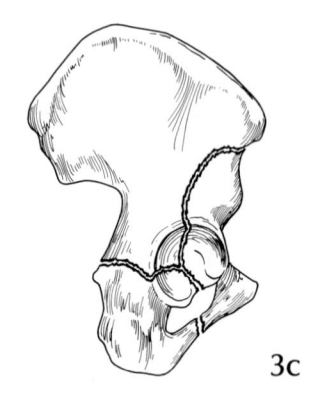

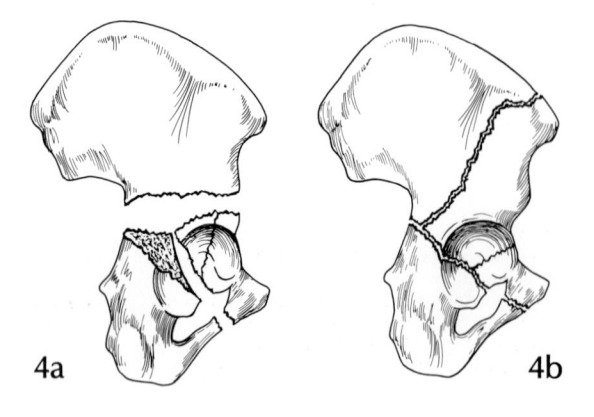

3a

3b

3c

4a & b

3. If the fracture affects the whole of both columns, the whole articular crescent of the acetabulum is detached in several pieces, so that only the back part of the ilium remains connected to the sacrum.

   A posterior approach may be used if the uppermost fracture line extends to the anterior edge of the iliac bone (a). Nevertheless we now feel it is much more convenient to use the extended lateral approach.

   When, as most frequently happens, the uppermost fracture line reaches the iliac crest (b), we choose the ilioinguinal incision in most cases, provided the posterior column fragment is in one piece (although a small additional posterior wall fragment may be neglected), and provided the case is operated within 15 days from the time of injury.

   The extended iliofemoral incision is preferred if the posterior column is detached in several pieces, if the sacroiliac joint is involved, or if the case is operated more than 15 days from the time of injury.

4a

4b

5a, b & c

4. In case of transverse fractures (*a*), T-shaped fractures (*b*), or associated transverse and posterior wall fractures (*c*), where the transverse fracture passes through the roof (transtectal types), the extended iliofemoral approach is advisable to get a complete and perfect control of the whole transverse fracture.

When opting to use the Kocher–Langenbeck or ilio-inguinal approaches, which lead respectively and more electively to the posterior and to the anterior column, one can never be sure of being able to perform the complete reconstruction of a complex case. A subsequent approach may be necessary and it is preferable to perform it during the same operation.

Anaesthesia

Any form of general anaesthesia can be used, but good relaxation is particularly useful during an anterior approach.

Equipment

Screws

Cortical screws from 20–120 mm long are necessary; 3.5 mm diameter screws are the best to fix the plates to the innominate bone and the author prefers the self-tapping ones.

Cortical screws of 4.5 mm diameter, spongiosa screws, and 6.5 mm fully or partially threaded screws are inserted between the two tables of the iliac wing or along the axis of the columns of the acetabulum.

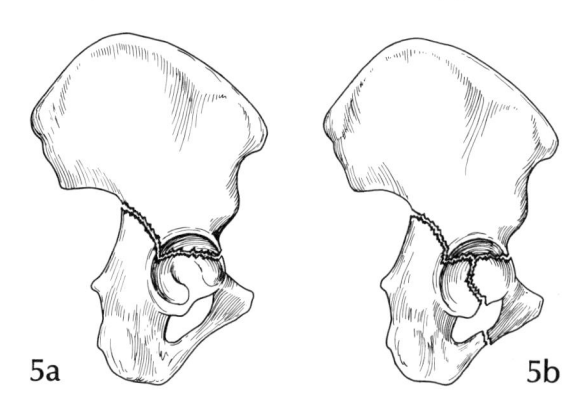

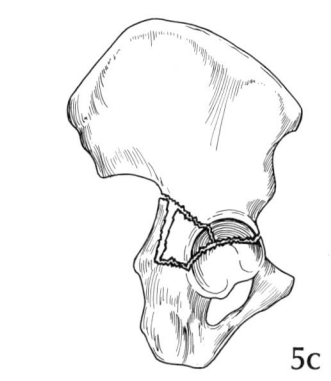

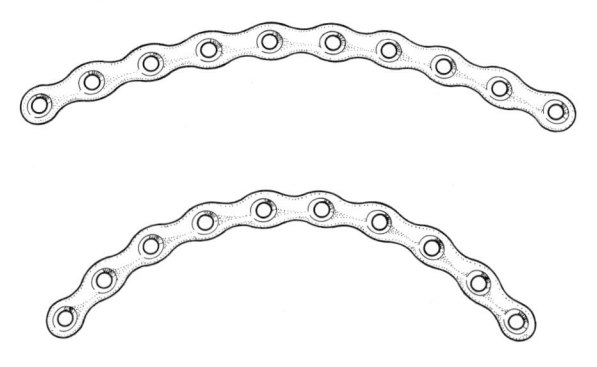

Plates

6

Straight Sherman-type plates with equidistant holes, either in vitallium or stainless steel, or AO reconstruction plates (3.5 or 4.5 mm) are adequate.

Letournel's curved acetabular plates with 6–12 holes are available in stainless steel or vitallium and their holes accept 3.5 or 4.5 mm screws. The 3.5 mm screws, where the heads lie flush with the plate, are preferred.

326 Pelvis and acetabulum

Operation

POSTERIOR APPROACH

The position of the patient, the equipment and the Kocher–Langenbeck approach are described in the chapter on 'Replacement and fixation of the posterior lip of the acetabulum' (*see* pp. 339–345).

The fracture lines divide the posterior column and the hip's capsule is more or less torn, giving access to the inside of the joint. This access may be improved by a capsulotomy along either the posterior wall or the lateral lip of the roof, depending on the existing damage. The joint is cleared of clots and loose fragments, so that the intra-articular track of the fracture lines can be identified.

Reduction and fixation

Principles

The centrally dislocated head of femur is extracted with the aid of traction allowed by the orthopaedic table and supplemented by a large hook placed around the femur just under its neck.

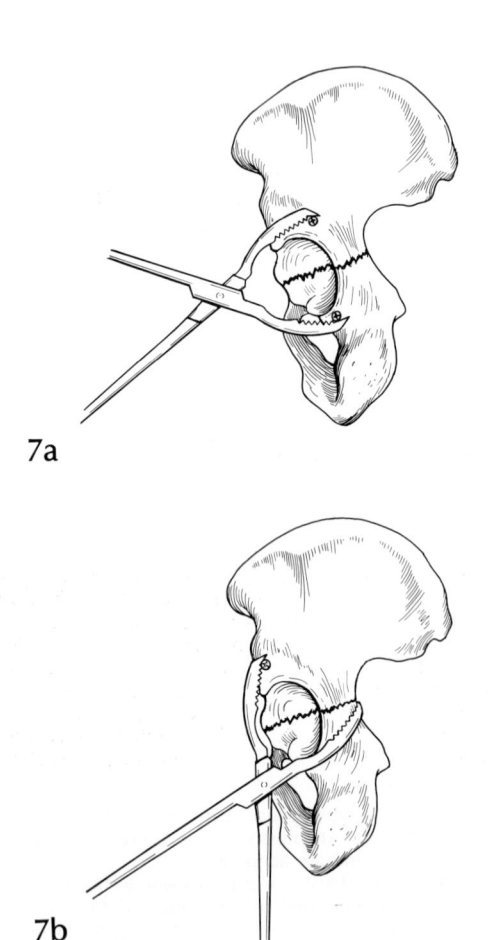

7a

7b

7a & b

The fractured bones are then restored to the correct position by direct manipulation, taking care to disturb their soft tissue attachments as little as possible. Repositioning is sometimes difficult to achieve or to maintain and it may be advisable to use forceps to grip one or two temporary screws, which must be inserted away from the intended site of the plate.

The procedure subsequently adopted depends on whether or not part of the roof of the acetabulum remains intact and undisplaced.

8

If part of the roof remains undisturbed under the blade of the ilium, the head is replaced under it, taking care to get a perfect fit. The head is kept in place by traction or in some cases by temporary transfixion.

The means of reduction and fixation of the fragments depend on the type of fracture.

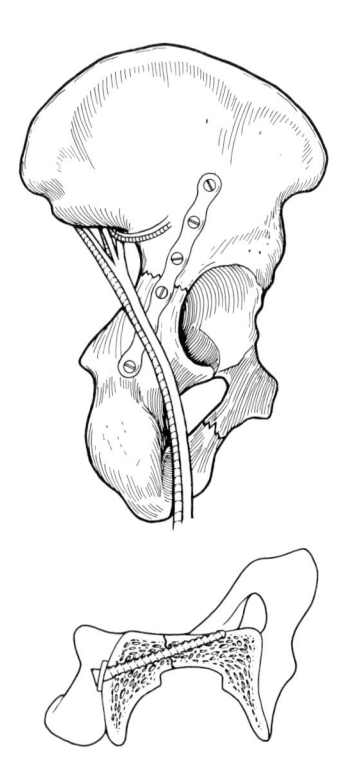

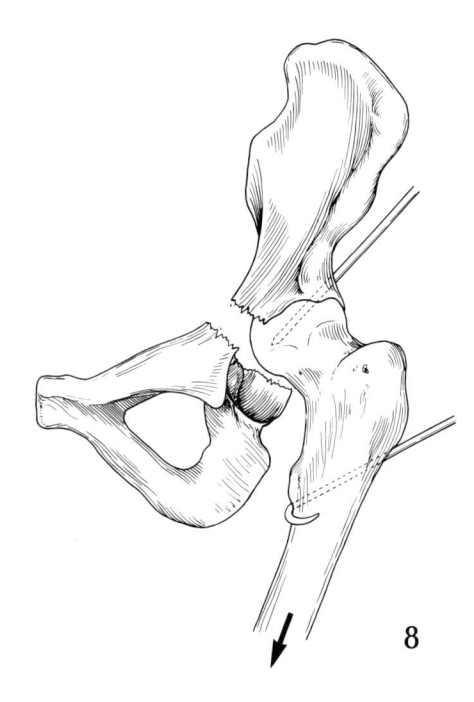

Posterior column fracture

9

The large fragment is manipulated by forceps with one jaw inside the greater sciatic notch, the other taking hold of the outer aspect of the ilium or on a temporary screw. A plate is shaped so as to lie perfectly on the posterior aspect of the column from the upper pole of the ischial tuberosity up to the blade of the ilium, with at least three screws above the fracture line. One must be careful to avoid leaving the column twisted out of line; this is done by control exercised from inside the pelvis, working through the greater sciatic notch.

Infratectal or juxtatectal transverse fractures

10a & b

The inferior part of the innominate bone is manipulated and plated as above, but there is often difficulty in dealing with the anterior part of the fracture at the level of the iliopectineal line. A finger introduced through the greater sciatic notch controls the manipulation, which can be further aided either by pushing the ischial tuberosity inwards or by inserting a femoral head extractor into it to act as a temporary handle. A 10–12 cm screw may be driven across the fracture line to reach the superior aspect of the iliopectineal line; it is parallel to the quadrilateral surface and its insertion is guided by a finger applied along the quadrilateral surface through the greater sciatic notch.

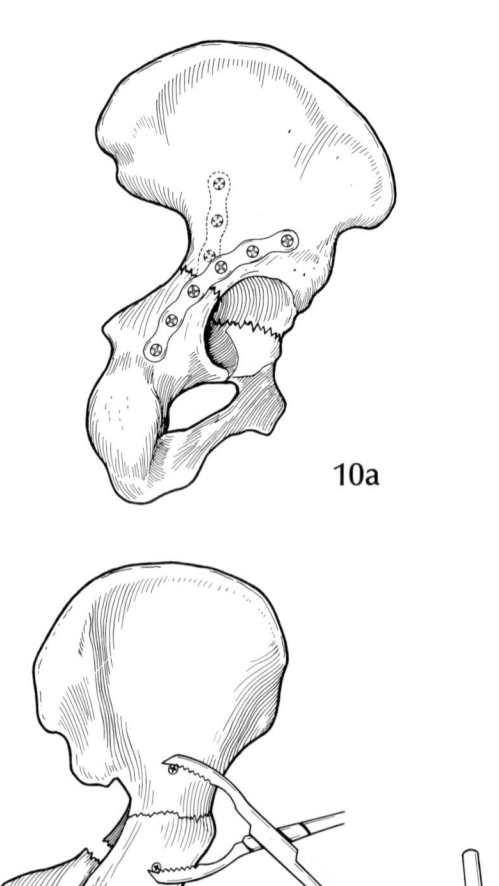

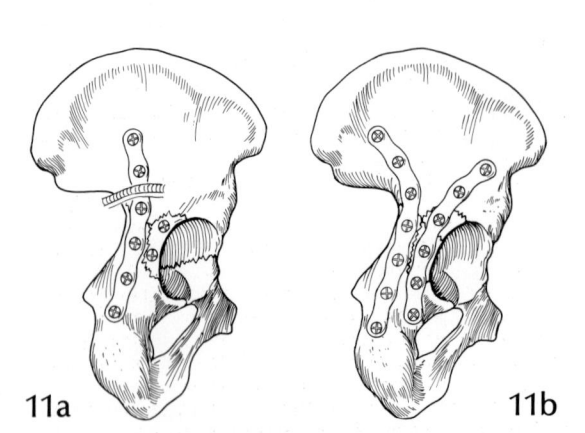

Associated transverse and posterior acetabular fractures

11a & b

The transverse component is dealt with as above and fixed by a plate which is placed near the greater sciatic notch and passes under the neurovascular bundles of the gluteal muscles to be screwed into the posterior part of the ilium.

A large posterior acetabular fragment is fixed by isolated screws or, more safely, by a curved plate, as already described for this fracture alone (*see Illustrations 10a and b*).

T-fractures

12a & b

The head of femur is placed and held under the roof and the fragment of the posterior column is set in place and plated as above, but one must avoid long screws which could reach the still displaced fragment of the anterior column and so hold it out of place.

Working through the greater sciatic notch, it may be possible to replace the anterior column and then to fix it with at least two long screws inserted from behind. If this is not possible this component must be approached from in front, using the ilioinguinal incision (see *Illustration 12b*).

In some cases it may be best to fix the segment of the anterior column first. With the posterior column segment retracted, the anterior column is reduced and fixed with lag screws. Then the posterior column is repositioned and plated as described.

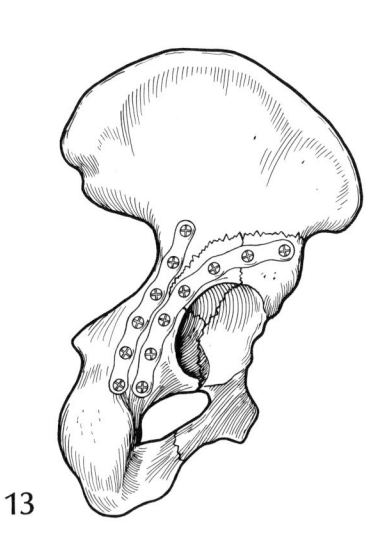

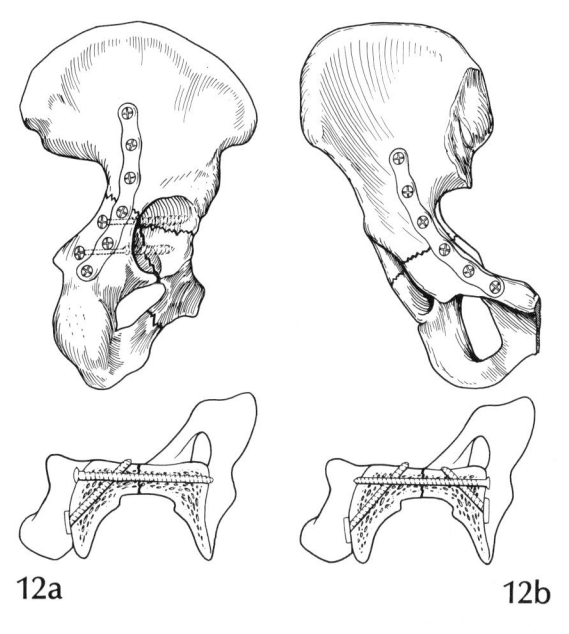

12a 12b

13

If none of the roof of the acetabulum remains attached to any part of the ilium that is still connected to the sacrum, the operation is more difficult. This is a pattern that affects the whole of both columns.

Firstly the head of femur is extracted from the pelvis and maintained by traction in a position which allows the surgeon to reduce the posterior column fragment.

The placement of the posterior column fragment must be perfect and should be controlled both from inside the pelvis and on the outer aspect of the bone. If one accepts a small imperfection at this stage, it will be impossible to deal accurately with the other fracture lines and the error will increase from step to step. The posterior column fracture is plated as if it were an isolated fracture of this part but avoiding screws long enough to reach and fix the displaced anterior column before it has been correctly repositioned.

Then, by freeing the inferior part of the ilium, up to its anterior border if necessary, the upper part of the anterior column fragment is replaced either by using forceps to take hold of a temporary screw or by a lever introduced into the fracture line.

A curved acetabular plate fixes the upper part of the anterior column to the posterior one; it should, if possible, cross the inferior angle of the iliac fracture line.

If the repositioning of the anterior column segment appears very difficult or impossible, it may be advisable to extend the incision by transforming it into a Dana Mear's triradiate approach. From the angle of the Kocher–Langenbeck incision, the skin is incised up to the anterior inferior iliac spine. The glutei muscle tendons are divided close to the greater trochanter, or the top of the trochanter is sectioned together with the gluteal tendons and the inferior part of the iliac wing is elevated to allow visualization of the fracture line separating the anterior column.

13

330 Pelvis and acetabulum

ILIOINGUINAL APPROACH

Position of patient

The patient lies supine on an orthopaedic table unless there is a vertical anterior fracture line of the opposite innominate bone, in which case traction would push the two pubes upwards and would prevent complete re-positioning.

Operative area

14a & b

The operative field has to extend (a) upwards for four fingers'-breadth above the iliac crest; (b) inwards for three to four fingers'-breadth beyond the midline; (c) inferiorly from the level of the superior border of the symphysis, sideways to the femoral vessels and then obliquely to below the vastus lateralis crest of the greater trochanter; and (d) laterally to just behind the line of the femur. The patient must therefore be draped accordingly.

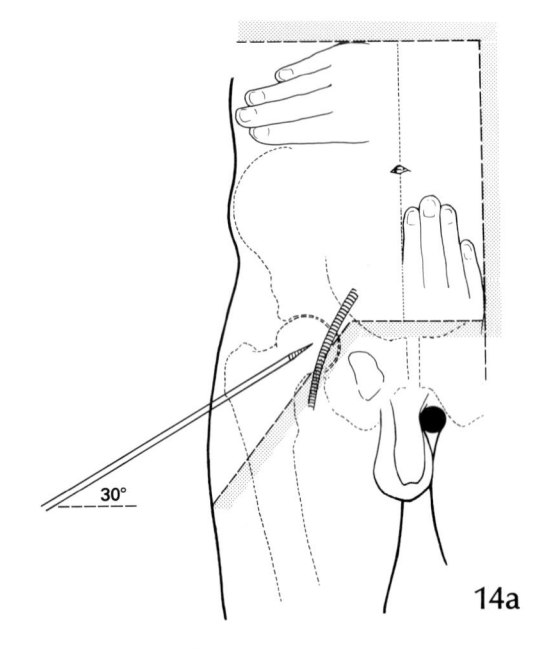

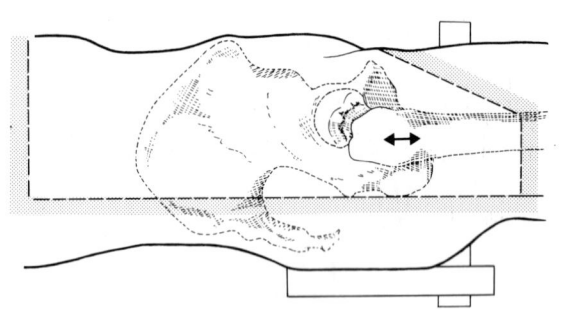

14a

14b

Approach

15a, 15b & 16

An incision is made along the anterior two-thirds of the iliac crest and then from its anterior superior spine towards the midline, two fingers'-breadth above the pubic symphysis.

Along the iliac crest the anterior abdominal muscles are detached and stripped in continuity with the iliacus from the inner aspect of the iliac wing. Beyond the fracture the rugine reaches the brim of the true pelvis. The iliac fossa is packed with a large swab.

The external oblique aponeurosis is incised 2 cm above the superficial inguinal ring and the inguinal canal is opened; the spermatic cord is then isolated and a tape is passed round it.

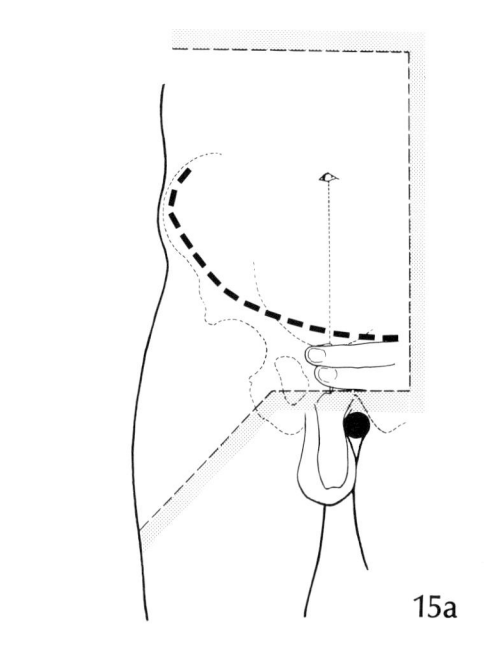

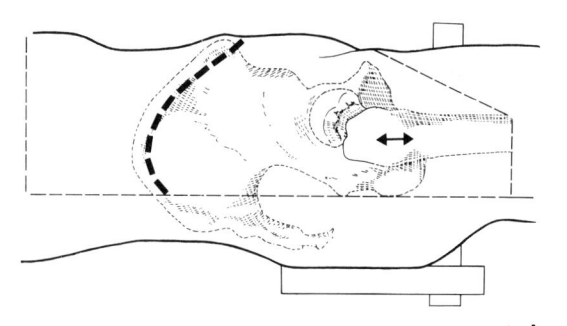

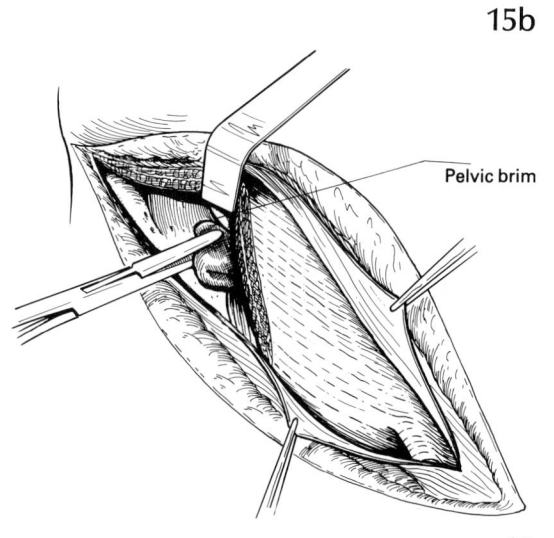

17

The short tendinous fibres of the origin of the internal oblique and transversus abdominis from the inguinal ligament are identified and cleaned. The scalpel divides either the tendinous fibres or the inguinal ligament itself, leaving above it enough fibrous tissue for the later repair. It enters the sheath of the iliopsoas muscle, where the femoral nerve must be located and safeguarded.

Near the anterior superior iliac spine the incision into the origin of internal oblique and transversus abdominis muscles is performed with great care, and further dissection in this region reveals and safeguards the lateral cutaneous nerve of the thigh, whose position is a little variable.

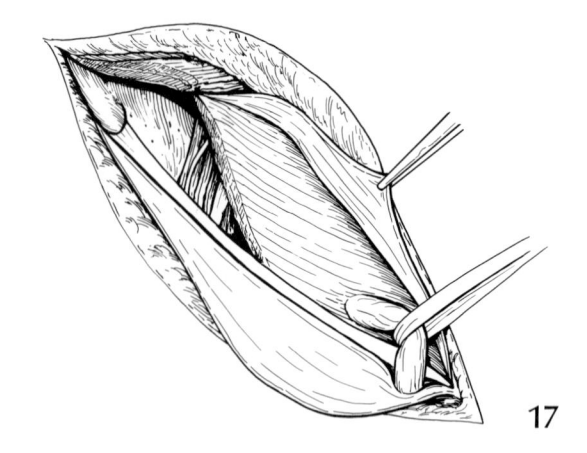

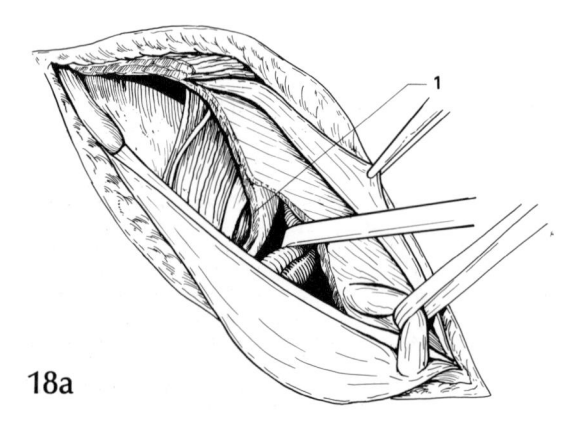

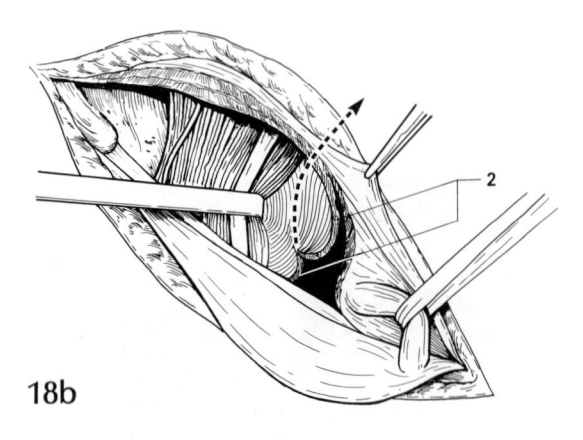

18a & b

A normal thickening (1) of the psoas fascia between the inguinal ligament and the anterior border of the iliac bone is then isolated by sharp dissection and is cut with care, because it separates the femoral nerve from the external iliac artery. This step is essential and has to be followed by the detachment of the iliac fascia along the brim of the true pelvis (2), in order to provide wide access to that cavity.

The iliopsoas muscle, the femoral nerve, and the lateral cutaneous nerve of the thigh are encircled with a second tape.

Display, correction and fixation of stove-in hip joints 333

19

Medial to the femoral vessels, the conjoint tendon and the transversalis fascia are divided and the retropubic space is entered and packed with a swab.

The vessels are mobilized gently with the finger in order not to damage lymphatics unnecessarily. The great vessels are encircled with a third tape.

When necessary, the tendon of the rectus abdominis can be divided about 1 cm from the pubis.

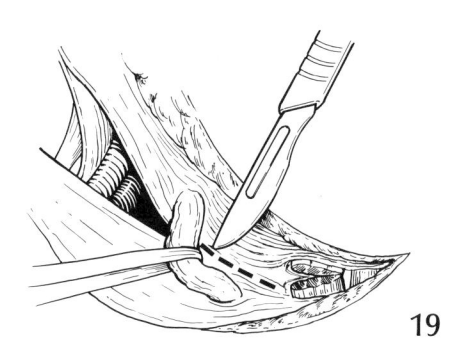

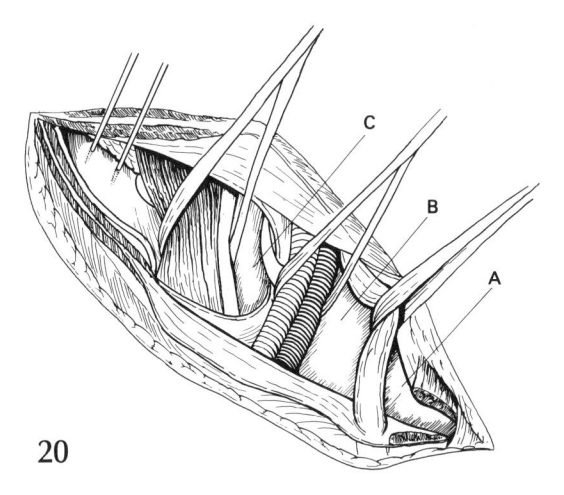

20

One or two Steinmann pins are driven into the bone in front of the sacroiliac joint to act as abdominal retractors.

By manipulating the tapes one can gain access to different parts of the pelvis: A, medial to the spermatic cord one can reach the inner part of the pubic ramus and the pubic symphysis; B, between the cord and the vessels, the outer part of the pubic ramus and the obturator vessels and nerve are accessible; and C, between the vessels and the iliopsoas the middle part of the iliopectineal line can be reached, and deep to this the quadrilateral surface that extends to the greater sciatic notch. Finally, lateral to the iliopsoas, the iliac fossa is widely exposed, the sacroiliac joint can be reached and the anterior aspect of the sacrum can also be freed.

21

In most cases it is not difficult to extract the head of femur from the pelvis, but the best way to keep it steady while assembly and fixation of the fragments are performed is to apply lateral traction. This can be done by making a small cut over the ridge between the gluteus medius and vastus lateralis muscles and fixing a femoral head extractor into the bone here; it should be inserted and pulled on in the line of the neck of the femur; traction is maintained by an assistant or a device attached to the table.

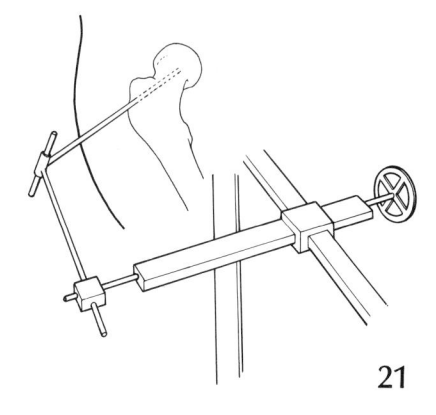

334 Pelvis and acetabulum

Replacement and fixation of fracture

If there is still a part of the articular crescent in its correct position and attached to the wing and it consists of the whole or a part of the posterior wall and a more or less important part of the roof, the fracture is of the anterior column type, either isolated or associated with a transverse fracture of the posterior column.

The head is replaced against the remaining part of the articular crescent, aided by both longitudinal and lateral traction.

22a, b & c

The fragments of the anterior column are then manipulated by means of forceps, or pushed directly into their normal position; a lever inserted in a fracture line may facilitate this. A large fragment of the anterior column may be seized by a forceps astride either the crest of the ilium or the anterior border of the ilium between the anterior spines.

The correction achieved, a few screws are inserted from the anterior fragments to the intact posterior part of the roof or to the posterior column. Then the plates must be shaped. The anterior column may be fixed by one or more plates screwed along the superior or inner aspect of the iliac crest, in the iliac fossa, or along the superior aspect of the iliopectineal line from in front of the sacroiliac joint to the pubic symphysis if necessary (a & b).

If a fracture line divides the posterior column, the reduction of its inferior fragment is achieved by direct manipulation of the fragment deep to the brim of the true pelvis, between the vessels and the iliopsoas muscle. Two 90–110 mm long screws are used to fix the fragment; they run parallel to the inner aspect of the bone and they may be used without a plate or to hold one of the plates in place (c).

If the whole articular crescent is broken and detached from the wing, the fracture is a combination of both the anterior and posterior column types.

Combined lateral and longitudinal traction extracts the stove-in hip and keeps the head in approximately the right place; slight over-traction does not matter.

Next, the fragments of the anterior column must be assembled as in the case described previously (p. 326).

Very often replacement is achieved by gripping the anterior column with forceps and using a lever in the fracture line to restore the displaced pieces of bone to their proper relationships.

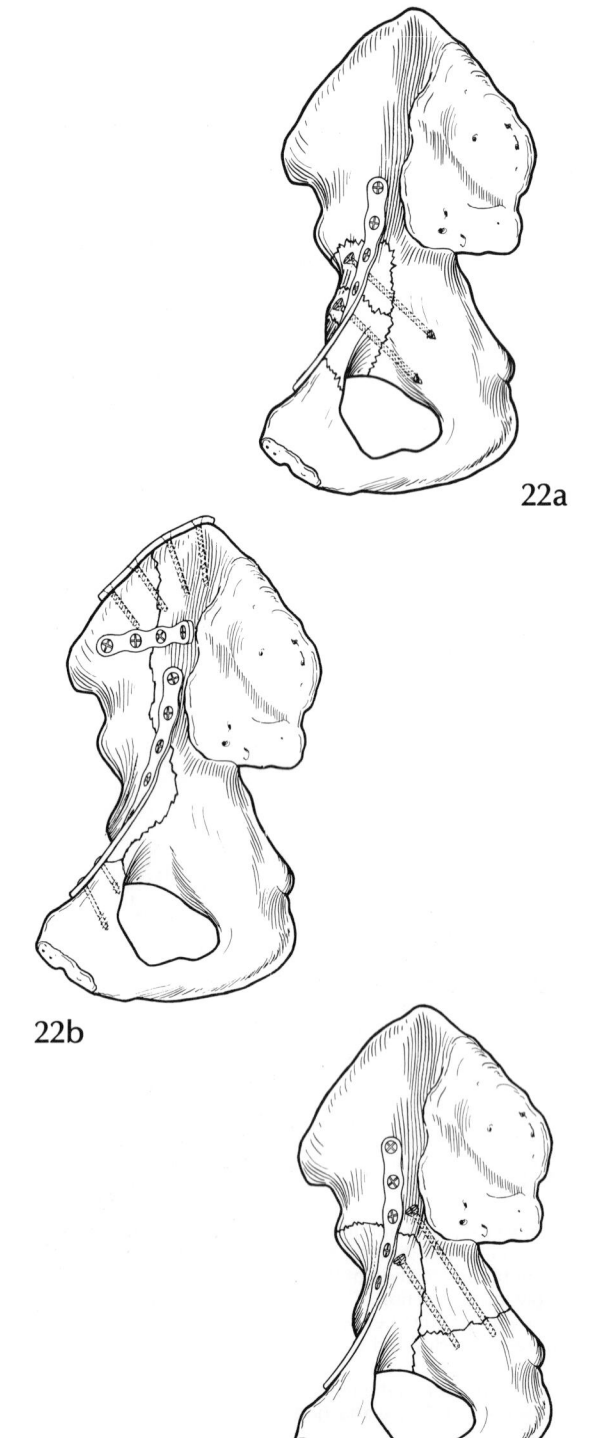

23

The first steps in fixation are achieved by isolated screws, but it is nearly always necessary to use plates as well. One must at this stage take care not to insert screws that can reach the still displaced posterior column and so hold it out of place. When traction is released the head should be in perfect contact with the reconstructed anterior column and the roof.

When this is done, in most cases the posterior column remains displaced, but its displacement has been lessened and, by working either between vessels and muscle or between vessels and cord, the posterior column can be pushed outwards and downwards and set perfectly or nearly perfectly in place. Screws to fix the posterior column can be inserted through the plate or apart from it. They need to be 90–120 mm long, passing from the iliac fossa or the pubic ramus either parallel to the inner aspect of the bone, reaching the posterior aspect of the posterior column, or obliquely to reach the quadrilateral surface.

By moving the hip before closure one can ensure that there are no screws in the joint.

If a satisfactory position of the posterior column is impossible to achieve, the anterior incision is closed. The patient must then be placed prone, but this must not be done until the circulation has been stabilized by the replacement of any lost blood. The posterior column is then exposed and fixed from behind in the way that has already been described.

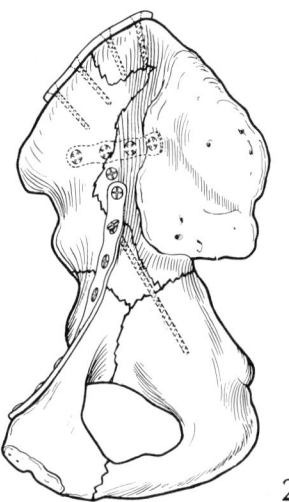

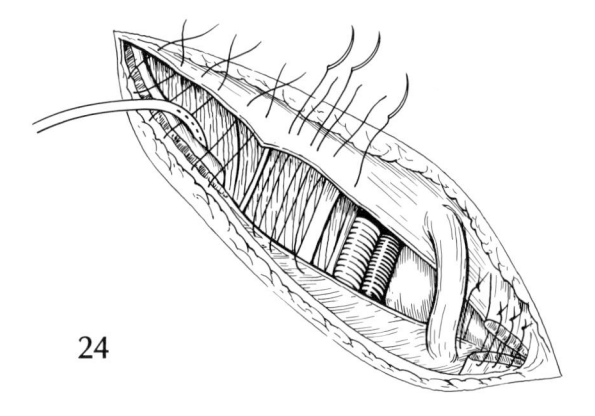

Closure

24

Closure of the ilioinguinal incision is anatomical and straightforward, but it must be done with care. Suction drains are inserted into the retropubic space and into the iliac fossa. The abdominal muscles are reattached. If divided, the anterior sheath of rectus abdominis, the conjoint tendon and the transversalis fascia are sutured. The tapes are removed, and one must see that the artery still pulsates and that the nerves are undamaged. The origins of the internal oblique and transversus abdominis are sutured to the inguinal ligament, using a fish-hook type of needle. The spermatic cord is put in place and the external oblique repaired. The inguinal canal, which has been so widely opened, is thus securely repaired.

336 Pelvis and acetabulum

LATERAL APPROACH OR EXTENDED ILIOFEMORAL APPROACH

25

This is performed with the patient on his side on an orthopaedic table. The pelvic support inserted between the thighs of the patient can be moved downwards and upwards and this adjustment, combined with longitudinal traction, allows one to extract the head of femur from the pelvis and keep it in the right position while rebuilding the acetabulum.

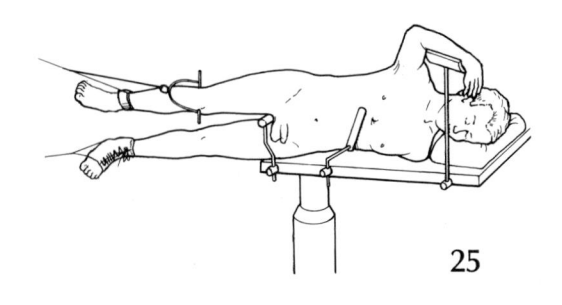

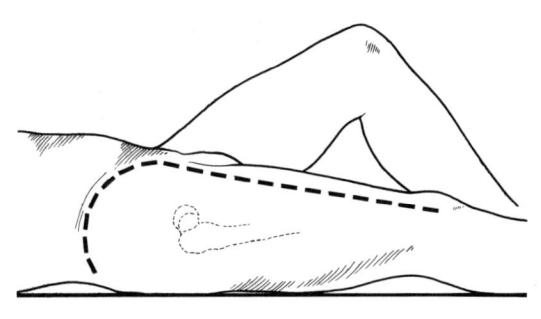

26

The skin incision is J-shaped and runs along the whole length of the iliac crest from the posterior superior spine, and then downwards from the anterior superior spine to the middle of the thigh in the direction of the lateral side of the patella.

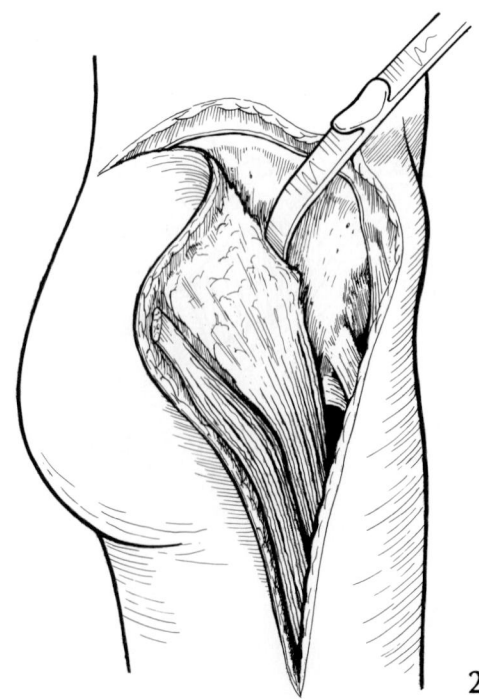

27

The gluteus muscles and the tensor fasciae latae are stripped from the outer aspect of the ilium, but from the anterior superior spine one should work within the sheath of the tensor, along the anterior border of the muscle, in order to avoid most of the branches of the lateral cutaneous nerve of the thigh. The fascia lata is split down to the end of the incision.

28

As the stripping of the gluteus muscles from the ilium progresses, the articular capsule is reached along its anterior and superior aspects; these are also stripped, giving access to the anterior border of the greater trochanter. The tendon of gluteus minimus is then cut close to the greater trochanter, followed by the tendon of gluteus medius, which is cut close to the lateral aspect of the greater trochanter. This makes a large, thick flap containing the three gluteus muscles, the tensor fasciae latae, their blood and nerve supplies. The flap is retracted backwards to give access to the posterior part of the hip joint, which is covered by the lateral rotators. Piriformis and obturator internus are cut and marked by a stitch, as in a posterior approach, and the special retractor can then be inserted into either sciatic notch.

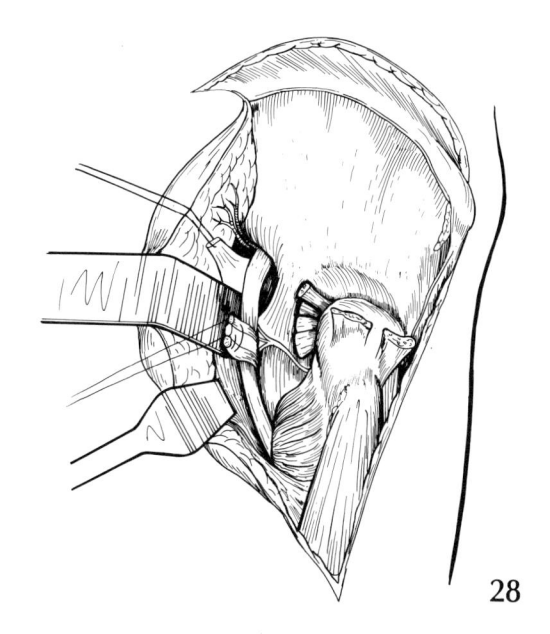

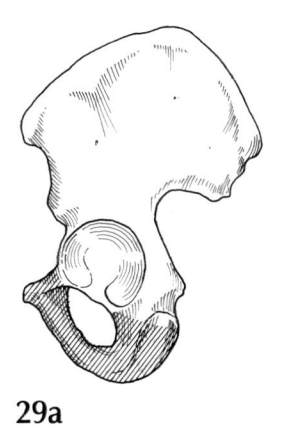

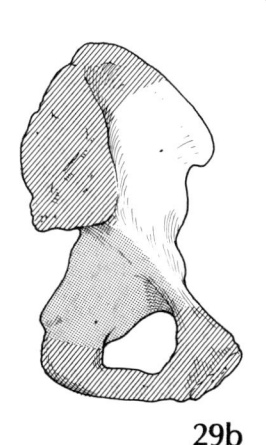

28

29a & b

This approach gives access to the entire blade of the ilium, the whole posterior column up to the upper pole of the ischial tuberosity and to the anterior column, but not beyond the body of the pubis.

If it appears necessary, one can elevate the abdominal muscles from the crest and elevate in continuity with them the iliacus from the internal iliac fossa, in order to gain access up to the sacroiliac area and the pelvic brim. The author restricts this approach to the internal iliac fossa to what is needed in each individual case.

29a 29b

30a & b

In cases of both column fractures, reduction and fixation of fracture lines are performed one after the other, taking care to perform an anatomical reduction of each fracture line, because if we accept a defect in an initial reduction it will be impossible to compensate for it while reducing the other fracture lines. Isolated screws, often inserted as lag screws between the two tables of the iliac wing, together with plates, allow rebuilding of the acetabulum and the innominate bone, but the inferior part of the anterior column, below the iliopectineal eminence, is not accessible.

In cases of transverse fracture, T-shaped fracture, or transverse fracture associated with the posterior wall, when the fracture component is transtectal, this approach appears to be the best.

In fact we control perfectly both extremities of the transverse fracture and the entire roof of the acetabulum by performing a capsulotomy along the acetabular lips.

The best way to fix the transverse fracture component is to insert a long screw along the axis of the anterior column, and to apply a plate along the posterior column. The long screw (often inserted as a lag screw) penetrates the bone along the posterior aspect of the pillar of the iliac wing, 3–4 cm above the acetabular lips. A finger applied against the iliopectineal eminence acts as a guide, and the endoarticular control allowed by the capsulotomy prevents penetration of the joint. This screw is either a 4.5 mm or 6.5 mm screw.

In cases of T-shaped fracture, fixation can begin with either the posterior or the anterior column segment, according to the case. The anterior column is fixed with a long screw as above. The posterior column fragment is plated as already described.

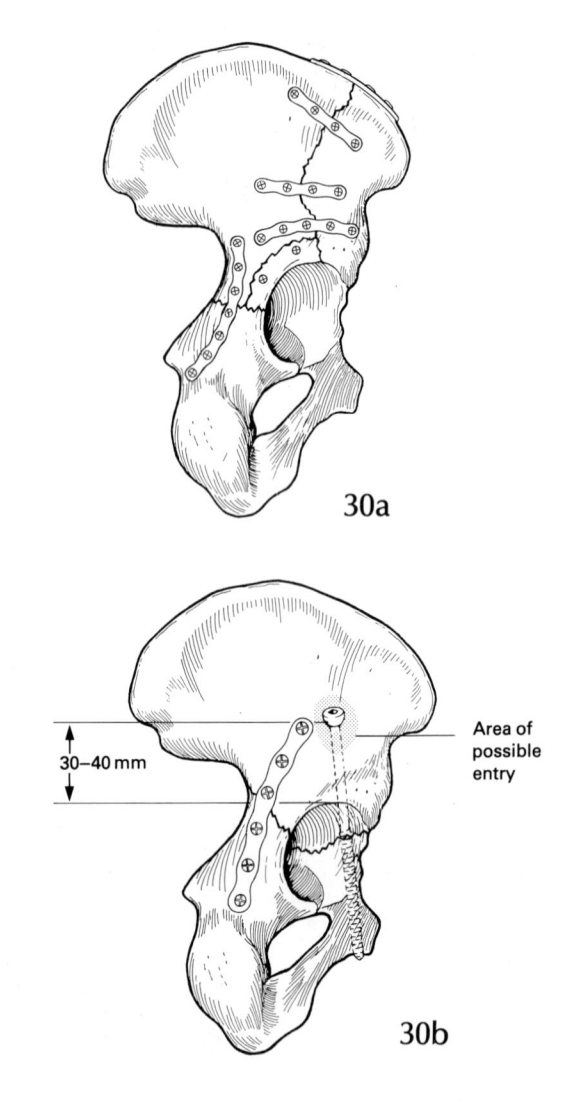

Wound closure

The wound is closed by reattaching the lateral rotators, the glutei tendons, to their trochanteric stumps and the aponeurosis of the glutei to the iliac crest.

Suction drains should be used.

Postoperative management

The patient stays in bed for 10–15 days. Passive exercises of the reconstructed hip begin on the third day. Antibiotics are given for 2 days before and 8 days after an ilioinguinal or a lateral approach. Anticoagulants are used in all cases. Walking without weight-bearing is allowed from the fifteenth day. The return to full weight-bearing usually requires 75–90 days according to radiographic appearances.

Illustrations by Peter Cox after G. Lee

Replacement and fixation of the posterior lip of the acetabulum

E. Letournel MD
Professor of Orthopaedic Surgery and Traumatology, Centre Medico-Chirurgical de la Porte de Choisy, Paris, France

Introduction

Indications

After a fracture dislocation of the acetabulum, the replacement and fixation of a fracture of the posterior lip of the acetabulum is advisable. This restores the articular crescent and thus the stability of the joint, and allows a natural distribution of intra-articular pressure, thereby preventing post-traumatic osteoarthrosis.

Furthermore the surgical correction allows one to clear the joint of any small fragments which are not visible with standard radiographs or even tomograms. Nevertheless they can be detected by a CT scan if the cuts are of 5 mm or less. Surgical exposure also enables the surgeon to recognize the fractures in which the external part of the posterior wall is separated into one or more fragments, whereas the inner part is impacted into the underlying cancellous bone and has to be dislodged and replaced in contact with the femoral head. We call this fracture a 'marginal impaction'; it is in fact met in all kinds of acetabular fractures. Good fixation allows early walking without weight-bearing and avoids all kinds of postoperative immobilization.

The only contraindication to surgery is when the size of the displaced fragment is so small that only one screw would be used to fix it. The post-traumatic incongruence resulting from this situation is very small and does not influence the long-term prognosis.

Preoperative

Timing of operation

The dislocation must be reduced as soon as possible after injury. Usually the femoral head is stable, but the fragments remain displaced. Rest in bed with slight lateral rotation of the limb avoids recurrent dislocation; traction is not necessary.

If the hip cannot be reduced (because, for example, of a big intra-articular fragment) or is unstable after reduction because of the extent of the fracture, operation should be carried out as an emergency.

Another indication for emergency surgery is the presence of an associated segmented fracture of the femoral head which precludes any attempt at reduction of the dislocation of the femoral head as the risk of adding a subcapital fracture is very high.

Provided the reduced head remains in the joint, replacement of the posterior fragment can be easily performed during the first 6 or 8 days after injury, so there is plenty of time in which to prepare the patient.

Anaesthesia

General anaesthesia is necessary and blood for transfusion should be available.

Position of patient

1

The patient is placed prone on an orthopaedic table.
   To relax the sciatic nerve and avoid damaging it during the posterior approach, the knee should be flexed about 45° and a transcondylar Steinmann pin inserted to allow traction on the limb. Flexing the knee more relaxes the sciatic nerve more, but induces a side-effect from the excess traction on the rectus femoris.

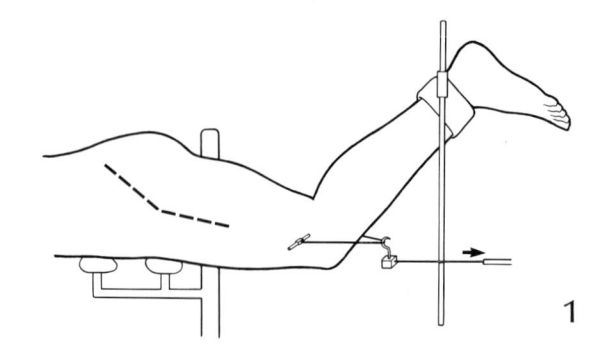

2a

2b

2c

2d

2e

Devices

2a-e

Screws are used; plates are often necessary.
   The plates do not need to be very thick and wide and they must be capable of being shaped to lie perfectly on the reconstructed posterior wall. Sherman-type plates, with equidistant holes, are satisfactory because they can be easily shaped in all directions. Vitallium plates (b) were used for many years. Stainless steel plates (c) are now available. There are also curved Letournel acetabular plates with 6, 8, 10 or 12 holes and of two curvatures available in vitallium (d) or stainless steel (e). The AO 3.5 reconstruction plate is also adequate, but more flexible.
   To give the plates the desired shape they can be bent using special benders or, more commonly, two large forceps. It is essential to shape the plate to follow perfectly the contours of the posterior column where it must lie; it is easy to curve the plate too much or too little and thus spoil the position of the fragment(s) when the screws are driven home.

Replacement and fixation of the posterior lip of the acetabulum 341

Special tools

3a & b

It is helpful to have an instrument to push fragments into place and it should be protected by a shield 4 mm from its end.

A special retractor may be inserted in either sciatic notch; it takes a good hold because of its distal hook, and it presents a convex surface to the nerve, but it must be kept close against the bone (sciatic spine upwards, ischial tuberosity downwards) in order to avoid compression of the nerve by one or other side of its hook.

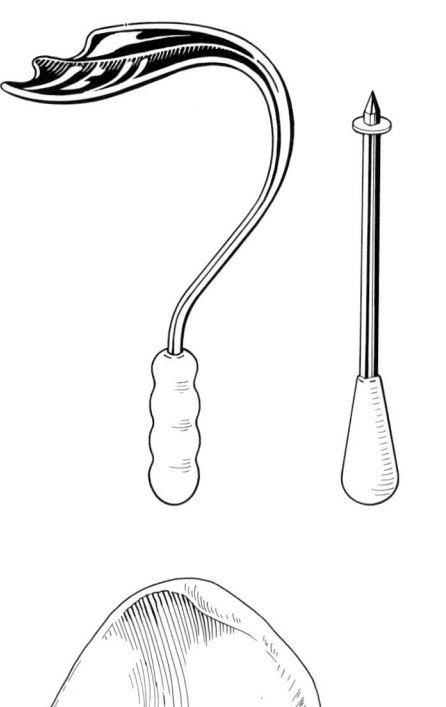

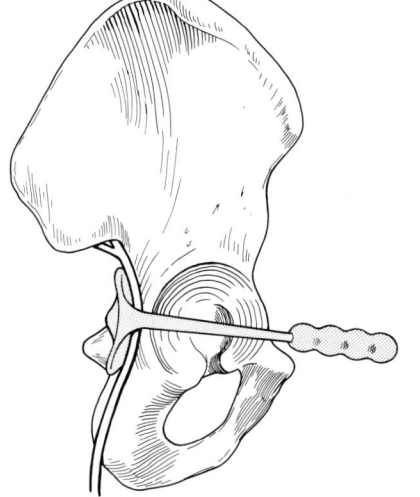

3a

3b

Operation

Kocher–Langenbeck approach

4a

The skin incision has two limbs centred on the superior part of the greater trochanter; the upper runs two-thirds of the way towards the posterior superior iliac spine and the lower passes down the lateral aspect of the thigh.

The gluteus maximus and the fascia lata are split in the line of the incision. The gluteus maximus is split only as far as the first important vascular pedicle.

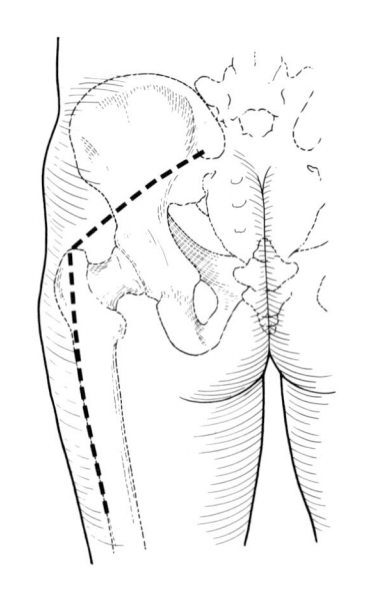

4b

The tendon of piriformis is divided, lifted up and attached by a stitch to the internal lip of the incision. Lifting the muscle exposes the sciatic nerve and gives access to the greater sciatic notch and to the neurovascular pedicle of the gluteal muscles.

The obturator internus and the gemelli are also divided through their terminal tendons, secured with a stitch and freed carefully from the bone. The underlying synovial bursa is opened and gives access to the lesser sciatic notch, into which the special retractor can be inserted and where it will remain separated from the nerve by the obturator tendon. The whole of both sciatic notches must be reached and exposed.

The upper pole of the ischial tuberosity has to be clearly identified but it is useless to divide the quadratus femoris.

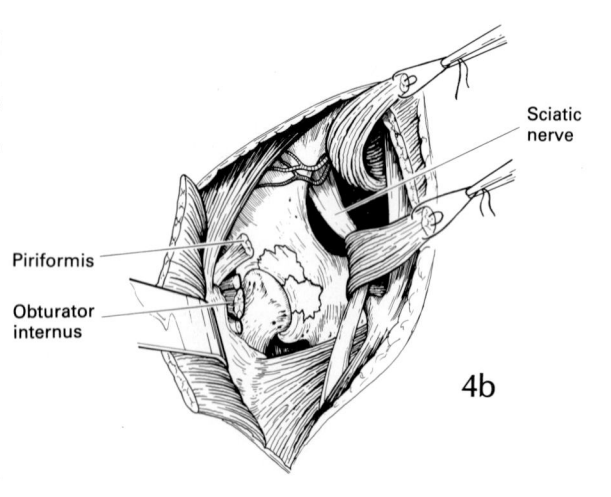

Posterior wall fracture

5a

The posterior wall fracture can then be displayed. It varies from case to case. The most typical is separate fragments with a part of the articular surface and a part of the retro-acetabular surface; these fragments may or may not remain attached to the capsule and other soft parts. Fragments of an associated marginal impaction may be embedded in the underlying cancellous bone and must be carefully looked for. Sometimes there are isolated fragments of the articular or the posterior cortical surface. Both the extent of the posterior wall avulsion and the number of fragments vary greatly from one case to another. The displaced fragments and the tear of the capsule allow access to the joint. Although it is difficult to avoid some stripping of the soft tissues from these fragments, such dissection should be kept to a minimum.

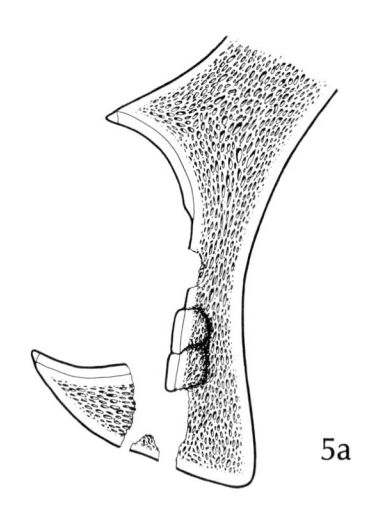

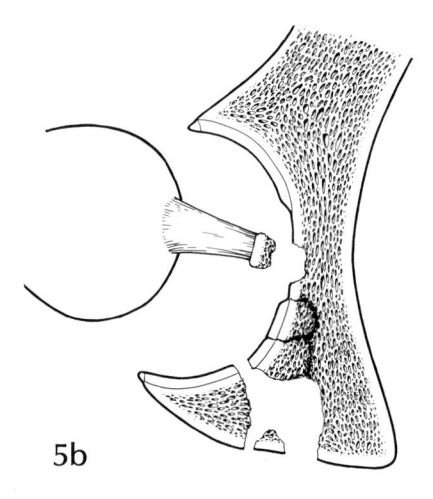

Clearing the joint

5b

The joint must be cleared of any fragments that are in the acetabular fossa and one must not forget to remove the fragment that is sometimes attached to the ligamentum teres, which generally remains attached to the head.

With the aid of traction one gains an excellent view of the joint and should easily recognize both free and impacted fragments.

Reduction

6a & b

When traction is released the head takes its place under the roof and the anterior part of the articular crescent, but perfect contact must be ensured. The fragments are then replaced. First, any impacted fragments are gently mobilized with a chisel or a lever, while trying to keep their cancellous part intact, and they are set in place upon the head of the femur. The posterior fragments are then replaced. It is easy when there is only one fragment, but is more difficult when there are several pieces which have to be put in their right places as carefully and perfectly as the pieces of a jigsaw puzzle. This takes time and may require many trials and errors. When there is a combination of separated and impacted fragments there may be a gap after they have been re-assembled; if this is likely to impair the stability of the reconstruction it should be filled with cancellous bone from the ilium or from the greater trochanter of the femur.

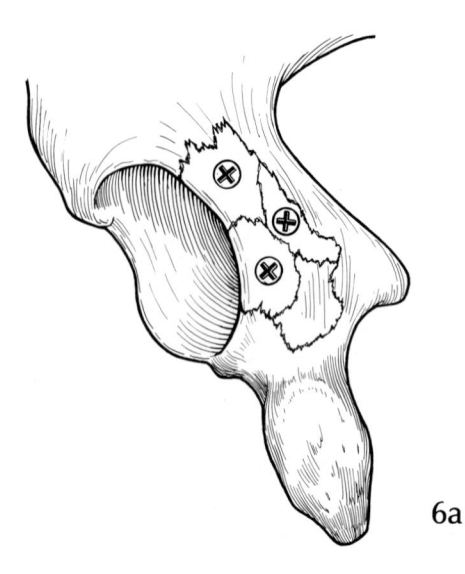

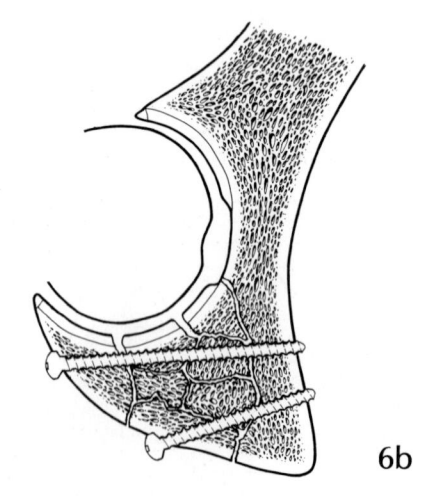

6a

6b

Fixation

7a, b & c

In the case of small fragments, two or three isolated screws may suffice; this will generally be when the fragments bear only a small portion of articular surface. A single big fragment may be fixed by several screws inserted in diverging directions. These screws are inserted into the posterior aspect of the fragment and are directed to the quadrilateral surface of the iliac bone where they obtain a good hold. Care must be taken to avoid the joint and the head and it is wise to test the movement of the head in its socket so as to be sure that there is no grating. A finger passed through the great sciatic notch may test the length of the screws.

When single screws are used I prefer those with a 3.5 mm diameter; the 4.5 mm are less commonly used. The technique of the 'lag screw' may be applied. I prefer the 'self-tapping screws', as tapping appears unnecessary to fix the innominate bone.

In most cases plates are needed as well as screws. Two or three screws are used to hold the fragments in place. Then a plate has to be fitted to the posterior column, from the upper pole of the ischial tuberosity to the posterior part of the wing or above the roof of the acetabulum, depending on the size and the exact site of the posterior fracture(s). The plate follows the long axis of the articular fragments. Whether straight or curved, the lower end of the plate is given a sharp bend to follow the contour of the 'infra-acetabular groove'. The rest of the plate is shaped to follow exactly the contours of the posterior column so as to be in perfect contact with the bone. The pedicle of the gluteal muscles is very carefully freed from the bone if it is necessary to insert the plate under it. The plate is then screwed down, taking care not to enter the joint. The lowest screw is inserted into the ischial tuberosity, where it finds a very strong hold and may be 40 or 45 mm long. The screws over the roof may be 30–40 mm and those into the posterior part of the wing, 25–35 mm. The intermediate screws, like the separate ones, take hold of the quadrilateral surface. If possible, one should insert two screws beyond each extremity of the fracture site.

With the stainless steel plate the 3.5 mm screw is preferable as their heads are flush with the plate and they do not interfere with the tissues gliding along the plate. After plating the freedom of the joint must be tested.

Closure

Piriformis and obturator internus are reattached to their tendons and sewn together side-to-side in order to provide a muscular pad between the sciatic nerve and the plate. One or two suction drains are required. Gluteus maximus is sutured and the skin closed. The transcondylar traction pin is then removed.

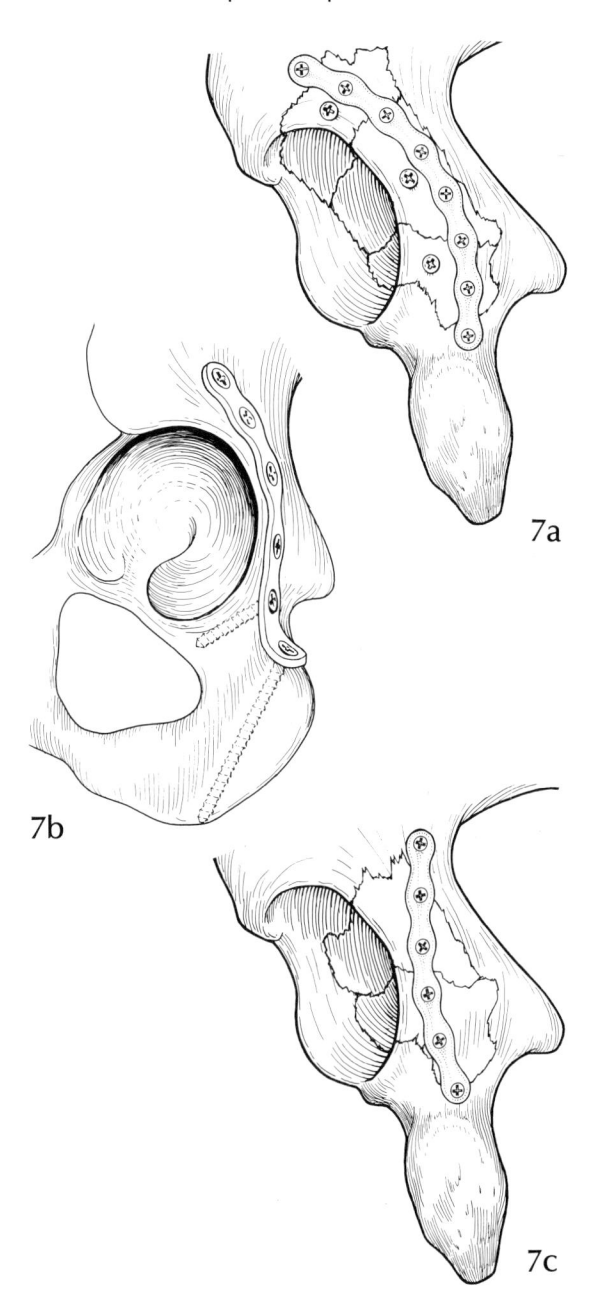

Postoperative management

No plaster, splint or traction is required, only bed rest. Prophylactic antibiotics and anticoagulant therapy are routine. Suction drains are removed after 5 or 6 days.

The patient is allowed to move his limb, and passive exercises are started on the second or third day. Walking without weight-bearing is allowed on the eighth to the tenth day. Full weight-bearing is allowed after 75 days.

Illustrations by Peter Cox after G. Lee

Exposure and fixation of disrupted pubic symphysis

E. Letournel MD
Professor of Orthopaedic Surgery and Traumatology, Centre Medico-Chirurgical de la Porte de Choisy, Paris, France

Introduction

Disruption of the pubic symphysis is usually caused by a major crushing injury to the pelvis. It is often associated with serious visceral injuries, in particular to the male urethra, and these must be considered before fixation is performed.

Even though there may appear to be merely a disruption or overlapping of the symphysis pubis there is inevitably sacroiliac ligament damage as well, resulting in an opening of the sacroiliac joint on one or both sides. This can be corrected by reduction and fixation of the pubic symphysis.

Indications for operation

Operation is advisable: (1) when the pubic bones overlap; and (2) when the pubic interval is greater than 1.5 cm. Only very small disruptions are treated conservatively.

Furthermore, this surgical treatment avoids all kinds of postoperative immobilization and allows walking with crutches sometimes only 10 days after operation.

Preoperative

This is not an emergency and delay of a few days allows: (1) the spontaneous arrest of bleeding from pelvic veins disrupted at the time of injury; and (2) preparation of the skin for incision through the region of the pubic hair.

Anaesthesia

General anaesthesia is used.
 The urinary bladder has to be evacuated either spontaneously or by catheter.

Position of patient

The patient may be placed upon an ordinary operating table, but an orthopaedic table may be useful to facilitate the reduction of the more severe disruptions by allowing asymmetrical traction on the limbs and medial rotation of both hips.

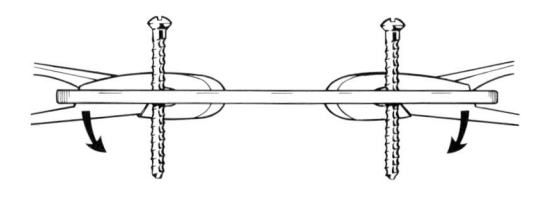

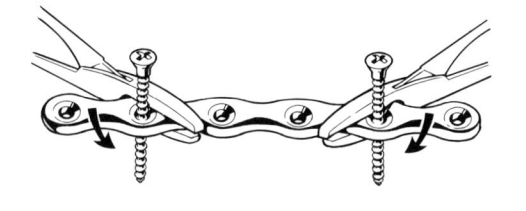

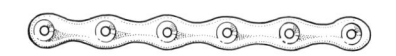

Apparatus

1

There is no special device. One can use a vitallium or stainless steel modified Sherman plate with equidistant holes. As it is to be applied on the superior aspect of the pubic bones it has to be bent along its long axis posteriorly.
 A plate of four or six holes is used. Thick and wide plates are not suitable; Sherman plates are adequate as they can be shaped so as to lie perfectly on the bone.
 To give the plate its posterior concavity one can use any bending apparatus. To obtain the desired amount of posterior curvature, the plate is grasped with strong forceps on either side of the midline and short screws inserted into the outer holes. An AO reconstruction plate with four to six holes is suitable. There are also now available precurved acetabular plates which are very convenient (see chapter on 'Display, correction and fixation of stove-in hip joints,' pp. 321–338).

1

Operation

Exposure

2a & b

In a case of simple disruption of the pubic symphysis, a vertical median incision is adequate. It should be 10–12 cm long and extend distally to the level of the superior border of the symphysis, i.e. crossing the pubic hair margin.

The recti abdomini are separated along the linea alba. Retzius' space is opened, the bladder is pushed back, and the posterior surfaces of the pubes are exposed.

The tear of the pubic symphysis is always asymmetrical. On one side the bone has been cleared of all its muscular and ligamentous insertions, and the rectus itself is attached only to the prepubic soft parts. On the other side the rectus is normally attached, and the capsule and the cartilage remain attached to the bone.

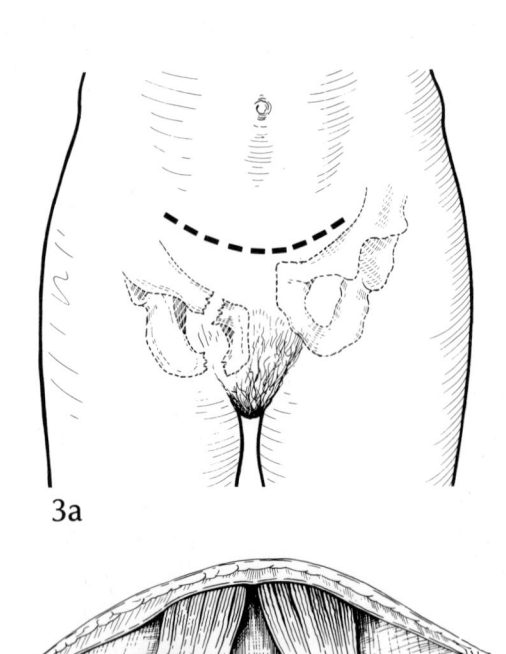

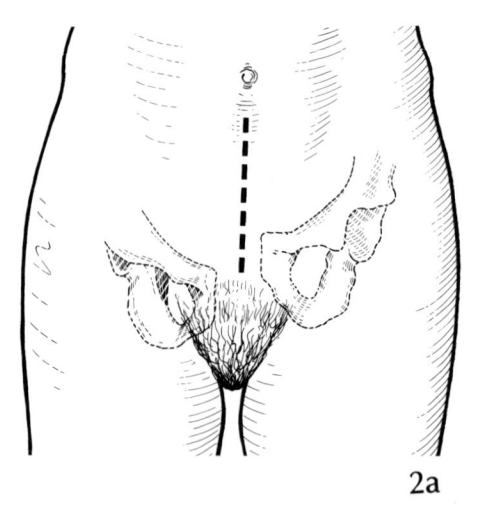

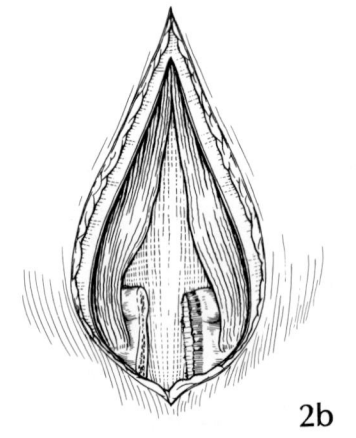

3a & b

In some cases, a disrupted symphysis is associated with a vertical fracture through one obturator foramen, dividing both the pubic and ischiopubic rami. If this fracture is displaced it is necessary to reduce the displacement and plate it at the same time as the symphysis. In this case a vertical incision is not suitable and a horizontal approach such as a Pfannenstiel incision is more appropriate. If necessary, one rectus abdominis is cut transversely near its pubic insertion and repaired later.

4a & b

In any case it is necessary to free the superior aspect of the pubic rami where the plate will be inserted. As a rule, one side is already more or less freed by the injuring force; on the other side the superior aspect has to be cleared from back to front, but the rectus must remain attached to the anterior border of that surface.

If the cartilage is uninjured and well-attached to one pubis it is left in place, as no attempt is made to get an arthrodesis of the joint in fresh cases.

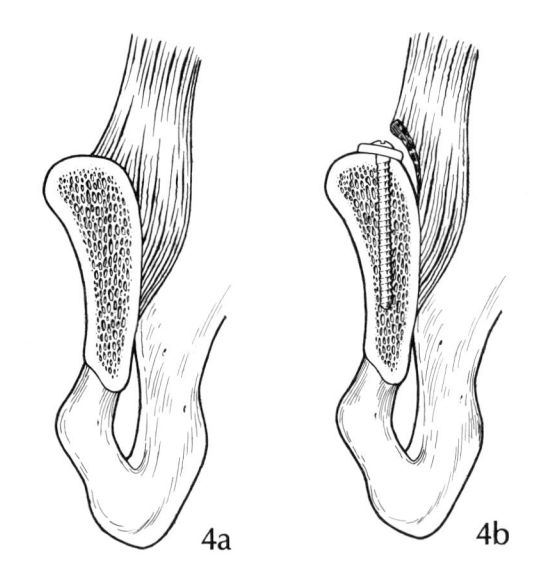

Reduction

5a, b & c

Medial rotation of both lower limbs, axial traction and hyperextension of the hip, allowed by the orthopaedic table, facilitate the reduction but a direct manipulation of the pubic bones is always necessary. The author uses Farabeuf's forceps to take hold of the anterior aspect of the pubic angle, or, better, inserting them into the obturator foramina (see Illustration 6a). To achieve this, the soft parts anterior to the pubis are elevated from the pubic angle in a downwards and outwards direction until the forceps enter the foramen.

Often the reduction is not achieved in one stage; when several stages are needed, a few minutes should be allowed between successive stages. The symphysis must fit in all directions and not only its superior aspect; a possible twist of the ilium has to be corrected to align the posterior aspects of the pubic bones correctly.

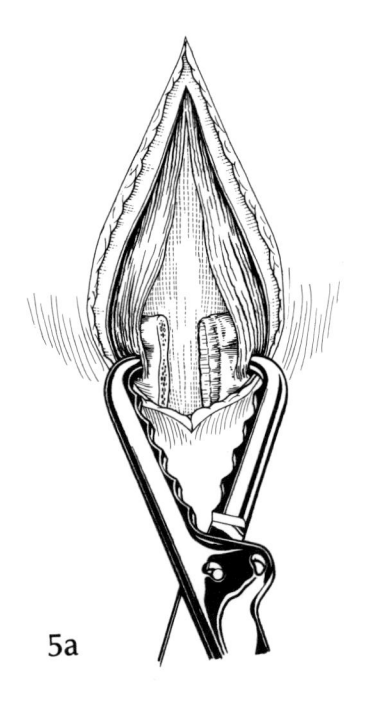

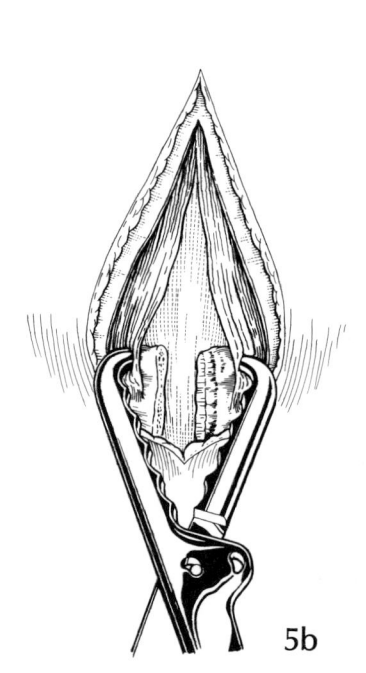

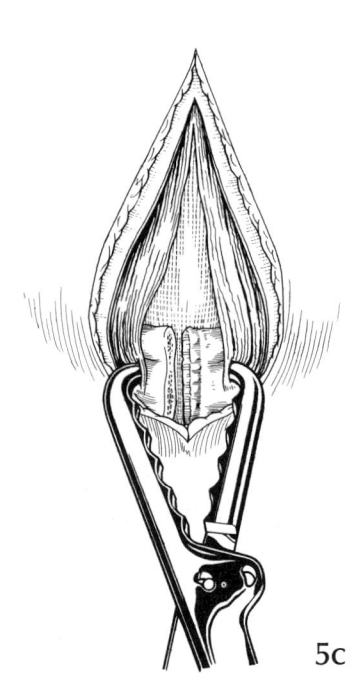

Fixation

6a & b

As the reduction is achieved a four- or six-hole plate is shaped to lie perfectly on the superior aspect of both pubic rami.

Two screws (35 mm or 45 mm) can be inserted in the body of each pubis. These screws should be parallel to the posterior surface of the pubis, i.e. directed obliquely backwards and downwards. From in front they look vertical and parallel or slightly divergent.

If a six-hole plate is used, the outer screws will be inserted into the superior pubic rami; they have to be shorter and must avoid the obturator vessels and nerve, but being screwed into two cortices they have a firm grip.

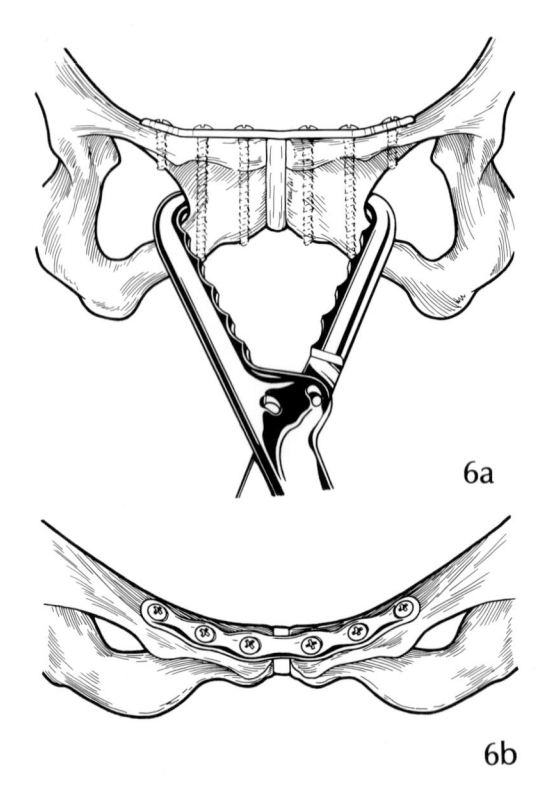

7

If it is necessary to span a disrupted symphysis and a fracture in the obturator foramen, the problem is more difficult and it is more important to understand the objective than to describe the procedure in detail. Usually I reduce the symphysis pubis and while reduction is maintained by the forceps, the fracture of the superior pubic ramus is reduced and fixed with a single screw. Then a long enough plate must be used to allow each fragment to be gripped by at least two screws and it must be made to fit all fragments accurately while they are held in place.

Closure of the wound

One or two suction drains are inserted, one in front and one behind the repaired symphysis. If the rectus has been cut across it is repaired carefully. The linea alba is sutured. The skin incision is then closed.

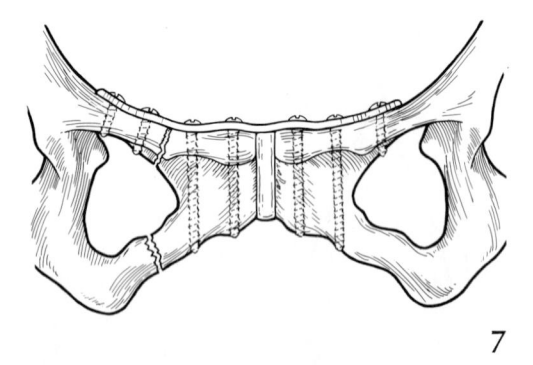

Postoperative management

As the area of the pubic hair has been incised prophylactic antibiotics are used, 1 day before the operation and 6 days afterwards. Suction drains are removed after 4–6 days. The patient remains in bed without any type of immobilization. Walking with partial weight-bearing and crutches is allowed after 10 days. Full weight-bearing is allowed after 6 weeks.

Illustrations by Peter Cox

Operative treatment of children's fractures

I. J. Leslie   MChOrth, FRCS
Department of Orthopaedic and Traumatic Surgery, Bristol Royal Infirmary, Bristol, UK

Introduction

The bones of children are different from those of adults in anatomy, physiology, and biomechanics and also they have the ability to grow and remodel. Deformity can be overcome, shortening can be self-corrected, children are not prone to stiffness even after extended periods of immobilization and articular cartilage appears to reconstitute itself. Therefore the indications for operative treatment are fewer than in adult fractures.

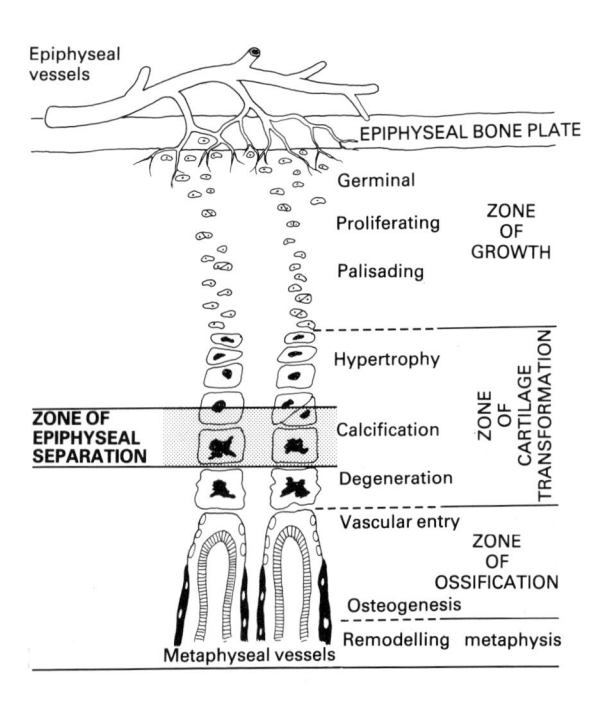

However, the presence of a growth-plate causes special problems. It is weaker than adjacent ligaments which do not rupture but which avulse the epiphysis if put under strain. Fractures in the metaphyseal or epiphyseal region usually involve the growth-plate which is injured in a third of the children with skeletal trauma.

Indications for operation

The indications for operative intervention are therefore the following.

1. Displaced fractures of the epiphyses
2. Diaphyseal fractures which cannot be maintained in an acceptable alignment
3. Unstable fractures with neurovascular complications.

General anaesthesia is necessary for operative treatment of fractures in children.

Injuries of the epiphysis

1

The growth-plate is a cartilaginous disc lying between the epiphysis and the metaphysis. In certain anatomical sites the epiphysis is subjected to traction forces by ligaments or tendons and is then called an apophysis. The germinal layer of cells is attached to the epiphysis from whence it receives its blood supply. Fractures usually occur at the junction between the calcified and uncalcified cartilage where it is weakest owing to the small amount of matrix present. If the epiphysis is accurately apposed to the metaphysis, the cleavage line heals rapidly and continues growing. However, failure to achieve apposition may lead to unequal growth or growth arrest.

Salter–Harris classification[1]

2a–e

The classification is in widespread use and provides a good guide to prognosis for the growth-plate: the higher the grade the higher risk there is of growth disturbance.

(a) Type I

The epiphysis separates completely from the metaphysis, the germinal layer remaining with the epiphysis. If undisplaced, these injuries may be interpreted as a sprain. However, as a guiding rule, children do not sprain their ligaments but suffer Type I epiphyseal fractures in which there is tenderness over the growth-plate. When the plate is fractured in the horizontal plane the germinal cells continue to grow, provided that the blood supply to the epiphysis is maintained. Avascular necrosis may be a problem in the femoral head. An apophysis is usually avulsed completely but maintains its blood supply through the ligamentous attachments.

(b) Type II

This is the commonest type of injury and the prognosis for subsequent growth is good. The major part of the fracture is in the plane of the growth-plate with a small vertical fracture through the metaphysis. The periosteum is torn on one side and is usually hinged on the side of the triangular metaphyseal fragment. The opposite metaphyseal edge may buttonhole through the periosteum and prevent reduction, for example, at the upper end of the humerus. Open reduction and fixation may occasionally be necessary.

(c) Type III

This is an intra-articular fracture in which one part of the epiphysis becomes separated from the remainder of the epiphysis and the metaphysis. It occurs most commonly at the lower end of the tibia when the growth-plate is partially closed.

(d) Type IV

This is an intra-articular fracture and the fracture line is vertical through the epiphysis and the metaphysis. The most common type is a fracture of the lateral condyle of the elbow.

(e) Type V

Originally this was described as a crush injury of the epiphysis due to excessive vertical loading. This may be misinterpreted as a Type I injury and will only be described as Type V when growth arrest occurs. Attention should be focused on the healing process of any epiphyseal injury. If an injury occurs evenly across the growth-plate and if in the race to effect healing, bone forms, then complete growth arrest will occur. If only part of the epiphysis is crushed, bone may bridge that part only, producing growth disturbance. When a growth-plate is damaged, a repair process ensues and the area may be filled with cartilage allowing growth to continue, or the area may fill with bone. This can occur with any type of epiphyseal injury including Type I and therefore all growth-plate injuries should be followed up for at least 6 months.

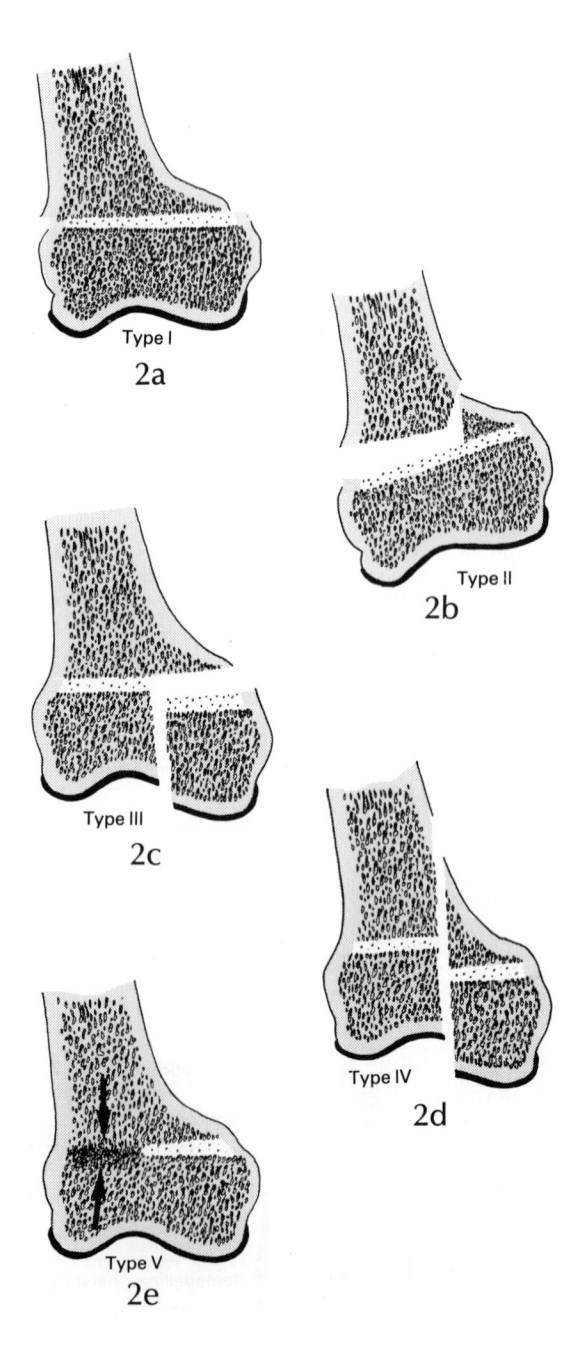

Treatment of epiphyseal injuries

Types I and II can generally be treated by closed reduction and although anatomical reduction is desirable, it is not essential. Remodelling will take place. Soft tissues may become interposed and prevent closed reduction and in those cases open reduction may be necessary.

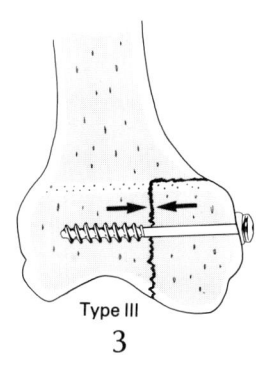

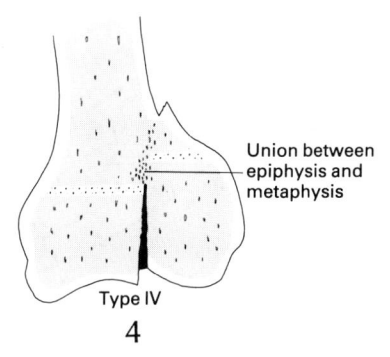

Types III and IV are intra-articular fractures and need accurate reduction. This usually means open reduction and internal fixation.

3

Accurate reduction is necessary to align the joint surface and internal fixation should compress the epiphyseal fragments together. Care should be taken to avoid damage to the epiphyseal blood supply. A neutralizing plate may be applied across the growth-plate if necessary but should be removed by 3 months.

4, 5a, b & c

In Type IV fractures the metaphyseal fragment may be excised to make reduction of the epiphysis more accurate. A growth-plate can be destroyed by infection and this is a risk with all open reductions. Kirschner wires should be buried beneath the skin as this reduces the risk of infection.

This fracture must be accurately reduced to align both the articular cartilage and the epiphyseal cartilage. Failure to achieve accurate reduction results in bony ridging and subsequent growth deformity (*see Illustration 4*). Open reduction is necessary, care being taken to avoid damage to the blood supply of the fragment. Using a washer on the screw, the epiphyseal fragment should be compressed against the epiphysis and the metaphyseal fragment compressed against the metaphysis. However, a compression screw should not cross the growth-plate (*see Illustration 5a & b*). A neutralizing plate can be applied provided it is removed later. Kirschner wires usually provide adequate fixation and may cross the growth-plate. However, they should be removed within 3 months (*see Illustration 5c*).

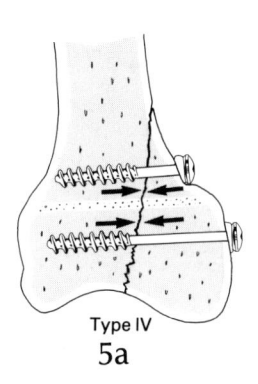

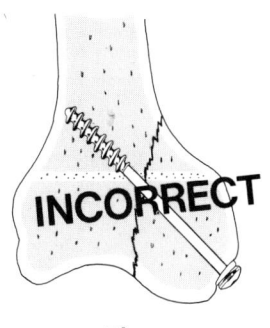

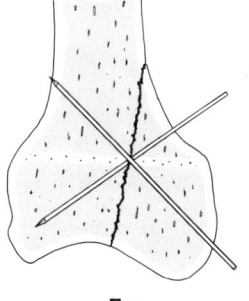

354 Fractures in children

THE ELBOW

While most fractures in this region are diagnosed on two standard radiographs, there will be some where doubt will exist. In such cases a true anteroposterior view of the humerus is essential and a radiograph of the opposite normal elbow will clarify the status of the epiphyseal centres. Only a small number of fractures around the elbow joint require operative treatment.

FRACTURE OF THE LATERAL CONDYLE OF THE ELBOW

6

This is a Salter–Harris Type IV fracture which passes vertically through the epiphysis and the metaphysis. It must not be called a fracture of the lateral epicondyle which has not usually ossified. The fracture of the condyle is intra-articular and the size of the fragment of bone seen on a radiograph is much smaller than the surprisingly large fragment of cartilage seen at operation. Undisplaced fractures require an above-elbow cast followed by check radiographs, as displacement may occur owing to the pull of the common extensor tendon if the wrist is not included in the cast. Since this is an intra-articular fracture with the possibility of non-union, malunion and growth arrest, then open reduction and internal fixation are necessary for all lateral condyle fractures with any displacement. The degree of displacement is difficult to determine when the ossific nucleus is small; if there is doubt it is better to perform an open reduction and internal fixation as results are generally better than those managed conservatively.

Position of patient

The patient should be placed supine with a tourniquet as high up the arm as possible. The arm is abducted to 90° and the forearm and hand are rested on a side-table.

Exposure

7 & 8

A straight vertical incision based on the lateral epicondyle is extended proximally over the supracondylar ridge and distally to the level of the head of the radius. The subcutaneous fat is incised and the fracture haematoma is washed out. The supracondylar ridge is palpated and incised accurately along its length. Using a scalpel, the origin of extensor carpi radialis longus and brachioradialis are lifted; a periosteal elevator is used to displace these muscles anteriorly, taking with them the radial nerve. Undue traction should not be exerted on this area as prolonged and powerful traction can cause a radial nerve palsy.

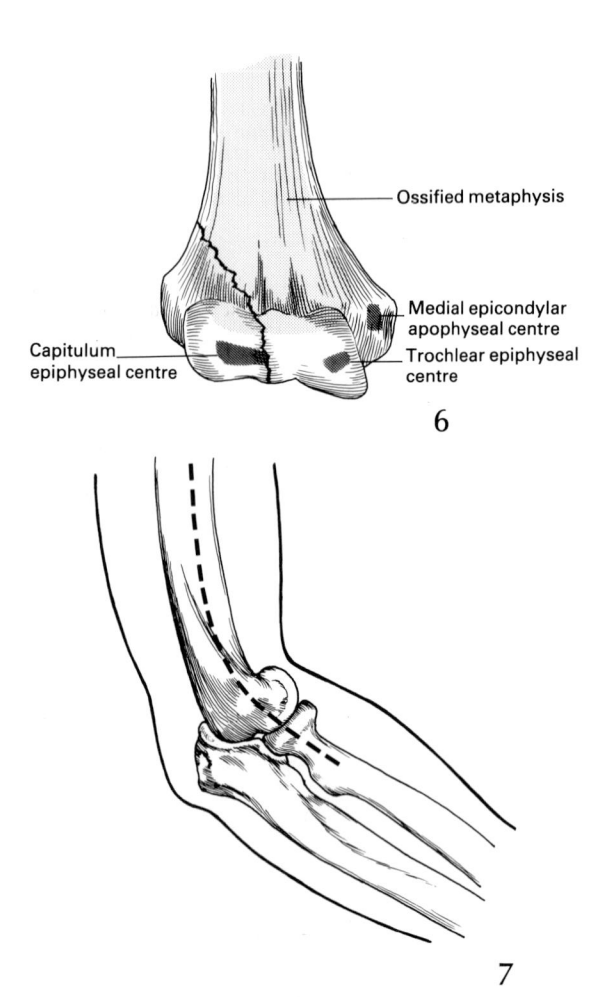

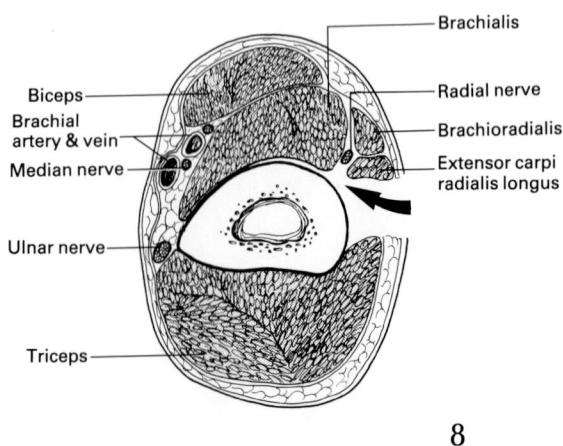

9

Posteriorly the medial head of triceps is elevated off the posterior surface of the supracondylar ridge. The proximal extent of the fracture is exposed and the soft tissue attachments to the fractured fragment are retained as much as possible in order to preserve the blood supply. This bony fragment may have been rotated through 180° and orientation may be confusing.

Division of the synovium anteriorly may be necessary to expose the joint into which a long-bladed retractor may be placed. This will expose the fracture of the metaphysis after washing the blood out of the joint. The fracture fragment is mobilized by blunt dissection and the fractured surface cleaned of all clots. The articular surface of the fragment will be visualized, thus helping with orientation. When both fracture surfaces have been cleaned, using a small curette and irrigation, they should be reduced and held with pointed bone-reduction forceps. It is easy to align a fracture surface along the supracondylar ridge, but it is also essential to check the alignment of the articular surface by looking across the anterior aspect of the exposed joint.

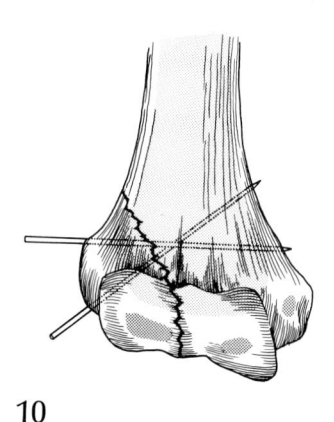

Internal fixation

10

A small longitudinal incision is made over the epicondyle, splitting the common extensor origin. Using a powered K-wire driver in one hand and steadying the fragment with the other, a wire is inserted into the lateral epicondyle and driven proximally and obliquely across the fracture into the medial cortex of the metaphysis. The position of the fracture is checked visually. A second Kirschner wire is inserted into the supracondylar ridge of the fragment a short distance above the other wire and it is driven more transversely across the metaphysis so that the wires cross. The bone-reduction forceps are removed, stability and reduction are checked, then the wires are cut off short, leaving them about 1 cm proud of the bone. They should not be so long that they protrude through the skin. A radiograph is taken to check the position of the pins.

Wound closure

The deep fascia is closed with interrupted absorbable sutures, as is the subcutaneous fat. The skin is closed with a subcuticular non-coloured absorbable synthetic suture. The tourniquet is released. A well-padded plaster of Paris backslab is applied from the upper arm down to include the wrist joint.

Postoperative management

The plaster backslab, if sufficiently strong, should be left in place for 3 weeks when mobilization is begun using a full-arm sling until the child is comfortable. The pins should be removed after 6 weeks. This may require general anaesthesia; however, occasionally they protrude through the skin and can easily be removed in the clinic.

FRACTURE OF THE MEDIAL EPICONDYLE

The medial epicondyle is an apophysis and is fractured by a valgus strain on the elbow joint associated with a contraction of the common flexor muscle. It is an extra-articular fracture and the radiograph may be confusing. It should not be confused with the rare intra-articular medial condyle fracture which transgresses the trochlea and which should be treated in a similar fashion to the lateral condyle fracture.

Fracture of the medial epicondyle occurs when the forearm is abducted. Initially the epicondyle is avulsed, further abduction may tear the medial capsule ligaments, the joint may then open up on the medial side and the bone fragment with its attached muscles may be dragged into the joint. If the joint then closes rapidly, the fragment is trapped. On an anteroposterior radiograph this fragment may be interpreted as an ossific nucleus for the trochlea; however, it must be remembered that the medial epicondyle appears before the trochlea and therefore if a trochlear nucleus is present on the radiograph there must be a medial epicondyle somewhere. Comparison with a radiograph of the other elbow is essential. The medial epicondyle lies slightly posteriorly and may be obscured by the metaphysis of the lower end of the humerus. The final event in the injury is complete abduction which produces a lateral dislocation of the joint.

These avulsion fractures may be subdivided into four groups for the purpose of treatment.

I. Minimal displacement
II. Displacement more than 3 mm
III. Medial epicondyle trapped within the joint
IV. Lateral dislocation of the elbow joint.

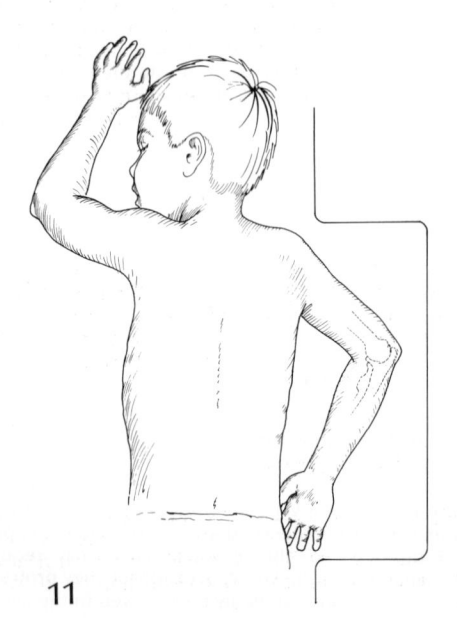

Indications for operation

Group I

In these injuries no operative treatment is necessary. A plaster of Paris backslab can be applied for 3 weeks.

Group II

A displaced fragment may indicate that the ligaments of the capsule and the stability of the joint have been disrupted. A general anaesthetic should be administered and the elbow stretched into valgus. If the displacement opens up, operation is indicated.

Group III

Although a trapped fragment may be retrieved from the joint by manipulation, the joint will still be unstable as the capsular ligaments will, by definition, be torn.

Group IV

Dislocation requires reduction and stabilization of the medial fragment.
Neurovascular damage is an indication for exploration.

Position of patient

The most commonly used position is with the patient supine, the table tilted towards the injured side and the arm resting on a side-table. The shoulder must be abducted, the arm laterally rotated and the elbow flexed to about 70°. However, this position can be quite awkward.

11

An alternative position is to have the patient prone with the arm abducted and medially rotated and resting on a table. The palm lies uppermost and the elbow is flexed about 50°–60°. It is essential to apply the tourniquet high on the arm and exsanguinate the limb by elevation before the patient is turned over to the prone position.

Some surgeons find it easier with the patient prone and the arm in a 'half-nelson' position resting across the back of the patient. In this case there is no necessity for a side-table.

11

Approach

12

The incision should be longitudinal and posterior to the epicondyle, so that it is hidden from view. The incision is started 2–3 cm proximal to the epicondyle and follows the bend of the elbow to a point overlying the common flexor muscle 2–3 cm distal to the epicondyle. The subcutaneous fat is divided down to the fascial layer overlying the flexor muscle. Using curved blunt scissors, the fat is dissected off the fascial layer to develop this plane which will be blood-stained. Working proximally the fragment will be found covered in haematoma unless it is trapped in the joint. Further proximally the medial supracondylar ridge is identified. The ulnar nerve is palpated with a finger and the fascia overlying it proximally is split. The nerve is followed proximally into the posterior aspect of the elbow and then distally into the flexor muscles. Extensive dissection of the nerve is not necessary; it only needs to be clearly identified, which can be done by gently passing a yellow 'vessel loop' around the nerve. If the bone fragment is locked in the joint, then extension of the elbow and a gentle valgus strain will allow the fragment to be retrieved. Throughout the procedure it is helpful to irrigate the joint to aid the identification of structures.

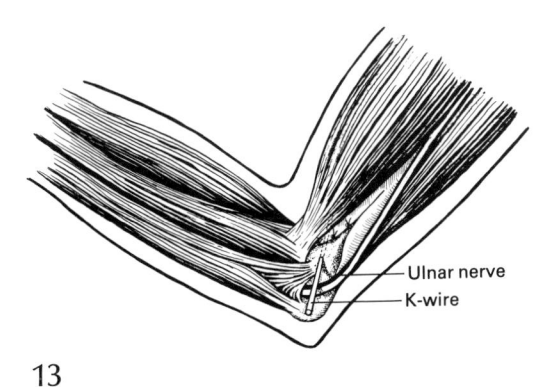

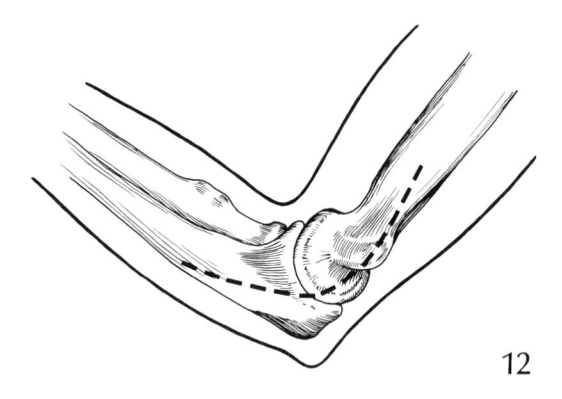

Reduction and fixation

13

The bone fragment usually falls back into position once it has been retrieved from the joint. Orientation is aided by the direction of the fibres of the flexor muscles. The elbow is flexed to relax the flexor muscles and the fragment is held in place with pointed bone-holding forceps. Care must be taken to ensure that the ulnar nerve is clear of the fracture line. A single Kirschner wire is mounted on a power-driven wire driver and, steadying the bone with one hand, the wire is driven obliquely through the fragment and into the metaphysis to lodge in the opposite cortex. The wire is cut short so that it does not protrude through the skin. One wire is usually sufficient to hold this fragment. Some surgeons prefer to suture the medial epicondyle back to the metaphysis using absorbable sutures, but a Kirschner wire is considered to be more stable.

Wound closure

The subcutaneous tissue is sutured with interrupted absorbable material. A subcuticular absorbable suture is used for the skin. A well-padded plaster back-slab is applied from the upper arm down to the palm of the hand, holding the elbow at 90° of flexion, the forearm pronated and the wrist joint minimally flexed.

Postoperative management

The plaster is removed at 3 weeks and the arm is rested in a full-arm sling until the child is confident enough to start mobilization. The Kirschner wire will need removing at about 6 weeks, if it has not worked loose through the skin before.

NECK OF THE RADIUS

The ossification centre for the head of the radius appears at 5 years and the growth-plate closes between 14 and 17 years. A fracture through the articular surface is rare and virtually all fractures involve the neck of the radius. This may be either a Salter–Harris Type II passing through the growth-plate together with a small piece of the metaphysis, or a complete metaphyseal fracture. The latter is more common since the cartilaginous growth-plate hugs the metaphysis like a cap. The blood supply to the growth-plate enters the metaphysis proximal to the usual level of fracture and consequently avascular necrosis of the head is rarely seen[2].

Two types of deformity can be identified[3].

A lateral tilt of the radial head is caused by a valgus strain. This may be associated with an injury on the medial side, for example rupture of the medial ligament, avulsion of the medial epicondyle or a fracture of the olecranon.

A 90° backward tilt of the radial head usually occurs through the growth-plate and is associated with posterior dislocation of the elbow.

Associated fractures occur in 50 per cent of injuries and a careful search must be made of the olecranon, shaft of the ulna, medial epicondyle and the capitulum.

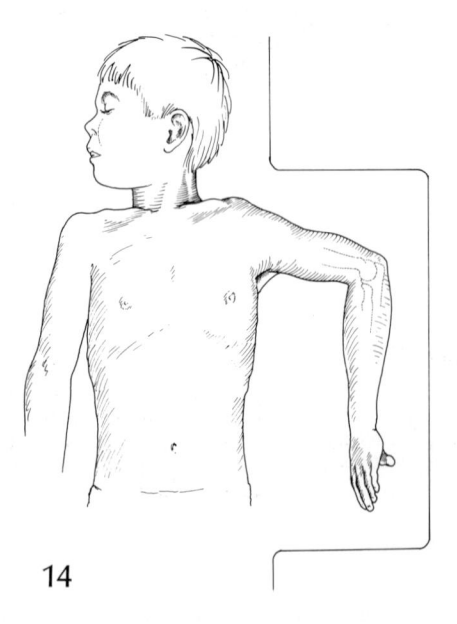

Treatment

Treatment depends mainly on the degree of displacement and/or angulation of the head of the radius.

1. For angulation of up to 30° in children under 10 years and up to 20° in those over 10 years, reduction is not necessary. The arm is protected in a full-arm cast for 3 weeks.
2. Angulation greater than the above should be treated by early manipulation followed by a long-arm plaster cast for 3 weeks.
3. Completely displaced fractures and those rare fractures that cannot be reduced to under 45° of angulation require open reduction[4,5]. The results of manipulation and surgery after 5 days are uniformly poor[4,5,6].

After open reduction, internal fixation is not necessarily required as most fractures are now stable. Since internal fixation is difficult and may produce problems, it is prudent to fix only those that appear unstable[5].

Operative hazards

The posterior interosseous nerve is vulnerable during the exposure. It may be divided or may undergo a traction lesion owing to the heavy use of retractors. Care must be taken to ensure the assistant is paying due attention to this nerve. It is helpful to pronate the forearm during the operation as this relaxes the associated muscles. It is important not to continue the incision more distally than the neck of the radius.

Position of patient

14

The patient lies supine, the shoulder is abducted to 90° and the elbow flexed to 90° with the arm resting on a padded table. The forearm is pronated. A pneumatic cuff is applied as high as possible on the arm.

Incision

15

The incision starts over the supracondylar ridge of the humerus and extends distally to the tip of the lateral epicondyle. It then curves forward to cross the posterior aspect of the head of the radius and may continue 1–2 cm distally through the skin only.

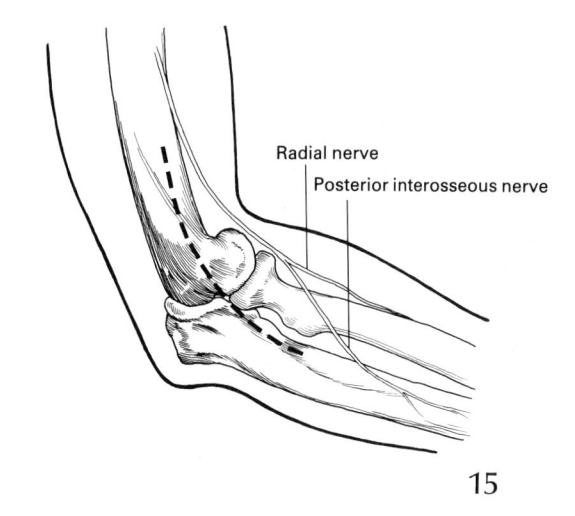

Exposure

16

The fascia is cleared of the overlying fat by blunt dissection. The incision along the supracondylar ridge is deepened through the fascia extending distally to the lateral epicondyle. The musculotendinous attachments are reflected anteriorly by sharp dissection. Distally the line between the extensor carpi ulnaris and the anconeus is followed. It is important not to dissect distally beyond the annular ligament which is not divided unless it is necessary to achieve reduction. The fibres of the supinator which cross the neck may be *gently* retracted distally. The surgeon should be constantly aware of the proximity of the posterior interosseous nerve. The synovium is opened to expose the radio-ulnar joint.

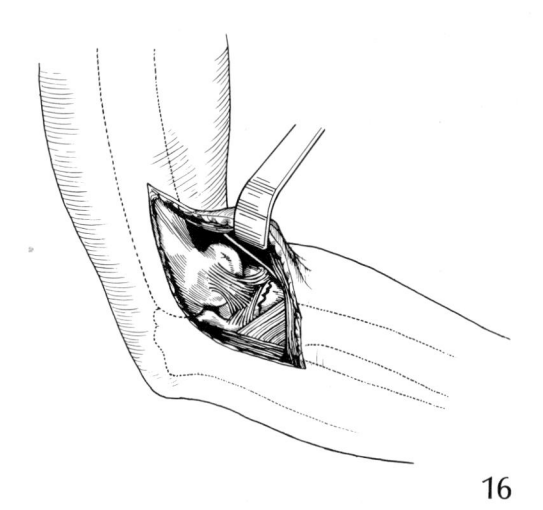

Reduction

The forearm is supinated from its hitherto pronated position to allow the maximum tilt to be exposed. Gentle pressure with the thumb while rotating will reduce the fragment. Occasionally it may be necessary to lever the radial head back into position using a MacDonald dissector. The stability can be tested by moving the elbow joint under visual control. If it is stable, then no more need be done although it is possible to pass an absorbable suture through the periosteum in order to ensure stability of the fracture.

Wound closure

Interrupted absorbable sutures are used to close both the musculofascial layer and the subcutaneous layer. An absorbable suture is used for the skin. A plaster backslab is applied which includes the wrist joint, and holds the elbow at 90° and the forearm in mid-rotation.

UNSTABLE OR SEVERELY DISPLACED FRACTURES

If the head of the radius can be reduced but is unstable, it will be necessary to provide some means of internal fixation. This is difficult.

17

After reduction of the fracture, a 2 mm Kirschner wire may be driven into the posterior aspect of the capitulum and, with the elbow flexed at 90°, the wire should be passed through the radial head and down the shaft of the radius for about 5 cm.

It is difficult to ensure that the wire exits from the anterior aspect of the capitulum in the correct position. In order to achieve some accuracy, small bone-holding forceps (or a towel clip) can be used as a guide. One arm of the forceps is placed in the elbow joint resting on the capitulum at the desired point of exit and the other arm of the forceps is used to indicate the entry point into the posterior aspect of the capitulum. The wire is driven through the capitulum in the plane of the forceps; it should exit at the tip of the forceps, and is then driven across the radial head and down the radius. The wire is cut short and the end bent to 90° to stop distal migration. A plaster cast must be applied otherwise the wire will bend and may break.

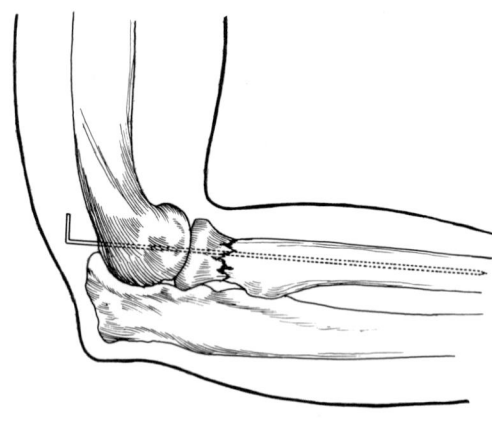

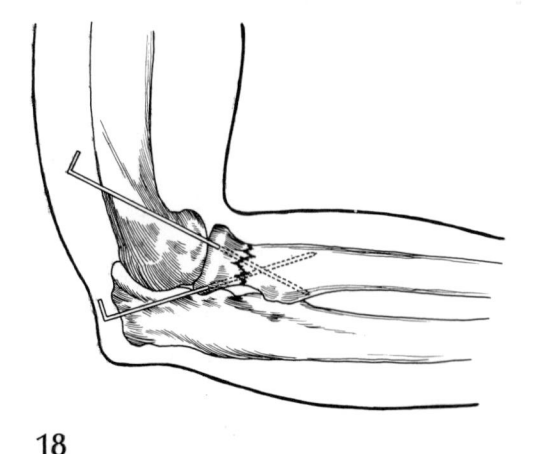

18

In view of the possible risk of the wire breaking as the elbow joint is moved, another method of fixation is described, although the accurate placement of these wires is difficult. With the forearm in neutral rotation an oblique wire is passed across the distal surface of the capitulum so that it enters the posterior aspect of the radial head, crosses the fracture and enters the anterior cortex of the metaphysis. A second wire is passed from the lateral side, along the lateral epicondyle and enters the radial head on its lateral side, passing across the fracture and entering the metaphysis of the radius on the medial side.

Postoperative management

An above-elbow cast, which includes the wrist, held in neutral rotation, is maintained for 3 weeks when a closed reduction or an open reduction without fixation has been performed. The use of absorbable skin sutures in children makes suture removal unnecessary. After removal of the cast, a radiographic assessment should be made to establish the state of union of the fracture. If progress is satisfactory, then a full-arm sling is applied for a further week, allowing gentle rotation of the forearm. If the radiograph does not show adequate union, then the cast must be maintained for a further 2 weeks.

If internal fixation has been performed, then union may be delayed. The wires are removed at 3 weeks and an above-elbow cast maintained for a further 2 weeks, followed by a sling for 2 weeks, encouraging active rotation of the forearm.

Complications

Complications are much less common in fractures managed by closed reduction. Restriction of rotation is more common after internal fixation and it is for this reason that the forearm should always be immobilized in the mid-rotation position, which is a more useful position if stiffness does occur.

Synostosis

This is uncommon. However, the proximal ends of the radius and ulna are extremely close and surgical interference in this region may be a factor in this complication.

Avascular necrosis

Avascular necrosis of the whole of the head of the radius is rarely seen, even in completely displaced fractures; however, necrosis of part of the head may be more frequent[2]. Open reduction is associated with a higher incidence[5]. When an open reduction is performed, care must be taken not to displace the radial head further. Excision of the radial head should not be performed in a child; it may be undertaken after growth has ceased and this may increase the rotation of the forearm.

Non-union

This is rare and may be due to soft tissue interposition or the radial head being placed back to front at open reduction.

362   Fractures in children

FEMORAL NECK

Fracture of the femoral neck in the child is uncommon and is usually caused by significant violence, for example falling from a height or a road accident. Other injuries must, therefore, be suspected.

Classification

19

The fractures are classified according to the anatomical location.

Transepiphyseal   An acute traumatic separation of a previous normal epiphysis.

Transcervical   A fracture across the mid-portion of the femoral neck.

Cervicotrochanteric or basal   A fracture across the base of the femoral neck.

Pertrochanteric   A fracture between the base of the femoral neck and the greater trochanter.

Undisplaced transcervical and basal cervical fractures are treated by a one-and-a-half hip spica for 8–12 weeks. However, repeat radiographs are essential to check that displacement is not occurring.

Pertrochanteric fractures are treated on traction followed by a one-and-a-half hip spica.

Indications for operation

1. Displaced transcervical and basal cervical fractures.
2. Transepiphyseal fractures.

The aim of surgical treatment is to obtain an anatomical reduction and to hold that reduction with multiple small pins. A trifin nail, as was commonly used for adult femoral fractures, must not be used in the child because the bone is particularly hard and the nail will separate the fracture fragments.

If adequate reduction cannot be achieved or maintained or if, on reduction, Pauwels' angle is greater than 60° then a primary valgus subtrochanteric osteotomy is recommended[7,8].

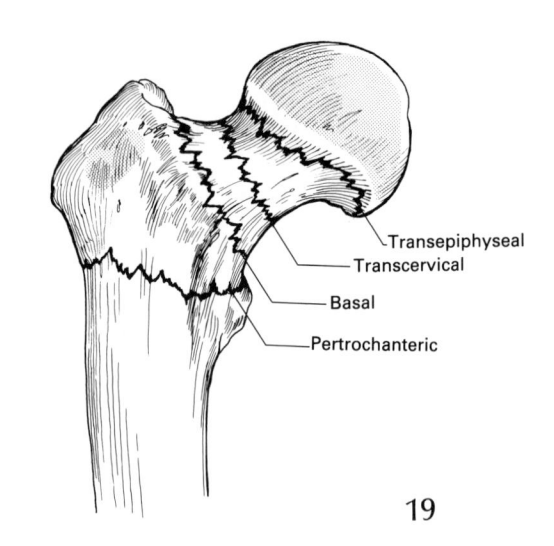

19

Transepiphyseal
Transcervical
Basal
Pertrochanteric

Position of patient

The anaesthetized child is placed on a fracture table. The uninjured limb is strapped into the foot support. The fractured limb is held with the hip and knee flexed, gentle traction is applied and the limb is gently rotated medially. It is held in this position by the foot support. The image intensifier is used in the anteroposterior and lateral positions to check the reduction. Repeated manipulation is not advised and if a good reduction cannot be achieved by closed means, then it is necessary to open the joint and reduce the fracture under direct vision.

Incision

A straight incision is made centred over the greater trochanter starting about 2 cm above the tip of the trochanter and extending distally for 10–12 cm. The fascia lata is incised longitudinally in the distal part of the wound and then a finger is introduced beneath this fascia to separate it from the underlying vastus lateralis muscle. Scissors are used to split the fascia lata proximally and a self-retaining retractor is inserted to hold the two sides of the fascia apart. The vastus lateralis is now exposed and it is split in the line of its fibres to expose the underlying upper part of the femoral shaft. If further exposure is required then a transverse incision is made across the base of the greater trochanter to form a T-shaped incision. Two small bone levers may be placed around the femoral shaft to provide retraction of this muscle.

20

If the fracture has not been reduced by closed methods, then the anterior capsule of the hip joint should be exposed. The position of the femoral neck is palpated. A periosteal elevator is used gently to lift the reflected head of the rectus femoris and the psoas muscle off the anterior capsule which is incised in line with the neck of the femur. This will release the haemarthrosis and the fracture can then be palpated. The femoral shaft is distracted laterally, the foot may have to be released from the foot support by an unscrubbed assistant and the femoral neck is reduced onto the femoral head.

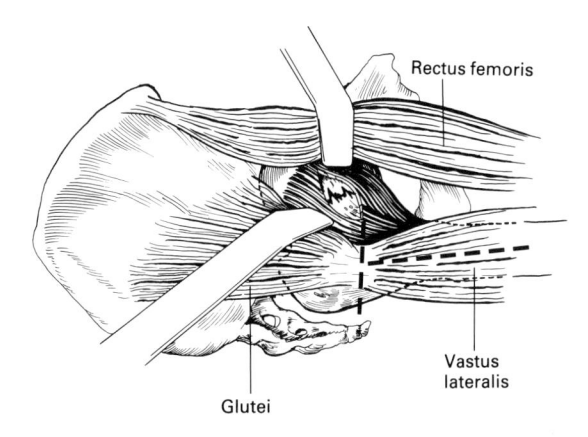

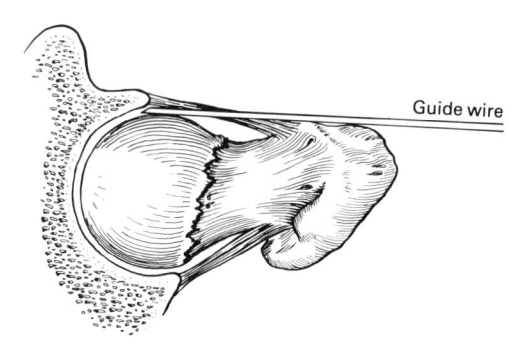

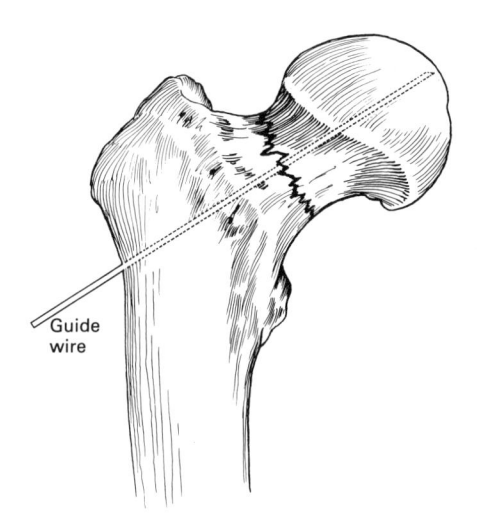

21a & b

A guide wire is mounted on a T-handle and, resting on the anterior edge of the femur, the wire is passed along the centre of the anterior surface of the femoral neck. The point of the wire will pass gently onto the femoral head. This wire will give an indication of the anteversion in the horizontal plane, and an anteroposterior view with the image intensifier will allow this wire to be placed centrally over the femoral neck. Another guide wire is now mounted on a power drill. The lateral surface of the upper femoral shaft is exposed and, using the first wire as a guide, the second wire is driven through the centre of the upper femur parallel to the first wire. If the fracture is transepiphyseal or a high transcervical fracture, then the wire should be driven across the epiphyseal plate into the epiphysis. It should not enter the hip joint. If the fracture is basal cervical then the wire should stop just short of the epiphyseal plate. The length is checked with the image intensifier and a lateral view is now taken to check its position in the horizontal plane. The first wire is now removed.

The lateral surface of the upper femur is mapped out so that three pins can be evenly placed in a triangular fashion. A threaded pin (Knowles pin) is now mounted on a power drill and inserted through the lateral cortex in the pre-planned position, and driven up to the fracture site parallel to the guide wire. The power drill is now taken off the Knowles pin and the pin advanced using a hand chuck. If the fracture is transepiphyseal or a high transcervical fracture, then this pin will have to cross the epiphyseal plate but must not penetrate this joint. Owing to the spherical nature of the femoral head, a pin can be protruding into the joint but appear on the radiograph as if it is in the head. To safeguard against this possibility, the point of the pins should be at least 5 mm from the bony margin[9]. If the fracture is a low transcervical or basal type then the pin should not cross the epiphyseal plate. A second Knowles pin is inserted parallel to the other one and the guide wire using the same technique. The guide wire is now removed and replaced with a third Knowles pin by the same technique. Each pin is inserted under radiographic control.

Knowles pins

22

Wound closure

If the capsule of the joint has been opened it is not closed. The fascia over the vastus lateralis is sutured with an absorbable suture, reattaching it, if necessary, to the greater trochanter. A small suction drain is inserted. The fascia lata is repaired with a continuous absorbable strong material. The subcutaneous layer is sutured with interrupted absorbable material and the skin is closed with a subcuticular absorbable suture. A well-padded one-and-a-half hip spica is now applied.

Postoperative management

A check radiograph is taken in the Radiology Department (in order to obtain high-quality films). The hip spica is left in place for 10–12 weeks. The child should not bear weight during this period. A second check radiograph should be taken 2 weeks postoperatively to see that the fracture has not displaced, despite the insertion of pins.

At 10–12 weeks the plaster may be bivalved, the child taken out of the cast, anteroposterior and lateral radiographs taken, and the child placed back in the posterior half of the hip spica until a decision has been made concerning mobilization. If the fracture appears sound then mobilization, initially with partial weight-bearing, should be started. However, if union is not complete, then a further period in plaster without weight-bearing should follow. Union of the transcervical fractures may be slow. The pins should be removed once union is complete and before 12 months.

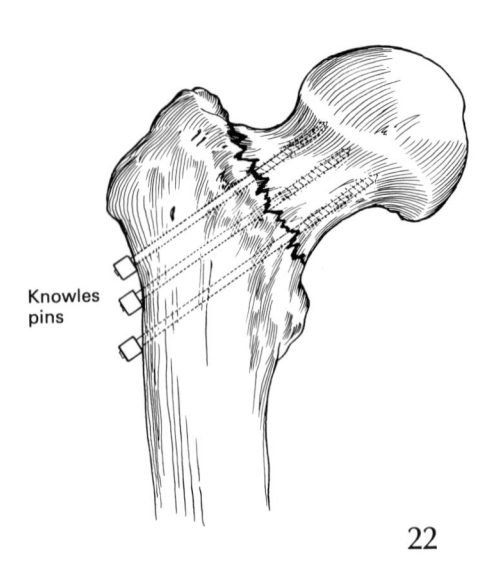

Complications

Despite meticulous care, a complication rate of 60 per cent is reported when multiple papers are combined.

Avascular necrosis

Displaced transepiphyseal fractures have a poor prognosis with 80 per cent undergoing avascular necrosis. However, transcervical and basal fractures have an incidence of 34 per cent and 27 per cent respectively[8]. Extreme abduction of the hip must be avoided as this will interfere with an already compromised blood supply to the femoral head.

Coxa vara

This is common and may be caused by the following.

1. Failure to reduce the fracture
2. Loss of alignment owing to inadequate immobilization or delayed union
3. Premature closure of the epiphysis.

Premature epiphyseal fusion

This results in total leg shortening and also in coxa vara.

Delayed union and non-union

These develop commonly in transcervical fractures when Pauwels' angle is greater than 60°. Primary subtrochanteric osteotomy will reduce this risk.

The pins used for internal fixation may hold the fracture apart if they are crossed. The pins should be parallel to each other.

THE ANKLE

FRACTURES AROUND THE MEDIAL MALLEOLUS

These fractures involve the articular surface to varying degrees and they may be classified as Salter–Harris Types II, III or IV. It is necessary to restore joint congruity and to realign the epiphyseal plate so that growth deformity does not occur. This may be done by closed reduction but failure to achieve the above aims necessitates operation. In the triplane fracture, growth disorder is not a problem as the fracture occurs when the growth-plate is partially closed; however, it is more difficult to achieve a good alignment of the fragment which is necessary to restore joint congruity[10].

Indications for operation

23

1. A large medial malleolar fragment.
2. Fractures through the articular surface where, after closed reduction, a gap or a step greater than 2 mm remains.
3. Salter–Harris Type IV fractures where the growth-plate of the fragment does not align with that of the tibia.

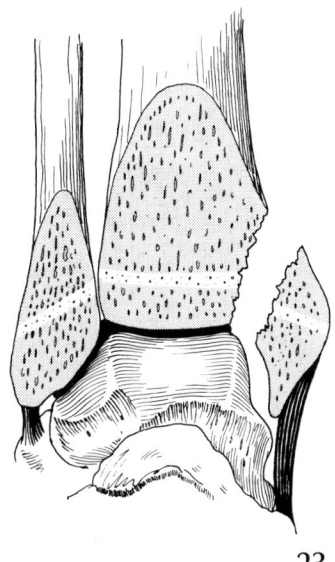

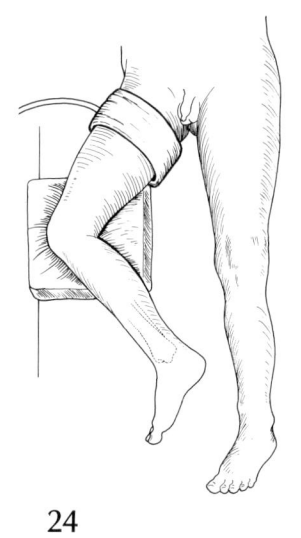

Position of patient

24

A pneumatic tourniquet is applied to the thigh. The patient lies supine with the knee flexed at 45° and the hip laterally rotated. The medial side of the ankle then lies uppermost. The knee rests on a well-padded support.

366 Fractures in children

Incision

25a

The usual incision is J-shaped and commences along the posterior border of the lower tibia and curves anteriorly distal to the tip of the malleolus. It follows the line of the posterior tibial vessels and nerve. It is carried distally as far as the navicular bone. The incision is deepened to the deep fascia and then the flap of skin is dissected anteriorly staying on the fascial layer. Care should be taken to lift the saphenous vein and nerve forward with the skin flap.

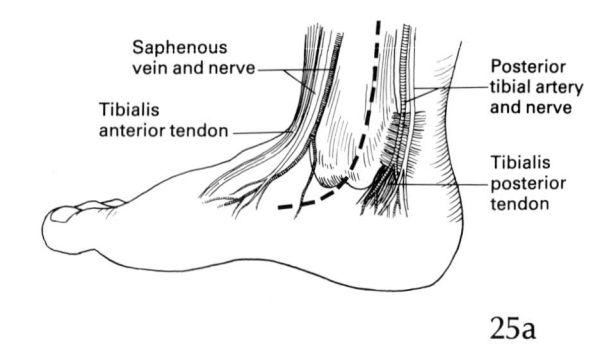

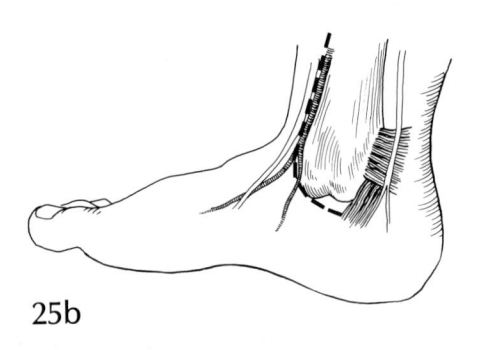

25a

25b

The incision may be reversed so that it starts on the anterior border of the medial malleolus and curves backwards below the tip of the malleolus. This gives better exposure of the fracture and allows entry into the anterior aspect of the joint. However, particular care should be taken to avoid the saphenous vein and nerve.

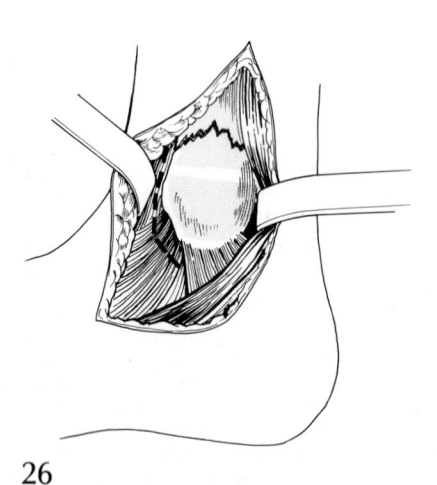

26

The medial malleolus is now exposed and the fracture will be obvious. It may be necessary to mobilize the tibialis anterior by incising along the medial border of the extensor retinaculum. If the posterior aspect needs to be displayed, then the flexor retinaculum is incised along the posterior border of the medial malleolus. A periosteal elevator is used to elevate the tendons and a bone lever is placed on the posterior surface of the tibia. The tendons will protect the neurovascular structures. It is necessary to open the joint to visualize the articular surface. This is done anteriorly along the line of the tibialis anterior. The capsule is opened in a longitudinal direction and the incision can be carried a short distance across the anterior aspect of the deltoid ligament. By plantarflexion of the ankle the articular surface will be exposed. It is important not to detach the deltoid ligament from the medial malleolus as the blood supply to that fragment of bone is contained within that ligament.

The joint is washed out and the edges of the fracture cleaned with a periosteal elevator and a fine curette. Reduction is then achieved. It is sometimes useful to use a small bonehook to pull the fragment back into position.

Fixation of the fragment

27

The fracture is held in place with pointed bone-holding forceps. A Kirschner wire is mounted on a powered K-wire driver. The wire is introduced near the anterior aspect of the tip of the malleolus and it is passed obliquely proximally, laterally and in a slightly posterior direction to gain a good fixation within the metaphysis. A second Kirschner wire is introduced slightly more posteriorly on the tip of the medial malleolus and passed laterally and in a more horizontal direction than the first Kirschner wire. If there is a large metaphyseal fragment then a horizontal wire can be passed through this fragment into the lateral cortex of the tibia as well. A check radiograph is taken on the operating table to ensure that reduction is adequate and that the wires are correctly placed.

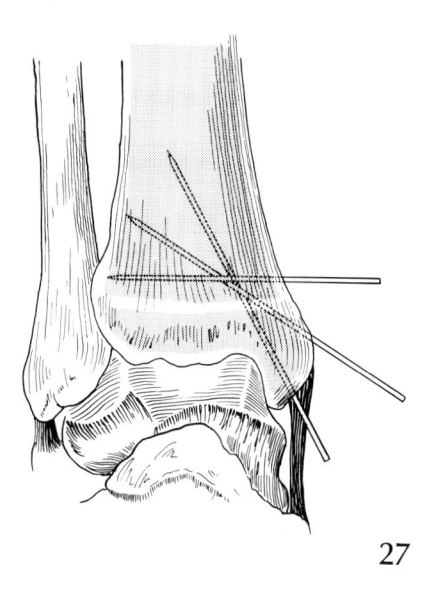

28

If the fracture of the medial malleolus is a Salter–Harris Type III, then only two wires will be used. One will pass across the growth-plate into the metaphysis, the other should pass transversely into the epiphysis.

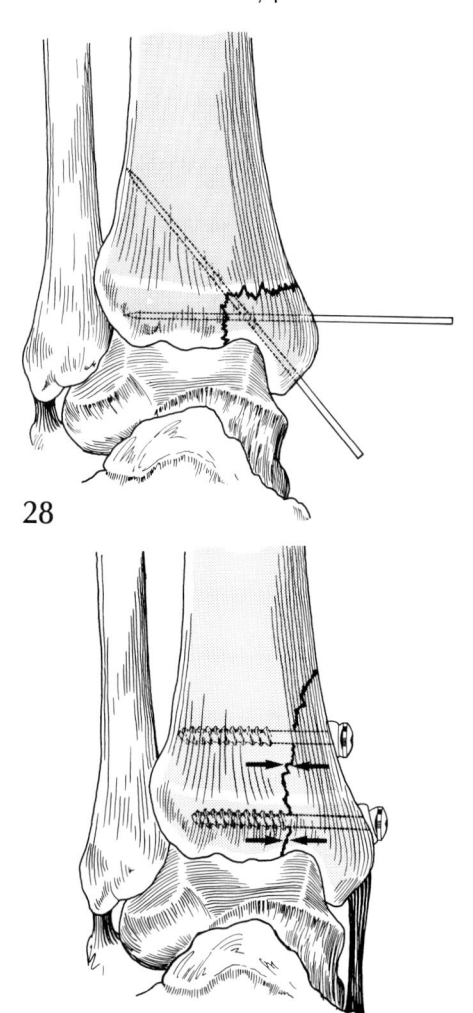

29

In the older child where there is a large metaphyseal fragment, two compressions screws may be used. The AO 3.5 mm screw is ideally suited for this purpose. The fragment is reduced and held with pointed bone-holding forceps. A 2 mm Kirschner wire is inserted through the metaphyseal fragment into the metaphysis in a horizontal direction and at right angles to the fracture line. This wire is left in place. A second 2 mm Kirschner wire is inserted through the epiphyseal portion of the fragment into the epiphysis of the tibia, parallel to the joint surface. It must not cross the epiphyseal plate nor must it enter the joint. A radiograph is taken to check the reduction and the position of the wires. The bone-holding forceps are reapplied and the proximal Kirschner wire is removed leaving a 2 mm hole. The depth is measured, the hole is tapped, the near cortex only is overdrilled with a 3.5 mm drill, and a 3.5 mm screw of the appropriate length, with washer, is inserted. This will compress the metaphyseal fragment using the lag-screw principle. The distal Kirschner wire is now removed and the procedure repeated.

Wound closure

The capsule and synovium are closed with an absorbable suture. The skin is closed with interrupted fine absorbable material. A well-padded plaster backslab is applied with the foot held in a plantigrade position.

Postoperative management

The foot is elevated for 48 hours. A check radiograph is performed. The child is then allowed to mobilize but without weight-bearing. The wound is inspected at 7–10 days and then a below-knee plaster cast is applied and the child remains without weight-bearing for a total period of 6 weeks from operation. The cast is then removed, a check radiograph is taken to assess union and mobilization with weight-bearing started if union is sound. The metal work should be removed after 12 weeks or when union is complete.

Complications

Non-union

Soft tissue interposition in the fracture gap may lead to non-union. Failure to reduce the fragment accurately by closed means indicates that soft tissue may have become interposed and operation is necessary.

Partial growth arrest

This may lead to cessation of growth on the medial side with subsequent varus deformity of the ankle. It is essential to realign both the epiphyseal cartilage and the articular cartilage in the Salter–Harris Type IV injury. However, there may have been some crushing element to the growth-plate and therefore follow-up of this fracture is essential.

References

1. Salter RB, Harris RW. Injuries involving the epiphyseal plate. *J Bone Joint Surg [Am]* 1963; 45-A: 587–622.
2. Rang M. *Children's fractures*, 2nd ed. Philadelphia: Lippincott, 1983.
3. Jeffrey CC. Fractures of the head of the radius in children. *J Bone Joint Surg [Br]* 1950; 32-B: 314–24.
4. Tibone JE, Stoltz M. Fractures of the radial head and neck in children. *J Bone Joint Surg [Am]* 1981; 63-A: 100–6.
5. Newman JH. Displaced radial neck fractures in children. *Injury* 1977; 9: 114–21.
6. McBride ED, Monnet J. Epiphyseal fractures of the head of the radius in children. *Clin Orthop* 1960; 16: 264–71.
7. Ratliff AHC. Fractures of the neck of the femur in children. *J Bone Joint Surg [Br]* 1962; 44-B: 528–42.
8. Tachdjian MO. *Paediatric orthopaedics*. Philadelphia: Saunders, 1972.
9. Pollen AG. Fallacies in the interpretation of radiographs during nailing of the neck of the femur. *Proc R Soc Med* 1965; 58: 329–31.
10. Spiegel PG, Mast JW, Cooperman DR, Laros GS. Triplane fractures of the distal tibial epiphysis. *Clin Orthop* 1984; 188: 74–89.

Illustrations by Paul Richardson

Delayed union, non-union and malunion of long-bone fractures

G. S. E. Dowd MD, MChOrth, FRCS
Consultant Orthopaedic Surgeon, St Bartholomew's and Homerton Hospitals, London, UK

George Bentley ChM, FRCS
Professor of Orthopaedic Surgery, Institute of Orthopaedics, University of London; Honorary Consultant Orthopaedic Surgeon, The Royal National Orthopaedic Hospital, Stanmore, Middlesex, and the Middlesex Hospital, London, UK

Introduction

Complications associated with fracture management are not uncommon. These problems include delayed union and non-union and also malunion of the fracture. While it is not possible to describe in great detail the management of these problems, the basic principles of treatment are described.

DELAYED UNION AND NON-UNION

There is no precise definition of delayed union of a fracture. In practical terms, a useful rule is that any fracture failing to unite at the average time for that specific fracture demonstrates delayed union. Clinically, the fracture fragments are mobile on stressing, and the appearance of the fracture line remains on the radiograph. Delayed union does not inevitably result in non-union; altering the stability of the fracture or revascularization of the ends of the fracture may lead to union.

Non-union may follow delayed union and is identified clinically, if mobile, and by radiography when a gap remains at the fracture site. There are two types of non-union: hypertrophic and atrophic. In the former, there is abundant callus from the fracture ends without bony bridging of the fragments, while in the latter there is no callus formation.

The most important causes of delayed union and non-union are inadequate immobilization for too short a time and avascularity of one or other end of the fracture. Other associated factors include soft tissue interposition in the fracture, distraction of the fragments by excessive traction, bone infection and gross periosteal stripping in high-velocity injuries.

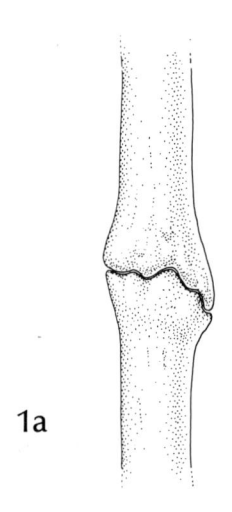

Hypertrophic non-union

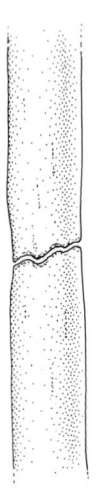

1a

A fracture in which delayed union or non-union occurs may have fracture ends with hypertrophic periosteal callus which has failed to bridge the fracture gap. The mechanisms of callus formation have been triggered, but because of excessive movement at the fracture site, the fracture bridging effect has failed.

By making the fracture fixation more rigid, a large percentage of these fractures will unite. In some cases, non-operative treatment should be prolonged, provided cast fixation can be improved. Full weight-bearing also facilitates healing. The disadvantages of this method of treatment include joint stiffness and disuse osteoporosis from prolonged immobilization. Also, prolonged hospitalization and absence from work may be significant factors in continued conservative treatment.

An alternative approach, is to reduce the period of conservative treatment by rendering the fracture site immobile by fixation using plates and screws or intramedullary nails. The advantages of this approach are that stability can be achieved and adjacent joints mobilized. The potential complications include infection and inadequate or inept fracture fixation.

Atrophic non-union

1b

A fracture in which very little callus can be seen and in which movement can still be identified despite an acceptable period of immobilization, is described as atrophic delayed union or non-union. The four mechanisms of periosteal, endosteal, medullary and cortical osteogenesis have failed. This type of non-union is frequently caused by avascularity of bone fragments and loss of the periosteal sleeve. While it is true that many fractures with atrophic delayed unions will proceed to union with prolonged immobilization, it is possible to stimulate union with onlay cancellous bone grafting. If fibrous ingrowth has made the fracture stable with regard to movement, then a cancellous bone graft with plaster fixation may be sufficient. If there is excessive movement at the fracture site, then internal fixation using a plate or intramedullary nail should supplement the bone graft.

1a

1b

Delayed union, non-union and malunion of long-bone fractures 371

Operative approaches

ANTEROLATERAL BONE GRAFTING OF THE TIBIA

Position of patient

2

The patient lies supine on the operating table with a sandbag under the buttock to allow medial rotation of the lower limb and to bring the iliac crest into prominence. Both the iliac crest and the leg are cleaned and draped. A tourniquet is applied to the thigh.

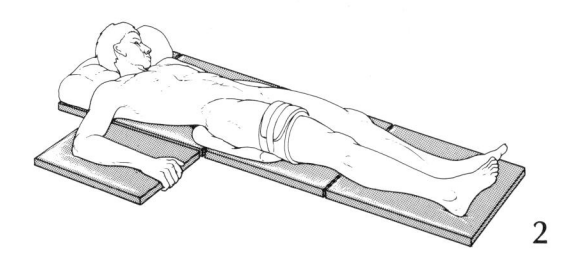

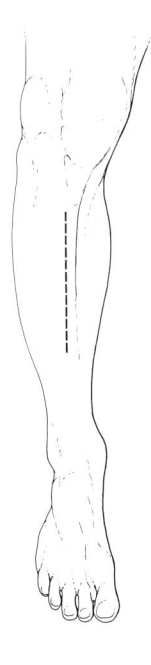

Incision

3

The skin incision is vertical, 1 cm lateral to the crest of the tibia.

Procedure

4a

The deep fascia is divided to the lateral side of the tibial crest, and the junction between the tibia and the tibialis anterior muscle identified. The periosteum is divided longitudinally anterior to the muscle, above and below the pseudarthrosis, and dissected off the bone. Two bone levers are applied round the posterolateral aspect of the tibia to retract the muscle and periosteum from the bone.

4b & c

Cancellous bone graft is taken from the ipsilateral iliac crest (see below) and stored in damp saline swabs. Strips of corticocancellous bone graft and also cancellous chips may be used to surround the site of non-union. There is still debate on whether removal of fibrous tissue from the fracture gap and replacement by cancellous graft is necessary. In general, with atrophic non-union the bone ends should be cleared of fibrous tissue and dead bone. The medullary cavity and the ends are packed gently with small cancellous bone chips, and corticocancellous strips are placed around the fracture. If stability is required then the fracture is fixed with a suitable plate. With a hypertrophic non-union the callus is trimmed to allow application of a six-hole compression plate, and a small amount of cancellous graft is placed around the fracture.

Closure

The periosteum is closed over the bone and graft with interrupted absorbable sutures. The deep fascia is loosely closed with interrupted absorbable sutures after insertion of a small-bore suction drain. Interrupted non-absorbable sutures are used to close the skin.

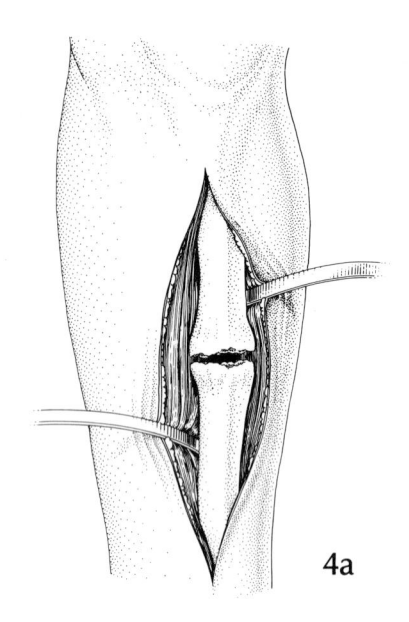

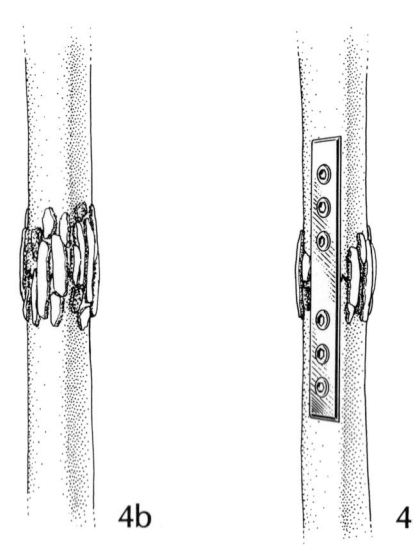

Postoperative management

The leg is placed in a well-padded above-knee plaster which is split to the skin to allow for swelling of the limb. The drain is removed at 24 hours. A further plaster is applied to the limb at about 10 days after operation, following removal of the sutures. Partial weight-bearing with crutches for 8 weeks is followed by full weight-bearing in a below-knee patellar tendon-bearing cast until union has occurred. Serial radiographs of the fracture should be obtained to show when union of the fracture has occurred.

Delayed union, non-union and malunion of long-bone fractures 373

POSTEROLATERAL (TRANSFIBULAR) BONE GRAFTING OF THE TIBIA

In many cases of delayed union and non-union of fractures of the tibia, the skin over the anterior middle two-thirds is either scarred or the site of a split-skin graft. In order to avoid a further skin incision into the damaged skin, the posterolateral approach to the tibia may be used for either bone grafting or plating the tibia.

Position of patient

5

The patient lies prone with a well-padded tourniquet around the thigh. The posterior iliac crest is prepared and draped as well as the leg and foot.

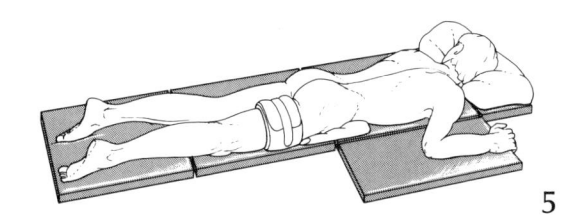

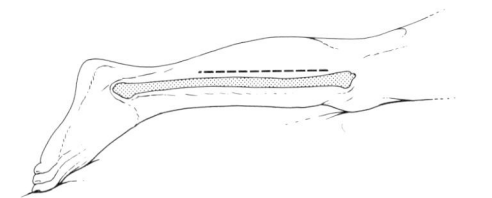

Incision

6

A vertical incision is made in the skin, behind and parallel to the posterolateral border of the fibula. The skin edges are raised about 2.5 cm along both sides of the wound to reveal the fascial line between the posterior intermuscular septum and the deep fascia.

Exposure

7a

An incision is made through the deep fascia behind the posterolateral intermuscular septum. The plane between gastrocnemius, soleus and flexor hallucis longus posteriorly, and the peroneal muscles and fibula anteriorly, is developed. The tibialis posterior is dissected off the posterior interosseous membrane until the lateral border of the tibia is identified. The posterior tibial nerve and artery are protected behind the tibialis posterior muscle. The anterior tibial artery is protected by the interosseous membrane.

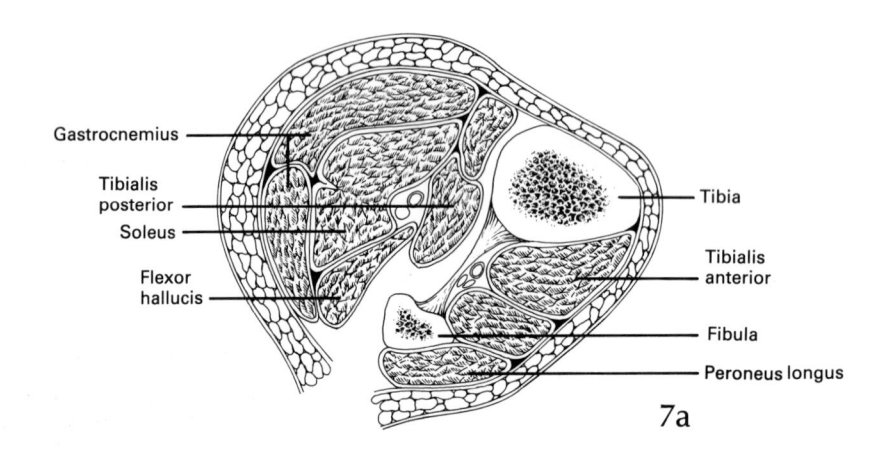

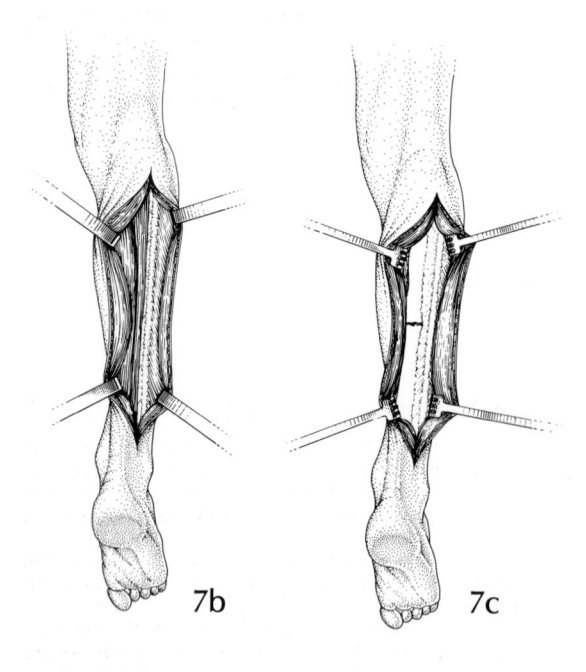

7b & c

The periosteum of the tibia is divided longitudinally and stripped off the bone together with part of the flexor digitorum muscle. Bone levers passed subperiosteally around the medial edge of the tibia allow the muscle mass to be retracted, enabling procedures on the posterior aspect of the tibia to be performed.

Bone grafting is then performed as for the anterior procedures.

Closure

The tourniquet is released and haemostasis secured. A small-bore drain is inserted through a separate skin incision. The deep fascia is closed with interrupted absorbable sutures and the skin with interrupted non-absorbable sutures.

Postoperative management

This is similar to management after the anterior approach to the tibia.

Bone grafting

The most frequently used sources of bone graft are from the patient's own iliac crest, upper tibial metaphysis, distal end of radius or from the ribs. The source of the greatest volume of cancellous bone is the posterior aspect of the ilium, but frequently the patient is lying supine to facilitate access to the fracture and, in these cases, the anterior iliac crest is more accessible. Bone graft is of two types, cortical and cancellous. Cortical bone has been used historically because it is strong and can be used to provide stability to the fracture by screwing it across the fracture gap. The disadvantage of cortical bone is that it is only weakly osteogenic and is dead bone which may undergo resorption and can only be very slowly revascularized. It is also more prone to infection. Cancellous bone is structurally weak, but is the most osteogenic, stimulating new bone formation across the fracture gap and, because of its open trabecular structure, is rapidly reossified.

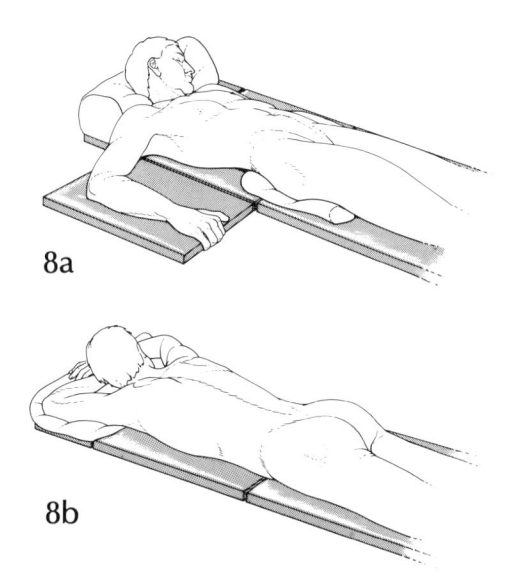

8a

8b

OBTAINING ILIAC BONE FOR GRAFTING

Position of patient

8a & b

This will depend on the position required to approach the fracture. If the patient lies supine, then a sandbag placed under the ipsilateral buttock will give access to the anterior part of the iliac crest. In the prone position, the posterior aspect of the iliac crest is easily accessible and provides large quantities of cancellous bone. The sacro-iliac joint should not be damaged. Occasionally both iliac crests require exposure to provide adequate amounts of bone graft. The use of Phemister grafts of cortical and cancellous bone leads to problems of postoperative pain, herniae etc, and is to be avoided whenever possible.

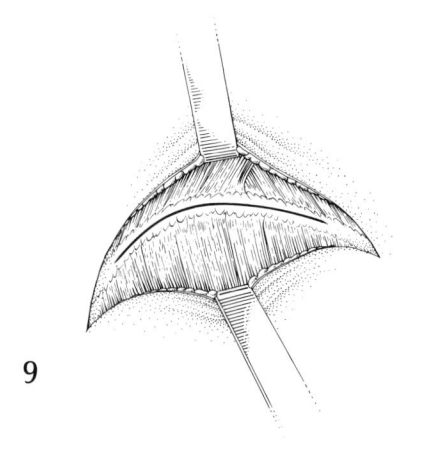

Incision

9

The skin incision is made just below the iliac crest, to avoid the scar being irritated by the band of the patient's trousers or skirt. The length of incision is dependent on the quantity of bone to be harvested. The posterior approach should be via a longitudinal incision to avoid damage to the cutaneous nerves supplying the buttock skin.

The lateral edge of the crest is defined and the line between the abdominal and gluteal muscles identified. An incision is made along the line and the gluteal muscles are dissected off the outer wing of the ilium to the required depth using a periosteal elevator. The gluteal muscles are held away from the wing of the ilium by a wide bone lever, taking care not to damage structures within the greater sciatic notch.

9

Delayed union, non-union and malunion

Procedure

10a & b

There are many methods of removing cortical iliac bone depending on the shape and size of the graft required. It is advisable to leave the bone at the upper edge of the ilium and the anterior superior iliac spine intact in order to maintain an acceptable cosmetic shape to the pelvis. In routine bone grafting longitudinal strips of corticocancellous bone, about 1 cm in width, can be removed from the outer wing of the ilium.

10c

Underlying cancellous bone chips are removed using a curette or gouge. Care should be taken not to penetrate the medial wall of the ilium. The cortical and cancellous bone should be kept separate and covered with gauze swabs moistened with saline. The bone is diced into small 0.5 cm fragments to facilitate vascular ingrowth.

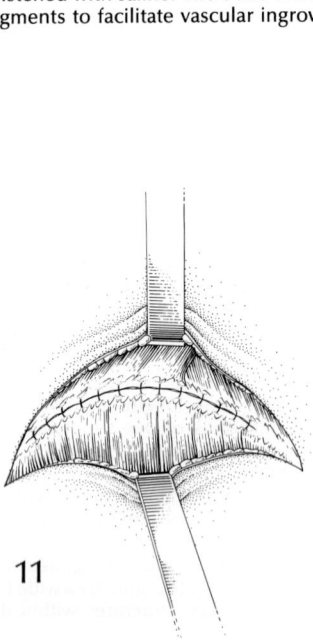

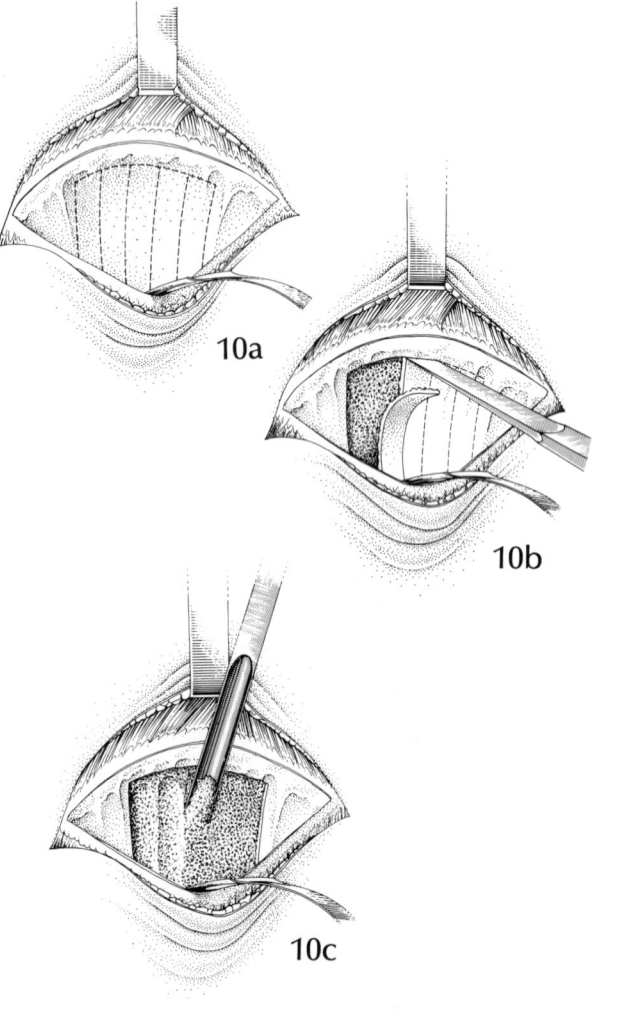

Closure

11

The area used to obtain bone graft is highly vascular, especially when a large area of raw cancellous bone remains. Excessive oozing can be controlled by pressing bone wax into the cancellous surface. The gluteal muscles are sutured back to the iliac crest and abdominal muscles with interrupted absorbable sutures. The skin is closed with interrupted non-absorbable sutures.

MALUNION

One of the principles of fracture management is to reduce the fracture fragments into as near an anatomical position as possible and to maintain the position until the fracture unites. Malunion is by definition fracture union in which alignment is any other than anatomical. In practice, mild degrees of varus or valgus of the main long bones are acceptable whereas gross malunion in excess of 30° may result in the risk of early degenerative change in adjacent joints. In the lower limb, a medial rotation malunion of the distal fragment of a tibial fracture will result in difficulty in walking. Marked loss of length in the long bones of the lower limb by overlap or angulation can also cause serious disability and an abnormal gait. In the upper limb, shortening of the humerus, while perhaps causing a cosmetic blemish, does not usually result in any serious functional disability. Rotational malunion can have serious effects in, for example, the forearm bones by restricting pronation and supination.

Where malunion is sufficient to require correction, specific operative treatment will depend on the type of deformity present and where it is situated. Angular deformity near to a joint in cancellous bone can usually be treated by a suitable wedge osteotomy, with or without internal fixation. In the mid-diaphyseal areas of long bones, an osteotomy at the site of malunion may be necessary to realign the fragments, followed by internal fixation by intramedullary nail or screws and plates. The fixation should be supplemented by a cancellous bone graft to avoid the further problem of non-union.

Shortening by overlap of fracture ends can be a very difficult condition to treat, since any attempt to lengthen the bone by osteotomy and distraction of the bone ends may be difficult without excessive soft tissue release and also excessive stretching of blood vessels and nerves. This may result in serious and irreversible complications. An alternative approach, for example in a short femur, after careful consideration, is to shorten the opposite limb.

METAPHYSEAL WEDGE OSTEOTOMY OF THE TIBIA FOR ANGULAR MALUNION

Slight but acceptable angular deformity in a long bone at the site of a metaphyseal fracture is not uncommon when the fracture is treated conservatively. Where the angulation is marked and is likely to predispose to significant alteration in the adjacent joint mechanics, then corrective osteotomy of the bone should be considered. The osteotomy should be made away from the joint but in a site which is suited to correct the deformity and at the same time will result in rapid bone healing. The metaphyseal area of the long bones is therefore a frequent site for this type of procedure, since it is mainly composed of well-vascularized cancellous bone. For example, in a fracture of the proximal third of the tibia, the osteotomy can be performed between the knee joint and the tibial tubercle. If there has been loss of length from the fracture, an opening wedge should be performed and a corticocancellous graft placed into the gap to maintain the position of the fragments. If length can be reconstituted by straightening the bone, then a closing wedge is performed, as in a high tibial osteotomy. Preoperative radiographs of the fracture should be taken to judge the site of the osteotomy and the size of wedge to be removed.

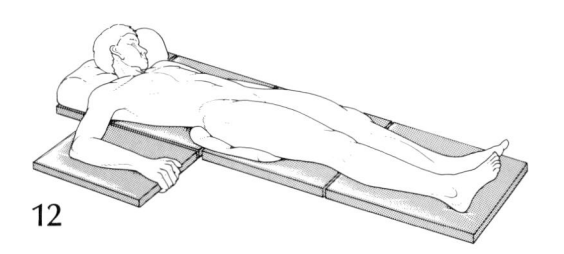

Position of patient

12

The patient lies supine on the operating table with a sandbag under the buttock of the affected leg. This allows medial rotation of the lower limb, resulting in easier access to the lateral aspect of the tibia and fibula.

Incision

13a & b

An incision is made from behind the biceps tendon approximately 4 cm above the knee joint and is carried downwards and forwards, over the head of the fibula to the upper border of the tibial tubercle. The subcutaneous tissue is divided down to the deep fascia in the line of the skin incision. The knee is then flexed to 90° to relax the popliteal artery.

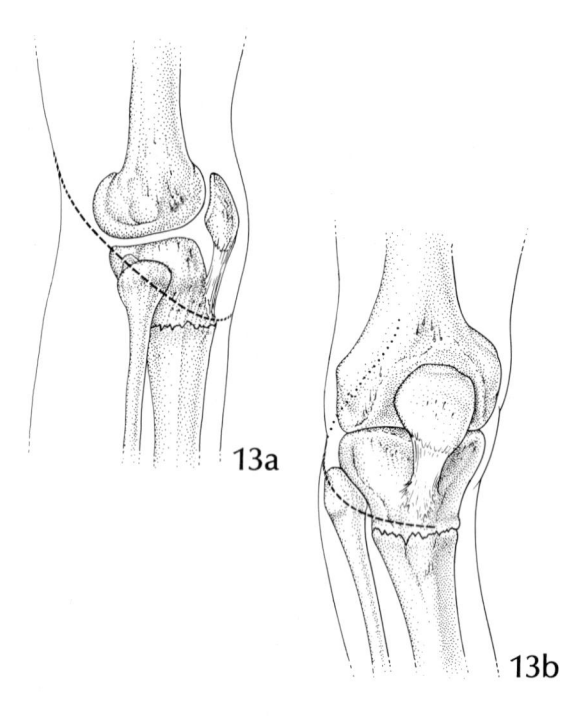

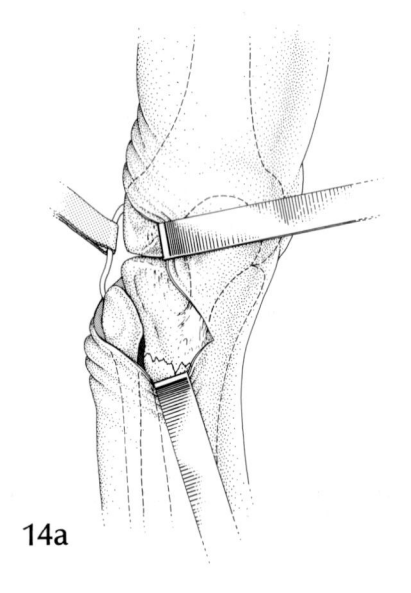

Procedure

14a

The deep fascia is divided in the line of the biceps tendon posteriorly and the common peroneal nerve is identified behind the tendon. The nerve is dissected free down to the neck of the fibula. Having exposed the nerve, a damp tape can be placed around the nerve to protect it during the osteotomy. The anterior part of the incision is deepened down to the bone at the point where the anterior tibial muscles insert into bone.

14b

The patellar tendon is identified and the tibial surface beneath the tendon proximal to its insertion is dissected free. The insertion of the tibialis anterior muscle is dissected off the bone for approximately 1–2 cm from anterior to posterior. Next, the head of the fibula is dissected free in its upper 1 cm and is removed with an osteotome. It is necessary to clear the posterior surface of the tibia in order to protect the popliteal artery. The knee is then extended. A guide wire is inserted across the tibia from the lateral to medial sides parallel with and about 1 cm below the joint line, above the tibial tubercle. A second guide wire is inserted across the tibia from the lateral side below the first and aimed to reach the first wire on the medial side of the tibia in such a position that it outlines the wedge of bone to be removed. The position of the two guide wires are checked by X-ray and their positions altered if necessary. (These guide wires may be inserted before the head of the fibula is dissected off.)

14b

14c

An oscillating saw is used to cut the wedge along the lines of the two guide wires, with the knee flexed to 90° to protect the popliteal vessels. The medial border of the tibia is preserved for the moment, as is the posterior cortex. The posterior cortex is divided with a sharp, wide osteotome under direct vision, again taking care not to damage the popliteal vessels. The wedge of bone is removed. The medial border of the tibia is divided by several drill holes in order to maintain the integrity of the periosteum and therefore improve the final stability of the osteotomy.

With gentle valgus pressure, the osteotomy should close with good apposition of the two cancellous bone surfaces. Care should be taken over this manoeuvre, otherwise the proximal tibia may fracture through into the joint causing haemarthrosis and stiffness postoperatively. Any resistance to closure should lead to a further check to see whether there is remaining bone at the site of the osteotomy resisting closure and to check that the posterior cortex has been completely divided. The final position of the tibia should be further checked by X-ray to ensure that the bone wedge was a satisfactory size and that the angular deformity has been corrected. The two guide wires are removed and the osteotomy stabilized with one or two offset staples. It is advisable to predrill the point of entry in the distal cortical fragment or the staple will tilt during insertion and may split the proximal fragment.

Closure of the wound

A small-bore drain is placed from the osteotomy site through a separate incision in the skin. The peroneal nerve is finally checked. The periosteal sleeve and muscle edge is closed with interrupted absorbable sutures, but the posterior fascia over the nerve is left open. The skin is closed with interrupted non-absorbable sutures. An

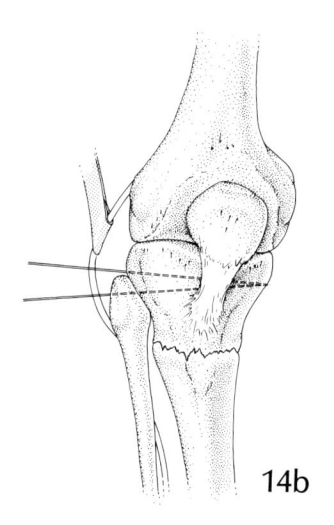

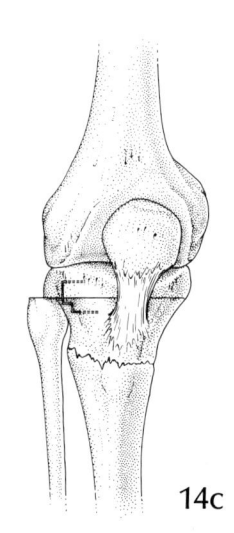

14c

occlusive dressing is applied to the wound and a well-padded cylinder cast is applied from ankle to groin after removal of the tourniquet.

Postoperative management

Providing the osteotomy is stable, the patient begins isometric quadriceps exercises as soon as possible. The plaster should be split if there is excessive swelling. The drain should be removed at 24 hours after the operation. The patient is mobilized weight-bearing at about 48 hours. At 3 weeks, the plaster and sutures are removed and gentle supervised knee flexion exercises begin in hospital. A backslab is maintained when walking until the patient has quadriceps control.

380 Delayed union, non-union and malunion

FEMORAL SHORTENING

Femoral shortening is a well-established method of limb-length equalization in adults. It is essential to ensure that the patient is fully aware that his final overall height will be less than the original. It is therefore a technique more applicable to individuals who are tall rather than of short stature. Shortening of the femur by 3 or 4 cm can be carried out at the subtrochanteric level without permanently weakening the thigh muscles. Full leg measurement radiographs are necessary preoperatively in order to decide on the amount of bone to be resected.

Position of patient

15

The patient is placed on an orthopaedic fracture table with gentle traction applied to both legs. The uninjured leg is abducted in order to obtain both anteroposterior and lateral radiographs of the femur on which the shortening is to be performed using the image intensifier. The leg and image intensifier are draped leaving access to the upper thigh.

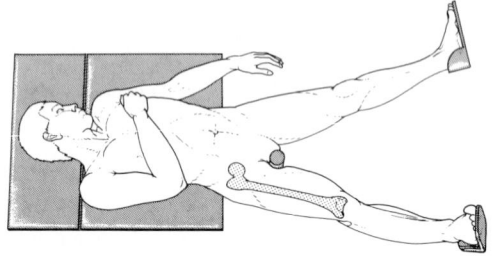

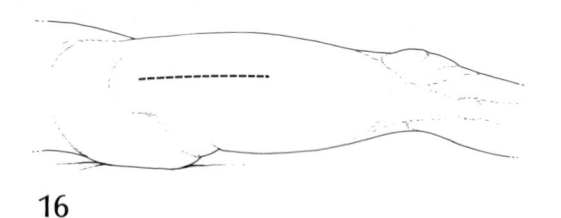

Incision

16

A mid-lateral incision is made from the tip of the greater trochanter distally 10–20 cm along the line of the shaft of the femur.

Procedure

The deep fascia is divided in the same line as the skin incision. The muscle mass of the vastus lateralis is lifted forward to identify the linea aspera. The vastus lateralis is divided near to the linea aspera, leaving enough tissue to resuture the muscle at the end of the operation. A bone lever is placed between the vastus lateralis and femur to allow a satisfactory exposure of the femur in its upper shaft and intertrochanteric region. A finger is placed over the front of the femur to identify the lesser trochanter.

17a & b

A guide wire (1) is drilled through the femur at right angles to the shaft and just below the lesser trochanter. A metal ruler is used to mark off the length of shaft to be resected distal to the guide wire and a further guide wire (2) is drilled across the femur at right angles to the shaft. The intertrochanteric region is now prepared for the right-angled blade–plate. A third guide wire is inserted at the upper edge of the flare of the greater trochanter approximately midway between the tip of the greater trochanter and the upper border of the lesser trochanter at right angles to the shaft of the femur. This engages the calcar femorale. The position of the guide wire should be checked by image intensifier and the length within the bone measured. The appropriate length of blade which will just engage the calcar is selected. The seating chisel for the 90° blade–plate is inserted through the cortex just below and in the line of the guide wire. This is very important since it is very difficult to insert the blade, especially into young, hard bone, once the femur has been divided. The position of the seating chisel is checked on the image intensifier in both planes and is removed. A longitudinal line is made on the femur with a saw to maintain the rotational plane.

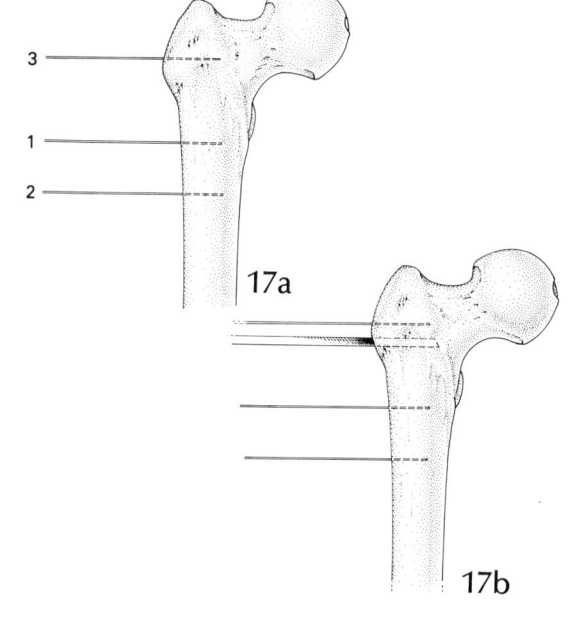

17c & d

Using an oscillating saw, the length of femoral shaft between the two distal wires is resected. The guide wires are removed. The 90° blade–plate is inserted into the channel made by the seating chisel and is driven into position using a mallet. The distal femur is reduced onto the proximal fragment ensuring that no rotational deformity has occurred, and is held with bone-holding forceps. The compression device is attached to the distal femoral fragment using a bicortical screw and is attached to the distal end of the plate. The two edges of the femoral fragments are compressed and the plate fixed into position using screws. The stability of the bone fragments are checked by direct vision and by image intensifier.

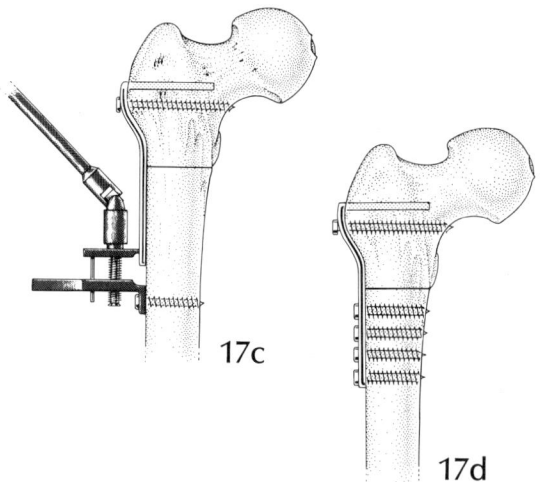

Closure

A small suction drain is placed along the femur and brought out through a separate skin incision. The vastus lateralis is sutured back to the thin layer of muscle attached to the linea aspera with interrupted absorbable sutures. The deep fascia is closed with a continuous absorbable suture. The subcutaneous tissue is closed with interrupted absorbable sutures and the skin with a continuous non-absorbable suture. A sterile occlusive dressing is applied to the wound.

Postoperative management

The suction drain is removed at 24 hours. At 48 hours the patient is allowed to touch-down using elbow crutches to walk. Sutures are removed at 10–14 days. Serial radiographs will show callus formation around the osteotomy site and at about 12 weeks from operation the state of bone union should allow full independent weight-bearing.

LENGTHENING OSTEOTOMY OF THE FEMUR FOR SHORTENING AND ANGULATION

Occasionally, conservative treatment of a mid-shaft femoral fracture may result in union of the fracture with overlap and angulation of the fragments. After careful consideration, it may be necessary to attempt to regain length and reduce angulation by osteotomizing the fracture callus and realigning the fracture ends. Up to 3 cm lengthening of the femur may occur without serious complications, provided an adequate soft tissue release is performed to mobilize the fracture ends. Preoperative radiographs should be carefully studied and the operation steps planned. A normal peripheral circulation and neurological status in the limb is essential.

Position of patient

The patient lies supine on the operating table with a sandbag under the buttock to allow access to the greater trochanter.

Incision

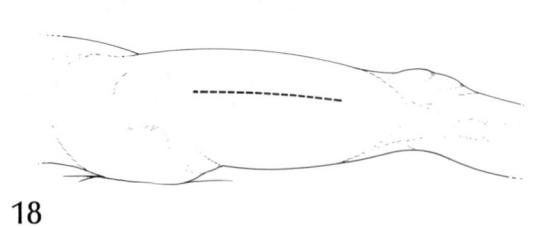

18

A longitudinal incision is made over the lateral aspect of the thigh overlying the malunion. The subcutaneous tissue and deep fascia are divided in the line of the skin incision.

Procedure

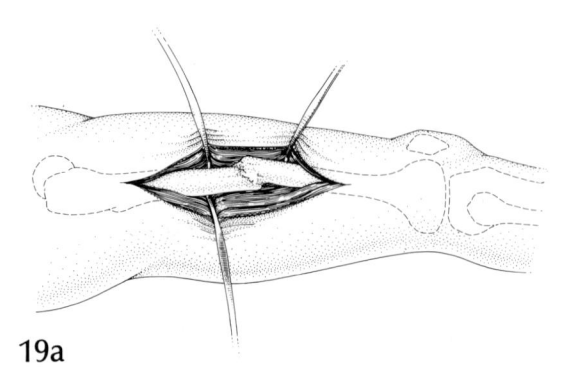

19a

The vastus lateralis muscle is identified and the posterior border attaching to the linea aspera is noted. The muscle is divided close to the linea aspera and using a periosteal elevator and sharp dissection, it is cleared from the femoral shaft and the site of malunion. Bone levers are placed over the femoral shaft towards the medial side to lift the muscle out of the way. The site of malunion is carefully examined and all soft tissue attachments are gently released from the bone in its circumference, including the linea aspera, for a distance of 5–7 cm each side. The soft tissue release is performed so that the limb can be lengthened without graft tension in the adjacent soft tissues.

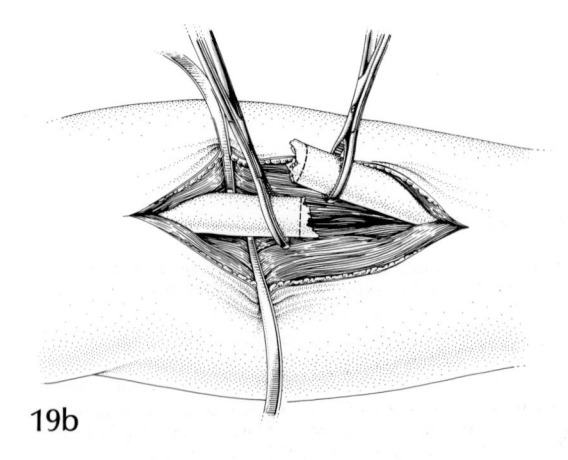

19b

The fracture callus is again examined and the bridge of callus joining the adjacent overlapping femoral cortices is carefully divided with an osteotome until the two fragments of the femur are free of one another. The soft tissues of the undersurface of fracture callus should be protected by a wide retractor or bone lever.

19c & d

Having mobilized the two fracture ends, they should each be divided cleanly across the two cortices at right angles to the shafts of the bones, taking as little bone as possibly initially. The site of the medullary canals should be identified and cleared of callus to allow passage of an intramedullary nail.

Traction should now be applied to the distal fragment and the two parts of the femur should be hitched and the bones aligned in their anatomical position. An AO femoral distractor may be fixed to the fragments to facilitate reduction. If reduction is not possible due to tight soft tissues, and providing the soft tissue release has been adequate, further slices of cortex should be removed until the two fragments can be reduced under reasonable tension. It should be constantly borne in mind that excessive soft tissue tension may result in sciatic nerve palsy or damage to the femoral artery.

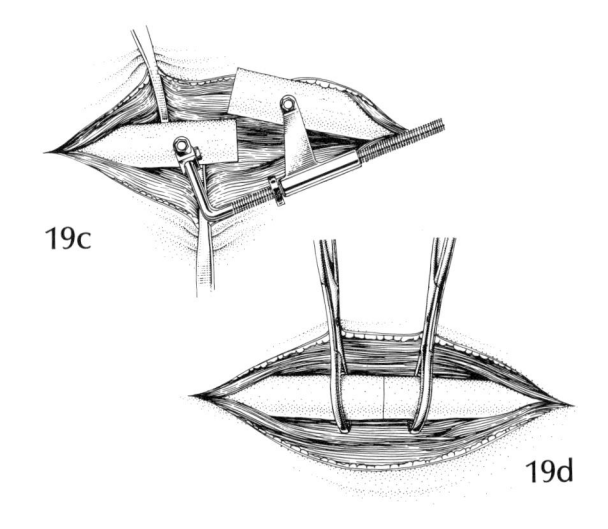

Fixation of the femoral shaft

20a & b

The fracture should be fixed by an intramedullary nail inserted from the greater trochanter in the usual manner (see the chapter on 'Küntscher's closed intramedullary nailing technique for the treatment of femoral shaft fractures, pp. 223–241). As large a nail as possible should be used after reaming of the medullary canal. In cases where stability cannot be guaranteed by an intramedullary nail, a locking nail should be considered. Because of the wide soft tissue stripping around the fracture site, corticocancellous bone grafts should be placed around the fracture site using the ipsilateral iliac crest.

Closure

The vastus lateralis is closed with interrupted absorbable sutures and the skin with non-absorbable sutures after insertion of a small-bore drainage tube. The skin is closed with interrupted nylon sutures.

Postoperative management

The wound is dressed with an occlusive dressing. The patient begins gentle flexion exercises of the hip and knee within 48 hours. Providing the fracture fixation is stable, the patient is allowed partial weight-bearing using crutches. Sutures are removed at 10–14 days. Further weight-bearing will depend on subsequent union of the fracture based on clinical and radiographic observation.

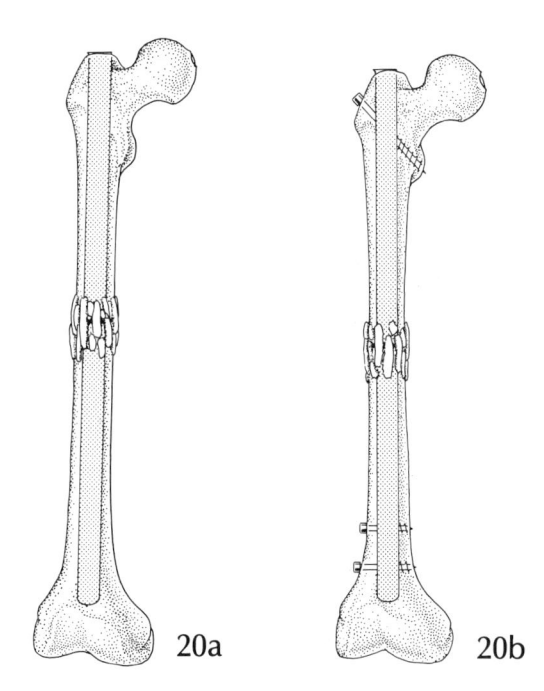

Further reading

Harmon PH. A simplified surgical approach to the posterior tibia for bone grafting and fibular transference. *J Bone Joint Surg* 1945; 27: 496–8.

McKibbin B. The biology of fracture healing in long bones. *J Bone Joint Surg [Br]* 1978; 60-B: 150–62.

Phemister DB. Treatment of ununited fractures by onlay bone grafts without screw or tie fixation and without breaking down of the fibrous union. *J Bone Joint Surg* 1947; 29: 946–60.

Illustrations by Peter Cox

Metastatic bone disease in the limb

Malcolm W. Fidler MS, FRCS
Consultant Orthopaedic Surgeon, Onze Lieve Vrouwe Gasthuis and Netherlands Cancer Institute, Amsterdam, The Netherlands

Introduction

The surgical techniques used for the internal fixation of fractures caused by metastases in the limbs are, in many ways, similar to those used in the treatment of non-pathological fractures. This chapter will accordingly be restricted to supplementary information relevant to the operative treatment of pathological fractures or their prevention. Some alternative techniques will be mentioned, for not every hospital has all the technical possibilities available.

Patients

Patients with fractures due to metastases require rapid relief of pain and restoration of function, so that they can become mobile and independent and return home as quickly as possible. Operations on the leg should allow full weight-bearing and those on the arm should allow adequate use of the hand. At the very least, pain must be relieved and nursing facilitated.

Where the prognosis is poor, the benefits of operation must outweigh the disadvantages of the procedure. In case of doubt, operation is probably preferable, at least psychologically. The advantages of operation in the leg are greater than in the arm, where, when the indication for operation is doubtful, a functional brace may be considered.

Operation

The chance of union following radiotherapy is enhanced by rigid internal fixation[1] and a favourable primary tumour[2]. However, bony union is not essential for success, but rigid, stable, durable and functional internal fixation is. Where necessary, this is achieved by (1) supplementing standard methods of internal fixation with polymethylmethacrylate bone cement[3], (2) by resecting diseased bone and accepting some shortening of the limb, or (3) by realigning the bone, as in the case of a subtrochanteric fracture, to achieve a more favourable weight-bearing situation. If the lesion is close to a joint, it can be resected and a normal or modified prosthesis inserted. The construction must survive the patient.

Any operation which transgresses a metastasis may theoretically increase local or general dissemination of tumour, though the benefits of operation far outweigh this theoretical disadvantage. Even so, careful wound toilet is essential.

Indications for operation

In a non-terminally ill patient fracture through a metastasis is the main indication. In a terminally ill patient or in a patient for whom operation is otherwise contraindicated, the upper limb can be protected in a splint or brace and the lower limb either in a splint or in traction.

Preoperative assessment

Blood profile

The haemoglobin, leucocyte count and platelet count may have been adversely affected by recent chemotherapy. Hypercalcaemia may be present.

Chest radiograph

This is essential to exclude metastases and pleural effusions.

Condition of the local tissues

Recent radiotherapy, provided that the soft tissues look and feel healthy, is not a contraindication to operation. The multiply operated, maximally irradiated, indurated limb must be viewed with care, and the patient warned of the possibility of amputation if infection or wound healing problems arise. Tumour ulceration usually requires amputation.

Technetium bone scan and radiographs

The radiographs should be taken in two planes and show the whole bone. An internal fixation device produces a concentration of stress at its ends. This stress point should not coincide with a weak spot in the bone due to another metastasis. If it does, a longer implant should be used to protect such a lesion from subsequent fracture. The bone scan also draws attention to any other metastases which may require radiotherapy, protection or prophylactic internal fixation.

Prophylactic antibiotics

The patient's resistance to infection is probably low due to the disease and any recent chemotherapy. Furthermore, a foreign body is being inserted and cement, if used, may adversely affect leucocyte metabolism.

An infected metal–cement implant is very difficult to remove and the patients, with limited life prognosis, do not have time available for subsequent lengthy healing and reconstructive procedures. Infection therefore usually requires amputation or at least involves a persistent sinus and lifelong antibiotics.

Prophylactic antibiotics are therefore used: e.g. intravenous cephamandole 2 g just prior to the operation and 6 hourly during the first 24 hours thereafter.

Blood transfusion

These patients are often anaemic. It is usually preferable to transfuse the patient during the operation rather than to attempt a rapid correction of the haemoglobin beforehand. Some pathological fractures bleed profusely (for example, if the primary is a carcinoma of the kidney). Although angiography and, if necessary, embolization are routine prior to operations on pathological fractures of the spine, the availability of these facilities and the logistics associated with the large number of cases usually preclude this technique with pathological fractures in the limbs. It is therefore essential that at least 3 pints of blood are available for operations carried out without a tourniquet.

Operation

The fixation must be stable in compression, bending and rotation. This will, in practice, also prevent translation. Apart from the use of a prosthesis, there are two basic techniques: plating and the use of an intramedullary nail.

PLATING

1

The final mechanical situation as shown in the illustration is doomed to failure. There must always be continuous bony support opposite the plate and preferably around the whole circumference of the bone. The best site for a plate is over the weakest part of the bone. If this is not feasible, the weak area must be reinforced with cement or the bone must be cut back and shortened.

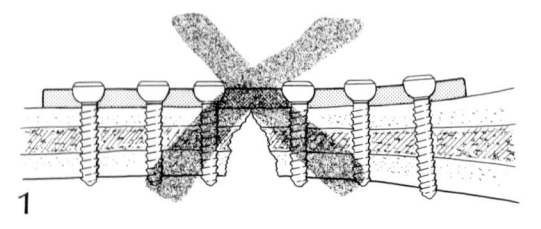

Preparation

The site of maximum bone destruction in the neighbourhood of the fracture can be seen on the preoperative radiographs and especially on those taken just prior to the fracture, if available. The patient is positioned accordingly and the fracture exposed. Careful haemostasis is essential; small vessels are cauterized and the larger vessels (for example, the posterior ends of the perforating vessels in the thigh) are ligated. Any muscle which has been severely damaged by the fractured bone-ends is excised.

Exploration and excision

The fracture is gently explored. Although much bone destruction may have occurred, it is usually possible to identify some corresponding points on the main fragments to facilitate restoration of normal rotation. Diseased bone and tumour tissue are removed, initially with a small sharp spoon and then with bone-nibblers until good, or at least reasonable, quality bone is encountered. If the whole circumference is eroded, this will require shortening of the bone ends. Intramedullary tumour is removed with sharp spoons of various sizes and shapes. As much as possible of the frequently thickening periosteum, especially on the opposite side, should be conserved to act as a restraint for any cement.

Pathology

The tumour tissue is always sent for pathological examination: the metastasis may be from a second unsuspected primary. In the case of a breast primary, determination of oestrogen receptors may aid the choice of hormonal therapy.

During the operation the wound is irrigated copiously with normal saline from a closed system, then with Dakin's solution and finally again with normal saline.

Application of plate

If good quality bone is present around the whole circumference of the fracture, and especially opposite the plate, then the plate is applied in the standard manner with use of the compressor. Dynamic compression plates alone usually provide insufficient compression for these often poorly defined fractures.

Cementing and compression fixation

2

More usually, there is good bony abutment in one area and defects elsewhere. In such cases, cement will be necessary. Plastic cement stops (as used during total hip replacement) are inserted in the proximal and distal fragments to just beyond what is considered to be normal bone. The fracture is reduced and stabilized with a contoured plate held in position by two Verbrugge bone clamps. The plate should overlie the defects and yet should leave room for the insertion of the nozzle of the cement gun. If necessary a defect can be enlarged appropriately to accommodate the nozzle.

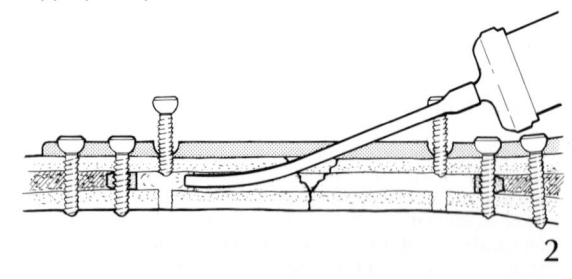

The bone is now drilled for the screws and compressor. The drill points should only just penetrate the far cortex so that the thickening periosteum remains intact to prevent later extravasation of cement. The plate is now screwed into place whilst compression is applied with the compressor. The screws between the plastic plugs are now unscrewed back to the near cortex. The cavity is again irrigated with cool saline and sucked dry.

Antibiotic-containing cement such as Allofix G (Streuli, Switzerland) in a fluid state is then injected into the cavity. If a thick periosteal cuff has been left in place, this will usually prevent excessive extravasation of cement. If such a cuff is not available, then any defects, apart from that for the cement nozzle, should be closed with strips of absorbable gelatin sponge supported by various pre-bent retractors and fingers. The nozzle is gradually withdrawn whilst more cement is pumped into the cavity. Finally cement is forced in with the thumb, which is used to close the cement hole.

The protruding screws are now driven home with a power screwdriver. All screws are checked by hand after the cement has polymerized. Any remaining bleeding vessels are coagulated. The operation site is again irrigated and the wound closed in layers with vacuum drains in each layer.

Plating with cement but no screws

An alternative method of fixation is to omit the screws in the fragment to which the compression device is attached. This fragment is held to the plate with a Verbrugge clamp, and the compressor tightened until it just begins to take effect. The liquid cement is injected as before and, when almost hard, the compressor is fully tightened, clamping the cement between the bone fragments. The remaining screws are then inserted. This method is somewhat more laborious as it entails drilling and tapping of the last holes through hard cement, but perhaps the fixation is slightly better.

If the defect in the bone is posterior and cannot be adequately blocked off to prevent injected low-viscosity cement running out, then high-viscosity cement (Palacos with gentamicin – Kulzer, West Germany) is moulded into the defect.

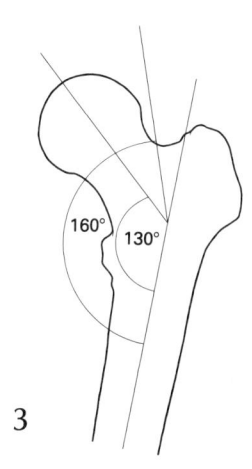

Realignment

Preoperative planning

3

Fractures of the proximal femur have the tendency to collapse into varus. The varus-deforming force can be considerably reduced by realigning the proximal fragment into a more vertical position. In practice, production of a neck–shaft angle of 160° results in a stable construction. The normal neck–shaft angle is approximately 130°. By realigning the fracture site into 30° of valgus, the desired situation is achieved.

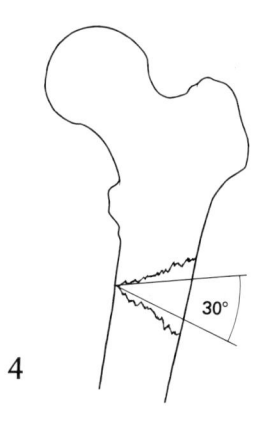

4

This technique is useful for the stabilization of subtrochanteric fractures, especially if more specialized equipment, such as Zickel instrumentation or a gamma nail, is unavailable. As the technique involves the removal of a lateral 30° wedge from the fracture site, it is particularly valuable when the lateral cortex is involved by tumour.

5 & 6

There are some important points. The junction of the screw–plate or blade–plate device must be against good bone cranial to the fracture so that the proximal fragment is supported by the cranial 2 cm of the plate and prevented from displacing laterally on the distal fragment. If the fracture is so far proximal that the screw–plate junction coincides with the fracture, there would be no lateral support, the weaker than normal medial cortex would collapse, the sliding screw would telescope or a fixed blade penetrate deeper into the head until either a new stable situation was reached or until the whole construction failed. With non-pathological fractures, stability is usually the final outcome; but with weak bone of pathological fractures, failure usually occurs.

Preoperative planning is therefore essential. The 135° dynamic hip screw provides excellent fixation. However, the plates are very strong and too thick for normal peroperative plate benders. It is advisable to determine the length of plate and the site at which it must be bent from the preoperative radiograph (the magnification factor is usually 1.2) and to bend it in the workshop beforehand.

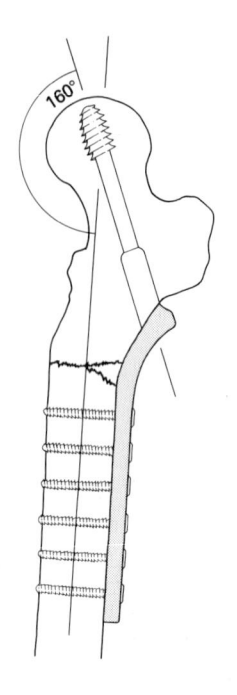

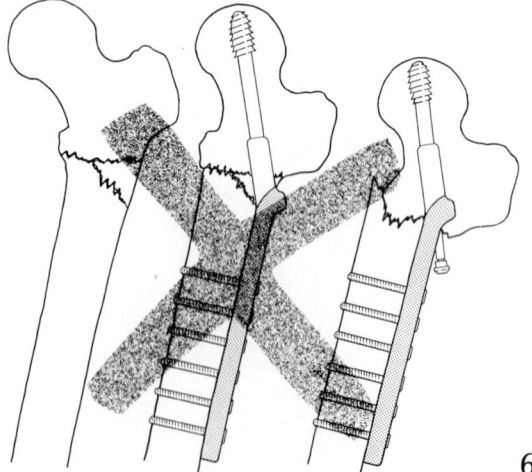

7

If the preoperative planning indicates that a 135° screw–plate will provide insufficient lateral support for the proximal fragment, a more proximal entry point is essential. This can be achieved by basing the reconstruction on an appropriate AO angled plate. If one of these plates with its thin blade is used, then the blade must be perfectly positioned just below the centre of a normal femoral head. If positioning is less than optimal, or the head is diseased, it will cut out. If such a situation is envisaged, a prosthesis would be preferable. AO plates can easily be bent during the operation.

Operative technique

The patient is positioned on the traction table with the leg in a few degrees of abduction and neutral rotation. Biplane image intensification, as for a routine 'hip screw' operation, is used. The fracture is exposed and diseased bone and tumour tissue removed as before. A 30° laterally based wedge is removed, taking away diseased bone by choice. If the use of cement is expected, a distal plastic medullary plug is inserted. The quality of the entry site is checked and the hip screw inserted in the routine manner, after placing a guide wire under biplane radiological control. The prebent plate is slipped over the screw. Traction is reduced and the leg abducted to approximate the distal fragment to the plate, which is then screwed in place. With good quality bone four screws are sufficient; if in doubt, six screws are inserted. Any remaining defect is filled with bone cement. The construction should be capable of bearing full weight.

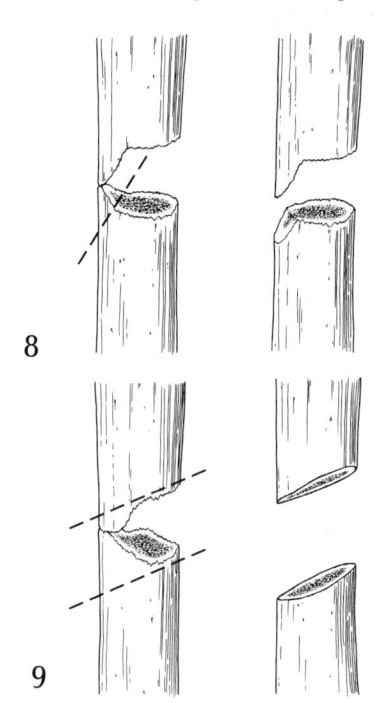

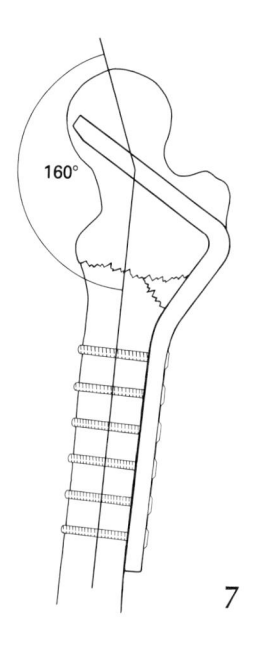

INTRAMEDULLARY NAILING

Intramedullary nails are inserted antegrade following removal of obviously diseased bone and tumour tissue, while temporary reduction and stabilization are achieved with a plate and Verbrugge clamps.

8 & 9

Reaming is essential to obtain a tight stable fit. However, when the nail is used to stabilize a fracture of the middle third of the femur, it is advisable to ream to an extra millimetre to avoid splitting the weakest bone in the vicinity of the fracture. Prior to inserting the nail, the medullary cavity is rinsed with copious amounts of Dakin's solution and normal saline. Usually the tight fit of the nail combined with partial interdigitation of the bone ends are sufficient to control rotation. A large residual cortical defect can be packed with cement, but if sufficient anchorage for the cement cannot be obtained it is better to resect the spike of good quality bone that holds the fracture out to length and accept some shortening in the interest of rigid stability. If good bone is resected then the resection lines should produce an antirotation effect.

10

As an alternative, if such shortening is undesirable, an antirotation plate, which also serves to hold a partial cement collar in place, can be used. After insertion of the nail, a small dynamic compression plate is applied loosely with unicortical screws. The 1.9 mm red offset drill guide is used so that the screws will produce maximal compression. The cement is packed into the defect and is left proud from the bone under the plate. As the cement becomes rubbery the plate is screwed home.

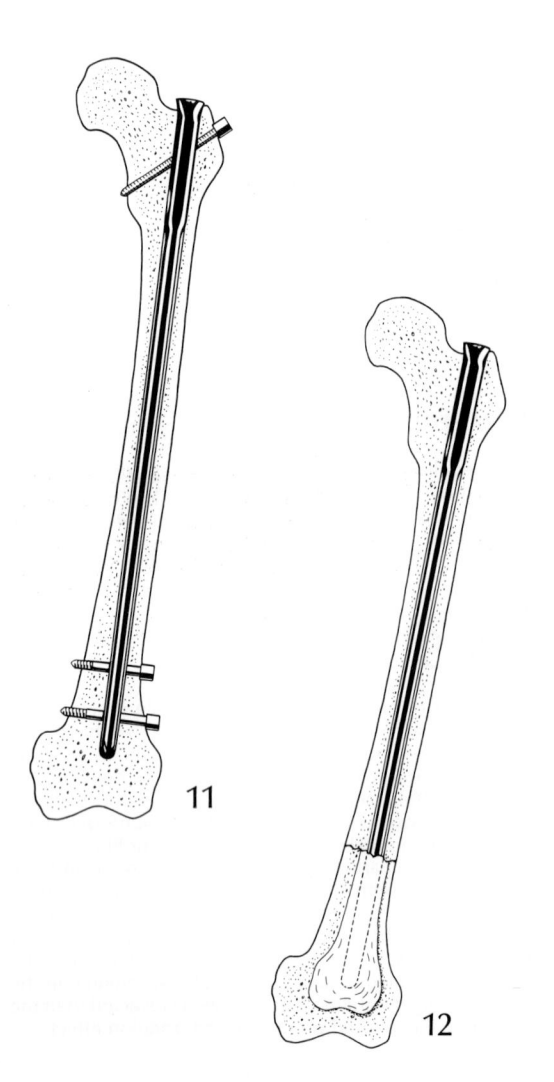

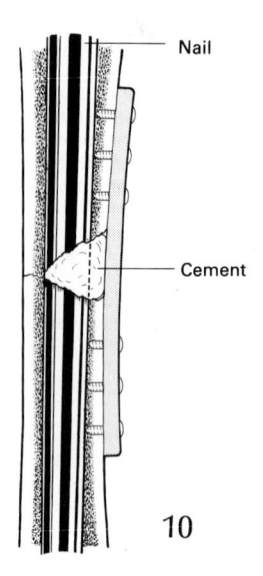

11

Rotational stability can also be maintained by using the Grosse and Kempf locking nail system[4], where necessary in combination with cement to fill defects at the fracture site. The bone may be shortened or held to length as required.

If the fracture is situated just proximal or distal to the middle third, a simple intramedullary nail gives poor control of the short fragment, especially with regard to rotational stability.

For proximal fractures, the locking nail system is useful. The distal transverse screws are not usually necessary because the nail is well gripped by the middle third of the femur. Any subsequent collapse of the fracture site is taken up by telescoping of the distal fragment along the nail: the nail should terminate far enough above the intercondylar notch. If there is any doubt about rotational stability, the distal transverse screws should also be inserted.

For distal fractures, the Grosse and Kempf system is also suitable, but this time usually only the distal locking screws are necessary.

12

An alternative for distal fractures is to use an ordinary intramedullary nail and cement. After reaming, the distal fragment is released from the temporary stabilizing plate and, with sharp long-handled spoons, is scraped out until firm cancellous bone is reached. The nail is now driven down to the fracture. Using the cement gun, the distal fragment is filled with liquid cement. The fracture is reduced and clamped and the nail driven down into the soft cement.

Use of bone graft

HOMOGRAFT

Although the techniques here described ensure immediate rigid fixation, the only absolute safeguard against late loosening is union. Frequently, cement will have been used to fill a defect, and in these areas direct union will be virtually impossible unless a periosteal bridge is present. At present, the impression exists that the addition of homograft bone chips from banked frozen femoral heads helps to stimulate new bone formation across and around the fracture site. Certainly, if bank bone is available, its use can do little harm. In contradistinction to the use of autograft, it does not involve a second incision, although of course the osteogenic potential is less.

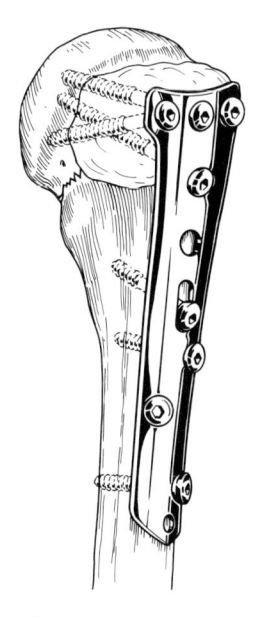

AUTOGRAFT

Occasionally a pathological fracture occurs through an area of radiation necrosis following the 'curative' irradiation of a metastasis. At operation the bone ends appear dead and avascular and there is no evidence of local tumour. A fragment of bone is taken for histology. There are two courses of action.

If one is certain about the diagnosis and if the patient has a good prognosis with no other bone metastases, especially none in the pelvis, then the fracture can be stabilized in the routine manner, with the addition of Phemister onlay grafts taken from the iliac crest, using new instruments, gowns and gloves.

The alternative is simply to stabilize the fracture. If the fracture fails to unite and becomes painful, and if the local and general situations remain favourable, then Phemister grafting can be added later.

Stabilization of fractures at different sites

HUMERUS

Neck

13

An anterior approach via the deltopectoral groove is used, just lateral to the cephalic vein which can be preserved. If necessary the medial fibres of deltoid are released from the clavicle. Tumour tissue and obviously soft bone are enucleated. The fracture is stabilized with a T-plate and cement. If the proximal fragment is insufficient for this technique, a Neer prosthesis can be inserted[5].

13

Shaft

Diffuse tumour involvement

An intramedullary nail is inserted from the greater tuberosity, either by a 'closed' technique with image intensification control or by an 'open' procedure after exposing and reducing the fracture. The patient is positioned on the side with the arm extended to bring the greater tuberosity forwards from under the acromion. A short anterior deltoid-splitting incision provides sufficient exposure for insertion of the guide wire, reamers and nail.

If sufficient bone stock is available for proximal and distal locking, a Seidel locking nail[6] (Howmedica, London, UK) can be used to advantage.

Localized lesion with fracture

Plate fixation with or without added bone cement is performed via an anterolateral incision. A femoral plate should be used. Resection of diseased bone and shortening up to 3 cm is quite acceptable (though the sleeves of clothing will need altering).

If operation is contraindicated, a Sarmiento splint is worthwhile.

Supracondylar

Medial and lateral semitubular plates are used with or without cement. Exposure is afforded via a pre-drilled olecranon osteotomy which is refixed with a screw, reinforced if necessary with a tension-band wire to guarantee immediate functional stability. An alternative approach is to release a tongue of the triceps. In exceptional circumstances, an elbow prosthesis with intramedullary stem fixation may be used.

RADIUS

The proximal 5 cm can be resected via a Boyd approach[7]. More distal fractures are amenable to plate and cement fixation.

ULNA

Proximal fractures can be treated with a plate and cement. The distal 5 cm can be resected if grossly involved.

WRIST

Metastases are rare. A carpal bone can be replaced with Silastic (Dow Corning, UK).

HAND

Metastases are rare. Stabilization of fractures is possible with the AO small fragment set, combined if necessary with cement. Occasionally, local amputation is preferable.

FEMUR

Head and neck

An endoprosthesis is used, replacing the femoral head and neck. If the acetabulum is also involved, then a total hip prosthesis is necessary. The depths of large defects in the pelvis can be filled with femoral head homograft from the deep-freeze bone bank. Any defects in the acetabular lip can be bridged with an Eichler ring. The acetabular component is then cemented in place. The anterolateral and posterior approaches to the hip are equally effective.

Trochanteric region

If the remaining bone stock is reasonable, a dynamic hip screw is used with or without cement. The proximal fragment should be brought into a more valgus position and the 150° plate used to improve weight-bearing mechanics.

14

If bone stock is poor, the head, neck and trochanteric region should be resected and replaced with a 'tumour' total hip prosthesis. A lateral osteoperiosteal flap can be left to provide attachment for the hip abductors. For the insertion of these large femoral prostheses, the posterior approach is preferable. If the whole of the proximal femur is to be removed, the shaft distal to the line of transection should be marked to aid rotational alignment of the prosthesis. Rotation should also be checked by reference to the linea aspera and the tibia with the knee flexed to 90°. Mistakes are very difficult to rectify.

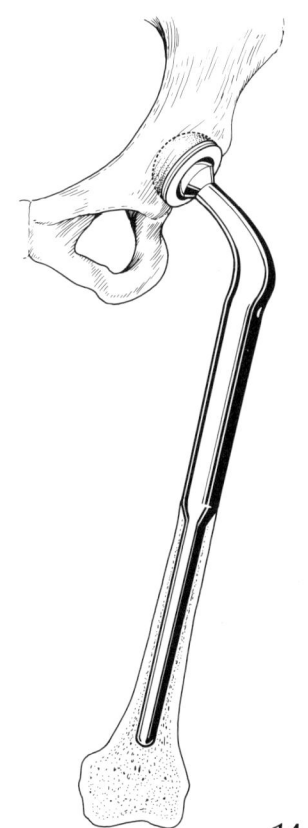

14

Metastatic disease

Subtrochanteric region

Zickel nail[8] or gamma nail

15

Diseased bone is removed and the procedure usually involves some shortening of the limb. Cement can be packed into residual defects but the grip is often poor; this is usually best avoided. If further necrosis and collapse occur the distal fragment can telescope. Rotation is usually well controlled by the signal arm proximally and the shape of the Zickel stem distally. Distal locking screws can be used in conjunction with a 'short' gamma nail, but this prevents any telescoping.

Homograft may be added around the fracture site.

16

The recently developed long gamma nail is particularly suitable for fixation of a subtrochanteric fracture and simultaneous prophylactic stabilization of a mid-shaft metastasis. If the more distal lesion is situated beyond the middle third of the femur, then additional stability can be obtained by inserting the distal transverse locking screws.

Distal shaft and supracondylar region

Intramedullary nailing techniques have been considered above (pp. 389–390). Supracondylar fractures may also be stabilized with Zickel supracondylar nails or blade–plates, reinforced if necessary with cement.

Condyles

Resection and replacement may be carried out with a modified total knee prosthesis provided that soft tissue cover, including the quadriceps mechanism, is adequate. The prosthesis must be constrained with intramedullary stem fixation.

A long anterior midline incision usually affords the best exposure.

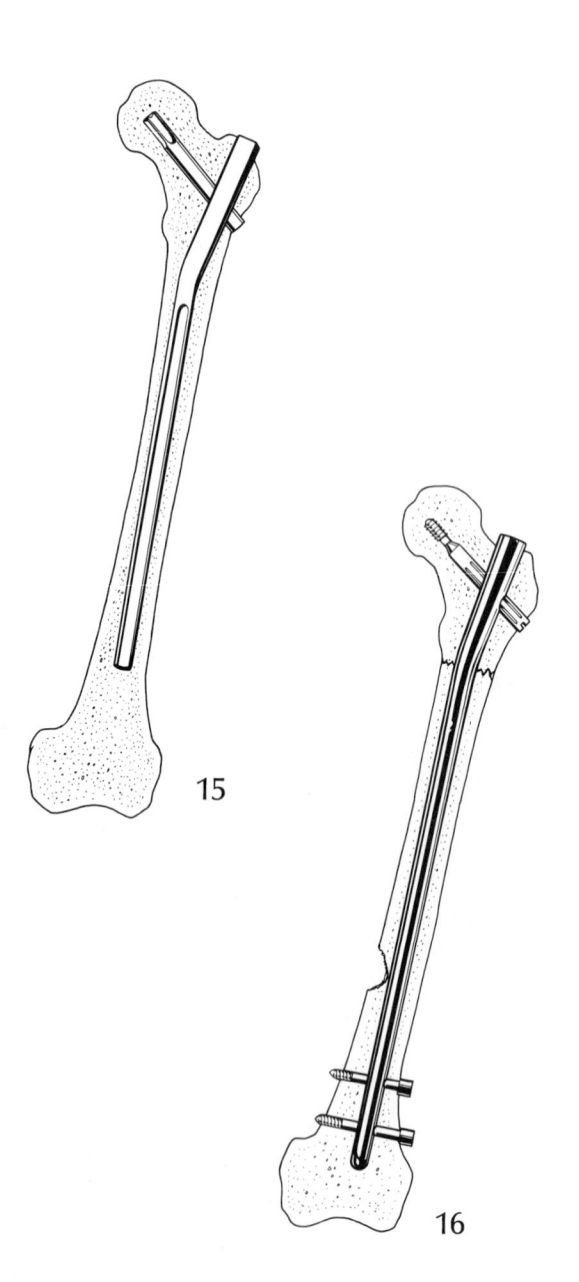

15

16

TIBIA

Plateau

Total knee replacement may be performed, provided soft tissue cover is adequate. Care must be taken to preserve the insertion of the patellar ligament.

Shaft

17

In the proximal third of the shaft, medial and lateral plates are used, usually augmented with cement. Screws should grip both cortices and some should be embedded in any cement. Screws used as bolts are often useful for optimal rigidity.

In the middle third, an intramedullary nail is used (see p. 390). In the distal third, the same techniques are used in the tibia as those for the distal third of the femur.

TARSUS

A fracture in the tarsus is treated by a weight-relieving tibial-bearing caliper. If this fails, then amputation and a prosthesis should be considered.

FOOT

Pathological fractures are rare in the foot and should be treated primarily conservatively.

Postoperative management

The operated limb is elevated and exercised as for non-pathological fractures.

The hip and the knee joints are mobilized with the aid of a patient-activated pulley and sling system, usually beginning on the day after the operation. If a total knee prosthesis has been inserted, continuous motorized passive movement is employed as soon as wound healing is seen to be satisfactory, usually after the fifth day. Full weight-bearing is usually possible after 48 hours, though crutches are usually required for some 2 weeks to minimize wound pain. A recent bone scan or radiographs should be consulted to make sure that the patient does not have dangerous metastases in the arm bones or other leg prior to the use of crutches.

Radiotherapy and chemotherapy may safely be administered after the fifth postoperative day, provided wound healing is satisfactory. Radiotherapy should include the whole of the operation field, including the ends of any intramedullary nails. The presence of metal slightly impairs the efficacy of radiotherapy but this can be disregarded. Radiotherapy does not appear to prevent direct fracture healing provided that the fixation is rigid[1].

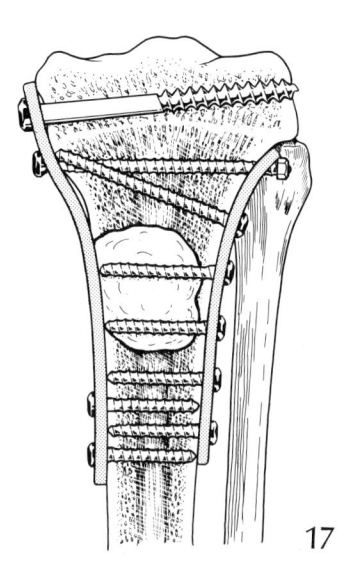

17

Some chemotherapeutic agents, namely methotrexate and adriamycin, probably impair fracture healing[9]. However, little is known about this, and as the general treatment of the patient takes precedence, this possible disadvantage of chemotherapy can be disregarded. In any case, the implant construction should be safe even in the absence of bony union.

PROPHYLACTIC FIXATION

The prevention of pathological fracture through a metastasis by prophylactic internal fixation spares the patient the pain and anguish of the fracture and usually substitutes a relatively minor operation for an otherwise more major procedure.

Indications

1. Destruction of more than 50 per cent of the cortex of a long bone[10,11].
2. Persistent pain following conservative treatment even if the lesion involves less than 50 per cent of the cortex.
3. The patient should not be terminally ill.

18a & b

Although, CT allows accurate measurement of the percentage of the cortex destroyed, CT is still not universally available. A simple method of estimating the percentage involvement on the basis of routine radiographs has been described[10]:

(a) A drawing of the metastasis is made on a rolled paper tube, corresponding to anteroposterior and lateral X-ray appearances.
(b) The paper tube is unrolled and the size of the metastasis as a percentage of the cortical circumference of the bone is given by $M/C \times 100$ per cent.

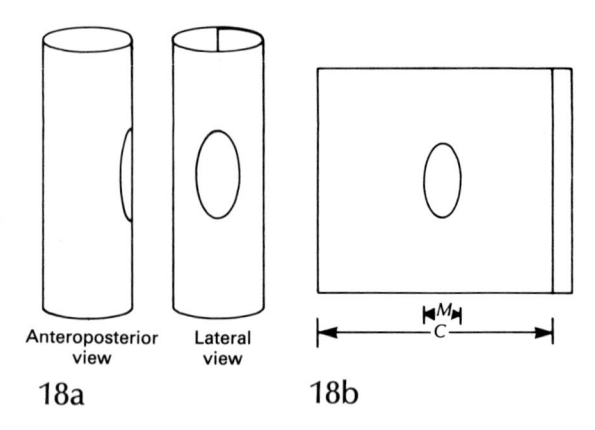

Anteroposterior view   Lateral view
18a   18b

OPERATIVE TECHNIQUE

Similar principles and methods are employed as for the treatment of pathological fractures, but the following points should be noted.
1. Lesions in the shafts of the humerus, femur and tibia are routinely stabilized with a closed intramedullary nail. If additional fixation is required, e.g. for lesions just proximal or distal to the middle third of the femur, the appropriate locking nail is used.
2. Metastases through which a fracture would necessitate a prosthesis, such as in the femoral neck, are not treated prophylactically unless painful because the prophylactic operation would be of the same order of magnitude as that for a fracture.

TOTAL EXCISION

Consideration should be given to total excision of a solitary metastasis from a thyroid or renal primary which has not broken through the periosteum. Careful preoperative assessment with radiographs, CT, bone scan angiography, and possibly NMR, is mandatory before embarking upon such a venture. The defect can be filled with a spacer fixed to the neighbouring bone with intramedullary stems[12]. In the vicinity of a joint, a modified total joint prosthesis can be used.

With other primary tumours, the indications for excision and replacement of a solitary metastasis are doubtful, but should be considered particularly if the site of the metastasis allows a relatively simple procedure in a patient with an otherwise good prognosis.

References

1. Bonarigo BC, Rubin P. Nonunion of pathologic fracture after radiation therapy. *Radiology* 1967; 88: 889–98.

2. Gainor BJ, Buchert P. Fracture healing in metastatic bone disease. *Clin Orthop* 1983; 178: 297–302.

3. Harrington KD, Sim FH, Enis JE, Johnston JO, Dick HM, Gristina AG. Methylmethacrylate as an adjunct in internal fixation of pathological fractures: experience with 375 cases. *J Bone Joint Surg [Am]* 1976; 58-A: 1047–54.

4. Kempf I, Grosse A, Beck G. Closed locked intramedullary nailing: its application to comminuted fractures of the femur. *J Bone Joint Surg [Am]* 1985; 67-A: 709–20.

5. Galasko CSB. Treatment of skeletal metastases. In: Galasko CSB, Noble J, eds. *Current trends in orthopaedic surgery.* Manchester: Manchester University Press, 1988: 72–97.

6. Seidel H. Humeral locking nail: a preliminary report. *Orthopaedics* 1989; 12(2): 219–26.

7. Crenshaw AH. Surgical approaches. In: Crenshaw AH, ed. *Campbell's operative orthopaedics* 7th ed. St Louis: Mosby, 1987: 100–2.

8. Zickel RE, Mouradian WH. Intramedullary fixation of pathological fractures and lesions of the subtrochanteric region of the femur. *J Bone Joint Surg [Am]* 1976; 58-A: 1061–6.

9. Burchardt H, Glowczewskie FP, Enneking WF. The effect of adriamycin and methotrexate on the repair of segmental cortical autografts in dogs. *J Bone Joint Surg [Am]* 1983; 65-A: 103–8.

10. Fidler M. Incidence of fracture through metastases in long bones. *Acta Orthop Scand* 1981; 52: 623–7.

11. Menck H, Schulze S, Larsen E. Metastasis size in pathologic femoral fractures. *Acta Orthop Scand* 1988; 59: 151–4.

12. Lempberg R, Ahlgren O. Prosthetic replacement of tumour-destroyed diaphyseal bone in the lower extremity. *Acta Orthop Scand* 1982; 53: 541–5.

General principles of amputation surgery

J. C. Angel FRCS
Consultant Orthopaedic Surgeon, Royal National Orthopaedic and Edgware General Hospitals, Middlesex, UK

Indications

Amputation is an operation for end-stage disease; it is important to ensure that the disease or injury necessitating the amputation has been fully assessed, and appropriate consultation with specialists in the disease necessitating the amputation have excluded alternative therapy.

Atherosclerosis

Atherosclerosis tends to affect the large and medium-sized arteries of the lower limb, leaving the distal vascular tree relatively intact. Thus gangrene of the toes in this condition indicates the presence of a much larger mass of disordered tissue. Demarcation of the gangrene is poor, and local amputations are unlikely to heal unless it is possible to relieve the proximal block by reconstructive arterial surgery. If there is no steep temperature gradient above the ankle, long posterior flap below-knee amputation is successful in the majority of cases[1]. Occasionally amputation is required for uncontrollable rest pain in the absence of gangrene.

Diabetes mellitus

In the diabetic patient requiring amputation there are three factors to bear in mind, each of which influences management.

First, the diabetic patient has both proximal and distal blocks in his arteries. The significance of this is that adequately perfused tissue is often to be found quite close to the area of gangrene. It means that the prognosis for a distal amputation is better than it would be for simple arteriosclerosis. At the same time, it must not be forgotten that vascular surgery may be able to salvage a limb with absent peripheral pulses.

Second, the majority of diabetics, by the time they manifest any kind of foot complication, have developed a peripheral neuropathy. This can lead to deformity and skin breakdown. The patient should be warned of this possibility threatening his remaining foot. Surgical footwear should be supplied if necessary.

Third, patients with diabetes have an altered response to bacterial infection. The connective tissues tend to form a slough which is slow to be cleared. Incision and drainage of such a lesion, instead of leading to a rapid resolution, frequently produces a chronically discharging cavity. The resulting wound should not be mistaken for the effects of ischaemia. Very often a simple, thorough surgical debridement is all that is required to bring about healing.

Venous insufficiency

The chronic debility associated with venous ulceration can sometimes be resolved only by ablation.

Injury

Amputation is required for trauma when conservative surgery does not offer a reasonable chance of restoring function. Where it may be acceptable to plan a prolonged course of reconstructive surgery and rehabilitation in a young person, the same may not apply in the elderly whose shorter life expectancy does not justify such a heavy investment of time and effort on the part of the patient. Severe compound fractures with neurovascular damage of the type classified as Group IIIC by Gustilo et al.[2] are best treated by immediate amputation.

In the case of burns and frostbite, much potentially viable tissue can be saved by allowing time for a clear-cut line of demarcation to appear before amputating. Electrical burns often involve the deeper tissues to a far greater extent than indicated by the superficial wound, thereby necessitating amputation at a higher level than at first anticipated.

Tumours

For those primary malignant tumours where the site and character do not allow local resection, amputation offers hope of a cure if no metastases have been found after a thorough search. The amputation may be justified even when distant metastases are known to be present if these tumours cause pain that cannot be relieved. It is important that the amputation flaps should be clear of the neoplastic process in order to prevent the extremely difficult problem of recurrence at the stump.

Infection

Now it is uncommon for acute infection to be the primary cause of an amputation. However, its presence not infrequently calls for a higher amputation than might otherwise have been the case and it is the reason for a number of revision amputations. Infection caused by gas-forming organisms has a particular capacity for rapid spread throughout the tissues. Of these *Clostridium welchii* is by far the most virulent but certain gas-producing coliforms and streptococci are dangerous, particularly in diabetic patients. The level of amputation should be high enough to exclude surgical emphysema from the stump, which should be left unsutured.

Chronic infection, usually osteomyelitis, may necessitate amputation because of chronic debility, associated deformity and functional loss or the development of malignant change. Except where malignant change has occurred, it is not essential to skirt the lesion by more than 1–2 cm as long as the amputation flaps have an adequate blood supply and are free from scarred and ischaemic tissue. Attempts to excise all oedematous tissue and secondary changes may result in unnecessary shortening of the stump.

Neurological disorders

These can lead to repeated skin breakdown and deformity. It may be possible to reduce the resulting functional deficit by amputation and prosthetic replacement. In paraplegic patients joint contractures of such severity may occur that they cause problems in nursing, and it may sometimes be better to amputate the limbs.

Congenital deformity

Some congenital deformities, particularly those associated with gross leg-length discrepancy and distortion of the foot, are best managed by amputation and prosthetic replacement. Congenital absence of the fibula or tibia and proximal focal femoral deficiency come into this category.

Preoperative assessment

Selection of level

Cosmesis

For some amputees cosmesis is of paramount importance while for others, particularly those of an independent nature who have to care for themselves, it is better to sacrifice cosmesis in favour of function and comfort. Such factors should be allowed to influence the level of amputation. For example, disarticulation, where technically possible, may be expected to provide a more robust and comfortable stump although the resulting prosthesis has poor cosmesis. Thus it is important to take a social history and form an impression about the degree and direction of the patient's motivation.

Where possible it should be established whether or not a patient is likely to be able to use a prosthesis before surgery. If it is clear that he is not, because of some severe disorder of the locomotor system, then it is appropriate to select a proximal level of amputation where there is a good chance of primary healing and less risk of difficulties arising through joint contracture. In making this assessment it is important not to be misled by a patient who is in severe pain or who is confused owing to infection.

Vascularity

In the patient with ischaemia of the limb, the level of amputation is determined largely by clinical criteria such as tissue appearance, hair growth and skin temperature. The presence or absence of peripheral pulses is generally less helpful. A number of supplementary investigations have been found to be of assistance and these include the measurement of distal blood pressure using Doppler ultrasound recordings, percutaneous oximetry, thermography and the measurement of blood pressure in the skin. Angiography cannot be used as an indicator of tissue perfusion.

Importance of the knee joint

The disadvantages of an above-knee amputation compared with one below the knee are as great as those between the below-knee amputee and a person with intact limbs. Thus it is worth exposing the patient to a moderate risk to try to save the knee and the upper few centimetres of the tibia. Reasonable function will usually be provided by 10 cm, but with less than 7 cm the residual limb will probably not be able to control the shank part of the prosthesis.

Investigations

In patients with ischaemia, haemoglobin, blood urea and fasting blood sugar estimations are desirable, together with electrocardiography. Swabs from septic areas in the part to be amputated must be sent for bacteriological culture and the sensitivity of any organisms to antibiotics must be noted. In diabetic patients a serum albumin below 35 g/l and a lymphocyte count under 1.5×10^9/l are bad prognostic signs for wound healing[3].

Preparation

Amputation has an irrevocable quality not shared by most surgical procedures. It is important that the patient understands why the operation is necessary. In the case of amputations performed as an elective procedure, for such conditions as chronic sepsis or congenital deformity, it is customary for the surgeon to seek a second opinion from one of his colleagues in order to confirm his decision and share the responsibility. When amputating on children, great care should be taken to explain the reason for the amputation to the parents as recriminations and feelings of guilt so often follow in the wake of a childhood amputation. Informed, written consent must be obtained. In the case of vascular disease or acute inflammation it is often desirable to obtain consent to proceed to a higher level of amputation should it prove necessary at operation. The limb to be amputated should be clearly marked.

Once the decision to amputate has been made, the patient should be encouraged to be as mobile as his condition allows. Smoking is forbidden. Diabetes is controlled and anaemia should be corrected. Blood is cross-matched to cover the possibility of haemorrhage. On the day of surgery the skin is shaved and infected areas on the extremity are sealed off inside a polythene bag.

Antibiotic therapy

Antibiotic therapy is commenced at the time of premedication in order to build up an adequate concentration in fat and bone. It is desirable to give penicillin to protect against clostridial infection and to supplement this with whatever antibiotics are required to deal with any organisms isolated distal to the amputation site. If the patient is sensitive to penicillin then erythromycin is a suitable alternative.

Gas gangrene, once a frequent complication of amputation surgery, has been virtually eliminated by good surgical technique and antibiotic cover[4].

Anaesthesia

General anaesthesia is preferable for all amputations other than the distal half of the digits. If this is prevented by toxaemia, or other factors, epidural anaesthesia is the next best choice. Intravenous regional anaesthesia can be used for distal amputations and infiltration anaesthesia may be suitable away from an infected area, particularly with disarticulations.

Tourniquet

Amputation surgery, except where there is marked ischaemia, is facilitated by the use of a pneumatic tourniquet, especially if a myoplasty is involved. Formal exsanguination of the limb is unnecessary. The limb can be drained satisfactorily by elevation for a minute or so.

Management of individual tissues

Many amputations have to be conducted according to the situation presented by the disease rather than according to set surgical procedures and it is important to grasp the principles involved.

Skin

The skin flaps are conveniently marked using a throat swab dipped in methylene blue. The relation of the bases of the flaps to the level of bone section varies according to age and tissue elasticity. In a child they should be located at the level of bone section, since the tension of the tissue will draw them up the limb. In an elderly person with flaccid tissues the flap will need to be located 2–5 cm proximally. The combined lengths of the flaps should be equal to the diameter of the limb. Where possible, the healthier, more durable flap is fashioned longer than the other: for example, if it comprises the skin of the back of the calf or the sole of the foot.

The skin is closed with interrupted, fine, simple sutures or with staples. Stitch marks rarely show in amputations. Where there is a particular risk of postoperative infection the skin edges should be apposed with two or three sutures over ribbon gauze soaked in aqueous proflavine emulsion. If the wound is clean in 5 days then the skin edges can be sutured as a delayed primary closure. If there is contamination then a later secondary closure may be more appropriate. It is rarely necessary or desirable to use skin grafting techniques in the closure of an amputation stump. There is usually a great deal of loss of bulk during the postoperative weeks and this allows wound contraction to work very efficiently. If skin grafts are applied this advantage is lost and innervated skin that initially retracts proximally cannot easily be brought down to be included in the stump at a later date.

Muscle (see Illustration 2, p. 423)

In general, muscle should be cut with a raked incision, the knife being angled towards the bone at the level of section. Here again, the level at which the cut should be made in relation to bone section is dependent on the tension within the tissues. Extra length is needed in children to compensate for the tendency for the muscle to be drawn proximally. The Syme's amputation knife cuts more effectively than a scalpel. It is best to cut muscle from the superficial to the deep layers. This automatically produces a raked incision. Cutting from within out has a tendency to form the rake in the wrong direction.

Bone

In deciding the level of bone section in the lower thigh and arm, consideration is given to allowing sufficient space between the cut end of the bone and the axis of the artificial joint immediately below the stump to accommodate a number of structures: the soft tissue covering the end of the bone, the end socket space or padding, the socket wall and the joint mechanism itself. The axis of the artificial joint is normally set at the level of the axis of the contralateral joint. If insufficient bone is removed then either the axis of the artificial joint must be set more distally, thus sacrificing cosmesis, or side joints must be used. These have a poor appearance, are weaker and tend to rub holes in clothes.

The level of bone section should be approached extraperiosteally. The periosteum is then divided circumferentially, care being taken not to strip it any higher. The bone is cut immediately distally. In most situations the Gigli saw is much the most satisfactory tool for this purpose. The fibula, which is often a difficult bone to divide cleanly, is best cut with an oscillating saw and the metaphysis of a long bone is cut with a tenon saw. The cut end of the bone should be rounded with a sharp rasp worked across the bone rather than up and down. During these procedures the soft tissues should be protected by covering them with saline-soaked swabs.

Vessels

Vessels of the size of the common femoral and the axillary artery should be doubly ligated with strong silk. More distally an absorbable transfixion ligature can be used. Below the elbow and the knee it is safe to ligate the artery and its venae comitantes as a bundle, having separated out the accompanying nerve.

Nerves

At any given level of section all named nerves should be sought, pulled down and divided with scissors. If a knife is used, the final part of the nerve to be divided is apt to form an elongated 'string' as the rest of the nerve retracts proximally. This can result in a painful, more distally located neuroma.

Closure

The muscle, or rather the deep fascia, is stitched over the end of the bone (myoplasty) using absorbable sutures. Where the subcutaneous surface of a bone is involved this must be bevelled, and its periosteum substitutes for deep fascia. To avoid the tendency in some situations for the sutured muscle to act with a stropping action over the end of the bone, an anchorage is made by passing one or two sutures through a small drill hole (osteomyoplasty). If too many holes are drilled there is a risk of forming a ring sequestrum at the distal end of the bone.

Drainage

All but the most minor amputations should be drained with a vacuum drain. This is brought out through the skin some distance from the wound. The dressings are arranged in such a way that they are not disturbed when the drain is pulled out in a proximal direction at the end of the second postoperative day.

Amputations in children

Amputations in children present special problems[5]. The amputated bone, especially in younger children, has a tendency to overgrow on its cut end by a process of accretion. Revisions are required to prevent the bone from ulcerating through the end of the stump. An infant undergoing an above-elbow or below-knee amputation may require three or more revision procedures before reaching maturity.

Every care should be taken to preserve epiphyseal lines[6]. For example, it is better to perform a disarticulation rather than amputate through the bone proximal to the joint. It is worthwhile even if skin grafting is necessary to achieve the extra length. On the whole, troublesome scar formation, neuromata and phantom limb pain are uncommon in children. As amputees, children require frequent prosthetic fitting to keep pace with growth.

Complications

Haematoma

The presence of a haematoma in an amputation wound predisposes to infection and greatly delays prosthetic fitting. Early surgical drainage is recommended.

Infection and flap necrosis

An amputation is one of the commonest wounds to become infected. This is because the tissues are often poorly vascularized, transection of the bacteria-laden lymphatics is inevitable if there is sepsis in the distal part of the extremity, and the wound often contains dead tissue such as a haematoma, denuded cortical bone or ligature material. When infection occurs it can sometimes be eradicated by antibiotics, together with incision and drainage of any collection of pus, but all too often a chronic sinus develops which persists until the focus is removed. This is often found to be a small sequestrum at the cut end of the bone or ligature material. In diabetic patients sloughed connective tissue is often responsible. If the infection or necrosis is localized, wedge resection can be very rewarding[7].

Joint contractures

These affect particularly the elderly and those in chronic pain. Hip contractures can be guarded against by regular prone-lying; and those in the knee by regular exercising and the constant use of a stump board which supports the distal part of the stump when sitting, and also discourages the formation of oedema.

Phantom limb sensation

It is usual for an adult amputee to feel that the missing part of the limb is still present. Reassurance about this strange feeling should be given and the patient made aware of the danger of attempting to use a limb that is not there, especially when getting out of bed half asleep.

Phantom pain

The majority of adult amputees complain of pain in the phantom limb and in some cases it is severe and persistent. It does not respond to drastic measures such as nerve division or even root section, indicating its origin to be either central or in the spinal cord. The phenomenon is more common in proximal than distal amputations and when there has been much severe pain before surgery.

Many methods of treatment have been advocated but none has been found to be consistently successful[8]. For a number of amputees the problem is very real. It can be quite relentless and on occasion it has driven amputees to suicide. Much pain is prevented by adequate postoperative analgesia and by a vigorous and well-planned rehabilitation programme.

Stump oedema

Amputation stumps are prone to becoming oedematous after surgery. The protein content of the interstitial fluid increases as a result of the postoperative inflammatory response and there is lymphatic stasis as a result of the muscle inactivity brought about by transection and pain. The tendency to oedema can be reduced by the delicate handling of tissues and the avoidance of a haematoma. Late oedema may occur as a result of negative pressure in the end-socket space or because of an overtight socket brim.

Rehabilitation

An amputation is but the first step of a rehabilitation process involving a multidisciplinary team.

The *physiotherapist* assists with the preoperative assessment of the patient. After the operation she prepares the stump for prosthetic fitting, guarding against joint contractures and minimizing the formation of oedema by means of bandaging and the use of a stump shrinker and a pneumatic walking aid. She encourages the patient to be as mobile as possible, providing whatever walking aids are necessary. When the first prosthesis arrives she teaches donning and doffing and undertakes gait training. Her services may also be required in dealing with stump pain using transcutaneous nerve stimulation (TNS).

The *occupational therapist* teaches the patient how to live independently with the artificial limb, providing gadgets and initiating home adaptations where necessary. She supervises the provision of a wheelchair if one is indicated. She also undertakes work assessment and trains upper limb amputees in the use of their artificial arms.

The *social worker* supports the patient and his family in adjusting to society. She acquaints him with what he is entitled to receive from the welfare services and puts him in touch with the appropriate authorities where necessary. The details of other national bodies are made available; for example, in the UK, the National Association for Limbless Disabled, the British Limbless Ex-servicemen's Association, the Royal Association for Rehabilitation, the Disabled Living Foundation, the British Amputee Sports Association and the British School of Motoring Disabled Driver's Teaching Centre. Similar organizations are available in most countries.

The *prosthetist*, working in conjunction with the prosthetic surgeon, works out the details of the artificial limb prescription and supervises its manufacture, fitting, alignment and maintenance.

Besides caring for the wound, the ward *nurse* has an important role in coordinating the team and adjusting the expectations of the patient and his family as regards the eventual outcome.

Ideally those involved should work in close contact with one another in the same environment but, since it is not practicable to site comprehensive prosthetic workshops in every hospital, the team is often fragmented, creating difficulties in communication and transport which are then exacerbated by bureaucratic factors. The surgeon is in the unique position of being able to monitor and influence the entire process and thus has a responsibility to ensure that the final outcome is, as far as possible, that planned at the time the patient consented to amputation.

References

1. Burgess EM, Romano RL, Zetl JH, Schrock RD. Amputations of the leg for peripheral vascular insufficiency. *J Bone Joint Surg [Am]* 1971; 53-A: 874–90.

2. Gustilo RB, Mendoza RM, Williams DN. Problems in the management of type III (severe) open fractures: a new classification of type III open fractures. *J Trauma* 1984; 24: 742–6.

3. Dickhout S, De Lee JC, Page CP. Nutritional status: importance in predicting wound healing after amputation. *J Bone Joint Surg [Am]* 1984; 66-A: 71–5.

4. Sonne-Holm S, Boeckstyns M, Menck H. et al. Prophylactic antibiotics in amputation of the lower extremity for ischaemia: a placebo-controlled, randomised trial of cefoxitin. *J Bone Joint Surg [Am]* 1985; 67-A: 800–3.

5. Jorring K. Amputation in children: a follow-up of 74 children whose lower extremities were amputated. *Acta Orthop Scand* 1971; 42: 178–86.

6. Aitken GT, Franz CH. The juvenile amputee. *J Bone Joint Surg [Am]* 1953; 35-A: 659–64.

7. Murdoch G. Amputation surgery in the lower extremity — part II. *Prosthet Orthot Int* 1977; 1: 183–92.

8. Sherman RA, Sherman CJ, Gall NG. A survey of current phantom limb pain treatment in the United States. *Pain* 1980; 8: 85–99.

Illustrations by Gillian Oliver after A. Barrett

Amputation through the upper limb

J. C. Angel FRCS
Consultant Orthopaedic Surgeon, Royal National Orthopaedic and Edgware General Hospitals, Middlesex, UK

Introduction

Indications

In the United Kingdom only one upper limb amputation is performed for every 20 through the lower limb. The principal indication is trauma but occasionally it is required for malignant tumours, gas gangrene, ischaemic gangrene, chronic infection, gross deformities and congenital abnormalities.

Contraindications

With complete traumatic amputations in which the area of tissue destruction is small as a result of a guillotine type of injury consideration should be given to reimplantation.

Preoperative preparation

General anaesthesia is preferred but a supraclavicular or brachial plexus block may be satisfactory. The patient lies supine, the arm is supported on a table and an inverted receiver is placed under the limb just proximal to the site of amputation.

Operations

BELOW-ELBOW AMPUTATION

Incision

1a & b

Equal dorsal and volar skin flaps are marked out, their bases at the junction of the middle and lower thirds of the ulna (approximately 17 cm distal to the tip of the olecranon process). During this the forearm should be in full supination otherwise the flaps, after being cut, are drawn into an oblique position by the natural elasticity of the skin. The deep fascia is incised just short of the same level.

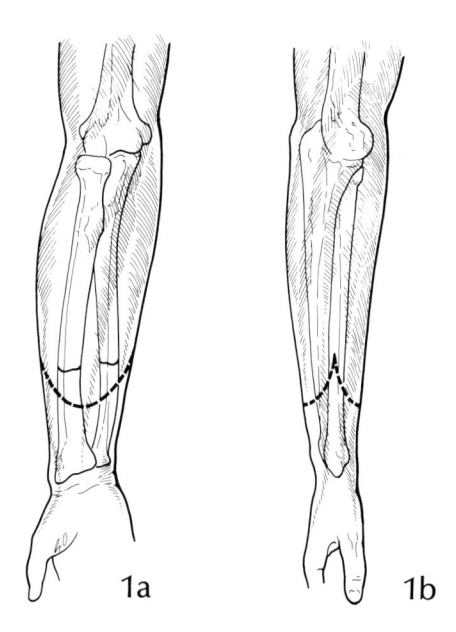

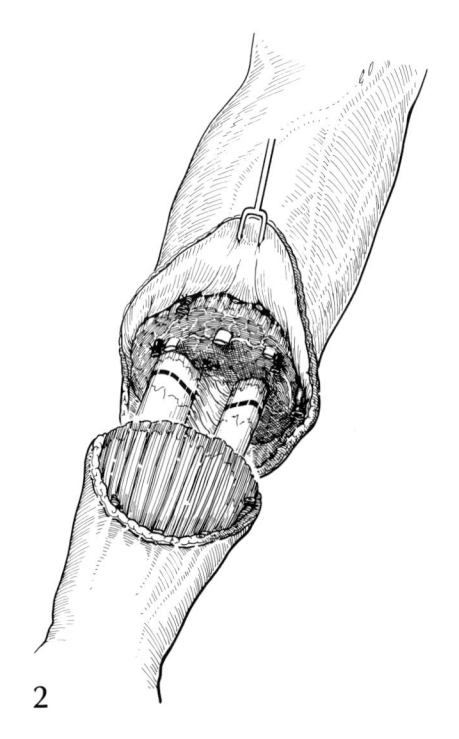

Exposure and division of soft tissue

2

The tendons, muscles and other soft tissues are cut with a slightly raked incision to meet the bone at the level of section. In practice it is found that the most suitable site is where the majority of the muscle bellies become tendinous. The radial and ulnar arteries and their accompanying venae comitantes are ligated with a non-absorbable transfixion ligature.

Division of radius and ulna

3

The ulna is cut a few millimetres more proximally than the radius and its subcutaneous border is bevelled. Both bones are smoothed with a rasp. The cut ends of the named nerves are then pulled down and cut high.

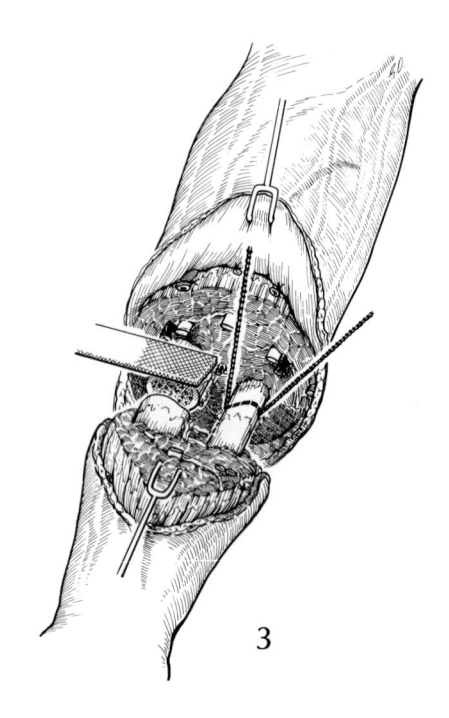

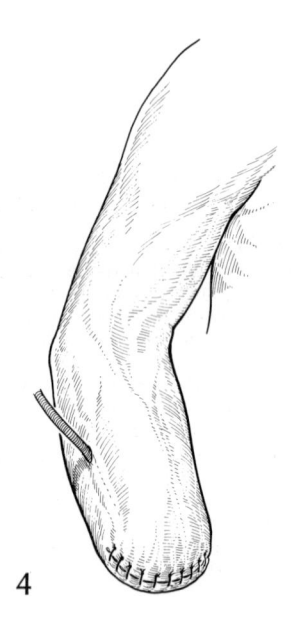

Closure and drainage

4

The drain is passed out through the muscle and skin on the lateral side of the forearm. The deep fascia is closed over the ends of the bones using a fine non-absorbable suture and the skin is approximated with either fine interrupted sutures or staples.

DISARTICULATION AT THE ELBOW

Skin flaps

5a & b

With the forearm in full supination equal anterior and posterior flaps are fashioned, their bases being level with the humeral epicondyles. The anterior flap extends just below the bicipital insertion with the elbow extended and the posterior flap to just below the tip of the olecranon with the elbow fully flexed.

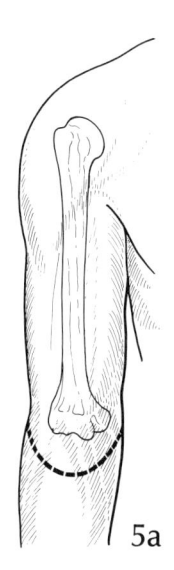

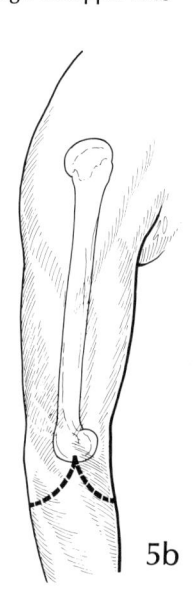

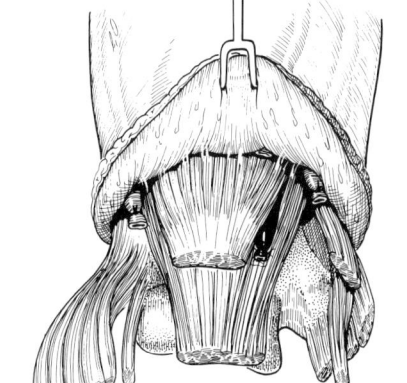

Division of soft tissues

6

The skin flaps are reflected proximally to the level of the epicondyles. The bicipital aponeurosis is divided and the flexor mass arising from the medial epicondyle is detached and reflected distally. This gives access to the main neurovascular bundle lying medial to the biceps tendon. The brachial vessels are individually ligated. The main nerves are drawn down and divided with scissors so that they retract at least 3 cm proximal to the level of the joint line.

Next the biceps tendon is detached from the radial tuberosity and the brachialis from the coronoid process of the ulna. The extensor musculature arising from the humeral epicondyle is divided at a level 6 cm distal to the joint line and reflected proximally. The triceps tendon is detached from the tip of the olecranon and the disarticulation is completed by dividing the anterior capsule and the collateral ligaments. The tourniquet is released and haemostasis is secured.

Soft-tissue covering for distal end of bone

7

The next task is to fashion soft-tissue covering for the distal end of the humerus, the articular surface of which is left intact. The triceps is brought forward and sutured to the distal ends of the biceps and brachialis. The remains of the extensor muscle mass is thinned by removing some of the deeper fibres and sutured to the remnant of the flexor mass at the medial epicondyle.

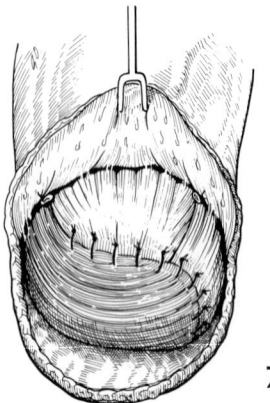

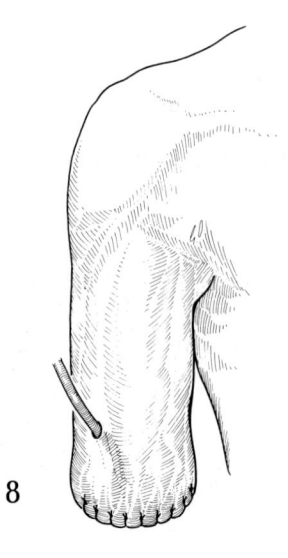

Closure

8

A suction drain is passed out through the skin on the lateral side of the arm, its tip being buried in contact with the articular surface. The skin flaps are closed with interrupted sutures.

ABOVE-ELBOW AMPUTATION

Incision

9a & b

Equal anteroposterior flaps are marked out, their bases being 20 cm from the tip of the acromion process of the scapula.

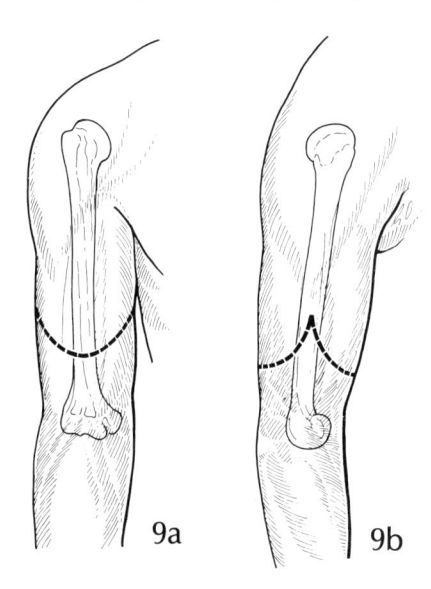

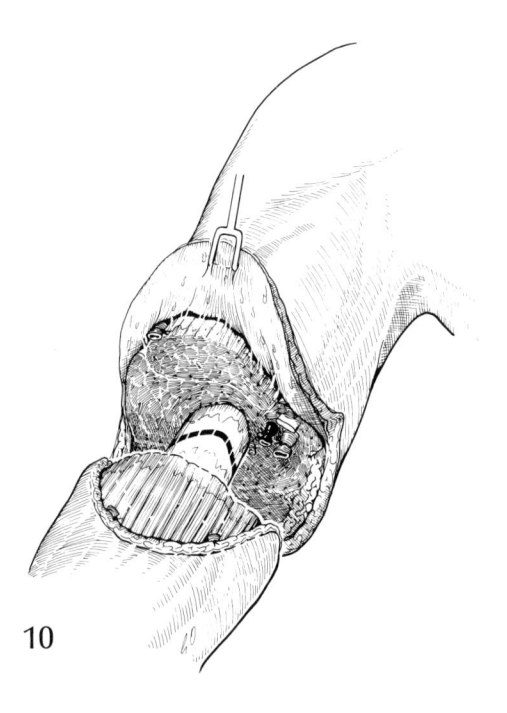

Division of soft tissues and humerus

10

The initial skin incision is continued through the deep fascia at a slightly more proximal level and through the muscle to meet the bone at the level of bone section. The brachial vessels are identified and doubly ligated with an absorbable ligature material. The periosteum is divided circumferentially at the level of bone section, 20 cm from the tip of the acromion, and the bone is cut with a Gigli saw and smoothed with a rasp. At this point the tourniquet can be deflated and any further bleeding controlled.

Closure

11

A drain is passed through the muscle and skin on the lateral side of the arm, and the fascia is closed over the cut end of the bone with interrupted non-absorbable sutures. The skin is closed with either sutures or staples.

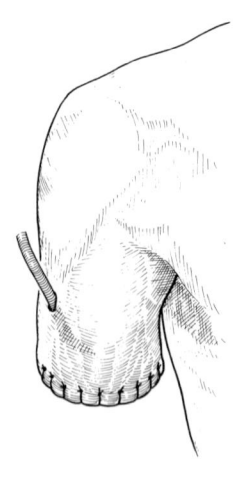

Postoperative management

The wound is dressed, protected with wool and bandaged. All this is kept in place with a stirrup of adhesive strapping. The drain is removed after 48 hours, at which time physiotherapy, to mobilize the remaining joints of the limb, is commenced.

Prosthetics

The minimum length of radius required to fit a below-elbow prosthesis projects 2.5 cm distal to the insertion of the biceps tendon. A forearm stump that retains more than 17 cm of ulna, and yet is not long enough to include the distal radio-ulnar joint, as in a wrist disarticulation, is not desirable from the prosthetic point of view and it should be avoided. With a stump of average length, the socket of the prosthesis is held in place by a harness which passes up the arm, behind the back and around the root of the opposite arm. A rotary device is fitted to the socket which allows the same function as forearm rotation. Into it can be connected a cosmetic hand, a functioning hand and a split hook or other terminal device. The hand or split hook is operated by a cord that is tensed by a forward shrugging movement of the shoulder.

Also available for below-elbow amputees are lightweight cosmetic hands that pull onto the stump in much the same manner as a glove, and myoelectric prostheses which make use of the electrical activity of the residual muscles of the forearm for the control of a motorized mechanical hand. These have considerable appeal, not least because they do away with the need for a cumbersome shoulder harness (appendage).

The advantage of the through-elbow disarticulation compared with the above-elbow level is that the stump is capable of transmitting shoulder movements, including rotation, to the prosthesis and also it provides a longer, stronger lever arm. The disadvantage is that the jointed side-steels have to be placed either side of the rather bulky socket, and the elbow joint locking mechanism is less robust and inefficient. The lower level of amputation is definitely advantageous to a man who works with his hands, particularly if the dominant hand has been lost. It is less useful in women whose sleeves tend to snag on the prosthesis, causing excessive wear to garments; also, they dislike the poor cosmesis.

Illustrations by Peter Cox after M. J. Courtney

Forequarter amputation

Paul C. Weaver MD, FRCS, FRCS(Ed)
Consultant Surgeon (Surgical Oncology), Portsmouth and South East Hampshire Group of Hospitals; Clinical Teacher, University of Southampton, UK

Introduction

The first successful forequarter or interscapulothoracic amputation was carried out in 1836. In 1887 Berger reviewed and standardized the anterior approach technique, which is used today with some variation. In this operation the main vessels and nerves are ligated early, as opposed to the posterior or Littlewood operation in which the quarter is dissected free before the vessels and nerves are secured.

When this amputation is carried out the whole of the upper limb is removed with the scapula and outer two-thirds of the clavicle (unless this bone is involved when the clavicle is disarticulated at the sternal joint).

Indications

Forequarter amputation is performed almost exclusively for malignant disease, with very minimal indication arising from trauma or war injuries. Forequarter amputation may be required in the management of malignant tumours of the shoulder girdle or soft tissues. Patients presenting with primary malignant tumours of bone and soft tissues are usually managed in multidisciplinary clinics and it is certainly very important to explore every avenue of limb conservation before embarking on radical ablative surgery. Providing the surgery is radical enough to remove the disease, it is certainly possible to manufacture prosthetic skeletal parts to support the arm. The arterial supply can likewise be replaced. The main limitation to conservation is involvement of the nerve supply to the arm and, in the case of soft tissue sarcomas, the necessity to adequately clear the compartment in which the tumour resides.

Contraindications

Amputation is contraindicated (1) in the presence of distant metastatic malignant disease or the inability to remove all tumour; (2) if the patient refuses to accept mutilation; and (3) if there is physical or mental unfitness for major surgery.

Preoperative

Clinical assessment

The patient should be carefully assessed, preferably in a multidisciplinary clinic with special emphasis on limb function, blood supply and neurological status. The previous treatment should carefully be reviewed and the possibility of less radical treatment considered, using either radiotherapy, chemotherapy, surgery or a combination.

Investigations

Radiography and computed tomography are essential to define the limits of disease and exclude possible metastatic spread, particularly to the lungs and liver. Nuclear magnetic resonance is particularly valuable in soft tissue disease for defining its limits. Ultrasound scanning is a rapid and cost-effective way of assessing the liver. Isotopic bone scanning may be required for detection of skeletal metastatic disease.

Biopsy

Unequivocal microscopic evidence is essential. Care must be taken with a biopsy incision not to encroach upon the skin flaps of the amputation.

Preoperative preparation

The patient and relatives are counselled. Limb-fitting surgeons are introduced to the patient with a view to discussing postoperative prostheses. The physiotherapist is introduced to the patient to discuss postoperative rehabilitation.

Any anaemia is corrected and 4 units of blood made available for the operation, although it is seldom necessary to use more than 2–3 units.

Bacteriology

If the patient has an open wound or a fungating lesion, preoperative swabs are taken so that the appropriate antibiotic cover can be given, but where there is no pre-existing infection, routine antibiotic cover is not necessary.

Anaesthesia

Endotracheal intubation is necessary. Hypotensive general anaesthesia helps reduce blood loss and contributes to the speed, accuracy and safety of surgery.

Operation

In general the classic Berger operation is used and requires a racquet-shaped incision with linear extension parallel to and above the clavicle. This is preferable to and safer than the Littlewood operation, because the large vessels are controlled early, reducing blood loss and, in addition, traction on the brachial plexus is minimized.

The posterior approach can be used when there is some doubt of operability and when exploration is deemed necessary before the major vessels and nerves are divided.

ANTERIOR APPROACH (Berger[1])

Position of patient

1

The patient is placed on the table on his side with the affected arm uppermost. A low sandbag or support is placed so that the trunk is inclined backwards to facilitate the initial approach to the clavicle and vessels. The affected arm is draped so that it is free and can be held by an assistant when required.

Incision

2

The skin flaps are marked out by drawing a line extending above and parallel to the inner two-thirds of the clavicle, and dividing into an anterior and posterior portion. The anterior incision passes obliquely downwards over the clavicle and coracoid process, then across the middle of the anterior axillary fold and obliquely across the axilla to the inferior angle of the scapula. The posterior portion passes over the outer part of the supraclavicular fossa and downwards across the scapula to its inferior angle. Modifications are made according to the site of the tumour and the state of the surrounding skin of the shoulder.

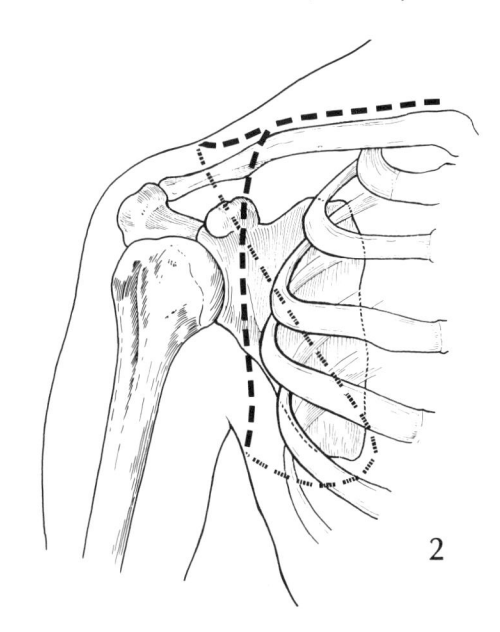

Division of clavicle

3

The supraclavicular incision is made to expose the medial two-thirds of the clavicle. The insertion of the pectoralis major and the outer edge of the sternomastoid are divided, using cutting diathermy; and a subperiosteal resection of the middle third of the clavicle is carried out using a Gigli saw. The axillary and subclavian vessels, and the brachial plexus, remain covered by the deep periosteum of the clavicle, axillary and cervical fascia, and the subclavius muscle.

Ligation of subclavian vessels and anterior dissection

4

The pectoralis major is now divided downwards from the clavicular bed to provide a wider exposure of the vessels. The deep periosteum and fascia are divided with care, exposing the axillary vein which is traced proximally to the first rib. Ligation of the suprascapular and cephalic veins will facilitate double ligation of the axillary vein at the level of the first rib. The axillary artery is now exposed, and after ligation of the superior thoracic and acromiothoracic vessels, the subclavian artery is doubly ligated at the level of the first rib. The trunks of the brachial plexus can now be cut across cleanly with the knife. The anterior skin incision is now completed, retracting the flap downwards and medially. The pectoral muscles are removed with the limb, dividing both pectoralis major and minor close to the chest wall. Axillary fat, lymphatics and clavipectoral fascia are dissected downwards and outwards *en bloc*.

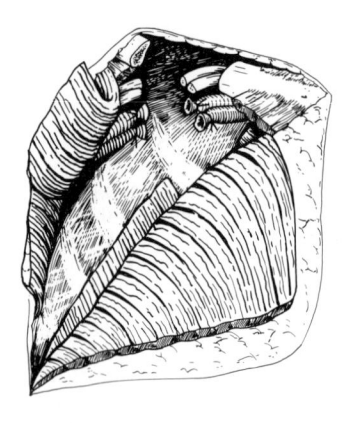

Posterior dissection

5 & 6

The posterior incision is made with the affected arm held forwards by an assistant. The suprascapular vessels are ligated. The flap is dissected backwards just posterior to the vertebral border of the scapula. Portions of the trapezius, latissimus dorsi and levator scapulae are resected according to the site and size of the tumour, using cutting diathermy. The rhomboid muscles, major and minor, are divided. By retracting the scapula away from the chest wall, the lower digitations of serratus anterior are divided close to the scapula. Traction on the arm is released and the patient allowed to roll gently backwards again. The arm is now lifted laterally and the upper digitations of serratus anterior and omohyoid are divided with their attached fascia.

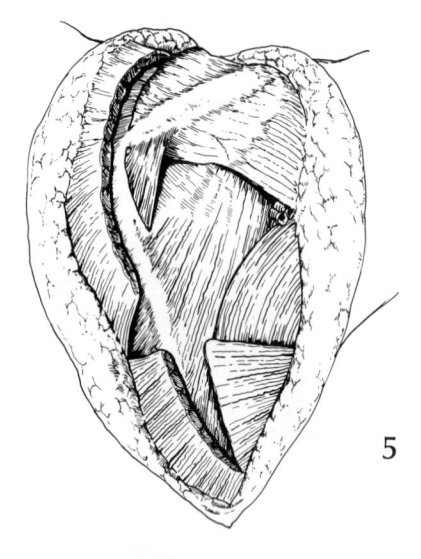

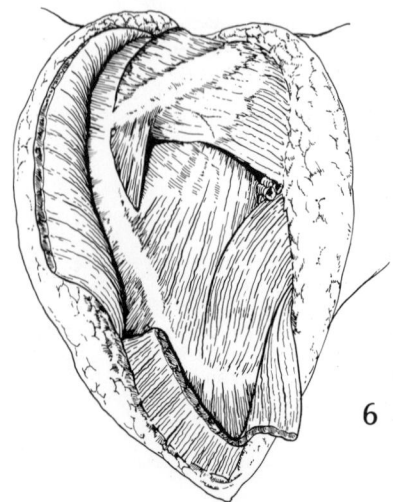

7 & 8

The forequarter is now removed and accurate haemostasis achieved. The wound is closed after introducing large suction drains. The skin only is closed using interrupted sutures or staples. The drains are connected to a sealed suction drainage system, or a closed underwater seal drainage bottle and thence to a Robert's pump. A wound dressing is applied.

POSTERIOR APPROACH (Littlewood[2])

This operation involves dividing the same structures as described in the previous operation but in a different sequence. The operation begins with the patient rotated forwards, completing the posterior dissection as described. The upper part of the anterior incision is then made and a subperiosteal resection of the middle third of the clavicle is carried out. This allows the quarter to fall away from the trunk, exposing the neurovascular bundle from behind, the limb and shoulder being supported by an assistant to prevent over-traction on the nerves. The trunks of the brachial plexus are divided, followed by ligation of the subclavian artery and vein. The anterior skin flap is then cut and the pectoral muscles are divided. The wound is closed and drained as previously described.

Postoperative management

The intravenous drip is only retained so long as a blood transfusion is required. Fluids may be given by mouth when the patient is conscious. Morphine analgesia by parenteral injection is usually required for the first 48 hours.

Care of the wound

The suction drains are left in place on suction until the drainage is less than 50 ml/24 hours and are usually removed about the fifth postoperative day, without removal of the pressure dressing which is left in place for 10 days. Sutures are removed on or about the fourteenth day, depending upon the state of the wound.

Prosthesis

In order to support normal clothing, the shoulder deformity is corrected with a light shoulder prosthesis, which is prepared by the limb-fitting surgeon using a cast made preoperatively. The patient may be provided with an artificial limb, once healing is complete, but in many cases the patient who asks for an artificial limb frequently stops using it, finding that its nuisance value outweighs the value of it as a cosmetic appliance.

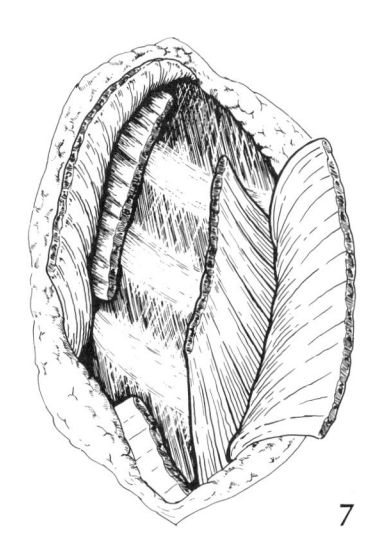

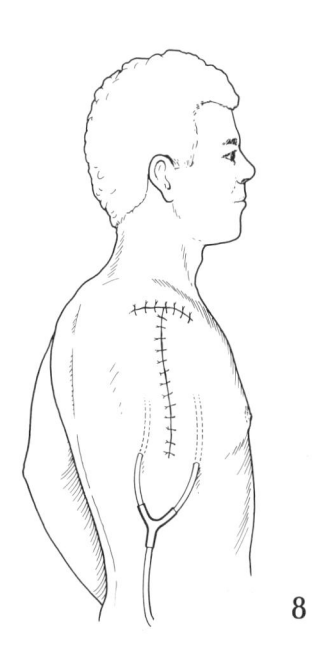

References

1. Berger P. *L'amputation du membre supérieure dans la configuité du tronc (amputation interscapulo-thoracique)*. Paris: G. Masson, 1887.

2. Littlewood H. Amputations at the shoulder and the hip. *Br Med J* 1922; i: 381–3.

Illustrations by Peter Cox after M. J. Courtney

Hindquarter amputation

Paul C. Weaver MD, FRCS, FRCS(Ed)
Consultant Surgeon (Surgical Oncology), Portsmouth and South East Hampshire Group of Hospitals; Clinical Teacher, University of Southampton, UK

Introduction

The indications for a full hindquarter amputation have declined with the ability of orthopaedic surgeons to replace sections of the pelvic girdle and hip. Hindquarter amputation was first carried out by Billroth in 1891 for soft tissue sarcoma; his patient died. The first recorded survival was in 1895 – a patient of Girard. The operation was developed in Britain by Sir Gordon Gordon-Taylor and the technique is based upon descriptions by Gordon-Taylor and Monro[1] and Westbury[2]. When the amputation is carried out part of the pelvic girdle and the whole lower limb are removed from the body.

Indications

Hindquarter and hip amputations are performed almost exclusively for malignant disease of the bone or soft tissues of the pelvis or thigh. In the main it is used as an attempt to cure the patient, although it can be of value in palliation when pain and massive fungation makes management impossible.

Very occasionally this major procedure is indicated in trauma[3]. Extended hemipelvectomy in continuity with adherent pelvic visceral cancer is described by Brunschwig[4].

In most instances patients with malignant disease of bone or soft tissue of the pelvis or thigh are managed in multidisciplinary clinics from the onset of their disease. Adequate management with radiotherapy and chemotherapy may prevent or delay the necessity for major surgery; where surgery is indicated it is now possible to replace parts of the pelvic girdle and hip, either by manufacturing these parts to the specific requirements of the patient or by an 'off-the-shelf' replacement system. Likewise the arterial supply to the limb can be reconstructed. The limiting factor in limb conservation is neurological involvement or extensive soft tissue sarcomas.

Contraindications

Amputation is contraindicated (1) in the presence of metastatic disease or the inability to remove all tumour; (2) when the patient refuses to accept mutilation; and (3) when there is physical or mental unfitness for major surgery.

Preoperative

Investigations

The patient being considered for hindquarter amputation must be reviewed by the multidisciplinary clinic to make certain that hindquarter amputation is the only alternative and that further therapy cannot be offered in the form of radiotherapy, chemotherapy or ablative surgery with reconstruction. Special attention is paid to bone and soft tissue involvement, the arterial blood supply and nerve function of the limb. Following clinical examination, radiography and computed tomography are used to define the limits of the disease and exclude possible metastatic spread. Nuclear magnetic resonance can be particularly useful, defining the limits of soft tissue malignancy. Ultrasound liver scan is a rapid and economic way of checking for liver metastases. An isotopic bone scan may be required to exclude possible skeletal metastases.

Biopsy

Unequivocal microscopic evidence is essential. Care must be taken with a biopsy incision not to encroach upon the skin flaps of the amputation.

Preoperative preparation

When the possibility of conservation surgery has been excluded, the patient and relatives are counselled and introduced to the limb-fitting surgeon and physiotherapist. If possible the patient is given arm exercises and balance training on the use of a single lower limb.

Any anaemia is corrected and 6 units of blood are made available. An enema or rectal washout is given prior to surgery to prevent early bowel evacuation and dressing contamination. The most feared bacterial complication of high lower limb amputations is contamination with clostridial bacteria from the bowel. Where there is no known allergy, intramuscular penicillin is given starting with the anaesthetic premedication. Preoperatively the thigh and buttock areas are treated and wrapped in dressings of povidone-iodine solution as protection against clostridial organisms.

Anaesthesia

Hypotensive anaesthesia, sometimes with the addition of spinal or epidural block, helps reduce blood loss and contributes to the speed, accuracy and safety of surgery.

After anaesthetic induction, a Foley catheter is passed to empty the bladder and left in place. The anus is excluded by a small woolpad and sealed round the natal cleft by an adhesive surgical drape.

Operation

Position of patient

1

The patient is positioned on his back with a long, narrow sandbag under the shoulder and buttock of the affected side. This gives good access to the major, anterior, extraperitoneal part of the dissection, and an assistant holding the leg can roll the patient towards the lateral position for the short time needed to cut the posterior flap and muscles.

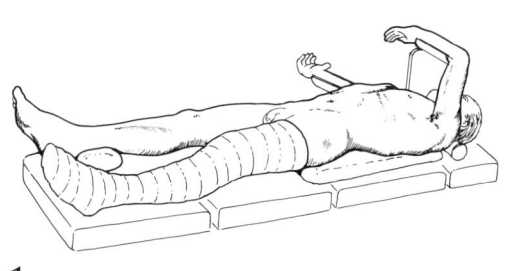

Incision

2

The outline of the skin flap is drawn. The anterior line passes immediately above and parallel to the inguinal ligament. The backwards extent depends upon the proposed site of section of the posterior pelvis. The posterior incision, made later in the operation, curves over the buttock in front of the greater trochanter, across the ischial tuberosity into the crease between the genitals and the thigh. Modifications are made where tumour is close and to avoid skin damaged by radiotherapy or by previous biopsy.

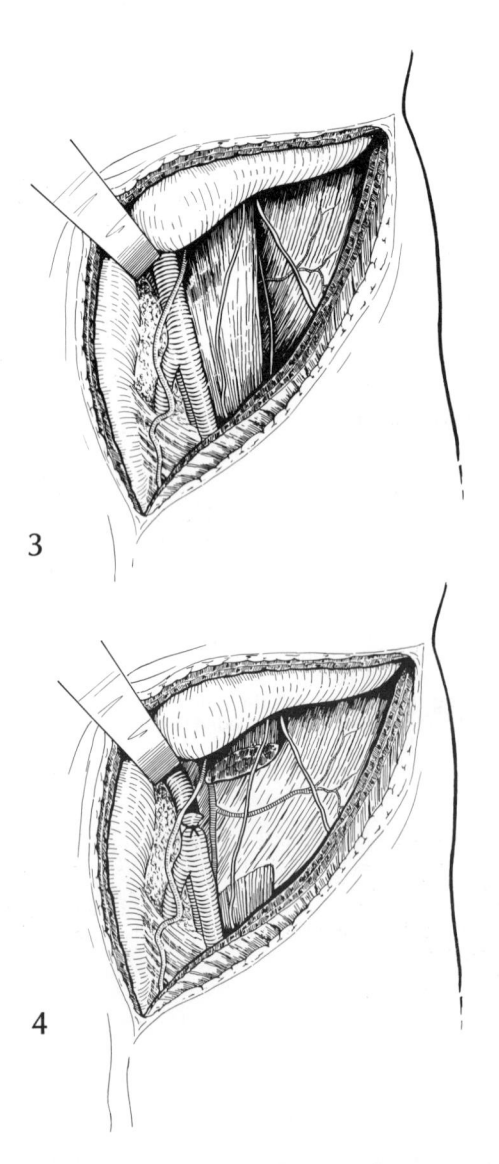

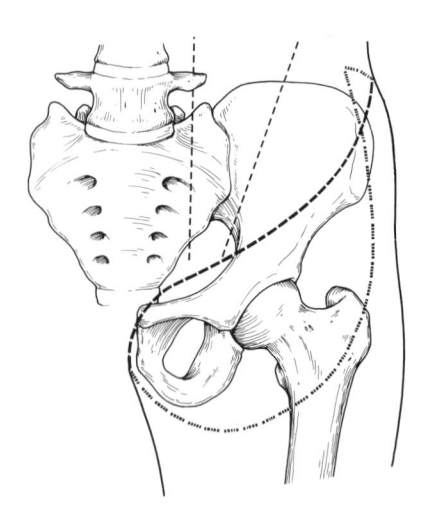

Exposure of iliac vessels and pubic disarticulation

3

The anterior incision is made and deepened through the abdominal wall muscles. The peritoneum of the iliac fossa is stripped medially and operability confirmed. The deep epigastric vessels are divided and the spermatic cord is mobilized and pushed medially. The rectus abdominis is cut across just above the pubis. The symphysis is divided at this stage, using a solid scalpel helped by a few blows with the osteotome. Monro's tubercle, the vertical ridge on the posterior aspect of the symphysis, is an invaluable guide to the plane of the articular cartilage.

After dividing the suprapubic ligament, with regard to the underlying membranous urethra, the symphysis opens. A gauze pack controls any venous oozing from this region while attention is turned to the crucial phase of the operation, division of the vascular pedicle of the limb. The peritoneum and ureter are swept medially to expose the iliac bifurcation.

Ligation of common iliac artery and vein

4

The common iliac artery is divided between silk ligatures followed by division of the psoas muscle with cutting diathermy. The nerves, femoral, obturator and lateral cutaneous nerve of the thigh (not shown), are cut cleanly with a knife. The ends of the psoas retract revealing the iliolumbar tributaries of the common iliac vein. These branches, between one and four in number, tether the main vein and must be divided carefully between silk ligatures, to permit the safe mobilization and ligation of the common iliac. If this step is omitted, the iliolumbar veins will tear out with the possibility of disastrous haemorrhage.

Division of the posterior ilium

5a & b

The posterior flap is developed, preserving a variable portion of gluteus maximus according to the site of the lesion. The divided vascular pedicle is gently pushed downwards to expose the greater sciatic notch. Both sides of the notch are now exposed and a large artery forceps is passed underneath this to draw through the end of a Gigli saw. The site of the pelvic section depends on the location and nature of the pathology. Division of the posterior part of the ilium involves minimal blood loss; the projecting remnant can be trimmed when the specimen is removed. Where necessary, section can be made through the ala of the sacrum in preference to sacroiliac disarticulation. The hindquarter is now lifted away from the trunk and the remaining soft structures divided: levator ani, perineal membrane, branches of the internal iliac vessels, sciatic nerve, piriformis, sacrotuberous and sacrospinous ligaments. Bleeding from the veins of the prostatic plexus and cavernous tissue may be troublesome and is best controlled by catgut stitches.

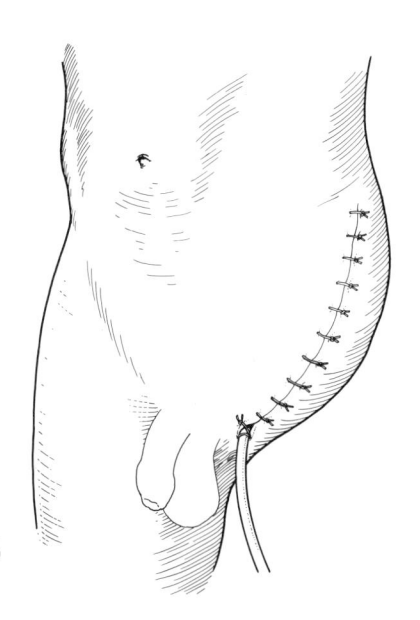

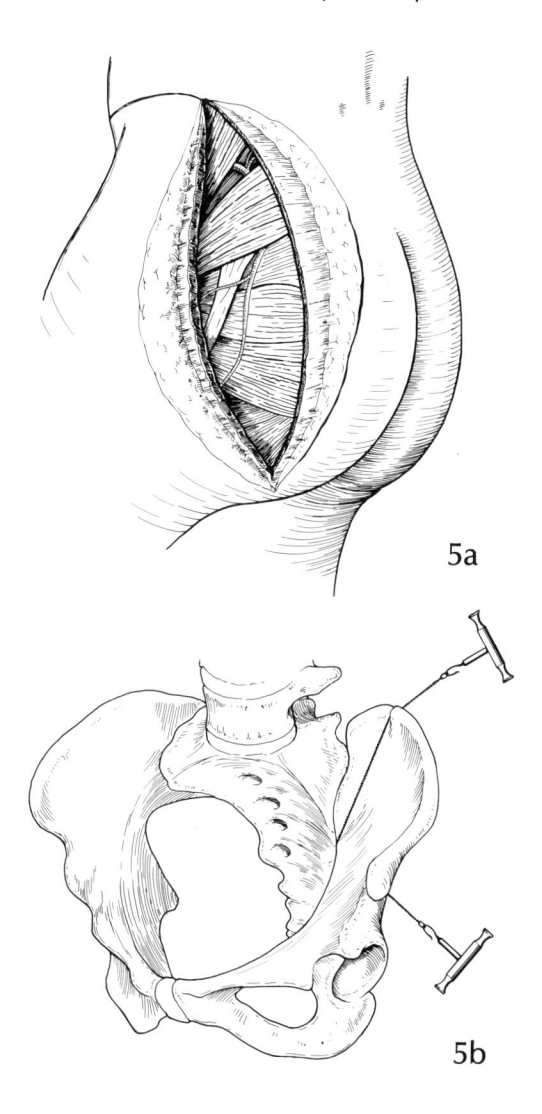

Wound closure

6

The wound is closed with non-absorbable skin sutures only, and suction drainage (via underwater seal drainage bottle and a Robert's pump) applied for 5–6 days. The bladder catheter is removed on the fifth postoperative morning. The wound is supported with gauze wool and strapping.

Postoperative management

General nursing

After the first 24 hours the patient's position is changed 4-hourly. Analgesia is given as frequently as necessary to keep the patient comfortable. Fluids and food can be given by mouth after 24 hours. An orthopaedic lifting chair is provided and active movement encouraged on the third day. Increased mobility is not encouraged until the drains are removed and these should be taken out with as little disturbance as possible to the support dressing, which is untouched for 14 days providing there is no unexplained pyrexia or excessive pain. Sutures are frequently left for 21 days as healing is slower than with most other wounds, particularly after radiotherapy.

After 14 days, walking with crutches is started where possible and a wheelchair is provided. After the removal of the sutures the possibility of a prosthesis is reviewed and ordered if necessary.

References

1. Gordon-Taylor SG, Monro R. Technique and management of the 'hindquarter' amputation. *Br J Surg* 1952; 39: 536–41.

2. Westbury G. Hindquarter and hip amputation. *Ann R Coll Surg Engl* 1967; 40: 226–34.

3. McLean EM. Avulsion of the hindquarter. *J Bone Joint Surg [Br]* 1962; 44-B: 384–5.

4. Brunschwig A. Hemipelvectomy in combination with partial pelvic exenteration for uncontrolled recurrent and metastatic cancer of the cervix: 5-year survival. *Surgery* 1962; 52: 299–304.

Illustrations by Gillian Oliver after A. Barrett

Disarticulation of the hip

J. C. Angel FRCS
Consultant Orthopaedic Surgeon, Royal National Orthopaedic and Edgware General Hospitals, Middlesex, UK

Introduction

Indications

The main indication for disarticulation of the hip is malignant disease that cannot be managed safely by a more distal amputation. Occasionally it may be called for in severe trauma, vascular disease and infection.

Preoperative preparation

Four to six units of blood should be available. The operation is performed under general anaesthesia with the patient lying supine, the sacrum being elevated on a large sandbag.

420 Amputations

Operation

Incision

1

The incision commences 6 cm lateral to the anterior superior iliac spine and just proximal to it. It curves anteriorly and then downwards to follow a line parallel to the inguinal ligament, some 2 cm below it. It then runs medially passing 5 cm below the root of the limb. Continuing posteriorly it descends slightly to a level 5 cm below the ischial tuberosity and then sweeps upwards in a broad curve crossing the greater trochanter (with the hip in neutral). Finally it turns slightly backwards to the starting point.

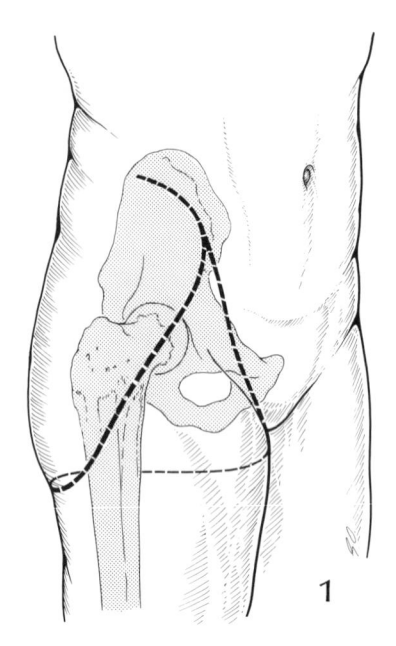

Flexors and adductors

2

The femoral vessels are exposed and ligated in the line of the incision. The femoral nerve and the lateral cutaneous nerve of the thigh are each pulled down gently and divided with scissors, the ends being allowed to retract proximally. The flexors are detached from the superior and inferior iliac spines. The pectineus muscle is divided in the line of the incision. The limb is then laterally rotated to bring the lesser trochanter into view. This allows the iliopsoas tendon to be transected close to its insertion. The adductors are cut close to their attachments to the pubis and ischium. The obturator externus is also dealt with at this stage. It must be cut some distance away from its origin which is encircled by the obturator artery because this vessel has a tendency to retract into the pelvis if cut accidentally.

Extensors and abductors

3

Next the limb is medially rotated and the gluteus medius and minimus are detached from the greater trochanter. The fascia lata and the distal fibres of gluteus maximus are divided in the line of the skin incision. The tendon of gluteus maximus is also released from its attachment to the linea aspera. The sciatic nerve is gently pulled down and cut with scissors. The short rotators are divided and detached from the region of the greater trochanter and the hip is disarticulated.

Closure

4

Two large suction drains are brought out posteriorly. The muscle and fascia of the posterior flap is brought anteriorly and sutured to the iliopsoas, pectineus and the remnants of the adductor muscles. Whilst doing this it is necessary to swing the flap in a cephalad direction to avoid a distally projecting protuberance of skin and subcutaneous tissue.

Postoperative management

The wound is dressed with gauze and an absorbent pad, which is held in position with adhesive plaster. The drains are removed after 48 hours at which time the patient can start to get out of bed.

Prosthetics

If the wound heals uneventfully work can be commenced on the first temporary artificial limb after 4 weeks. The conventional prosthesis is made up of a leather or plastic socket designed to fit snugly round the pelvis, most of the body weight being transmitted through the ischial tuberosity. For this reason it is important to avoid scars in the tuber area. The 'hip joint' is located directly under the socket and projects downwards from it. When the patient sits the pelvis tends to tilt towards the opposite side unless the normal buttock is supported on a cushion. The hip and knee joints each have hand-operated locks which make sitting down a rather awkward business.

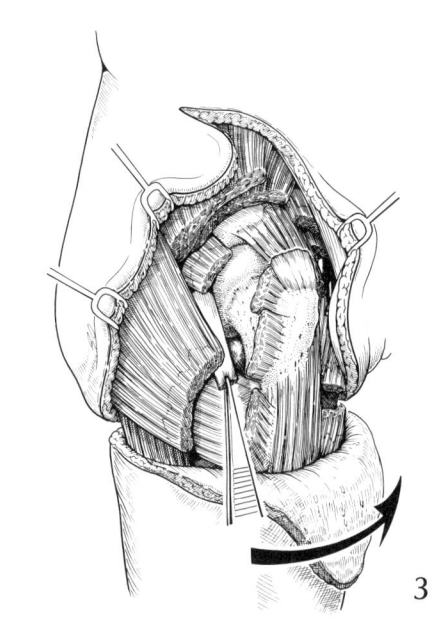

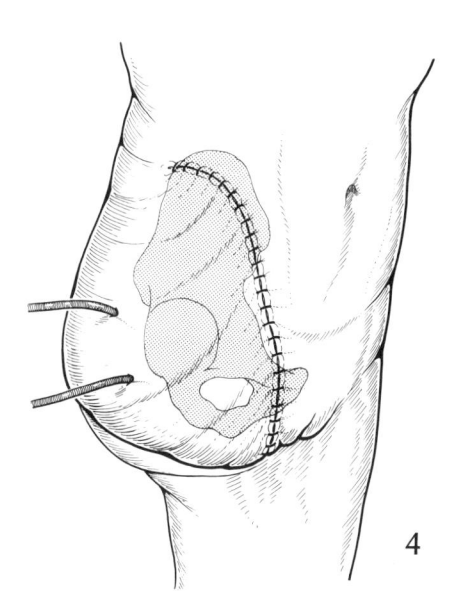

More modern prostheses use the 'Canadian' socket, in which the hip is located antero-inferiorly and both joints are freely moving. The surgical significance of this later type of prosthesis is that it may be precluded by an excessive amount of soft tissue at the distal end of the wound. It must be remembered that the energy required to walk in these prostheses greatly exceeds the requirements of crutch-walking so that few elderly people are able to use them.

Illustrations by Gillian Oliver after A. Barrett

Above-knee amputation

J. C. Angel FRCS
Consultant Orthopaedic Surgeon, Royal National Orthopaedic and Edgware General Hospitals, Middlesex, UK

Introduction

Indications

Amputation above the knee is usually the next level to be considered whenever a below-knee amputation is precluded. Occasionally amputation at intervening levels, such as the supracondylar or through-knee, may provide a suitable alternative but the decision to use them must be taken with due regard to prosthetic considerations.

Contraindications

The operation is contraindicated in children if it is possible, by any measure, to save the growing lower end of the femur.

Preoperative

The hip joint should be examined for fixed flexion deformity, the presence of which may require a shorter stump to be fashioned in order that the deformity may be accommodated in the socket of the artificial limb. Fixed adduction may indicate that the patient will need an overlong artificial limb in the same way that he may already have been wearing a shoe raise to correct apparent shortening.

It is reassuring to have a tourniquet around the root of the limb in case of emergency although this might not be practicable with a short conical thigh if it encroaches on the operative area. The buttock should be elevated on a sandbag.

Selection of level

The level of bone section varies according to the type of prosthesis to be worn (see p. 426) and the anticipated soft-tissue thickness distal to the end of the bone. The latter can vary from less than 1 cm to over 10 cm and is largely dependent on the thickness of the subcutaneous layer. Thus an active person of average build, who might be expected to have a soft-tissue thickness of 3 cm and ultimately wear a suction socket fitted with a stabilized knee mechanism, will need a level of bone section 15 cm above the knee or above the level of the prosthetic knee axis if that is likely to be different. On the other hand, a thin, elderly person who is likely to be fitted with a rigid pelvic band suspension and a simple, semi-automatic knee lock, needs a bone section only 8 cm above the knee if the anticipated soft-tissue thickness is only 2 cm.
 It is desirable to leave the residual femur at least 20 cm long to retain its function as a lever and to allow the fitting of a suction socket. With short fat people, these objectives could be incompatible and it may have to be accepted that they are not suitable for a suction socket or a stabilized knee or both. Patients who are not expected to be fitted with an artificial limb should be given the longest stump that is compatible with clearing the diseased tissue so that they have the best possible sitting balance.

Operation

Incision

1

The level of bone section is marked on the medial and lateral sides of the stump, using either a fibre-tip pen or a throat swab dipped in methylene blue. The equal anterior and posterior, semicircular skin flaps must then be marked on the skin. In children, whose soft tissues are highly elastic, the base of the flaps should be located at the same level as bone section but in the elderly whose soft tissues are inelastic, the base of the flaps should be 3 cm proximal to this level. This prevents undue laxity in the soft tissues and helps to reduce the risk of haematoma formation, as well as improve the shape of the stump.

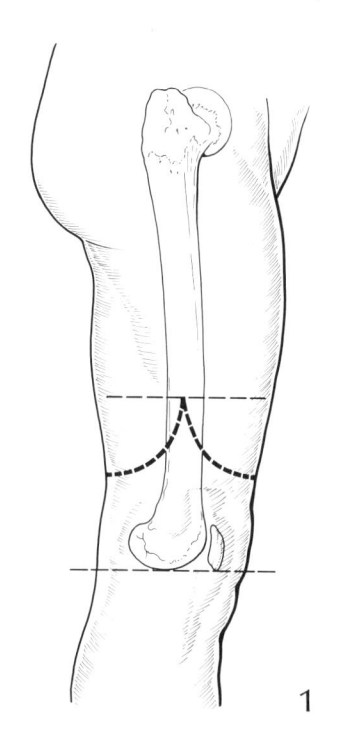

Dissection

2

The skin flaps should be cut with the knife moving from summit to base and the subcutaneous tissue is divided with a raking cut so that more fat is amputated than skin. Anteriorly, the cut is extended through the quadriceps muscle so that the deepest fibres are divided at the level of bone section or even slightly proximal to it. Posteriorly, the deep fascia is cut sufficiently distally to allow it to be wrapped around the distal end of the bone.

A finger is passed around the sartorius and it is freed by blunt dissection and then severed at the level of bone section. This permits access to the femoral vessels just as they pass through the adductor hiatus. They are divided after ligating each individually with 1/0 silk.

Bone section and removal of limb

3 & 4

The periosteum of the femur is divided circumferentially exactly at the point of section in order to prevent it from being stripped. The bone is cut with a Gigli saw. A bone hook is inserted into the distal femur and used to apply traction while the remaining soft tissues are divided. The sciatic nerve is gently pulled down and cut high with scissors. In dysvascular cases the arteria comitans nervi ischiadici, the small vessel running in the substance of the nerve, may cause troublesome bleeding and need attention. The tourniquet is released and haemostasis is secured. The cut end of the femur is rounded with a rasp. A slight bevel is made over the anterolateral aspect.

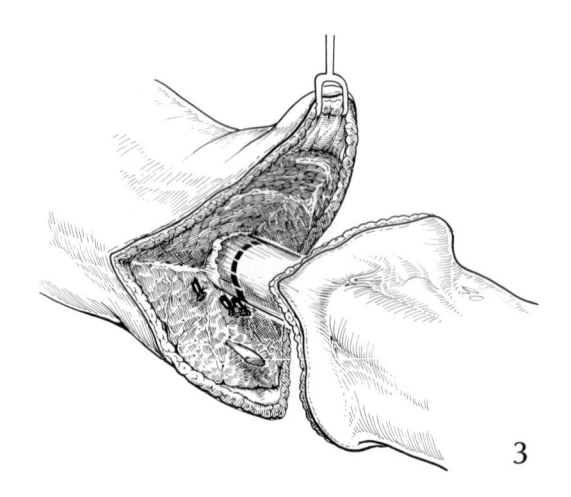

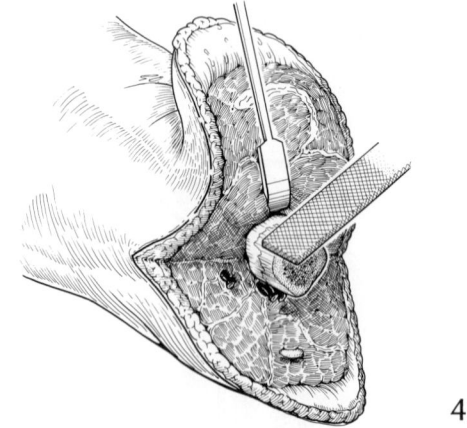

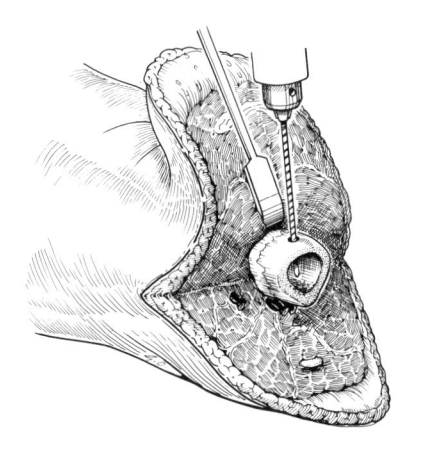

Myodesis

5a, b & c

The muscles are examined to ensure that the deep fascia can be closed over the end of the bone. It is usually necessary to shorten the deepest fibres and trim the muscle layer medially and laterally.

A small hole is drilled through the anterior femoral cortex a few millimetres above its distal end. Two nylon mattress sutures are then passed through the distal hamstrings and used to anchor them to the distal end of the bone. The remaining muscles are sutured to them and the deep fascia is closed. The aim is to have each muscle group under slight tension with the hip in the neutral position.

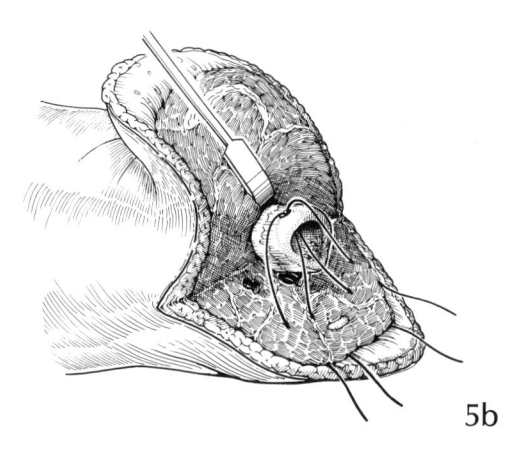

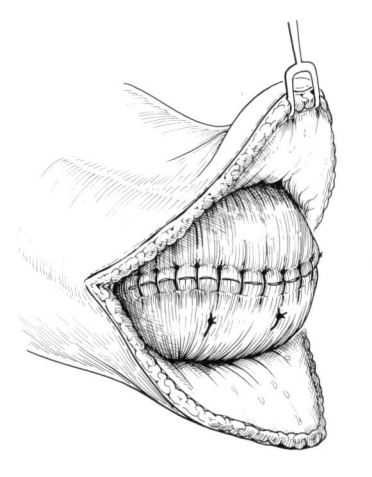

Closure

6

A drain is tucked down to the cut end of the bone and passed through the lateral musculature out onto the lateral side of the thigh. The subcutaneous layer is closed with interrupted sutures and the skin with staples.

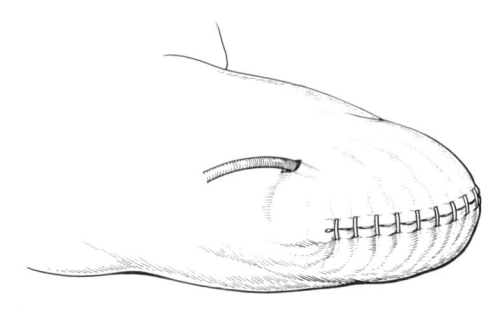

Postoperative management

The wound is dressed with spirit-soaked gauze and gentle pressure is applied by means of wool and crêpe dressing. It is important that this is held onto the stump by means of U-slabs of adhesive strapping brought up onto the lower abdomen and the buttock. The drain can usually be removed after 2 days and the patient is then encouraged to be as mobile as possible. Prone lying for 15 minutes twice a day prevents the development of a flexion contracture of the hip. The use of the Pneumatic Post Amputation Mobility aid (PPAM aid)[1] helps to restore the patient's general overall mobility. It is also a valuable means of assessing doubtful candidates for prosthetic fitting. If wound healing proceeds uneventfully it should be possible to fit the first temporary limb during the third or fourth postoperative week.

Prosthetics

7

Most above-knee amputees up to the age of 60 have the strength and agility to take advantage of a limb fitted with a suction socket and a stabilized knee mechanism which prevents the joint from buckling when the weight is applied in a bent position. All this requires an adequate gap between the prosthetic knee axis and the distal end of the amputation stump. Insufficient clearance will make it necessary either to lower the centre of the artificial knee, which is undesirable from the cosmetic point of view, or to modify the prosthetic prescription.

Older people require less sophisticated equipment, preferring the security of a lockable knee joint. Less clearance is needed and so a longer stump can be fashioned, as illustrated, in which, it must be stressed, the minimum clearance has been shown. Extra room for the knee mechanism eases the task for the prosthetist.

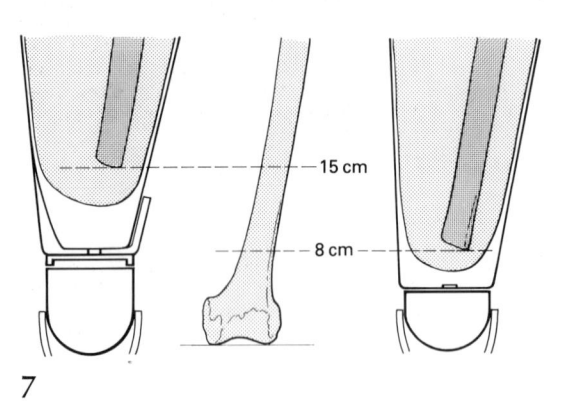

Reference

1. Redhead RG. The early rehabilitation of lower limb amputees using a pneumatic walking aid. *Prosthet Orthot Int* 1983; 7: 88–90.

Illustrations by Gillian Oliver after A. Barrett

Disarticulation at the knee

J. C. Angel FRCS
Consultant Orthopaedic Surgeon, Royal National Orthopaedic and Edgware General Hospitals, Middlesex, UK

Introduction

The two advantages of a through-knee disarticulation when compared with an above-knee amputation are that it provides a comfortable, robust stump capable of full end-bearing and the protuberant femoral condyles offer the potential for suspending the prosthesis without a waistband. The disadvantages include less reliable healing and the need either to place the prosthetic knee 5 cm below the normal level of the knee axis or to fit bulky, jointed side steels.

Kjølbye[1], reviewing a large series of amputations, noted the tendency for wound breakdown to occur at the through-knee level because the flaps were not fashioned sufficiently long to cover the bulky femoral condyles. He stressed that they must never be sutured under the slightest tension. Before selecting this level of amputation it should be borne in mind that the skin and soft-tissue cover required is little less than that needed to attempt a short below-knee amputation which can give a very much more satisfactory result.

Indications

It is indicated in situations where there is inadequate soft-tissue cover to perform a below-knee amputation or where the future use of a below-knee prosthesis is precluded by a knee flexion contracture of more than 45°, a range of knee flexion of less than 40° or the patient's poor long-term general condition. It is also useful in very ill patients as it can be performed rapidly, if necessary under infiltration anaesthesia. In children it should be used if at all possible in preference to an above-knee amputation, even if this means extensive skin grafting of the distal end of the stump.

Contraindications

An above-knee amputation should be performed in preference if the advantages of the robust end-bearing stump are outweighed by the uncertain healing, poor cosmesis and lack of proper knee control mechanisms.

Preoperative

General anaesthesia is preferred although epidural anaesthesia is an alternative. If a tourniquet is used it should be inflated with the knee flexed to 90°. The operation is most easily performed in the prone position unless there is a hip flexion contracture, restricted knee flexion, cardiopulmonary disease or obesity.

Operation

THROUGH-KNEE DISARTICULATION USING LATERAL FLAPS

Incision

1a & b

From a point midway between the lower pole of the patella and the tibial tubercle the lateral incision is curved downwards to mark a flap that extends 5 cm below the upper border of the tibial tubercle. The line then curves proximally to a point in the midline of the popliteal fossa 2 cm above the joint line with the knee extended. The medial flap needs to be 2 cm longer to cover the larger medial femoral condyle.

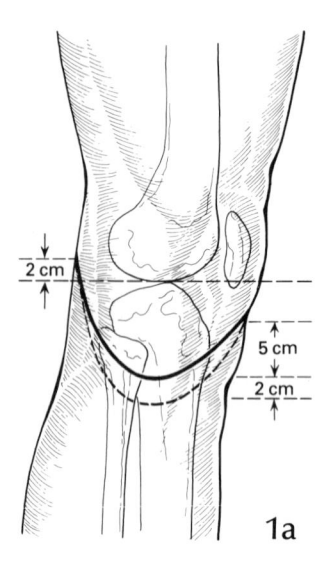

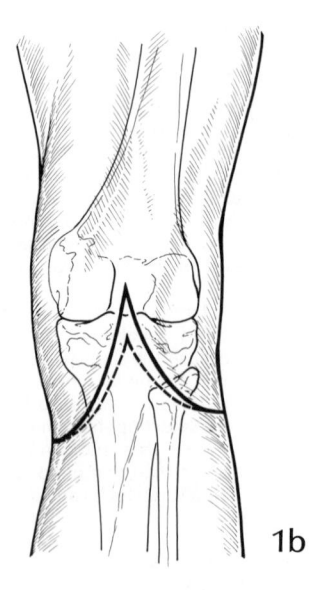

Disarticulation at the knee 429

Deep tissues

2

The incisions are carried down to bone and the flaps are raised, keeping close to the periosteal covering. Thus the patellar tendon and medial and lateral hamstrings are divided. The knee is then flexed to a right angle and the medial and lateral ligaments of the knee joint, together with the capsule, are freed from the margins of the tibia. The menisci and the cruciate ligaments are also detached. The popliteal vessels are identified, clamped, divided and ligated. The tibial and common peroneal nerves are pulled down and cut as high as possible with scissors. The gastrocnemius is sectioned close to its origin. The disarticulation is completed by dividing the remaining soft tissues, including the tendon of popliteus. The menisci are excised. Haemostasis is secured after releasing the tourniquet.

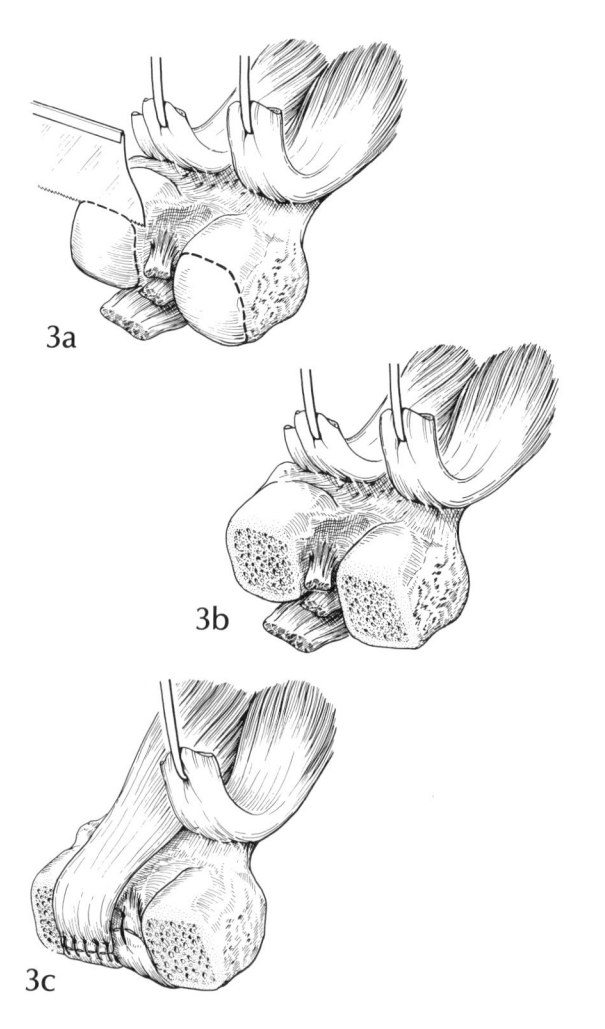

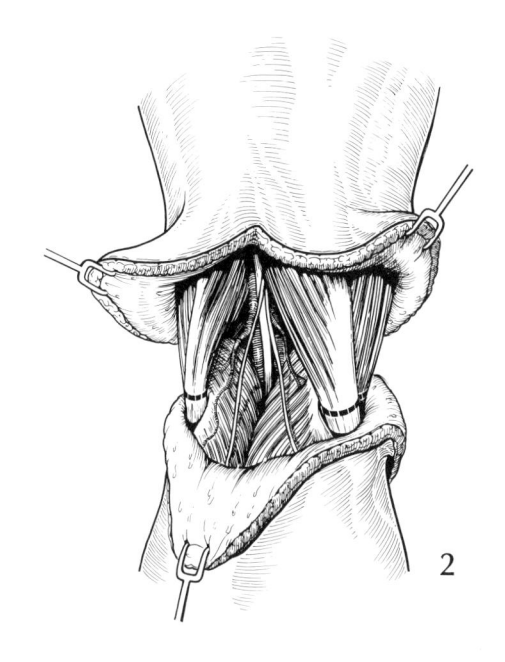

Preparation of femoral condyles

3a, b & c

The articular cartilage and subchondral bone are removed from the distal end of the femur using a tenon saw to fashion the distal flat surface[2]. It is most important that the plane of this cut lies at right angles to the eventual line of weight-bearing. The remainder of the subchondral bone is also removed.

The patellar tendon is sutured to the cruciate ligaments with No. 1 chromic catgut and the retinacula either side of the tendon are stitched to the hamstrings.

Closure

4

A suction drain is passed out laterally through the skin proximal to the level of the wound and the skin is closed with interrupted sutures or staples. Note that the patella is not removed. It is most important that the skin flaps fall comfortably together. With even slight tension the wound is likely to break down, exposing the femoral condyles, a situation that can be retrieved only by above-knee amputation.

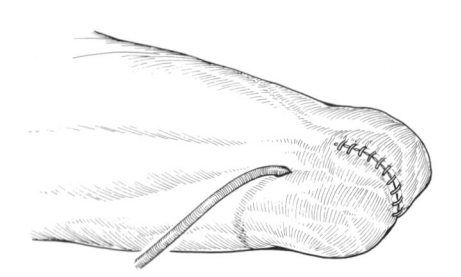

Postoperative management

The wound is covered with gauze and the stump is bandaged with orthopaedic wool and crêpe held in place with a U-shaped slab of adhesive plaster. The suction drain projects from the top of the dressing in such a way that it can be easily withdrawn after 48 hours.

Prosthetics

The traditional prosthesis has a moulded leather thigh corset and can be provided with a tuber-bearing seat if required. It is attached to jointed side steels which are fixed below to a shank of metal or wood. With this system the scope for providing swing and stance-phase knee controls is very limited. Also the protuberant joints tend to damage clothing. A more modern alternative makes use of a polycentric, four-bar linkage knee joint attached to the distal end of the socket, which swings the shank up behind the femoral condyles as the knee is flexed.

References

1. Kjølbye J. The surgery of the through-knee amputation. In: Murdoch G, ed. *Prosthetic and orthotic practice*. London: Edward Arnold, 1970: 255–7.

2. Burgess EM. Disarticulation at the knee: a modified technique. *Arch Surg* 1977; 112: 1250–5.

Illustrations by Gillian Oliver after A. Barrett

Below-knee amputation

J. C. Angel FRCS
Consultant Orthopaedic Surgeon, Royal National Orthopaedic and Edgware General Hospitals, Middlesex, UK

Introduction

Indications

Wherever possible, preserve the all-important knee joint![1]

Amputation below the knee is indicated in peripheral vascular disease, trauma, chronic infection and certain deformities. In these conditions the long posterior flap operation is generally suitable. Below-knee amputation may also be indicated in severe acute infection and tumours where equal flaps are often preferable.

Contraindications

The operation is usually contraindicated if the disorders of the locomotor or nervous system, or the patient's general condition, preclude the future use of a prosthesis, especially if there is any doubt about the wound healing. The residual length of the tibia needs to be more than 7 cm long if it is to control the prosthesis adequately, although in some circumstances 5 cm will suffice. The knee joint must have a functional range of movement. Flexion deformities of up to 40° can be accommodated by the alignment of the socket of the artificial limb. Stubborn deformities greater than this are a contraindication.

Preoperative

If the foot is grossly contaminated it should be covered with absorbent dressings and sealed inside a polythene bag before the patient enters the theatre environment. General anaesthesia is preferred, but where this is not suitable epidural or some other form of regional anaesthesia can be used. The performance of the operation is facilitated by the use of a tourniquet but this may not be appropriate in peripheral vascular disease, especially where bleeding is being used to assess the level of section. The skin should be shaved from the mid-thigh level downwards. A large sandbag is placed under the ipsilateral buttock.

Operations

LONG POSTERIOR FLAP BELOW-KNEE AMPUTATION

Incision

1

The level of bone section is marked on the front of the shin. Ideally the level of amputation should be assessed by preserving 2.5 cm of tibia for every 30 cm in height of the patient (ie, 1 inch per foot). This means that a residual tibia of 15 cm is appropriate for a patient who is 2 m tall. A ruler is used to measure the distance from the knee joint line with the knee extended. This can be achieved by measuring one hand's breadth (the patient's) below the most distal part of the tibial tubercle.

On the same circumference two points are marked medially and laterally almost two-thirds of the way back to the mid-posterior point. From these points a short anterior flap of 2 cm is marked and an overlong posterior flap, the sides of which are parallel when it is laid out flat. A common error is to taper the sides and it is worth checking this point by elevating the foot and examining the calf from behind.

Where it is known that the vascular supply to the area is seriously compromised the level of bone section should be raised to 10 cm below the knee joint line to enhance the prospects of healing.

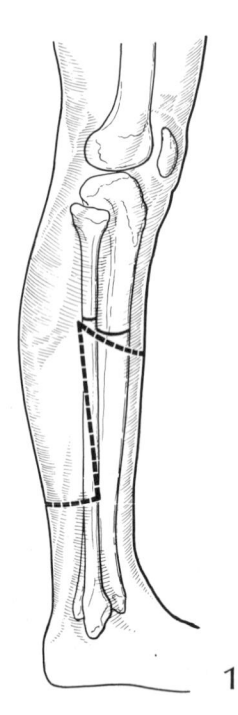

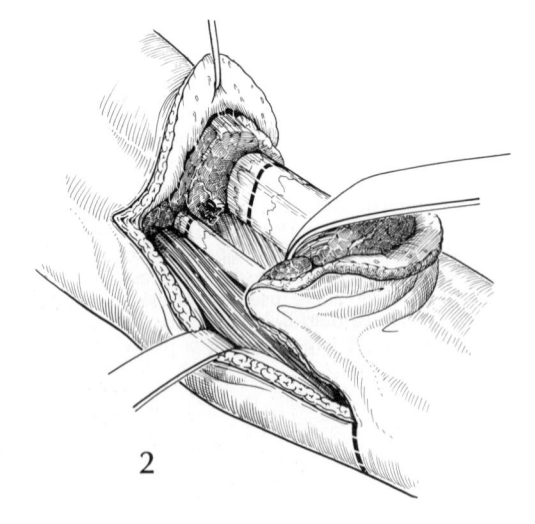

Dividing the bones

2

The lateral incisions are deepened to include the deep fascia. The anterior incision is taken cleanly down to bone and interosseous membrane, clamping the anterior tibial vessels on the way. The periosteum on the front of the tibia is raised proximally for a short distance to where the bevel is to be formed. The level of bone section is checked once again with a ruler. The tibia is divided with a Gigli saw. For the last few cuts the hands are drawn proximally to form the bevel. The fibula is conveniently sectioned using a powered oscillating saw at the same level as the tibia with a view to making the definitive trim once the limb has been removed.

Removal of the limb

3

The proximal calf is supported on a receiver and the assistant distracts the distal tibia with a bone hook. The soft tissues are divided in a long oblique cut using Syme's amputation knife. If the blade is run down the length of the back of the fibula it will find its way automatically into the two incisions made earlier through the deep fascia. Distally the knife blade is turned through 90° to cut through the skin and muscle of the distal calf.

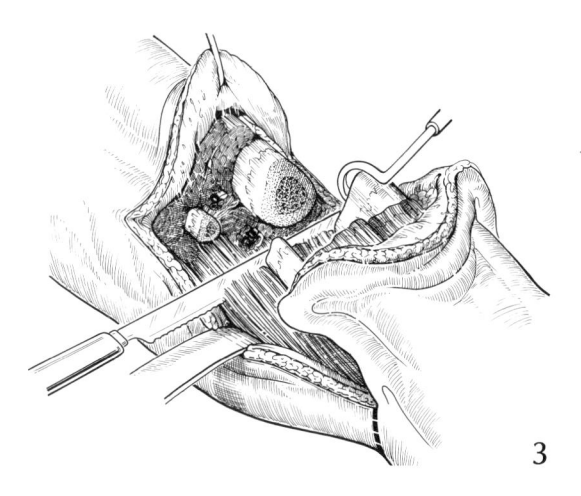

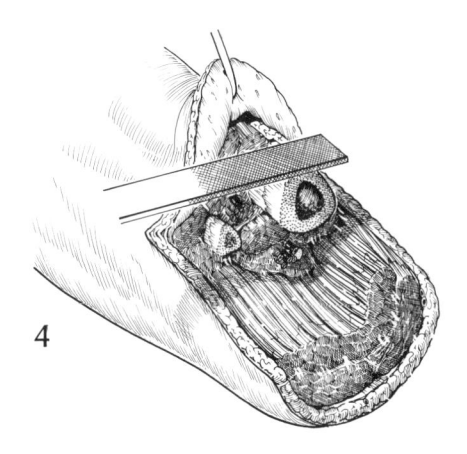

Trimming of the bones

4

The fibula is cut for the second time at a point 1.5 cm proximal to the cut end of the tibia. It is trimmed obliquely as if rounding off a composite bony structure formed by the tibia and fibula together. The tibia is rounded off with the aid of an osteotome and mallet and then a rasp. It must be borne in mind that the bevel and the area of the tibial crest above it will be in intimate contact with the socket of the artificial limb and any lack of smoothness could be a permanent source of discomfort to the patient.

Shaping the muscle

5

The posterior tibial nerve will be seen emerging from behind the muscles of the posterior compartment. On each side of it will be found the peroneal and posterior tibial groups of vessels. These, together with the anterior tibial vessels, are ligated with an absorbable transfixion ligature at a level proximal to the cut end of the tibia.

The receiver is removed and the posterior flap is laid out on the flat surface of the operating table. The soleus is removed from the posterior flap[2]. It is first separated from the gastrocnemius with a finger, starting from the medial side. Sharp dissection may be required to complete this process on the lateral side of the calf. The anatomy of this area is prone to variation and it may be necessary to leave some of the posterior fibres of the soleus on the lateral side in order to have sufficient depth of muscle in the posterior flap. The reflected fibres of soleus and also the muscles of the posterior compartment are sectioned at the same level as the tibia.

The muscle flap is then wrapped around the distal tibia to gauge the optimum length. It should just meet the anterior periosteum. It is then laid back down on the operating table and, *under no tension,* it is cut to length. It is then a simple matter to taper and thin the muscle so that the final stump is free of any bulbous shape.

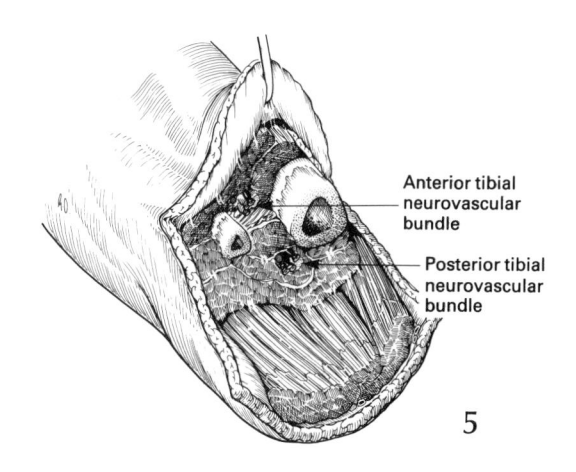

Trimming the nerves

6

The anterior and posterior tibial, peroneal, saphenous and sural nerves should each be gently pulled down and, with scissors, cut high to allow their terminal neuromata to form in their fatty connective tissue tunnels away from the main wound.

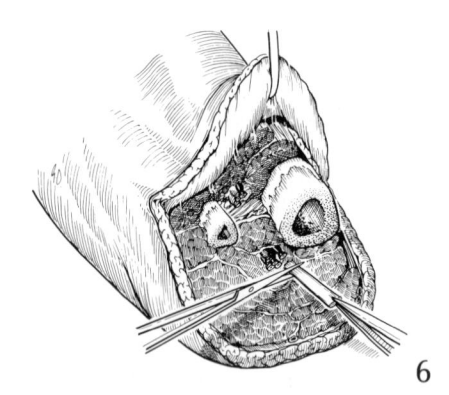

Wound closure

7

The tourniquet is released and the bleeding is controlled with diathermy. Sometimes a venous sinus in the calf requires to be underrun with an absorbable suture. A drain is passed up the peroneal compartment and brought out on the lateral aspect of the leg.

The assistant supports the flap while the muscle layer is sutured to the anterior periosteum of the tibia and the adjacent deep fascia of the anterior compartment. The skin on the posterior flap is grasped with tissue forceps and held up to overlap the anterior flap. It is trimmed to allow it to be closed under very slight tension. If there is a deep subcutaneous layer it is important that the incision be adequately raked to avoid an unnecessarily long posterior skin flap. A number of sutures may be required in the subcutaneous layer. The resulting skin wound usually has unequal skin edges for which skin staples provide a useful and rapid means of closure.

BELOW-KNEE AMPUTATION WITH EQUAL ANTERIOR AND POSTERIOR FLAPS

Incision

8

Equal anterior and posterior flaps are marked with their bases at about the level of bone section and their lengths half the diameter of the limb. The incisions are taken down to include the deep fascia. The periosteum is stripped from the subcutaneous surface of the tibia with a rugine and the combined layer of periosteum and deep fascia is raised off the bone to the point where it is proposed the bone will be divided.

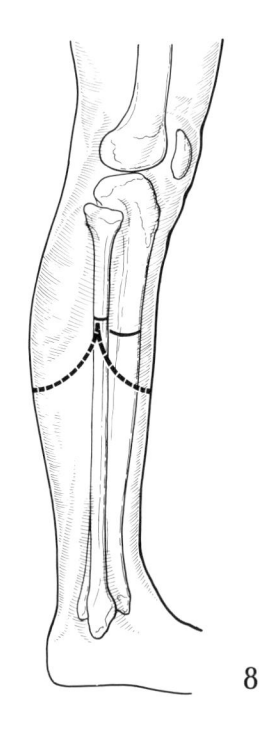

Deep tissues

9

The muscles are divided to allow them to retract to the level of bone section. The bones, vessels and nerves are handled in much the same way as for the long posterior flap operation.

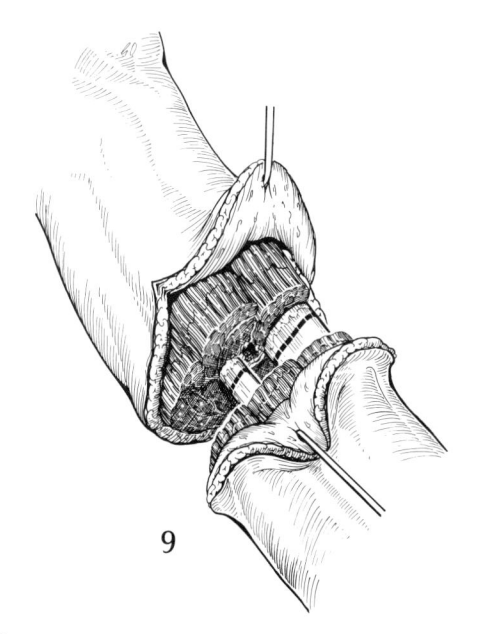

Closure

10

A suction drain is brought out through the lateral compartment onto the lateral side of the limb. The deep fascia is sutured with interrupted, absorbable sutures and the skin is closed with staples.

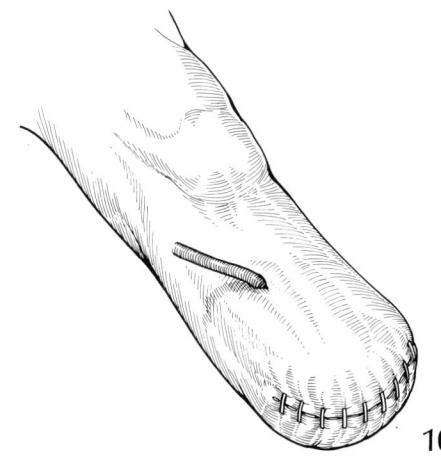

Postoperative management

Rigid dressing

11

A spirit-soaked gauze dressing is placed over the wound and the limb is covered with a padded plaster up to the mid-thigh level. Firm moulding just above the femoral condyles is necessary to hold the cast in position. The drain emerges from the top of the plaster and can be removed after 48 hours by simple traction. The use of plaster protects the amputation wound, limits postoperative swelling and prevents the development of a knee flexion contracture.

The patient is allowed up after 3 or 4 days as the danger of haematoma formation recedes. The plaster can be removed after 5–10 days to allow inspection of the wound and the use of the Pneumatic Post Amputation Mobility aid (PPAM aid)[3]. At this point the wound needs a light bandage, held in place by a U-shaped strip of adhesive strapping passing up either side of the thigh. Once wound healing is fairly certain the shape of the stump can be controlled by means of a Juzo stump shrinker (Julius Zorn, Aichach, Germany), a device which, if properly fitted, is far more reliable than the more traditional stump bandage. The skin staples or sutures should remain in place for 2 to 3 weeks, depending on the degree of ischaemia of the stump.

Prosthetics

The below-knee stump provides proprioception and good control over the position of the foot, something that is denied the above-knee amputee. From the functional point of view the difference between the below-knee amputation and the above-knee is as great as that between having an intact limb and a below-knee amputation. The below-knee stump is usually fitted with a patellar-tendon-bearing prosthesis. The walls of the snug-fitting socket are made so as to direct pressure to those areas that are best able to withstand it, such as the lower pole of the patella, the medial tibial condyle and the back of the calf. The prosthesis is suspended by a leather cuff that grips the femoral condyles.

Another type of prosthesis is available for those engaged in heavy manual labour on rough ground, those who need to kneel to do their work and for patients with unstable knees. This consists of a thigh corset which receives most of the body weight from the inverted cone of the thigh, jointed side-steels and a below-knee socket that plays a relatively small part in load transmission although it is important in detecting and controlling the position of the foot.

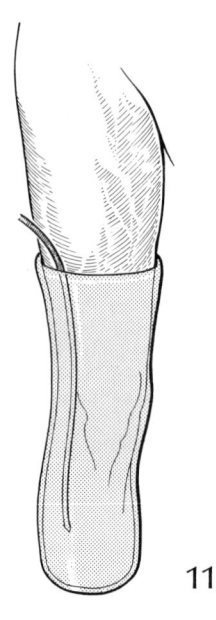

References

1. Gerhardt JJ, King PS, Zettl JH. *Amputations: immediate and early prosthetic management.* Berne: Huber, 1982.

2. Murdoch G. Amputation surgery in the lower extremity. *Prosthet Orthot Int* 1977; 1: 72–83.

3. Redhead RG. The early rehabilitation of lower limb amputees using a pneumatic walking aid. *Prosthet Orthot Int* 1983; 7: 88–90.

Illustrations by Gillian Oliver

Syme's amputation

J. C. Angel FRCS
Consultant Orthopaedic Surgeon, Royal National Orthopaedic and Edgware General Hospitals, Middlesex, UK

Introduction

Syme's amputation produces a stump with end-bearing properties and good proprioception. It allows walking with a low energy consumption and a minimum of initial gait training. Some patients are able to walk without a prosthesis. These points add up to a clear functional advantage over below-knee amputation.

Indications

It is indicated in trauma, diabetes, other vascular disorders involving the distal vascular tree, frostbite and immersion foot, uncorrectable deformities of the foot, certain cases of gross leg-length discrepancy and intractable sepsis associated with a neurological deficit.

Alternatives

In some circumstances consideration may be given to slightly more distal levels of amputation such as the tarsometatarsal (Lisfranc) and midtarsal (Chopart) levels. These will only succeed if there is adequate plantar skin to cover the front of the stump, and if the ankle and subtalar joints can be kept mobile or at least protected from developing a subsequent deformity. Achilles tenotomy and subtalar fusion at a later date may be necessary. Another amputation that is useful in the presence of marked shortening, especially in children, is the Boyd amputation in which the plantar half of the os calcis is fused to the tibia.

Contraindications

These include ulceration of the heel, cases of gangrene associated with a sharp skin temperature gradient in the hindfoot or proximal to it. For cosmetic reasons it is not generally suitable in women. Complete anaesthesia of the stump is not a contraindication, a fact that confirms the robust nature of the stump.

A number of factors have been identified as being prejudicial to wound healing after Syme's amputation. For example, a serum albumin of below 35 g/l and a total lymphocyte count[1] of below 1.5×10^9/l and a pressure index[2] of below 0.45.

Preoperative

The operation is performed with the patient supine. A pneumatic tourniquet is applied and inflated after elevating the limb for approximately a minute. The leg is supported on a receiver to allow the ankle to be moved freely. The surgeon seats himself at the end of the table.

Operation

Incision

1

From the tips of the malleoli two lines are projected distally, perpendicular to the sole of the foot. They are then joined by a slightly oblique line running across the sole. The anterior flap is marked on a line taking the shortest distance across the front of the ankle.

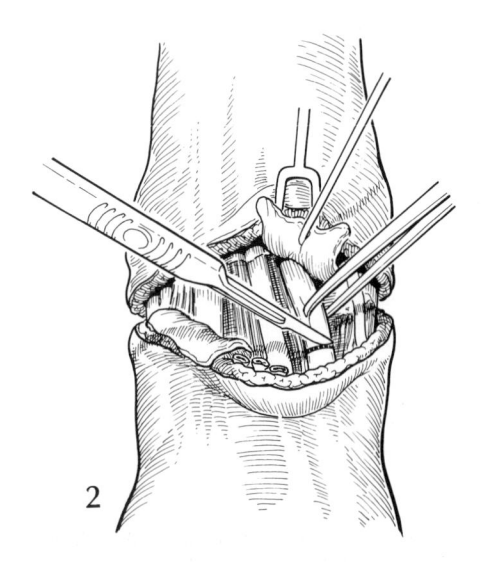

Extensor tendons

2

The plantar incision is deepened directly down to bone using a slightly raked cut. Anteriorly the extensor retinaculum is divided transversely. The extensor tendons are each pulled down and divided as high as possible. The distal stumps of the tendons are also cut off to prevent them from getting in the way. The ankle joint is then entered through the anterior capsule, and the medial and lateral ligaments are divided from within.

Dissecting off the heel pad

3

Attention is then turned to the posterior flap. A subperiosteal dissection of the os calcis is begun and continued posteriorly as far as it comfortably can be. Returning to the dorsal incision, the posterior capsule of the ankle is divided and the dorsal surface of the os calcis is exposed, taking care to keep close to bone. This part of the dissection can be facilitated by drawing the tarsus forward with a bone hook driven first into the talus and then subsequently into the back of the os calcis. As the posterior pole is approached the heel pad is gradually dissected off the bone, working from the sides and from above and below in a systematic manner. After removing the foot the malleoli are cleared of soft tissue by extraperiosteal dissection. The various tendons, held in tissue forceps, make useful retractors at this stage.

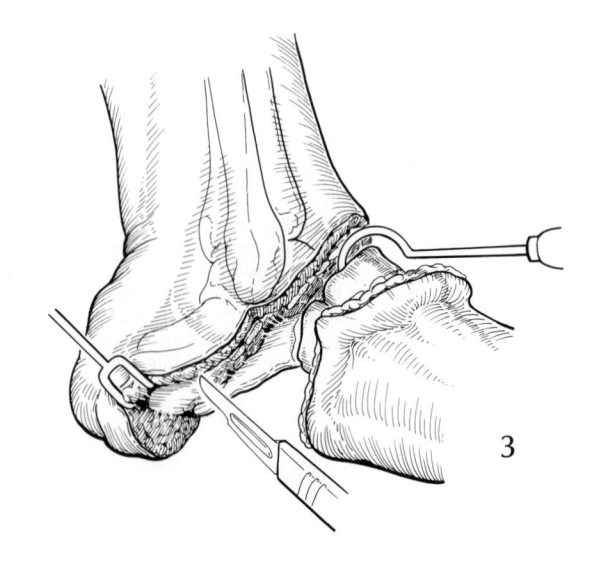

Bone section

4

Next the medial and lateral plantar and the anterior tibial vascular bundles are ligated. The tourniquet is released and the bleeding controlled. The nerves are pulled down a short distance and cut. A tenon saw is used to cut off the malleoli and the distal end of the tibia. Great care must be taken to ensure that the plane of section is at right angles to the long axis of the bone. The level is such as to just remove all the articular cartilage. The cut edges are lightly smoothed with a file.

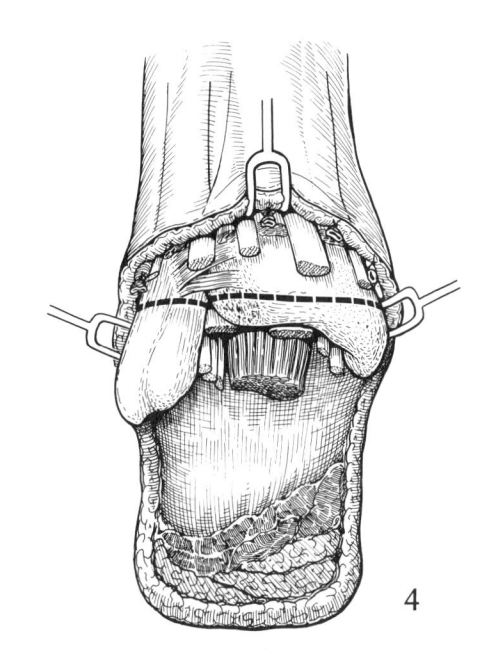

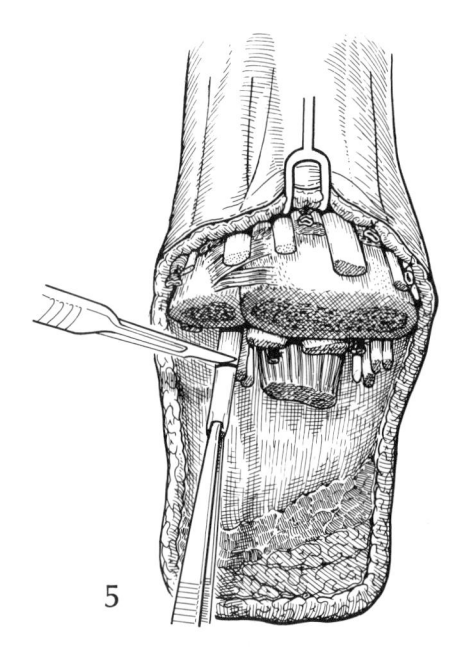

Preparing the flaps

5

The flexor and peroneal tendons are pulled down and divided as high as possible. The flaps are trimmed to fit comfortably together. Loose pedicles of fibrous tissue are trimmed. The remaining muscle fibres in the heel pad are left intact as they help to fill the dead space of the final wound with viable tissue. A suction drain is driven up behind the inferior tibiofibular joint and brought out on the lateral aspect of the leg 7.5 cm above the level of the wound.

Closure

6

The plantar fascia is sutured to the soft tissue on the front of the tibia with absorbable sutures, making sure that the heel pad is located centrally under the cut surface of the bone[3]. Skin closure must be meticulous despite the difference in thickness between the two flaps. The wound is dressed and a rigid dressing of plaster of Paris is applied. As the plaster sets it is moulded round the heel pad to ensure that its central position is maintained.

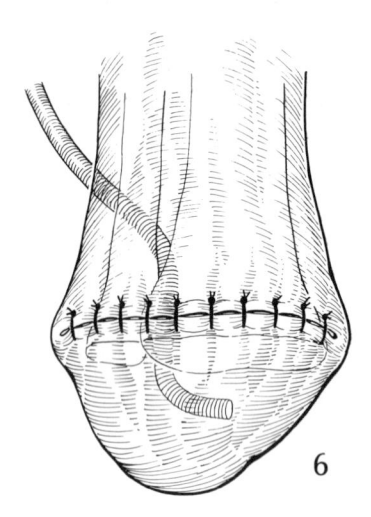

Postoperative management

The drain is removed after 48 hours. At 5 days the plaster is changed to allow an inspection of the wound. It is changed again during the third week. If the wound is satisfactory at this stage, weight-bearing can be permitted.

Stump bandaging has to be performed with extreme caution after Syme's amputation. There is a tendency for the bandage to constrict the limb immediately proximal to the bulb. This risk can be diminished by building up the narrow part of the ankle with orthopaedic wool and suspending the bandage with a stirrup of adhesive tape.

Prosthetics

The Syme's prosthesis, in accommodating the bulb of the stump, usually has an unsightly appearance. The exceptions to this occur where the overall shortening allows the bulb to be accommodated in the 'calf' of the prosthesis.

The traditional prosthesis, comprised of a leather, lace-up corset and side-steels, is durable and capable of off-loading some of the weight from the end of the stump. A better appearance and greater ease of donning and doffing is achieved with a limb fitted with an enclosed plastic socket, nitrogen foam liner and low-profile, solid ankle cushion heel (SACH) foot.

References

1. Dickhout S, DeLee JC, Page CP. Nutritional status: importance in predicting wound healing after amputation. *J Bone Joint Surg [Am]* 1984; 66-A: 71.

2. Wagner FW Jr. The dysvascular foot: a system for diagnosis and treatment. *Foot Ankle* 1981; 2: 64–122.

3. Harris RI. Syme's amputation: the technical details essential for success. *J Bone Joint Surg [Br]* 1956; 38-B: 614–32.

Illustrations by Gillian Oliver

Transmetatarsal amputation

J. C. Angel FRCS
Consultant Orthopaedic Surgeon, Royal National Orthopaedic and Edgware General Hospitals, Middlesex, UK

Introduction

Indications

Transmetatarsal amputation is indicated for severe trauma involving the toes and forefoot. Recently, amputations through the bases of the metatarsals have proved useful in dealing with the complications of diabetes mellitus[1].

Contraindications

The operation is unlikely to succeed when performed for gangrene if the major cause is a proximal arterial block unless this has been relieved by vascular surgery.

Preoperative

Local infection should be controlled as far as possible. In the case of frostbite, ample time should be allowed for demarcation to appear. A pneumatic tourniquet is applied to the thigh and a sandbag is placed under the ipsilateral buttock to control the position of the foot. The operator sits at the end of the table.

Operation

Incision

1

The dorsal incision commences towards the sole on either side of the foot and it passes convexly across the dorsum 1 cm distal to the anticipated level of bone section. The plantar incision fashions a longer flap roughly parallel to the flexion crease of the toes. It needs to be slightly longer medially in order to cover the greater thickness of the foot on this side.

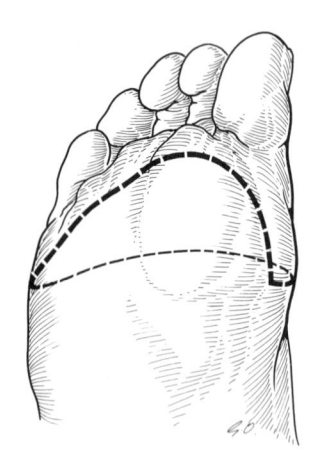

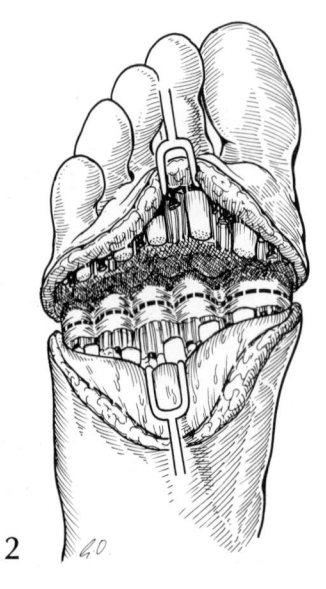

Fashioning the plantar flap

2

The plantar incision is carried down to bone and a flap is raised back to the level of bone section.

Fashioning the dorsal flap and bone section

3

The dorsal incision is taken down to bone, making a small flap. Using a power saw, the blade of which is kept cool with saline, the metatarsal bones are divided at the chosen level of section (which is largely determined by the viability of the flaps). The direction of the cut is made parallel to the tarsometatarsal joints. The fifth metatarsal bone is shortened and the outer side bevelled.

The tendons are grasped with forceps, pulled down and cut short with scissors. The remaining soft tissues are trimmed to allow the flaps to fall comfortably together. The metatarsal arteries and other vessels are ligated and the tourniquet is released.

Closure

4

After haemostasis has been secured, the fascia is sutured with interrupted catgut and the skin is closed with nylon or staples.

Postoperative management

The wound is dressed and lightly bandaged. The foot is elevated for a few days. The patient is then allowed up on crutches with the limb in a below-knee plaster which is moulded to maintain the foot and subtalar joints in a neutral position. The plaster can usually be dispensed with at the time of suture removal at the end of the third week.

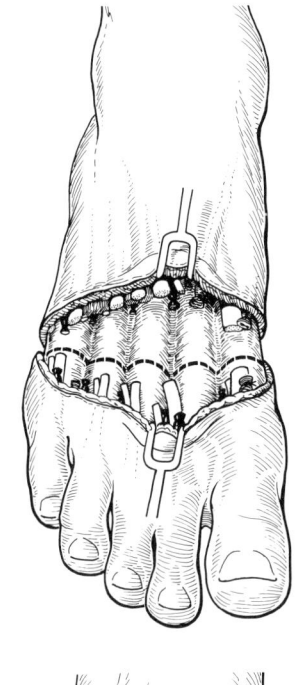

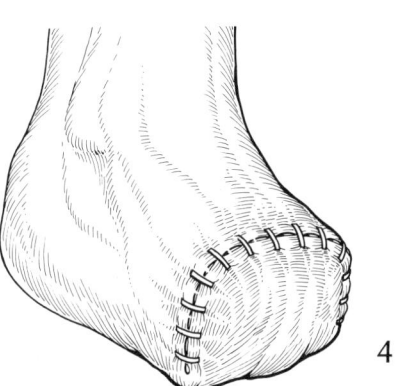

Prosthetic fitting

The residual part of the foot functions reasonably well in normal footwear with the toe filled, but the heel has a tendency to escape from the back of the shoe. This can be guarded against by the use of a fairly rigid insole to which an ankle strap has been fitted. Even so, the step lacks spring and a limp is inevitable when walking faster than a stroll.

Reference

1. Pinzur M, Kaminsky M, Sage R, Cronin R, Osterman H. Amputations at the middle level of the foot: a retrospective and prospective review. *J Bone Joint Surg [Am]* 1986; 68-A: 1061–4.

Illustrations by Gillian Oliver

Amputation of the toes

J. C. Angel FRCS
Consultant Orthopaedic Surgeon, Royal National Orthopaedic and Edgware General Hospitals, Middlesex, UK

Introduction

Indications

One or more toes may need to be amputated for diabetic gangrene, uncorrectable deformity, severe bony infection or trauma.

Secondary effects

Collectively the lesser toes are important in running and in balancing in the squatting position. Individually they are of minimal biomechanical importance but single toes cannot be amputated with impunity because of the tendency for secondary deformities to develop.

Amputation of the second toe very commonly leads to the development of hallux valgus despite efforts to fill the gap with a toe spacer. Removal of the fifth toe leaves the head of the fifth metatarsal exposed to mechanical trauma and predisposes to the formation of a tender bursa. Partial amputation of the lesser toes is followed by a deformity in the remaining stump: a type of hammer toe developing after a middle phalanx amputation, and an extension deformity after amputations through the proximal phalanx. These deformities can, of course, be dealt with as they arise and, particularly in the case of the second toe, it may be preferable to do this rather than remove the whole toe.

Deformities are minimized by amputating through the base of a phalanx. If this cannot be achieved and it is necessary to disarticulate an interphalangeal or metatarsophalangeal joint, then the capsule should be carefully closed to prevent retraction of the short muscles. It is not desirable to amputate through the neck or shafts of the intermediate or proximal phalanges.

Ray resection

It is sometimes necessary for part of a metatarsal to be removed when a toe is amputated. This is especially so when dealing with diabetics in whom healing can be achieved in the case of the first or fifth rays, though it is less likely to prove successful with the middle three rays unless vascular reconstructive surgery has been undertaken or some other important factor mitigating against the control of gangrene has been eliminated.

Operation

Incision

1

A racquet incision is made with the blade sufficiently distal to the webs to allow the lateral flaps to fall naturally together. On the great and fifth toe it is placed obliquely to make a longer outside flap.

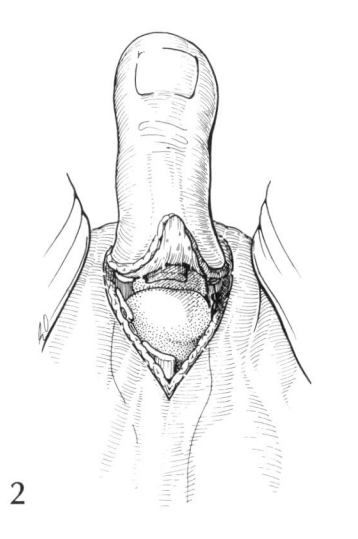

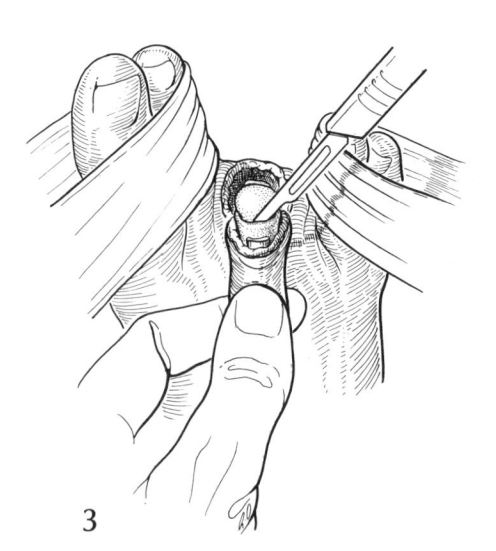

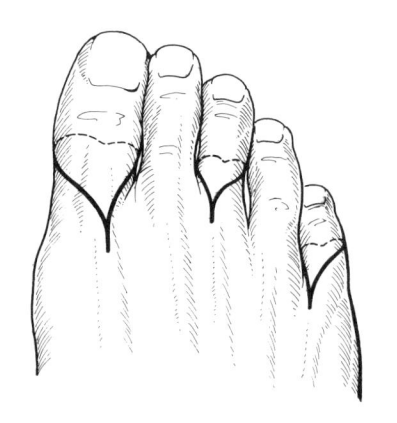

Dissection

2 & 3

The flaps are taken down to bone and then dissected off the phalanx. Where possible the base of the phalanx is preserved and the bone is divided just distal to the capsular insertion. Otherwise a disarticulation is performed, with care being taken to divide the capsule of the metatarsophalangeal joint as distally as possible in order to retain the transverse intermetatarsal ligaments and the insertion of the small muscles of the foot.

Closure

4, 5 & 6

Haemostasis is secured. It is not always necessary or desirable to suture the wound, especially if infected.

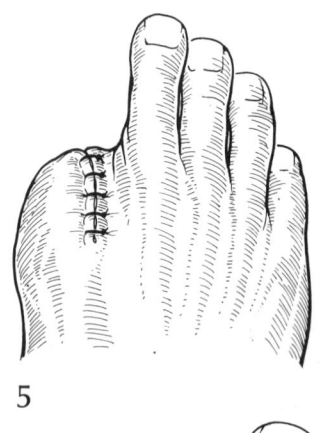

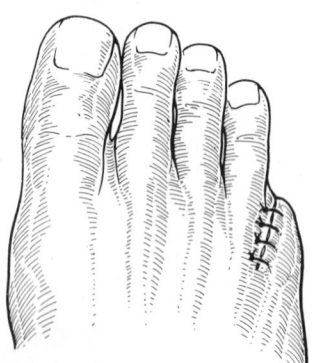

Postoperative management

Tulle gras is applied to the wound and the foot is wrapped in sterile orthopaedic wool and bandaged. A few turns around the ankle help to hold the dressing in place and apply gentle pressure to the amputation site. If stitches have been inserted they can usually be removed by the tenth day. When the wound has been left open it will very often be found to have healed with a linear scar in the same interval. The tendency for secondary deformities to occur in the remaining toes can be diminished by the use of a toe spacer, for which the patient may be referred to a chiropodist.

Illustrations by Gillian Lee

Axillary approach for thoracic outlet syndrome

Robert D. Leffert MD
Associate Professor of Orthopaedic Surgery, Harvard Medical School; Chief of the Surgical Upper Extremity Rehabilitation Unit, Massachusetts General Hospital, Boston, USA

Introduction

The diagnosis of thoracic outlet syndrome is clinical, and there are no objective tests that can provide absolute affirmation of the clinical impression.

A history of pain and paraesthesiae involving the entire limb or hand, most concentrated on the ulnar aspect and induced by positioning the hand overhead, is highly significant. Nocturnal pain and paraesthesiae are common. The Wright's manoeuvre, abducting and laterally rotating the arm while palpating the pulses at the wrist, should not be considered positive unless it reproduces the symptoms. Operations done because it is possible to obliterate a pulse in the absence of symptoms are doomed to failure in a high percentage of cases.

The neurological findings are usually confined to the ulnar-innervated intrinsic muscles in the hand and less commonly the deep flexors of the little and ring fingers. Sensory deficit most often affects these same fingers and the medial aspect of the forearm.

Indications

1. Intractable pain in a patient whose past medical history is well-documented and known to the surgeon.
2. The presence of significant neurological deficits in the hand.
3. Chronic sequelae of vascular compression in the limb such as swelling or trophic changes.
4. Failure of a carefully supervised programme of postural re-education and muscle strengthening for the suspensory muscles of the shoulder complex, including trapezius, rhomboids, and levator scapulae.
5. Impending acute vascular catastrophe.

Contraindications

It is necessary to evaluate carefully the symptoms of pain and paraesthesiae with which these patients present and to rule out the possibility that these are coming from other, more common, sources.

The differential diagnosis must include cervical radiculopathy, apical tumours of the lung and pleura, cardiac disease, ulnar neuropathy at the elbow, and carpal tunnel syndrome. Unless these have been ruled out, surgery in the thoracic outlet is contraindicated.

A severe degree of postural abnormality of the shoulder in the form of scapular ptosis due to disuse atrophy of the trapezius is a relative contraindication to surgery, since even with decompression of the outlet, these patients will suffer unrelieved traction on the nerves and vessels that will continue to cause discomfort. This is the major cause of failed surgery in those patients in whom a technically adequate operation has been done.

Severe and untreated emotional depression can make postoperative compliance with rehabilitative exercises more difficult and thereby detract from the ultimate degree of relief from surgery. In addition, the postural abnormality of the severely depressed patient will be additive to that which is found in many patients with thoracic outlet syndrome.

Significant obesity will contribute not only to the technical difficulty of the transaxillary approach to the thoracic outlet, but produce further drag on the shoulders. For this reason, gigantomastia is also a relative contraindication to thoracic outlet surgery, and such patients should undergo supervised weight loss and consider reduction mammoplasty before undergoing surgery on the thoracic outlet.

Preoperative

Anaesthesia

General endotracheal anaesthesia is employed for all surgery on the thoracic outlet. It is extremely important that profound muscular relaxation be available, especially for patients who are operated upon by the axillary route, since it is impossible to use that approach safely in a patient whose muscles are not relaxed. The anaesthetist should have discussed the conduct of the surgery with the surgeon prior to the incision to avoid either inadequate relaxation during surgery, or a prolonged period of being unable to extubate the patient postoperatively because of overdosage with relaxants. In some patients, this problem may occur in situations where the level of anaesthesia was inadequate and increasing doses of relaxants were given.

Because of the large blood vessels that are present in the operative field and the possibility of haemorrhage, it is suggested that blood be readily available.

Choice of procedure and operative approach

The thoracic outlet may be approached anteriorly, posteriorly or through the axilla. The operative procedure may vary, depending on the perceived needs of the patient. Although scalenotomy was historically advocated for many years, the high rate of recurrence has made it a procedure with few, if any, applications. Some surgeons prefer the anterior, supraclavicular approach for exploration of the thoracic outlet, but in my opinion it does not provide sufficient posterior access to justify its use, except where access to a difficult cervical rib is needed. It may be useful, though, where there is significant scarring, or a recurrence with anterior structures that require resection. Under such circumstances, scalenectomy, which has some advocates, may be performed.

For most of the cases, I believe that the transaxillary approach, with resection of the first rib that has been popularized by Roos, is preferred. The majority of this discussion will be concerned with it, although the other routes will be briefly discussed.

Operation

TRANSAXILLARY FIRST RIB RESECTION

Position of patient

The patient lies on the operating table in the lateral position with the affected side up. Kidney rests and blanket rolls or an inflatable 'beanbag' may be used to maintain the lateral decubitus, and a strip of carefully applied adhesive tape may be used across the buttocks and secured to the table on both sides to keep the patient from losing position during the course of the procedure. A folded sheet is placed beneath the downside hemithorax to lift it off the table and thereby to relieve pressure on the axilla and the non-operative arm, which will invariably be the site of the intravenous lines. Care must be taken to ensure that all bony prominences, such as the head of the downside fibula, are carefully padded. The head of the table is then raised about 20° according to the line of sight of the surgeon.

Position of the operating team

The surgeon stands behind the patient. Because of the depth of the wound in this approach, it will be necessary for the surgeon to wear a headlamp or to use lighted retractors to achieve an adequate level of illumination.

The patient's arm is draped free and held forward flexed and abducted, roughly perpendicular to floor, by a scrubbed assistant positioned on a standing platform; he raises and lowers the limb as the surgeon directs. It is inadvisable to suspend the arm from the ceiling or drip stand, since unremitting traction can result in injury to the brachial plexus. Two additional assistants with retractors are stationed between the surgeon and the head of the table on either side.

Skin preparation and draping

The axillary hair should have been shaved and a preliminary scrub with surgical soap done prior to arrival in the operating room. Standard skin preparation, according to the preferences of the surgeon, should include the base of the neck, ipsilateral hemithorax and back. The draping should allow access to these areas in the event of injury to major vessels.

Instruments

In addition to a general tray, chest and vascular instruments should be available. A rounded and blunt periosteal elevator, as well as a rib raspatory and the Roos rib cutter are extremely useful. The advantage of the Roos instrument is that its cutting surfaces are at an angle to the handles so that when inserted through the axilla, it produces a transverse section of the rib rather than the oblique one that a straight cutter would make.

Incision

1

The skin incision is made transversely between the pectoralis major and the latissimus dorsi over the third interspace, which is located just below the axillary hairline. Sharp, self-retaining retractors are spread across the wound for dissection of the superficial tissues and haemostasis. The deep fascia is incised vertically and care taken to protect the intercostobrachial nerve which comes from the second interspace. Dissection is carried down through the subcutaneous tissues to the ribcage while the pectoral and latissimus muscles are retracted. Profound muscular relaxation is required from this point to the beginning of the closure, or else the operation cannot be done with safety. The supreme thoracic artery and vein come off the axillary vessels lateral to the first rib and enter the intercostal space. They must be isolated and ligated for access to the superior surface of the first rib, which is gained by blunt dissection of the fascia.

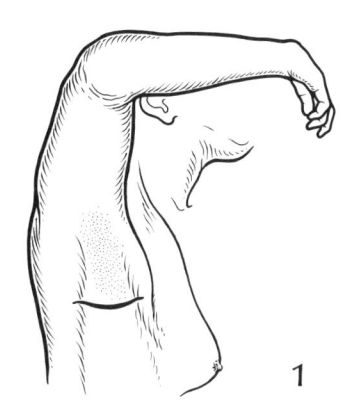

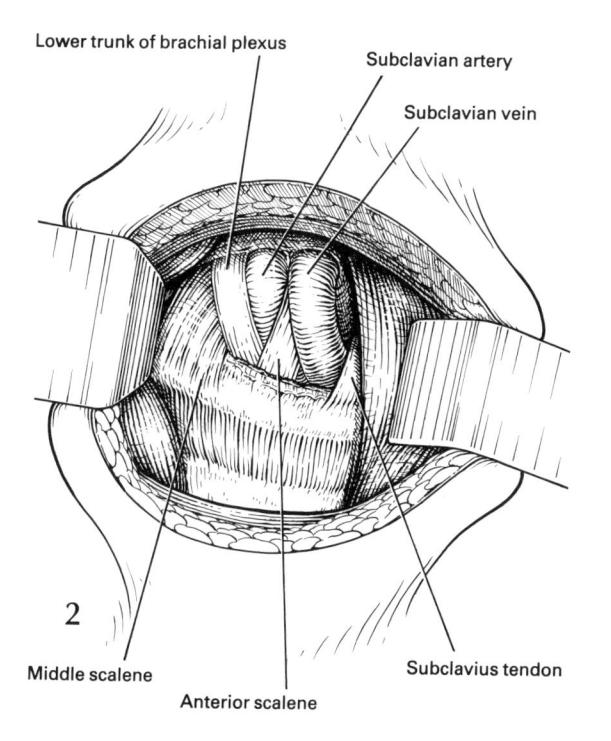

Identification of vital structures

2

The anatomy of the region must then be carefully identified as the arm is held up by the assistant to elevate the nerves and vessels off the surface of the first rib. The most anterior and medial structure in the field is the tendon of the subclavius muscle, behind and lateral to which may be seen the subclavian vein. It is a large, blue, fluttering structure that can sometimes be greatly enlarged if there has been significant and chronic compression. Lateral to the vein is the tendon of the anterior scalene muscle, which attaches to the scalene tubercle located on the medial edge of the first rib. Blunt dissection on either side of the tendon will better define it, and prior to detachment from the tubercle, it should be freed from the pleura which often adheres to it posteriorly. The phrenic nerve is not at risk here, since it is located 2–3 cm more proximally. Lateral to the tendon is the subclavian artery, and adjacent to it the lower trunk of the brachial plexus composed of C8 and T1.

Detachment of the scalene muscles and subclavius tendon from the first rib

3

It is prudent to detach half of the anterior scalene tendon thickness at a time while shielding the vessel on the other side with a gauze pledget or clamp. The middle scalene muscle has a broad attachment to the superior surface of the first rib, and it can be bluntly elevated from the bone with a periosteal elevator while the nerves and vessels are protected by traction on the arm. As much of the periosteum as possible should be left on the rib or disrupted so as to minimize the possibility or regrowth postoperatively. This is a particular risk in younger patients. The lateral edge of the rib can be freed of muscle by the use of an angled raspatory, and then the inferior surface of the rib may be separated from the suprapleural membrane with the periosteal elevator while care is taken not to puncture the pleura. Finally, the tendon of the subclavius muscle is sharply incised at the most lateral aspect of its attachment to the rib and then bluntly elevated with an elevator directed away from the subclavian vein so that if the instrument should suddenly slip, this structure would not be torn.

The field is irrigated with antibiotic solution and the integrity of the pleura is tested. If a rent in the pleura is present, either the pleural cavity can be aspirated just prior to closure, or a chest drain can be inserted and removed the next day.

A search for congenital bands that might have been causing compression is carried out as each structure is dissected, and they are dealt with as necessary.

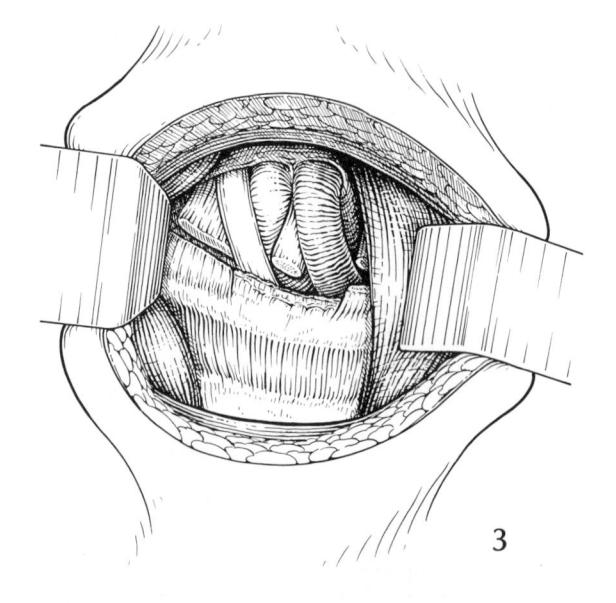

Section and removal of the first rib

4

When the muscles have been cleared, the Roos angled rib cutter is introduced into the wound. When used on the left side of the body, the cutter is turned so that the large steel tooth is pointing cephalad, while on the right side it points caudad. It is hooked around the rib anteriorly and then the jaws are cautiously closed under direct vision. The instrument is pushed posteriorly so that the cutting edges are behind the brachial plexus by about 2 cm, which puts them close to the costotransverse articulation. Again, under direct vision, the handles of the cutter are squeezed together and the rib is cut. The cutter is extracted by sliding it medially, still with the jaws almost closed to avoid injury to the vital structures, and then extracted from the wound. The rib is then grasped with a clamp or bone-holding forceps and pulled forward. A rib shears or rongeur is used to separate it from the costal cartilage as close to the sternum as possible with care to protect the subclavian vein from injury.

The posterior line of section of the rib must be inspected to verify that the nerves have been adequately and widely decompressed, and if not, this must be accomplished with a wide rongeur to avoid making a series of small sawtooth notches in the remaining bone. There should ideally be between 1 and 2 cm of bone retained, but in all cases the relationship between the nerves and the line of resection of the bone must be assessed. This part of the procedure is potentially injurious to the nerves, which must sometimes be gently retracted while the bone is removed. If this is done with anything less than the utmost care, there is a real risk of nerve injury, which could be permanent.

The pleura is again tested for leaks. The adequacy of the decompression is tested manually by placing two fingers in the outlet and putting the arm in the various positions that were provocative prior to surgery. In rare cases, there will be inadequate space between the clavicle and the second rib, so that the middle third of the second rib may have to be resected.

Closure

The retractors are removed and the muscles are allowed to approximate. The deep structures are inspected for the last time to verify their integrity and haemostasis. If a chest tube has been inserted, it is connected to underwater suction. The subcutaneous tissues are closed with interrupted gut suture, and the skin with a non-absorbable subcuticular suture that will be removed at 2 weeks. Since the wound should be absolutely dry before closure, no drains are needed. If it is not, it should be meticulously explored to find the source of bleeding.

A single layer of gauze is the only dressing that is required.

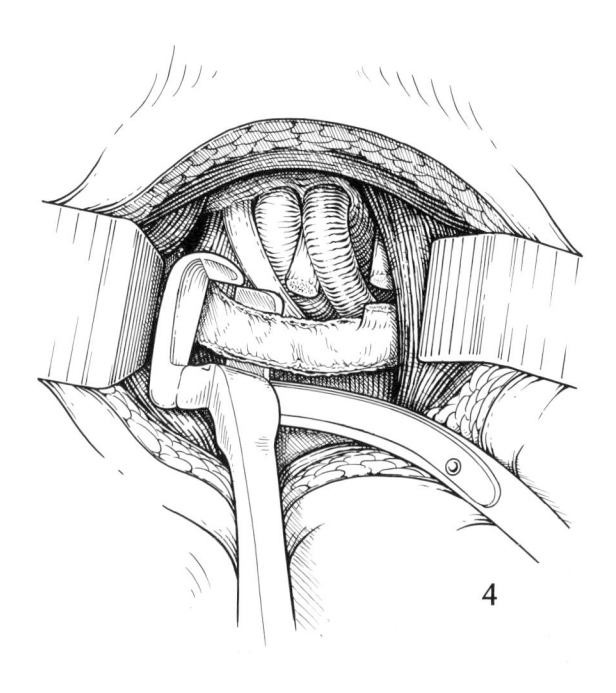

Postoperative management

The arm is placed in a sling for comfort in the first 2 or 3 postoperative days. A semi-sitting chest radiograph is made in the recovery room to assess the position of the chest tube, if one has been placed, and to detect the presence of a clinically unapparent pneumothorax.

The patient is usually allowed out of bed on the first postoperative day and is encouraged to move about and do deep breathing exercises. Smoking is prohibited. The sling may be removed *ad lib*. Discharge from the hospital is usually on the third postoperative day and the patient is advised to restrict activity for the next 2 weeks. The patient returns to the clinic for suture removal and begins gentle shoulder girdle exercises to prevent or treat postural abnormalities of the scapula which can lead to postoperative recurrence of symptoms. These exercises should be continued for as long as there is any tendency towards atrophy of the shoulder girdle muscles, particularly the upper trapezius. Unrestricted activities are permitted at 2 months.

Complications

Injury to nerves and vessels

Potentially serious complications from this procedure are those which occur as a result of injury to the nerves and vessels. These structures must be under constant and direct vision for the entire time they are exposed in the wound, and no cutting-edged instrument must be used in the operative field unless the entire extent of its cutting surfaces can be seen.

Injury to nerves, the lower trunk of the brachial plexus, can occur in several ways. The first of these is direct laceration. The rib cutter may close on the nerves, in which case a laceration occurs, and the prognosis for recovery of function is dismal even if it is possible to achieve a technical repair. The placement of a retractor on the plexus may be necessitated during the remodelling of the posterior stump of the rib if enough has not been taken with the rib cutter. This is done with the utmost care to avoid excessive local traction or compression on the nerves.

Not only the brachial plexus, but also the nerve to the serratus anterior may be injured, since its path may be quite variable and may bring it into harm's way. In addition to direct laceration, it is possible to injure the nerve in the field either by traction on the arm, as it crosses the first rib, or on the chest wall.

Laceration of the vessels during the procedure is the most significant potential complication, especially with the use of the axillary approach, since proximal and distal control of the vessels would be extremely difficult in the absence of additional incisions. Instruments for vascular repair and thoracotomy, as well as appropriate surgical back-up, must be available at a moment's notice should the need arise.

Intraoperative pneumothorax occurs in about one-third of the cases in my experience, and the management has already been described.

Injury to the intercostobrachial nerve may result in hypoaesthesia and in some cases, dysaesthesia over the posterior aspect of the arm. If the nerve has not been lacerated, the sensibility usually normalizes in time.

Inadequate decompression

Failure to achieve adequate decompression of the nerves will result from insufficient posterior resection of the rib, usually occurring with less experienced operators. This will be apparent as a failure to achieve clinical relief of the symptoms despite the reversal of the positive provocative manoeuvres, since the artery will have been decompressed. If there has been significant venous compression and the anterior stump of rib is too long, then a similar condition will prevail. In both cases, the reoperation will be a difficult and hazardous procedure, usually requiring a different anatomical approach, dictated by the structures most involved.

Recurrence

Recurrence of symptoms may occur after a variable period of time as a result of adhesion of the plexus to the posterior rib stump if it is too long, or if there has been regeneration of the rib due to failure to remove sufficient periosteum at the time of resection of the rib. In most cases, however, and in the absence of these factors, patients who develop postural ptosis of the scapula due to trapezius muscle atrophy will experience a recurrence of symptoms similar to those for which they had surgery. This condition should be treated by recognition of the pathogenesis and appropriate physiotherapy to strengthen the muscles rather than by surgery, in most cases.

OTHER SURGICAL APPROACHES

POSTERIOR APPROACH

This is identical with that used for upper-stage thoracoplasty. It is useful for decompression in patients who are extremely muscular or obese and in whom the axillary approach would be technically difficult, and it is the preferred route for reoperations in which a retained posterior segment of rib has become adherent to the nerves and is causing symptoms.

ANTERIOR APPROACHES

The supraclavicular, anterior approach to the structures of the thoracic outlet can be used for scalenotomy, scalenectomy and resection of cervical ribs. With this approach, access to the posterior portion of the first rib is limited.

The transclavicular approach may be used in reoperations wherein there is adherence of the subclavian vein or artery to the retained edge of the resected first rib.

Further reading

Adson AW. Cervical ribs: symptoms, differential diagnosis and indications for section of the insertion of the scalenus anticus muscle. *J Int Coll Surg* 1951; 16: 546–59.

Clagett OT. Research and prosearch. *J Thorac Cardiovasc Surg* 1962; 44: 153–66.

Peet RM, Henriksen JD, Anderson TP, Martin GM. Thoracic outlet syndrome: evaluation of a therapeutic exercise program. *Staff Meet Mayo Clin* 1956; 31: 281–7.

Roos DB. Transaxillary approach for first rib resection to relieve thoracic outlet syndrome. *Ann Surg* 1966; 163: 354–8.

Roos DB. Experience with first rib resection for thoracic outlet syndrome. *Ann Surg* 1971; 173: 429–42.

Roos DB. Congenital anomalies associated with thoracic outlet syndrome: anatomy, symptoms, diagnosis and treatment. *Am J Surg* 1976; 132: 771–8.

Sanders RJ, Monsour JW, Gerber WF, Adams WR, Thompson N. Scalenectomy versus first rib resection for treatment of the thoracic outlet syndrome. *Surgery* 1979; 85(1): 109–21.

Illustrations by Peter Cox

Transoral approach to the cervical spine

H. Alan Crockard FRCS, FRCS(Ed)
Consultant Neurosurgeon, The National Hospitals for Nervous Diseases, London, UK

Andrew O. Ransford FRCS
Consultant Orthopaedic Surgeon, Royal National Orthopaedic Hospital, London, UK

Introduction

With the complexity of development and the three-dimensional movements which are required of the spine at the craniocervical junction, it is not surprising that a spectrum of conditions arise which may secondarily compromise the neuraxis. A few of the more obvious abnormalities have been evaluated by conventional radiographic techniques, but the introduction of computed axial tomography (CT scanning) and magnetic resonance imaging (MRI) has allowed detailed investigations of the upper spine and the craniocervical junction, and has revealed other hitherto unsuspected abnormalities in the region. CT flexion and extension views have provided a functional assessment of the area and allowed guidelines on management for the various abnormalities. The operating microscope has provided illumination and magnification to improve the surgical results in an otherwise inaccessible area.

The normal anatomy and pathology of the area is described and recommended investigations reviewed in this chapter. A detailed discussion of the operative technique in the area will follow. The management of these problems is complex and requires a team approach. Surgery is unlikely to be fruitful for those involved on an occasional basis.

Development

The craniocervical junction is derived from the lower two occipital and the upper two cervical sclerotomes. The occipital condyles and the tip of the odontoid peg originate from 'occipital material': the first cervical vertebra and the body of the odontoid peg from the first cervical sclerotome; the second cervical sclerotome produces the rest of that vertebra. As the sclerotome responds to the neuraxial development, bone anomalies may indicate an abnormality of the neuraxis. Spina bifida is quite common in this area (3 per cent of all adults), as are anterior defects (2 per cent of all adults). The first cervical vertebra may fuse with the base of the skull (occipitalization/assimilation of the atlas). Occasionally there may be a third condyle between C1, or the tip of the odontoid peg, and the anterior margin of the foramen magnum. Such a situation is found normally in reptiles and rodents. The dens has several ossification centres and as the fusion between the tip and the main body of the peg does not occur until well after birth, failure of ossification may occur, leading to abnormal movement and repetitive injury to the brain stem.

Normal anatomy

Occipitoatlantal joints (O–C1)

These are a large pair of joints rarely commented on in routine radiographic reports and rarely, if ever, diagnosed as a source of pain. Nodding movements occur here and erosion of the joints in rheumatoid arthritis must be responsible for one form of vertical migration of the peg (cranial settling). Patients with this type of dislocation that survive merit case reports.

Atlas (C1)

The transverse ligament acts as a tie beam and prevents deformation of this ring of bone, with its lateral masses. As long as the transverse ligament is intact, anterior or posterior surgical interference (transoral removal anteriorly or laminectomy posteriorly) does not destabilize the C1–2 joint. The incomplete ring may burst open if the transverse ligament is pathological. Some sort of fixation or fusion will always be necessary if bone is removed in patients with a pathological transverse ligament. In Jefferson fractures, the mechanical integrity of the transverse ligament (as seen on CT scan) is likewise of importance as the odontoid peg may no longer be constrained in these patients.

Atlantoaxial joints (C1–2)

The anatomy here is familiar. Acute rotatory unilateral facet subluxation in children is still too often misdiagnosed as a wry neck.

Axis (C2)

The odontoid peg has a blood supply similar to the femoral head, and may be compromised in similar conditions, e.g. steroid therapy.

Movement

Seventy per cent of all head-on-neck movement occurs in the craniocervical region. Pure flexion and extension takes place at the atlantoaxial joint. Rotation occurs around the odontoid peg, held as an axle between the posterior aspect of the arch of C1 and the very thick transverse ligament. Extremes of rotation to either side are checked by the alar ligaments, reinforced by a second layer of defence, the cruciate ligaments. All these ligaments are taut in the mid-position when the head is facing forwards. The supplementary ligaments are so strong that division of the transverse ligament alone allows only minimal displacement of the odontoid peg. Pathological movement implies damage to the whole complex. Head rotation is a complex movement which occurs in at least two planes. The shape of the lateral masses of C1 and C2 results in an elongation of the neck as the head is rotated, tightening these ligaments. Basilar invagination (cranial settling) is secondary to metabolic bone disease or rheumatoid arthritis. Distortion or erosion of the joints allows shortening of the craniocervical region and passage of the odontoid peg into the foramen magnum.

When the head is flexed, the spinal cord moves anteriorly at the foramen magnum relative to the bones. The attachment of the dentate ligament and the filum terminali causes a lengthening force to be applied to the cord at the same time. If there is a subluxating dens, either fixed or intermittent, this will accentuate the forces applied to the neuraxis. It is our belief that the intermittent application of these forces associated with head movement is responsible for neurological deterioration, and is more important than the absolute dimensions of the foramen magnum or the spinal canal in the region.

Radiographic measurements

Various lines have been described but none is truly satisfactory. Distortion of the brain stem may only occur at extremes of movement. Currently the CT myelogram is the only investigation which demonstrates this adequately. The radiologist must look for it in different postures and when reconstructing the image in appropriate planes.

Pathology

Table 1 outlines some of the problems in the area. A more detailed description of the lesions can be found elsewhere[1].

The basic principles of evaluation in each case are as follows. Are the bones in the region of a normal configuration? Are there abnormal or exaggerated movements at any of the joints? Is there a bony deformity in the region, and, if so, is it fixed or mobile? Is there potentially a soft tissue mass which could distort the dura and the neuraxis in the region? What is the configuration of the neuraxis in the region and is it deformed during head and neck movements?

Table 1 Pathology of cervical spine

Congenital	Hypoplastic or absent dens Morquio's syndrome
Metabolic	Osteogenesis imperfecta
Traumatic	Jefferson fractures Odontoid fracture Hangman's fracture Rotatory subluxation
Degenerative	Osteoarthritis

Neoplastic	Primary
	  Chordoma
	  Osteoblastoma
	  Osteoclastoma
	Secondary
	  Breast carcinoma

Iatrogenic	Previous posterior fusion/ decompression Radiotherapy

Infective	Osteomyelitis
	  Pyogenic
	  Tuberculous
	  Fungal

Preoperative

Investigations

Plain radiographs

1a & b

True lateral flexion (a) and extension (b) views, and anteroposterior radiographs of the upper cervical spine and the base of skull, are a useful screening test to alert the clinician to the possibility of an abnormality in the region. They are a particularly useful screening device in patients with rheumatoid arthritis.

Computed tomography

Computed tomography, especially with metrizamide enhancement, and three-dimensional reconstruction currently provides information on the bones and joints in the area, and of the effect of the abnormality on the intradural contents. Flexion and extension views must be performed to allow a dynamic assessment of the situation.

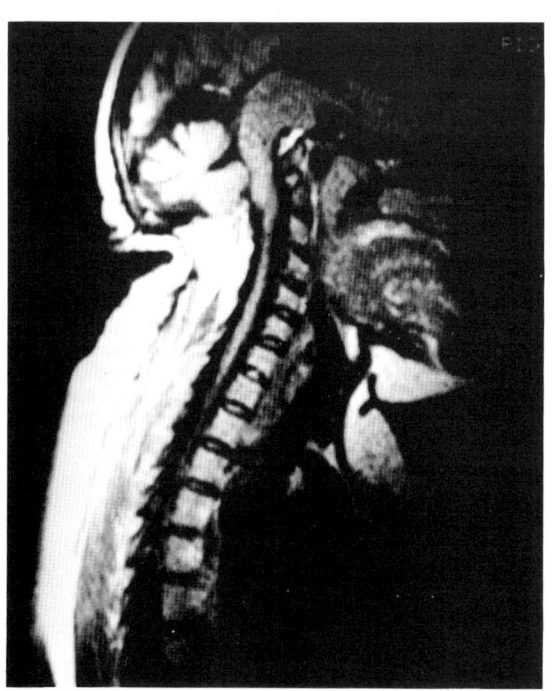

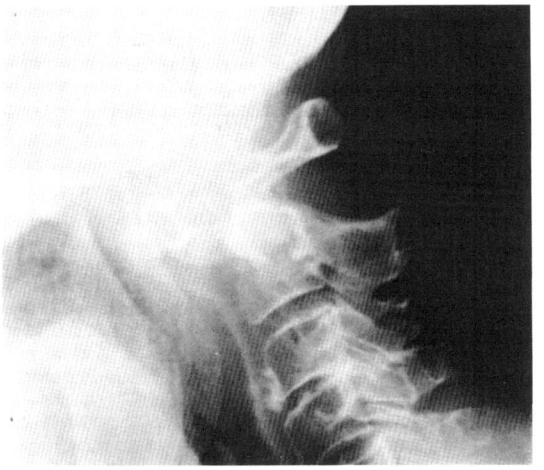

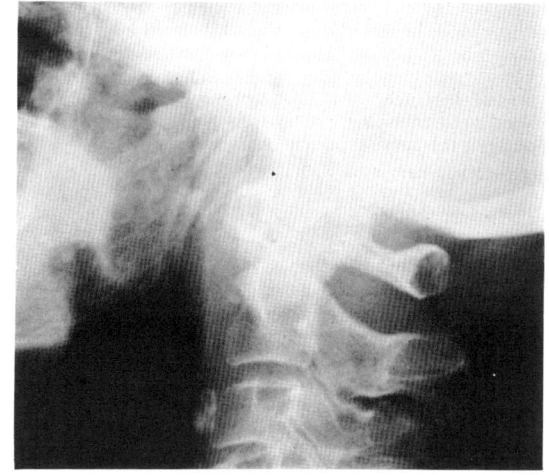

Magnetic resonance imaging

2

Magnetic resonance images provide excellent information of the neuraxial compression and soft tissue masses. *Illustration 2* demonstrates a case of osteogenesis imperfecta, in which the pontine and brain stem distribution is most dramatic.

With more powerful magnets and computer programs, the scan time will be reduced sufficiently to allow comfortable assessment of the situation in flexion and extension. The images again can be reconstructed in any plane. At present the bony abnormalities are not so well defined as with the latest generation of CT scanners. Soft tissue abnormalities, however, are outlined very much better.

Angiography

Angiography should be considered if extensive bone work is required. In congenital malformation there may be associated congenital vascular anomalies of the vertebral arteries.

Indications for an anterior approach

The general principles to which the clinician must address himself in the management of problems at the craniocervical junction and upper cervical spine will flow naturally from the understanding of the mechanisms producing the clinical picture. If there is a deformity which is totally reducible then there is a sound argument for a posterior fixation which is technically easier and which has stood the test of time over 50 years of clinical evaluation. With further experience there may be indications for an anterior fixation even in this situation. If there is anterior dural compression and distortion of the neuraxis by an anterior mass or by an irreducible dislocation of the bony elements in the area, then posterior fixation will at best limit further deterioration. With imaging techniques readily available, it would be unwise to correct a bony deformity without a detailed knowledge of the state of the underlying neuraxis. Table 2 outlines the general principles of management of a lesion in the region.

Table 2 Management of craniocervical problems

	No bony instability or deformity	Reducible bony instability	Bony deformity
No neuraxial compression	No surgery	Posterior fixation	No surgery
Anterior neuraxial compression	Anterior surgery	Posterior fixation	Anterior surgery and posterior fixation
Posterior neuraxial compression	Posterior decompression	Posterior decompression and fixation	Posterior decompression; and possibly posterior fixation

Assessment

Mouth

An obvious but easily overlooked assessment is surgical access through the oral cavity. In patients with rheumatoid arthritis or ankylosing spondylosis, the temporomandibular joints may also be involved, reducing mouth opening. If the interdental or intergum distance is less than 25 mm with the mouth fully open, it is unlikely that surgical access will be gained. Abnormal dentition or deficient dentition may affect the positioning of the transoral retractor.

Associated limb deformity

Limb deformity may make patient positioning on the operating table difficult. Care must obviously be taken of the pressure areas: skin degloving injuries can be prevented by application of orthopaedic wool.

Pulmonary function

Pulmonary function must be assessed and documented. Respiratory function may be reduced because of chest deformities, or owing to central depression associated with the neuraxial compression. It is vital to ascertain whether the patient will be able to breathe again after having been put on a ventilator for surgery.

Skull traction

In the unstable traumatized patient, skull traction will have to be applied to reduce and then to immobilize the dislocation (see chapter on 'The halo–body cast', pp. 486–490). In other cases, achieving improvement in neurological and respiratory function might be beneficial. A further consideration is whether the translocated dens can be brought down out of the foramen magnum. It must be said, however, that those who employ traction only do so when there is a frank instability, usually of traumatic origin, and it is not our practice to employ it for prolonged periods of time prior to surgery. Following operation it is rarely used as we prefer to use internal fixation following decompression.

Bacteriological culture

Many of these patients are quite ill; some are in an immunodepressed state. It is essential to be aware of the flora in the nose and throat prior to the transoral surgery so that appropriate antibiotics may be given should complications arise. It is our practice to give preoperative and postoperative antibiotics, usually cephalosporin and occasionally metronidazole.

Operation

Anaesthesia

Anaesthetic technique will be severely tested in these patients. The reader is advised to consult Calder[2] for details. Tracheostomy, not easy in these patients, can usually be avoided. Nasotracheal intubation is performed using a fibreoptic laryngoscope in the awake patient. The armoured Mallinckrodt nasotracheal tube is retained for 2 to 5 days following the surgery to divert pulmonary secretions from the operative area. A nasogastric tube is passed at the same time to divert the gastric contents. Both tubes are displaced from the operative field using a specially designed retractor. Controlled respiration is usually employed, but if there is any suggestion that the medulla is compressed or likely to be compressed during the procedure, then spontaneous respiration is used and a close watch kept on the respiratory trace. In our experience this provides the most sensitive guide to medullary compression and has been more reliable than somatosensory evoked response and cortical evoked motor responses in such patients.

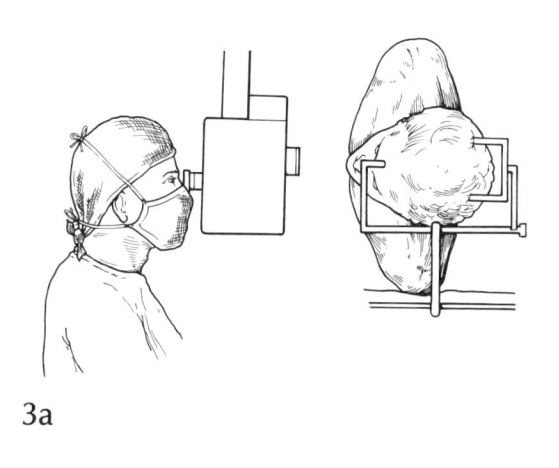

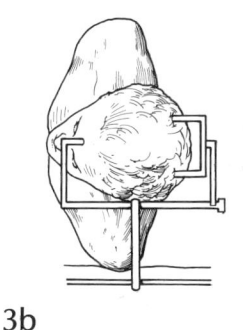

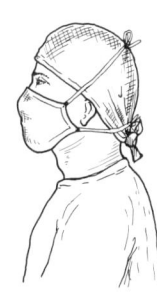

Position

3a & b

In general, all patients with intradural pathology or extensive extradural tumours are placed in the supine position. In those patients in whom an anterior decompression and a posterior fixation is contemplated, a lateral position is adopted. This allows anterior and posterior surgery while keeping the neck fixed and stable. *Illustration 3a* shows the transoral approach, and *Illustration 3b* occipitocervical fixation.

A Mayfield skull clamp with its three-pin fixation allows good head immobilization and permits minor adjustments to position. The head frame is now available in carbon fibre and peroperative radiographs can be obtained without interference. The exact position of the head is determined by the deformity, avoidance of brain stem compression and by any change in physiological monitoring. Extension improves surgical visibility for the transoral procedure, and flexion assists the passage of the sublaminar wires if these are used in the posterior fixation.

Surgical exposure

4a & b

Lighting is a major difficulty, as is the length of instruments. Incision of the soft palate is best avoided to reduce postoperative incompetence of the nasopharyngeal sphincter. Retraction, using a Jacques' catheter, has been employed, and, while this provides good midline exposure up to the rim of the foramen magnum, lateral exposure is limited. A specially designed retractor has been developed (Codman and Shurtleff, Randolph, Massachusetts, USA) which allows cephalad and lateral exposure without division of the soft palate, and which is useful for all procedures from the anterior rim of the foramen magnum down to the third cervical vertebra. The retractor incorporates a halo around the mouth to which other instruments, such as suction and additional fibre lights, can be applied by a universal locking system. The soft palate and the nasogastric and nasotracheal tubes are held out of the operative field. If the surgery is to be continued on to the clivus, then a palatal incision extending through the soft palate, and sometimes into the hard palate, will be required. A further attachment allows for this retraction. Tooth and gum protection is provided by sterilizable dental alginate.

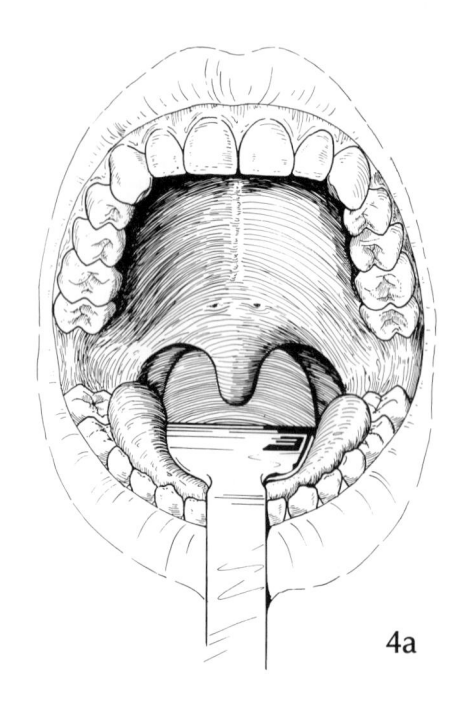

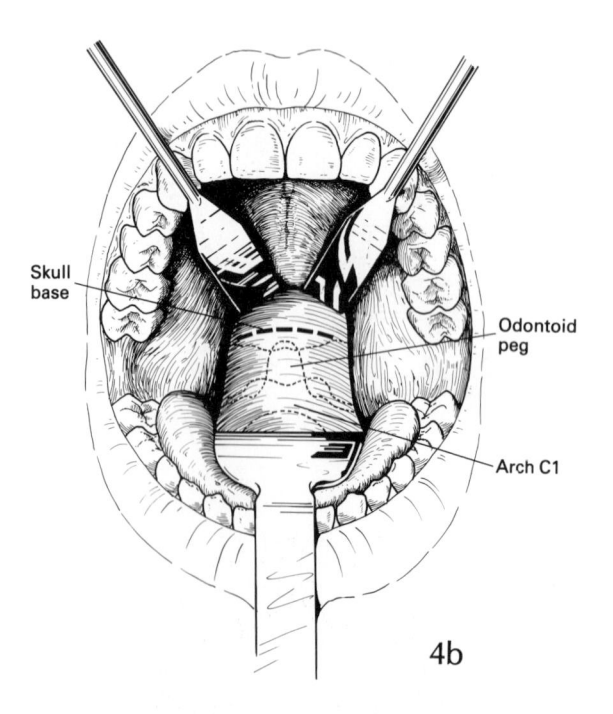

Procedure

The operating microscope, with a binocular eyepiece for the assistant, is helpful, if only to provide adequate lighting. The pharynx is infiltrated with adrenaline 1 in 200 000 and 1 per cent lignocaine to define the tissue planes and reduce bleeding.

5a & b

The spine may be exposed either by a midline pharyngeal incision or a square flap. The latter is theoretically attractive and useful when considering anterior bone grafting, but we have not experienced undue difficulty with the midline incision which is more easily closed. The bony midline is reasonably identified as the anterior longitudinal ligament is attached to the anterior tubercle on the arch of C1. The longus colli muscles are attached on each side and exactly in the midline only bone is detected. The pharyngeal wall is then retracted using the transoral pharyngeal retractor which not only retracts the posterior pharyngeal soft tissue but provides lateral protection to the mouth. The anterior longitudinal ligament is divided longitudinally using low-power cutting diathermy. Scout radiographs are helpful but, with experience, become unnecessary. The bone work is carried out using a 3 mm cutting burr until directly approaching the dura, at which point a diamond burr is employed.

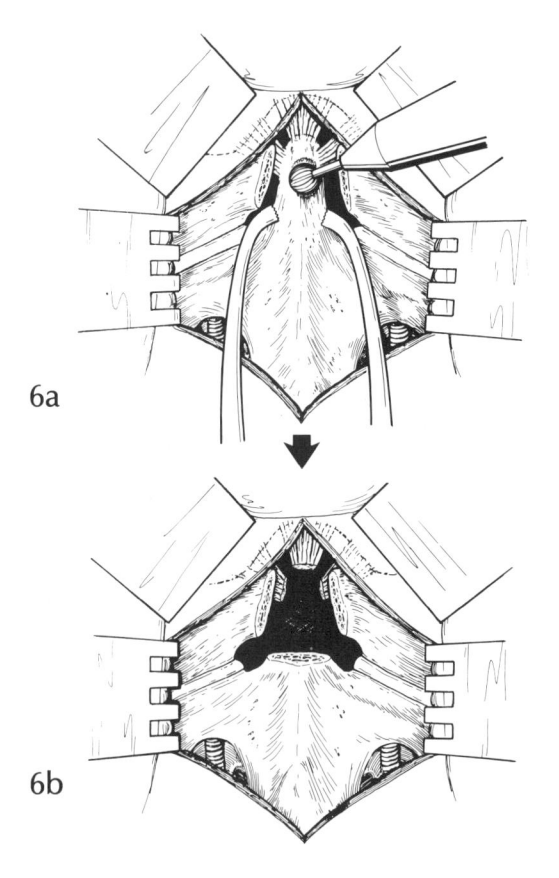

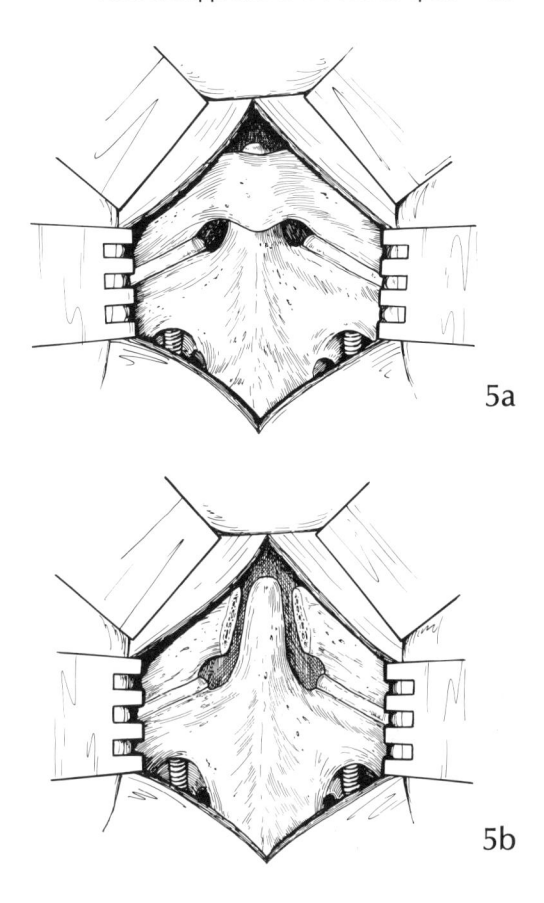

6a & b

The anterior arch of the atlas is resected to expose the odontoid peg. Posterior to this is a small synovial joint which may contain fluid under pressure. Odontoidectomy is carried out piecemeal. The odontoid peg is removed using the high-speed air drill (*a*). As it is enucleated, the apical and alar ligaments require sharp dissection with a knife. If the peg is loose it bounces about and needs to be held with specially designed offset graspers. The transverse ligament and cruciate ligaments are now apparent and behind is the dura, which is decompressed after removal of bone, tectorial membrane and associated ligaments (*b*). Any CSF leak must be sealed and CSF pressure reduced by a lumbar shunt to reduce the likelihood of a postoperative fistula.

7a & b

Closure is undertaken in two layers using interrupted absorbable Vicryl (Ethicon, UK) sutures. Muscles and fascia (a) are closed, followed by pharyngeal mucosal closure (b). The surgery requires skill and three-dimensional bimanual operative dexterity.

Craniocervical stabilization

After transoral surgery, instability is usually increased. The stability of the craniocervical junction will require protection either by an internal fixation device or an external halo-body jacket. Except in the terminally ill, bone grafting will be required for ultimate stabilization and this is usually inserted posteriorly, although we use transoral bone grafting occasionally without significant problems[3].

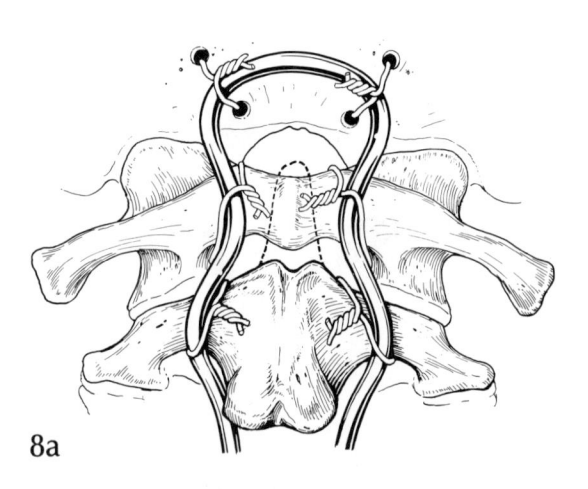

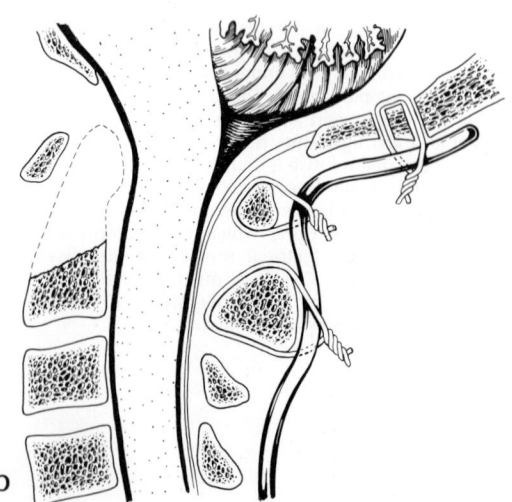

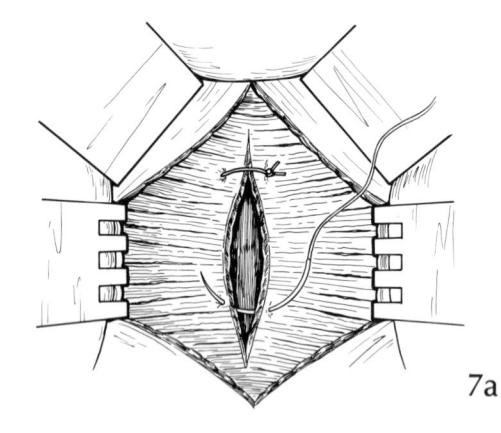

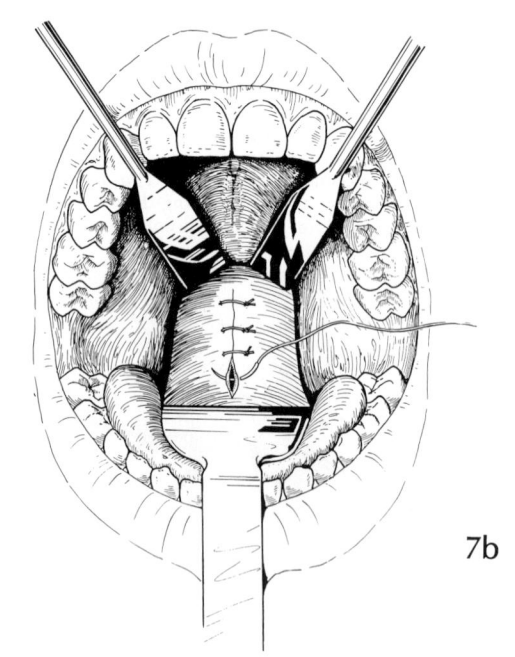

8a & b

In the rheumatoid patient[4] or those with malignancy, we prefer occipitocervical fixation and insert a Hartshill–Ransford loop (Surgicraft Ltd, Redditch, UK) held in place by sublaminar and occipital wires through drill holes[5].

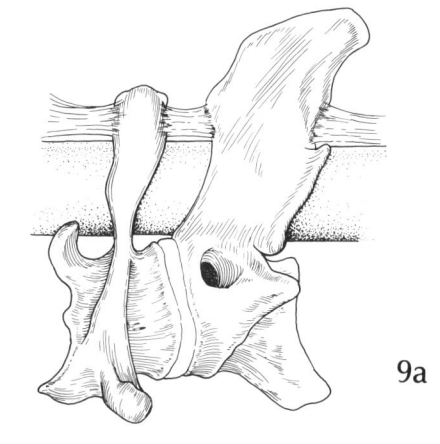

9a, b & c

The passage of sublaminar wires is potentially hazardous[6], especially when neuraxial compression persists. It is essential to remove the ligamentum flavum on each side and to use blunted or doubled wires (18- or 20-gauge) to prevent dural penetration and cord damage. An instrument has been devised (Codman and Shurtleff Instruments) which may strip the attachment of the ligamentum flavum and because of its grooved inner surface may act as a guide along which to pass the sublaminar wire, thereby protecting the underlying dura. Postoperatively, all that is required in terms of neck support is a soft cervical collar.

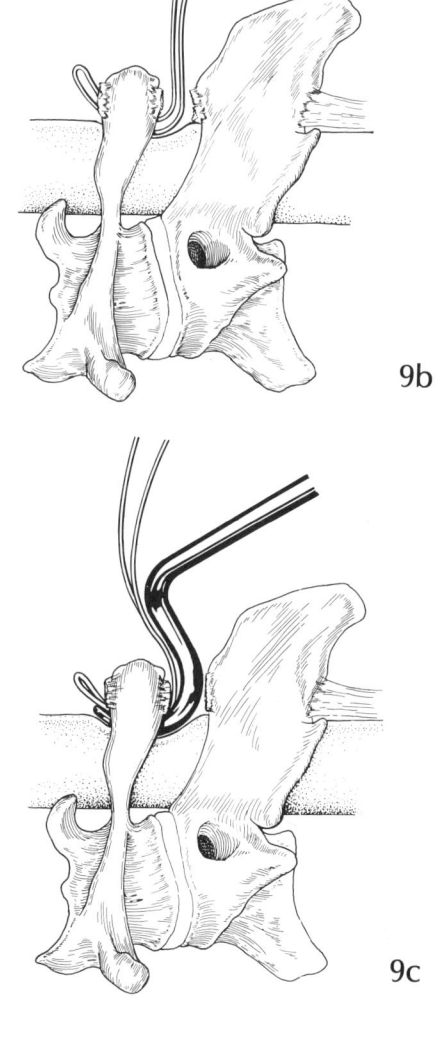

10

A postoperative radiograph is taken to show the loop in position.

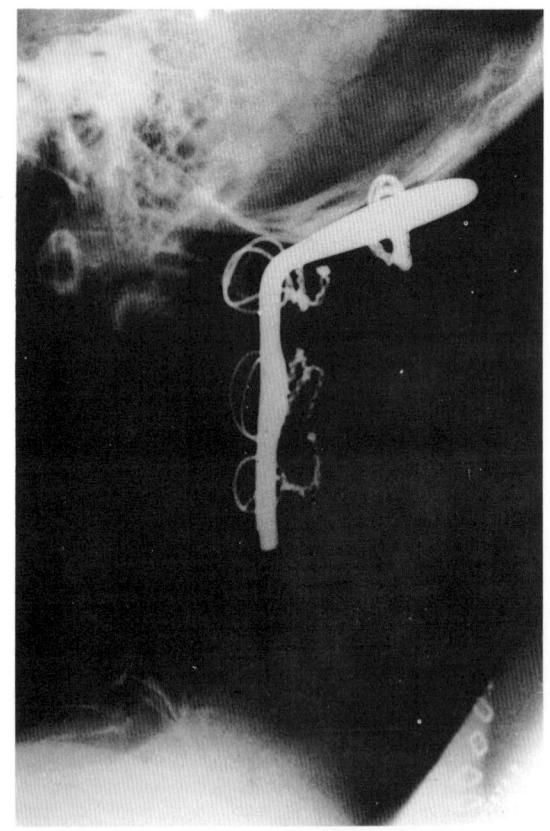

10

References

1. Crockard HA. Anterior approaches to lesions of the upper cervical spine. *Clin Neurosurg* 1988; 34: 389–416.

2. Calder I. Anaesthesia for transoral and craniocervical surgery. *Baillière's Clin Anaesth* 1987; 2: 441–57.

3. Ashraf J, Crockard HA. Transoral fusion for high cervical fractures. *J Bone Joint Surg [Br]* 1990; 72-B: 76–9.

4. Crockard HA, Calder I, Ransford AO. One stage transoral decompression and posterior fixation in rheumatoid atlanto-axial subluxation. *J Bone Joint Surg [Br]* 1990; 72-B: 682–5.

5. Ransford AO, Crockard HA, Pozo JL. Craniocervical instability treated by contoured loop fixation. *J Bone Joint Surg [Br]* 1986; 68-B: 173–7.

6. Crockard HA, Ransford AO. Stabilization of the spine. *Adv Tech Stand Neurosurg* 1990; 17: 159–88.

Illustrations by Patrick Elliott after P. Miles

Anterior fusions of the cervical spine

David L. Hamblen PhD, FRCS
Professor of Orthopaedic Surgery, Western Infirmary, Glasgow, UK

Introduction

The anterior approach to the cervical spine provides the most direct access to the vertebral bodies, permitting clearance of degenerate disc material from the intervertebral spaces and interbody fusion techniques. The anatomy of the region permits easy anterolateral exposure to the bodies of the third to seventh vertebrae. Above and below these levels the approach to the bodies is technically more difficult and requires a direct anterior transpharyngeal or trans-sternal approach.

Three techniques of interbody fusion have been described using this common approach. They utilize corticocancellous bone from the iliac crest in the form of a block[1], a dowel[2] or a 'keystone' strut graft[3].

Indications

The anterior interbody fusion may be used for the following indications.

1. To provide intervertebral stability following the operative removal of degenerate disc material through an anterior approach.
2. Post-traumatic instability following hyperflexion fractures or fracture-dislocations.
3. Cervical spondylosis confined to one or two levels associated with intractable pain, or progressive neurological impairment from cord or root compression.
4. Following resection of major portions of one or more vertebral bodies involved by infections or tumours of benign or low-grade malignancy.
5. To correct and stabilize late hyperflexion deformities following extensive posterior surgical laminectomies.

Preoperative

In the commonest indications of disc degeneration or spondylosis the selection of the level for fusion is usually made from the clinical features combined with information from plain radiographs. The most useful are lateral views in maximum flexion and extension, or dynamic cineradiography when this technique is available[4]. Discography may be indicated when the level of disc degeneration is uncertain[5], but it is not recommended as routine since it is a difficult investigation to perform and even more difficult to interpret. Cervical myelography is only of value in suspected cord compression.

When excessive spinal instability is present as a result of trauma or disease, fusion should be preceded by the application of 4.5–7.0 kg (10–15 lb) of skeletal traction through skull calipers. Preoperative stability may also be achieved by the application of a halo–jacket. Increased traction may sometimes be required to achieve reduction of dislocated articular facets in acute hyperflexion injuries.

Anaesthesia

General anaesthesia is preferred routinely and the insertion of an armoured endotracheal tube facilitates mobilization and handling of the tracheo-oesophageal structures while preventing obstruction to the airway. It also allows more adequate skin preparation and draping of the patient.

Operation

Special instruments

Special instrumentation is only required for the Cloward technique for dowel graft fusion. The other techniques of interbody fusion use general orthopaedic instrumentation. Useful additions are blunt-ended self-retaining retractors, a range of small curettes, fine pituitary rongeurs, a laminar spreader, angled osteotomes, and a bone punch.

Position of patient

1

The patient is placed in the supine position with a small sandbag between the shoulders. The head is supported in a cerebellar headrest in slight extension, with the chin turned away from the side of operation. Either side may be used, but the left is usually preferred because of the lesser risk of damage to the recurrent laryngeal nerve. However, the presence of the thoracic duct on the left should be kept in mind during the procedure.

After preparation of the skin a standard thyroid drape is used, which allows the anaesthetist access to the face if necessary. The iliac crest on the same side should be prepared and draped for removal of the bone graft.

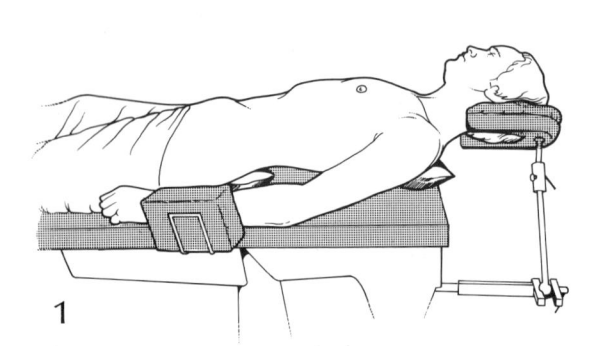

Incision

2

The level and technique of fusion determines the type of skin incision used. An incision in a skin crease, running from the midline to the anterior border of the sternomastoid muscle, at the level of the lower border of the thyroid cartilage, gives the best cosmetic result. When a more extensive exposure is required to allow clearance of bone disease, or to permit multiple-level fusion, a vertical incision along the line of the anterior border of the sternomastoid is recommended. This begins 2 cm below the mastoid process and ends just above the sternum.

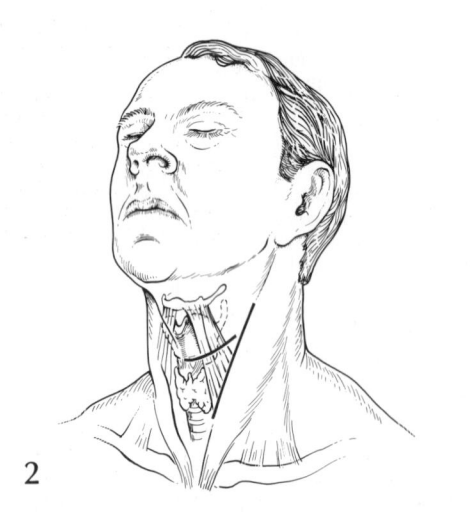

Exposure of the spine

3

The thin muscular layer of the platysma is divided in the line of the skin incision but preserved as a separate layer for repair. The flaps are retracted proximally and distally to allow vertical incision of the fascia along the anterior border of the sternomastoid muscle. Blunt dissection is used to develop the space between the strap muscle medially and the sternomastoid laterally after retraction or division of the omohyoid muscle distally.

Deep to the sternomastoid the carotid artery can be easily palpated and gently retracted laterally with the other contents of the carotid sheath. The trachea and oesophagus are separated from the prevertebral fascia and mobilized medially to allow the finger to palpate the anterior surfaces of the bodies of the midcervical vertebrae. Normally, only the middle thyroid vein requires ligation and division. In high exposure it may be necessary to ligate the superior thyroid artery and vein, with care to avoid damage to the superior laryngeal nerve running down the lateral wall of the pharynx.

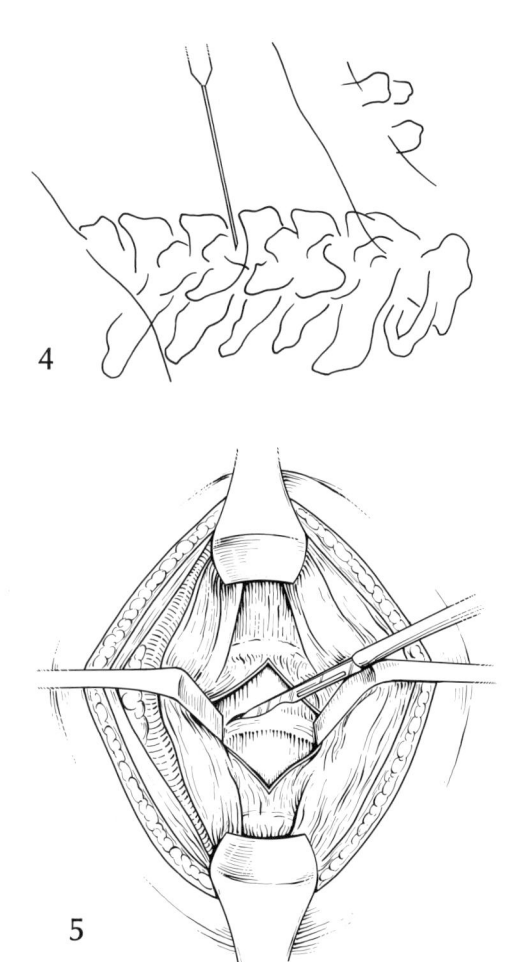

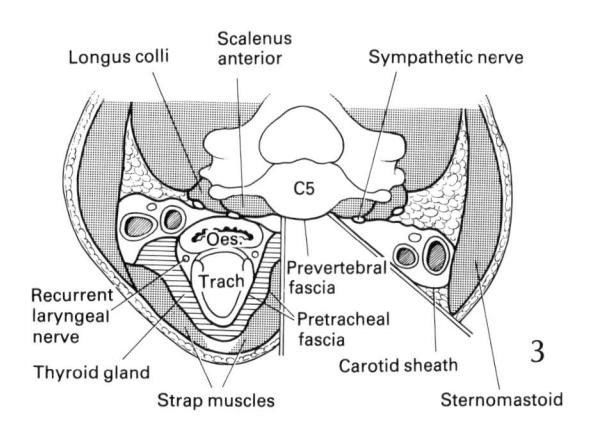

Identification of vertebral level

4

The midline of the bodies is easily recognized by the fascial strip running vertically between the two vertebral longus colli muscles. At this stage it is essential to confirm the proposed level of fusion using radiological control. A 26-gauge hypodermic needle is inserted into the midline of the selected intervertebral space and its position checked with a lateral radiograph or the image intensifier. The position of the needle also marks the angle of the intervertebral space, which runs upwards as well as backwards from the neutral position. After the correct level has been confirmed, the longus colli muscles are stripped laterally to allow wider exposure of the intervertebral space prior to disc removal. Any bleeding from the bony surfaces can be controlled with coagulation diathermy.

Disc excision

5

The anterior ligament and annulus are excised over the front of the intervertebral space with a long-handled scalpel, to allow clearance of disc material using curettes and rongeurs. Care must be taken not to dissect blindly into the space to a depth greater than 1.25 cm, to avoid accidental entry into the spinal canal and damage to its contents. When formal spinal decompression is required, the use of a vertebral spreader and magnification with an operating microscope facilitates safe removal of posterior osteophytes or prolapsed disc material. The vertebral end-plates should be left intact to prevent collapse of the vertebral bodies around the graft. The further stages in the operative procedure depend on which technique of fusion is chosen.

CLOWARD DOWEL PROCEDURE

Preparation of vertebral cavity

6a, b & c

After clearance of disc material the special drill guard (a) is inserted in the midline over the intervertebral space by tapping the teeth on its footplate into the bone of the two adjacent vertebrae. A broad 14 mm or 16 mm fluted drill (b), which has a collar at its base, can then be passed down the adjustable guard so that the tip passes through the hole in the footplate and a shallow 1 cm hole cut. To run in the line of the intervertebral space, the hole should have the disc running across its centre. The screw-thread on the drill guard is advanced 1–2 mm at a time to allow gradual deepening of the hole (c). Each time the drill is removed bony debris is cleared and the depth tested with an adjustable guage to avoid accidental penetration of the spinal canal. When the cortical wall is breached any remaining fragments of bone and disc can be removed from the canal with fine pituitary rongeurs.

Occasionally prominent posterolateral osteophytes cause nerve root compression and may require removal. This is not recommended as a routine procedure since osteophytes may resolve spontaneously following interbody fusion due to distraction of the intervertebral space and elimination of movement.

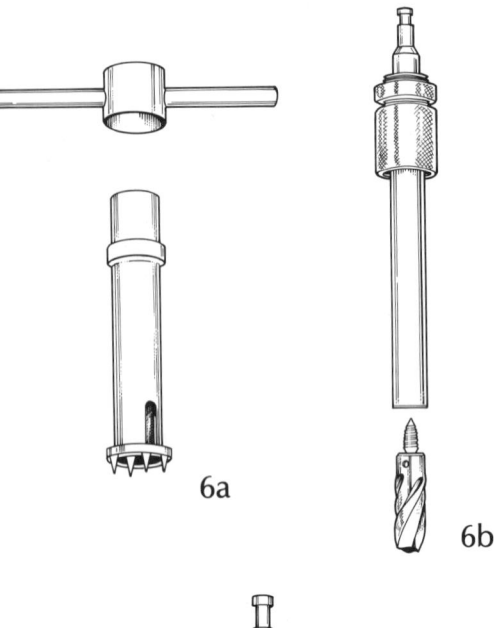

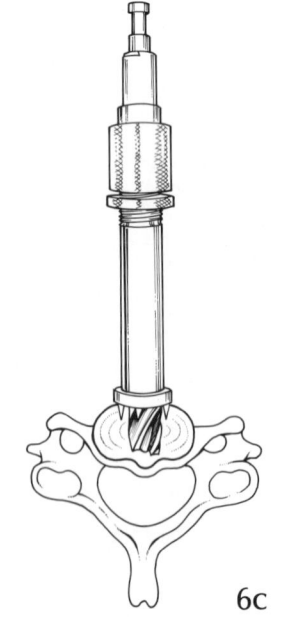

Removal of dowel graft from iliac crest

7

The outer table of the anterior portion of the iliac crest is exposed through a short transverse incision and the periosteum stripped from its surface. A matching size of dowel cutter with a centre pin is introduced on a Hudson brace and drilled completely through the ilium to give a cylindrical plug with a cortical surface at both ends. This is trimmed to size by reducing its length to 2 mm less than the depth of the drill hole, which can be measured from the graduations on the drill guide.

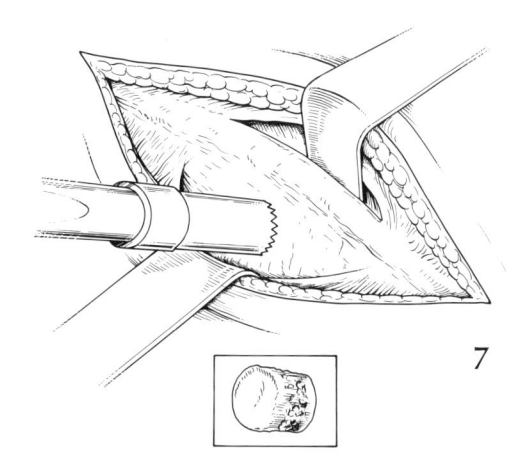

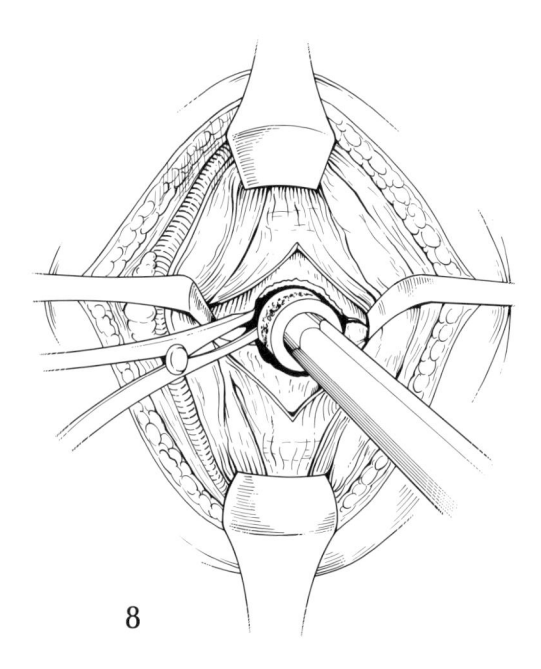

Insertion of dowel graft

8

The intervertebral space is distracted by traction on the head and insertion of the laminar spreaders. This allows the cylindrical graft to be tapped into the prepared cavity with a punch. It should be countersunk to a depth of 1 mm below the surface of the bodies to minimize risk of extrusion. When two adjacent spaces are to be fused, the cavities are prepared with smaller 10 or 12 mm diameter drills so that they do not communicate and thereby predispose to dowel extrusion. Matching small sizes of dowel cutters are also available to prepare the appropriate grafts.

ROBINSON BLOCK GRAFT TECHNIQUE

Preparation of intervertebral space

9

After complete removal of the intervertebral disc the laminar spreaders are inserted and the cartilaginous end-plates are curetted out, leaving the subchondral bone-plates largely intact. These may be perforated at a few sites to encourage bone ingrowth into the graft.

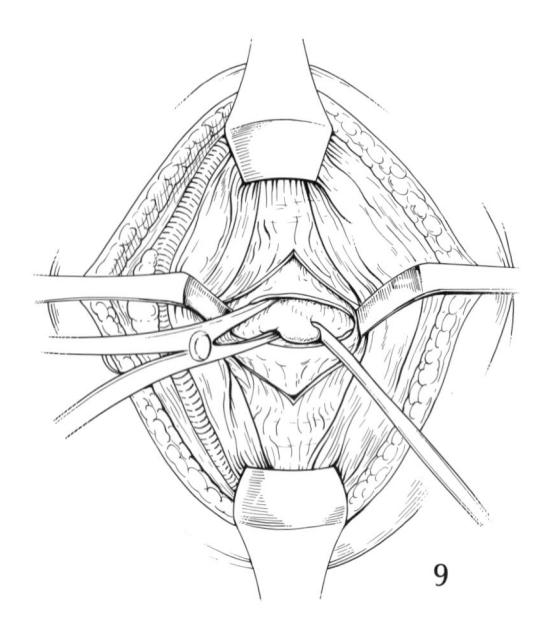

Removal of block graft

10

A full-thickness bone graft is removed from the anterior end of the iliac crest using two parallel cuts into its superior border. These should measure 1 cm in width and 2 cm in depth. The cortex is left intact on the superficial and deep surfaces of the graft, as well as on its free edge. The graft is then trimmed to be 5 mm less than the measured depth of the intervertebral space.

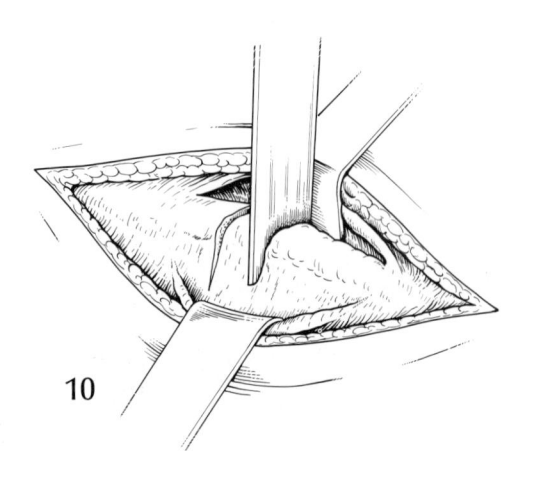

Insertion of block graft

11

The intervertebral space is distracted to its maximum extent by the insertion of laminar spreaders or by the anaesthetist pulling on the head. The graft is positioned in the midline of the space with its cortical surfaces lying vertically on each side to provide maximum resistance to collapse. It is tapped into position with a punch until it is countersunk 1–2 mm and the traction is then released to lock it under compression.

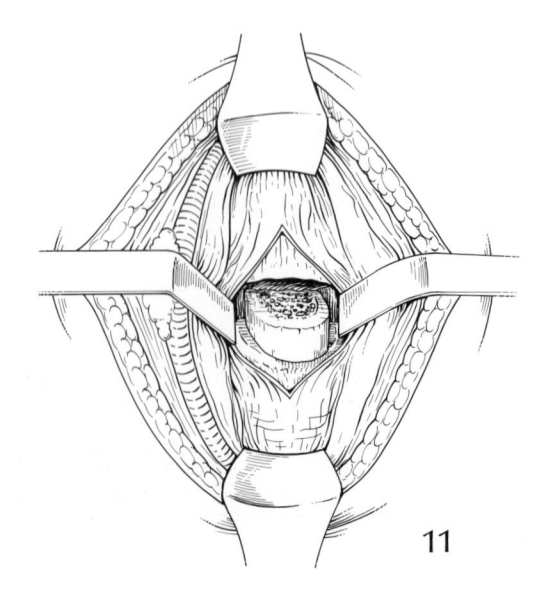

BAILEY STRUT GRAFT TECHNIQUE

Preparation of graft bed

12

After routine clearance of the intervertebral disc, the bed for the graft is prepared by cutting an anterior trough in the bodies to be fused. When neoplastic or infective tissue is to be removed this is included in the excised area. The proximal and distal ends of the trough are bevelled into the posterior bone of the vertebral body to produce a 'keystone' effect.

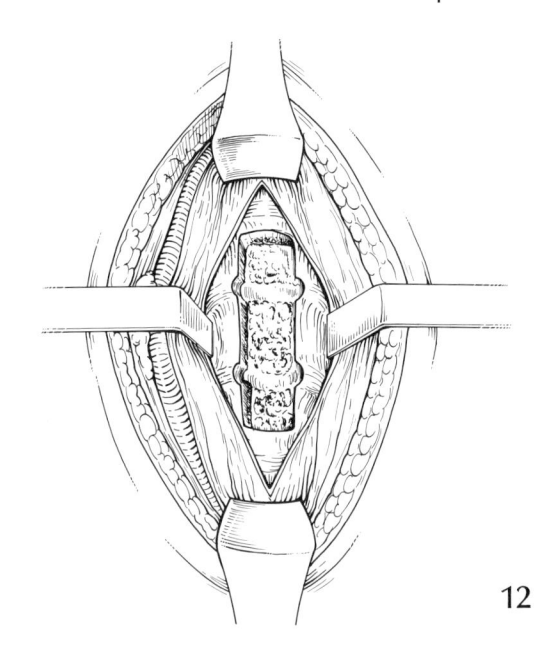

Removal of strut graft from iliac crest

13

A suitable slightly-oversized rectangular corticocancellous graft is then removed from the outer table of the iliac crest together with some cancellous bone chips.

Insertion of strut graft

14

After the cancellous chips are packed into the base of the trough and the intervertebral space, the vertebrae are distracted by traction and the rectangular graft tapped into position with a punch. The cortical surface should lie anteriorly and is locked in position by the anterior edges of the vertebrae proximally and distally once traction has been released.

Wound closure

The same wound closure is used following each type of intervertebral fusion. A single suction drain should be used for 24 hours to minimize wound haematoma formation. No deep sutures are required unless the longus colli muscle and prevertebral fascia require closure. For optimum cosmesis, the platysma muscle should be repaired as a separate layer and the skin closed with subcuticular suture.

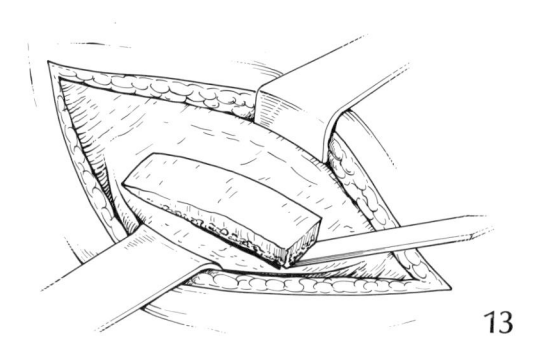

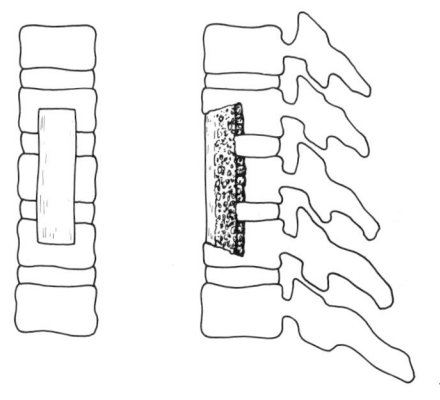

Postoperative management

This is dependent on the pathology present and the stability achieved following the insertion of the graft. After fractures and dislocations, or where portions of several vertebral bodies have been removed, it may be necessary to use a rigid cervicothoracic brace for 6–12 weeks until early radiological fusion is apparent. In patients undergoing fusion for disc degeneration, a soft rubber collar is all that is required until the wound is healed; splintage can then be discarded and normal mobility allowed.

References

1. Robinson RA, Smith GW. Antero-lateral cervical disc removal and interbody fusion for cervical disc syndrome. *Bull Johns Hopkins Hosp* 1955; 96: 223–4.

2. Cloward RB. Vertebral body fusion for ruptured cervical discs: description of instruments and operative technic. *Am J Surg.* 1959; 98: 722–7.

3. Bailey RW, Badgley CE. Stabilization of the cervical spine by anterior fusion. *J Bone Joint Surg [Am]* 1960; 42-A: 565–94.

4. Brunton FJ, Wilkinson JA, Wise KSH, Simonis RB. Cine radiography in cervical spondylosis as a means of determining the level for anterior fusion. *J Bone Joint Surg [Br]* 1982; 64-B: 399–404.

5. Kikuchi S, Macnab I, Moreau P. Localisation of the level of symptomatic cervical disc degeneration. *J Bone Joint Surg [Br]* 1981; 63-B: 272–7.

Illustrations by Patrick Elliott after P. Miles

Posterior fusions of the cervical spine

David L. Hamblen PhD, FRCS
Professor of Orthopaedic Surgery, Western Infirmary, Glasgow, UK

Introduction

The posterior aspect of the cervical spine is readily accessible from the occiput to the cervicothoracic junction. This approach allows fusion from the atlas to the seventh cervical vertebra and permits the fusion mass to be carried up onto the occiput or down to the first thoracic vertebra. After a midline incision the ligaments and muscles are stripped subperiosteally from the spinous processes and laminae. No dangerous structures are encountered except at the upper end of the spine where the vertebral arteries and dural sinuses are at risk.

Four different types of fusion can be performed using this same posterior approach. They are occipitocervical fusion, atlantoaxial fusion, interspinous fusion, and posterolateral facet fusion. The indications and techniques for each procedure differ but the preoperative care, anaesthesia and positioning are common to all.

Preoperative

Posterior fusions are frequently preceded by the application of skeletal traction to reduce dislocations or subluxations and to maintain stability. Either conventional skull calipers or a halo splint can be utilized and provide easy control of the position of head and neck when the patient is turned from the supine to the prone position.

Anaesthesia

General anaesthesia is used as routine and demands considerable skill to achieve endotracheal intubation while avoiding excessive flexion or extension of the cervical spine. An armoured, non-kinkable endotracheal tube must be used in all cases.

472　Cervical spine

Position of patient

1

After induction of anaesthesia the patient is placed in the prone position with the head supported by a neurosurgical cerebellar head-rest. This permits easy adjustment of the position of the spine in any plane while permitting access to the face for anaesthetic purposes. The spine is normally placed in the neutral position; though some flexion permits easier access to the suboccipital region, this is likely to result in redisplacement of vertebrae. The final position should be checked with a lateral radiograph before surgery is commenced and at the time of wire tightening.

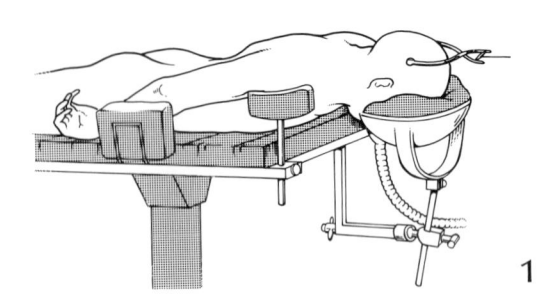

Operations

OCCIPITOCERVICAL FUSION

Indications

Fusion from the upper cervical vertebrae to the occiput may occasionally be required for the following indications:

1. Comminuted bursting fracture of the ring of the atlas (Jefferson fracture).
2. Atlantoaxial instability complicating rheumatoid arthritis or local sepsis, where access to the posterior arch of the atlas is inadequate to permit atlantoaxial fusion.
3. Following posterior surgical decompression for congenital anomalies in the craniovertebral region or for unreduced atlantoaxial dislocation.

Special instruments

Stainless steel monofilament wire of 18–20 swg or 1 mm braided cable is used to provide stability in all posterior fusions. Wire-handling instruments are required, including passers, tighteners and cutters. A small air-drill facilitates the placement of holes for vertebral wiring and can also be used with a dental burr for rapid decortication. If the graft is to be wired to the occiput, instruments for neurosurgical burr holes will be required and the assistance of a neurosurgeon, if available, is ideal.

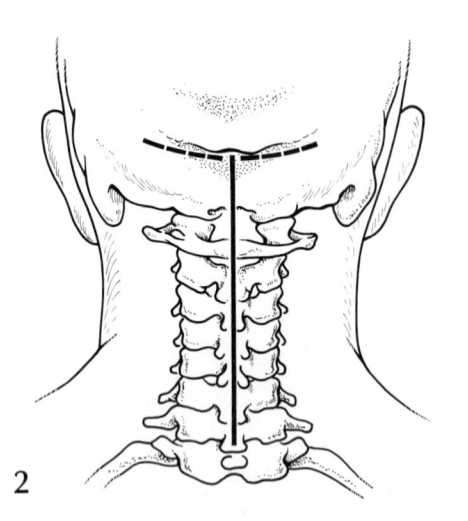

Incision

2

A longitudinal midline incision is used, extending from the external occipital protuberance to the spinous process of the most distal vertebra in the fusion. Occasionally, when access to the suboccipital region is difficult, this incision can be extended at its upper end for 5 cm on each side as a T-shaped Cushing incision.

Division of ligamentum nuchae

3

The dense ligamentum nuchae and intermuscular septum are incised using cutting diathermy to expose the occipital protuberance and the tips of the spinous processes. Care should be taken to remain in the midline as this will minimize bleeding.

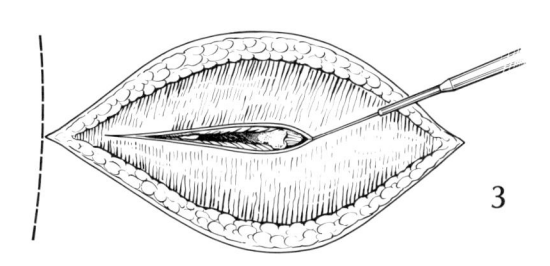

Muscle stripping from bone surfaces

4

The muscles are stripped subperiosteally from the spinous processes and laminae using a broad Cobb's elevator. Care must be taken not to extend the dissection laterally for more than 1.5 cm from the midline of the arch of the atlas to avoid damage to the vertebral arteries. To minimize bleeding, muscle stripping and packing with gauze swabs should be performed alternately on each side.

Exposure of bony surfaces

5

Self-retaining retractors are now inserted to expose the posterior aspect of the occiput up to the external protuberance, the posterior arch of the atlas, and the spinous processes and laminae of the distal vertebrae. Any remaining muscle and interspinous ligament can be removed with nibbling forceps prior to placement of the wires.

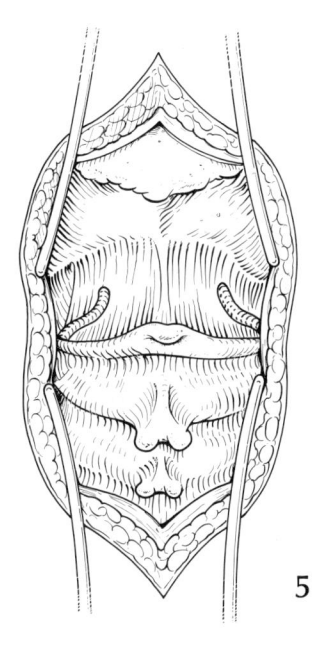

Placement of vertebral wires

6

By careful dissection of the posterior atlanto-occipital membrane from the anterior aspect of the posterior arch of the atlas, it should be possible to pass a wire loop around the bone. This can then be divided to provide a wire on each side of the midline. Distally it is sometimes difficult to pass wires around the laminae; as an alternative these may be passed through drill holes in the base of the spinous process on each side.

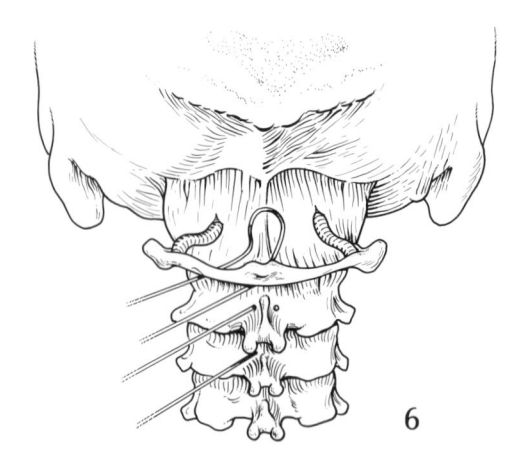

Placement of occipital wires

7

Proximal wiring of the graft to the occiput is not used routinely. Normally the grafts can be shaped to lie against the rawed surface of the occiput and would become incorporated after 2 to 3 months. When immediate stability is required, wires can be passed through occipital burr holes to anchor the graft proximally. Two burr holes are made on each side, at least 1 cm from the midline to avoid the dural sinuses. The alternative use of a single hole on each side to allow the wire to be passed into the epidural space and out over the posterior lip of the foramen magnum demands more difficult dissection and is not recommended.

Removal of bone graft

8

The bone graft can be removed from the posterior iliac crest without altering the position of the patient. Through a curved incision along the iliac crest the muscles are stripped from the lateral aspect of the ilium. Using several broad osteotomes the outer table is then removed as a large corticocancellous graft. The rectangular graft, measuring about 8 × 5 cm, can be split into two longitudinally, after preliminary holes for the wires have been made with an awl. Additional cancellous chips are removed prior to wound closure over a suction drain.

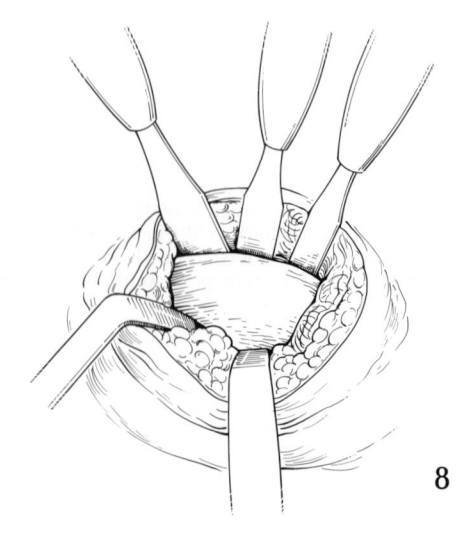

Preparation of graft bed

9

After the wires are in position the bone in the fusion bed is cleaned of all soft tissue and cancellous bone is exposed. On the occiput the bone can be rawed with a dental burr on an air drill; but for the laminae and spinous processes, rongeurs are much safer.

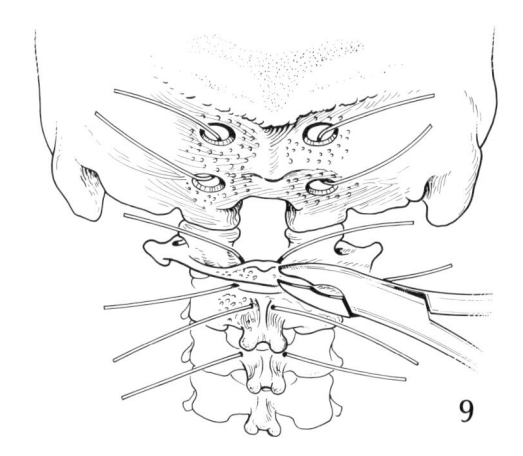

Fixation of graft

10

After the wires have been passed through the prepared holes, the two corticocancellous grafts are placed in position. The natural curve of the ilium allows these grafts to conform to the laminae and spinous processes on each side of the midline. The wires are then tightened and twisted with suitable wire tighteners. Additional cancellous bone chips are then inserted around the main graft to reinforce the fusion mass. To avoid any risk of cord compression, bone chips should not be used where wide laminectomy has been performed.

In an alternative technique described by Newman and Sweetnam[1] cancellous bone chips are applied directly to the raw bone surfaces without wiring or block grafts. This will still produce fusion, but postoperative stability is poor and requires prolonged external splintage.

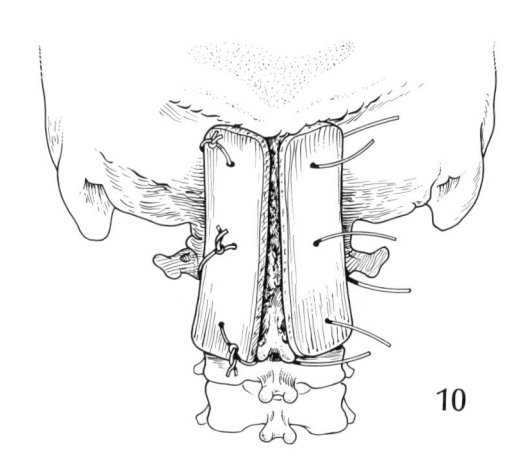

Wound closure

The wound is closed in layers using absorbable sutures to close the muscles, taking care to cover the graft completely. A single suction drain used for 24 hours will reduce wound haematoma formation, which might lead to cord compression or wound breakdown.

Postoperative management

Skull traction is normally continued for 2 weeks until the wound is healed. During this period the patient is nursed on a turning frame or in a split cardiac bed with a traction pulley placed at its head. If a radiograph shows satisfactory stability at this stage the patient can be sat up for application of a moulded cervicothoracic orthosis. When a halo splint has been used in combination with a plaster or polythene body jacket, walking may be permitted earlier. After 6 weeks the halo can be changed to a deep moulded Plastazote (Smith & Nephew, Hull, UK) cervicothoracic support with polythene reinforcements, which is worn until radiological union is complete.

ATLANTOAXIAL FUSION

Indications

A localized posterior fusion of atlas to axis is indicated for:

1. Unstable fractures through the base of the odontoid process, except in the very young or very old where conservative treatment will suffice.
2. Congenital anomalies of the odontoid such as hypoplasia, absence or separation, which may result in atlantoaxial dislocation.
3. Atlantoaxial dislocation from rupture or softening of the transverse ligament associated with chronic rheumatoid disease, or more rarely following local sepsis. Surgical stabilization is usually reserved for dislocations complicated by signs of spinal cord compression or vertebral artery ischaemia.

Special instruments

These are the same as for occipitocervical fusion.

Incision

A midline incision is used extending from the occipital protuberance to the midcervical region. The ligamentum nuchae is incised and the muscles stripped subperiosteally from the first three cervical vertebrae as in the occipitocervical fusion.

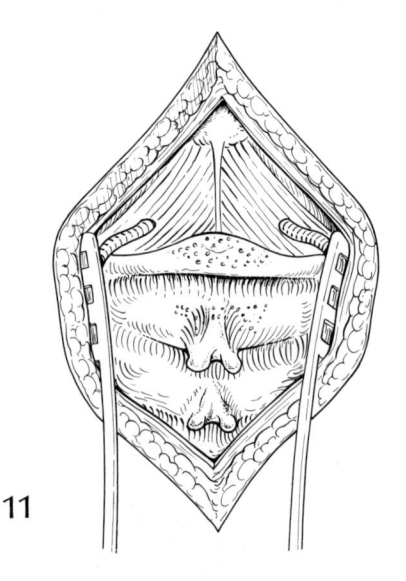

Exposure of atlas and axis

11

The posterior arch of the atlas may be very thin and needs to be exposed with care. Dissection is carried laterally from the tubercle with a small periosteal elevator for no more than 1 cm to avoid damage to the vertebral arteries. These can normally be palpated as they emerge above the arch about 1.5 cm from the midline. The spinous process and laminae of the axis are then cleared of soft tissue and nibbled down to expose raw cancellous bone.

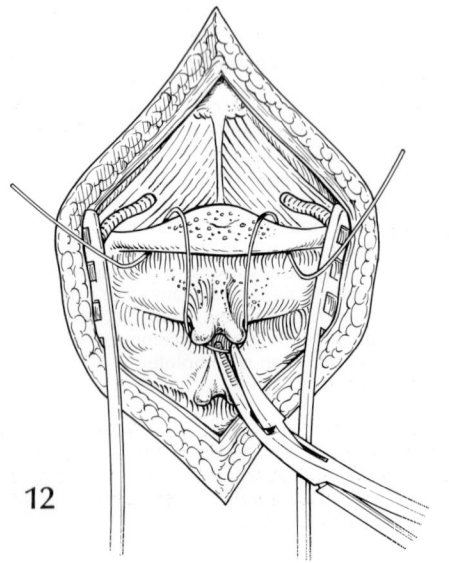

Placement of wire loop around atlas

12

The posterior atlanto-occipital membrane is carefully dissected from the superior and inferior margins of the posterior arch of the atlas in the midline. A loop of 18–20 swg stainless steel wire or 1 mm braided cable can then be inserted from below to pass anterior to the arch and posterior to the membrane. The wire can be drawn out above the arch with fine curved forceps and looped back down over the spinous process of the axis to lie around its base.

Fixation of graft

Two alternative techniques have been described for bone graft fixation in atlantoaxial arthrodesis.

13a

In the method of McGraw and Rusch[2] a corticocancellous graft measuring approximately 3 × 4 cm is removed from the posterior iliac crest using the technique described for occipitocervical fusion. It is trimmed and a notch cut on its inferior edge to allow it to sit securely on the spinous process of the axis. Two shallow notches cut in the lateral edge will allow the free ends of the wire to be tied over the graft without slipping. Extra cancellous bone chips are packed under the main graft before final tightening of the wire.

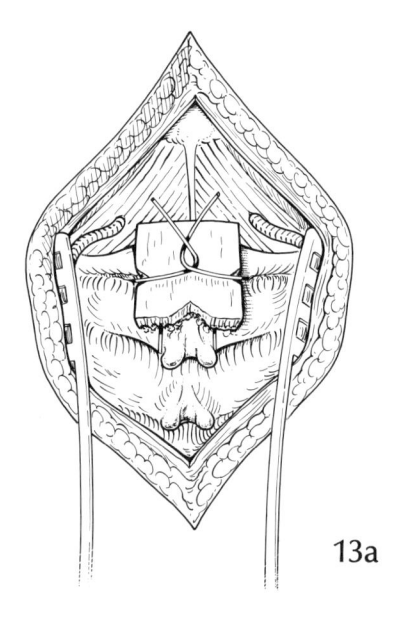

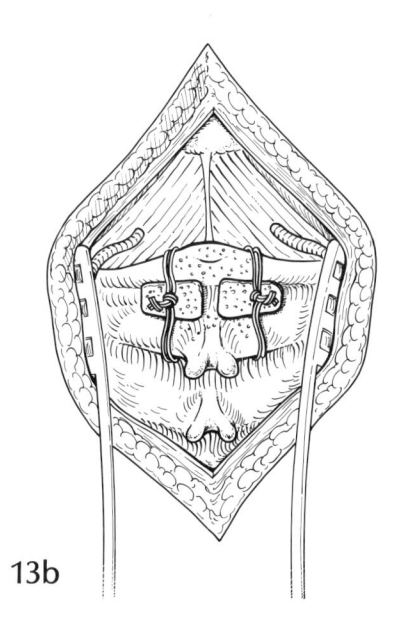

13b

For the method of Brooks and Jenkins[3] two smaller corticocancellous grafts measuring 1.25 × 3.5 cm are used, one in the interlaminal space on each side of the midline. Prior to insertion they are bevelled on their inner surfaces to allow them to be wedged under compression between the atlas and axis and secured with a doubled wire loop. This technique has been shown experimentally to give a much stronger biomechanical fixation, but is more difficult to perform. The technique of McGraw and Rusch is simpler, gives equivalent clinical results, and is safer for the less experienced surgeon.

Wound closure

Closure is performed in layers as for occipitocervical fusion.

Postoperative management

When skull traction is used preoperatively it is continued after surgery until the wound is healed. If fixation appears satisfactory on a radiograph the patient can be mobilized wearing a moulded reinforced Plastazote support or a rigid cervicothoracic brace.

INTERSPINOUS FUSION

Indications

Stabilization of the posterior vertebral complex is most efficiently achieved by interspinous fusion and is indicated for instability following:

1. Fracture and fracture-dislocations of the cervical vertebrae associated with gross disruption of the posterior ligamentous complex, or where open reduction is required for locked facets.
2. Limited decompressive laminectomy at one level.
3. Failed anterior interbody fusion.
4. Multiple-level subluxation due to rheumatoid arthritis or other inflammatory disease when associated with neurological impairment.

Incision

A midline incision is used along the tips of the spinous processes from one level above to one level below the fusion. A lateral radiograph with a wire marker could be used to check, if the vertebral level is in doubt.

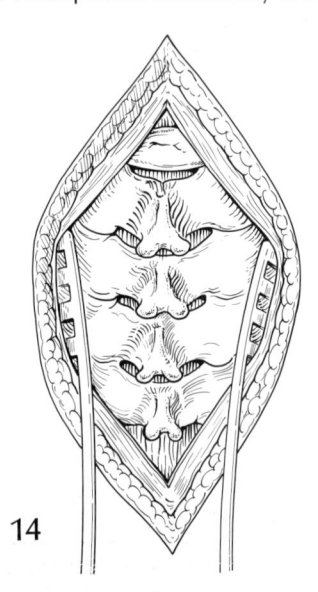

Exposure of spinous processes

14

After incision of the ligamentum nuchae in the line of the incision, the muscles are stripped subperiosteally from the spinous process and laminae on each side. Dissection is carried out laterally to the articular facet joints and self-retaining retractors inserted. The posterior elements are cleared of all soft tissue including the interspinous ligaments over the segment to be fused.

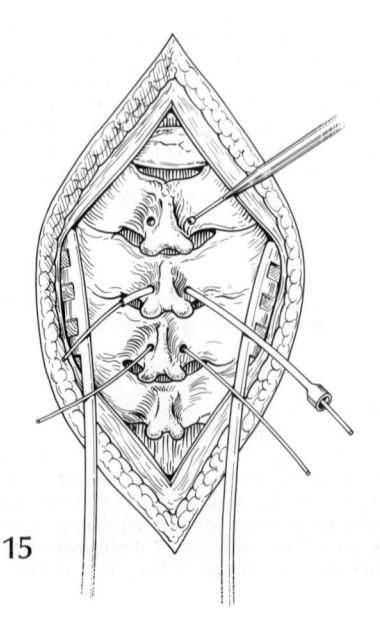

Drilling of spinous processes

15

Drill holes are made through the cortical bone at the base of the mid-portion of the spinous processes on each side. The holes are joined transversely by the use of a wire passer or sharp towel clip. The use of a hollow wire passer facilitates the introduction of the steel wires across the midline. One loop of wire is used for each two consecutive vertebrae to be included in the fusion mass. When more than three levels are to be fused an additional wire is used to encircle the whole length, passing through the spinous processes of the proximal and distal vertebrae. The wires are then tightened and twisted to secure fixation. Where the bone is very soft, as in rheumatoid arthritis, it may be necessary to pass the wires beneath the laminae to lessen the risk of them cutting out.

Decortication of fusion bed

16

It is preferable to defer decortication until the wires have been inserted and tightened. This provides more stability and resistance, as well as ensuring that the sites of cortical bony support for the wire are not prejudiced. The cortical bone of the lamina is removed conveniently with fine nibbling forceps or rongeurs down to bleeding cancellous bone. For the spinous processes this can be performed more speedily with a dental burr on an air drill, with less risk of accidental cord damage.

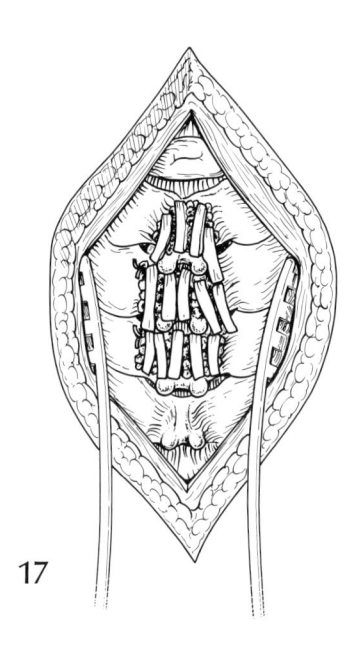

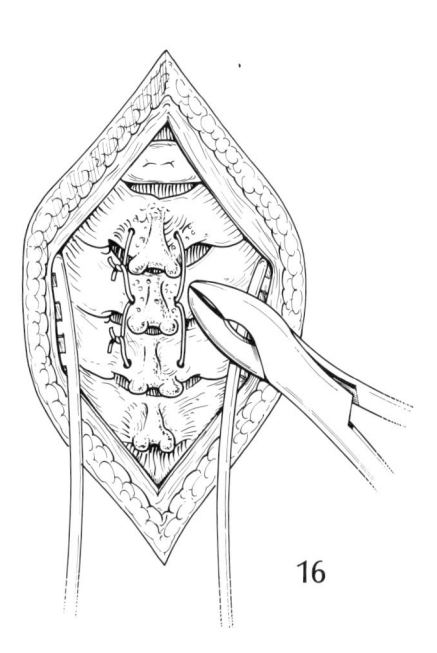

Insertion of bone graft

17

As the wires provide stability in the interspinous fusion the use of corticocancellous strips and chips is preferred to large grafts. These can be conveniently removed from the posterior iliac crest and provide the best osteogenic stimulus to fusion. They are packed on and around the prepared laminae and spinous processes.

In rheumatoid arthritis with multiple-level subluxations and osteoporotic bone, it may be necessary to provide more rigid stability to prevent further collapse and recurrence of cord compression. Posterior stability can be improved by the addition of bilateral corticocancellous grafts, a unilateral graft combined with methylmethacrylate bone cement, or a contoured metal loop.

Wound closure

The wound is closed in layers over the graft, with suction drainage to limit haematoma formation.

Postoperative management

Skull traction, when used, is continued until the wound has healed and radiographs have shown intact wires giving satisfactory stability. The patient can then be mobilized in an extended plaster, or reinforced Plastazote collar until radiological union is complete. When a halo splint is used with a body corset, earlier walking may be permitted.

480 Cervical spine

POSTEROLATERAL FACET FUSION

Indications

Posterolateral facet fusion is mechanically less efficient and technically more difficult than interspinous fusion but is indicated for:

1. Primary stabilization immediately after extensive decompressive laminectomy for cord compression at multiple levels.
2. Late instability following previous multiple-level laminectomy when this causes severe pain or neurological impairment.

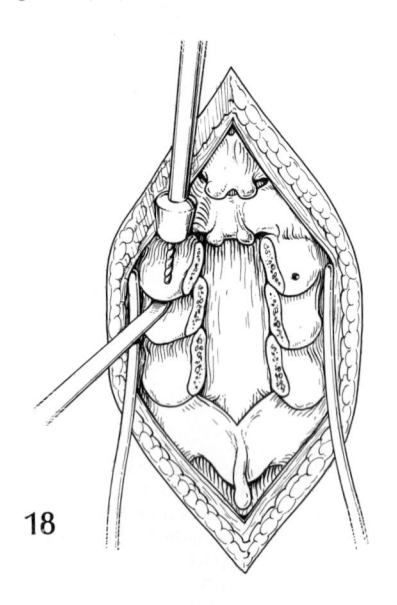

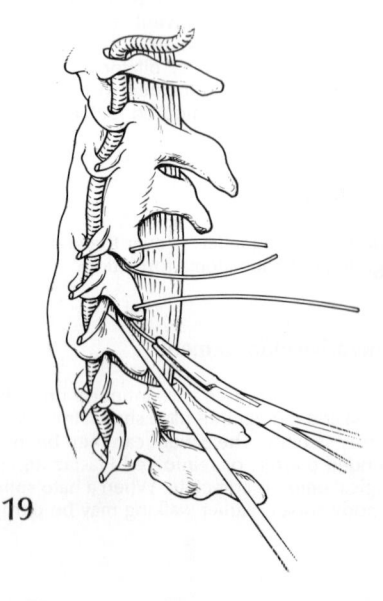

Incision

A long midline incision is used to allow generous exposure of the area, particularly for revision surgery. When previous laminectomy has been performed, great care is required in deepening the incision because of the danger of damage to a dural prolapse or the underlying cord. If possible the dissection should begin both proximally and distally from any intact spinous processes until the margins of the laminectomy defect can be defined. The central soft tissues are left undisturbed and subperiosteal clearance of the lateral remnants of the laminae and facet joints can be performed without risk.

Preparation of facet joints

18

The articular facet joints are exposed from one level above to one level below the laminectomy defect. The capsule is excised to permit distraction of each joint by insertion of a narrow osteotome or dissector. The articular cartilage can then be curetted from the surface of the facets. An 2.8 mm (7/64 inch) drill hole is made through the centre of each inferior facet at right angles to the plane of the joint.

Insertion of wires

19

An 18–20 swg wire loop is then passed through the hole in each inferior facet to provide anchorage for the graft. To facilitate this the joint is again distracted by 2–3 mm to allow the insertion of the jaws of fine artery forceps to seize the end of the wire as it is passed through the hole.

Insertion of bone grafts

20

A large corticocancellous graft is obtained from the posterior iliac crest using the technique described for occipitocervical fusion. This is split longitudinally and trimmed to appropriate length for the number of joints to be fused. Before insertion of the grafts the remnants of the laminae and the facets are decorticated as much as possible without prejudicing the wire fixation. The two grafts are placed in position laterally and the loop of wire in each facet tightened and twisted over them and then cut short.

Wound closure

Wound closure is routine, being performed in layers with suction drainage for 24 hours.

Postoperative management

Because of the poor mechanical stability, more rigid postoperative splintage is required than with interspinous fusion. When skull traction is used preoperatively it can be continued for up to 4 weeks and the patient then mobilized with a rigid cervicothoracic plaster cast or brace. This immobilization is continued until radiological union occurs, which may take 3 to 4 months.

References

1. Newman P, Sweetnam R. Occipito-cervical fusion: an operative technique and its indications. *J Bone Joint Surg [Br]* 1969; 51-B: 423–31.

2. McGraw RW, Rusch RM. Atlanto-axial arthrodesis. *J Bone Joint Surg [Br]* 1973; 55-B: 482–9.

3. Brooks AL, Jenkins EB. Atlanto-axial arthrodesis by the wedge compression method. *J Bone Joint Surg [Am]* 1978; 60-A: 279–84.

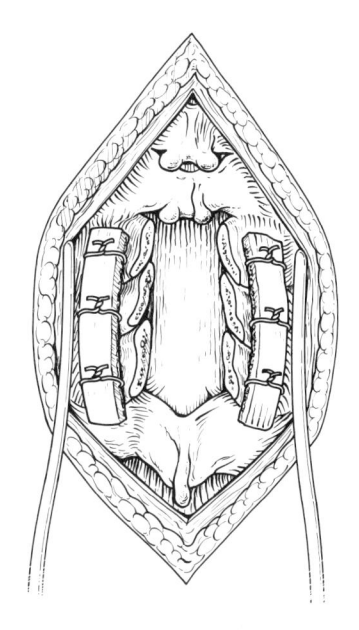

Illustrations by Peter Cox

Halofemoral traction

J. C. Dorgan MChOrth, FRCS
Consultant Orthopaedic Surgeon, Royal Liverpool Children's Hospital and Royal Liverpool Hospital, Liverpool, UK

Introduction

Halofemoral traction is a means whereby preoperative correction of a spinal deformity may be obtained. The use of halo skull traction was first described by Perry and Nickel in 1959[1]. The use of the halo device coupled with femoral traction was first described by Moe in 1963 and the first results of its use published in 1967 by Kane and Moe[2]. Its routine use in idiopathic scoliosis[3] has been discontinued but in severe scoliosis it still provides a relatively safe, effective and comfortable method of achieving preoperative correction of the deformity. It is particularly useful in staged procedures to correct a rigid scoliosis where it can be used following the initial soft-tissue release or osteotomy to obtain a gradual correction before the spine is fused[4]. It may also be used to determine the operability of poor-risk cases with cardiopulmonary failure.

Procedure

Application of the halo

The selection of an appropriate halo may be carried out on the ward preoperatively. It is also useful to decide which holes in the halo give the best pin placement and that the correct pins are available.

In children a general anaesthetic with endotracheal intubation is used but in adults the procedure may be carried out using local anaesthesia. The patient is positioned supine on the operating table with the head and neck suspended over the end of the table. The easiest way to achieve this is to have an assistant seated at the head of the table supporting the patient's head.

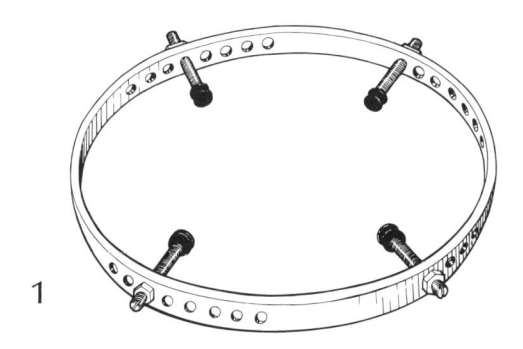

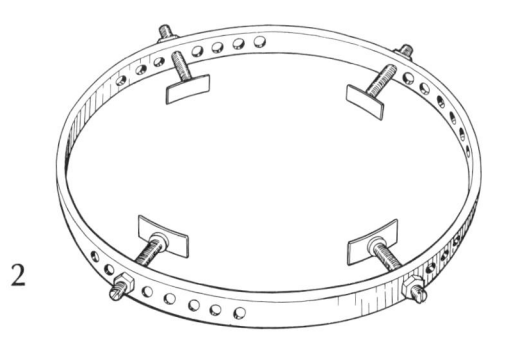

1 & 2

The halo is then positioned. The tips of the pins may be protected with the rubber pistons from 2 ml or 5 ml syringes. This allows the halo position to be adjusted and held without penetration of the scalp by the pins and it also keeps the tips of the pins sterile until they are ready to be inserted. Alternatively, the commercially available halo, using extra pins fitted with flat plates, may be used to position the halo prior to pin insertion.

3–5

The halo should be positioned so that there is a clearance all the way round of approximately 1.5 cm between the ring and the scalp. The lower rim of the halo should be placed about 2 cm above the superior orbital margin and 1 cm above the pinna of the ear. The pins are positioned so that they lie perpendicular to the skull and will engage the frontal and parietal eminences. The anterior pins are positioned so that they will lie in the hairline if at all feasible. One should try to avoid the temporalis muscle, however, as pin insertion through the muscle is a cause of pain and possible pin loosening during traction. Diagonally opposite pins are then tightened using a torque screwdriver until all four pins are securely fastened. Torques should not exceed 0.04 Pa (6 lb/in^2) in adults and 0.03 Pa (5 lb/in^2) in children. If there is a sudden decrease in resistance the pin has penetrated the outer table of the skull. If this happens the pin should be removed and inserted through an adjacent hole in the halo. Once the pins are securely fastened the halo can be locked into position by tightening the nuts with a spanner.

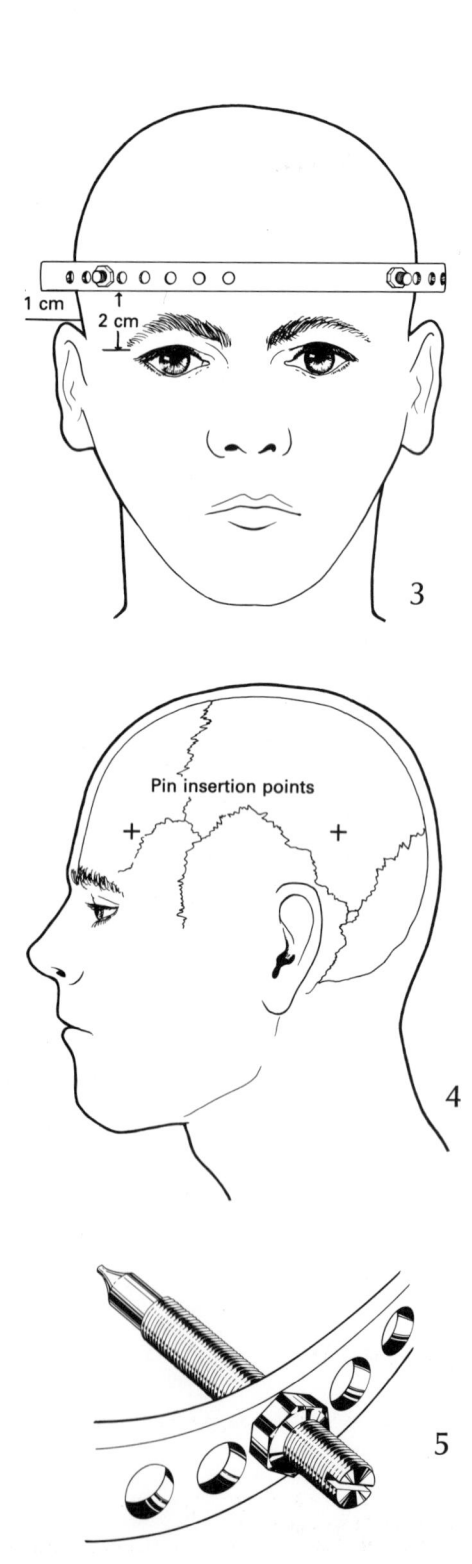

Insertion of the femoral pins

6

The patient is repositioned on the operating table and the area around both knees prepared and draped. On each side a small stab wound is made and a Denham pin inserted from medial to lateral just above the flare of the condyles. The advantage of the Denham pin over a Steinmann pin is that the self-tapping thread on the Denham pins engages the cortex and stops pin migration. This reduces the risk of pin-tract infection.

Postoperative management

7

The pins are checked for any signs of loosening and are re-tightened using the torque screwdriver at 48 hours. The head end of the bed is elevated slightly and the halo is fixed to the bed with wire loops. Weights are applied to the femoral pins via stirrups.

Traction is commenced after 48 hours with 3 kg on each leg initially. The weights are increased daily by 1 kg on each leg until a maximum of one-third of body weight is obtained. A careful examination of the cranial nerves and neurological assessment of the arms and legs must be carried out each day.

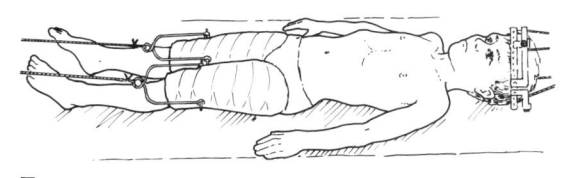

Complications

The following complications of halofemoral traction may occur.

Halo
1. Infection of pin sites leading to osteomyelitis of skull
2. Loosening and slippage of the halo
3. Penetration of the skull with extradural abscess formation

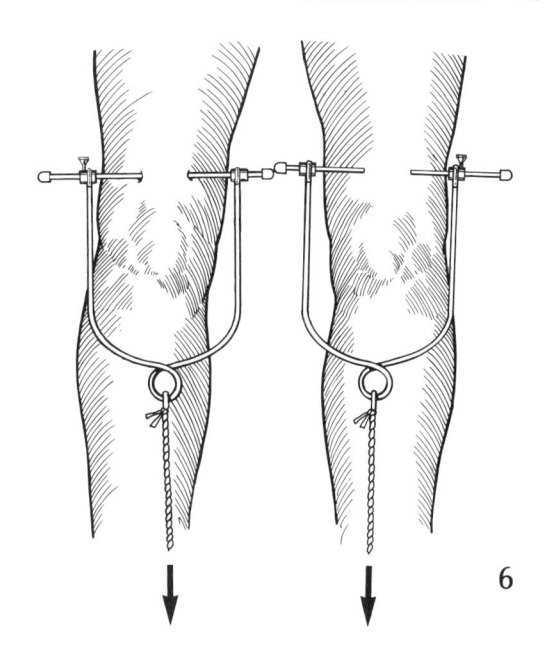

Femoral pins
1. Pin-tract infection
2. Loosening

Neurological
1. Cranial nerve lesions: VIth nerve palsy is the commonest
2. Brachial plexus lesion, especially T1 root
3. Paraplegia or tetraplegia.

Pressure sores

Deep vein thrombosis

Vascular compression of the duodenum – the 'cast syndrome'.

References

1. Perry J, Nickel VL. Total cervical spine fusion for neck paralysis. *J Bone Joint Surg [Am]* 1959; 41-A: 37–60.

2. Kane WJ, Moe JH, Lai CC. Halo-femoral pin distraction in the treatment of scoliosis. *J Bone Joint Surg [Am]* 1967; 49-A: 1018.

3. Moe JH. Complications of scoliosis treatment. *Clin Orthop* 1967; 53: 21–30.

4. Perry J. The halo in spinal abnormalities: practical factors and avoidance of complications. *Orthop Clin North Am* 1972; 3: 69–80.

Illustrations by Peter Cox

The halo–body cast

Sean P. F. Hughes MS, FRCS
Professor of Orthopaedic Surgery, University of Edinburgh; Clinical Research Unit, Princess Margaret Rose Orthopaedic Hospital, Edinburgh, UK

Introduction

Perry and Nickel introduced the halo system in 1959 for the treatment of patients with poliomyelitis[1]. However, it was James[2] who was the first to report on the use of the halo–body fixation for the treatment of fractures when he described its application in patients with fractures of the odontoid process.

Since then there has been an increasing interest in the applications and design of such a system. The original apparatus was indeed fairly cumbersome, and consisted essentially of a halo linked to a plaster jacket by means of a four-poster frame. This system could be difficult to apply, so other devices were introduced using three or four posts to link the halo to the body plaster. However, because of the method of attaching the vertical rods to the halo and to plates incorporated into the plaster these systems were used in only a few centres where expertise was available.

In 1979 Cooper et al.[3] reported their results using the halo–vest for the treatment of patients with cervical spinal injuries. The halo–vest does not rest upon the iliac crest as was originally described by Perry and Nickel. In this chapter the Princess Margaret Rose Orthopaedic Hospital halo–body fixation system is described. Its value lies in its relative simplicity of application and the fact that the plaster rests upon the iliac crest, ensuring a stable system which is important for unstable injuries of the cervical spine[4].

Indications

1a & b

The main purpose of halo–body fixation is to stabilize the cervical spine and to allow the patient to be upright and mobile. This may be required:

1. In instability from fractures or ligamentous damage
2. In rheumatoid arthritis
3. Where there is bone destruction from metastatic disease or following infection or surgery.

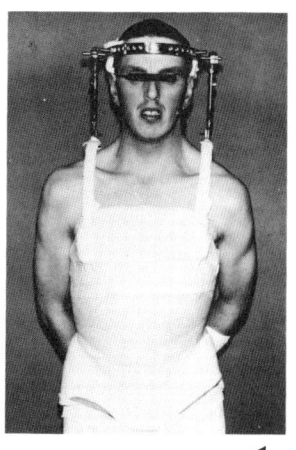

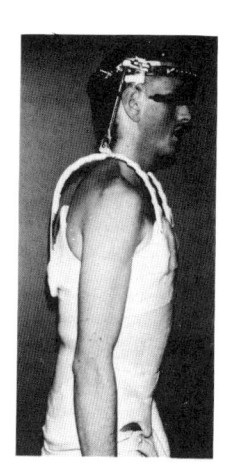

1a   1b

Fractures

Most fractures of the cervical spine are the result of road traffic accidents. The levels involved are usually the upper or lower cervical spine.

1. Fracture-dislocation of C1 on C2.
2. Fracture-dislocation of C2 on C3.
3. Fracture-dislocation of C6 on C7.

In patients with ligament disruption the neck can be stabilized in a halo–body fixation system as a prelude to surgery.

Rheumatoid arthritis

In patients who have atlanto-axial subluxation to such a degree as to cause cord compression, halo–body fixation can be applied to control the spine prior to surgery.

Bone destruction

Metastatic disease Extensive bone destruction may occur with carcinoma of the breast in an otherwise reasonably healthy patient.

Infection Destruction of vertebral bodies may follow infection associated with previous injury.

Surgery Rarely, the neck is totally unstable following anterior and posterior decompression prior to surgery.

Stability of the cervical spine is achieved by linking the skull to the fitted plaster jacket which rests on the iliac crests. Through such a system it is possible to undertake both anterior and posterior surgery of the cervical spine.

Design of the halo–body system

The system was designed by Mr T. Cairns, Past Head of the Orthotics Unit at Princess Margaret Rose Orthopaedic Hospital.

2, 3 & 4

The halo consists of a standard single-size stainless steel ring which has two 50 mm long stainless steel horns attached centrally on each side. The ring is perforated to allow four threaded screws to be fixed to the skull. Malleable plates are incorporated into a plaster jacket and are linked to the halo ring by means of shoulder pieces and hollow vertical struts containing a threaded rod. The plaster jacket itself can be made of any material, from plaster of Paris to the newer synthetic materials. The rods allow for adjustments in the height of the shoulder rests and the halo, whilst also allowing for the movements of flexion and extension, as well as rotation at the metal joints. A certain degree of rotation is also permitted at the swivel joints which link the vertical struts with the shoulder rests. These planes of movement are needed when applying the device.

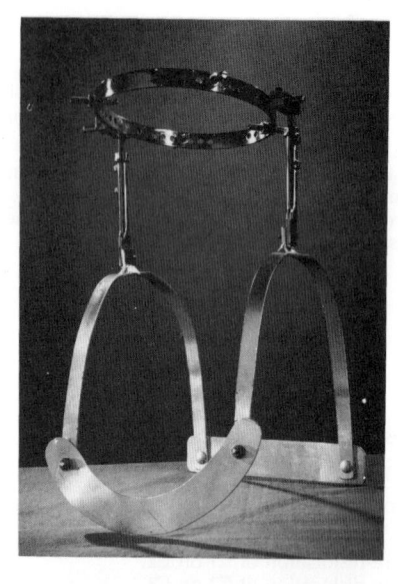

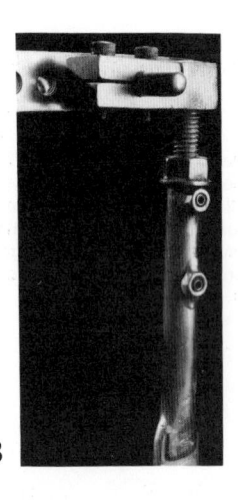

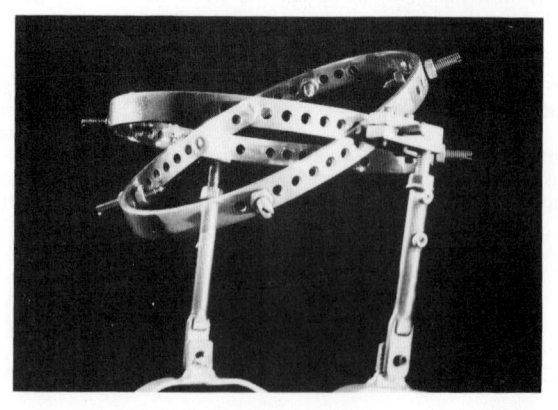

Procedure

5

The patient is initially placed in a well-fitting plaster jacket using the Oxford Cotrel table, which enables the patient to be suspended horizontally by the shoulders and buttocks, leaving the trunk completely free for the cast to be applied. The jacket extends from the thorax to well below the iliac crests and is attenuated over these crests, as with a Milwaukee brace. This is so that the jacket does not rise up when the system is linked together, which could occur when the patient is sitting.

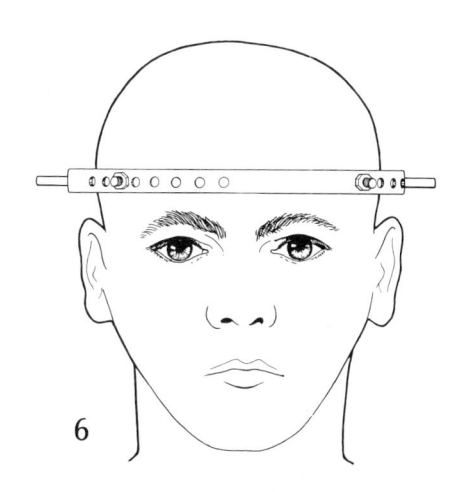

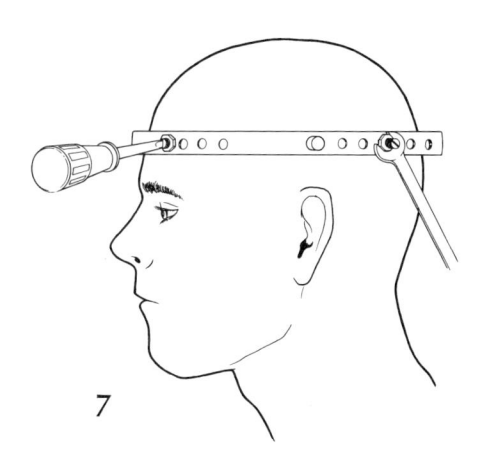

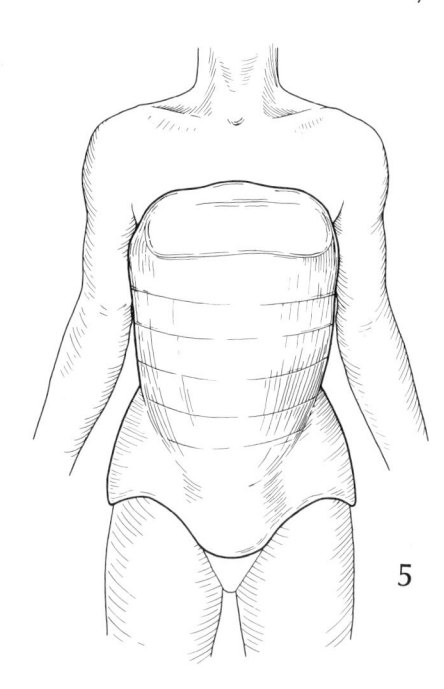

6, 7 & 8

When the plaster cast has set the halo is then applied to the skull. Unless the fracture needs manipulation because of locked facets it is unnecessary to give a general anaesthetic. Local anaesthesia is applied by infiltration with 1–2 per cent lignocaine with adrenaline. The ring is aligned against the skull using four pads. The setting should be above the ears. The four threaded pins are then inserted into the vertex of the skull and tightened with a torque screwdriver set at $41 \, kN/m^2$. The nut washers are secured into place, the vertical struts are attached to the ring and to the shoulder pieces, and the malleable plates incorporated into the jacket.

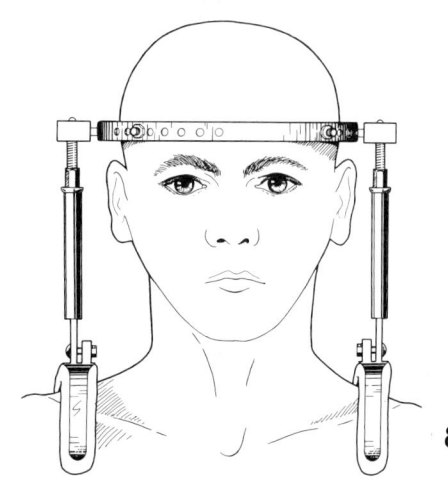

Post-application management

It is important that the patient is fully informed about this procedure, both before, during and after application of the device. Once the patient has the halo–body device applied, his field of vision is restricted as he cannot turn his head; therefore his attention must be sought from the front. Because the neck is held rigidly, the patient can be safely and indeed confidently mobilized usually within 24 hours of application.

If no further treatment is contemplated, the patient can be allowed home, wearing the fixation system, provided he is reviewed regularly and there is adequate support from the family and the general practitioner.

If operative treatment is considered, the frame need not be removed: it is possible to approach the cervical spine anteriorly from C3–T1 and posteriorly from the occiput to T1, provided the frame is draped carefully.

9

After the halo has been removed the patient can be fitted into a four-poster collar.

Our experience with this system has produced few complications, although the shape of the patient is important. Obese short patients are not ideal for this system as it is difficult to apply the plaster cast accurately, and moulding over the iliac crest may not be ideal. The result is that the system can move when the patient sits, and this leads to loosening and to pin-tract infection. However, most patients fit the dimensions required.

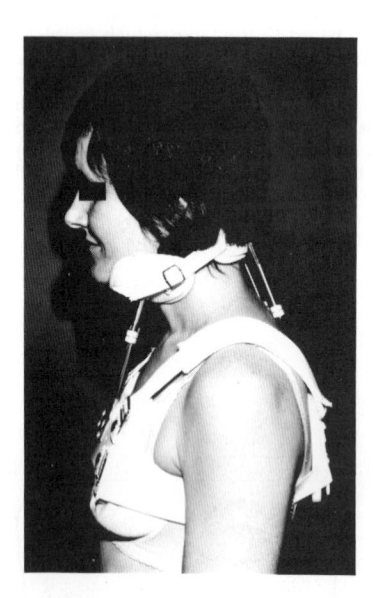

Conclusion

The Princess Margaret Rose Orthopaedic Hospital halo–body fixation goes a long way to fulfilling the criteria laid down by Nickel, Perry and Garrett[5] as essential for a successful halo system.

1. Precise control of the position of the cervical spine in three planes.
2. Progressive and adjustable longitudinal traction.
3. Rigid stabilization.
4. Simple application.
5. Freedom from complications during the prolonged period which is necessary for spinal fusion.
6. Minimum discomfort.

References

1. Perry J, Nickel VL. Total cervical spine fusion for neck paralysis. *J Bone Joint Surg [Am]* 1959; 41-A: 37–60.

2. James JIP. Fracture dislocation of cervical spine. *J R Coll Surg Edinb* 1960; 5:232–3.

3. Cooper PR, Maravilla KR, Sklar FH, Moody SF, Clark WK. Halo immobilization of cervical spine fractures: indications and results. *J Neurosurg* 1979; 50: 603–10.

4. Hughes SPF, Cairns T, Iyer V, Liston J, Thomson JD. Halo-body device. *Paraplegia* 1984; 22: 260–6.

5. Nickel VL, Perry J, Garrett A, Heppenstall M. The halo: a spinal skeletal traction fixation device. *J Bone Joint Surg [Am]* 1968; 50-A: 1400–9.

Illustrations by Peter Cox

Posterior procedures for idiopathic scoliosis

Michael Edgar MChir, FRCS
Consultant Orthopaedic Surgeon, The Middlesex Hospital, London, and The Royal National Orthopaedic Hospital, Stanmore, UK

Introduction

Development of Harrington instrumentation

The procedure described below in detail is the Harrington–Luque instrumentation combined with a standard posterior spinal fusion. This represents a stage in the development in the use of Harrington instrumentation.

The system was first used by Paul Harrington in 1958, and its early development subsequently reviewed by him[1]. In order to strengthen the fixation, a transverse bar system was added at the apex of the curve to provide a three-point fixation for the rod[2,3]. Harrington also supplemented the distraction rod on the concave side by using a compression system on the convex side. Because most idiopathic scolioses are lordotic, a multiple-level distraction system was developed[4]: this uses a large diameter, threaded Wisconsin rod and Keene hooks on the convex side, combined with a standard Harrington distraction rod on the concave side.

The simplicity of the Luque segmental instrumentation with sublaminar wires[5] became very popular in the early 1980s, tending to replace alternative more complex instrumentation systems. Combining the Luque sublaminar wires with the Harrington rod provided a straightforward technique for excellent stability of the fusion area; this combination has been widely adopted with various modifications[6,7]. There is slight concern about the passage of sublaminar wires, and it is wise to monitor the spinal cord while performing the Harrington–Luque technique. Currently, trials of the new Cotrel–Dubousset or CD instrumentation[8] are taking place in the United Kingdom, and it has become popular elsewhere, but it is expensive and has not yet been shown to be superior to previous systems. Therefore, it is not in general use.

Finally, as a further modification of the Luque system there has been the development of the Hartshill rectangle, where two rods are joined at their ends to form a rectangle which can be contoured to the corrected scoliosis with sublaminar wire fixation[9].

Indications for posterior fusion

The indications for corrective posterior spinal fusion and instrumentation in idiopathic scoliosis are as follows.

1. *Adolescent patients* who have a major thoracic curve with a Cobb angle over 50°, particularly if:
(a) the curve is deteriorating with skeletal growth remaining and
(b) if the deformity is not being controlled by a brace or
(c) where the deformity is not cosmetically acceptable, either because of imbalance or because of marked vertebral rotation and associated rib hump.

2. *Mature patients with curves over 55°*, including double structural deformities and lumbar curves. Even if maturity has been reached, these deformities should be stabilized surgically because there is now good evidence that scoliosis of this magnitude can deteriorate quite considerably during adult life[10].

Indications for anterior and posterior fusion

As a precursor to a second-stage posterior spinal fusion, it may be necessary to perform an anterior disc excision and spinal fusion (see next section). This is indicated as a preliminary multiple interbody operation in the following situations.

1. *Patients who are skeletally immature* at the start of their adolescent growth spurt, that is with the iliac apophyses absent or only just appearing (Risser Grade 0 or 1). This is particularly important if lordosis or marked rotation is present. In these cases, if posterior spinal fusion and instrumentation alone is carried out there will be continued growth anteriorly, which will result in lordosis and, more important, an increasing rotation of the previously operated vertebrae with secondary deterioration of the rib hump[11]. Clearly, in early curves of less than 50° conservative measures, such as serial corrective plaster casts and bracing, should be tried. Once a curve has deteriorated beyond 50°–55° in the immature child, two-stage anterior and posterior fusion must be undertaken.

2. *Rigid or severe curves over 80°*. These can be better managed by an initial anterior fusion especially in the thoracic spine providing respiratory function allows excision of the discs and the anterior longitudinal ligament. This allows better correction and a more solid fusion mass when the second stage of posterior spinal fusion and instrumentation is undertaken. Between the two stages in these cases, particularly if the curve is very marked (over 100°), halo-femoral or halo-tibial traction facilitates the posterior instrumentation.

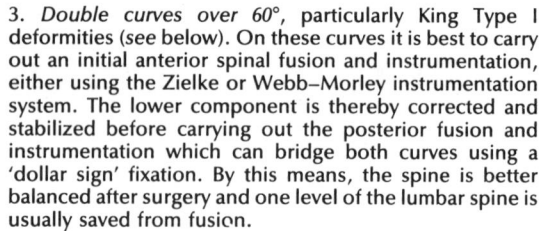

3. *Double curves over 60°*, particularly King Type I deformities (see below). On these curves it is best to carry out an initial anterior spinal fusion and instrumentation, either using the Zielke or Webb–Morley instrumentation system. The lower component is thereby corrected and stabilized before carrying out the posterior fusion and instrumentation which can bridge both curves using a 'dollar sign' fixation. By this means, the spine is better balanced after surgery and one level of the lumbar spine is usually saved from fusion.

4. *Kyphosis associated with the 'idiopathic' curve*, either due to an apparent kyphosis in infantile scoliosis or an associated Scheuermann's true kyphosis. Occasionally it is best to carry out an anterior release and fusion over the kyphotic zone anteriorly, before the second-stage posterior fusion and instrumentation.

Preoperative

Investigations

Before planning surgery, a thorough clinical evaluation, including cardiorespiratory assessment and haematological tests to investigate basic renal and metabolic function, is required. Respiratory function tests with instruction in the use of a triggered positive ventilation system, which will be used postoperatively, is carried out by the physiotherapist. Electrocardiography is performed if there is any concern about the cardiac status, with referral to a cardiologist as required.

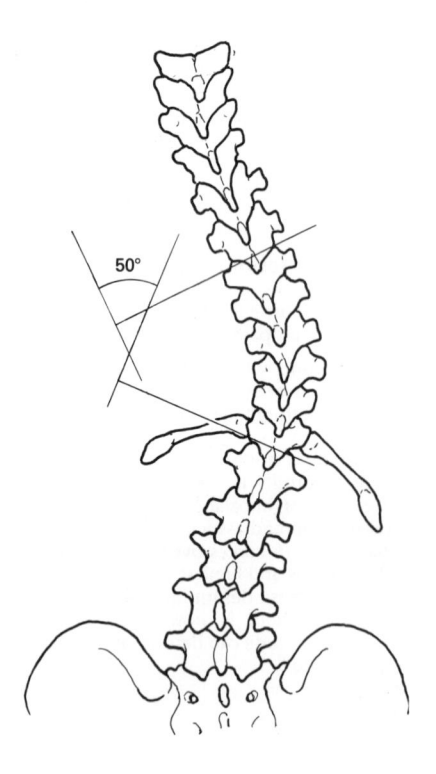

1

The mobility and balance of the spinal deformity must be assessed with a plumbline and the rib hump measured using either a 'gibbometer' or else an inclinometer. Erect anteroposterior and lateral radiographs are taken and the Cobb angle measured. A small metal strip is placed over a transverse skin mark at the level of one of the upper lumbar spinous processes and a supine anteroposterior view of the spine is then taken; this marker film is then used at operation to judge the levels of fusion.

Planning the fusion levels

The instrumented portion of the spine should be as short as possible but long enough to provide a corrected and balanced spine so that ideally the end vertebrae holding the hooks are square and in the midline. It is best if they are in neutral rotation, but this is secondary to balance. As a general rule, the Harrington rod extends two levels above and below the limits of the Cobb angle in the average single thoracic curve (King Type III, *Illustration 2c*). The correctibility of the curve is judged either by supine passive side-bending anteroposterior radiographs of the spine or by a supine anteroposterior film taken with the patient being stretched with traction.

2a & b

Selection of the fusion levels depends on the curve type. Curve types I–V according to the classification of King et al.[12] are illustrated. In Type I curves a 'dollar sign' Harrington rod can be used, but instrumentation is likely to extend down to L4 and with distraction there is the risk of unbalancing the spine to the side of the lower major deformity. Therefore, these are the ideal curves for two-stage surgery with anterior instrumentation being undertaken in the first stage (as described above). Type II curves are double structural deformities, where the thoracic curve predominates and a 'dollar sign' rod is ideal for these, with or without a preceding anterior procedure for the lower curve. Good balance is usually achieved, although the lower hook will usually need to be at L4 in a single-stage procedure.

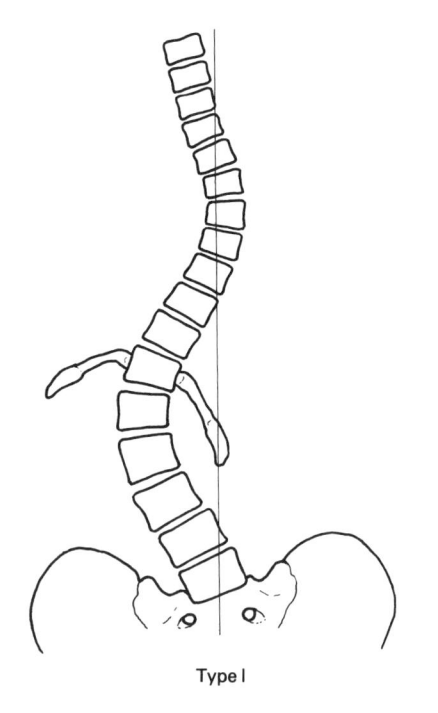

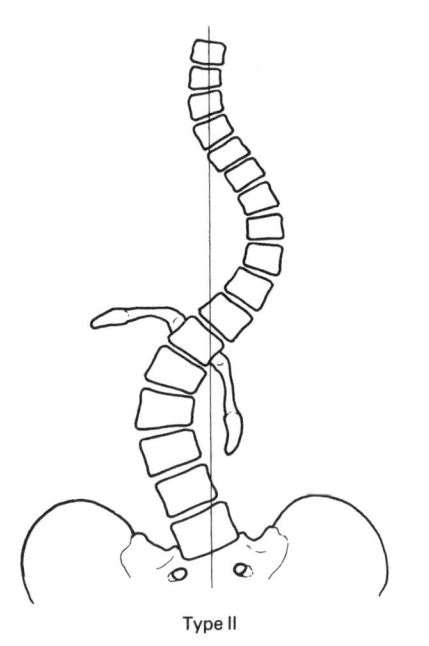

494 Thoracic and lumbar spine

2c

The Type III curve is a classic single right thoracic deformity discussed above.

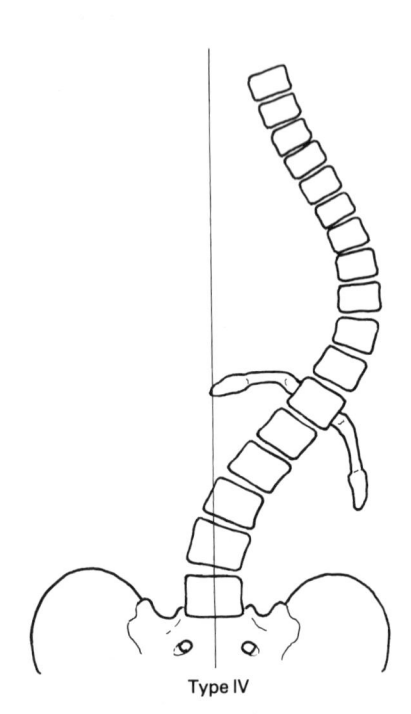

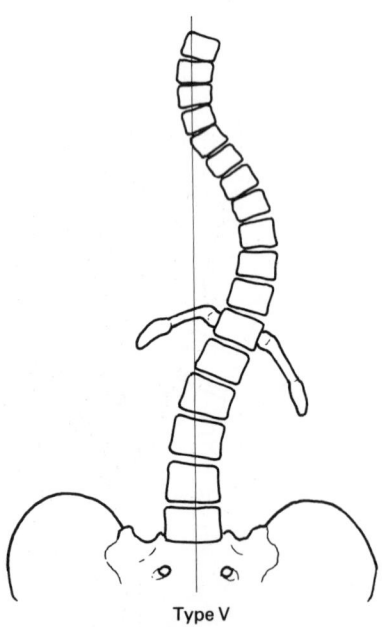

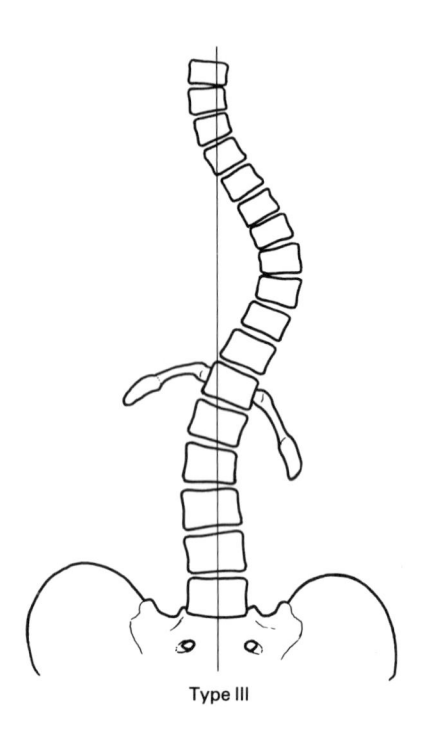

2d Type IV

Type III 2c

2d & e

Type IV scoliosis presents a trap for the unwary in that the long lower compensatory curve is associated with imbalance of the spine. Therefore instrumentation must be sufficiently far distal to restore this balance. In Type V deformities, there is a minor structural curve in the left upper thoracic region above the major right lower thoracic curve. Unless instrumentation is continued in a 'dollar sign' fashion well up into this curve, any distraction is likely to exaggerate the effect of this upper structural component, unbalancing it and resulting in the left shoulder being higher than the right.

2e Type V

Operation

Position of patient

3

After general anaesthesia with endotracheal intubation and essential monitoring devices involving electrocardiograms, intra-arterial cannula and rectal thermometer recordings, the patient is placed in the prone position on one of the available spinal supports. The Montreal mattress, Toronto frame, double Renton rest or Gardner frame (Downs Ltd, Mitcham, UK) are suitable. The overriding principle is the same, namely that the abdomen should be free from pressure and the chest supported carefully without any concentration of pressure anteriorly that might cause dangerous narrowing of the anteroposterior diameter of the chest in those cases with marked lordosis. Positioning of the arms is important and they need to be anterior, that is below the line of the trunk, and it is probably wise not to elevate the shoulders more than 90° for fear of traction on the brachial plexus.

Incision and splitting of spinous process tips

4 & 5

Using the indelible skin mark (see marker film in preoperative investigations above) as a reference point, the spinous processes are palpated to identify the levels of the planned length of fusion. It is wise to extend the incision to include two further spinous processes proximally and to include one further spine distally. At the proximal end, the epidural electrode of the spinal cord monitor will need to be passed through the interspace above the fusion.

It is important that the longitudinal incision is straight and placed in the midline. After dividing the skin, cutting diathermy is recommended as it gives the best haemostasis. Once the subcutaneous fat has been traversed in the line of the incision, the deep fascia and tips of the transverse processes are exposed. The cartilaginous epiphyseal caps on the tips of these are then split longitudinally with scalpel or cutting diathermy, and the intervening spinous and interspinous ligaments similarly divided. Each half of the epiphyseal cap is then pulled off to the underlying spinous process using a Cobb spinal elevator. This exposes the actual bony spine and with further stripping, using the Cobb instrument, the periosteum can be elevated quite easily to the base of the spinous process. Once again, the levels are checked at this stage.

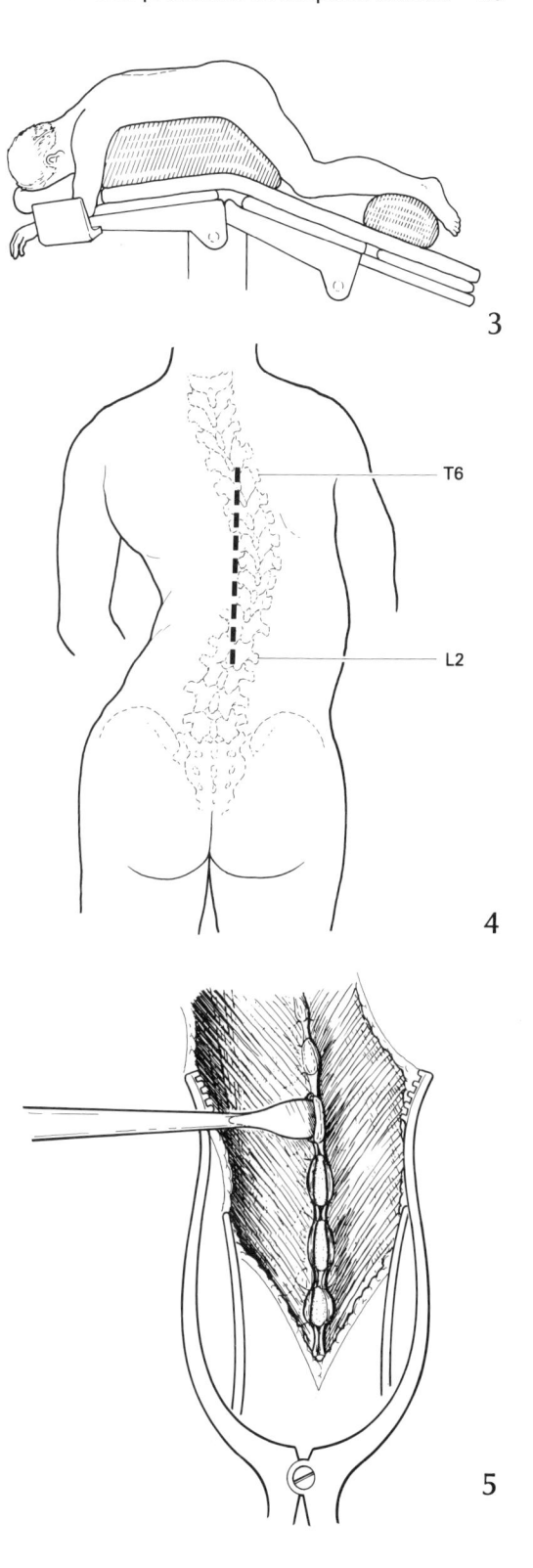

Exposure of the laminae and transverse processes

6a & b

Starting at the proximal end of the incision, the spinal elevator is used to extend the periosteal stripping down to the laminae and then the transverse process. This can be achieved in one gentle sweep. This is repeated at the adjacent level on the same side. The intervening muscle attachment to the trailing edge of the lamina and facet joint is then carefully dissected off before this space deep to the muscle is packed firmly with a gauze swab. It is easier to start on the concave side, and this process is repeated on the convex side until the entire posterior thoracic elements are exposed.

In the lumbar region, the facet joint capsule projects further posteriorly and this forms a ridge between the lamina and transverse process so that it is not possible to expose the whole posterior surface in one sweep. Once exposed, the facet joint capsule is incised and the cartilage cap on the tips of these facets is removed; after some soft tissue dissection the periosteum can be elevated laterally from the outer side of the facet to the transverse process. The wound is again packed. Haemostasis along the spine is then achieved and any soft tissue remnants, particularly those obscuring the facet joints, are removed.

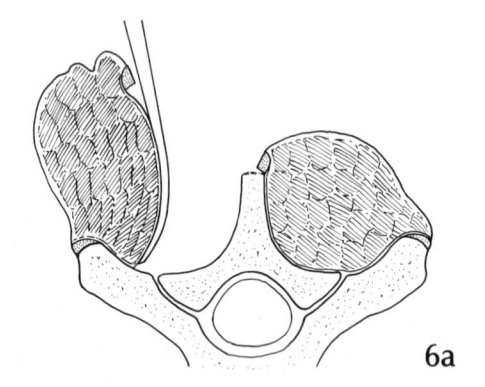

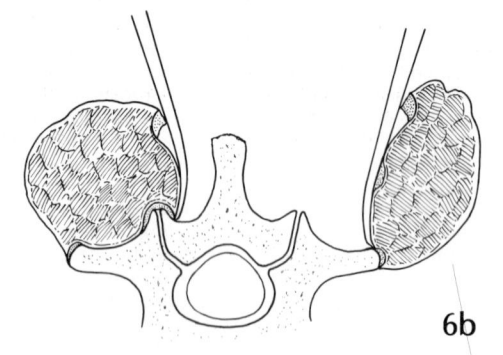

Insertion of the upper Harrington distraction hook

7a,b & 8a,b

The most proximal facet joint on the concave side, which receives the top hook, is cleared of any remaining soft tissue and its curved trailing edge straightened transversely using a small osteotome. After gentle proximal traction on the spinous process using a Kocher's forceps to expose further the plane of the joint and its medial border with the ligamentum flavum, a No. 1251 Harrington hook with a sharp forward edge is inserted into the joint so that its medial edge overlaps the ligamentum flavum. It is important not to disturb the deep lateral capsule of the facet joint which acts as an anchor preventing the hook rotating out laterally. The hook insertion is carried out using a standard hook clamp and large curved hook driver with the hook angled downwards at about 60° as it enters the joint. Otherwise, the hook will split the lamina and its hold will be weak. After entering the joint, the hook is gradually brought into its correct neutral position and gently tapped into place so that it is embedded into the pedicle. This hook is removed and is replaced by a No. 1253 blunt hook (see *Illustration 8a*), which remains. The curve of the hook must fit snugly round the lamina. If it is too large there is risk of cord pressure. In juvenile patients or when the lamina is narrow, a narrow hook (No. 77-6454) or a paediatric hook (No. 8500 418) should be used.

If spinal cord monitoring is being used with somatosensory evoked potentials from popliteal electrodes then the epidural recording electrode is best inserted at this stage through a fenestration one level proximal to the hook insertion.

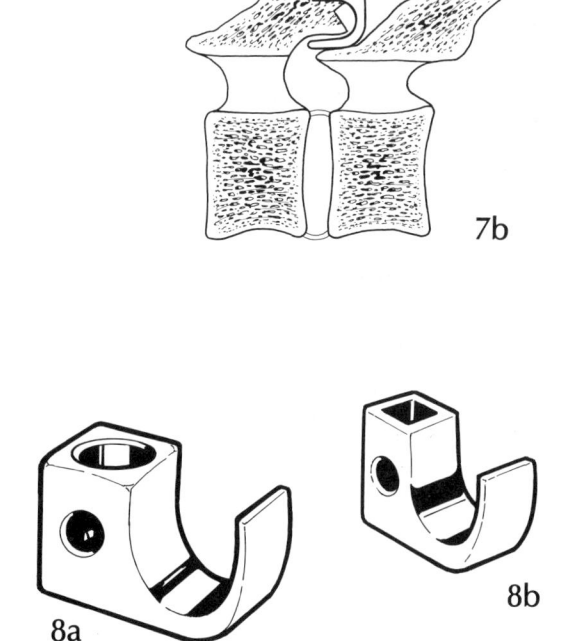

498 Thoracic and lumbar spine

Insertion of lower Harrington distraction hook and attachment of outrigger

9

The distal vertebra in the fusion is located and a fenestration of the ligamentum flavum just above this is performed in a routine manner on the concave side. In single curves this will be on the same side as the top hook but in double curves on the opposite side, i.e. 'dollar' sign. Using the laminectomy punch forceps, the ligamentum flavum and the rostral edge of the distal vertebra are trimmed and squared to receive the distal hook (see *Illustration 11a*). A blunt square-holed Harrington hook (No. 1201-50, see *Illustration 8b*) is carefully inserted around the lamina, taking care that it is not impinging the underlying dura. It may be necessary to trim the lamina in thickness to provide this hook with a snug fit. Outrigger extension pieces are then fitted to top and bottom hooks and the outrigger is then attached (Üllrich standard gauged outrigger is the best.) The deformity is corrected by distraction with a force, in the first instance, up to 20 kg. This facilitates subsequent excision of the facet joint. The spinal cord monitoring response is watched carefully at this stage. (The epidural electrode is shown in the illustration.)

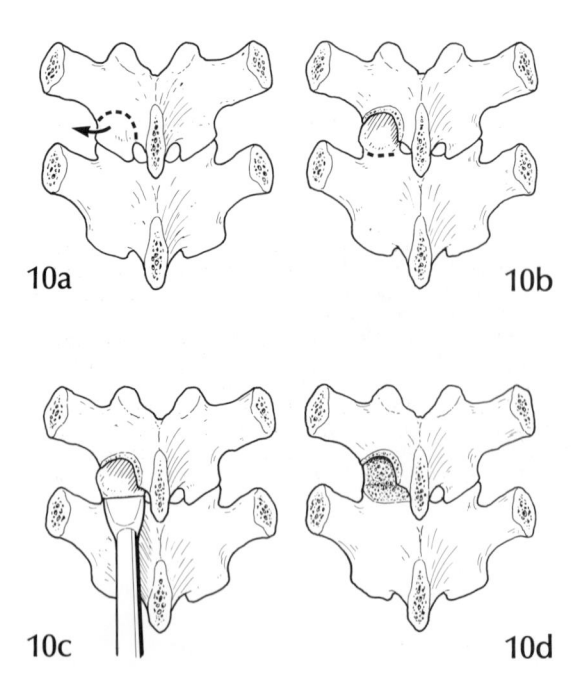

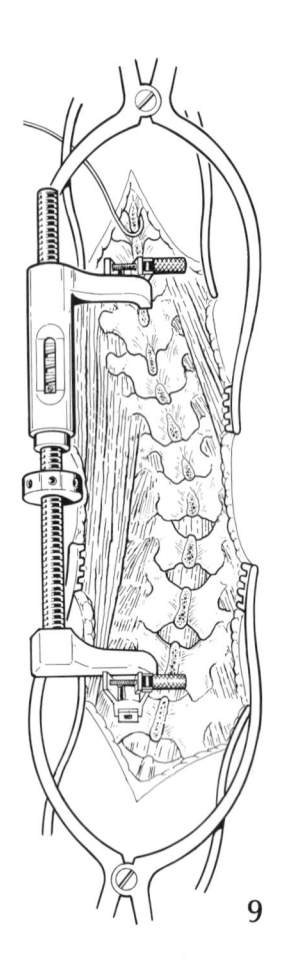

9

10a   10b

10c   10d

Excision of the thoracic facet joints

10a–d

The inferior facet which covers the superior facet of the adjacent level posteriorly is identified as a rounded prominence lying in the angle between the bases of the transverse and spinous processes. A small Capener or Moe gouge is used to remove the inferior facet (*a*) as an ellipse. The superior facet (*b*) of the vertebra below is then exposed. With the gouge directed horizontally in a rostral direction, this articular surface is then excised (*c*) and discarded. Once the articular surfaces are removed, these small pieces of bone can be added to the bone graft stock. Care should be taken not to miss the convex facet joint opposite the top hook.

Excision of the lumbar facet joints

11a & b

The lumbar facet joints lie almost in a sagittal plane. The articular surfaces of these facets are excised with a slightly larger gouge than that used for the thoracic joints. Narrow bone rongeurs (Pennybacker or Üllrich) can be similarly used to excise these lumbar facet joints. At the distal end of the fusion, the facet joint adjacent to the Harrington hook is excised with care so as not to weaken the hold of this hook.

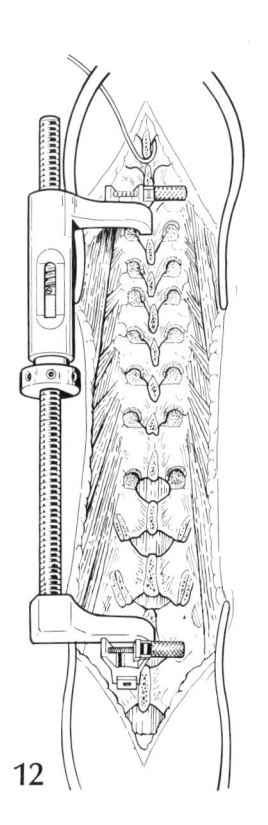

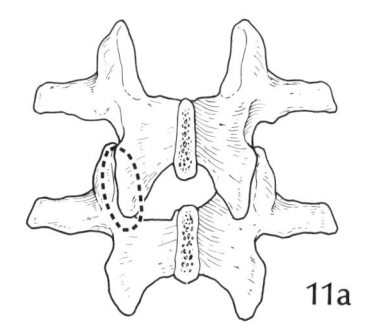

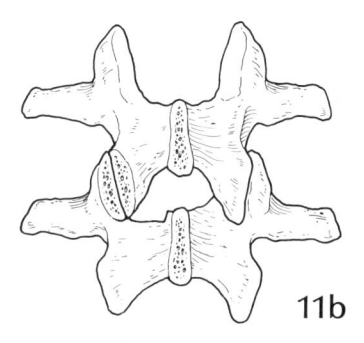

Decortication of laminae and transverse processes

12

The spinous processes are excised at their bases with angled bone cutters. This removed bone is fragmented and added to the bone graft stock. Using a large Capener gouge, the laminae and transverse processes are then decorticated. Again these thin strips of bone are removed and added to the bone graft. It is important that the transverse processes at each level are thoroughly decorticated; but where sublaminal wires are being used, care must be taken not to weaken the superior and inferior margins of the laminae because of the cheesewire effect that the Luque wire will produce if the lamina is too weak.

Insertion of sublaminar wires

13a–d

The doubled wire (American gauge 18) needs to be pre-bent into a semicircle shape as shown (a), the diameter of which corresponds to the width of the lamina. An adequate fenestration must be made at each level, and the wire gently and carefully passed. It is probably best hand-held and passed from the distal side in a cephalad direction around each lamina with the looped end of the double wire leading. When the looped end appears in the fenestration aperture above the lamina (b), it is carefully grasped with wire-holding forceps and then gently pulled through so that each limb of the wire loop is equal in length (c). Each limb is then contoured around the posterior side of the lamina (d) by kinking the loop. This prevents any disturbance of the wire which would cause back pressure on the spinal cord. The wire is then bent over the wound edge and left free or held in wire-holding forceps, the handles of which may be run on to a metal rod to keep the wires in order.

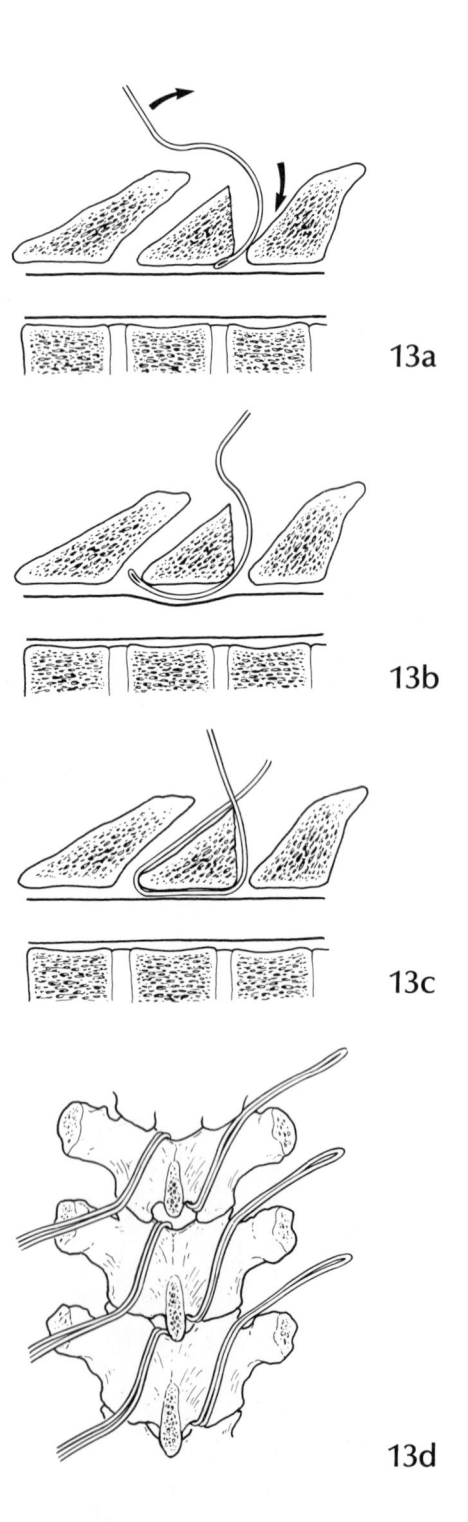

Insertion of Harrington rod and final correction

14

Usually the Harrington rod needs contouring to shape it to the required kyphosis angle along the thoracic spine and lordosis angle below. It is best to use a rod which has a square shape at its collar end, fitting into a square hole in the lower hook. The Harrington rod of appropriate length is chosen with the outrigger reading between 25 and 30 kg for the average adolescent patient. If the laminae are small, then it is best to reduce the distraction force to 20 kg. The appropriate size of rod is then contoured and the ratchet end slid through the upper rod before being slid down to engage the lower hook. During this procedure the rod is held in a rod clamp with a gentle side-to-side and rotatory manoeuvre. After final distraction, it is important that not more than three ratchet notches of the Harrington rod take part in the tension zone below the top hook; if more are involved, the rod is weakened to the point where a stress fracture may occur later. It may be necessary to release the outrigger distraction during rod insertion in order to make the hooks more mobile.

After the initial distraction, using either the 'ticket punch' spreader or the Gaines distractor, the extension clamps for the hooks and outrigger are removed before the final distraction of the Harrington rod. It is usually possible to achieve one more ratchet notch than was measured with the outrigger, and this should be allowed for. The C-ring washer (No. 1273) is then placed on the rod just distal to the top hook and fixed by means of the C-ring crimper.

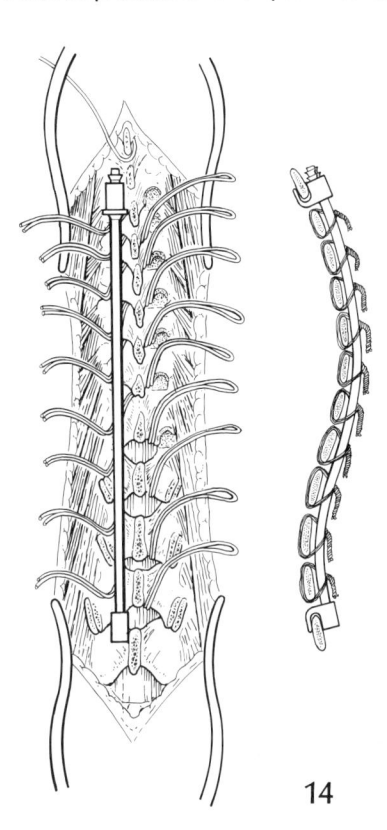

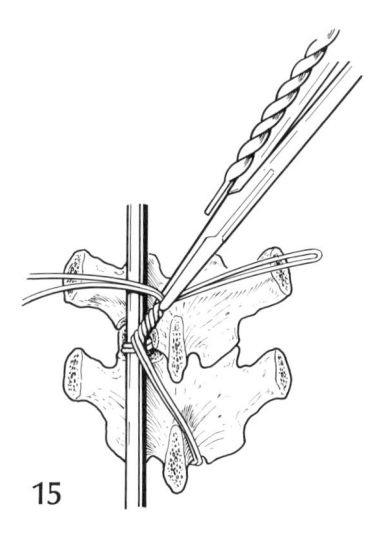

Tightening and trimming of the sublaminar wires

15

The wires are tightened in sequence using a jet-spin twister, which rotates the doubled wires in a clockwise direction, a process which is continued until the wire begins to twist on itself. Twisting must stop at this stage or the wire will break. Wire tightening starts distally, commencing with the lamina adjacent to the bottom hook. The wire tightening then continues proximally until half-way along the fusion length. At this point, it is best to tighten the wire around the lamina adjacent to the top hook before completing the process to provide support to counter the increasing force on the upper hook due to the corrective effect. Once the wires are tightened they should be rechecked as some degree of loosening may have been provoked by further correction. The wires are then divided, leaving a free end 1 cm long, which is then bent down to clear the muscle layer and to strengthen the actual twist (see *Illustration 16*).

Addition of bone graft and wound closure

16

The bone graft already harvested and added to the bone stock is usually sufficient in the average case of adolescent idiopathic scoliosis, in which case the slivers of bone are placed longitudinally along the fusion length on both convex and concave side, taking care to tuck fragments along each side of the Harrington rod.

Supplementary bone graft can be obtained from the posterior ilium through a separate oblique incision, taking care not to disturb the muscle attachment to the iliac crest. It is wise to close this wound with a suction drain to prevent a painful haematoma. In addition to autogenous bone, allograft from a carefully supervised bone bank can be successfully added to the wound in small cancellous fragments. Femoral heads are a fertile source for this.

In closing the main wound, it is not necessary to use a suction drain. The muscle and fascial layers are closed with interrupted absorbable sutures. After placing a stitch in the subcutaneous fat, which needs to be put in with care so as not to distort alignment of the skin edge, a fine subcuticular continuous suture is used to bring the skin together, and this is supported by adhesive wound closure strips. The amount of care that is required in careful skin closure cannot be over-emphasized.

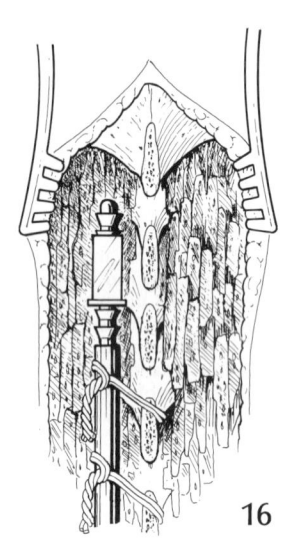

Postoperative management

Patients are left free in a firm bed, to be log-rolled every 2–4 hours, with supportive pillows along the spine when they are in the lateral position. Careful analgesia with morphine derivatives is required for the first 2 or 3 days, and this is probably best administered with an intravenous pump to maintain adequate levels of analgesia. Over the first few days, careful physiotherapy is also needed with assisted positive pressure ventilation, as discussed under the preoperative section.

At 48 hours, anteroposterior and lateral radiographs of the spine are taken using a portable machine to check that the instrumentation is in its correct position. This is also the best time to carry out a postoperative haemoglobin check and to consider removal of intravenous infusion in the light of the patient's condition and any impending ileus. A fluid balance chart must be kept strictly over the first 5 days.

On the fifth day, these patients can usually be carefully mobilized, being taught by the physiotherapist to sit on the edge of the bed and then stand for increasing periods, and also to sit in an upright chair.

Once the wound is healed, the patient can take a shower and be cast for a Subortholene front-opening underarm brace (Tuesel, Germany). It is best for this to be worn for 6 months after discharge, primarily as a protection rather than as a necessity. Certainly, adolescents returning to school feel more secure over this period in such a brace. At 6 months the patient may gradually increase activities, returning to normal at about 9 months, when the fusion mass should be quite sound.

References

1. Harrington PR. The history and development of Harrington instrumentation. *Clin Orthop* 1973; 93: 110–2.

2. Armstrong GWD, Connock SHG. A transverse loading system applied to modified Harrington instrumentation. *Clin Orthop* 1975; 108: 70–5.

3. Ransford AO, Edgar MA. A transverse bar system to supplement Harrington distraction instrumentation in scoliosis. *J Bone Joint Surg [Br]* 1982; 64-B: 226–7.

4. Ross KR, August AC, Edgar MA, Ransford AO. Multiple level distraction instrumentation for adolescent idiopathic scoliosis. *J Bone Joint Surg [Br]* 1986; 68-B: 670.

5. Luque ER. Segmental spinal instrumentation for the correction of scoliosis. *Clin Orthop* 1982; 163: 192–8.

6. Winter RB, Anderson MB. Spinal arthrodesis for spinal deformity using posterior instrumentation and sublaminar wiring: a preliminary report of 100 consecutive cases. *Int Orthop* 1985; 9: 237–45.

7. Dickson RA, Archer IA. The surgical treatment of late-onset idiopathic thoracic scoliosis: the Leeds procedure. *J Bone Joint Surg [Br]* 1987; 69-B: 709–14.

8. Dubousset J, Graf H, Miladi L, Cotrel Y. Spinal and thoracic derotation with CD instrumentation. *Orthop Trans* 1986; 10(1): 36.

9. Dove J. Preliminary report on the Hartshill rectangle. *J Bone Joint Surg [Br]* 1986; 68-B: 681.

10. Edgar MA, Mehta MH. Long-term follow-up of fused and unfused idiopathic scoliosis. *J Bone Joint Surg [Br]* 1988; 70-B: 712–6.

11. Hefti FL, McMaster MJ. The effect of the adolescent growth spurt on early posterior spinal fusion in infantile and juvenile idiopathic scoliosis. *J Bone Joint Surg [Br]* 1983; 65-B: 247–54.

12. King HA, Moe JH, Bradford DS, Winter RB. The selection of fusion levels in thoracic idiopathic scoliosis. *J Bone Joint Surg [Am]* 1983; 65-A: 1302–13.

Illustrations by Philip Wilson

Anterior procedures for spinal deformity

T. R. Morley FRCS
Consultant Orthopaedic Surgeon, King's College Hospital, London, and The Royal National Orthopaedic Hospital, Stanmore, UK

P. J. Webb FRCS
Consultant Orthopaedic Surgeon, The Hospital for Sick Children, Great Ormond Street, London, and The Royal National Orthopaedic Hospital, Stanmore, UK

Introduction

With improvements in anaesthesia and in postoperative care, the anterior approach to the spine has rapidly developed. Although the indications and benefits of the anterior approach in tuberculosis have long been known, the hazards were dissuasive.

Indications

The anterior approach to the spine is indicated either because the pathology is anterior, or to improve correction, or where it is important to shorten the bony canal. The indications may be absolute or relative.

Absolute indications

1. If the deformity is associated with kyphosis, particularly if there is cord compression, the cord may require decompression and the canal shortening. Distractive forces across a kyphosis must be applied with great care.
2. Where there are deficient posterior elements, anterior fusion increases the fusion mass. It is indicated in congenital spina bifida, and after laminectomy.
3. With congenital posterior hemivertebrae, which carry a high risk of neurological complications, decompression as well as fusion is often indicated.
4. In growth-arrest procedures, where the growth imbalance is anterior due to congenital anomalies, anterior surgery is indicated.
5. In neurological scoliosis, which is unstable with posterior fusion alone, all-round fusion is needed to improve the fusion mass.

Relative indications

1. In lumbar scoliosis, particularly with lordosis, the correction achieved by anterior surgery is better in both planes, and also derotates the spine.
2. Where it is important to keep the length of fusion to a minimum, the anterior approach is indicated. Fusion to L4 and below is associated with a significantly greater risk of developing back pain in adult life.
3. For the lumbar component of double curves, this approach achieves a better correction and saves extensive fusion.
4. In stiff and major scolioses, anterior release is used before the second-stage traction or posterior fusion.

Preoperative

Timing of surgery

The timing of surgery is dependent on the severity of the deformity, the rate of progression and the neurological status. The skeletal maturity of the child and the size of the vertebrae also require consideration.

Evaluation

The preoperative evaluation of a deformity considers four aspects. The bony deformity is defined by plain radiology, lateral bending films and tomography. Its relation to the spinal cord is shown by a computed tomographic scan. The spinal cord and roots are assessed by contrast radiology and nuclear magnetic resonance. Finally the blood supply is visualized by angiography. In addition to the evaluation of the deformity, the patient may require cardiovascular, pulmonary and renal investigation.

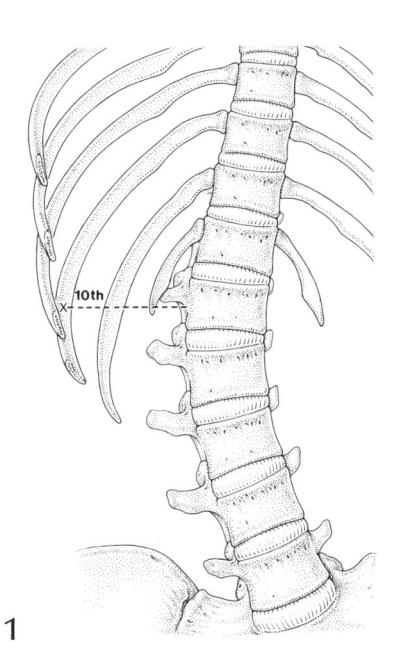

Choice of levels for instrumentation

Surgery should extend over the full length of the deformity and leave the spine stable in both planes. After release procedures, traction may occasionally be indicated to achieve slow, controlled reduction in the deformity. Traction has to be skeletal, and undertaken slowly. Stiff kyphotic deformities are a relative contra-indication to traction.

1

Choosing the levels to be instrumented is done on the basis of lateral bending films. The aim is to achieve a full and stable correction but at the same time limit the length of fusion. The lateral flexion view into the concavity demonstrates the ability of the lower lumbar vertebrae to correct into the zone of stability and also demonstrates the flexibility of the compensatory curves. The bending view into the convexity demonstrates the ability of the primary curve to correct and to derotate. The fusion must include the levels where the disc spaces do not open on the concavity when flexed into the convexity.

After the area for fusion has been selected, a standing anteroposterior film is studied to decide on the incision site: a line is drawn from the apical vertebrae to the mid-axillary line, and the rib which bisects this line is chosen. The incision is marked before preparing the skin.

Anaesthesia

Moderate hypotension only is necessary. The cord blood supply is maintained above 70 mm of mercury.

Spinal cord monitoring

Because most anterior procedures shorten the bony canal the risks of neurological damage are reduced. An exception to this is where the spine is kyphotic, and is being lengthened, or where bone is being excised, in which case care and the use of cord monitoring is advisable.

506 Thoracic and lumbar spine

Position of patient

2

The patient is operated upon in the lateral position, with the convexity uppermost. In order to facilitate the approach and later correction, the patient is positioned with the table broken at the apex of the deformity. The patient needs to be firmly held to make certain there is no loss of position during the operation. Where the approach is above the fifth rib, under the scapula, the arm should be left free to avoid damage to the brachial plexus.

A spinal cord monitor lead may be placed in the epidural space percutaneously, if any distraction force is to be used.

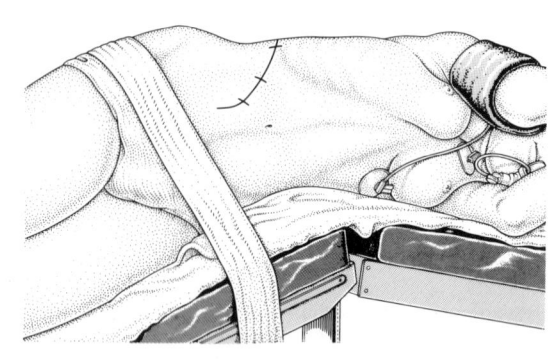

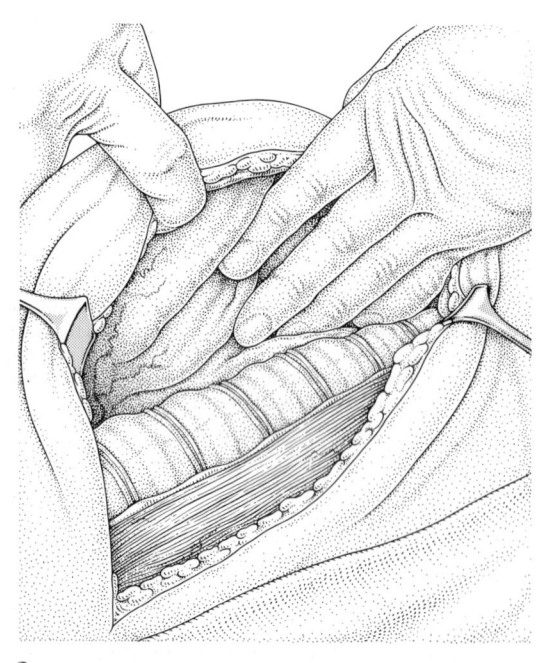

Operation

Approach

3

The spine is most commonly exposed by a thoraco-abdominal approach. The incision starts at the angle of the rib and is carried forward to the rectus sheath but not beyond. If a wide exposure is required the incision is curved caudally.

The rib having been exposed subperiosteally, it is cut and is used later as graft. The abdominal muscles are divided in the line of the incision. The retroperitoneal space is easily identified at the costal margin and the peritoneum is then stripped, exposing the psoas muscle, spine and diaphragm. The kidney and ureter are carried forward.

Anterior procedures for spinal deformity 507

Splitting the diaphragm

4

The diaphragm is split peripherally, leaving a 1 cm cuff. The parietal pleura is then split along the mid-lateral border of the vertebrae and the incision extended caudally through the attachments of the diaphragm and along the anterior border of the psoas. This exposes the segmental vessels and the sympathetic chain.

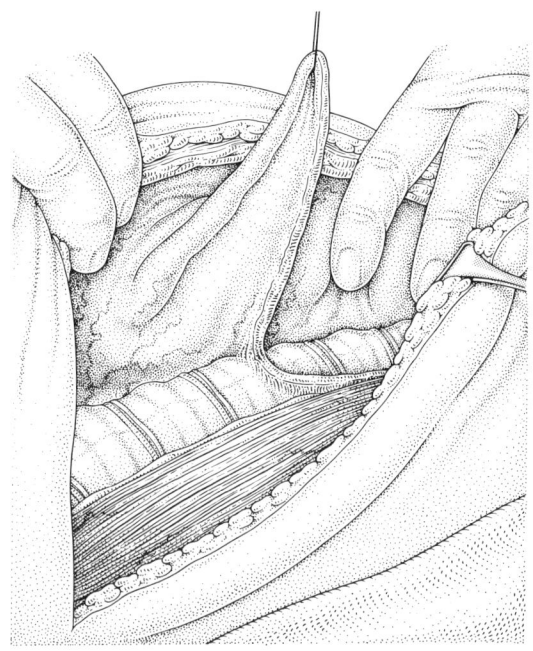

Division of segmental vessels

5

The segmental vessels are not divided if a simple release is being performed, but if the spine is being instrumented these are divided at every level. The artery and vein are clearly identified and then divided either between ligatures or with diathermy, avoiding diathermy near the foramen. The exposure of the vertebrae can then be completed extraperiosteally, detaching the arcuate ligaments and sweeping the diaphragm and great vessels into the concavity. The psoas muscle arches over the vessels and is attached to the annulus and body of a vertebra on either side of the disc. This muscle is detached from its extensive attachments and retracted into the convexity, completing the exposure of the vertebrae.

Where there are no other specific indications, it is safer to approach the spine from the left side, thus avoiding the inferior vena cava, which is more easily damaged. If the common iliac vein is being mobilized anteriorly, the iliolumbar vein must be identified and divided to avoid avulsion from its root.

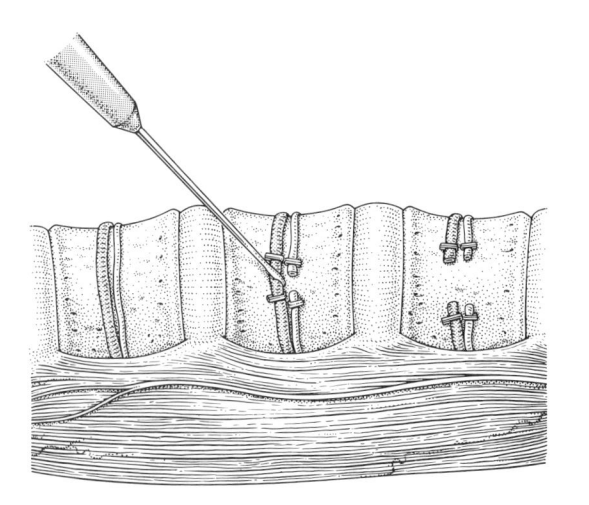

508 Thoracic and lumbar spine

Excision of the disc

6a & b

It is important to excise the disc as completely as possible. Derotation is not achieved by force, but by a release sufficient to allow the vertebrae to realign with ease. The disc is incised transversely and then cut into segments. The disc material, both nucleus and annulus, is then removed with nibblers. Posteriorly, the removal is continued until there is a change in direction of the fibres, denoting the posterior longitudinal ligament. It is particularly important to remove all the disc material on the convexity posteriorly as this will allow the vertebrae to approximate closely after the instrumentation.

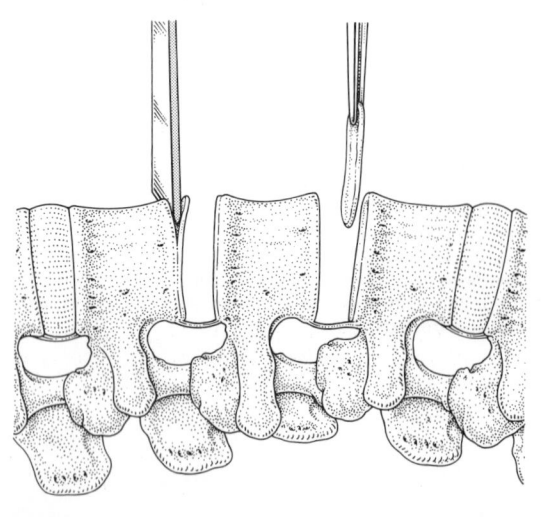

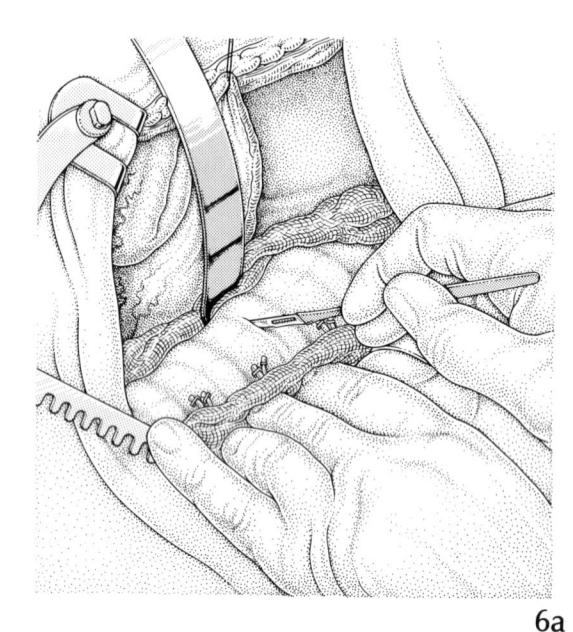

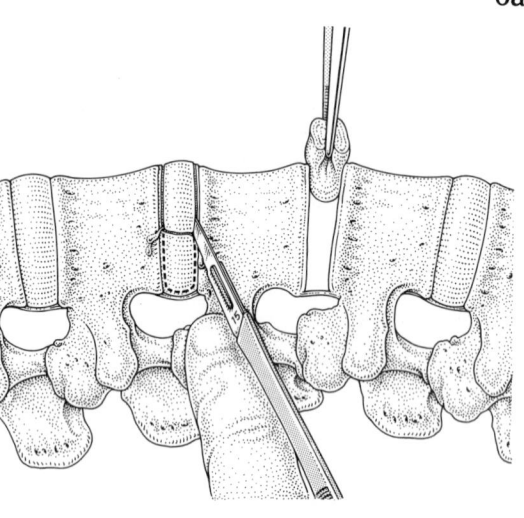

6a

6b

Excision of growth-plate

7

The growth-plates or, in the case of an adult, the end-plates are removed carefully with either an osteotome or a Cobb elevator. After the excision, bleeding cancellous bone is exposed. Again, this dissection must be carried well posteriorly to achieve a complete release and to enhance subsequent fusion.

7

Anterior procedures for spinal deformity 509

Instrumentation

Anterior instrumentation is based on the principle of joining cancellous screws, inserted transversely across the vertebral bodies, either by a cable, a threaded rod or a solid rod.

Placement of screws

8

Screws are placed transversely across each vertebra. The screws enter laterally but are placed more posteriorly at the apex of the curve. This encourages the spine to derotate during the final phase of correction.

9

Exact placement of screws is important. A finger is placed in the concavity with the fingertip on the transverse process and the screw then directed towards the pulp. If the screw is placed too far anteriorly the hold is inadequate, whilst posterior placement risks entering the spinal canal. The length of the screws should be such that the tip is just through the far cortex but should not be too long, as this could cause subsequent erosion of the great vessels.

The vertebral screws can either be compressed, to correct lateral deformity, or distracted carefully to correct kyphosis.

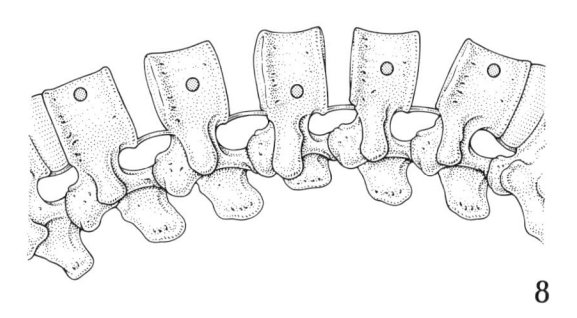

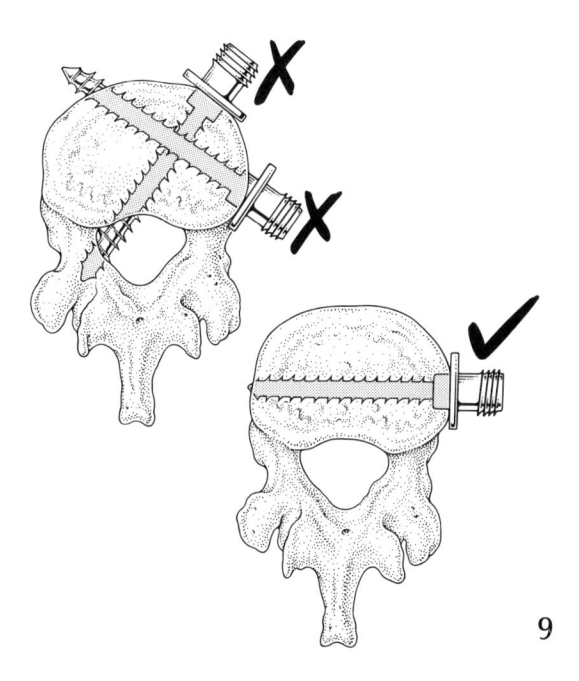

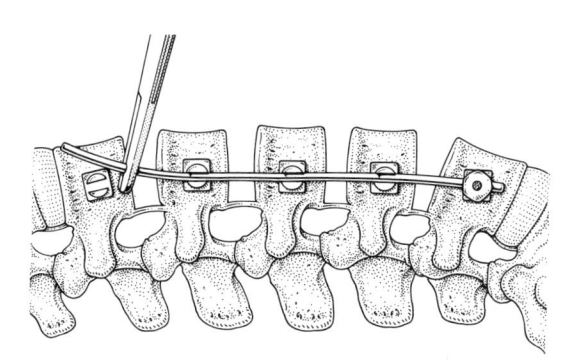

Rod placement

10

The rod is placed in the slots in the head of the screws. Two rod types are available, a soft rod for compression and a hard rod for distraction. The rod is held loosely by a collet and screw cap.

510 Thoracic and lumbar spine

Graft placements

11

The inherent problem associated with the anterior approach and instrumentation is a tendency to cause kyphosis. This is prevented by placing bone grafts anteriorly and in the concavity, and then closing the disc space over the graft. The rod itself can also be contoured.

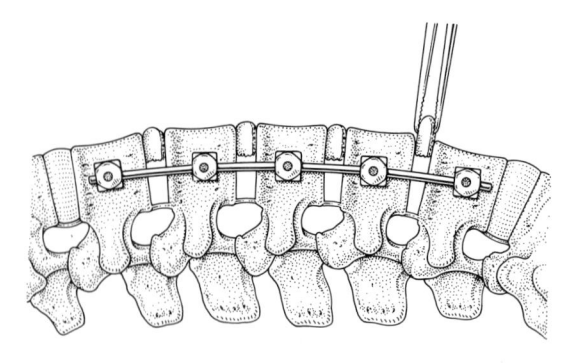

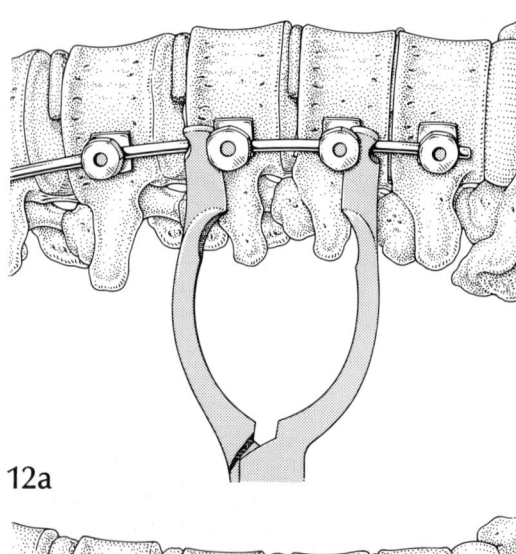

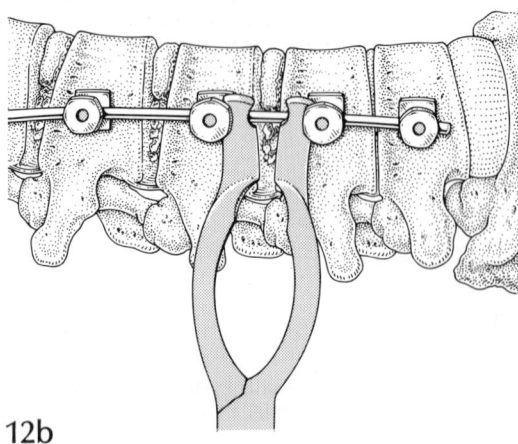

11

12a

Correction of deformity

12a & b

The correction of a lateral deformity is achieved by shortening the convexity by bringing together the screw heads which grip onto a smooth rod. The screws grip by indenting the rod with a small collet and this can then be adjusted as often as necessary in order to achieve a full correction.
  If the deformity is kyphotic, distraction of the screw heads is equally possible placing the graft anteriorly but needs to be cautious as the bony canal is being lengthened.
  The operating table is unbroken at this stage to facilitate correction.

12b

Closure

13

After careful haemostasis the rod is trimmed and the parietal pleura and diaphragm repaired. The chest is closed over a drain and the abdominal muscles closed in layers.

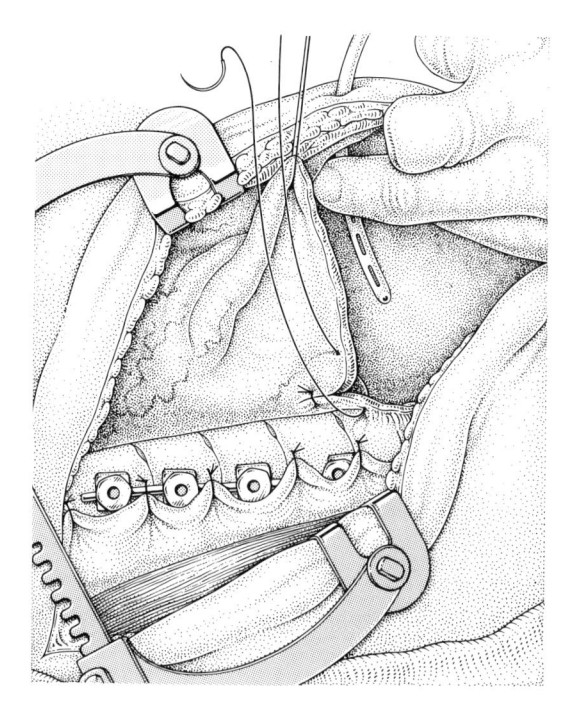

Postoperative management

The patient is nursed lying flat and is rolled into the half-lateral position. Neurological status is carefully observed.

A chest radiograph is taken to demonstrate the position of the drain and to check that the lung has fully expanded. Chest physiotherapy may be given.

The patient is mobilized after one week in a simple external underarm support. Braces are used occasionally to give added protection and are worn for 6 months.

Check radiographs need to be taken in the standing position to confirm the placement of the instrumentation and the stability of the correction.

Illustrations by Peter Cox

Luque instrumentation for neuromuscular scoliosis

George Bentley ChM, FRCS
Professor of Orthopaedic Surgery, The Institute of Orthopaedics, University of London; Honorary Consultant Orthopaedic Surgeon, Royal National Orthopaedic Hospital, Stanmore, and The Middlesex Hospital, London, UK

Julian Jessop FRCS
Lecturer, University Department of Orthopaedic Surgery, The Institute of Orthopaedics, Royal National Orthopaedic Hospital, Stanmore, UK

Introduction

Neuromuscular scoliosis represents only 7 per cent of all scoliosis but it is often relentlessly progressive, leading to severe deformity and respiratory failure. The underlying disorders include Duchenne's muscular dystrophy, spinal muscular atrophy, cerebral palsy and poliomyelitis. Other less common conditions are limb girdle dystrophy, facioscapulo humeral dystrophy, Emery–Draphous syndrome, Prader–Willi syndrome, arthrogryposis and congenital muscular dystrophy.

Indications

In Duchenne muscular dystrophy the patients are too weak to stand by the age of 8–10 years. They then develop a progressive kyphoscoliosis in 95 per cent of cases and this is exacerbated by the adolescent growth spurt. Surgical stabilization is now recommended at this early stage since total correction of the deformity can be achieved by an operation that is technically easier than later in the disease, involves less blood loss and is safer for the patient who will have better respiratory function. In other forms of dystrophy and poliomyelitis the patients may continue to walk independently and have a normal life prognosis. Here the emphasis is on maintaining spinal stability to facilitate walking. It is important to assess the spinal movement required for walking since these patients may have difficulties if fusion is performed which abolishes that movement.

The aim of surgical stabilization in these children is to treat established spinal deformity, especially when severe and uncontrolled by bracing. Often such patients find the brace is extremely uncomfortable and difficult to wear and most cite the ability to abandon the brace as the greatest benefit of surgical stabilization. In addition surgery can help to slow down the otherwise inevitable deterioration in spinal curvature and lung function which affects these patients, who become progressively more debilitated due to recurrent infections and respiratory failure. It may therefore contribute to increased longevity. At the very least, it improves the cosmetic appearance of the patients, allowing them to sit upright in a chair without using an arm for support, and freeing them for more productive activity.

The indications for surgery are therefore:

1. A progressive neuromuscular scoliosis which is not being controlled by bracing.
2. In Duchenne muscular dystrophy, any scoliosis which has progressed beyond 20°.

Preoperative

Careful clinical examination and assessment of peripheral neurological state and fixed flexion deformities must be performed before operation. It is important to explain to the parents the risks and benefits of surgery. The risks include death during or after anaesthesia, failure to correct or hold the spine, wound infection, spinal cord injury and pneumohaemothorax.

All children require assessment of cardiac function by echocardiography and respiratory function since both cardiac and diaphragmatic muscle may be affected in Duchenne muscular dystrophy. Children with a vital capacity and FEV_1 of less than 20 per cent of that predicted are considered unfit for surgery.

1 & 2

Anteroposterior spinal radiographs are taken with the patient in the sitting position and when suspended by the shoulders. The Cobb angle is measured in both views and the limits of the curve determined. Pelvic tilt is also measured since this affects sitting stability and comfort.

Adequate quantities of crossmatched blood are essential. Blood loss in these cases is commonly high owing to excess capillary fragility. In Duchenne patients it is not unusual to lose 80 per cent of the estimated blood volume and on occasion this may be as high as 200 per cent.

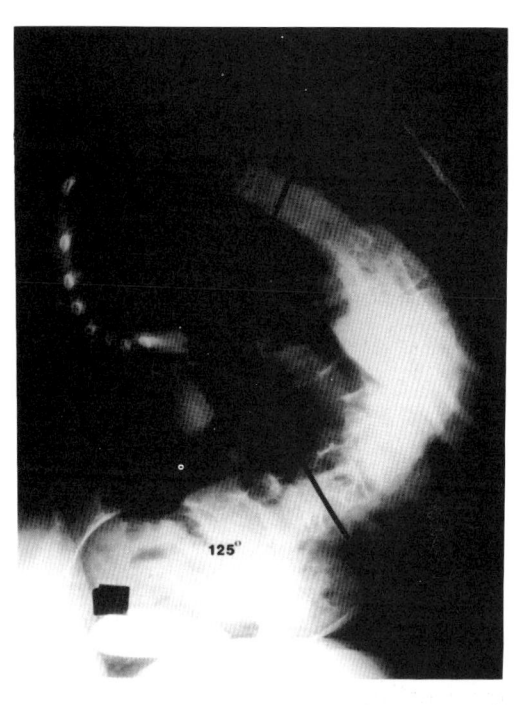

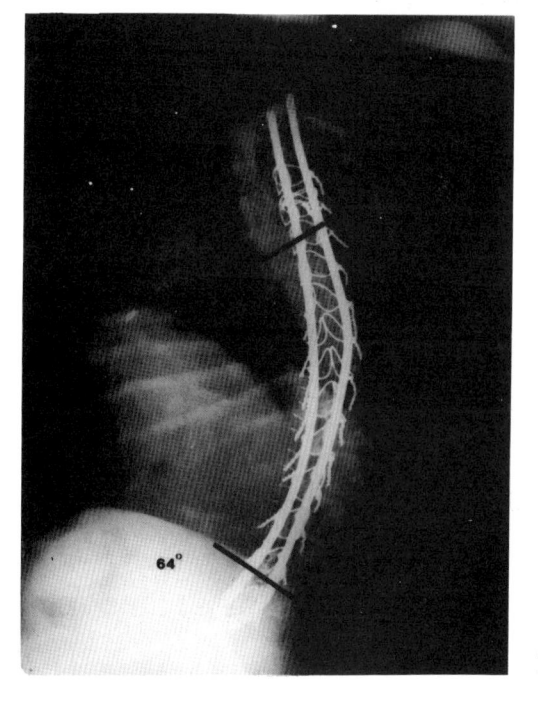

514 Thoracic and lumbar spine

Choice of procedure

For children who are wheelchair-bound, Luque instrumentation without formal fusion is an effective form of treatment. For patients with less severe neuromuscular disorders who are likely to remain ambulant, Harrington rod fixation augmented by Luque segmental laminar wires and posterior fusion is the procedure of choice.

LUQUE INSTRUMENTATION

Anaesthesia

General anaesthesia is induced. After intubation central venous and intra-arterial lines are set up and continuous monitoring of pulse, blood pressure, electrocardiogram and body temperature is performed. Intravenous antibiotics (flucloxacillin and amoxycillin) are given intravenously. Stimulating electrodes for spinal evoked potentials are applied over the medial and lateral popliteal nerves in the popliteal fossa of each leg. A urinary catheter and rectal thermometer are introduced.

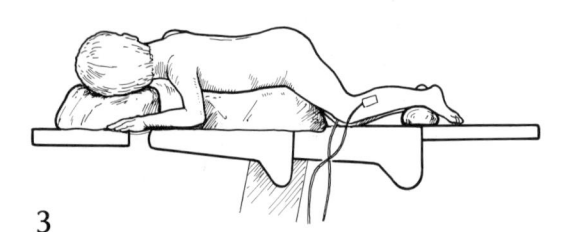

Position of patient

3

The patient is placed prone on a Montreal mattress. A clean air enclosure is desirable. The skin of the entire back from neck to buttock is thoroughly cleaned with Hibitane (ICI Pharmaceuticals, UK) and spirit. Adhesive transparent drape is then applied.

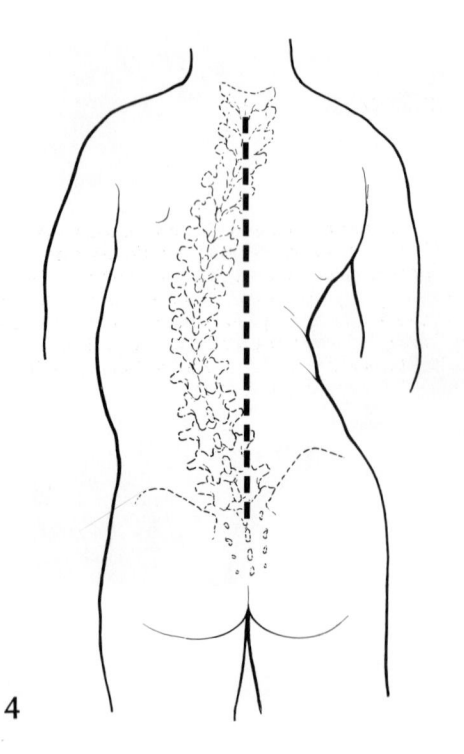

Incision

4

The location of the highest vertebral level involved in the curve (established from the preoperative radiograph) is determined by palpation of the spinous processes. A straight longitudinal incision is made from this point down to the centre of the back at the level of the sacrum. It is important that this incision should not stray into the natal cleft, as this can produce a painful scar.

Exposure of the spinous processes and laminae

5

The incision is deepened through the subcutaneous fat to expose the deep fascia and haemostasis obtained. Using cutting diathermy, the supraspinous and interspinous ligaments are divided. The paraspinal muscles are then reflected, using subperiosteal dissection with a mixture of cutting diathermy and the Cobb spinal elevator. Haemostasis is meticulous and as each area is exposed and bleeding vessels cauterized, it is packed with rolled-up gauze swabs. Further dissection using the Cobb elevator exposes the laminae and bases of the transverse processes. Self-retaining retractors are now inserted.

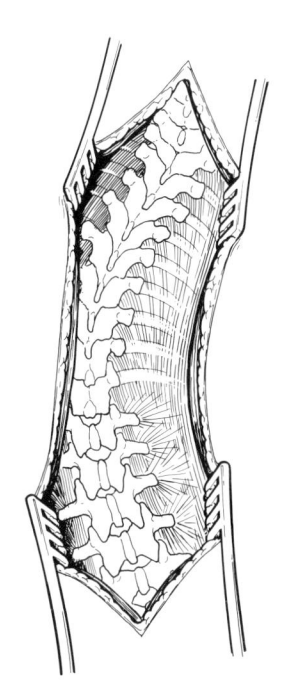

Spinal monitoring

6

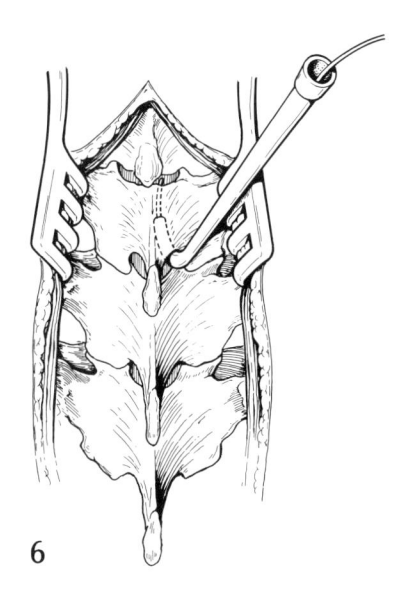

The spinal monitoring electrode is now placed above the top vertebra of the curve. A small cannula with its sharp central trocar is inserted through the ligamentum flavum in the midline. The trocar is then withdrawn and, provided there is no leak of cerebrospinal fluid, the monitoring lead is introduced for a distance of about 5 cm. The lead is marked to facilitate this. An adequate trace should be secured before proceeding further.

516 Thoracic and lumbar spine

Insertion and contouring of the Luque rods

7

The vertebral levels are again checked and the sacroiliac joints are identified. The sharp introducing instrument is then driven into the bone in this region to produce a foramen into which the distal end of the rods can be buried. In large children it is possible to place the rods between the cortices of the pelvis, but in small children the rods will pass through the joint and exit the posterior cortex. Great care must be taken to avoid penetrating the inner cortex and entering the pelvis.

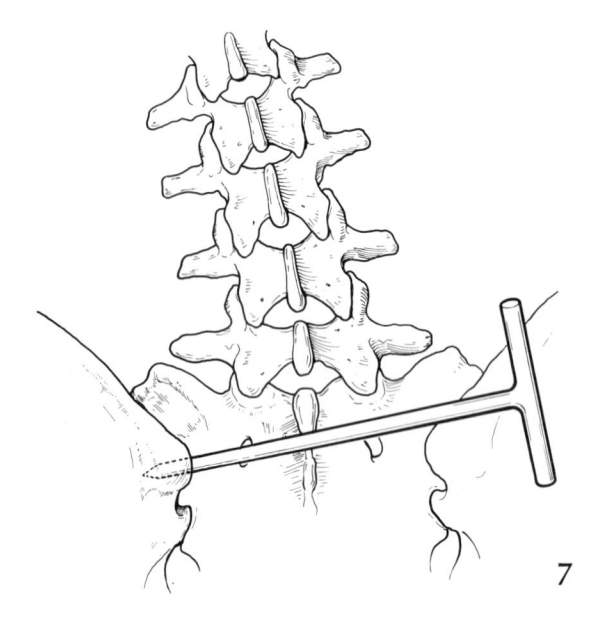

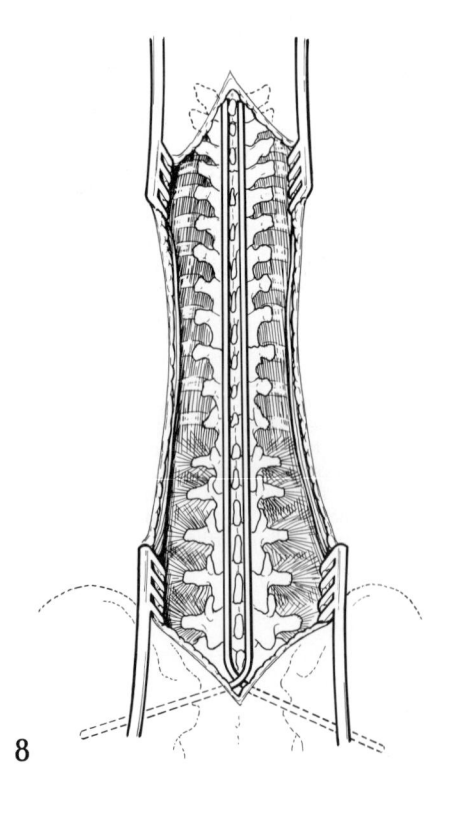

8

The distance between the point of entry of the rod and the upper point of the curve is estimated. The rod is then bent to accommodate the sharp curve where it will turn laterally into the sacroiliac region, and trimmed at the appropriate proximal level using large bolt-cutters. The curve is corrected as much as possible by manipulation. The rod is then contoured carefully in the sagittal and coronal planes so that it will lie on the laminae on the convex side of the curve, on the opposite side to its insertion point into the pelvis, producing appropriate correction. The second rod is introduced into the other sacroiliac area, crossed over or under the convex rod, and contoured to lie on the laminae on the concave side.

It is important to assess the fixed flexion deformity in the hips preoperatively and contour the rods to give adequate lordosis. If the lordosis is reduced by the rods the fixed flexion deformity at the hips will be increased and walking or sitting may be very difficult and painful.

Insertion of sublaminar wires

9 & 10

The supraspinous and interspinous ligaments are then removed using scalpel and nibblers, starting at the top of the incision and working downwards. The rods are temporarily removed. The space between the neural arches is carefully enlarged and the dura mater exposed by careful division of the ligamentum flavum with a scalpel in the midline. A MacDonald dissector is passed into the spinal canal to ensure free passage. A Cloward punch is used to enlarge the space if necessary. In the thoracic region it is often necessary to excise the tip of the spinous process to gain access. Double (18 gauge) Luque wires are contoured appropriately and then introduced carefully beneath the neural arches from top to bottom of the curve. It is important to maintain tension on the wire throughout and to bend the wire down over each side of the neural arch when it has been successfully passed. This prevents impingement on the dura which can lead to neurological damage. The wires are then divided and one of each pair is turned on itself on each side of the neural arch so that there will be one wire holding each rod at each level.

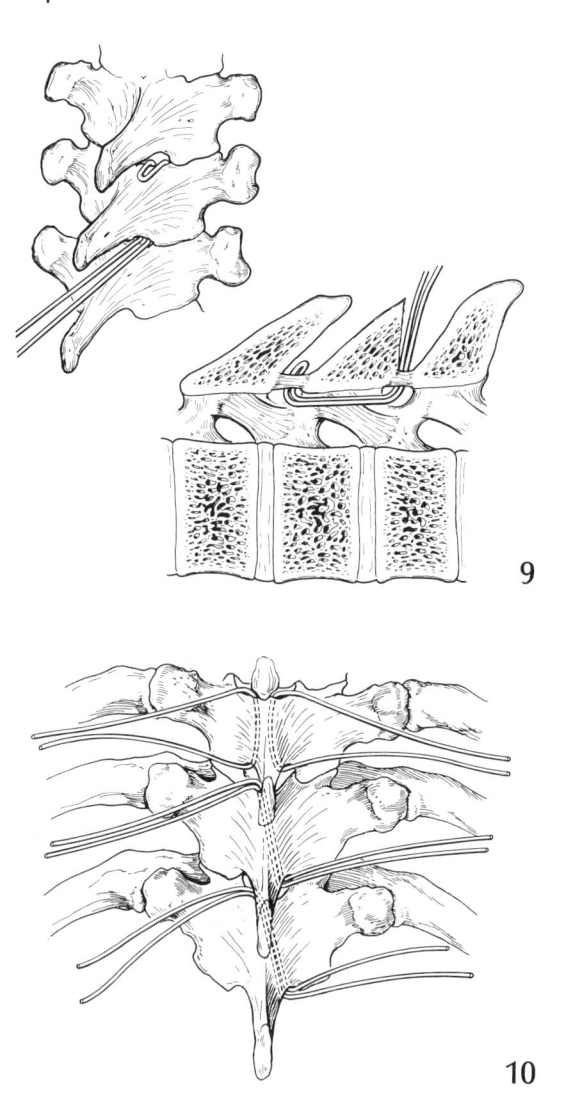

Tightening of wires over the rods

11

The rods are again inserted and secured by tightening the wires. The convex wires are tightened first, working from distal to proximal; then the concave wires are tightened, the rod being controlled by a rod-holding forcep. Sometimes it is necessary to secure the most proximal wires before the distal, depending on the 'fit' of the rod to the spine. The spinal monitoring trace must be carefully watched during this procedure as abnormalities are common. If the trace disappears and there has been no apparent trauma to the spinal cord, it is usually safe to proceed and the trace will then return within 15 minutes. If, however, the trace does not return, it is necessary to loosen the wires until the trace recovers, as this will represent the point at which impingement has occurred.

12

The wires are then checked for tightness. They should be tightened until it is no longer possible to slide them on the rod. They are then trimmed. Finally the posterior spinal joints are exposed with a gouge using the Moe technique, the neural arch of L5 and S1 vertebrae are decorticated and the bone from the spinous processes placed across the gap.

Wound closure

Continuous absorbable sutures are used for all layers. Sutures are placed in the paraspinal muscles, the deep fascia, and the subcutaneous fat. A continuous intradermal suture is finally placed in the skin and reinforced with adhesive wound-closure strips.

HARRINGTON–LUQUE INSTRUMENTATION

In mobile patients with limited curves the Harrington–Luque procedure is used as described previously. Double sublaminar wires are passed beneath alternate vertebrae and are tightened after maximal distraction of the Harrington rod. Moe fusion and posterior decortication are performed from top to bottom of the curve, and corticocancellous bone from the iliac crest is placed in each posterior joint and over the whole of the neural arches and transverse processes in the curve. Postoperatively these patients remain in bed for 7–10 days and mobilize using a plastic spinal support with Velcro (Apilx, France) fastenings, which is retained for 6 months except for showering or bathing. At this stage stability and fusion of the spine can be confirmed radiologically and the patient is gradually weaned from the support over 3 months.

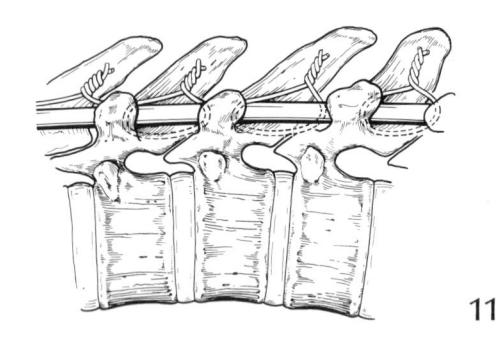

Postoperative management

Blood loss is noted and appropriate replacement given. An immediate chest radiograph film is taken to exclude pneumothorax. Lower limb function, i.e. sensation and toe movements, are monitored hourly. The patient is nursed supine and log-rolled 45° in each direction every 2 hours. Antibiotics are continued for 1 week postoperatively. At the end of 1 week, if the wound is satisfactory, the patient may begin to sit up and may usually leave hospital after 14 days.

References

1. Luque ER, Cardoso A. Treatment of scoliosis without arthrodesis or external support; preliminary report. *Orthop Trans* 1977; 1: 37–8.

2. Moe JH, Winter RB, Bradford DS, Lonstein JE. *Scoliosis and other spinal deformities*. Philadelphia: Saunders, 1978.

Illustrations by D. Howat and L. Butler

Surgical management of lumbar disc prolapses

H. V. Crock *AO*, MD, MS, FRCS, FRACS
Honorary Consultant, Royal Postgraduate Medical School, Hammersmith Hospital, London, UK

Introduction

In the English-speaking world the term 'laminectomy' is used commonly to describe any operation for the removal of prolapsed disc tissue. Laminectomy means excision of a lamina and implies its total removal. Properly, this term should be replaced by the phrase: 'operation for the excision of disc fragments'. Differing methods of surgical approach will depend on factors such as the size of the spinal canal, the height of the disc space and on the site, size and distribution of the prolapsed disc tissue.

Types of lumbar disc prolapse

The characteristics of prolapses vary with the physical qualities of the affected disc tissue[1]. In young persons, discrete small rounded, firm or fluctuant protrusions are found with stretched, but intact, annular fibres covering the prolapse. When these fibres are incised, a small quantity of disc tissue exudes. The consistency of such discs is often described as rubbery. Some degenerate annular fibres are usually found with the extruded nuclear tissue.

Extrusion of variable quantities of disc tissue (1–20 g) into the spinal canal may occur when gross degenerative changes have affected the disc as a whole. These sequestrated disc fragments include nuclear, annular and end-plate cartilage components. Between these two extremes a variety of pathological changes occur, such as incomplete sequestration with marked perineural fibrosis, due to physicochemical changes in the disc[2], calcification of the nucleus pulposus and calcification in prolapsed tissue, followed by erosion of the dural sac[3].

A sequestrated fragment may migrate to another level from the disc of its origin, leaving a clearly defined defect in the posterior annulus. Sequestrated disc tissue may present posterior to the dural sac[4].

Rarely, disc tissue prolapses into a vertebral body and re-enters the spinal canal, pushing ahead of it a small fragment of vertebral end-plate bone and cartilage. Knowledge of the varying relationships which prolapsed disc tissue bears to the neural contents of the spinal canal is essential to the understanding of the varied clinical pictures which may present.

In a subrhizal prolapse, the disc fragment which lies anterior to the affected nerve root usually causes severe pain, with objective motor and sensory signs distally in the part of the limb supplied by the compressed nerve. Axillary prolapses situated between the dural sac and the nerve root sheath, or pararhizal prolapses, lying on the outer side of the nerve root sheath, may produce symptoms of severe sciatica without abnormal objective physical signs.

1

The illustration shows six types of disc prolapses in the lower lumbar region. At L4–5 on the left side migrating *sequestrated disc fragments* (a), with a small circular annular defect above them, are shown and below this at L5–S1 a *pararhizal prolapse* (b). In the midline a large *central sequestration* is depicted (c). On the right side an *axillary prolapse* is illustrated (d) at L4–5 and further laterally, outside the intervertebral foramen, a *far lateral disc prolapse* (e). Finally, on the right side at L5–S1, the common *subrhizal disc prolapse* is shown (f).

Centrally placed prolapses or large migrating sequestrated fragments in the spinal canal can give rise to physical signs which vary from day to day and from one leg to the other. Cauda equina claudication, with the onset of buttock or leg pain after walking short distances, may also be found[5,6].

Indications for operative treatment

Many intervertebral disc prolapses recover with non-operative treatment. The indications depend on the severity and duration of symptoms and signs. Absolute indications are as follows.

1. Profound neurological deficit, e.g. complete foot drop
2. Central disc prolapse with bladder paralysis
3. A history of severe nerve root pain, paraesthesiae and numbness exceeding 6 months with or without motor deficit
4. Recurrent severe pain, paraesthesia and numbness in the legs.

Preoperative management

Preoperative preparation

The accuracy of diagnosis of disc prolapse has improved dramatically in recent years with the wider use of computed tomographic (CT) scanning, with or without water-soluble radiculography, and most recently with magnetic resonance imaging. Plain radiographs of the spine have maintained an important role in diagnosis. These films should always be available in the operating theatre, along with the results of other special investigations.

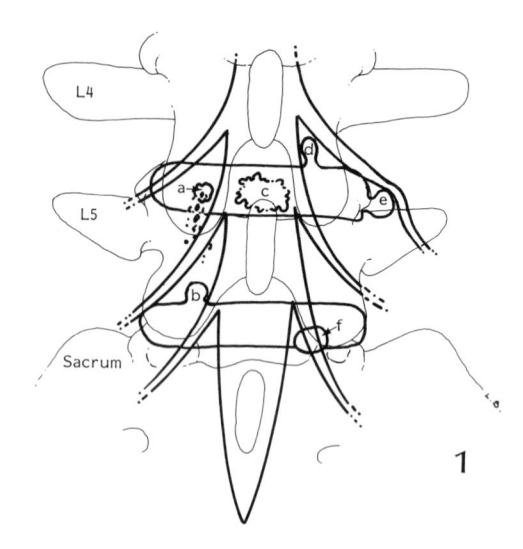

Full blood examination, including blood grouping and erythrocyte sedimentation rate, should be performed. It is wise to insert an intravenous infusion in all patients before operation for disc disorders, though blood transfusion is rarely indicated. The use of prophylactic chemotherapy may be indicated if there is an antecedent history of serious infection, or of previous wound infections.

Anaesthesia

General anaesthesia with muscular relaxation and mechanical ventilation is most commonly employed. Continuous monitoring of cardiopulmonary function has become routine.

Position of patient

2 & 3

A variety of suitable postures is shown in the illustrations. The most versatile and easily managed is the prone position. The supporting sponge rubber U-piece is simply constructed and inexpensive. The right arm is shown dependent and supported on the well-padded arm rest, which is suspended below the level of the table to prevent stretching of the brachial plexus and ulnar nerve injury. The left arm rests by the patient's side. The table is angled in the centre. The surgeon's assistant and other observers will have unobstructed views of procedures throughout the course of the operation. The entire range of surgical manoeuvres that may be required for the execution of even the most complex operation, including transdural excision of prolapsed disc tissue, can be accomplished in comfort and without undue restraints on its duration.

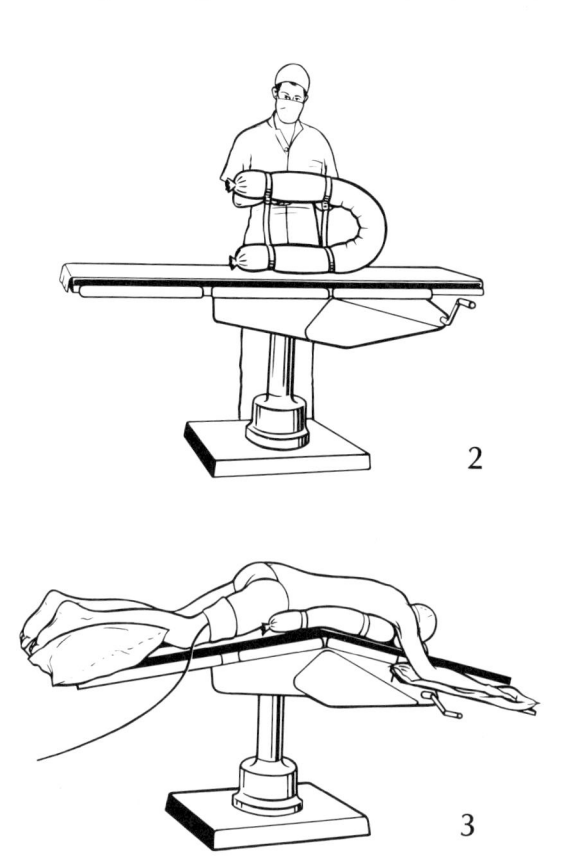

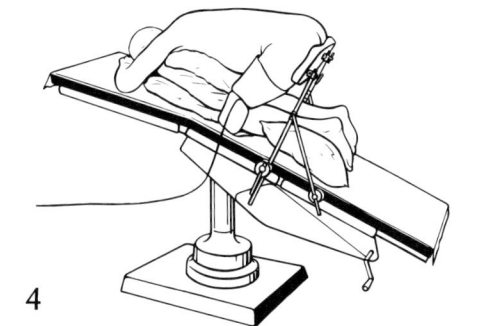

Jack-knife or kneeling position

4

In this position, with the use a simple frame to support the buttocks, excellent operating conditions are provided. Alternatively, the patient can be placed in this position with pillows under the chest so the the abdomen is unsupported. A pillow is placed under the patient's feet and a restraining strap across the legs, though venous obstruction in the lower limbs is then likely to occur. The table is angled. It is more difficult to set patients in this position, and potentially difficult to move them quickly to deal with an emergency, such as circulatory collapse, should it arise. Elbows must be cushioned to avoid excessive pressure on the ulnar nerves. Generally this position should be avoided.

Lateral position

5

This position can be recommended only in special circumstances, for example when the patient is extremely obese or when there are special chest problems which may complicate anaesthesia. Note the pillow between the patient's legs, the restraining strap crossing the iliac crest and the sandbag placed under the loin above the dependent iliac crest. The table is angled in the centre. There are drawbacks to the routine use of this position: the assistant surgeon is rarely comfortable and has a restricted view; lighting of the operative field is often inadequate and blood tends to pool on the dependent side of the spine making access to the nerve root canal more difficult.

Instruments

Recommended instruments and disposable supplies are listed below.

1. Self-retaining retractors
2. Fine sucker
3. Bayonet forceps
4. Long-handled carrier for size 11 or size 15 scalpel blade
5. Watson Cheyne dissector
6. Nerve root retractor, such as a Scaglietti probe (25 cm long)
7. A range of bone rongeurs
8. A range of pituitary rongeurs, straight, angled outwards at 45° and at 90° with cutting cups of varying dimensions
9. Hammer
10. Fine osteotomes and chisels
11. Ring curettes
12. 6/0 suture material on fine cutting needles with a fine needle holder
13. Surgical patties and haemostatic gauze or sponge materials
14. Bone wax
15. Bipolar coagulator
16. Cobb elevator.

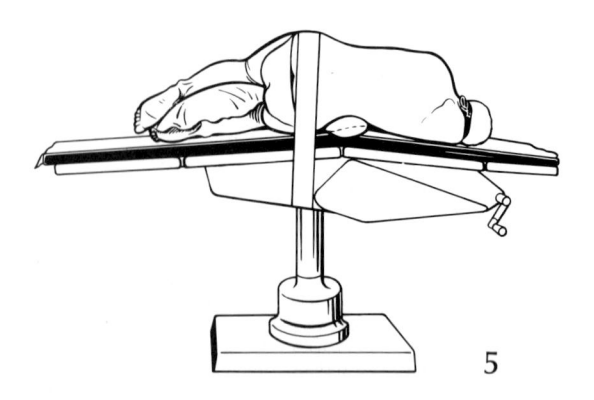

Operation

Skin incision

Before the skin incision is made the surgeon should once again inspect the patient's radiographs, paying attention to vertebral anomalies, such as spina bifida occulta and sacralization, and noting certain lesions such as spondylolisthesis or isolated disc resorption[1]. The level of the planned exposure of the spine should be noted. Radiographs of the lumbar spine taken in the operating theatre are often of poor quality and cannot, therefore, be relied upon to identify a particular spinal level.

The skin incision is made in the midline or slightly right or left of the spinous processes, extending longitudinally a short distance above and below the vertebral interspace to be explored. It is deepened at once through the subcutaneous fat layer to the level of the thoracolumbar fascia. In extremely obese patients the depth of the subcutaneous fat layer between the skin and this fascia may be 12 cm or more. This tissue should be handled carefully, and the use of coagulating diathermy reduced to a minimum.

Separation of the paraspinal muscles

An incision is made in the thoracolumbar fascia on one side of the tip of the spinous process, using the cutting current diathermy, passed through a suitable blade-shaped end. The incision continues downwards and upwards immediately adjacent to the side of the spinous process, parallel to the adjacent interspinous ligaments and then to the sides of the related spinous processes. Bleeding occurs at this stage from posterior branches of the lumbar arteries related to the middle of the side of each spinous process. The muscle mass may be retracted with closed dissecting forceps placed into the depth of the space, so that the diathermy blade may cut the musculotendinous attachments from the inferior surfaces of the spinous processes and from the interspinous ligaments near their bases. Throughout this procedure the smoke generated by the diathermy cutting tip can be evacuated with the sucker.

The muscle mass is next separated from the outer surface of each lamina using an appropriate 'elevator', such as the Cobb. Following the use of the muscle elevator which raises the paraspinal muscles laterally to the level of the apophyseal joint capsules, further bleeding may be encountered from posterior branches of the lumbar arteries in the area. This bleeding is readily controlled by inserting cotton swabs bearing X-ray markers (Raytec, Johnson & Johnson, Ascot, UK) packed into the depths of the wound along its length.

The same approach is repeated on the opposite side of the spinous processes until the paraspinal muscle mass has been similarly separated from the roof of the spinal canal. Cotton Raytec swabs are again inserted and the self-retaining retractors of the surgeon's choice then prepared for insertion.

Some surgeons favour muscle stripping on one side of the spine only[7]. Limited approaches of this kind can be recommended for the removal of clearly defined disc prolapses causing unilateral sciatica. Special retractors are available for use in this circumstance.

Bilateral laminal exposure is indicated when stenosis of the spinal canal is present and in cases of isolated disc resorption associated with unilateral disc fragment prolapse.

Considerable blood loss may occur even during this preliminary stage of the approach to the disc prolapse. The technique described above will reduce this haemorrhage to a minimum.

The cotton Raytec swabs are removed from the lower end of the wound on either side of the spinous process. Hand-held retractors are used to expose the back of the sacrum, allowing the first self-retaining retractor to be inserted and fixed in place. This procedure is repeated at the upper end of the wound and the second self-retaining retractor inserted.

At this stage, cotton Raytec swabs are again packed firmly along one side of the spine while attention is focused on the opposite side to identify the lumbosacral junction. Soft-tissue remnants of muscle fibres and fat are then removed from the interspace to be opened. This cleaning-up process can be accomplished rapidly and neatly using a straight pituitary rongeur with a 4 mm cup, taking off first the muscle remnants from the interspinous ligament and then all the soft tissues from the posterior surface of the ligamentum flavum.

Bleeding is not a problem during these manoeuvres at the lumbosacral junction until the extrasynovial fat pad of the apophyseal joint is removed, if this is necessary. On avulsing this fat pad, quite brisk arterial and venous haemorrhage will occur. Using a sucker and cotton Raytec swab, the bleeding vessels are readily identified. The vessels are picked up with the bayonet forceps and coagulated with diathermy. When exposure at the L4–5 interspace is required, the initial clearing procedure is performed and the pars interarticularis of the fifth lumbar lamina is exposed. The sucker tip may be used as a dissector at this stage, sucking up remnants of fatty tissue. The main stem of the posterior branch of the lumbar artery with its accompanying venae comitantes is found constantly at the middle of the outer edge of the pars interarticularis. From it, arcuate branches pass upwards and downwards across the capsule of the apophyseal joint. Bleeding points are easily identified, though care must be taken not to use diathermy on the main stem of this artery anterior to the anterior margin of the pars interarticularis. Damage at the intervertebral foramen to arteries which are destined to supply the regional nerve roots is thereby avoided[8]. In cases where exposure of both sides of the interspace is required, the detailed clearing process, just described, is then completed on the opposite side.

6

Capsular fibres extend medially onto the ligamentum flavum for some distance at its upper margin where it passes beneath the inferior margin of the superior lamina of the interspace. Note (a) the extension of capsular fibres onto the posterior surface of the ligamentum flavum, and (b) the extrasynovial fat pads. The capsular extension should be removed with a straight pituitary rongeur so that, if necessary, portions of the inferior surface of the superior lamina at the interspace may be excised, using an outward-angled rongeur. Some surgeons prefer to use chisels or gouges for this purpose. Bone wax is applied to the bleeding cut surface of the cancellous bone.

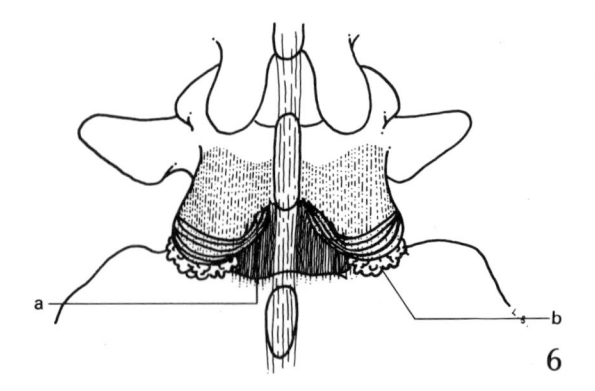

Opening the spinal canal

The ligamentum flavum should be incised vertically in the midline using a scalpel with either a No. 11 or No. 15 blade. The cut edge of the ligamentum flavum is picked up with a fine-toothed forceps and the incision deepened until the epidural fat or the dura itself is exposed.

The blunt end of the Watson Cheyne dissector is then used to widen the opening into the spinal canal. Through the vertical slit in the ligamentum flavum thus created, a small moistened cotton patty is inserted between the ligamentum flavum and the epidural fat, using the curved end of the Watson Cheyne dissector. The ligamentum flavum is then cut in a lateral direction, first at the upper edge of the interspace and later at the lower edge of the interspace, until a flap is raised and turned out laterally.

Even at this early stage of opening the spinal canal, the presence of a large prolapse can be suspected if it is difficult to insert a patty, particularly when attempting to push it laterally under the ligamentum flavum, as the flap in enlarged.

The ligamentum flavum is turned laterally as a flap to the level of the medial edge of the apophyseal joint, and excised using a vertical incision.

Following this opening into the spinal canal, certain landmarks should be identified using a Watson Cheyne probe. Either the blunt or curved end may be inserted, depending on the size of the protrusion at the affected level. If the prolapse is small, the blunt end is inserted laterally, so that the pedicle on the inferior side of the intervertebral disc space can be palpated. The regional nerve root is then palpated. Moving upwards, the posterior surface of the disc may be felt and the disposition of a prolapse assessed.

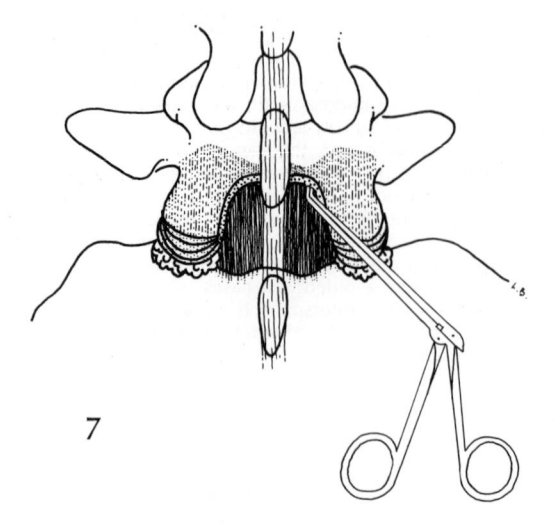

7

If wider exposure is required, it is usually easily achieved by using a 45° outward-angled rongeur. Assuming, for example, that it is necessary to remove more of the outer edge of the ligamentum flavum, then the sucker, with a moistened patty on its tip, may be used to retract the dura and nerve roots towards the midline, while the rongeur is inserted beneath the edge of the ligamentum flavum under direct vision. Depending on the size of the prolapse, it may or may not be possible to insert the angled rongeur. If attempts are made to force the foot-plate of the rongeur between the ligamentum flavum and the nerve root which is being pressed backwards by a large disc prolapse, the root may be bruised or crushed. On occasions, even a thin rongeur cannot be inserted. The interspace, then, will need to be enlarged either superiorly or inferiorly or in both directions, until sufficient space has been created to allow identification of the nerve root as it traverses the vertebral interspace.

8

When dealing with large subrhizal prolapses at the L5–S1 level, for example, enlargement of the interspace may be necessary by removal of part of the superior border of the lamina of S1, commencing initially in the midline and passing laterally. It may be necessary to perform a decompression of the S1 nerve root canal by removing the medial portion of the S1 facet flush with the inner margin of the S1 pedicle. The illustration shows a fourth lumbar vertebra from behind. On the right side of the specimen the fifth lumbar nerve root canal has been unroofed and the inner margin of the pedicle is shown. In the operation of nerve root canal decompression, the apex of the facet also needs to be removed.

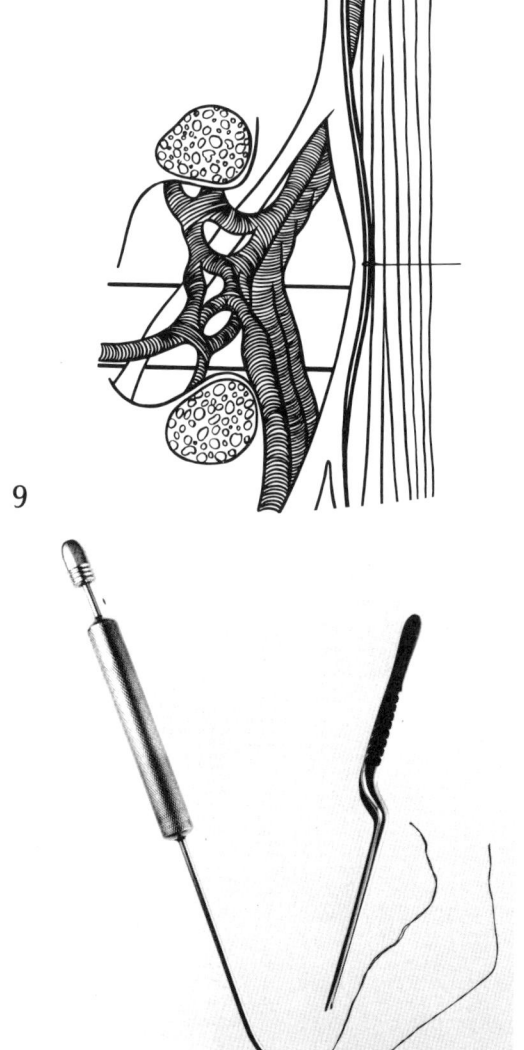

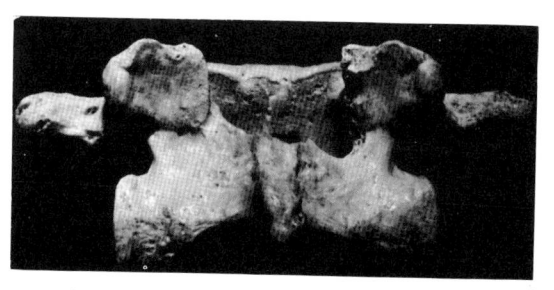

(Reproduced by Courtesy of J. B. Lippincott Co. from Clinical Orthopaedics and Related Research Vol. 115, 1976)

9 & 10

During complicated manoeuvres of this type, haemorrhage may occur from the posterior internal vertebral venous plexus surrounding and lateral to the nerve root. This is usually not troublesome when the patient is in the prone position. On occasions, however, the plexus may be distended, and brisk venous haemorrhage can occur following damage to some of its small branches. *Illustration 9* shows the detailed anatomy of the internal vertebral venous plexus in the lumbar region. The cut edge of the dural sac has been retracted slightly towards the midline. Note the radicular vein which emerges from the dural sac, medial to the nerve root, to join the plexus. Venous haemorrhage is always readily controlled using a patty and sucker as shown in *Illustration 10*.

Bleeding from several points of this plexiform system of veins can be controlled by light packing of a haemostatic substance held in place with a moistened patty. Use of the coagulating diathermy is rarely necessary.

Good exposure of the field with minimal bleeding must be obtained before the nerve root is retracted away from the prolapsed disc material.

Techniques required for different types of disc prolapses

Special points of technique will be described in relation to individual types of disc prolapse.

SMALL SUBRHIZAL PROLAPSE

11

Partial excision of the ligamentum flavum on one side will afford satisfactory access to the canal. Initially, identification of the pedicle, disc and affected nerve root is made using the sucker and patty as a medial retractor, and the blunt end of the Watson Cheyne dissector in the lateral part of the canal. The photograph is a dissection of the lower lumbar spine in an adult and shows some of the relations of the lumbar nerve roots. Note especially the origins of the nerve root sleeves from the dural sac and the courses of the nerve roots in relation to the pedicles.

Blunt dissection will free the epidural fat, and the nerve root can usually be easily retracted medially. The discrete rounded prolapse with intact annular fibres is outlined and a suitable nerve root retractor inserted. The sucker with a moist patty on its tip can be used as a retractor laterally in the interspace, while the assistant holds the nerve root medially. In a dry field, it should be possible to incise the annular fibres over the prolapse in a cruciate fashion, using a No. 11 or No. 15 scalpel blade. The prolapsed tissue then begins to emerge spontaneously and it may be picked out with a straight pituitary rongeur of appropriate dimension.

Only a small volume of disc tissue can be removed in such cases and curettage of the interspace is not recommended. Cases of this type are ideally suited for the use of an operating microscope – for so-called microdiscectomy.

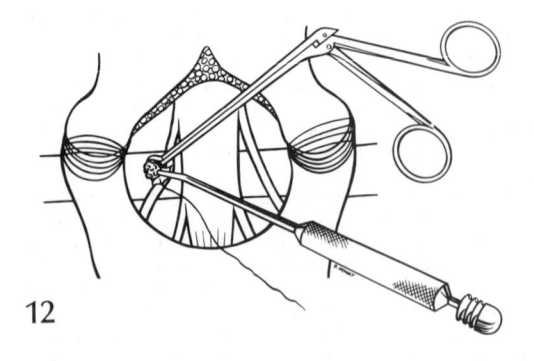

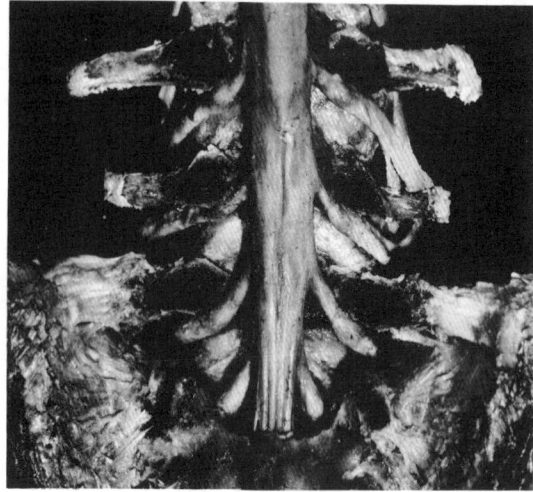

Dissected by Dr M. C. Crock. 11

LARGE SUBRHIZAL PROLAPSE

Adequate exposure on the side of the prolapse is essential. Technical details for the enlargement both superiorly and inferiorly have been outlined above. If the affected root is flattened, its lateral margin is difficult to distinguish from the disc tissues beneath it. The nerve root sleeve should be identified at its junction with the dura above, or the nerve root itself should be defined at the level of the inferior pedicle. By either method, with the use of an appropriate nerve root dissector, the nerve root can be identified and retracted off the prolapse either to its medial or lateral side. Very fine straight and curved pituitary rongeurs will be required to remove the first of the fragments of prolapsed tissue, possibly through an incision in intact annular fibres. Only after the removal of initial fragments with small instruments will it be possible to complete the dissection and retraction of the nerve root from the bulk of the prolapse.

12

As the tension on the nerve root is released it can be easily retracted. The opening in the annular fibres may be enlarged under vision, and rongeurs of increasing cup size inserted for removal of free disc fragments from the interspace. The disposition of the instruments during removal of prolapsed disc tissue is shown. The sucker with a patty on the end of it may be used as a retractor held by the surgeon in his left hand while, with the rongeur in his right hand, disc fragments are lifted out from the interspace.

12

13

When large amounts of disc material can be removed easily, the risk of penetration of a rongeur deep into the interspace, with the possibility of damage to intra-abdominal structures, is high. The use of ring curettes is recommended in these circumstances for removal of loose disc fragments and vertebral end-plate cartilage. Bilateral root canal and foraminal decompressions should be performed by completing the removal of the ligamentum flavum laterally along with the inner and superior margins of the superior articular facets of the inferior vertebra at the interspace. Excision of the whole facet joint should be avoided.

SEQUESTRATED DISC FRAGMENTS

When free fragments of disc tissue are found at the lumbosacral level, yet the posterior annular fibres of the L5–S1 disc space are intact, exploration of the higher interspace is essential. In these circumstances careful palpation of the L5–S1 disc with the blunt end of the Watson Cheyne dissector, beneath the dural sac towards the midline, will be necessary before it can be safely assumed that the disc tissue has not arisen from that interspace.

If, on the other hand, the L4–5 interspace has been exposed and a rather adherent nerve root retracted from the back of the disc to reveal a circumscribed rounded defect in the annulus, then free sequestrated disc material may be found at the lower interspace.

CENTRAL DISC PROLAPSE

If a central disc prolapse is present, it is usually, though not always, suspected in the early stages of opening the spinal canal. For example, the canal may be opened on one side and the nerve root which comes into view cannot be retracted towards the midline, though the disc beneath it and lateral to it appears normal. In such a case, digital palpation of the dural sac confirms the diagnosis.

Wide exposure may be required, even involving excision of the spinous process and the arch of the lamina on the superior side of the interspace. Careful attention should be paid to removal of the laminal arch, so that the pars interarticularis on each side is left intact. Once adequate exposure of the spinal canal has been achieved, the size of the central disc prolapse can be estimated by digital palpation. Access to the prolapse is then usually possible from one or other side of the dural sac.

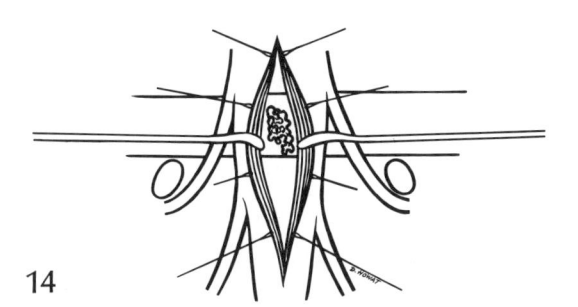

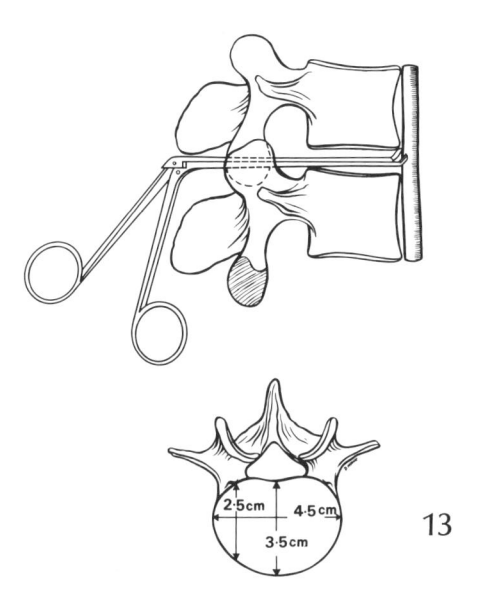

14

Rarely is it necessary to open the dural sac in the midline. Should such a course be followed, use of low vacuum suction is essential, the sucker tip being guarded by a small patty. Filaments of the cauda equina can be retracted easily to either side using smooth rounded instruments. At no time should an unguarded sucker be placed within the dural sac as filaments of the cauda equina may be avulsed. The actual process of removal of disc tissue is easily and rapidly accomplished by the transdural route after incision of the dura anteriorly. It is likely that the prolapse will have emerged on one side of the posterior ligament. If large quantities of disc material can be easily removed, it is wise to use a ring curette to clear other loose disc remnants from the interspace. Uncontrolled forward movements with rongeurs or curettes introduce the added risks of major vessel or gut injury should the instruments slip into the abdominal cavity. Some authors recommend closure of the anterior layer of the dural sac following this procedure but this is not always necessary. However, the posterior layer should be closed with a continuous fine dural stitch, care being taken to avoid trapping filaments of the cauda equina in the closing suture.

When many fragments of intervertebral disc tissue have been removed, bilateral nerve root canal decompressions and foraminotomies should be performed. This involves excision of part of the upper edge of the inferior lamina. The inner border and the tip of the superior articular process should be removed flush with the medial border of its supporting pedicle. The whole of the ligamentum flavum is excised. The most effective instruments for this purpose are 45° outward-angled pituitary rongeurs of appropriate sizes.

EXTRAFORAMINAL DISC PROLAPSE

This type of disc prolapse is uncommon, though it can be readily indentified with CT scanning, CT discography or MRI examination of the spine.

The level of disc prolapse should be confirmed with control radiographs in the operating theatre. A short incision is made over the middle of the appropriate sacrospinalis muscle mass. The thoracolumbar fascia is split in the line of the skin incision. The muscle fibres are split by blunt dissection and retractors inserted to expose the vertically orientated fibres of the intertransverse muscle. The medial border of this muscle is identified between the two transverse processes at their junctions with the pedicles. The fibres are separated from the upper surface of the inferior transverse process and retracted laterally. The nerve root is then seen where it lies outside the intervertebral foramen. An operating microscope is useful in deep dissection of this type, but is not essential. With careful blunt dissection, the nerve root may be separated from the disc prolapse, which is removed in the usual manner, under vision. Haemorrhage should not be a problem if the main branches of the lumbar artery and its veins are preserved[8].

Disc prolapses associated with other special problems

With spinal canal stenosis

This should be recognized preoperatively in most instances, if myelography or MRI examinations have been performed. Disc prolapses found in these cases are often small. Adequate spinal canal decompression with bilateral nerve root canal and foraminal decompressions must be performed following excision of the disc prolapse.

With nerve root and other anomalies

Recognition of anomalies of the nerve roots or of the regional blood vessels demands careful exposure[8]. A conjoined nerve root which arises from the dural sac at right angles, passing directly laterally through the intervertebral foramen across the posterior surface of the disc, may, at operation, easily be mistaken for a prolapse. It may therefore be incised, excised or avulsed in error.

With isolated disc resorption

Unilateral sciatica in cases of isolated disc resorption[1] is not common. The most important part of the surgery for this condition is bilateral nerve root canal decompression and foraminotomy. The disc prolapse in such instances usually consists of a small fragment of vertebral end-plate cartilage situated under the root to which it may be adherent, requiring careful dissection, especially as the root may be flattened.

With spondylolisthesis

Disc prolapse may occur at the level of the spondylolisthesis or above it. The prolapsed disc fragments should be removed and a decision made on the use of supplementary procedures such as spinal fusion or spinal canal decompression.

Upper lumbar disc prolapses

Prolapses may occur in the L1–2 and L2–3 area. Operations at these levels are potentially hazardous. Providing the dural sac is retracted gently and rongeurs of small calibre are used, injury to the conus medullaris should not occur.

Preserving the bony canal

In the past it has been common practice to remove either half of one side of a lamina, or to cut a narrow channel between two disc spaces across half of a lamina while attempting to locate an elusive disc prolapse. This interference with the roof of the spinal canal should be avoided, particularly in cases with spinal canal or nerve root canal stenosis. Exploration of an intervertebral disc space can be performed satisfactorily through a limited exposure, carried out along the lines recommended above. If no lesion is found at one level, due to error, then it is better to look at the next level upwards or downwards from the primary exploration without disturbing the integrity of the lamina.

Care of the dural sac

Dural tears are most likely to occur in complicated cases, for example, in spinal canal stenosis, where opening of the canal proves difficult, or again, in the course of separating an adherent root from a disc prolapse. They may be inflicted even before the ligamentum flavum has been opened, if a rongeur slips into the dural canal. Dural defects should be identified carefully and repaired using fine sutures.

Wound closure

Suction drainage may be used but should be avoided if the dura has been repaired. The thoracolumbar fascia is reattached to the midline ligaments on each side, thereby restoring the extensor function[9]. Deep muscle sutures are avoided unless a spinous process has been excised. Subcuticular plain catgut or polyglycolic acid sutures are used and tied carefully to avoid crushing the fatty tissue. In extremely obese patients, excessive use of diathermy in the fatty layer and rough handling of this tissue will result in the leakage of liquefied fat from the wound, with subsequent infection in this layer. Deep tension sutures passed through the skin, and tied over rubber tubing may be necessary. Skin closure is best effected with subcuticular sutures.

References

1. Crock HV. Traumatic disc injury. In: Vinken PJ, Bruyn GW, eds. *Handbook of clinical neurology*. Vol. 25: Injuries of the spine and spinal cord. Pt. 1. Amsterdam: North Holland, 1976: 481–511.

2. Nachemson A. Intradiscal measurements of pH in patients with lumbar rhizopathies. *Acta Orthop Scand* 1969; 40: 23–42.

3. Blikra G. Intra-dural herniated lumbar disc. *J Neurosurg* 1969; 31: 676–9.

4. Hooper J. Low back pain and manipulation. *Med J Aust* 1973; 1: 549–51.

5. Verbiest H. Further experience on the pathological influence of a developmental narrowness of the bony lumbar vertebral canal. *J Bone Joint Surg [Br]* 1955; 37-B: 576–83.

6. Verbiest H. *Neurogenic intermittent claudication with special references to stenosis of the lumbar vertebral canal*. Amsterdam: North Holland, 1976.

7. Finneson BE. *Low back pain*. Philadelphia: Lippincott, 1973.

8. Crock HV, Yoshizawa H. *The blood supply of the vertebral column and spinal cord in man*. New York: Springer Verlag, 1977.

9. Crock HV, Crock MC. A technique for decompression of the lumbar spine canal. *Neuro-Orthopaedics* 1988; 5: 96–9.

Illustrations by Gillian Oliver

Chemonucleolysis for herniated intervertebral disc

Michael Sullivan FRCS
Consultant Orthopaedic Surgeon, Royal National Orthopaedic Hospital, London, UK

Introduction

Chemonucleolysis is the technique of injecting an enzyme into the nucleus of a prolapsed disc to reduce the tension. The most commonly used enzyme is chymopapain. This is a proteolytic enzyme acting on the proteoglycan of the disc. It breaks down the water-binding capacity of the proteoglycan molecules. Thus the technique of chemonucleolysis is not useful in the old degenerate disc.

Indications

This technique should ideally be used only on a patient under the age of 40 years who has a ruptured intervertebral disc. To make this diagnosis there must be the following features.

1. Normal plain radiographs.
2. More leg than back pain, the leg pain being distal to the knee.
3. Straight-leg raising limited in the affected leg, with or without cross-leg pain.
4. A positive neurological sign or symptom: an absent ankle jerk or typical paraesthesia in the lateral foot and toes for the S1 nerve root.
5. A positive neuroradiological investigation, including a radiculogram, computed tomography, magnetic resonance imaging and a venogram.

Contraindications

1. Previous injection of chymopapain. Whereas 0.75 per cent of patients will suffer acute anaphylaxis at the first injection, 12 per cent will be affected at subsequent injection.
2. Pregnancy.
3. Disc prolapse above the conus medullaris. The cervical discs have been injected, but it is unwise to do so.
4. Severe cardiac disease. Adrenaline may be needed in a case of anaphylaxis.

Preoperative

Anaesthesia

The procedure must be undertaken where there is excellent biplanar image intensification. This may be the operating theatre or radiology department. General or local anaesthesia may be used; the latter is safer. With general anaesthesia, no 'volatile' gas such as halothane (Fluothane) should be used. These gases sensitize the heart to adrenaline which will be needed if anaphylaxis occurs.

The patient is premedicated with papaveretum, scopolamine, promethazine hydrochloride and hydrocortisone, whether for local or general anaesthesia. In the anaesthetic room the patient is given phenoperidine and midazolam, and a wide-bore intravenous cannula is inserted. It is unwise to do this without an anaesthetist present. The patient must have a cardiac monitor.

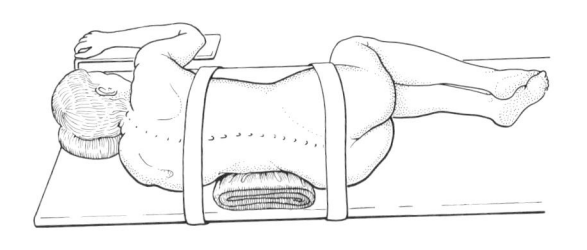

Position of patient

1

The patient is placed in the left lateral position, on the radiolucent table. A wedge is put under the loin to get a reverse curve to the spine. The back must be kept absolutely vertical by putting the right arm on a rest and strapping the buttocks. The hips and knees are at 90°/90° flexion.

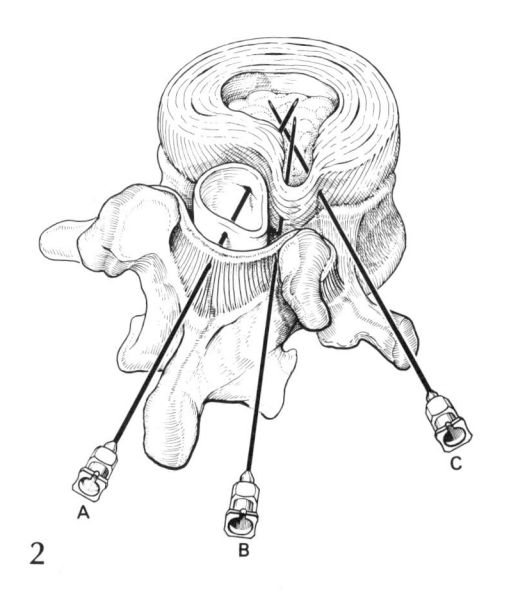

Technique

2

Local anaesthetic is injected into the skin. The needle is placed 8–10 cm from the midline. The correct position is shown by needle C; needle A would cross the dura, while needle B would cross the root sleeve.

532 Thoracic and lumbar spine

3 & 4

For the L4–5 disc the needle is advanced in the coronal plane at 45° to the plane of the back, but at L5–S1 it must also pass 30° caudal.

5

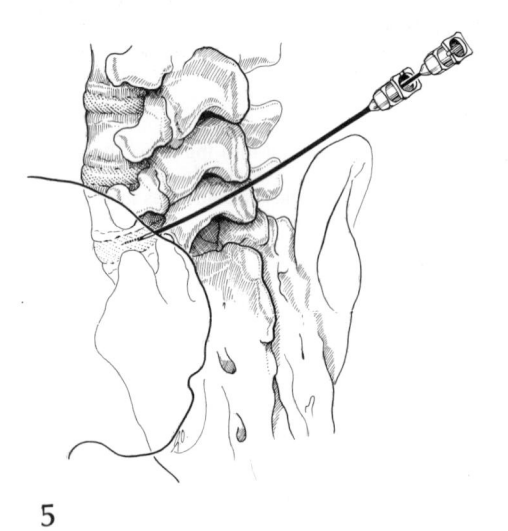

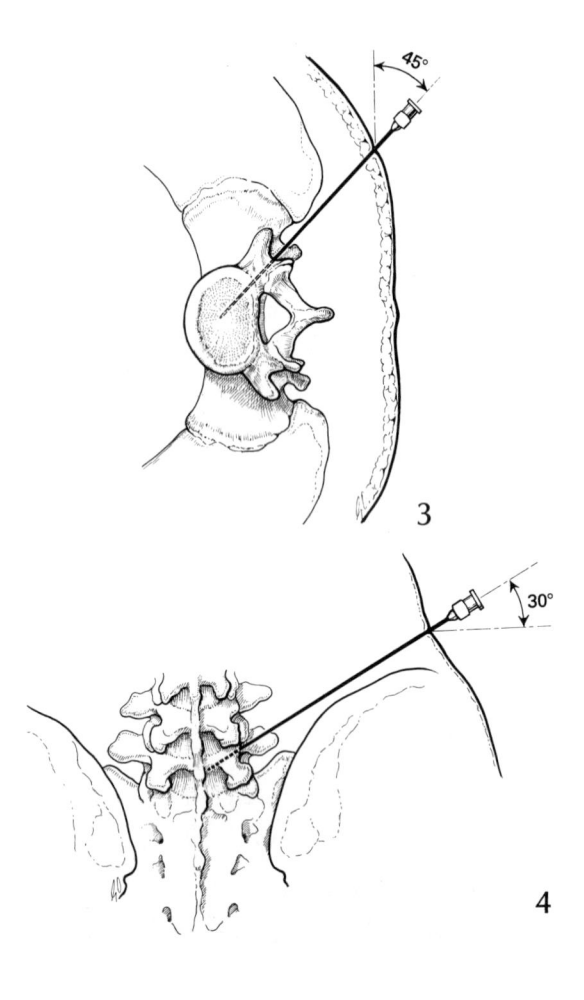

It may be extremely difficult to get the needle into the L5–S1 space, and this is helped by passing a curved 22-gauge needle down the 18-gauge needle.

6

The needle must lie in the middle third of the disc, and be checked with biplanar radiography. It is possible to slide the needle down the side of the annulus, and if the radiograph is taken in only one plane the needle appears to be in the centre of the disc when it is not. When the needle is correctly placed it should not be necessary to use discography but, if there is doubt, 1 ml of water-soluble contrast can be injected.

When the needle is in position, 8 mg of chymopapain is injected. The enzyme comes in a vial containing 20 mg in the dried state; this is dissolved in 5 ml of water. It is extremely rare that one needs to inject more than one disc space. A soft disc prolapse at more than one level rarely occurs.

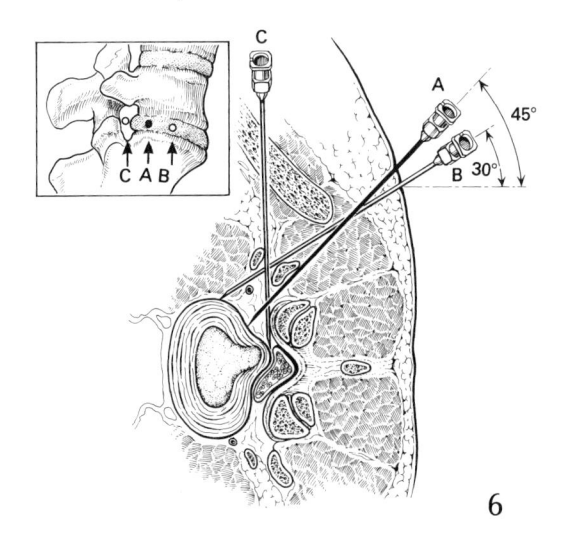

6

Postoperative management

The patient must be kept in the operating environment for 3 hours to be watched for signs of anaphylaxis. If this occurs it is treated with adrenaline, hydrocortisone and intravenous fluids.

The patient is then kept in bed for 2 days and then discharged wearing a spinal corset. Depending on occupation, the return to work may be 1 to 6 weeks later.

Complications

1. Acute anaphylaxis. This is not a problem as long as the contraindications are observed.
2. Ascending transverse myelitis. This has occurred in some patients who have been injected intrathecally in error. The paraplegia is permanent. Every one of the patients who have had this complication have been injected by a doctor doing his first ten injections.
3. Disc space infection.
4. Transient cauda equina loss.

Illustrations by Gillian Oliver

Posterior decompression for spinal stenosis

Michael Sullivan FRCS
Consultant Orthopaedic Surgeon, Royal National Orthopaedic Hospital, London, UK

Introduction

The word stenosis means 'narrowing of a tube', and therefore any spinal canal which is narrowed could be defined as having spinal stenosis. This would include virtually every person over the age of 70 years. The proper medical definition is narrowing of the whole or part of the spinal canal leading to pain in one or both lower limbs. It does not include patients who experience back pain at night and also have a narrow canal. To decompress a spine simply for back pain is almost always a mistake.

Preoperative

Presentation

The syndrome presents most commonly in men after the fifth decade. The leg pain may be present continuously but much more commonly on exercise. The pain may be bilateral or unilateral and can easily be confused with vascular claudication. Both occur in older men.

In neurogenic claudication the patients develop pain at a certain walking distance; if they continue beyond that distance they will develop numbness and paraesthesia; and occasionally motor dysfunction such as a drop foot. The patients have a simian stance which flexes the lumbar spine and eases the root tension. They will find it easier to walk uphill than downhill, and much easier to ride a bicycle as the spine is flexed.

On examination the patients may or may not have motor, reflex or sensory loss. They invariably have full straight-leg raising.

Spinal stenosis may be unilateral, involving one nerve root, or segmental; extremely rarely it involves the whole canal. This is a very important distinction as only a minimum of surgery should be performed to relieve the patient's symptoms. Massive laminectomies are disastrous. The patients invariably become back cripples who need spinal fusions. The end-result is that the patient wishes he was back with his claudication, which he could at least relieve with rest. The essence of treatment is minimal surgery.

Classification

Spinal stenosis is classified into 2 types:
1. Congenital
   (a) Idiopathic
   (b) Achondroplastic
2. Acquired stenosis
   (a) Degenerative
       (i) Central canal
       (ii) Peripheral canal and lateral recess
       (iii) Degenerative spondylolisthesis.
   (b) Combined – e.g. degenerative with disc prolapse
   (c) Spondylolisthetic
       (i) Dysplastic
       (ii) Isthmic
   (d) Iatrogenic
       (i) After laminectomy
       (ii) After spinal fusion (anterior or posterior)
   (e) Post-traumatic (late changes).

The most common type is the peripheral canal degenerative stenosis and the most difficult to treat is the iatrogenic type.

Assessment

Once the clinical diagnosis is made, investigations are needed to confirm the level of involvement and to plan the surgery.

The most useful investigations are a water-soluble myelogram and magnetic resonance imaging. They will give an overview of the state of the canal. However, spinal stenosis is not a diagnosis made from a myelogram alone: a narrowed column of contrast medium is not a reason for decompression.

The exact root or roots involved must be accurately assessed. This can often be found from the history and examination but electromyograms and nerve root injections will help. Once it is decided which roots are involved then computed tomography (CT) can be used to visualize the site of compression accurately. A CT scan should not be the first line investigation.

It is seldom necessary to decompress more than one segment and never necessary to do a laminectomy. The only exception to this is in achondroplasia.

Decompression

Position of patient

1a & b

The patient is placed prone on a firm rubber mattress strapped on the operating table. There is a hole in the mattress for the patient's abdomen, to stop pressure on the lumbar veins. The table is broken in order to extend the patient's lumbar spine.

Incision

2

A midline incision is made from the upper sacrum to just above the level of the stenosis.

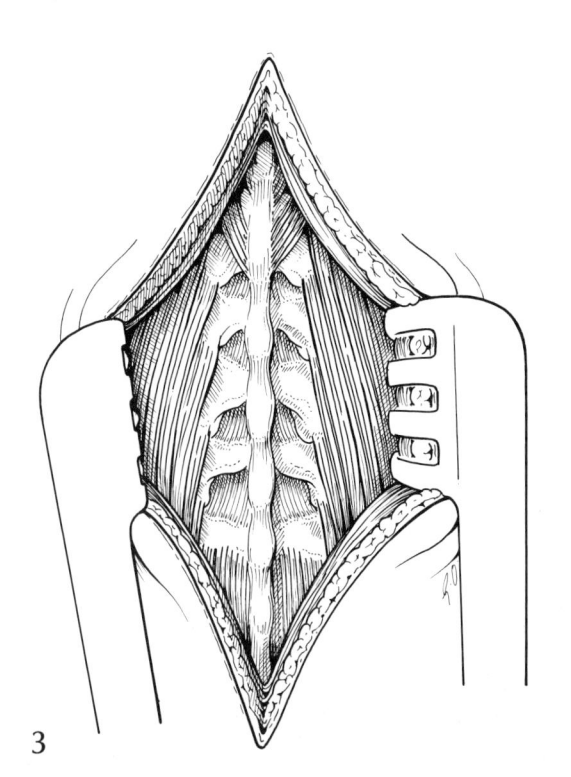

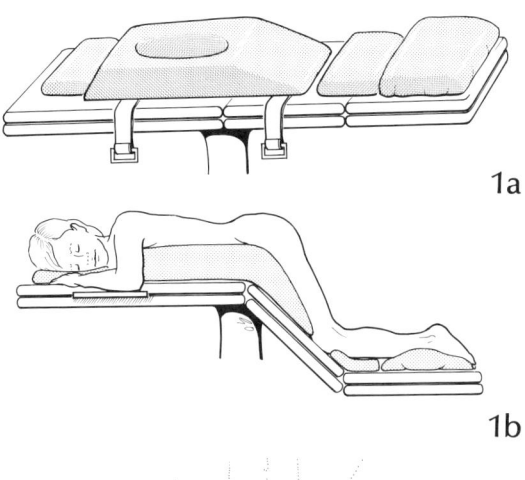

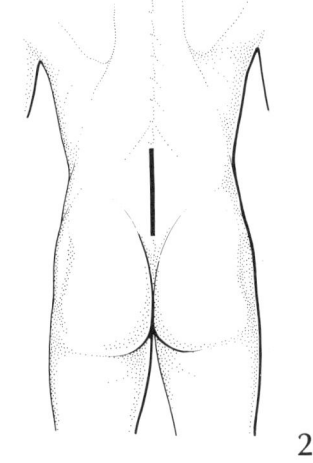

3

Using a cutting diathermy the fascia and muscles are divided from the spinous processes. This cannot be done if the patient has had a previous laminectomy. A knife is then used.

536 Thoracic and lumbar spine

Exposure of the spine

4

The muscles are then stripped laterally with a Cobb's elevator to just lateral to the facet joints. As long as the stripping is kept close to bone the bleeding is minimal. The area can be packed with swabs for 3–4 minutes, which will stop the bleeding. A strong self-retaining retractor, e.g. a Harris, is then placed in position.

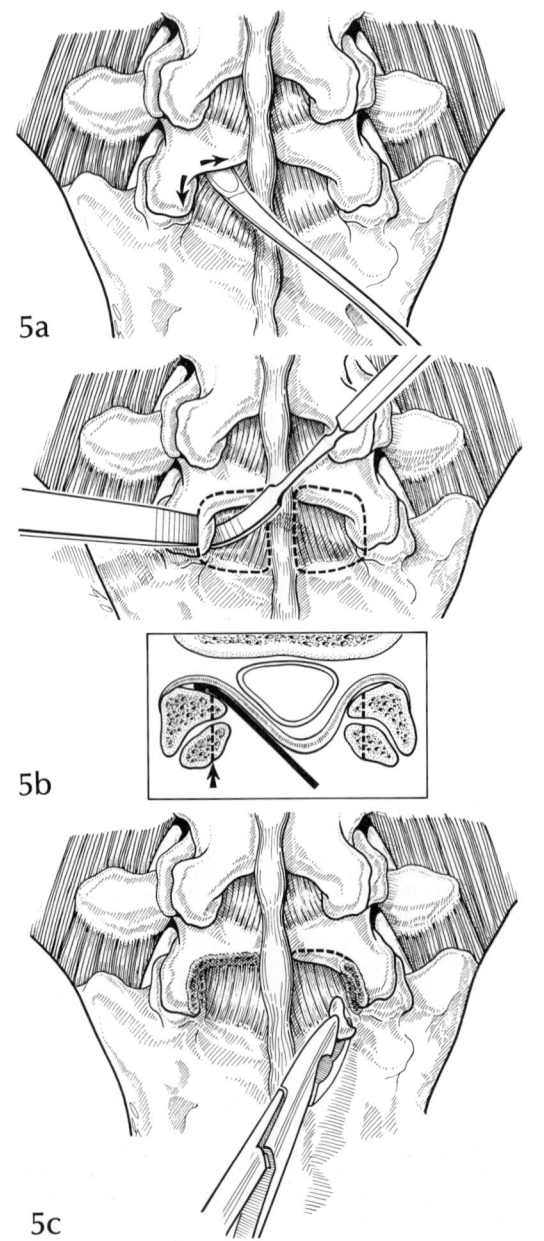

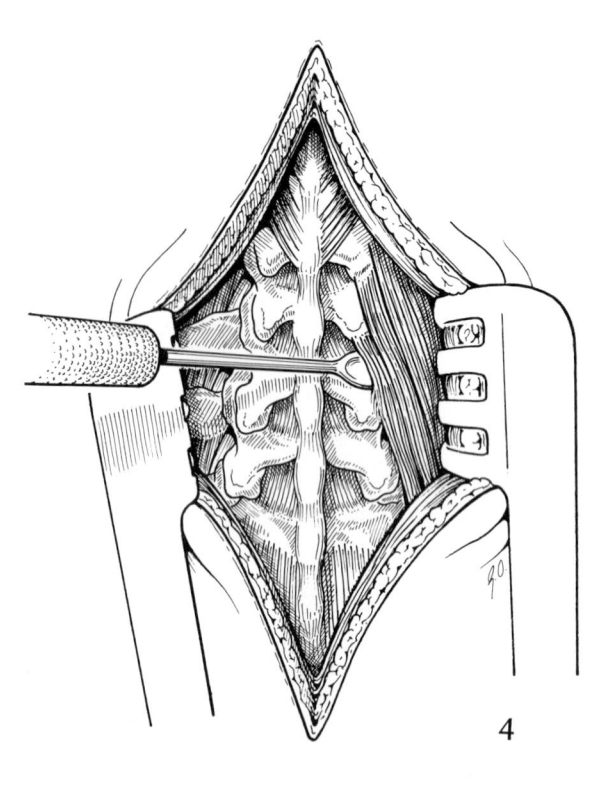

Dissection of the vertebra

5a

An Adson's elevator is then passed under the lamina to free the ligamentum flavum, and worked laterally under the facet joint. The deep (or anterior capsule) is continuous with the ligamentum flavum. It is important to begin the dissection laterally and work medially. Starting medially in a very tight canal can cause a lesion of the cauda equina.

5b

A MacDonald's dissector is passed under the facet joint and the lateral lamina. The bone is then cut with a sharp narrow osteotome.

5c

The bone is removed with narrow rongeurs. The ligamentum flavum should not be opened until all the bone work is done: it acts as an excellent protection to the dura.

Partial excision of lamina and facet joint

6

The ligamentum flavum is then opened and removed as one piece, working from lateral to medial. A MacDonald's dissector should always be passed between ligamentum and dura. It is possible for the dura to be stuck to the ligamentum flavum.

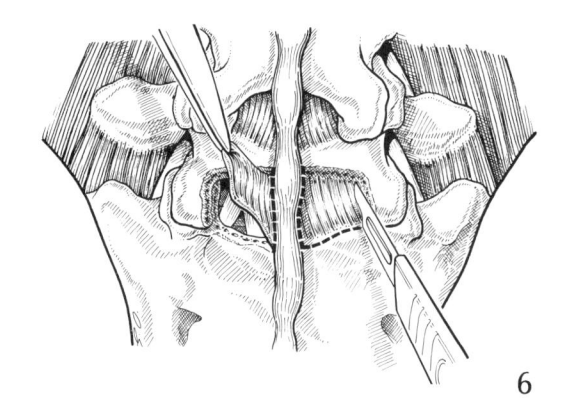

7

The classic way of performing this procedure should not be used: if punches are used under the lamina or facet joint they will bruise the nerve root and lead to intraneural fibrosis. The 'battered nerve root' will lead to intractable root pain.

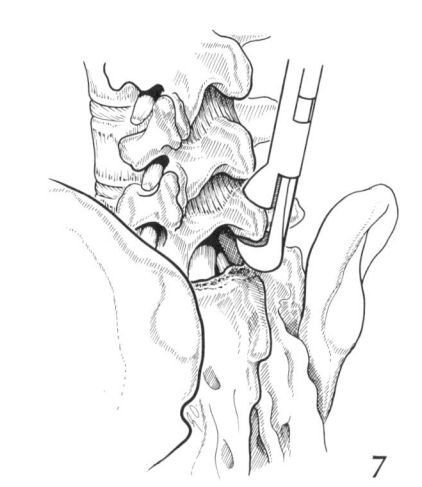

8

The manoeuvre shown in illustrations 5a, b, c and 6 can be undertaken at as many levels as is necessary, either bilaterally or unilaterally. It is unnecessary to do a laminectomy. A narrow bridge of lamina can always be left. It is most important to leave the midline structures which will maintain the tenting of the dura. The nerve roots must be completely freed by undercutting the facet joints. A complete facetectomy should not be done, nor any damage to the pars interarticularis, which will lead to an unstable spine. The lamina is a shingled structure so that the cutting back of the leading edge will decompress the midline structures.

The deep part of the interspinous ligament can be excised. At the end of the operation the nerve roots and central dura should be quite free.

A sucker should not be used during the operation as it only causes more bleeding of the epidural veins. It is better to pack swabs to control the bleeding. Hypotension is unsafe in the elderly.

538   Thoracic and lumbar spine

Multiple level decompression

9

A multiple-level interlaminar decompression can be very difficult and time-consuming. If a classical laminectomy is done, excision should still begin laterally and proceed medially. The most important part of the surgery is still the decompression of the lateral recess.

The worst possible result is a large laminectomy with failure to decompress the nerve roots. The patient then has the iatrogenic back pain plus the original root stenosis.

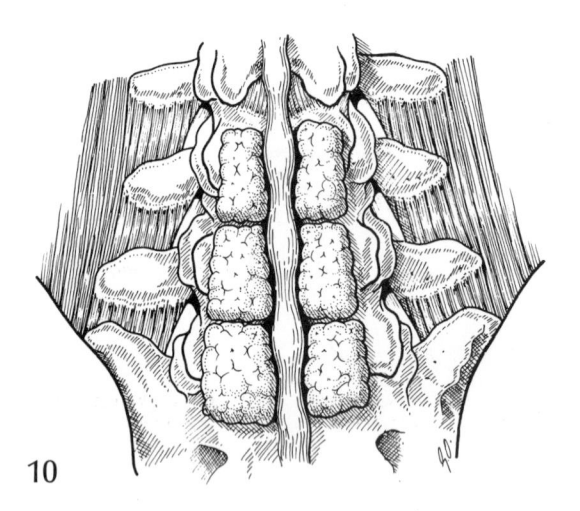

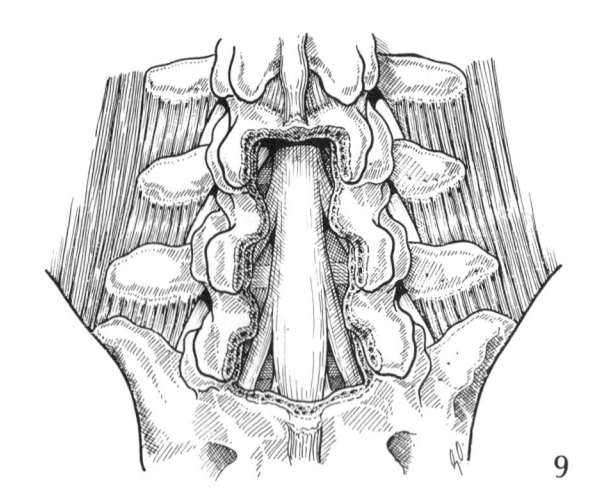

Closure

10

A thick fat graft is cut from the subcutaneous layer and laid on the exposed theca and nerve roots. Foreign material should not be used. It is not necessary to drain the wound. Haemostasis should be complete. If there is a dural leak the wound must not be drained. The wound is then closed in layers.

Postoperative management

The patient is nursed free in bed and can get up after 48 hours. Activities increase within the limits of discomfort. The symptoms may not resolve for 6 weeks because of local oedema of the nerve roots. Full activities begin after 3 months.

Illustrations by Paul Richardson after A. Barrett and F. Price

Posterior lumbar spinal fusion

E. O'Gorman Kirwan MA, FRCS, FRCS(Ed)
Consultant Orthopaedic Surgeon, University College Hospital and Royal National Orthopaedic Hospital, London, UK

Introduction

Indications and contraindications

The posterior spinal elements must be intact, thereby excluding lytic spondylolisthesis with a defect in the pars interarticularis or cases when extensive laminectomies have been performed.

The advantage of this technique is that it facilitates combined exposure of the neural canal and subsequent removal of discs or facetectomy with arthrodesis in one exposure and thereby preserves the segmental neurovascular supply to the dorsal musculature. It can also provide internal fixation with consequent earlier mobilization and comfort to the patient and does not necessarily require a brace or plaster of Paris.

Preoperative

No special preparatory measures are necessary.

Anaesthesia

General anaesthesia with intratracheal intubation is essential. Blood transfusion may be necessary.

Position of patient

The patient is placed in the prone position on a spinal support which allows the abdomen to hang freely in order to prevent pressure on the intra-abdominal veins. The anterosuperior spines should be over the break in the table to allow flexion and extension under vision.

Operation

Incision

1

The skin incision extends from above the third lumbar spine to the first sacral spine and then curves to one side, producing a flap in order to facilitate exposure of the posterior iliac crest.

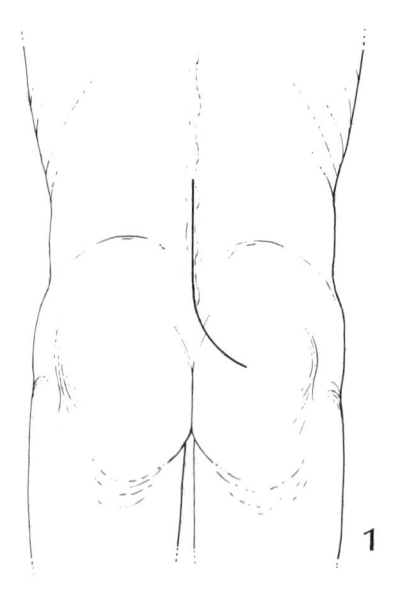

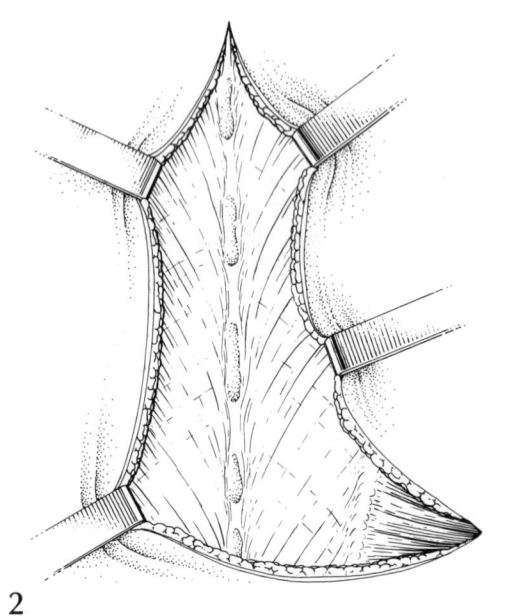

Exposure of iliac donor site

2

The flap consisting of the skin and superficial fascia is elevated, exposing the donor crest; care must be taken to avoid damage to the structurally important thoracolumbar fascia at its insertion into the iliac crest.

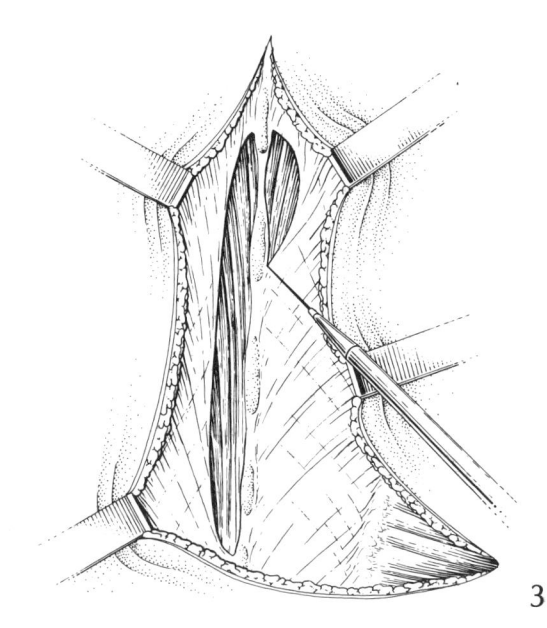

Stripping of muscles

3 & 4

The fascia is divided in the midline on either side of the spinous processes using cutting diathermy. The muscles are elevated and stripped from the spinous processes, laminae and articular facets using a Cobb's elevator and not an osteotome, in order to avoid damage to the articular facet capsules at higher levels.

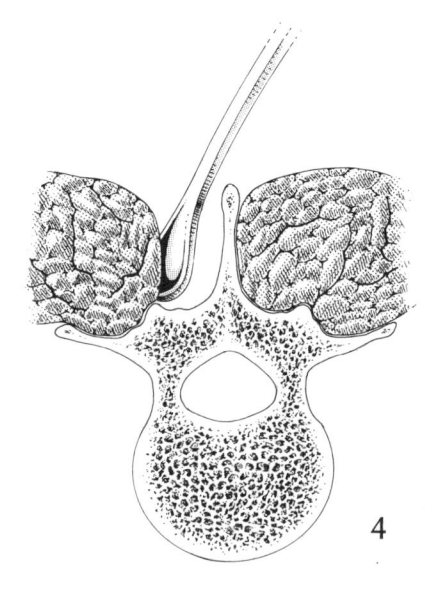

Decortication of laminae

5 & 6

Further dissection is needed to clear soft tissues from the laminae, spinous processes and capsule of the articular facets. A bone-nibbling forceps is useful for this. The bone is then decorticated using a Capener gouge.

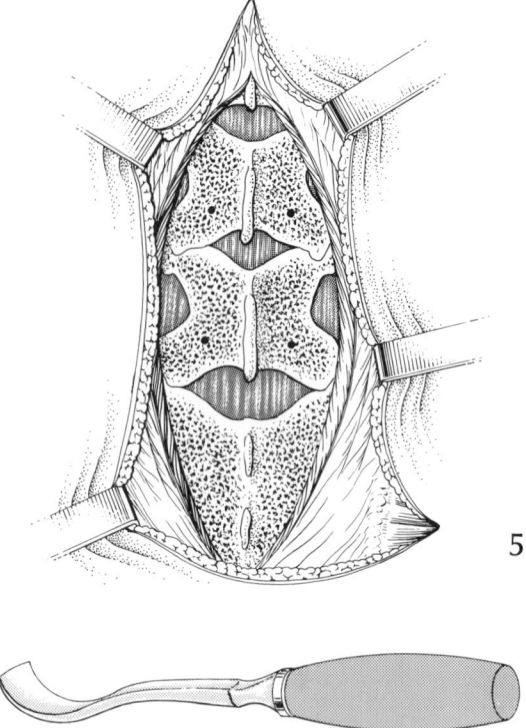

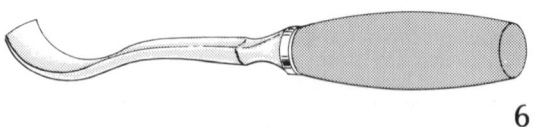

Insertion of screws

7

Holes are drilled into the laminae of the vertebra above the level to be fused using a hand drill; the drill, 3 mm in diameter, is directed at an angle varying with the segmental level so as to lie in bone and avoid damage to the nerve roots.

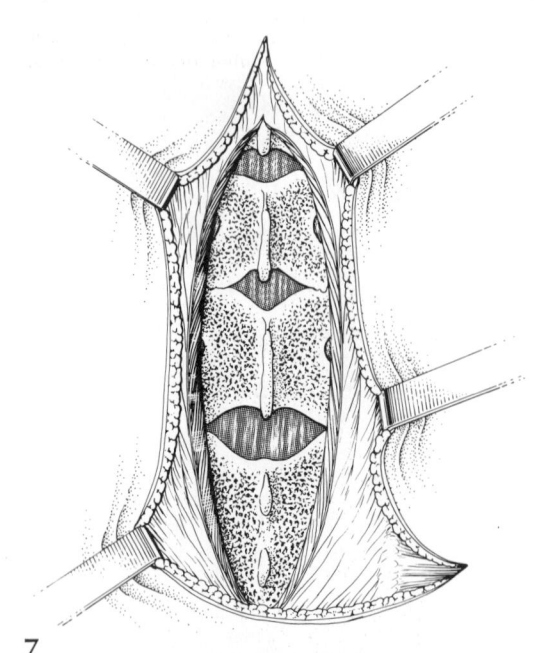

Direction of screws

8

The screws must travel from the vertebra above, across the joint and enter the pedicle and body of the vertebra below.

Angle and length of screw

L4–L5	10–15° degrees from midline 30° upwards from horizontal Length 3–4.5 cm
Lumbosacral level	30° outwards from midline 30° upwards from horizontal Length 4–5 cm

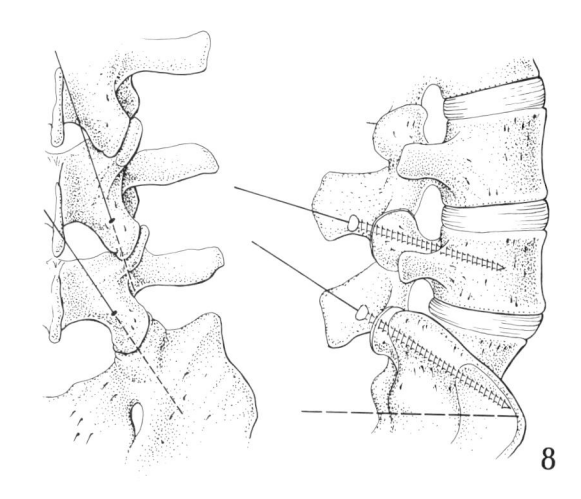

Removal of bone from the ilium

9

Bone must be taken from the outer table of the iliac crest, avoiding any damage to the insertion of the thoracolumbar fascia and the small cutaneous nerves. The gluteal fascia and gluteus maximus are elevated from the outer table and the graft taken as cancellous slivers after removal of the cortical lid. The gluteus maximus and fascia are then resutured to the iliac crest.

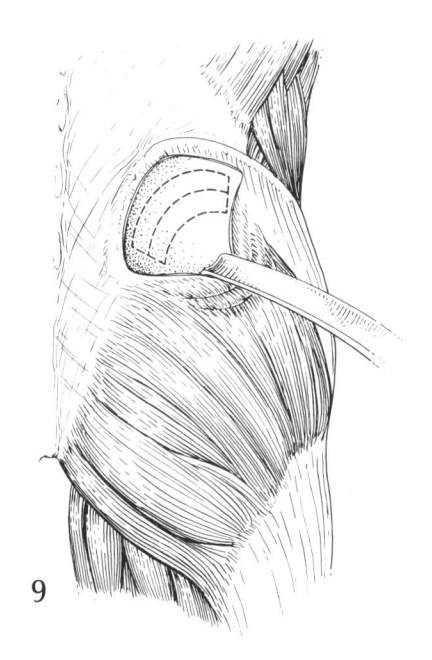

Insertion of graft

10

The slivers are placed on the decorticated laminae and chips inserted around them.

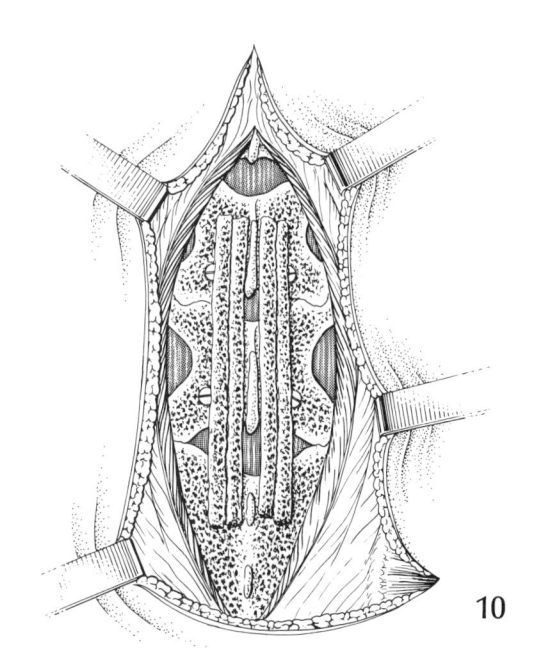

Suture of thoracolumbar fascia

11

The thoracolumbar fascia is sutured across the midline, replacing the muscles in their correct position. Closure of the wound is completed with interrupted subcutaneous and skin drainage.

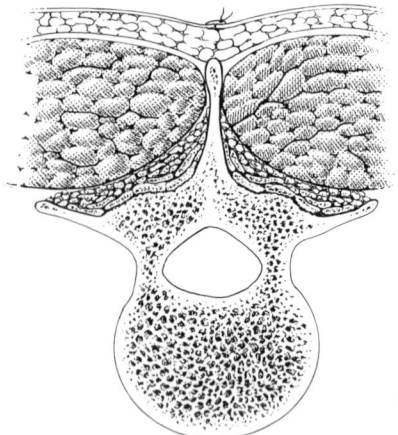

Drainage of wound

12

A vacuum drain is inserted into the donor site and crosses the midline deep to the superficial fascia.

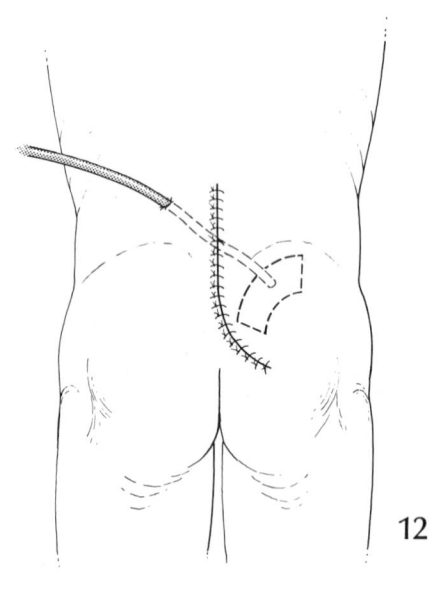

Postoperative management

A gauze and wool dressing is applied and the patient is nursed in an ordinary bed. The drain is removed after 48 hours.

The patient is mobilized out of bed when muscle control has returned. The patient should be able to turn freely in bed and do extension, abdominal and straight-leg raising exercises before being allowed to walk. This is usually accomplished within a few days. Thereafter the patient is supported in a light plaster of Paris lumbosacral support or corset for 12 weeks when increased activity may be allowed.

Illustrations by Paul Richardson after A. Barrett

Intertransverse fusion for spondylolisthesis and lumbar instability

E. O'Gorman Kirwan   MA, FRCS FRCS(Ed)
Consultant Orthopaedic Surgeon, University College Hospital and Royal National Orthopaedic Hospital, London, UK

Introduction

Spondylolisthesis is a mechanical derangement which has a number of very different aetiological types.

Surgery may be required to:

1. relieve the symptoms caused by compression of the neural elements on the spinal canal (decompression);
2. relieve the pain of instability (arthrodesis); or
3. a combination of both.

If there are no neural compressive symptoms the dorsal midline muscles may be preserved and an intertransverse fusion performed by splitting the erector spinae muscles bilaterally in their lateral two-thirds.

Conversely, if a combined procedure of decompression and fusion is required, a midline approach with extensive muscle retraction as far as the tips of the transverse processes will be required.

546 Thoracic and lumbar spine

Operations

INTERTRANSVERSE FUSION WITHOUT DECOMPRESSION

Incisions

1a & b

Two curved vertical incisions extending across the posterior iliac crest and about 7.5 cm from the midline are normally used.

A transverse skin incision just below the iliac crest produces a more cosmetic scar and can be used if the patient is not very large or the extent of the fusion is limited.

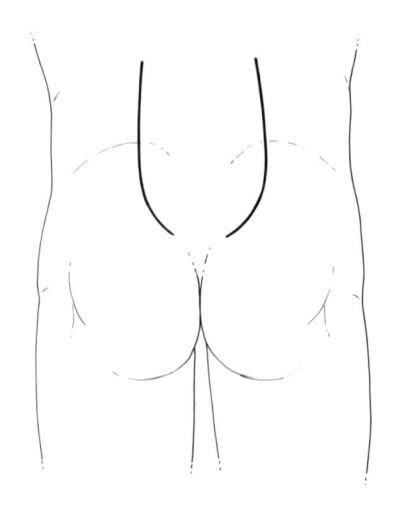

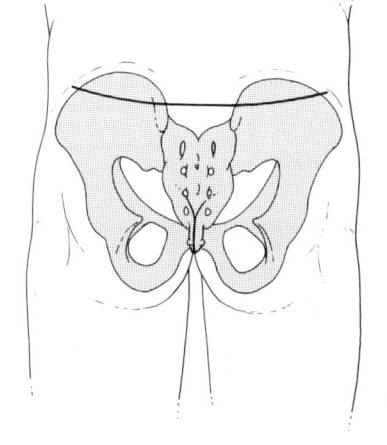

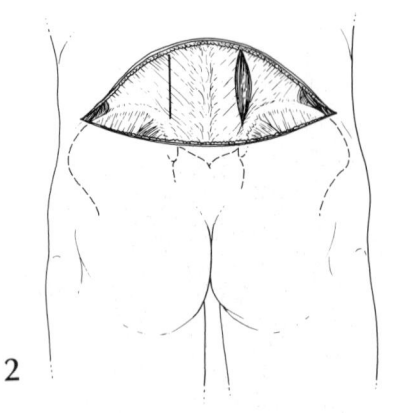

Division of thoracolumbar fascia

2

The thoracolumbar fascia is split vertically in its lateral two-thirds and the erector spinae muscles are split in the same plane.

Stripping of soft tissues

3

The wound is deepened until the transverse processes, upper surface of the ala of the sacrum and facet joints are exposed.

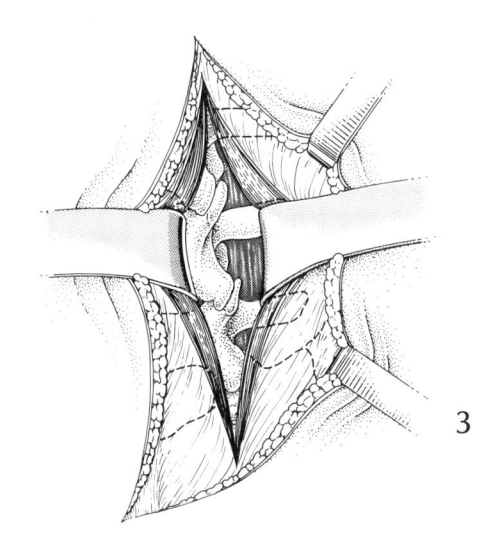

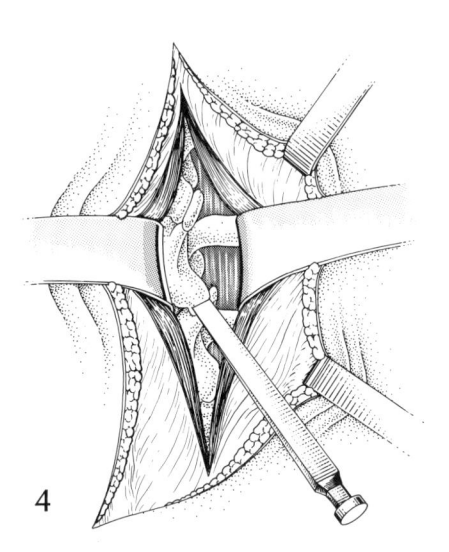

Clearing of articular surfaces

4

The joint surfaces should be excised with a small osteotome.

Decortication

5

Meticulous decortication of the upper surface of the sacrum, the lateral aspect of the articular facets and the transverse processes should be done using a gouge and nibbler.

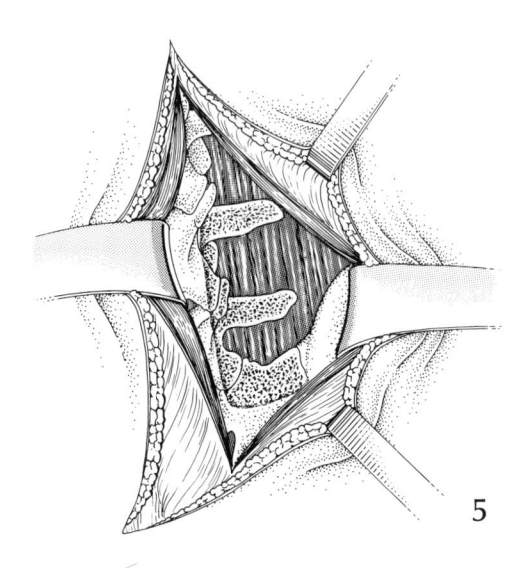

Grafting

6

Cancellous slivers taken from the posterior iliac crest are packed into the area.

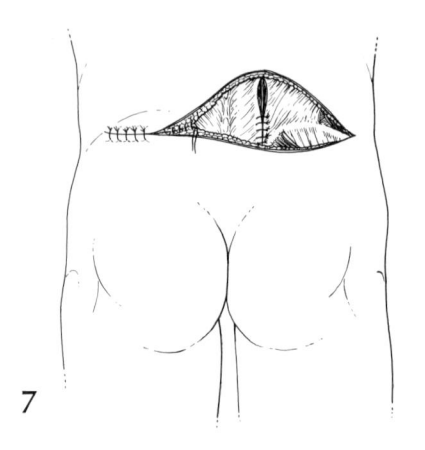

7

INTERTRANSVERSE FUSION WITH DECOMPRESSION

8

Through a curved midline incision the sacrospinalis muscle is reflected from each side of the sacrum, exposing the alae lateral to the articular facets. The muscle is retracted manually on each side. After decompression of the spine, the outer side of the superior articular processes of L4 and L5 are exposed and decorticated. Cancellous grafts are placed in the lateral gutter lying on the transverse processes and alae of the sacrum.

Postoperative management

A gauze and wool dressing is applied and the patient is nursed in an ordinary bed. The drain is removed after 48 hours.

The patient is mobilized out of bed when muscle control has returned. The patient should be able to turn freely in bed and do extension, abdominal and straight-leg raising exercises before being allowed to walk. This is usually accomplished within a few days. Thereafter the patient is supported in a light plaster of Paris lumbosacral support or corset for 12 weeks when increased activity may be allowed.

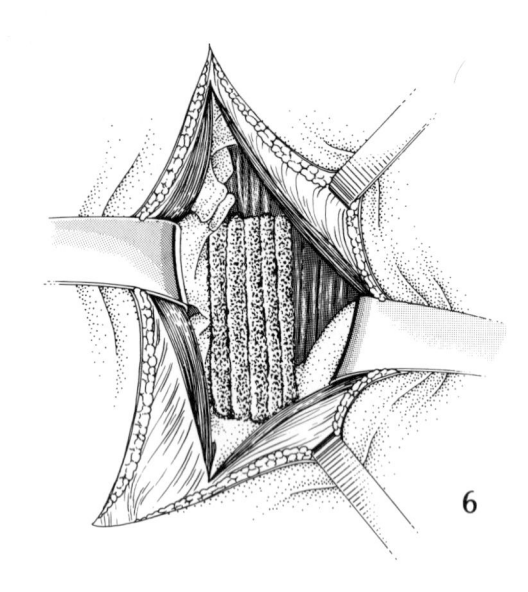

Closure

7

Interrupted sutures to thoracolumbar fascia, subcutaneous fat and skin are inserted.

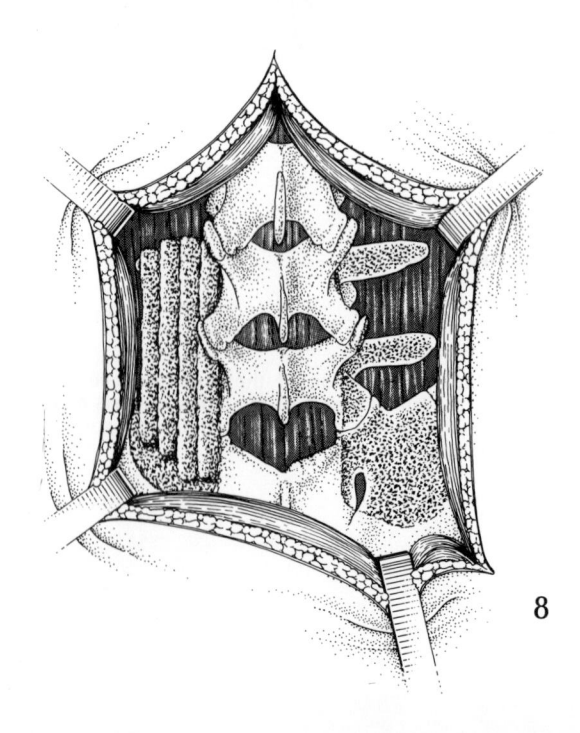

Illustrations by Peter Cox

Surgical reduction of severe spondylolisthesis

J. P. O'Brien PhD, FRCS(Ed), FACS, FRACS
Consultant Surgeon in Spinal Disorders, 149 Harley Street, London;
Lecturer in Spinal Surgery, The Academic Neurosurgical Unit, The Royal London Hospital, London, UK

Introduction

This chapter describes a technique for the reduction of severe spondylolisthesis of grade 3, or greater, in severity. There are many causes of spondylolisthesis; the most severe varieties are usually of the dysplastic type and our experience in the evolution of this technique has been more commonly with the adolescent age group although some patients were treated in their early 30s. It is not, however, advisable for older age groups where the displacement, usually at the lumbosacral joint, has become stiff and often ankylosed, if not actually spontaneously fused.

550 Thoracic and lumbar spine

Historical background

1 & 2

The first reported reduction of a severe spondylolisthesis was by Jenkins[1] in 1936 in which he used strong longitudinal traction, achieved very good correction and performed an anterior lumbosacral fusion. Before surgery, advanced lumbosacral spondylolisthesis included scoliosis, kyphosis, lordosis and forward trunk shift (*Illustration 1*). One year after surgery the patient showed excellent correction of the trunk deformity. Unfortunately, the reduction with traction was treated with anterior fusion alone and complete recurrence of the deformity occurred. Combined anterior and posterior fusion is essential in severe fixed spinal curves.

With the advent of techniques of posterior instrumentation and fusion in the 1960s, Harrington instrumentation was used. However, this aggravated the kyphos and increased the forward shift of the patients so that they were fused in a permanently flexed position, often so unbalanced as to lose the ability to walk without support[2].

The earliest literature on anterior lumbar fusion was described in the treatment of spondylolisthesis as a cause of back pain[3-5]. This work was published in the early 1930s but did not gain popularity because of the difficulty with surgical access to the front of the spine. Anterior fusions became more controversial in the 1960s when it was demonstrated that damage to the presacral nerve which crosses the lumbosacral disc results in retrograde ejaculation in the male. However, from the biomechanical point of view, a spondylolisthesis is an unstable deformity and the principles of treating a fixed spinal curve such as this are as follows.

1. Mobilize the deformity
2. Reduce the deformity
3. Fuse the spine, both from the anterior and posterior aspects.

This presentation is based on experience with over 30 cases treated in the past 15 years. It remains controversial because the literature abounds with the merits of accepting the deformity and, if symptoms persist, merely fusing it *in situ*. It remains one of very few spinal deformities, and in fact orthopaedic deformities, where it is generally felt that ignoring the deformity is acceptable.

This has largely been based on the literature which has documented cases of neurological deficit, in particular cauda equina lesions, produced as a result of injudicious traction in attempts to correct the spondylolisthesis. It cannot be stressed too greatly that severe spondylolisthesis, apart from being inherently an unstable deformity, is, by definition, a high-risk deformity because of the compression of the dural sac which is tented over the back of the sacrum. Only recently has it become evident that even fusion *in situ* can be hazardous and may produce permanent neurological deficit[6]. Wiltse recently confirmed knowledge of 10 cases of fusion *in situ* which have led to cauda equina lesions in recent years (personal communication).

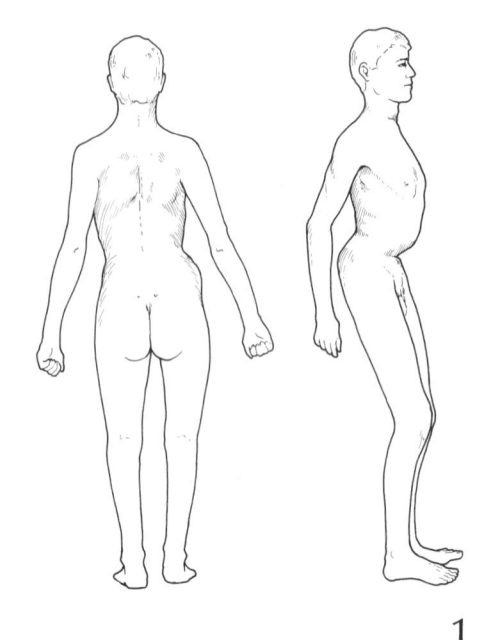

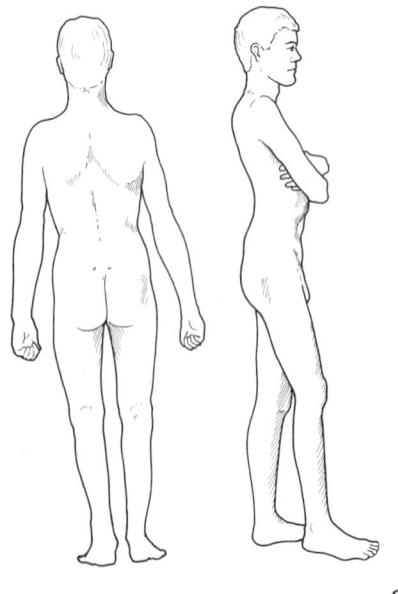

Anatomical lesion

3

The primary defect in severe spondylolisthesis of the dysplastic variety, which is the common severe type, is a poorly developed hypoplastic lamina of L5 which is the invariable level of the displacement. With the adolescent growth spurt, increasing activities and rapid increase in weight, the dysplastic lamina, particularly if the lumbosacral angle is rather steep, does not protect the joint. Pars interarticularis defects develop and there is forward shift with disruption of the lumbosacral disc. The extent of shift can be mild or severe and was classified by Meyerding[7] into grades 1, 2, 3 and 4. Grade 5 severe spondylolisthesis which is actually intrapelvic is termed spondyloptosis.

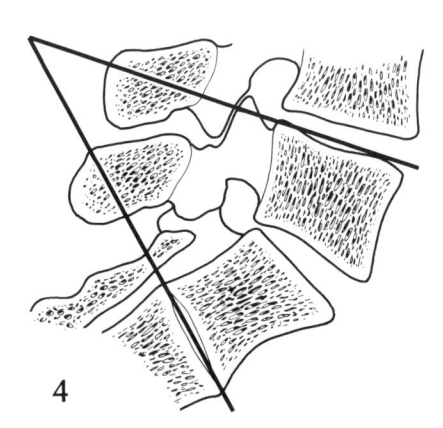

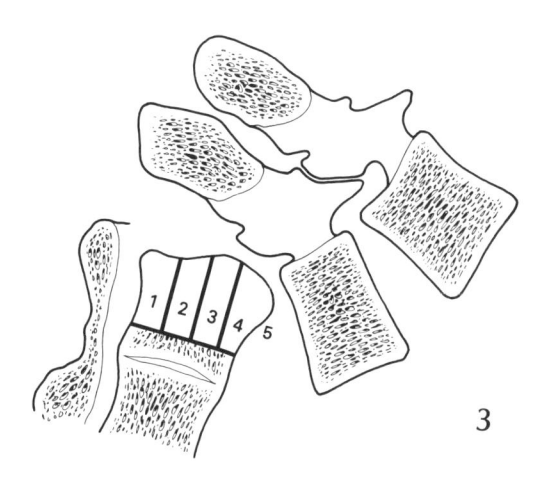

Measurements in severe spondylolisthesis

Several important measurements have been identified amongst the myriad of angles and measurements available.

The degree of slip

The classification described by Meyerding has been mentioned above. This chapter concentrates mainly on the Meyerding grades of slip 3 and above, including the most severe form, or spondyloptosis. Spondylolisthesis of grades 1 or 2 in severity is relatively minor in terms of deformity and can invariably be reduced easily with anterior surgery, including radical removal of the annulus and distraction of the deformed disc space, and maintenance of that correction with interbody grafts.

The angle of kyphosis

4

In normal circumstances, the angle subtended by a line drawn along the top of the body of L5 and the disc between the first and second sacral bodies is an angle formed behind the lumbar spine. With continuing forward shift of the body of L5 at about the grade 3 stage of shift, there is rotation of the body of L5 around the sacrum. This produces a kyphosis at the lumbosacral joint and the angle of kyphosis, if drawn between the top of the body of L5 and the S1–2 disc space, now meets anterior to the lumbar spine.

It is the correction of the angle of kyphosis which is essential in obtaining major correction of the deformity in this difficult displacement.

Indications for surgery

These are usually fairly clear-cut. The patient, usually a teenager, will present with severe pain in the back and with unilateral or bilateral sciatica. There will be difficulty with walking because of tight hamstrings. On examination, the patient is obviously in severe pain, and there may be an associated scoliosis[8]. (This scoliosis will usually spontaneously resolve if and when the spondylolisthesis is reduced and fused, see *Illustrations 11* and *12*.)

There is usually a palpable knob at the lumbosacral level. Bilateral straight-leg raising is severely impaired and there may be motor loss, usually of the L5 motor root which is tightly stretched around the forwardly displaced L5 pedicle.

Development of combined traction and fusion technique

This technique has evolved over the past 15 years. It was evident from the literature that posterior instrumentation and fusion was inadequate, certainly with the posterior fusion and the implants available in the 1960s. Bone graft is designed to function optimally under compression. If it is placed under distraction, it resorbs or pseudarthroses develop. Placement of bone posteriorly or laterally with a severe spondylolisthesis is fraught with the possibility of failure of the bone graft and increase in severity of the deformity.

Anterior fusion itself was attempted by Jenkins in the mid 1930s (see *Illustrations 1* and *2*) and has been repeated but it is inadequate to hold two-thirds of the body weight. Our own experience with the first two cases was that after reduction of the spondylolisthesis and anterior lumbosacral fusion, complete recurrence of the deformity occurred.

Against this background of literature and personal experience, it was obvious that, once correction had been achieved by *gradual* traction, both posterior fusion and anterior fusion were required.

Preoperative

Investigations

Plain radiographs

Routine anteroposterior and lateral radiographs will reveal the extent of the spondylolisthesis. It is important to take a lateral film coned on the displaced vertebra. Lateral tomography will also provide a good anatomical definition of the deformity. The presence or lack of chronic osteoarthritic changes in the region of the spondylolisthetic segment should be looked for. These include osteophytes, lipping, arthritic changes in the facet joints, excessive sclerosis beneath the cartilage end-plate; such changes indicate a chronic displacement and suggest that it is stiffer than the more acute variety and will therefore require more traction to reduce the displacement. In this group of patients, because of the stiff deformity, neurological deficit occurs more commonly.

Many adolescent patients with severe lumbosacral spondylolistheses are, in the author's opinion, in an acute stage and this will be apparent from the relative lack of the chronic radiological changes mentioned above, although there is always wedging of the body of L5. The usual more acute adolescent deformity is seen in *Illustrations 8, 9* and *10*.

Measurement of the extent of spondylolisthesis is important. Measurements of the extent of forward shift according to Meyerding's classification, i.e. grades 1, 2, 3, 4 or spondyloptosis, and also the angle of kyphosis, which is the single most important measurement of this deformity, are taken[9].

5 & 6

The anteroposterior film will confirm the presence or absence of scoliosis. This is usually a long thoracolumbar curve, originating at the deformed L5 segment and invariably, if present for any length of time, associated with structural rotation. *Illustration 5* shows severe spondylolisthesis before operation, while *Illustration 6* shows satisfactory reduction which is solid 2 years later.

Radiculogram

A radiculogram is essential to define the extent of compression of the dural sac at the level of the deformity. Some authors have stated that this is not necessary, but in the author's view such an approach means that crucial information is unavailable. It is very important to elucidate the factor causing the compression of the dural sac. It may be the back of the posterior part of the sacrum or it may be the upper tilted aspect of the fifth lumbar lamina, as demonstrated by Buirski *et al.*[10].

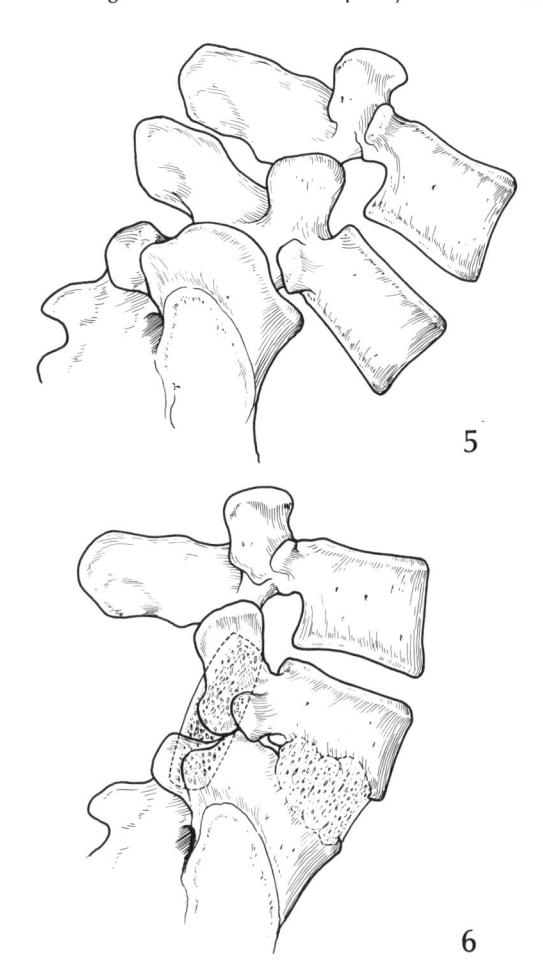

Discography

7

Discography at the L4–5 level is important. It is surprising how often, even in the teenager, this can be torn and, if the disc is torn, it should be removed and replaced with bone graft as for the lumbosacral disc. When this is confirmed, the L4–5 fusion must be included at the time of anterior surgery.

Gait studies

If these are available they provide an accurate documentation of the patient's posture and mobility, and forward shift of the upper trunk. They provide valuable dynamic documentation of the spondylolisthesis and its effects.

Operations

ACUTE REDUCTION OF SEVERE SPONDYLOLISTHESIS

Acute reduction may be performed either by forcible reduction on a traction table or by acute reduction during operation. Both methods risk damage to the cauda equina.

GRADUAL REDUCTION OF SEVERE SPONDYLOLISTHESIS

8

Gradual reduction takes the form of skeletal traction applied to the skull and lower limbs while the patient is conscious and over a period of 10–14 days, with close monitoring of the neurological system, close observation of the patient and regular lateral radiographs of the deformity to show the correction occurring. Preoperative severe spondylolisthesis in the lumbosacral joint is shown.

The present staged technique is as follows.

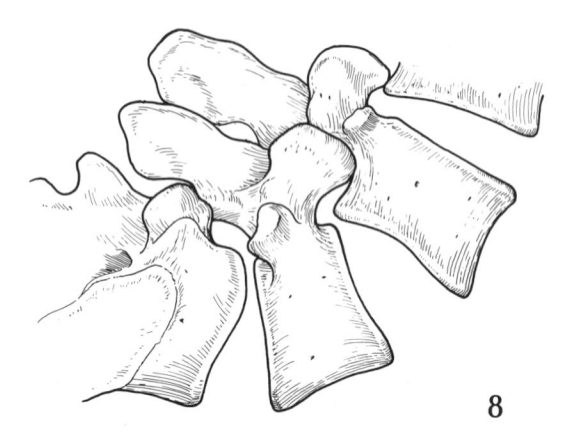

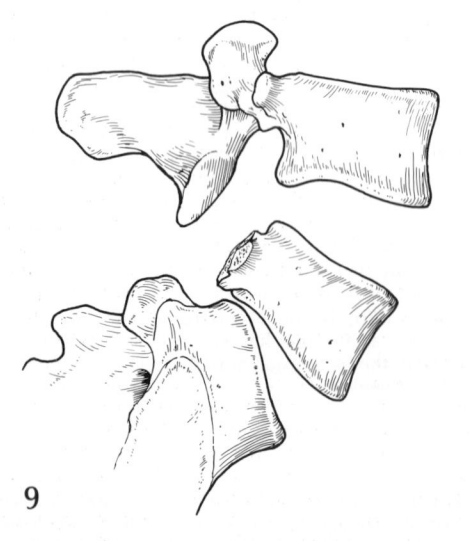

Laminectomy of L5

9

This allows the body of L5 to be reduced with traction back on to the sacrum. At the same time as laminectomy of L5, the L5 nerve roots, which are most vulnerable, must be adequately, widely and totally decompressed, otherwise they will be damaged during reduction of the body of L5. After laminectomy of L5 with nerve root decompression, gradual traction over 10 days has produced the degree of correction shown here. At the same operation, alar–transverse fusion is performed. Bone is put into the lateral gutters; this is a technically difficult procedure because the lateral gutters are so deep and blind. A bulk of bone is available in both lateral gutters so that when the body of L5 is reduced with traction, the transverse processes of L5, dysplastic though they may be, are pulled back into the bony mass of cancellous autograft; this provides the lateral fusion.

Skull–femoral traction

At the time of the first-stage operation, a skull halo or Gardner–Wells tongs are applied and pins are placed into the lower aspect of the femoral shafts, taking care that they are approximately 2.5 cm proximal to the lower femoral growth-plates. With the patient supine and still anaesthetized on the operating table, the mobility achieved by the laminectomy can be tested with pressure over the front of the body of L5 using a lead-lined glove and obtaining a lateral radiograph of the situation achieved. Sometimes it is surprising that the body of L5 will reduce by 50 per cent or more with this manoeuvre. This is a reliable indicator that an excellent reduction will be achieved.

Traction is commenced when the patient is comfortable. Weights are increased by several pounds on the skull halo and the femoral pins each day, with the patient in a hyperextended position, usually obtained by breaking the bed in the middle. The principle of this is that the deformity is a flexion deformity and traction should be applied with the spine in extension to be maximally efficient.

Radiographs are taken every 3 days. A simple lateral radiograph centred on L5 will show whether progress and reduction is taking place.

A basic neurological examination for patients undergoing distraction has been reported elsewhere[11] and all staff dealing with the patient should be familiar with this practice which is repeated twice daily (Table 1). Further detail on neurological assessment is available elsewhere[12].

Reduction will take place in the large majority of patients when the weights have been increased adequately. In some cases, however, the deformity is quite stiff and the strongest weights will achieve only slight reduction. A close look at the lateral radiograph of the spondylolisthesis in these patients will reveal, providing the laminectomy of L5 has been complete, that there are osteophytes and chronic bone changes present. In these, it appears that the slip has been quite chronic and the adjacent ligaments have shortened and have stiffened the deformity, often making it hazardous to correct the deformity without the serious risk of neurological damage. In these patients, a decision must be made within 2–3 weeks that further increase in weights is unlikely to obtain the desired result. Fortunately, this is an uncommon situation but its presence can be catastrophic.

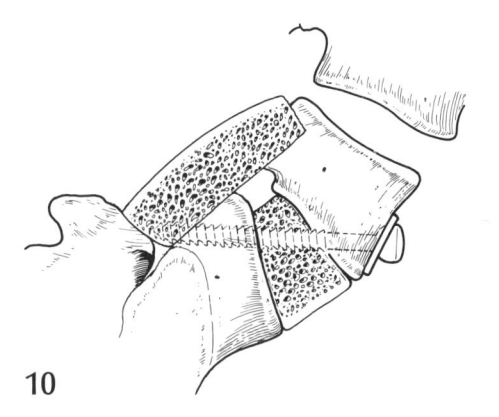

Table 1 Basic neurological examination of patients undergoing distraction

Spinal cord
  Questions 1. Any weakness in the legs?
             2. Any numbness in the legs?
             3. Any loss of bladder function?
  Tests   1. Up- or down-going toes?
             2. Any clonus of ankles or knees?

Cranial nerves (tests for VI, IX, X, XII)
  Questions 1. Any double vision?
             2. Any difficulty with swallowing?
             3. Difficulty coughing?
             4. Any change in voice?
             5. Any tongue weakness?
  Tests   1. Eye movements (VI)
             2. Palate reflex (IX)
             3. Explosive cough (X)
             4. Quality of speech, nasal? (IX or X)
             5. Extend tongue, is it midline? (XII)

Upper limbs
  Questions 1. Difficulty in moving hand, arm or shoulder joint?
             2. Any numbness or weakness of the hand?
  Tests   1. Abduct the shoulder (C5,6)
             2. Flex the forearm (C5,6)
             3. Test grip of hand
             4. Test sensation of fingertips (C6–T1)

Anterior lumbosacral fusion

10

The day before anterior lumbosacral fusion is performed, the patient receives an enema, and, during induction, a catheter is inserted into the bladder. When reduction has been achieved, the corrected position of the spondylolisthesis is maintained by an anterior lumbosacral fusion. *Illustration 10* shows anatomical reduction restored 5 months after lumbosacral fusion. An AO screw maintains the reduction and enhances the anterior lumbosacral graft. The posterior fusion is solid. It should be clear that posterior techniques will not suffice because of the inherent instability of the deformity. Operative discography is performed at the time of surgery to establish that the L4–5 disc is intact (if it is not, it must be included in the fusion). If the disc at the spondylolisthesis level is injected with a radio-opaque dye and a lateral picture taken during the operation, it will be seen that a huge cleft is present throughout the disc; it has therefore lost its inherent properties of mechanical strength and stability (see *Illustration 7*).

The anterior fusion operation is performed with the patient lying supine and with the table broken so that the hips are hyperextended. A lower left paramedian incision is performed and the approach is transperitoneal, as popularized by Freebody[13]. It is much safer altogether to approach the deformity through the peritoneum rather than retroperitoneally because it is intrapelvic and access is usually technically difficult, especially when the displacement has not been completely anatomically reduced.

10

Presacral nerve

The anatomy of the presacral nerve must be clearly understood and must be visualized. To help see the nerve, the technique described by Freebody[13] is used to avoid damage to it. Adrenaline-in-saline, 5–10 ml of 1:500 000, is injected into the posterior peritoneal tissues in the region of the lumbosacral disc. This balloons out the peritoneum from the areolar tissues surrounding the spine, and the presacral nerve can be seen in the balloon of fluid. It is seen over the middle and crosses the lumbosacral disc from the left to right side. It is a thick nerve, easily seen and palpated. A midline vertical incision in the peritoneum is made to the right side of the presacral nerve and with small dry swabs, the wet prevertebral tissues are moved both to the left and to the right side, the presacral nerve being moved with the left flap of peritoneum to the left side.

The presacral artery and vein will need to be ligated to gain clear access to the lumbosacral disc.

Disc excision

It cannot be overstated that the ease of access depends very much on how much reduction has been achieved over the previous 10–14 days.

Steinmann pins are used to retract the tissues, including the bifurcation of the common iliac vessels. The pins are driven into the body of L5, are excellent and safe retractors for the vessels. They can also be used on the sacrum, depending on its slope, particularly pins with a bend at the lower 2.5 cm.

The disc is excised with sharp scalpels and O'Brien disc knives. Correct instrumentation at this stage is of the utmost importance. The O'Brien range of anterior spinal instruments is invaluable in removing the entire disc back to the posterior vertebral rim. The lateral annulus is removed with large rongeurs and curetting of the cartilaginous end-plate carried out until raw bleeding cancellous bone is exposed. This can only be checked with an angled dental mirror, kept in hot water to prevent it steaming up. It is held in the angled deep lumbosacral disc space and is used in a similar manner to its use in dental surgery. Remnants of white cartilaginous end-plate are clearly seen and must be more thoroughly curetted. This is a fundamental practical technique in this operation, if pseudarthrosis and loss of reduction is to be avoided.

Further reduction at time of surgery

It is tempting to lever the body of L5 further back on the sacrum at this stage of the procedure if preliminary traction has not achieved anatomical reduction. A bone hook is the ideal instrument for this but excessive extension and forcible further reduction is to be avoided at all costs, tempting though it may be.

Bone graft

A separate incision is made over the left iliac crest and, using spine elevators, muscles are stripped from the iliac crest in the region of the tubercle which is the strongest and thickest part of the bone. When the iliac crest has been stripped, the disc space must be measured for height and depth so that accurately fitting plugs of tricortical iliac crest may be cut with osteotomes. In a patient without deformity the anteroposterior length of safe graft is of the order of 30 mm. This will vary from level to level and from patient to patient, but accurate measurement of the depth and height in the deformed motor segment is essential. The cauda equina has already been subject to previous surgery 2 weeks beforehand and has been stretched for a period of time, and is therefore more vulnerable than a primary fusion case.

Appropriately cut blocks of tricortical iliac crest are removed with osteotomes and impacted into the lumbosacral disc space.

Further reduction at this stage will occur if a wide annulectomy has been performed and if firm impaction of the bone grafts is carried out.

Internal fixation of the bone grafts

Cancellous AO screws are ideal for fixing the cancellous grafts in position. Radiographic control is essential and the screws may be passed through the body of L5, through the grafts (for two grafts, two screws are ideal) and gaining a firm hold into the first sacral body, ensuring that the end of the screw does not penetrate the spinal canal and catch the dural sac.

A check radiograph will confirm that the grafts are satisfactory, that the AO screws are in position and that they compress the cancellous graft in between the body of L5 and the sacrum.

Integrity of the L4–5 disc

Operative discography, of the L4–5 disc, performed as a preliminary procedure before disc removal will show whether the L4–5 disc is torn. If so, it should also be removed and grafted. This will require removal of the Steinmann pins from the body of L5, retraction of the vessels to the right side and access to the L4–5 disc between the sympathetic trunk and the common iliac vessels.

Closure

The posterior peritoneum is sutured and the wound is closed in anatomical layers without drainage. The iliac crest wound has a vacuum drain inserted and is closed in layers.

Postoperative management

Removal of the traction system

It is wise to leave the skull and femoral traction system in position until this stage because if, for some reason, instability with the grafts is apparent, a further period of several weeks' traction may be required until they become firm enough for the traction to be removed.

In most cases, however, the skull halo and the femoral pins may now be removed.

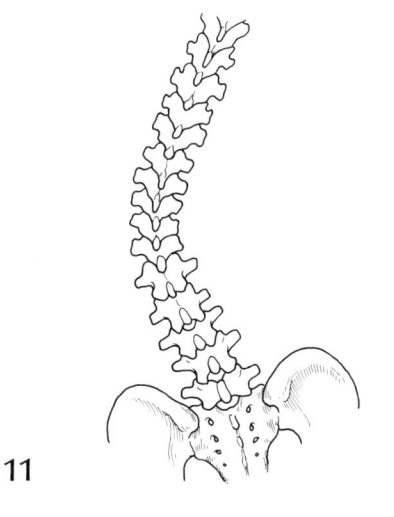

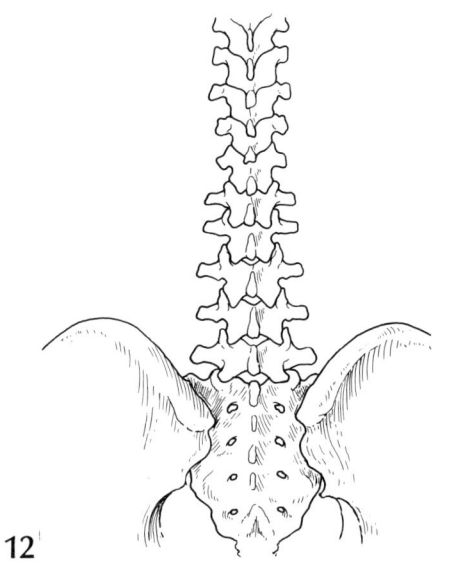

Postoperative nursing

Ileus and pain relief are the main issues at this stage. A routine nasogastric tube is advisable with transperitoneal surgery. The ileus usually lasts a couple of days and nil by mouth is allowed until strong bowel sounds have recurred.

Postoperative immobilization

A 'Scotch cast' double hip spica is applied, extending from the nipple line down to the knees, and this should be kept in position with the patient in bed for 3 months, at which stage radiographs are taken. It is only when the grafts have consolidated, and this is confirmed by clear lateral radiographs, that protected weight-bearing may be permitted. Loss of correction at this stage is a disaster and must be avoided at all costs, even if it does mean an added period of time without weight-bearing. Later rehabilitation is aimed at restoration of the abdominal and trunk muscles and should extend over 6–12 months. Height gain is usually of the order of 5 cm.

11 & 12

The scoliosis apparent before surgery is usually spontaneously corrected by the time the patient has commenced walking and regained his normal proprioceptive reflexes.

Complications

The most catastrophic problem is a complete cauda equina lesion. This has not been seen in the author's experience but it does occur with overenthusiastic use of new and attractive traction and instrumentation systems. It must be emphasized that to carry out this type of spinal surgery requires a team approach, ideally in a specialist spinal unit. The surgeons involved must have expert working knowledge of the following.

1. Posterior surgery and nerve root decompression
2. Systems of traction
3. Expertise with anterior approaches to the spine, handling of the gut, vessels, etc.
4. Additionally, if internal fixation is used, a thorough working knowledge of the AO system and its principles.

In a recently reviewed series of 30 patients, only two had minimal loss of motor power in L5. None required foot drop splints and there were no cauda equina lesions. The most disappointing problems were seen in the first two patients treated by the author, in whom posterior fusion was not added to the anterior fusion and postoperative immobilization was not thorough so that complete loss of correction occurred. This is a complication which is easily avoidable if due care is taken.

Conclusion

This chapter briefly presents a combined surgically staged technique for the reduction of severe spondylolisthesis, usually of the dysplastic variety seen in the teenager and invariably at the lumbosacral level. It has not been attempted in patients over the age of 30 years. The technique rests basically on gradual reduction with the patient conscious over a period of 2 weeks, commencing initially with:

1. laminectomy of L5, nerve root decompression and alar–transverse fusion;
2. gradual increasing traction over the following 2 weeks, using radiographic control and close monitoring of the neurological system;
3. when reduction has been achieved, anterior lumbosacral fusion through a transperitoneal approach.

The experience is based on 30 patients treated over a 15-year period, in whom, on review, the reductions were excellent in all but a few patients and the complication rate very low.

While it might be argued that fusion *in situ* is an acceptable method of treatment of this deformity, recent literature has pointed out that even fusion *in situ* is associated with an unacceptable incidence of late cauda equina lesions, thus stressing the potentially dangerous deformity presented by this condition, no matter how conservative the surgical treatment may be. Fusion *in situ* is also associated with an unacceptable cosmetic appearance.

References

1. Jenkins JA. Spondylolisthesis. *Br J Surg* 1936; 24: 80–5.
2. Harrington PR, Dickson JH. Spinal instrumentation in the treatment of severe progressive spondylolisthesis. *Clin Orthop* 1976; 117: 157–63.
3. Capener N. Spondylolisthesis. *Br J Surg* 1932; 19: 374–86.
4. Burns BH. An operation for spondylolisthesis. *Lancet* 1933; i: 1233.
5. Mercer W. Spondylolisthesis: with a description of a new method of operative treatment and notes of ten cases. *Edinburgh Med J* 1936; 43: 545–72.
6. Maurice HD, Morley TR. Cauda equina lesions following fusion in situ and decompressive laminectomy for severe spondylolisthesis. Four case reports. *Spine* 1989; 14: 214–16.
7. Meyerding HW. Spondylolisthesis. *Surg Gynecol Obstet* 1932; 54: 371–7.
8. McPhee IB, O'Brien JP. Reduction of severe spondylolisthesis – a preliminary report. *Spine* 1979; 4, 5: 430–4.
9. McCall IW, O'Brien JP, Speck GR. Terminology and measurement spondylolisthesis. *J Bone Joint Surg [Am]* 1984; 66-A: 631 (correspondence).
10. Buirski G, McCall IW, O'Brien JP. Myelography in severe lumbosacral spondylolisthesis. *Br J Radiol* 1984; 57: 1067–72.
11. O'Brien JP, Yau AC, Hodgson AR. Halo pelvic traction; a technic for severe spinal deformities. *Clin Orthop* 1973; 93: 179–90.
12. O'Brien JP. *The halo pelvic apparatus*. PhD Thesis, Gothenberg, 1975.
13. Freebody D, Bendall R, Taylor RD. Anterior transperitoneal lumbar fusion. *J Bone Joint Surg [Br]* 1971; 53-B: 617–27.

Illustrations by Anthony C. S. Yiu

Operations for infections of the spine

John C. Y. Leong FRCS, FRCS (Ed), FRACS
Professor of Orthopaedic Surgery, University of Hong Kong

Introduction

This section deals with the commoner spinal infections, including pyogenic infection and tuberculosis. Other rare conditions such as typhoid, brucellosis, actinomycosis and hydatid disease, will not be discussed.

Surgical treatment for pyogenic and tuberculous spondylitis is complementary to the use of the appropriate antibiotics and antituberculous chemotherapy. Both conditions can be treated conservatively. The indications for surgical treatment will be explained below, but rarely is surgery an absolute necessity. It also depends upon the availability of good anaesthesia, and surgeons with proper training in the required surgical skills.

For tuberculosis of the spine, the controversy between conservative treatment as advocated by Konstam and his co-workers in Africa, and radical excision of the disease focus followed by anterior spinal fusion as advocated by Hodgson and his co-workers in Hong Kong, was taken up by the Medical Research Council of Britain, which organized a series of controlled clinical trails of the two methods of treatment. The longest follow-up period is now 15 years. The conclusion is that, whilst conservative treatment is effective in the treatment of tuberculosis of the spine, surgical treatment offers the following advantages: (1) more rapid return of patients to a favourable status, (2) a much shorter period required for radiological fusion, and a higher percentage of fusion even at 10 years after treatment, (3) less loss of vertebral height, (4) better correction of kyphosis, and significantly lower percentage of patients with severe deformities, and (5) more rapid and better recovery of paraplegia. One other important advantage not mentioned is immediate relief of preoperative pain by the surgical procedure.

In pyogenic spondylitis, it has been shown that the following risk factors increase the likelihood of paraplegia: (1) age greater than 35 years, (2) cervical spine more likely than thoracic, and thoracic more than lumbar, (3) concomitant medical conditions such as diabetes mellitus or rheumatoid arthritis, and (4) steroid therapy.

It is also established that autogenous bone grafts used in pyogenic spondylitis will survive and not be destroyed by the disease process, provided the appropriate antibiotics are used intravenously over at least a period of 6 weeks, followed by another 6 weeks or longer of oral administration.

Preoperative assessment

Indications

1. Pain in the presence of a large paraspinal abscess shadow on a plain radiograph of the spine, not responding to the appropriate antibiotics or chemotherapy.
2. Site of the disease: surgery more strongly indicated in the cervical spine, especially in children.
3. Extent of the disease: disease affecting more than two consecutive vertebral bodies.
4. Severity of deformity: either on presentation, or becoming progressively severe during conservative treatment.
5. Presence of paraplegia.
6. Impending rupture of the abscess into surrounding structures.
7. When the diagnosis is in doubt.

Pain with unresponsive abscess

A sizable abscess, in our experience, may take a long time to resolve. Pain and the general condition of the patient improves rapidly after operative treatment.

Site

In the cervical spine, there is no splintage by the surrounding rib cage as there is in the thoracic spine. Marked collapse and deformity is common, with destruction of bone and intervertebral disc. This leads to spinal cord compression. Our experience shows a high incidence of paraplegia in cervical tuberculosis in those over the age of 10 years. The treatment of choice is therefore surgical excision of diseased tissue followed by grafting.

Extent

Involvement of more than two vertebral bodies often leads to significant kyphosis, even if healing occurs by conservative means. This kyphosis is undesirable, and can be prevented by excision of diseased tissue followed by anterior spinal fusion.

Severity

The same argument holds true for deformities which are severe on presentation, or progress during the course of conservative treatment.

Paraplegia

Paraplegia secondary to tuberculosis of the spine may be divided into two main groups.

Paraplegia of active disease This is due to compression of the spinal cord by abscess, caseous material, and sequestra. In a severe form the disease penetrates through the dura, resulting in pachymeningitis externae: this causes a spastic type of paraplegia. Rapid decompression and evacuation of diseased material is desirable, and in our experience results in rapid and better recovery of neurological function.

Paraplegia of healed disease This occurs gradually, as a result of a progressive kyphosis during healing following treatment by conservative measures. Although the spinal column may in time become very stable by spontaneous fusion at the site of deformity, a bony ridge forms at the internal kyphus, and presses on the spinal cord. Progressive ischaemia as well as mechanical pressure will lead to progressive paraplegia. Surgical treatment of such patients involves multiple staged procedures, and will not be described in this section.

Impending rupture of the abscess

The lung, oesophagus, and aorta may be the site of impending rupture of a tuberculous abscess. When such is recognized, surgical treatment of the abscess and the primary disease focus is the rational treatment.

Doubtful diagnosis

Obtaining tissue for diagnosis and for identification of the organism is an important consideration, especially where such infections are uncommon.

Preoperative preparation

For young children, a plaster bed is made to facilitate nursing and turning in the postoperative period. A Stoke Mandeville turning bed, or a Stryker turning frame, should be available for older children and adults. In patients presenting with significant kyphosis with active disease, a period of preoperative halo traction to reduce the deformity is advisable. Antibiotics or antituberculous therapy should be started at least a week before surgery.

Anaesthesia

General anaesthesia with endotracheal intubation is required. Occasionally one-lung anaesthesia is useful to enable complete collapse of the lung on the operated side when a transpleural approach is used. Absence of pressure on the abdomen must be ensured. Although blood loss of more than 500 ml is unusual, at least 2 units of blood should be cross-matched and available.

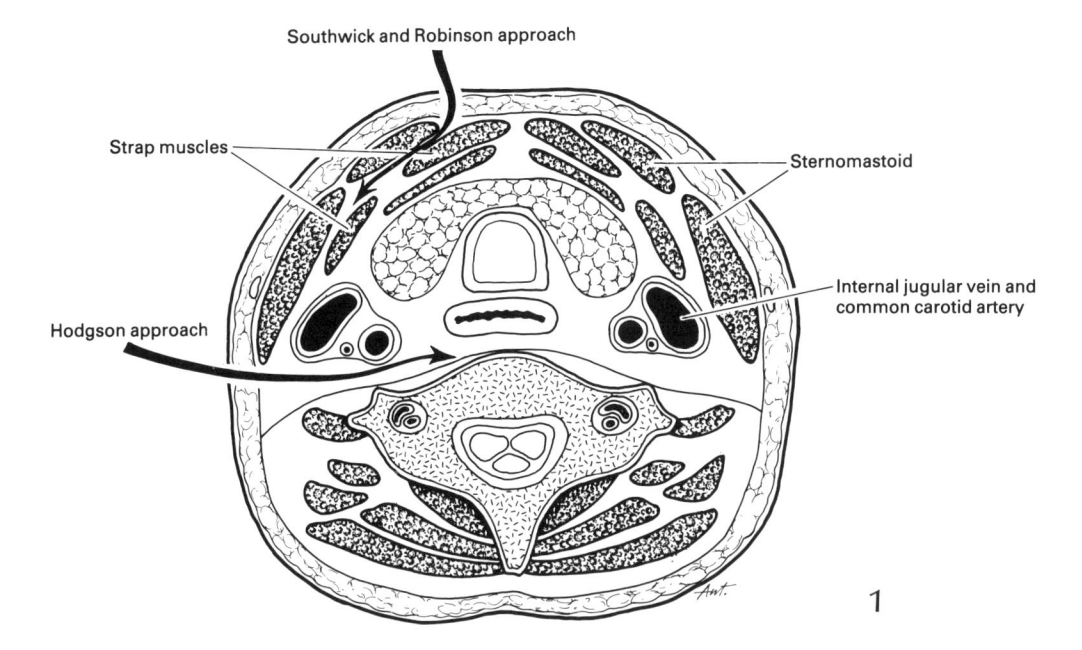

Operations for infections of the spine 561

Southwick and Robinson approach
Strap muscles
Sternomastoid
Internal jugular vein and common carotid artery
Hodgson approach

1

Operations

CERVICAL SPINE

Position of patient

The patient should be supine with a roll of soft padding underneath the shoulders, and a ring underneath the head. The cervical spine should be slightly extended to facilitate the surgical exposure with the head either in a neutral position or turned to the opposite side.

Approach

1

The approach may be anterior to the sternomastoid muscle (Southwick and Robinson), or posterior to that muscle (Hodgson). The former can give exposure from C3 to C7, but is less convenient for the lower part of the cervical spine, exposure of which is facilitated by the latter approach.

Special instruments

2

S-shaped retractors with blunt teeth are useful for retracting the longus cervicis muscles and midline structures. Angled Kerrison rongeurs are useful to reach the posterior half of the vertebral body. A small vertebral spreader increases access between vertebral bodies.

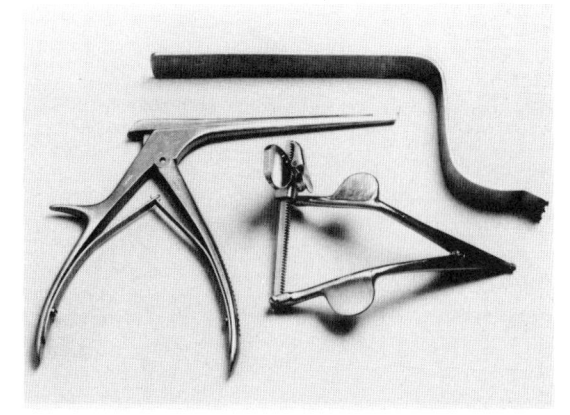

2

Incision

3a & b

For exposure to one or two levels, a hemi-collar incision is adequate. For more extensive involvement, an oblique incision along the anterior margin of the sternomastoid muscle is preferred. This can be lengthened at will. In the Southwick and Robinson approach, the hemi-collar incision starts 1 cm lateral to the anterior margin of the sternomastoid muscle and ends at the midline. In the Hodgson approach, the hemi-collar incision starts at the anterior border of the sternomastoid muscle and extends laterally to the anterior edge of the trapezius muscle. The superficial fascia and platysma are divided in the line of the skin incision.

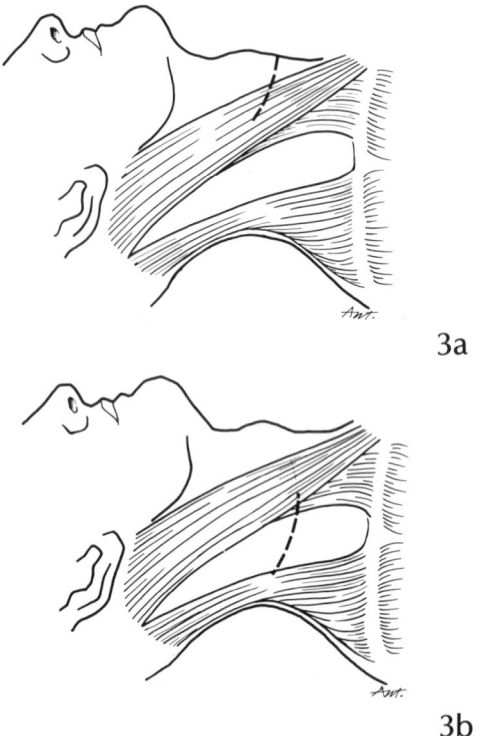

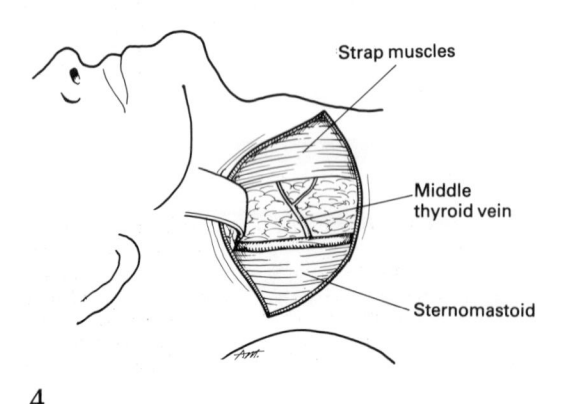

Deep dissection

Southwick and Robinson approach

4

The sternomastoid muscle is identified. The interval between the anterior edge of the muscle and the midline structures (including the strap muscles, the trachea, thyroid gland, and oesophagus) is developed by blunt dissection or spreading with a pair of scissors. In this interval, the middle thyroid vein or the inferior thyroid may be encountered, depending on the level of the incision. These should be divided between ligatures. Occasionally, longitudinal trunks of the ansa cervicalis are also encountered. These can be pushed to one side. If the lower cervical spine is being exposed, the omohyoid muscle is encountered, and it can be divided to give better access. The carotid sheath can be palpated deep to the sternomastoid muscle, and lateral to the interval developed.

Hodgson approach

5

This approach is through the posterior triangle. The external jugular vein, if in the way, is ligated. The sternomastoid muscle is identified, and if particularly broad, is divided in its posterior third. The common carotid sheath comes into view. By blunt dissection in the fat pad behind the sheath, a plane is developed overlying the prevertebral fascia of the posterior triangle. It is further developed medially across the vertebral bodies. The carotid sheath and midline structures are retracted forward. Care is needed to avoid damage to the oesophagus.

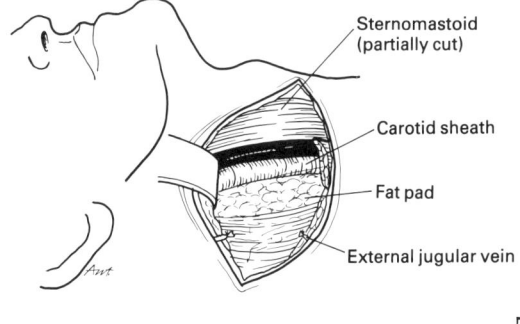

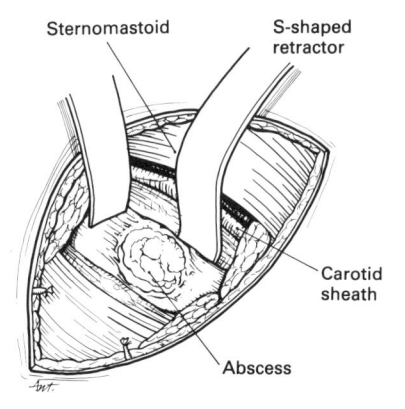

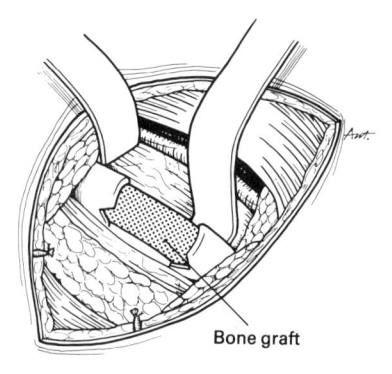

Excision of diseased tissue and bone grafting

6a & b

The prevertebral fascia is next seen covering the anterior aspect of the spinal column, and the longus cervicis muscles on either side. At the level of involvement, there is an abscess and surrounding oedema. Sometimes, the disease process has not involved the anterior longitudinal ligament. However, palpation of the ligament along its length will reveal an area of 'bogginess'.

The wall of the abscess is incised, and thorough evacuation of the diseased tissue is done, until bleeding bone is exposed. The cervical vertebral bodies are small, and therefore careful preparation of the recipient site is needed, to ensure that the bone graft is mortised in with exactness. Iliac crest graft is used. The prevertebral fascia is closed if possible.

Postoperative management

If a short fusion of one level is done, the patient lies in bed for 2 weeks and is allowed up with a well-moulded Plastazote (Smith & Nephew, Hull, UK) or Orthoplast (Johnson & Johnson, New Milton, UK) cervical collar. If the bone graft spans across two or more levels, the patient can get up only with the use of a halo–cast which is maintained for 8 weeks or until radiological fusion is apparent.

THORACIC SPINE

Approach

A transpleural anterior approach is recommended in most instances. This will serve the whole thoracic spine, and facilitates evacuation of diseased material through the abscess wall, as well as anterior spinal fusion. An alternative is the costo-transversectomy approach, which is more applicable to patients with a significant kyphotic deformity, but the exposure is limited and makes preparation and placement of interbody grafts difficult. It is useful as a lesser procedure mainly to decompress the spinal cord.

Transpleural approach

Position of patient

The patient is placed in the full lateral position, either with the right side up or the left side up. The level of the lesion should be placed over the kidney bridge of the operating table, so that the bridge can be raised during the operation to spread open the intervertebral space.

Incision

7a & b

A J-shaped parascapular incision is used for the upper thoracic spine (T1 to T3).

For the lower thoracic spine an incision is made along the rib, extending from the lateral border of the erector spinae muscle forwards to the costochondral junction. The rib chosen should be such that in the mid-axillary line it lies opposite the centre of the lesion. This is usually two ribs higher than the centre of the vertebral lesion.

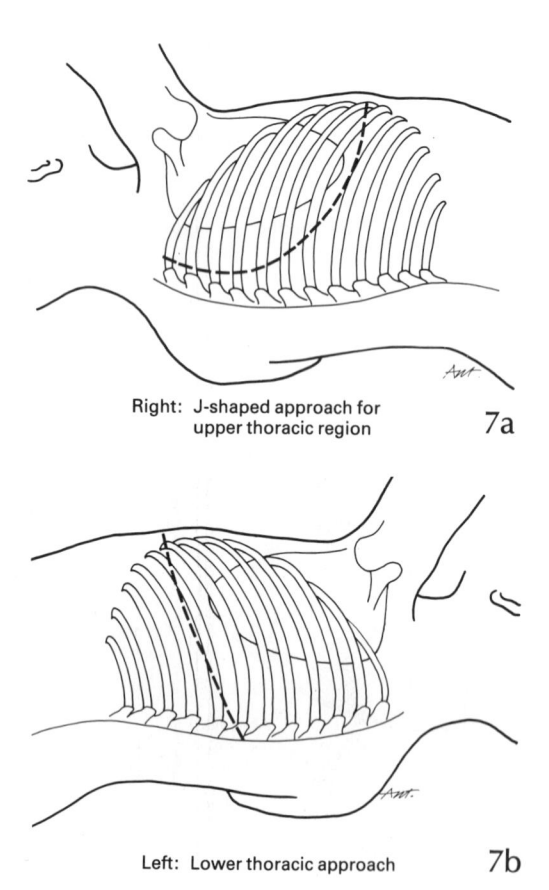

Right: J-shaped approach for upper thoracic region 7a

Left: Lower thoracic approach 7b

Deep dissection

8a & b

The chest wall muscles are cut in layers with diathermy, and the rib removed subperiosteally. The chest is entered, the lung gently retracted and the abscess is usually obvious. Sometimes, there is only oedema and thickening of soft tissue surrounding the involved vertebrae.

For the upper thoracic spine, the right-sided approach is easier, as the azygos vein is less in the way than the arch of the aorta. The intercostal vessels can be divided between ligatures, and if necessary the azygos vein itself can be ligated.

For the rest of the thoracic spine, the side to be chosen depends on where the main abscess is situated. Once the intercostal vessels overlying the abscess are divided between ligatures, the abscess wall can be opened with a diathermy needle, and pus and diseased tissue can be thoroughly evacuated.

Not infrequently, adhesions may occur between the lung and the parietal pleura. These are best separated by blunt dissection. Similar adhesions between the lung and the aorta should be dealt with in the same way. If a marked kyphosis is present, the aorta may be kinked and the intercostal vessels supplying the destroyed vertebrae are found bunched together at the apex of the curve. Mobilization of the aorta then becomes more tedious and requires care.

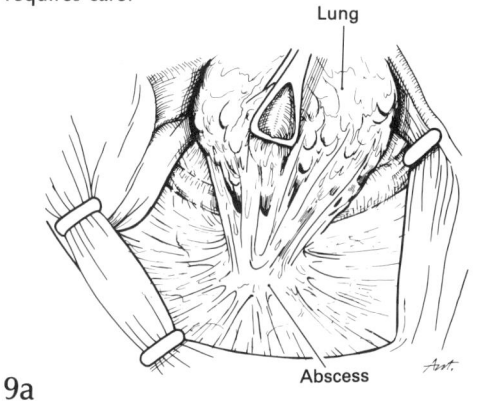

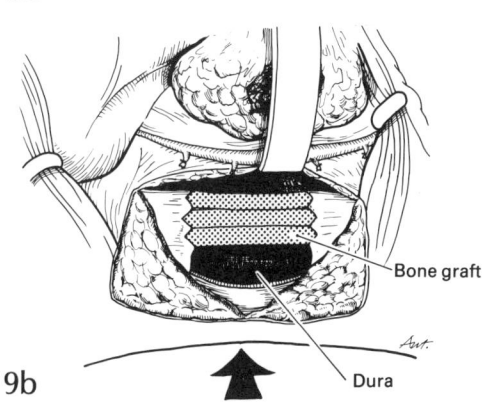

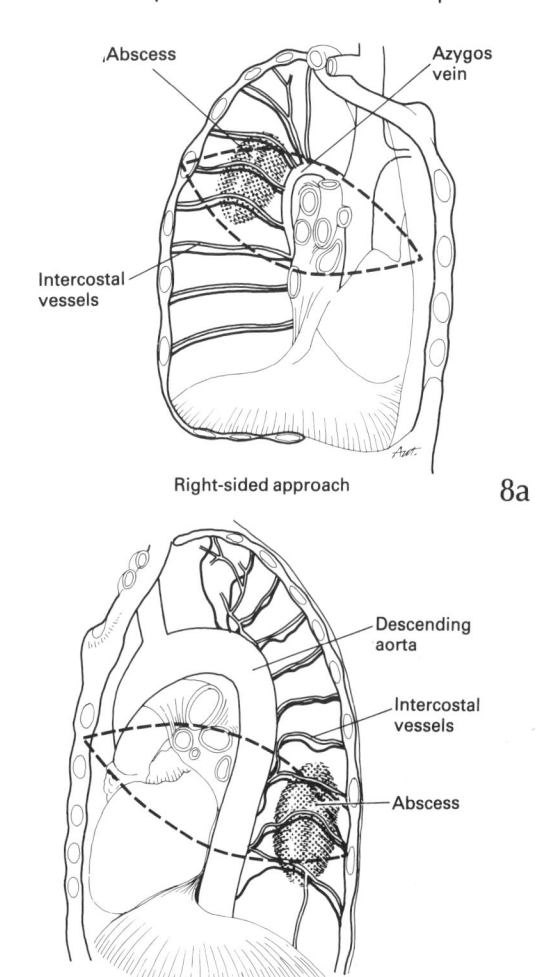

Removal of diseased tissue and bone grafting

9a & b

Removal of diseased tissue is performed until bleeding bone is seen. The posterior longitudinal ligament is visualized and removed carefully, exposing the dura. Then the recipient site is prepared by cutting grooves in the normal vertebral bodies in the coronal plane to receive the bone graft. Pressure is applied on the kyphus so that the spine is sprung open enabling measurement to be made of the required height of the bone grafts, which can be obtained from the excised rib. This ensures stability of the grafts in compression. The abscess wall is closed over a piece of absorbable gelatin sponge, which has been impregnated with 1 g streptomycin and 200 mg isoniazid powder. The usual chest drain is inserted.

Costo-transversectomy approach

Position of patient

The patient is placed prone on a spinal frame, to ensure that there is no pressure on the abdomen.

Incision

10

A posterior slightly curved longitudinal incision is made to one side of the midline.

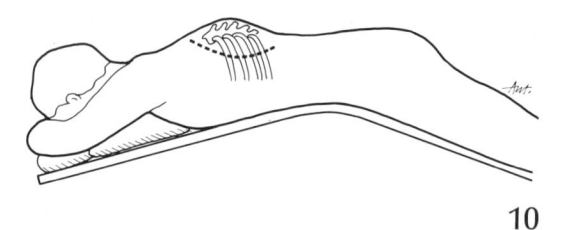

Deep dissection

11a & b

Subperiosteal exposure is made of the posterior elements, laterally to the tips of the transverse processes, and continuing laterally to expose 2 to 3 cm of the ribs on the side of the exposure. This length is removed from two ribs proximal and two ribs distal to the apex of the kyphus. The intercostal nerves are protected. Extrapleural dissection then enables an approach to the anterolateral aspect of the spine. Debridement and decompression of the anterior aspect of the spinal canal can then be done.

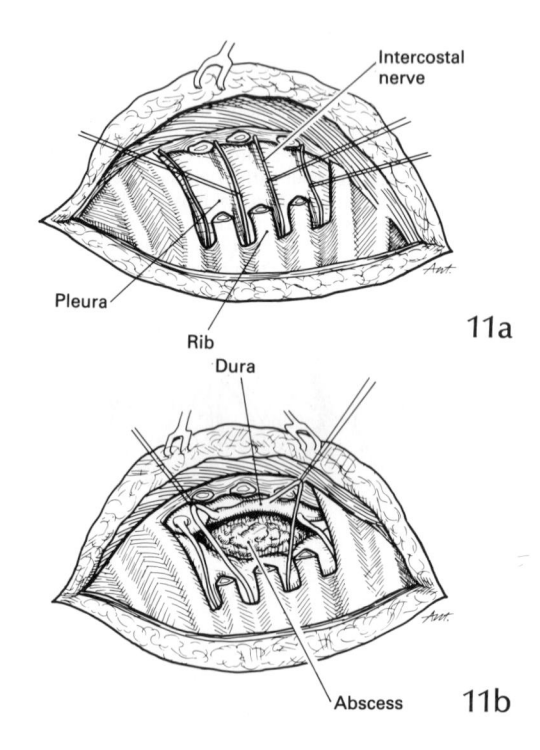

THORACOLUMBAR SPINE

The position of the patient is the same as for surgery of the thoracic spine.

Incision

12

The incision is made along the left tenth rib extending into the left upper quadrant for about 4 cm.

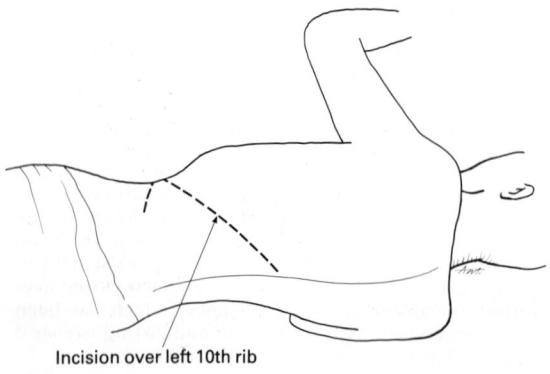

Deep dissection

13a & b

The left tenth rib is removed. The anterior end of the rib is still usually cartilaginous. This is split longitudinally, and the tissue deep to it spread with a pair of scissors to enter the extraperitoneal space. The chest cavity is entered.

14a & b

The peritoneum is stripped from the under surface of the diaphragm anteromedially. The diaphragm is incised, leaving about 2.5 cm of its posterior margin for resuturing later. The spine is then exposed intrapleurally and extraperitoneally. If the eleventh rib is removed, the parietal pleura can be dissected off the diaphragm carefully and the approach kept extrapleural and extraperitoneal. A chest drain is inserted and a vacuum drain for the retroperitoneal space.

Postoperative management

Full expansion of the lungs must be ensured by taking serial chest radiographs. The chest drain can usually be removed at 48 to 72 hours postoperatively. If a short fusion of one level is done, the patient lies in bed for 2 weeks and is allowed up with a plaster jacket. If long grafts are used, the patient should remain in bed for up to 6 weeks, so that the bone grafts become more sticky, before getting up with a plaster jacket which is retained for at least 3 months.

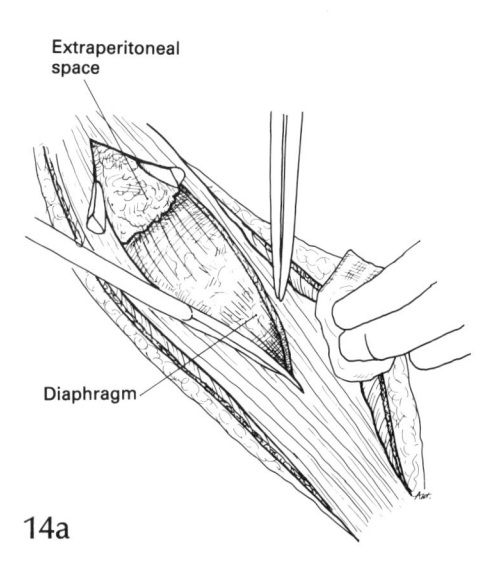

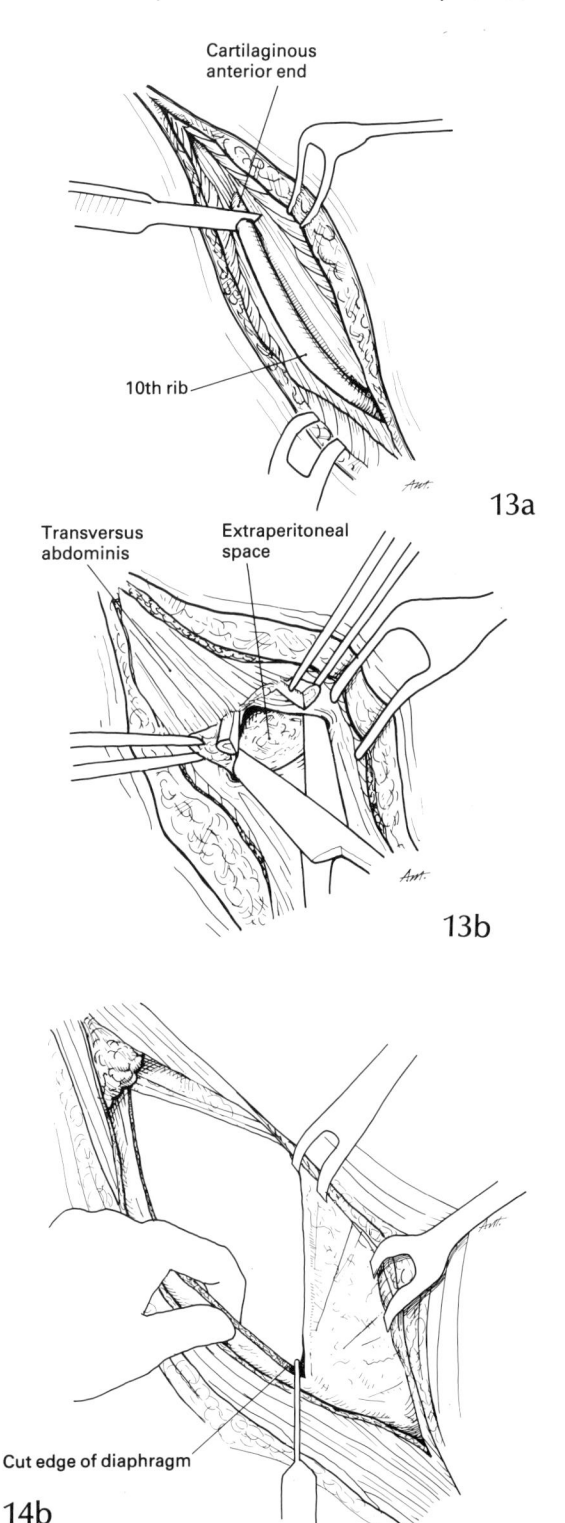

568   Thoracic and lumbar spine

LUMBAR SPINE

Position of patient

The patient lies in the full lateral position with the left side up, with the kidney bridge centred under the level of the lesion. For L4 to S1 lesions, a semi-lateral position may be used. A left-sided approach is preferable because mobilization of the aorta and common iliac artery to the right side is easier than mobilizing the corresponding veins to the left.

Incision

15

For lesions of L1 to L3 (not illustrated), an oblique flank incision is made, extending backwards to the lateral border of the erector spinae muscle and forwards to the linea semilunaris. For L4 to S1, an oblique incision is made in the left lower quadrant, extending from a point mid-way between the subcostal margin and the anterior superior iliac spine to a point in the midline between the xiphisternum and the pubic symphysis.

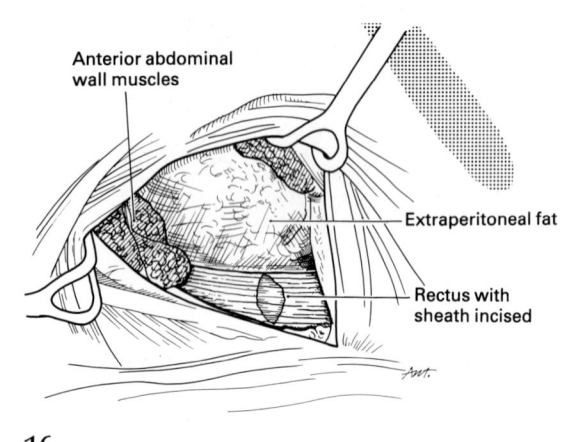

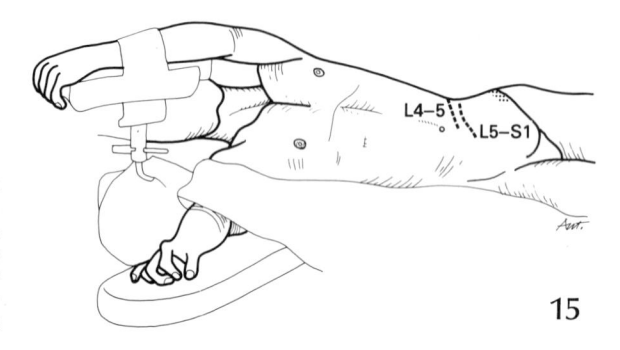

Deep dissection

16

The anterior abdominal wall muscles and anterior rectus sheath are divided with diathermy in the line of the skin incision. The extraperitoneal fat is identified, and the peritoneum stripped medially and cephalad from the left iliac fossa. It is also separated carefully from the posterior rectus fascia, which is divided transversely after identifying and protecting the inferior epigastric vessels.

17 & 18

This exposes the left psoas muscles, with the genito-femoral nerve lying on it. The ureter, recognized by its peristaltic movements, is reflected together with the peritoneum. Further blunt dissection is used to identify the segmental vessels and the iliolumbar vessels. These vessels must be carefully ligated and divided over the relevant levels to be approached.

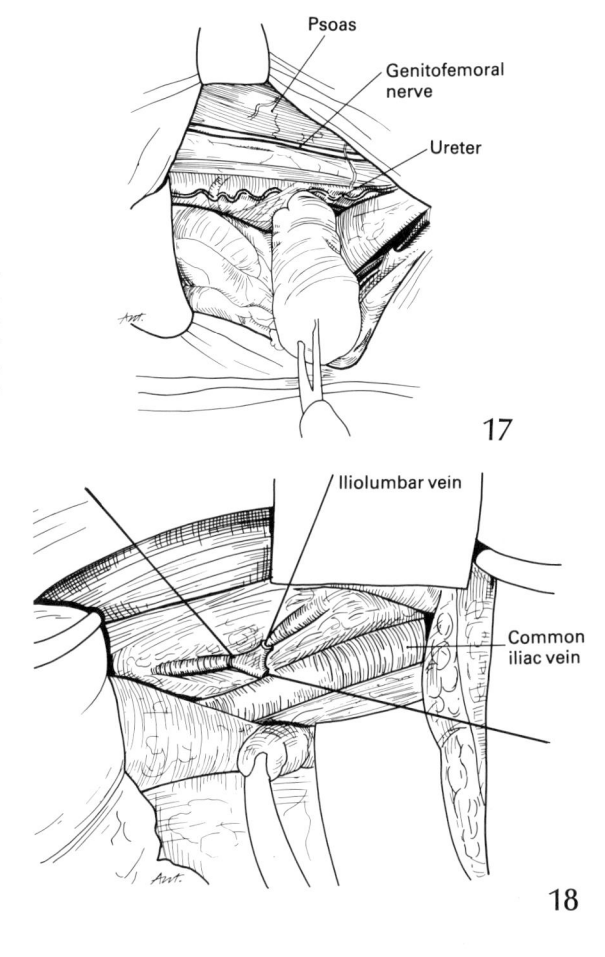

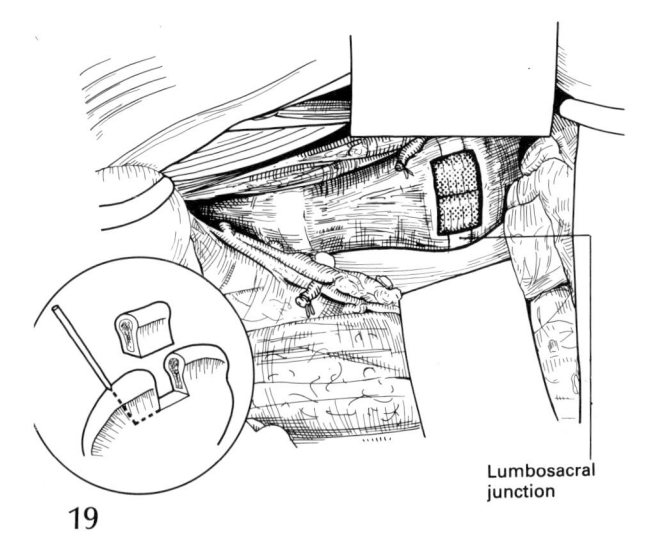

Removal of diseased tissues and bone grafting

19

This is done in the manner described previously. In the lumbar spine, the bodies are bigger, and a tricortico-cancellous iliac crest graft is preferred. The graft can be harvested through the same incision, with a little undermining of the subcutaneous tissues. A vacuum drain is used for the diseased area.

Postoperative management

Paralytic ileus commonly occurs for the first one to two days postoperatively. Nothing is given by mouth. Ryle's tube suction is continued, if necessary, until good bowel sounds return. The period of bed rest and immobilization with a plaster jacket is the same as for the thoracic spine.

Further reading

Hodgson AR, Stock FE. Anterior spinal fusion: a preliminary communication on the radical treatment of Pott's disease and Pott's paraplegia. *Br J Surg* 1956; 44: 266–75.

Hodgson AR, Stock FE, Fang HSY, Ong GB. Anterior spinal fusion: the operative approach and pathological findings in 412 patients with Pott's disease of the spine. *Br J Surg* 1960; 48: 172–8.

Hodgson AR. An approach to the cervical spine (C-3 to C-7). *Clin Orthop* 1965; 39: 129–34.

Hsu LCS, Leong JCY. Tuberculosis of the lower cervical spine (C2 to C7): a report on 40 cases. *J Bone J Surg [Br]* 1984; 66-B: 1–5.

Leong JCY, Hodgson AR. Surgical treatment of tuberculosis of the spine. In: Leach R, Lowell D, Reisborough E, Hoaglund FT, eds. *Controversy in orthopaedic surgery*, Chapter 16. Philadelphia: Saunders 1982.

Medical Research Council Working Party on Tuberculosis of the Spine. Eighth report. A 10-year assessment of a controlled trial comparing debridement and anterior spinal fusion in the management of tuberculosis of the spine in patients on standard chemotherapy in Hong Kong. *J Bone Joint Surg [Br]* 1982; 64-B, 393–8.

Southwick WO, Robinson RA. Surgical approaches to the vertebral bodies in the cervical and lumbar regions. *J Bone Joint Surg [Am]* 1957 39-A: 631–44.

Illustrations by Peter Cox

Metastatic bone disease of the spine

Malcolm W. Fidler MS, FRCS
Consultant Orthopaedic Surgeon, Onze Lieve Vrouwe Gasthuis and Netherlands Cancer Institute, Amsterdam, The Netherlands

Introduction

The routine approaches to the spine and methods of stabilization, such as rectangles with laminar wires and pedicle screws with plates, are covered in the chapter on 'Spinal injuries' (see pp. 624–669). Details relevant to the treatment of metastases and pathological fractures alone will be described in this chapter.

Aim

Patients with metastases have limited life expectancies. Surgical treatment should restore adequate neurological function, relieve pain and ensure immediate and permanent spinal stability so that the patient can be mobilized and return home as soon as possible.

Indications

1. Spinal cord, cauda equina or nerve root compression caused by a bone or disc fragment, or by tumour which is radioresistant, or after a maximum dose of radiotherapy has been given (or where the rate of progression of a cord lesion is such that radiotherapy can not be expected to be successful).
2. Severe pain despite adequate conservative treatment.
3. An unstable fracture which threatens the integrity of the spinal cord or cauda equina.

The neighbouring vertebrae must be capable of supporting the reconstruction.

A rapidly growing uncontrollable malignancy is a contraindication to surgery.

Basic principles

Decompression

1

The spinal cord is very vulnerable to pressure. Retraction, especially if the cord is already compromised, must be avoided. Decompression is carried out from the direction of the spinal cord compression. In particular, anterior compression is treated by anterior decompression. Access is best gained through the shaded area shown in the illustration: the cause of the compression can be withdrawn comfortably, safely and under direct vision without retraction of the dura or pressure on the cord.

Laminectomy for anterior spinal cord compression requires dural retraction and almost always results in neurological deterioration[1]; it should be avoided. It also further jeopardizes spinal stability.

The cauda equina is less vulnerable to pressure and the dura may be gently retracted during a posterior approach. However, if the dura is taut because of displaced vertebral body fragments or tumour, further neurological damage may result.

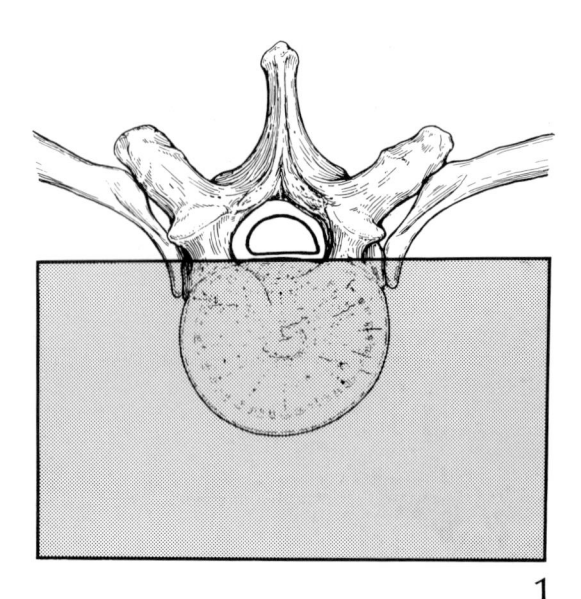

Stabilization

On biomechanical grounds, the part of the spinal column which has failed should be restored[2]. In particular, this means that vertebral body collapse should be treated by anterior reconstruction.

Flexion/compression

2

Optimum mechanical advantage for the correction of a kyphosis associated with a pathological fracture of the vertebral body is obtained by anterior distraction and optimal stabilization by an anterior reconstruction. The strongest part of the vertebral body in patients over 40 years of age is at the periphery[3]. Any anterior reconstruction should support the whole of the vertebral end-plate and especially its anterior rim.

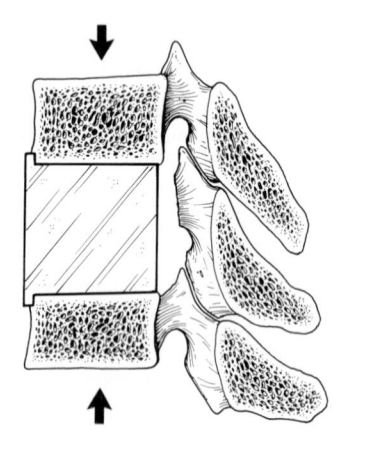

Rotation

This is best controlled by pedicle screws and plates or by a rigid snug-fitting posterior rectangle construction fastened to the vertebrae with laminar wires and reinforced with cement. Addition of an anterolateral paravertebral strengthened Zielke system to an interbody construction also effectively controls rotation[4] and prevents hyperextension, though the Kaneda[5] device, as tested by Gurr et al.[6] should be even better.

Translation

This must also be controlled by any reconstruction.

Stabilization at various sites

In the cervical spine and particularly in the upper spine where rotatory stability is important, posterior stabilization is probably advantageous, especially when bridging more than two diseased vertebrae.

In the thoracic and lumbar spines, where compression forces are maximal, anterior stabilization is essential.

Anterior stabilization following vertebral body resection may be achieved with bone graft or various metal or ceramic implants reinforced with bone cement[7-15].

Posterior stabilization principally involves rectangle/laminar wires or pedicle screw/plate systems, where necessary reinforced with bone cement[16-20].

Although pedicle screws can be inserted at all levels, it seems reasonable to use laminar wiring techniques above the midthoracic spine where the pedicles are small, and pedicle screw fixation more caudally where the pedicles are larger. A combination of the two techniques, namely pedicle screws which can be used in conjunction with rectangles, is currently being developed by Dove (personal communication) and may prove useful in bridging midthoracic disease.

Cement

It must be stressed that cement is excellent at withstanding compressive loads, but poor with regard to shear or tensile stresses. It is therefore especially suitable for anterior interbody reconstruction where compressive loads predominate.

As part of a posterior reconstruction where an implant is fixed to the vertebrae with laminar wires, cement is used only to reinforce the metal construction, chiefly by acting as a grout between metal and bone in order to spread the contact load, and prevent movement and loosening of the wires. Cement should not be used as the prime posterior stabilizer.

Cement studs should be short (4 mm) and broad (at least 6 mm diameter).

Incisions

Incisions must take into account any previous incisions as well as any areas severely affected by radiotherapy. If necessary, the spine can usually be exposed from the other side.

Preoperative

Investigations

Blood examination

Depression of bone marrow activity by recent chemotherapy or radiotherapy will be elucidated by blood examination. Hypercalcaemia may be present.

Radiographs

Anteroposterior and lateral radiographs of the spine and chest should be taken.

Bone scan

A bone scan should be taken to identify lesions in neighbouring vertebrae as well as in remote areas.

Myelogram

A myelogram will delineate the extent of the obstruction. If there is a complete obstruction to the passage of contrast, contrast should also be introduced by suboccipital puncture to determine the cranial extent of the lesion. The myelogram also reveals any epidural skip lesions.

Computed tomography (CT)

After myelography, CT defines the extent of vertebral body destruction and the precise zone of neural compression. Sagittal reconstructions or, if unavailable, lateral tomograms help to complete the three-dimensional picture of the lesion.

Nuclear magnetic resonance (NMR)

NMR can supplant CT and myelography but, in Europe, is still not generally available for emergency use.

Selective angiography

This reveals any vascular abnormalities near the tumour. If hypervascular, the tumour bed is embolized with Ivalon (Polystan Benelux, Almere Haven, The Netherlands). Any segmental artery which also gives rise to a medullary feeder artery, e.g. the artery of Adamkiewicz is, of course, not embolized. Angiography and embolization are carried out within 2–3 days of surgery. If performed earlier, there is a risk of collaterals opening up or recanalization occurring.

Angiography is not routinely performed for lesions in the neck as embolization would be too dangerous. The disadvantages of angiography would then outweigh the advantages unless a major anterior resection is contemplated.

Biopsy

If there is any doubt about the nature of the lesion, biopsy is essential. A percutaneous posterolateral approach is used for the vertebral body. (If a resectable primary lesion is suspected, open percutaneous transpedicular biopsy is advisable[21].) With a purely posterior lesion, needle biopsy may be dangerous unless the spinous process is also involved. Open biopsy is usually simple and safer.

Material removed during operation is always examined histologically; a second unsuspected type of tumour is occasionally found.

When emergency decompression is necessary and the diagnosis is unknown, biopsy is combined with the definitive operation (see section on 'Timing of surgery' below).

Antibiotics

Cephamandole (2 g) is injected intravenously just before surgery and repeated 6-hourly during the first 24 hours.

At present the advisability of preoperative selective intestinal sterilization is being assessed.

Expectations of surgery

With even a severe paraparesis, recovery sufficient for walking can usually be expected. Recovery of a paraplegia has been described when the onset was slow and some sensation was still present[22].

Restoration of spinal stability almost invariably leads to a gratifying relief of pain.

The postoperative survival, however, is related more to the nature of the primary tumour and its response to any possible radiotherapy and chemotherapy, as well as to the extent of dissemination of the disease.

Timing of surgery

In general, the sooner surgery is performed the better. With a slowly progressive neurological lesion (over a few days), operation can be planned for the next convenient list. Rapid progression should be treated as an emergency. The myelogram/CT is essential. The angiogram/embolization is usually possible within a few hours; if not, it can be omitted. If the diagnosis is in doubt, the decompression provides good biopsy material and a frozen section should confirm the presence of tumour; if not, infection should be considered before inserting an implant and cement.

If possible, operation should be postponed until the blood picture has returned to normal if chemotherapeutic agents have recently been given.

Operations

Cervical spine

Preliminary halo traction is applied when the patient is admitted if it is necessary to relieve severe pain, to correct a severe kyphosis or to stabilize an unstable fracture. Careful neurological control is essential.

ANTERIOR CORD DECOMPRESSION

This is effected by removal of the involved vertebral body or bodies.

Application of halo

If a halo is not already in place, one is applied after induction of anaesthesia. Although anterior surgery for pathological fractures can be carried out with the help of various self-retaining retractors in the absence of a halo, halo traction allows the head to be easily and safely manoeuvred, if necessary, during the operation.

Position

3

The operating table is assembled with its pedestal as far away from the head-end as possible to allow lateral C-arm image intensification. When not in use, the C-arm can conveniently be moved away towards the pedestal.

It is usually easier for a right-handed surgeon to approach the cervical spine from the right-hand side, although danger to the recurrent laryngeal nerve in the presence of an anomalous right subclavian artery should not be forgotten.

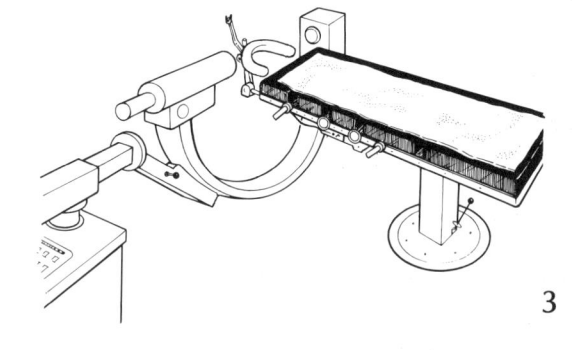

4

The patient is positioned supine with the head initially turned slightly to the left and supported on the appropriate operating table extension with 3 kg traction. A larger weight can be applied if necessary. The shoulders are gently pulled caudally and fixed to the operating table with adhesive tape.

The anaesthetic tube is positioned along the non-operated side of the patient to the foot end of the table.

The alignment and curvature of the cervical spine are checked with the image intensifier. The level of the diseased vertebra(e) is identified with the aid of a metal marker and marked on the skin with indelible ink.

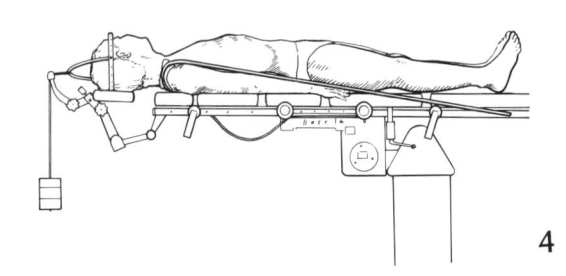

Incision

For single vertebral body excision, an oblique skin crease incision is made, centred at the level of the lesion, from the lateral border of the sternomastoid almost to the midline. If more exposure is envisaged, an incision along the anterior border of the sternomastoid is used, also centred on the level of the metastasis. The spine is then approached between the carotid sheath laterally and the pharynx and larynx, or oesophagus and trachea, medially, as described in the chapter on 'Anterior fusions of the spine' (pp. 463–470).

Tumour removal

The prominent diseased vertebra(e) is usually easily identified. In case of doubt, a needle is inserted and the position checked with the image intensifier. The longus colli muscles are separated in the midline and are mobilized laterally by a combination of sharp and blunt dissection. A Cloward self-retaining retractor is inserted. Medially the smooth-edged blade is used; if it slips superficial to longus colli, its smooth edge is unlikely to damage the oesophagus. Laterally, the crenellated blade is used.

For cranial and caudal retraction, a second self-retaining Cloward retractor may be inserted at right angles to the first, but one or two 2-cm wide Langenbeck retractors of appropriate length may be more useful.

With a needle, the intervertebral discs are identified cranial and caudal to the diseased vertebra(e) which is then removed piecemeal along with the discs. As dissection proceeds, the neighbouring vertebrae can be distracted to correct any kyphosis and improve exposure by inserting appropriate self-retaining retractors. This can be done more simply by adding weight to the halo traction. Any doubt as to the depth of the cavity should be resolved using the image intensifier.

The posterior longitudinal ligament should be removed to gain access to epidural tumour. Laterally, on both sides of the central cavity, tumour is removed gently with appropriate long-handled, angled sharp spoons. This is done gently because of the presence of the vertebral artery and, to a lesser extent, emerging nerve roots. The location of any lateral tumour extension can be seen on the CT.

The wound is irrigated copiously with Dakin's solution and then saline, preferably from a closed irrigation system.

ANTERIOR STABILIZATION

This is only practicable following resection of the vertebral bodies of C3 and below.

The head is returned to the neutral position. If necessary, the alignment and curvature of the vertebrae are checked with the image intensifier.

5a, b & c

A piece of vitallium mesh is cut and bent to shape (a,b). It is narrow where it is in contact with bone and wide where it turns onto and protects the dura. It extends along the front of the cranial vertebra, flush along the middle of the vertebral end-plate, along the full width of the dura, the middle of the caudal vertebral end-plate and the anterior surface of the caudal vertebra (c). A suitable 'AO small fragment set' plate is selected to bridge the defect. If the correct length is not available a longer one can be cut to length and the cut edge dulled with a sterile file. Two screws cranially and caudally should be used although one screw proximally is enough when the plate is used to bridge only one vertebra. Caspar plates may be used instead of AO plates if available.

The plate is positioned and the sites for the screw holes and slits in the mesh noted. The slits facilitate positioning of the mesh. It is easier to make these holes or slits if the mesh is temporarily removed.

The plate is loosely screwed in place with two AO 3.5 mm screws in 2.5 mm tapped drill holes which include the posterior cortices. The other holes are drilled and tapped. The plate is removed, the mesh reinserted with a layer of absorbable gelatin sponge (Gelfoam, Allen & Hanburys, Greenford, UK) to protect the dura and the plate screwed into position. The image intensifier is now used to check the final alignment and in particular the length of the screws which should grip the posterior cortices. If all is well, the screws are backed off a couple of turns.

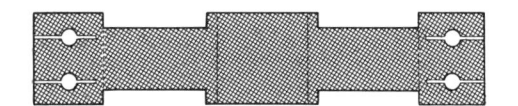

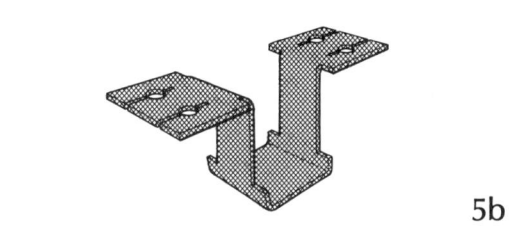

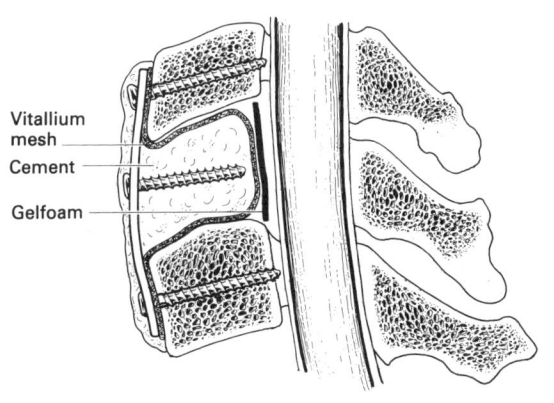

Cement

Pressure cannot be applied for fear of forcing cement against the dura. Cool, low viscosity cement (Allofix G, Streuli, Uznack, Belgium) is injected into the cavity while still fluid. The cement syringe should be fitted with a suitable nozzle, e.g. a piece of a catheter which reaches to the bottom of the cavity. The cavity must be dry to avoid mixing cement and blood. When oozing is troublesome, packing the cavity and waiting for 10–15 minutes is usually effective. If necessary, a fine sucker is inserted in the depth of the cavity whilst the first portion of the cement is injected.

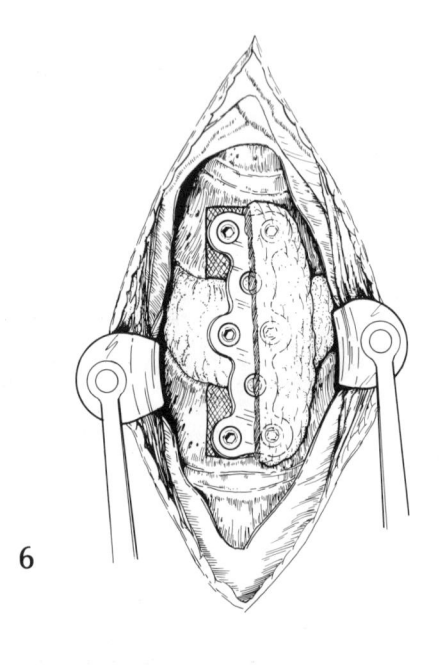

6

The cement is allowed to flow over the edges of the adjacent vertebrae. While still soft, the screws are tightened and an extra screw is inserted to bond the cement and plate together. A thin layer of cement is moulded over the plate and the screws. There must be no sharp cement edges which might harm the oesophagus or pharynx. The wound is irrigated with cold saline during polymerization of the cement.

The longus colli muscles are approximated: closure is never possible. A piece of Gelfoam is inserted between the oesophagus/pharynx and the construction. A mini vacuum drain is inserted. Only the platysma and the skin require suturing.

7

If vitallium mesh is unavailable, the cement can be anchored by making 6 mm diameter pits in the end-plates of the adjacent vertebrae with a dental drill and burr, or manoeuvring a piece of threaded rod through the end-plates. The anterior plate is screwed in place as before. The dura is protected with a layer of Gelfoam before cement is added.

Postoperative management

The halo is removed before the patient wakes and the neck is supported in a Philadelphia collar or Somi brace. This is worn day and night for 6 weeks, except for washing when the neck is kept straight; it is then worn at night or while travelling by car for a further 6 weeks until a firm fibrous capsule envelops the prosthesis. The patient can usually be mobilized on the day following operation depending on the neurological situation.

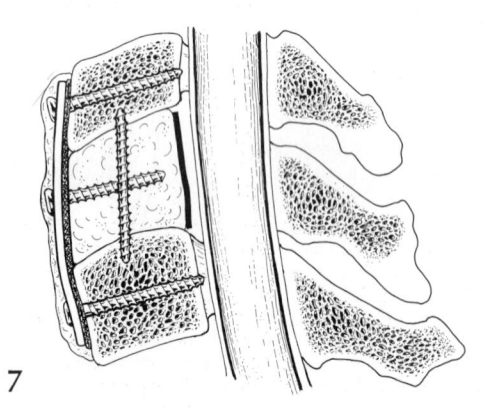

POSTERIOR DECOMPRESSION

Posterior or lateral cord compression is treated by removing the appropriate parts of the laminae and facets, and any epidural tumour.

Nerve root compression can be relieved by the posterior or anterior approach.

During operations on the upper cervical spine, the massive spinous process of the axis is an unmistakable reference point.

POSTERIOR STABILIZATION

Indications

1. Stabilization of C1 and C2 with or without anterior decompression.
2. Stabilization in conjunction with posterior nerve root decompression, or posterior or lateral cord decompression.
3. Stabilization of any number of cervical vertebrae.
4. Supplementary stabilization following anterior decompression and stabilization of three or more vertebrae.

Atlas and axis

For stabilization of C1 and C2, a special plate has been developed.

The plate is screwed to the occiput in the midline, where the AO screws gain a firm grip in the thick strong internal occipital crest. Fixation to the cervical laminae is with the well-proven double 1 mm laminar wires. Bone cement and autograft enhance fixation.

The plates are available in three lengths; two healthy vertebrae caudal to the diseased vertebra or the unstable segment must be included in the construction.

If the special plates are not available, a steel loop such as that designed by Ransford[23] can be used.

Position

8

The operating table is assembled as for the anterior approach. The patient is positioned prone with the head supported in halo traction on the operating table extension.

Lateral image intensification or radiographs are taken to check reduction and spinal curvature.

Incision

A midline incision is made. The occiput, from the foramen magnum to the superior nuchal line and for 3 cm on each side of the midline, as well as the laminae and facet joints of the appropriate cervical vertebrae, are exposed. The exposure is described in detail in the chapter on 'Posterior fusions of the cervical spine' (see pp. 471–481).

When exposing the cranial edge of the atlas, it is important that the operator should keep within 1.5 cm of the midline to avoid the vertebral artery.

A malleable template is used to check the curvature of the plate. The plate can be contoured if necessary.

Bilateral double cold drawn 1 mm laminar wires are passed. Preliminary passage of a thread loop using aneurysm needles of various sizes is often helpful. Healthy spinous processes are not removed as they help to contain, and afford fixation for, the cement.

Positioning of plate

Holes of 3.2 mm are drilled in the midline of the occiput, i.e. in the internal occipital crest which is usually 1–1.5 cm thick. A drill guard (or adjustable stop) is used. A drill which protrudes 11 mm out of the drill guard is used initially, and especial care is taken when drilling the inner cortex. The screw length (size 14 mm is usual) is measured, and the threads for the standard AO 4.5 mm screws are tapped. (An inadvertent CSF leak can be plugged with the screw.)

9

The plate is screwed into position; the screws should just grip the apex of the internal occipital crest. The laminar wires are twisted and tightened.

Exposed dura or nerve root is protected by a free fat graft; where cement will be added, additional protection is provided by a layer of Gelfoam.

Cement or autograft is added from the posterior iliac crest as indicated. A thin layer of cement should be applied over the screws to prevent loosening.

Bone cement is used as a grout on both sides when the prognosis is less than 6–12 months. When the prognosis is longer, bone cement is added on one side and tumour-free autograft on the other. (The presence of donor site metastases should be excluded by referral to the preoperative bone scan.)

If tumour tissue has been exposed during decompression, the cement is used on this side and a graft, when indicated, on the intact side. This improves the chance of bone union and reduces the chance of tumour invading the graft.

A strip of moist Gelfoam placed laterally effectively prevents the cement escaping into the muscles.

Closure

Routine closure of the wound (over a vacuum drain), paying special attention to the ligamentum nuchae, is performed. The halo is removed.

Postoperative management

The patient can be mobilized on the following day. (Most patients appreciate a Philadelphia collar or Somi brace during the first 2 weeks while the wound heals.) Thereafter the support is worn when the patient travels by car.

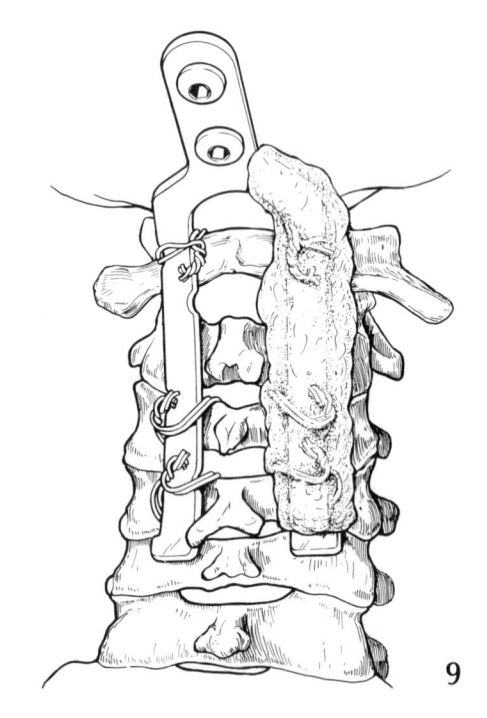

Metastatic bone disease of the spine 581

C3 and below

10

At these levels a rectangle is applied from two levels above to two levels below the diseased vertebrae. Fixation is by double cold drawn laminar wires augmented by cement and autograft (as for the occipitocervical plate). Healthy spinous processes are not removed.

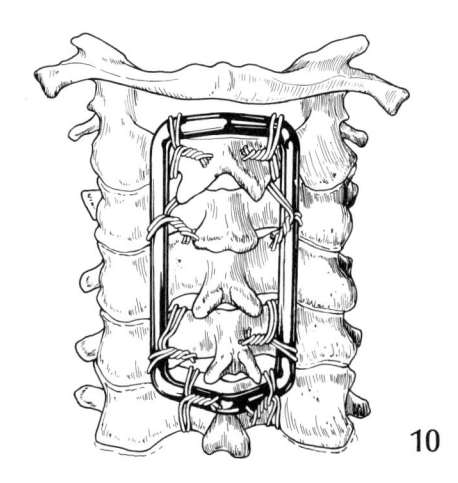

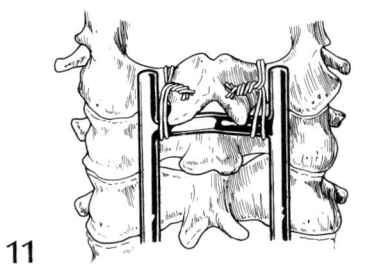

11

When the stabilization extends up to the axis, the origins of the inferior oblique and rectus capitis posterior major muscles can be spared by using a rectangle as shown: the laminae of C3 must also be wired to the rectangle. Otherwise a collar is advisable until the resutured origins of these muscles heal.

Thoracic and lumbar spines

ANTERIOR DECOMPRESSION (THORACIC SPINE)

Position

12

The patient is placed in the lateral thoracotomy position with the affected segment of the spine over the operating table bridge which is raised to improve access. An inflatable cushion some 10 cm in diameter is positioned transversely under the appropriate ribs to prevent the cranial segment of the spine falling away laterally after resection of the diseased vertebral bodies. The cushion is particularly useful for female patients.

Although the thoracic spine can be approached from either side, a left-sided approach is preferable as it facilitates identification and ligature of the segmental arteries as they arise from the aorta. If a large left paravertebral tumour mass would render a left-sided approach unduly hazardous, or if the cord is compressed from the right as well as anteriorly, a right-sided approach is used. In the presence of a large medullary feeder artery (the artery of Adamkiewicz is on the left in 80 per cent of cases with a predilection for T9/T11[24]), one would tend to approach the spine from the other side. If one approaches from the same side, great care is necessary in the region of the intervertebral foramen and any diathermy should be bipolar.

Supports are positioned against the right anterior superior iliac spine, the left posterior superior iliac spine or buttock, and the back of the upper chest. This last support can be omitted in the case of a high thoracotomy. The left arm is supported on a standard arm rest.

Supports should not interfere with any necessary radiographs.

Anaesthesia

For lesions above T9, a double-lumen tube is helpful so that the lung can be collapsed to facilitate exposure of the spine. For lesions below T9, a standard endotracheal tube is sufficient.

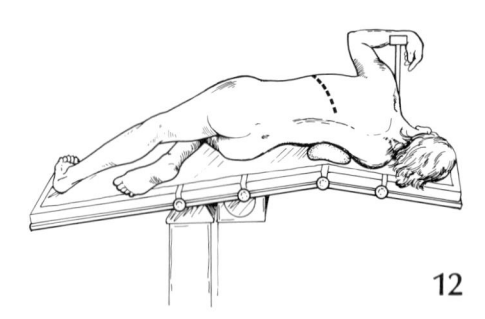

Incision and exposure

The ribs increase in obliquity from above down. The levels for the thoracotomy incisions to expose the cranialmost diseased vertebra are listed below. These incisions also allow exposure of the adjacent healthy cranial vertebrae and several more caudal vertebrae.

T1 Anterior via the neck. A left-sided approach is used in view of the normal position of the right recurrent laryngeal nerve. One must beware of the thoracic duct. If a metastasis in T1 is hypervascular and embolization is unsuccessful, then it should be approached as for T2 so that any bleeding can be controlled. Care is necessary so that the T1 anterior primary ramus is not injured.

The upper thoracic vertebrae may also be exposed anteriorly as described by Sundaresan et al.[25] and Birch et al.[26]

T2 Above the third rib: if necessary excise the third rib
T3 Above the third rib: if necessary excise the third rib
T4 Above the fourth rib
T5 Above the fifth rib
T6 Above the sixth rib
T7 Above the sixth rib
T8 Above the sixth rib
T9 Above the seventh rib
T10 Above the eighth rib
T11 Above the ninth rib
T12 Above the tenth rib. The diaphragm should be released slightly to expose the cranial half of L1 for insertion of the DKS screw (Ulrich, Ulm, Germany).

The incision normally stretches along the rib from the lateral edge of the erector spinae to the anterior axillary line. If necessary it can be extended anteriorly. (For a complete description of the exposure of the thoracic spine, see the chapter on 'Approaches to the spine', pp. 597–623.)

The proposed posterolateral thoracotomy incision is marked on the skin and identified with a metal marker. The level is checked radiographically. The radiograph also shows whether the fractured spine is straight or not.

The level of the rib is confirmed before the periosteum is incised. The upper ribs can be counted by passing a hand up under serratus anterior. The uppermost rib which can be comfortably palpated is usually the second, and the first rib can usually just be tipped with gently exploring fingers. The periosteum along the chosen rib is cut with diathermy and rasped upwards along with the intercostal muscles. Subperiosteal resection of a 2 cm long segment of the rib close to the angle facilitates separation of the ribs and improves exposure of the spine. In the upper chest, a similar segment of rib can also be removed from a neighbouring rib to improve exposure further. Resection of a rib is usually unnecessary.

The pleural cavity is palpated and the lung is either collapsed or retracted forwards to expose the spine, where an obvious swelling will usually be found corresponding to the site of the tumour.

The mediastinal pleura is incised longitudinally along the anterior margin of the affected vertebral bodies and then posteriorly across the middle of the affected segment. The flaps of this T-incision are elevated and held aside by stay sutures. The sympathetic chain should be spared whenever possible. Branches to the splanchnic nerves need to be divided at the level of the vertebral body resection.

The ipsilateral segmental vessels crossing the diseased vertebrae are divided between ligatures in the interval between aorta and spine. The aorta is retracted forwards to expose the contralateral segmental vessels, which are ligatured or clipped in continuity. During dissection between aorta and spine, a bloodless field is essential. Any vessels entering the anterior surface of the affected vertebrae are coagulated, tied or clipped before division. The source of any lymph leak must be identified and closed. The ipsilateral segmental vessels are again ligatured just anterior to the intervertebral foramina.

13a & b

A window is made in the middle third of the affected segment and deepened in the coronal plane to form a tunnel across the spine. The posterior wall of the tunnel is then removed. Palpation of the anterior wall of an intervertebral foramen with a dural elevator or a Watson–Cheyne dissector guides the operator to the plane of the dura, as does exposure of the appropriate intercostal nerve or palpation along the end-plates of the intact cranial and caudal vertebrae as these are exposed.

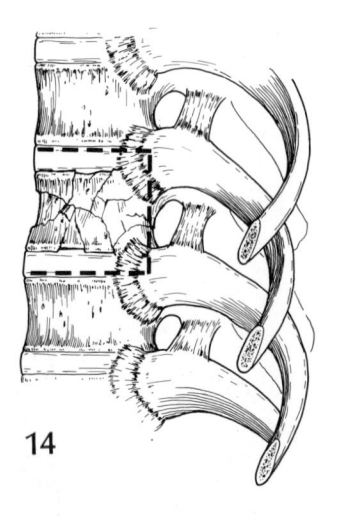

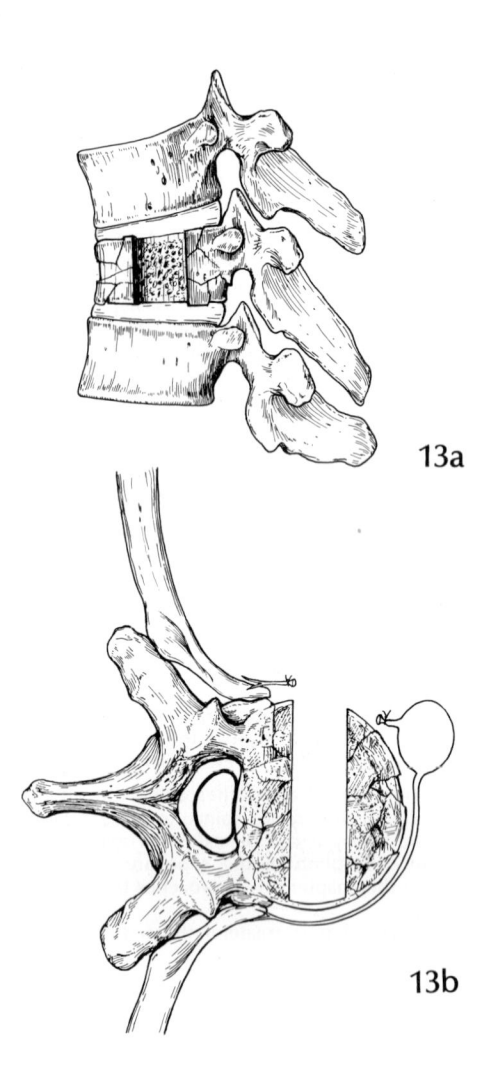

14

The head of the rib is removed at the same time as the intervertebral disc.

Removal of tumour

15a–d

Soft tumour and bone fragments can be removed using a circular motion of a variety of long-handled, angled, sharp spoons. The fragments are caught with the edge of the spoon and rotated or pulled into the coronal tunnel, i.e. away from the dura (a). Normal bone and firm compressed diseased bone can be removed using a slightly curved 1 cm wide osteotome as follows. Slivers of bone and bone mixed with tumour are removed in the coronal plane (b) until the spinal canal is just opened or until a thin flexible remnant of bone separates the osteotome and canal. (A power burr may be used instead of the osteotome.) The canal is then opened with a strong dural elevator (c). The thin remaining bone can then be prised forwards and removed with the osteotome and a variety of fine punches and bone nibblers (d). It is advisable to concentrate on decompressing the dura first on the contralateral side. If the uppermost side is first completely decompressed, the dura bulges out and obscures the far side. The hand holding the osteotome must be well supported at all times. A Cobb elevator is particularly useful for exposing the end-plates of the adjoining healthy vertebral bodies.

The posterior longitudinal ligament is often intact but should be removed, at least partially, to allow access to any epidural tumour which, if present, can usually be peeled off the dura. If such peeling is difficult then it is better to leave a thin layer of tumour than to inadvertently tear open the dura.

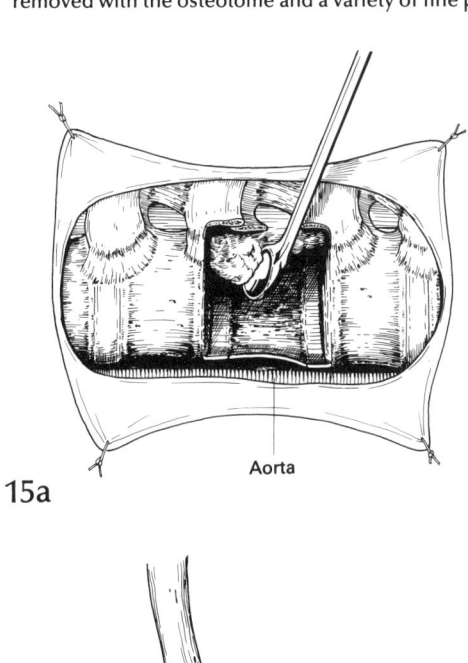

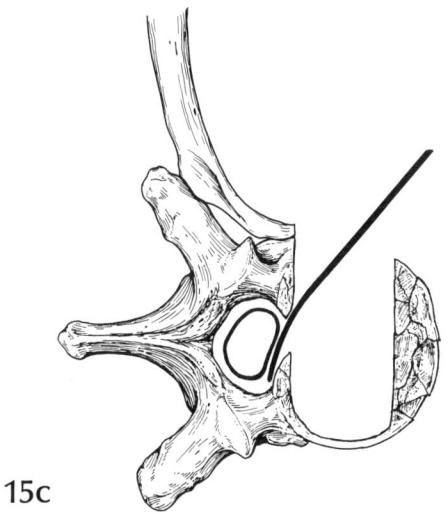

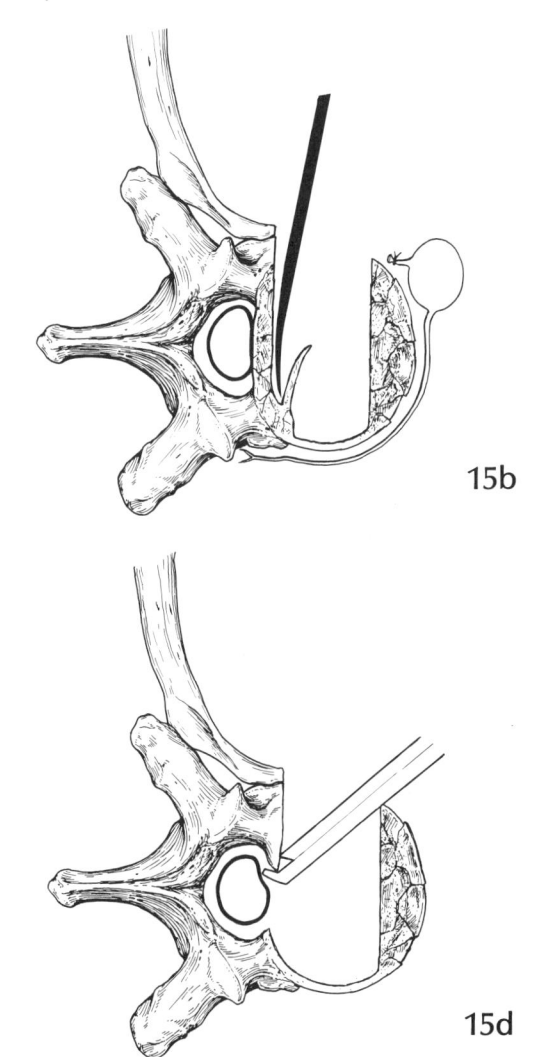

16

If necessary, the pedicle and the base of the transverse process can also be removed to give access to lateral and even posterolateral epidural tumour tissue. During such a manoeuvre one must be especially careful of the emerging nerve roots which leave the dura anterior to the coronal diameter. Bleeding in the vicinity of the intervertebral foramen should be carefully identified and coagulated with bipolar diathermy.

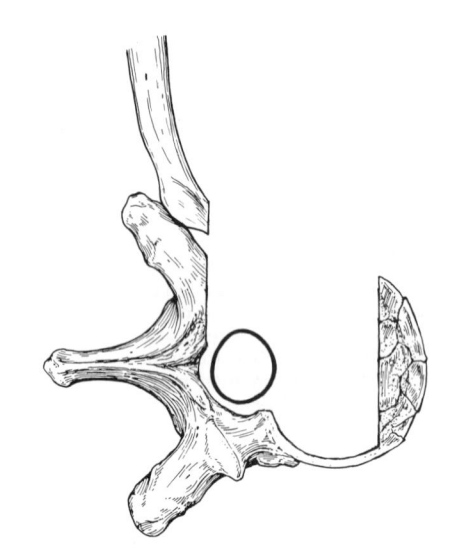

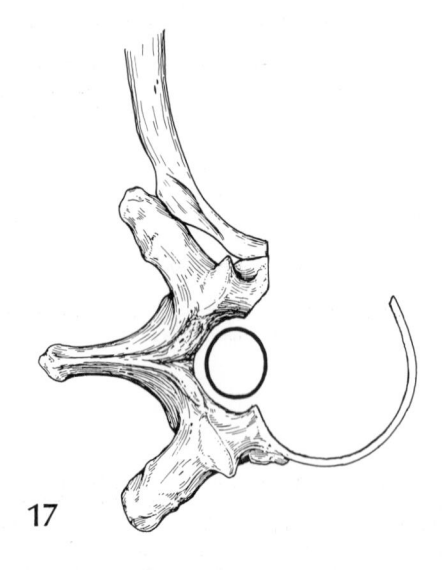

17

The anterior portion of each diseased vertebral body is then removed until only the anterior longitudinal ligament and an osteoperiosteal shell remain anteriorly and on the far side. Osteotomes, various sizes of bone nibblers, long-handled sharp spoons and power burrs can all be used to advantage.

After the dural decompression is completed, the pleural cavity and the operation site are rinsed with warmed Dakin's solution and then with saline.

ANTERIOR DECOMPRESSION (LUMBAR SPINE)

The cord usually terminates at L1 and so the same respect for the dura is necessary here as in the thoracic spine. Below this level, as mentioned above, a posterior approach may be used to relieve anterior compression, but as anterior stabilization is, in any case, necessary on mechanical grounds, it seems logical to carry out both decompression and stabilization anteriorly.

Incision and exposure

The lumbar spine is approached retroperitoneally and the levels of incision are as below.

With the patient in the lateral position:
L1 Above the tenth rib with release of the diaphragm
L2 Through the bed of the twelfth rib
L3 Parallel to and under the twelfth rib
With the patient in the three-quarter position:
L4 Oblique incision halfway between the twelfth rib and the iliac crest
With the patient supine:
L5 Oblique or long left paramedian incision and then retroperitoneal approach.

(These exposures are described in detail in the chapter on 'Approaches to the spine', pp. 597–623.)

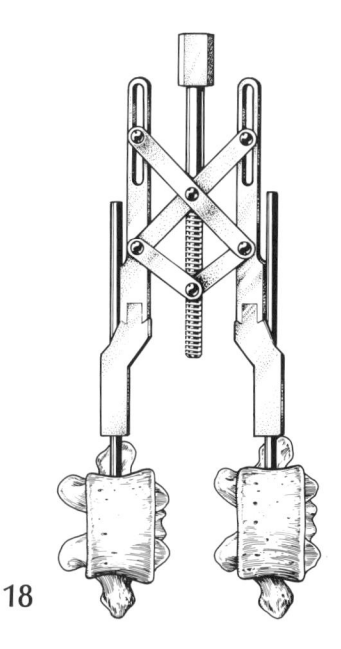

During exposure of the spine, the vena cava and, more caudally, the left iliac vein must be mobilized to the right, along with the aorta. They must not remain obscured and tethered to the front of the spine by tumour.

Once the spine is exposed, the diseased vertebrae are removed in the same way as the thoracic vertebrae (see above). As a guide to orientation, the intervertebral foramen can be palpated with a curved dural elevator, passed gently backwards around the intervertebral disc under the psoas muscle which is progressively released.

At L4, because of the position of the patient, the initial tunnel in the vertebral body is directed posterolaterally into the vertebral body rather than in a coronal plane; at L5, the vertebral body is removed piecemeal from in front.

ANTERIOR STABILIZATION (THORACIC AND LUMBAR SPINES)

To facilitate spinal stabilization after resection of a thoracic or lumbar vertebral body, a range of special prostheses has been designed.

When more than one vertebral body has been removed, a modular telescopic prosthesis is used. The primary interbody device is optimally suited to support the vertebral bodies and also to minimize interference with the paravertebral tissues. The prosthesis initially supports the anterior vertebral body rim (see above). Addition of cement is essential to support the vertebral end-plates and also to reinforce the modular prosthesis.

Following resection of the vertebral body of T1, anterior stabilization may only be possible in favourable circumstances, otherwise posterior stabilization with a rectangle is carried out.

Technique

After removal of one vertebral body

After one vertebral body has been removed, the vertebral body prosthesis is inserted as follows.

18

Steinmann pins 5 mm thick are inserted transversely and anteriorly into the vertebral bodies (away from the sites of the subsequent vertebral body screws). The modified Morscher spinal spreader is applied. (If difficulty is experienced in using the modified Morscher spreader during stabilization of the upper thoracic vertebrae, the spine can be distracted by head traction).

The kyphosis is corrected gently with the spreader until the anterior longitudinal ligament is fairly taut. Pressure with the hand over the apex of the kyphosis helps to straighten the spine. It is important that it is not overdistracted.

19a & b

With the awl, or a burr mounted on a dental drill, a shallow (4 mm), 8 mm-diameter cement pit is fashioned in the centre of the vertebral end-plate (*Illustration 19a*). Where the vertebrae are of sufficient width (caudal to T9), two anti-rotation cement pits are fashioned with the burr, 6 mm in diameter and 4 mm deep to left and right in the end-plates (*Illustration 19b*).

The size of the gap is measured and the prosthesis of the nearest size is chosen. If necessary, the gap can be reduced, or slightly distracted. In the upper thoracic spine, if the gap is too small for the smallest prosthesis, reconstruction as in the cervical spine (*see Illustrations 5, 6 and 7*) is carried out, though the plate is applied more laterally.

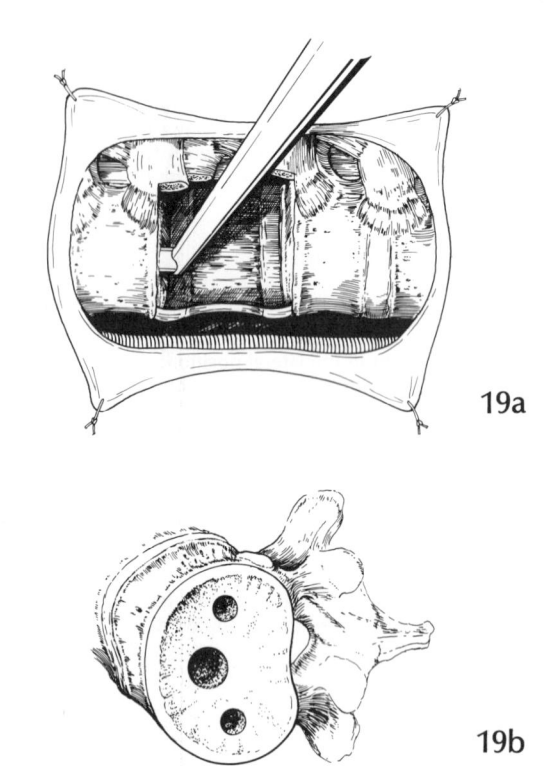

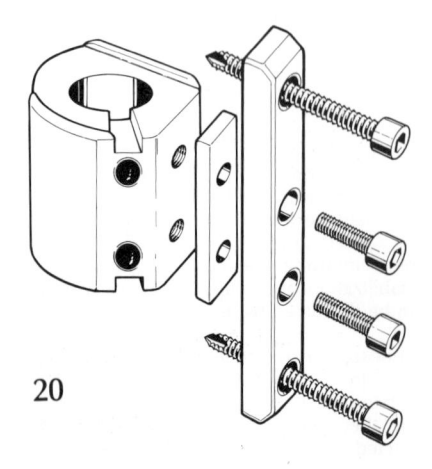

20

The prosthesis is assembled. The width can be increased by using the 5 mm spacer. Sometimes it is more convenient to add the paravertebral plate after removal of the Morscher spinal spreader (*see below*).

The prosthesis is inserted with its anterior lips around the anterior edges of the neighbouring vertebrae: the anterior longitudinal ligament is first transversely incised opposite the vertebral body edges.

The modified Morscher spinal spreader and Steinmann pins are removed.

Because of the obliquity of the ribs and the incision, the rib spreader may have twisted the spine. If necessary, the rib spreader is relaxed.

A control anteroposterior radiograph is taken; if necessary, the inflatable cushion or the operating table bridge can be adjusted to obtain a straight spine.

Holes are drilled for the self-tapping vertebral body screws. The lengths of the screws are measured and they are then inserted. The screws should grip the opposite cortex.

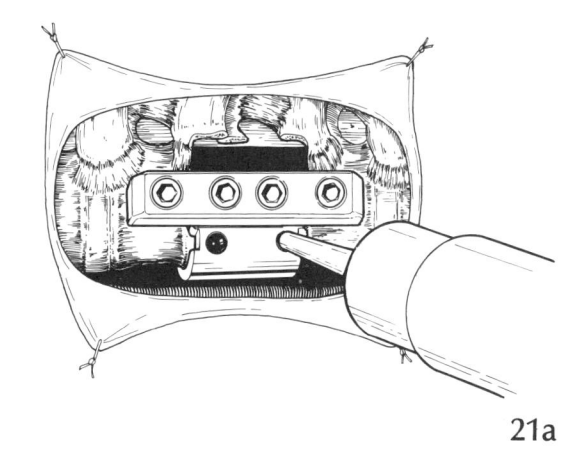

21a & b

Liquid cement is pumped via the holes in the prosthesis (a) to fill the holes in the vertebral end-plates and to act as a grout between the vertebrae and the prosthesis (b).

To minimize postoperative pain, the intercostal nerves above and below the incision are infiltrated posteriorly with 0.5 per cent bupivacaine hydrochloride. An epidural catheter is not inserted for fear of introducing infection.

22

The mediastinal pleura is loosely approximated. There must be direct continuity between the epidural space and pleural cavity to allow free drainage of any epidural bleeding. The chest is closed routinely with one water-seal drain emerging from the chest inferolaterally.

When replacing L4, the prosthesis cannot be used if the paravertebral plate will come to lie under and against the iliac vessels. The modular interbody distractor (see below) with its central fixation is used instead, but the paravertebral DKS system cannot be added. Rotation and hyperextension must be controlled by adding a posterior pedicle screw and plate fixation system (see below). For similar reasons, anterior and posterior stabilization are routinely employed at L5. The posterior operation is carried out either at the same time or 2 weeks later, depending on the condition of the patient.

For improved stabilization of the lumbar spine a modified interbody prosthesis is currently being assessed. At L1–L3 it is bonded with cement to a Kaneda or similar paravertebral device, but at L4 and L5 posterior stabilization is added instead

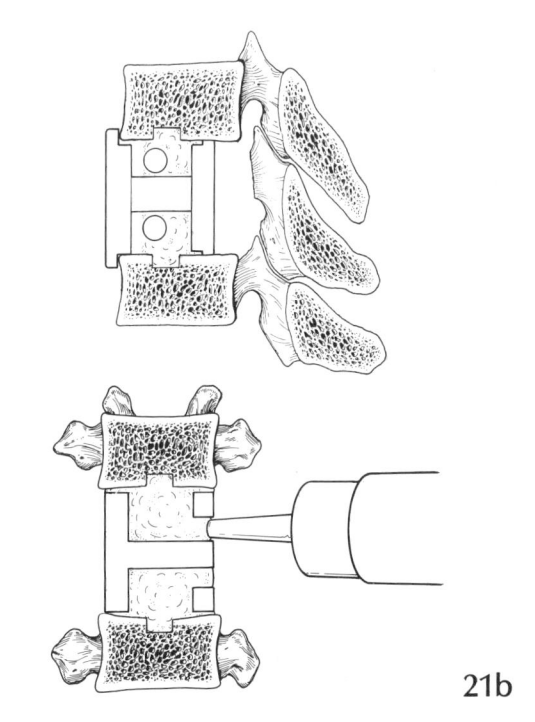

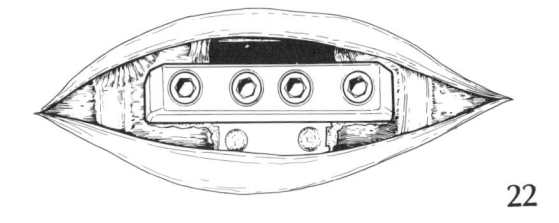

Thoracic and lumbar spine

After removal of more than one vertebral body

After removal of more than one vertebral body, the modular interbody distractor/prosthesis, reinforced with the DKS system or the Kaneda device, is used.

23

Zielke staples are inserted in the sides of the neighbouring healthy vertebral bodies.

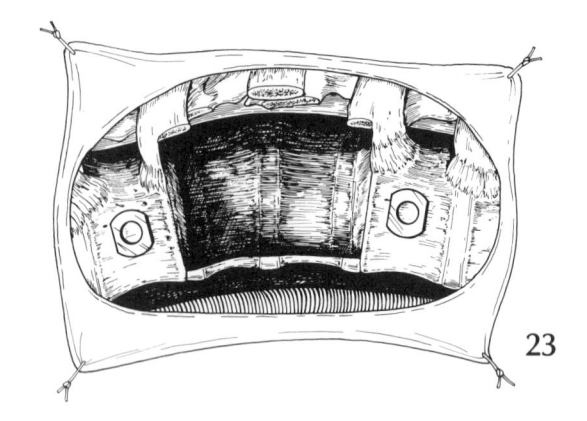

24

The central holes for the prosthesis are made in the vertebral end-plates with the awl. The distance from the anterior cortex is determined with the guide. The centre in the coronal plane is measured with a ruler. Where appropriate, anti-rotation cement pits are fashioned as described above.

The 5 mm Steinmann pins are inserted through the staples: the pins will be subsequently replaced with the DKS screws. The Zielke staples, Steinmann pins, Morscher spreader and the DKS system are not used if the upper thoracic vertebrae are too small (*see above*), or if the Kaneda device will be added (*see below*).

25

The kyphosis is corrected with the modified Morscher spinal spreader until the anterior longitudinal ligament is fairly taut. It is important that it is not overdistracted. (If the defect is too large for the spreader, the interbody distractor can itself be used to correct the kyphosis.)

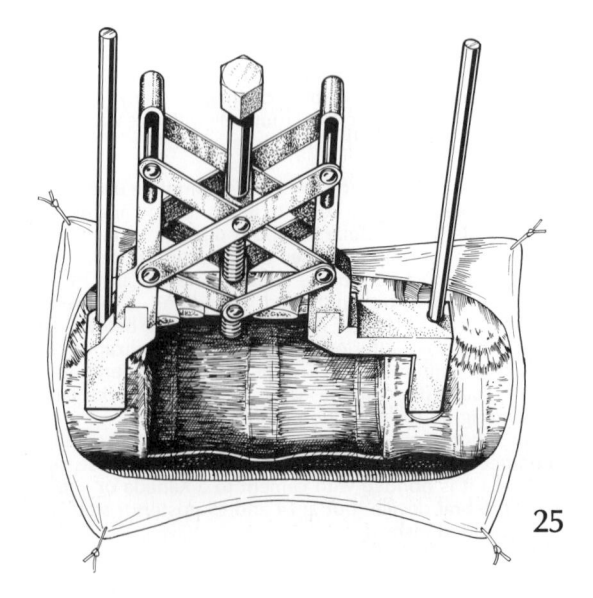

26

The height of the space is measured and the appropriate length of central threaded distractor, lateral telescopic stabilizer, and appropriate support plates are chosen.

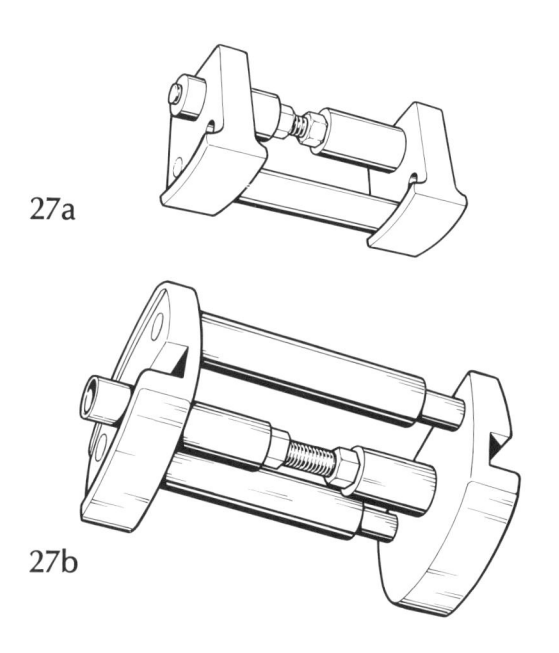

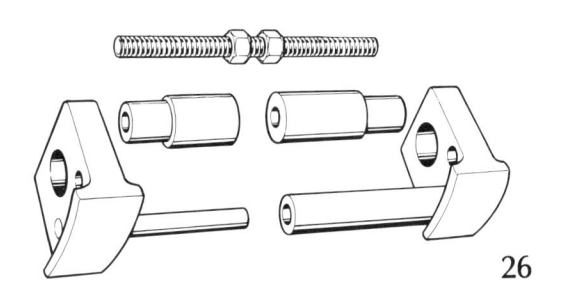

27a & b

The interbody distractor is assembled (a). The larger version can be used for the lower lumbar spine (b).

28

The interbody distractor is inserted. The anterior lips of the support plates must fit round the anterior edges of the intact vertebrae, which are exposed by elevating or transversely incising the anterior longitudinal ligament.

The interbody device is gently distracted to seat the central studs.

The modified Morscher spreader and the Steinmann pins are removed. Any further distraction can be achieved with the interbody screw distractor. It is important that it is not overdistracted. In the lumbar spine the lordosis should not be restored as this produces a potential unstable anterior open wedge configuration.

DKS screws and rod are inserted. The screws should grip the opposite cortex.

A control radiograph is taken. If necessary, the DKS nuts, inflatable cushion and operating table are adjusted to obtain a straight spine. The DKS lock nuts are tightened. The rib spreader may have to be relaxed as mentioned previously.

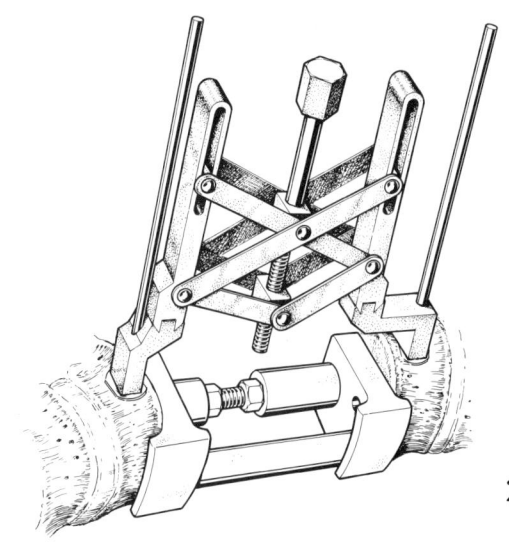

29a & b

The dura and aorta are protected with layers of Gelfoam and a piece of vitallium mesh or malleable retractors.

Liquid cement is injected into the defect.

30

The cement is moulded to incorporate and smooth around the DKS system. Cold saline is used to cool the system during polymerization.

Closure

Closure is performed in the same way as after removal of one vertebral body.

Addition of the Kaneda device[5]

31

The Kaneda device, rather than the DKS system, is currently used to reinforce the anterior interbody construction following anterior decompression and replacement of two or more vertebral bodies below T9. Where necessary, the Kaneda device can be extended by joining two rods together with a threaded sleeve.

If the Kaneda device is unavailable, the DKS system is still a good alternative, where necessary supplemented with posterior instrumentation (*see* below).

Postoperative management

Drains are removed between 24 and 48 hours after surgery.

After vertebral body replacement at the thoracolumbar junction or in the lumbar spine where there are no ribs to provide ancillary support, external support is advisable when the patient is out of bed until a firm capsule develops around the prosthesis. If a vertebral body prosthesis has been used, a canvas corset with steel stays is recommended. With multiple level replacement, a Boston overlap brace is worn for 3 months; thereafter, a canvas corset is worn for at least 3 months.

The patient can be mobilized as soon as possible within the limits imposed by any pre-existing neurological deficit.

Additional posterior spinal fusion in patients with a good prognosis is discussed below.

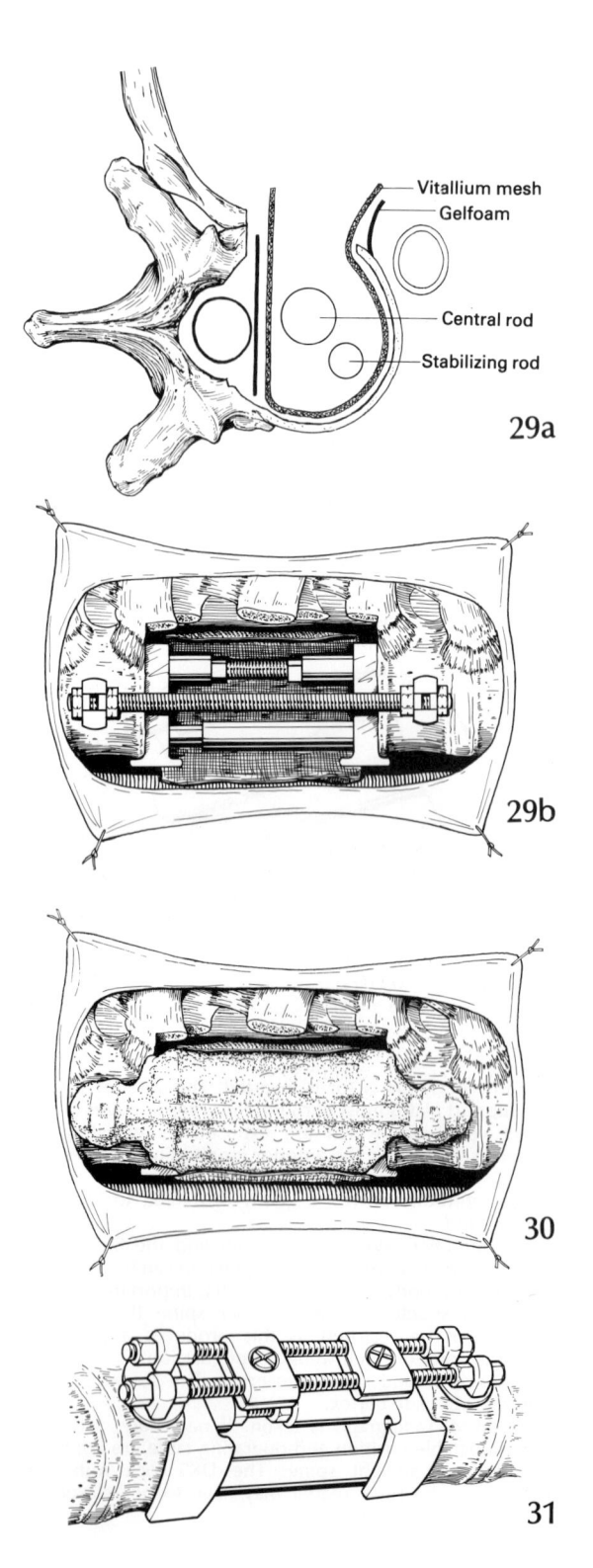

SUPPLEMENTARY POSTERIOR INSTRUMENTATION AFTER ANTERIOR STABILIZATION

Indications

1. Stabilization of L4 and L5. (At these levels an anterior paravertebral device could impinge against the iliac vessels.)
2. If there is doubt about the efficacy of the anterior stabilization.
3. Obviously osteoporotic spine (see below).
4. After anterior decompression and replacement of three or more vertebrae, including or below T10, if the Kaneda device has not been used.

With a lesion from T2 to T9, where the reconstruction is supported by the rib cage, supplementary posterior fusion rather than instrumentation is usually preferred.

If the condition of the posterior tissues following radiotherapy makes posterior instrumentation too hazardous, posterior fusion is carried out and a brace is worn until the fusion is solid.

Technique

32

Stabilization is achieved with pedicle screws/plates or rectangle/laminar wires/cement, if necessary supplemented with autograft (see also Introduction).

If it is not necessary to open the spinal canal, the estimated entry points for pedicle screws are checked with image intensification.

No attempt should be made to restore a lumbar lordosis by contouring the plates as this could lead to loosening of the anterior construction. The supplementary posterior construction must produce slight compression of any anterior interbody construction.

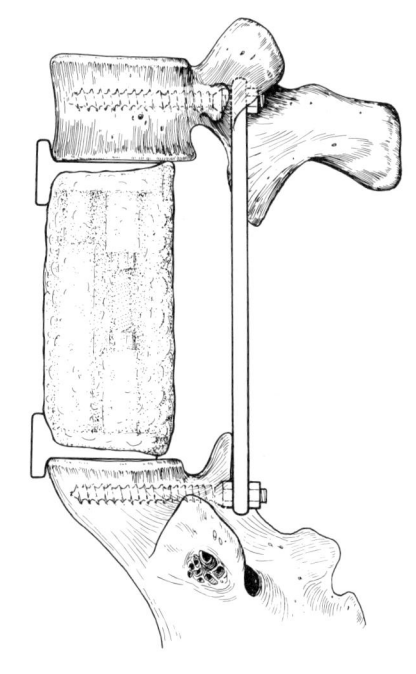

POSTERIOR DECOMPRESSION AND STABILIZATION OF THE THORACIC AND LUMBAR SPINES

When the myelogram/CT shows that cord or cauda equina compression is purely posterior or lateral, with involvement of the laminae, then decompression by laminectomy/facetectomy is indicated. If necessary, one or more thoracic nerve roots (except T1) may be ligatured or clipped and divided to aid gentle mobilization of the cord during removal of lateral epidural tumour. The spine is then stabilized with a rectangle or pedicle screw construction depending on the spinal level (see above).

LAMINAR REMOVAL AND REPLACEMENT

33

Occasionally cord compression and pain are caused by posterior or lateral epidural metastases with only minimal bone involvement. Exposure is gained by cutting the laminae, including the medial portions of the facets, with a fine oscillating saw as shown. An osteotome is then inserted into each saw cut to lever the laminae free.

After removal of the epidural tumour, the laminae are screwed back into position with a thin bone graft to compensate for, or even enlarge upon, the bone lost during sawing[27]. This technique not only protects the cord and, when the laminae have united, restores spinal stability, but also provides a simple and sound basis for any posterior fusion.

POSTERIOR STABILIZATION ALONE FOR PATHOLOGICAL FRACTURES OF THE THORACIC AND LUMBAR SPINES

This technique has been reported by Flatley et al.[16] Although posterior reduction of an anterior fracture can sometimes lead to neurological improvement, considering the mechanical superiority of anterior stabilization and its suitability after anterior decompression, it would seem that posterior techniques alone should be reserved for use in poor-risk patients and preferably those suffering from pain rather than anterior cord or cauda equina compression. The presence of several non-adjacent pathological fractures makes posterior instrumentation more attractive.

The thoracolumbar and lumbar regions should probably also be supported with a brace or corset after the posterior operation.

SUPPLEMENTARY POSTERIOR SPINAL FUSION

As patients survive longer with better methods of treating their underlying tumours, so must the durability of spinal stabilization techniques improve. Rigid, stable fixation is still essential for immediate relief of pain and early mobilization. Where the prognosis is more than 1–2 years, posterior or posterolateral spinal fusion is added for long-term security in the following situations.

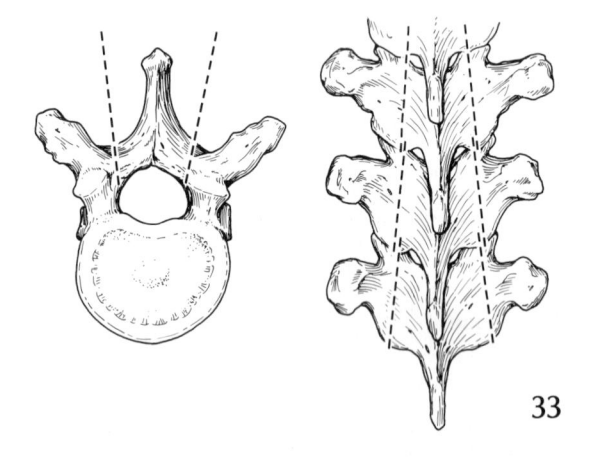

33

Indications

1. Cervical spine and T1, or below T9: following replacement of two or more vertebral bodies.
2. T2–T9, where the ribs add some measure of stability: following replacement of three or more vertebral bodies; or following replacement of two or more vertebral bodies if the posterior column has also been destroyed by laminectomy and facetectomies.
3. In association with posterior instrumentation.

The availability of tumour-free autograft is determined from the bone scan. If tumour-free autograft is not available, homograft or irradiated autograft may be used though with less certainty of success.

The bone grafts are added after radiotherapy or chemotherapy.

Bone graft is not used if it would come in contact with, and be invaded by, tumour; then posterior instrumentation should be considered instead.

After single vertebral body replacement, an expectant policy is at present followed.

When the indications for supplementary posterior instrumentation or fusion after anterior stabilization are doubtful, a temporary brace and an expectant attitude should be adopted, and posterior surgery only carried out if the anterior construction begins to loosen.

Complications

Bleeding

Severe bleeding from the tumour is uncommon after embolization and ligation of the segmental vessels. Continuous oozing can be troublesome. Perseverance in removing the tumour is usually rewarded by an abrupt end to the oozing. Collagen sponge or thrombin-soaked Gelfoam is useful for packing the depths of the cavity.

If oozing persists, it is essential to check the clotting mechanism and especially the thrombocyte count.

Bleeding epidural vessels should be cauterized with bipolar diathermy.

The operation site should be dry before adding any cement. If necessary, the wound should be packed and left for 15 minutes before addition of cement.

Cerebrospinal fluid leak

Leakage may be from the nerve root sleeve in which case it usually plugs itself. If not, a thoracic nerve root (T1 excepted) can be ligated. A lumbar root should not be sacrificed, but the dural sleeve sutured.

Alternatively, leakage may be from the dural sac. Any leak should be carefully repaired, the more so if the local tissues are indurated after radiotherapy. Suture with fine, 8/0 polypropylene is usually effective. A persistent leak can be repaired using Lyodura (B. Braun Melsungen, Melsungen, Germany) and thrombin 'two component' glue. If access is insufficient for suture or glueing of an anterior dural tear, the defect should be covered with Lyodura and Gelfoam after the wound has been finally irrigated.

When simple suturing alone is ineffective or not possible, the CSF pressure is temporarily reduced during the following 10 days with a subarachnoid drain inserted through a healthy interlaminar space. The patient is nursed in the Trendelenburg position.

Infection

Despite the underlying condition of the patients, infection is fortunately rare. Any infection must be vigorously treated with reoperation and debridement.

In posterior wounds, gentamicin chains should be inserted and renewed or removed 2 weeks later. Appropriate intravenous antibiotics followed by oral antibiotics should probably be continued until 3 months after the erythrocyte sedimentation rate has returned to normal. If in doubt, lifelong antibiotics should be given to minimize the chance of recurrence; these patients do not have the time for prolonged reconstructive procedures.

Late failure of stabilization

In the neck, progressive destruction of neighbouring vertebral bodies can lead to failure of a posterior construction and recurrence of pain. The construction can be extended.

Surprisingly, although some tumour tissue must always remain after anterior decompression and stabilization, there have, so far, been no cases of failure of the construction because of local recurrence.

Osteoporosis

In one elderly patient, the neighbouring cranial osteoporotic vertebral body collapsed with recurrence of pain and the danger of further collapse and cord damage. Supplementary posterior stabilization restored stability and relieved pain. If such a problem is anticipated, the thoracolumbar spine should be supported with a brace or supplementary posterior stabilization.

Miliary metastases in neighbouring vertebrae

These are not an absolute contraindication to anterior surgery, but prolonged postoperative bracing is wise.

Painful exacerbation of degenerative changes adjacent to a fused segment

This has been encountered once below an occipital–C4 fusion. Anterior C4–5 fusion relieved the pain.

Multidisciplinary approach

For these often difficult problems, a multidisciplinary approach with close cooperation between radiologist, radiotherapist, oncologist and spinal surgeon is essential. The assistance of thoracic and general surgical colleagues can be of considerable help in the presence of severe paravertebral infiltration.

Postoperative treatment

Radiotherapy can begin when wound healing is satisfactory, usually from the fifth postoperative day. Chemotherapy is usually delayed until after the tenth day.

If bone chip autografts have been added, radiotherapy and chemotherapy should probably be delayed for 6 weeks.

References

1. Black P. Spinal metastases: current status and recommended guidelines for management. *Neurosurgery* 1979; 5: 726–46.

2. White AA, Panjabi MM. *Clinical biomechanics of the spine.* Philadelphia: J. B. Lippincott, 1978: 394–5.

3. Rockoff SD, Sweet E, Bleustein J. The relative contribution of trabecular and cortical bone to the strength of human lumbar vertebrae. *Calcif Tissue Res* 1969; 3: 163–75.

4. Fidler MW. Anterior and posterior stabilization of the spine following vertebral body resection: a postmortem investigation. *Spine* 1986; 11: 362–6.

5. Kaneda K, Abumi K, Fujiya M. Burst fractures with neurologic deficits of the thoracolumbar spine: results of anterior decompression and stabilisation with anterior instrumentation. *Spine* 1984; 9: 788–95.

6. Gurr KR, McAfee PC, Shih C-M. Biomechanical analysis of anterior and posterior instrumentation systems after corpectomy. *J Bone Joint Surg [Am]* 1988; 70-A: 1182–91.

7. Polster J, Brinckmann P. Ein Wirbelkörperimplantat zur Verwendung bei Palliativoperationen an der Wirbelsäule. *Z Orthop* 1977; 115: 118–22.

8. Clark CR, Keggi KJ, Panjabi MM. Methylmethacrylate stabilisation of the cervical spine. *J Bone Joint Surg [Am]* 1984; 66-A: 40–6.

9. Siegal T, Siegal T. Vertebral body resection for epidural compression by malignant tumors; results of forty-seven consecutive operative procedures. *J Bone Joint Surg [Am]* 1985; 67-A: 375–82.

10. Fidler MW. Anterior decompression and stabilisation of metastatic spinal fractures. *J Bone Joint Surg [Br]* 1986; 68-B: 83–90.

11. Harrington KD. Metastatic disease of the spine. *J Bone Joint Surg [Am]* 1986; 68-A: 1110–15.

12. Kostuik JP, Errico TJ, Gleason TF, Errico CC. Spinal stabilization of vertebral column tumors. *Spine* 1988; 13: 250–6.

13. Ono K, Yonenobu K, Ebara S, Fujiwara K, Yamashita K, Fuji T, Dunn EJ. Prosthetic replacement surgery for cervical spine metastasis. *Spine* 1988; 13: 817–22.

14. Turner PL, Prince HG, Webb JK, Sokal MPJW. Surgery for malignant extradural tumours of the spine. *J Bone Joint Surg [Br]* 1988; 70-B: 451–6.

15. Manabe S, Tateishi A, Abe M, Ohno T. Surgical treatment of metastatic tumours of the spine. *Spine* 1989; 14: 41–7.

16. Flatley TJ, Anderson MH, Anast GT. Spinal instability due to malignant disease: treatment by segmental spinal stabilization. *J Bone Joint Surg [Am]* 1984; 66-A: 47–52.

17. Fidler MW. Pathological fractures of the cervical spine: palliative surgical treatment. *J Bone Joint Surg [Br]* 1985; 67-B: 352–7.

18. Steffee AD, Biscup RS, Sitkowski DJ. Segmental spine plates with pedicle screw fixation: a new internal fixation device for disorders of the lumbar and thoracolumbar spine. *Clin Orthop* 1986; 203: 45–53.

19. Bridwell KH, Jenny AB, Saul T, Rich KM, Grubb RL. Posterior segmental spinal instrumentation (PSSI) with posterolateral decompression and debulking for metastatic thoracic and lumbar spine disease; limitations of the technique. *Spine* 1988; 13: 1383–94.

20. Galasko CSB. Spinal instability secondary to metatstatic cancer. *J Bone Joint Surg [Br]* 1991; 73-B: in press.

21. Fidler MW, Niers BBAM. Open transpedicular vertebral body biopsy. *J Bone Joint Surg [Br]* 1990; 72-B: 884–5.

22. McBroom RJ, Reiss B, Perrin R. *Surgical decompression for paraplegia due to metastatic cancer.* Paper read at the Annual Meeting of the International Society for the Study of the Lumbar Spine, Miami 1988.

23. Ransford AO, Crockard HA, Pozo JL, Thomas NP, Nelson IW. Craniocervical instability treated by contoured loop fixation. *J Bone Joint Surg [Br]* 1986; 68-B: 173–7.

24. Domisse GF. The arteries, arterioles and capillaries of the spinal cord: surgical guidelines in the prevention of postoperative paraplegia. *Ann R Coll Surg Engl* 1980; 62: 369–76.

25. Sundaresan N, Shah J, Foley KM, Rosen G. An anterior surgical approach to the upper thoracic vertebrae. *J Neurosurg* 1984; 61: 686–90.

26. Birch R, Bonney G, Marshall RW. A surgical approach to the cervicothoracic spine. *J Bone Joint Surg [Br]* 1990; 72-B: 904–7.

27. Fidler MW, Bongartz EB. Laminar removal and replacement: a technique for the removal of epidural tumour. *Spine* 1988; 13: 218–20.

Illustrations by Gillian Oliver

Approaches to the spine

J. K. Webb FRCS
Consultant Orthopaedic Surgeon, Queen's Medical Centre, Nottingham, UK

Introduction

Indications

The indications for various approaches depend mainly on the type and site of pathology, as well as the experience and expertise of the operator. To treat spinal disorders adequately, a thorough knowledge of both anterior and posterior approaches is required. Most of the indications for each approach can be found among the following:

1. Spinal deformity
2. Trauma
3. Tumours
4. Infection
5. Degenerative disorders.

Anterior approaches

TRANSORAL APPROACH TO C1–C2

Anaesthesia

General anaesthesia, with an endotracheal tube, is required (a tracheostomy is not essential).

Position of patient

1 & 2

The patient is supine with the head slightly hyperextended. A self-retaining mouth retractor (McIver with an accessory blade) is used to hold the mouth open and retract the endotracheal tube to one side.

A suture may be placed through the tongue to retract it away from the surgical field. The soft palate may obscure the posterior pharynx. Exposure is facilitated by placing a suture through the uvula, and securing it to the junction of the soft and hard palates, or by splitting the uvula and suturing each half to the respective lateral oropharyngeal wall.

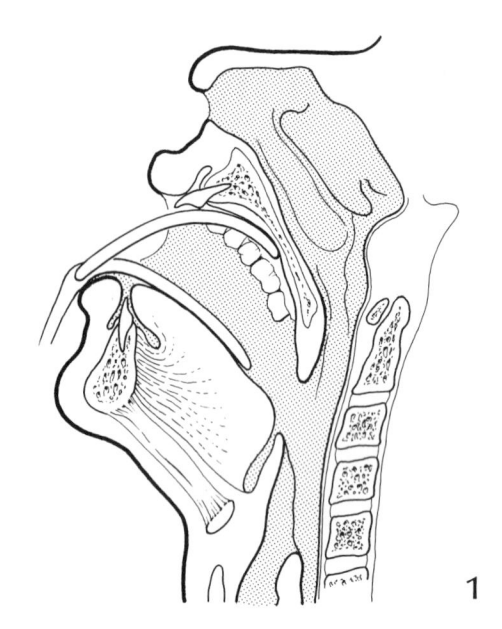

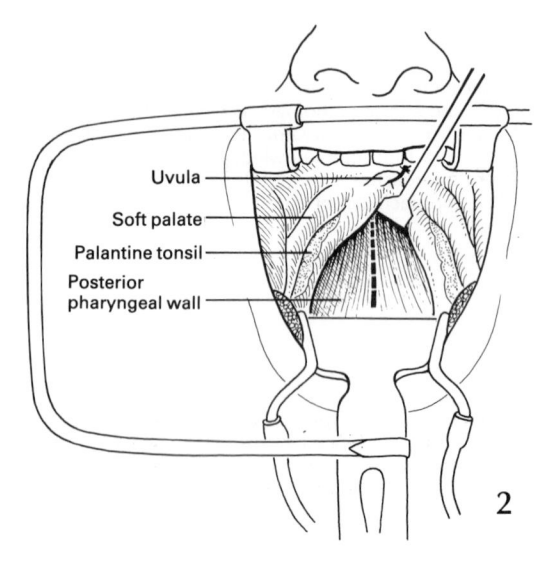

Incision

3

The anterior tubercle of the atlas is palpated. The pharyngeal raphe is incised longitudinally in the midline, splitting the four midline structures: the posterior pharyngeal mucosa, the superior constrictor muscle, the prevertebral fascia overlying the longus colli muscle, and the anterior longitudinal ligament.

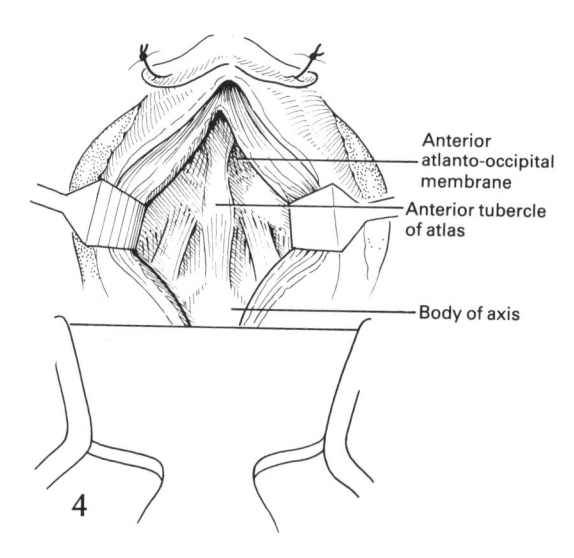

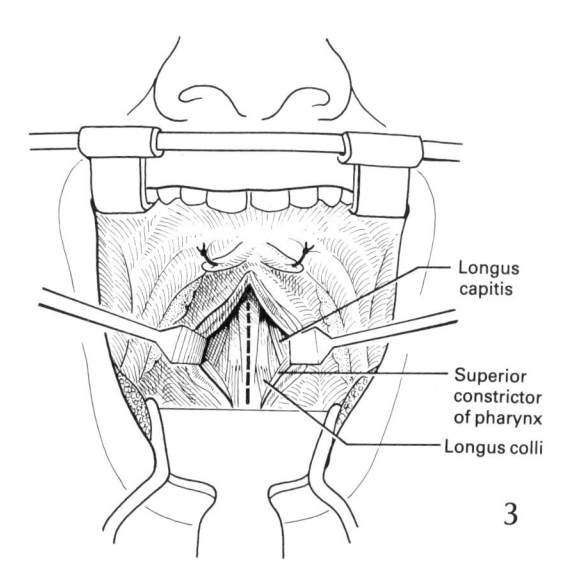

Exposure

4

The soft tissues are stripped laterally with a swab. The atlas and axis can be exposed to approximately 1.5 cm from the midline; lateral to this the vertebral artery is vulnerable (particularly at the inferior border of C2).

5

This allows adequate exposure from the base of the skull to the junction of C2–3. To facilitate exposure of the base of the skull, the soft palate may be split anteriorly, and part of the hard palate removed.

Precautions

1. The vertebral artery is at risk if the dissection is too lateral.
2. Care must be taken to avoid penetration of the retromandibular fossa lateral to the atlas, where the ninth and tenth cranial nerves are at risk.
3. The stay suture should not be placed too deeply in the lateral pharyngeal wall, where the internal carotid artery is at risk.

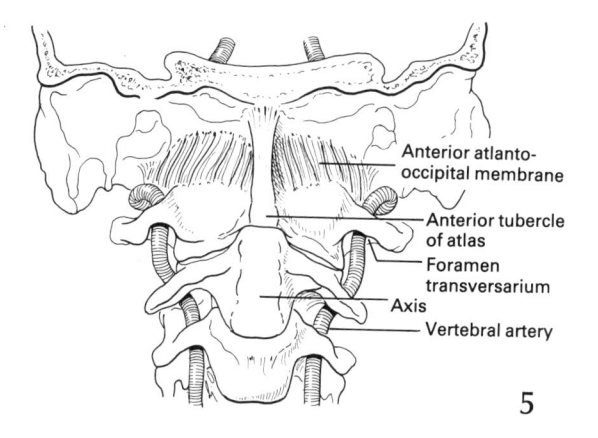

TONGUE-SPLITTING APPROACH

6

An extension of the transoral approach is the mandible- and tongue-splitting approach first reported by Kocher[1] in 1911, and applied to spinal surgery[2] in 1977. This approach is useful if a wide direct exposure to the cervical vertebrae is required from the clivus to C6. Disadvantages are that a tracheostomy is mandatory, and, as with other transoral approaches, there is a high risk of infection. The epiglottis must not be damaged.

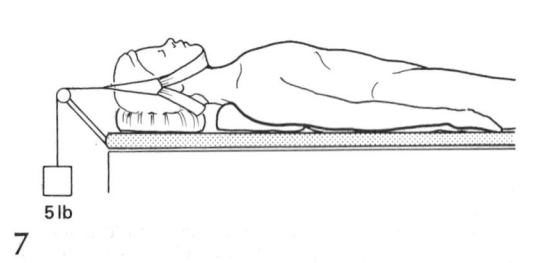

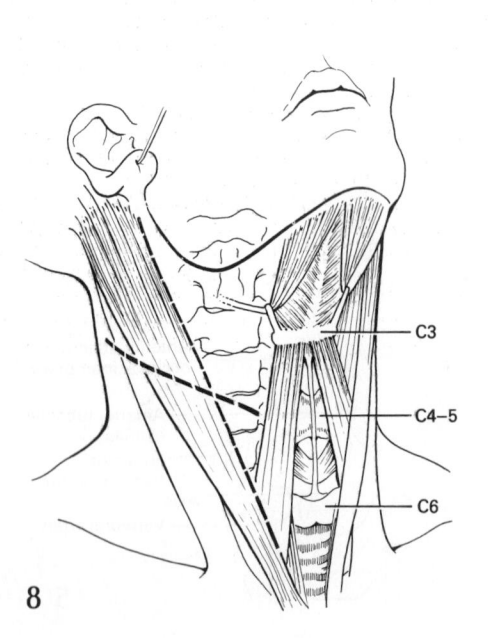

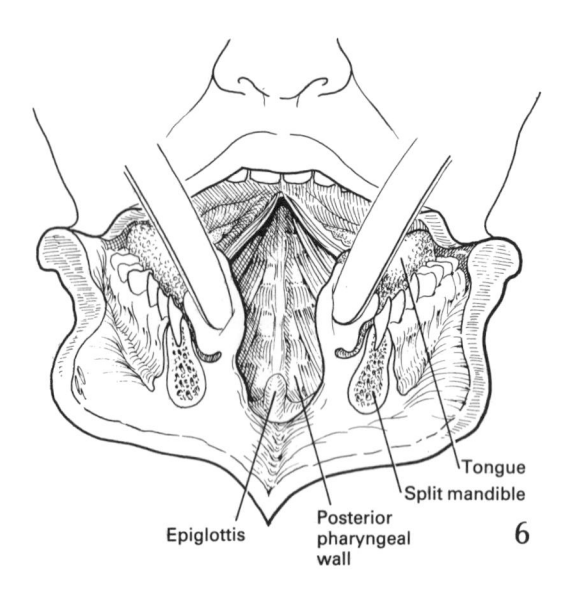

ANTERIOR APPROACH TO C3–T1

Position of patient

7

The patient is placed supine with a sandbag between the scapulae to extend the neck. Halter traction with 2.27 kg (5 lb) may facilitate head extension. The head is rotated 20°–30° to the contralateral side.

The ideal side to approach is debated. The recurrent laryngeal nerve is more at risk on the right side, especially below C6, while the thoracic duct is at risk on the left. Most surgeons recommend approaching from the side of pathology.

Incision and level

8

The type of incision depends on the extent of vertebral exposure. Exposure of one to two vertebrae can be accomplished by a transverse incision parallel to the skin creases. Several palpable structures help in identifying the level:

C2–3 – the lower border of the mandible
C3   – the hyoid bone
C4–5 – the thyroid cartilage
C6   – the cricoid cartilage and the carotid tubercle.

For exposure of several segments, a longitudinal incision along the anterior border of sternomastoid is preferred.

Dissection

9

Dissection is made through subcutaneous tissue to the platysma muscle. The platysma is opened in line with its fibres at the anterior border of sternomastoid to expose the superficial cervical fascia. Branches of the external jugular vein or transverse cutaneous nerves may require dividing.

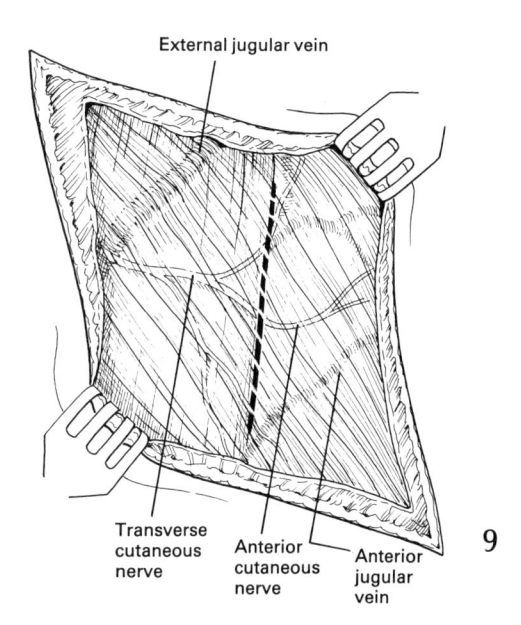

10

Dividing the superficial cervical fascia along the anterior border of sternomastoid allows the plane between sternomastoid laterally and the strap muscles (sternohyoid and sternothyroid) medially to be developed.

Division of the pretracheal fascia allows the carotid sheath (laterally) to be separated from the trachea, thyroid and underlying oesophagus medially.

The upper belly of the omohyoid muscle may obscure the field at the level of C6, and may require division, while the middle thyroid veins deep to the pretracheal fascia may also require ligation at this level.

The oesophagus is mobilized from the midline by blunt dissection to expose the cervical spine. The prevertebral fascia is divided and the longus colli muscle retracted laterally, to expose the cervical spine covered by the anterior longitudinal ligament. The sympathetic chain lies on the longus colli, just lateral to the vertebral bodies.

The appropriate cervical level must be confirmed radiologically.

Extension

11

This approach can extend superiorly to C2 by dividing the superior thyroid artery and vein, but the stylohyoid and digastric muscles, as well as the hypoglossal and superior laryngeal nerve, prevent further superior extension. The base of the odontoid can be reached by dividing the superior thyroid, lingual and facial branches of the external carotid artery, but places the superior laryngeal nerve at risk.

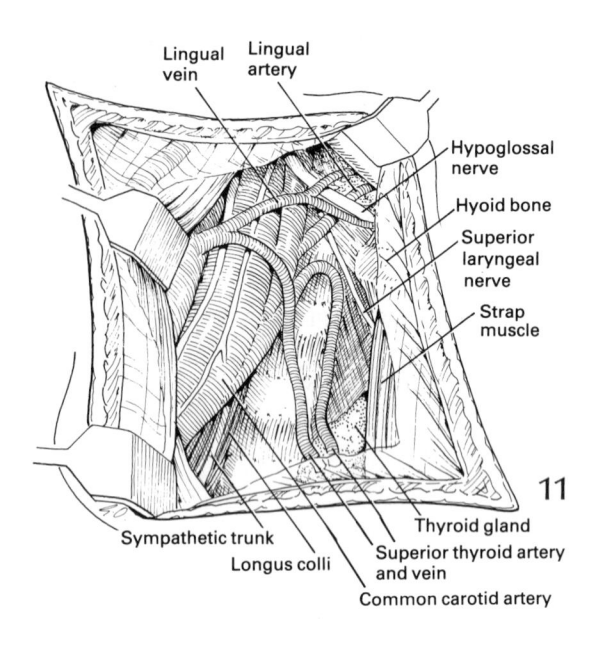

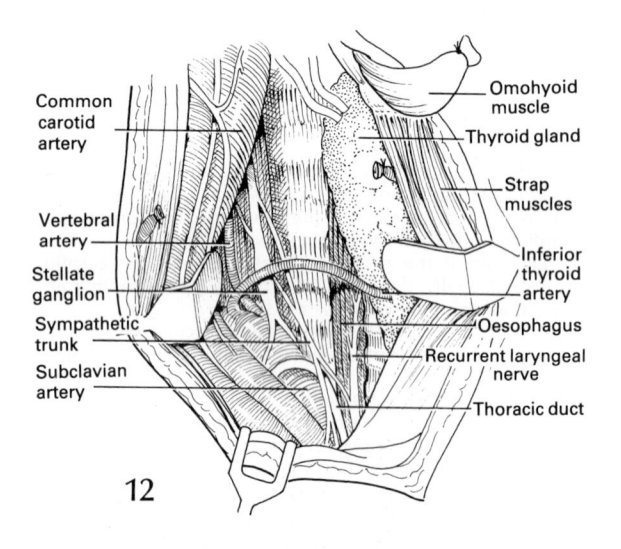

12

It is possible to extend this approach inferiorly, as far as T2, by dividing and ligating the inferior thyroid artery. Other structures which must be protected at this level include the sympathetic trunk and stellate ganglion (on the anterior aspect of longus colli), the thoracic duct and the recurrent laryngeal nerve.

Precautions

1. Care should be taken not to damage the carotid sheath and its contents (common carotid artery, internal jugular vein, vagus nerve).
2. The recurrent laryngeal nerve is more at risk on the right side, where it runs irregularly and at a higher level, having coursed below the subclavian artery, compared to the aortic arch on the left.
3. The hypoglossal nerve is at risk in the upper cervical spine.
4. Superior laryngeal nerve injury may result in hoarseness.
5. Sympathetic trunk injury may result in Horner's syndrome.
6. The thoracic duct should be protected in lower cervical approaches. It courses centrally across the subclavian artery, and opens into the venous angle.

APPROACH TO CERVICOTHORACIC AREA

The cervicothoracic area is difficult to approach anteriorly. The low anterior cervical approach provides access as low as T2, but places several structures at risk.

For equal exposure of the cervical and thoracic spine from C4 to T4, the sternal splitting approach commonly used in cardiac surgery has been recommended[3].

Exposure of the upper thoracic spine is achieved by a modification of the standard thoracotomy[4].

ANTERIOR APPROACH TO UPPER THORACIC SPINE

Position of patient

13

The patient is placed in the lateral position with the uppermost arm supported. The right-sided approach is preferable, as the straight course of the brachiocephalic artery, compared with the curved course of the left subclavian artery, reduces the likelihood of injury. However, if the pathology is on the left side, a left-sided approach is preferable.

Incision

A curved incision is made from the inferior angle of the scapula to opposite the spinal process of C3.

Dissection

14

Trapezius is divided in line with the skin incision, as medially as possible, to minimize denervation. A small portion of latissimus dorsi is divided, including those fibres inserting into the inferior angle of the scapula.

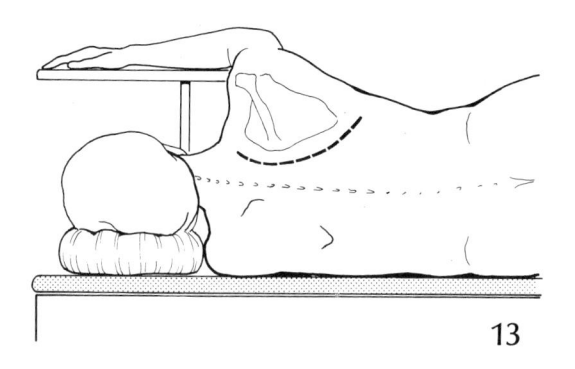

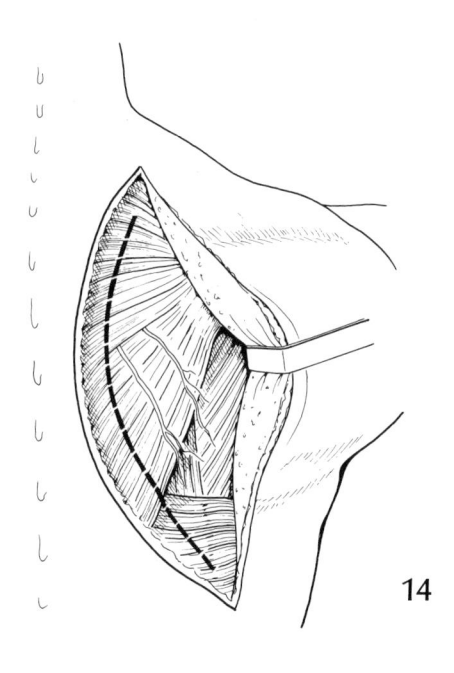

15

The trapezius is retracted laterally and the rhomboids and levator scapulae muscles are divided just short of their insertion into the medial border of the scapula.

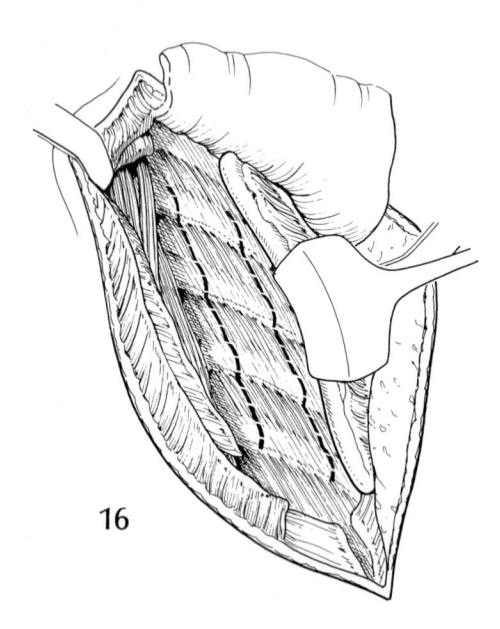

16

The scapula is now retracted laterally to expose the upper chest wall. The posterior 7–10 cm of the second to fifth ribs are exposed subperiosteally and removed, leaving the head and neck of each rib. Usually, the first rib can be left intact, unless exposure of T1 is required.

17

The pleura is divided in the bed of the fifth rib, and then vertically along the medial cut ends of the ribs. This L-shaped incision creates a pleuromuscular flap, which is retracted laterally with the underlying lung, to expose the upper thoracic spine.

The pleura overlying the vertebrae is split longitudinally, and the segmental vessels ligated at the appropriate levels.

Postoperative management

The arm is rested in a sling for 2 weeks, then gradually mobilized.

Precautions

When dissecting around the neck of the first rib, care must be taken to avoid damaging the anterior root of T1 as it crosses to join the brachial plexus.

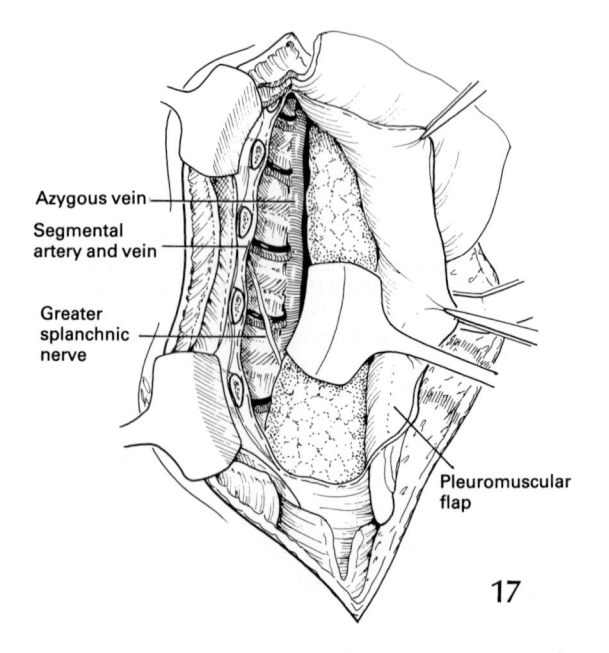

ANTERIOR APPROACH TO T4–11

Position of patient

18

The patient is placed in a lateral position with the upper arm supported.

A left-sided approach is often preferable, as it is simpler to deal with vessels arising from the aorta than those draining into the inferior vena cava with a right-sided approach (as illustrated). However, the approach for scoliosis is from the side of the convexity.

Incision

To determine the level of approach, the rib horizontal to the vertebral level at the mid-axillary line on a chest radiograph is resected. This is usually two ribs above the required vertebral level. The incision is from the midline posteriorly to the costal cartilage anteriorly, in the line of the rib.

Dissection

19

The muscle layers are then divided in the line of the skin incision using cutting diathermy. This usually involves partial division of latissimus dorsi and serratus anterior.

20

Resection of the appropriate rib facilitates exposure and provides bone for grafting if required. The periosteum of the rib is split longitudinally, and elevated, avoiding damage to the intercostal vessels and nerve at the inferior border of the rib.

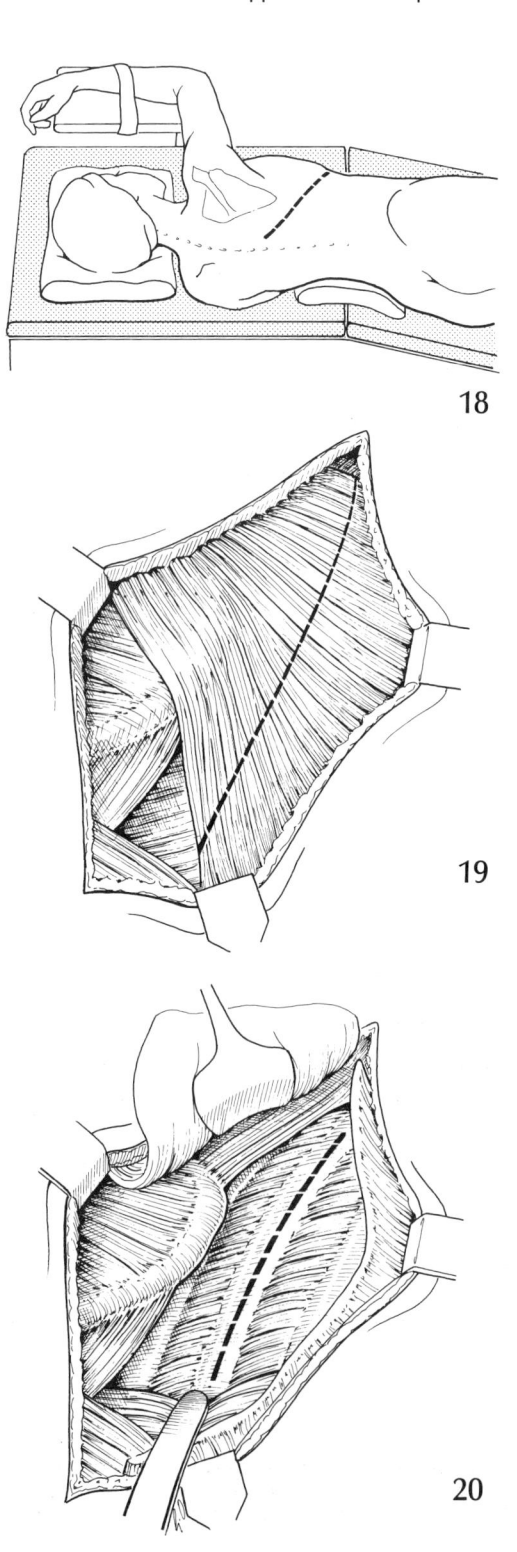

21

Using a Doyen elevator, the periosteum is stripped from the undersurface of the rib. The rib is transected anteriorly at the costochondral junction, and posteriorly 2 cm lateral to the costotransverse articulation. The rib is then removed.

An alternative is an intercostal thoracotomy, particularly in children, where only a few vertebrae need exposing, and where a rib graft is not required.

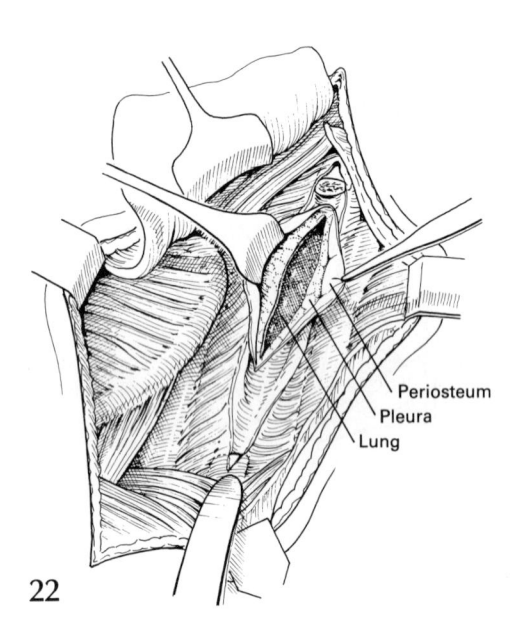

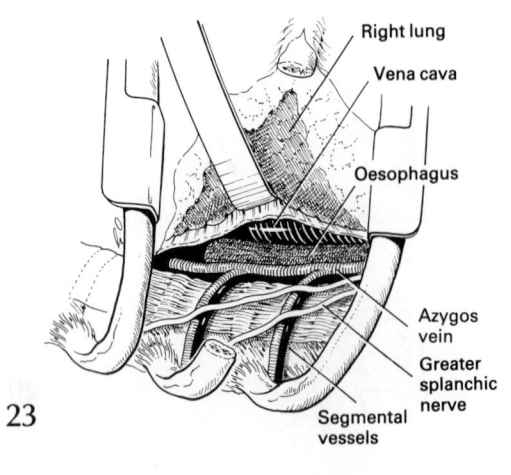

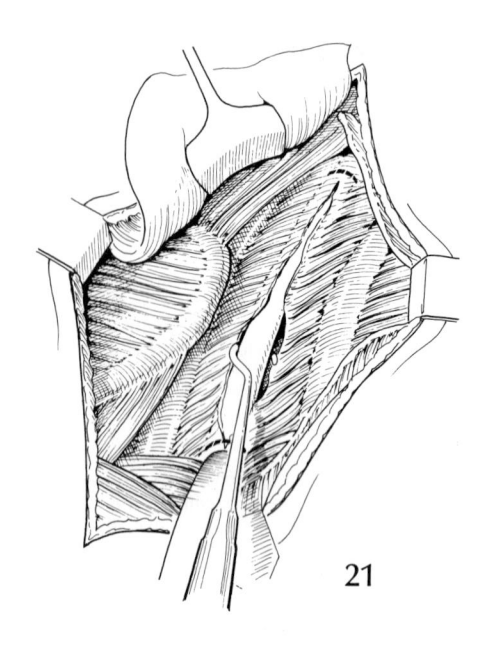

22 & 23

While the lung is deflated, the parietal pleura and periosteum is elevated with fine forceps, incised and split in line with the rib. The lung is then retracted with a moist swab, and the ribs spread. The vertebral bodies can now be seen, covered with parietal pleura, beneath which lie the segmental arteries and accompanying veins.

The parietal pleura is gently split longitudinally, protecting the segmental vessels, which can then be isolated, ligated and divided. To preserve the arterial arcades which supply the spinal cord, the segmental arteries should be divided as anteriorly as possible, and dissected posteriorly for a short distance only.

Closure

The would is closed in layers with at least one pleural drain.

Precautions

1. The neck of the rib must not be removed, otherwise damage might occur to the dorsal branch of the posterior intercostal artery.
2. Diathermy must not be used near the intervertebral foramen as it could damage the spinal artery.

ANTERIOR APPROACH TO THORACOLUMBAR JUNCTION

Level of approach

If pathology allows, a left-sided approach is preferred, as a right-sided approach is hampered by the liver and more friable vena cava.

The level of approach is determined by choosing a rib in the mid-axillary line, opposite the vertebrae to be exposed. This allows adequate proximal exposure to 'work down' to the lesion. For maximal exposure of T11–12, the ninth rib is resected; for T12–L1, the tenth rib. The eleventh rib approach is the highest practical, extrapleural, retroperitoneal anterior approach to T12–L2 in high-risk patients, i.e. it avoids cutting the diaphragm.

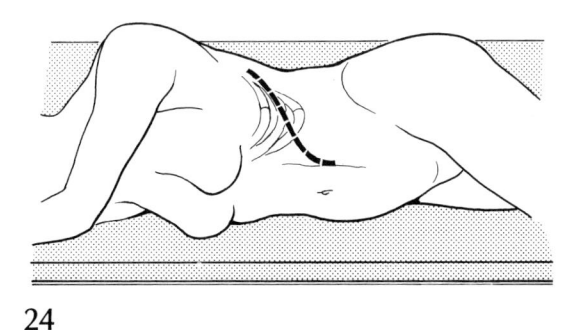

Tenth rib approach

Position of patient

24

The patient is placed on the right side.

Incision

An oblique incision is made from the posterior aspect of the tenth rib to the costal cartilage, then curved anteriorly to the umbilicus.

608 Thoracic and lumbar spine

Dissection

25

The underlying muscle layers are divided in line with the skin incision down to the appropriate rib. The periosteum is divided along the axis of the rib with diathermy, and the periosteum stripped from the deep surface of the rib. The rib is removed by dividing as far anteriorly and posteriorly as possible, leaving the head and neck.

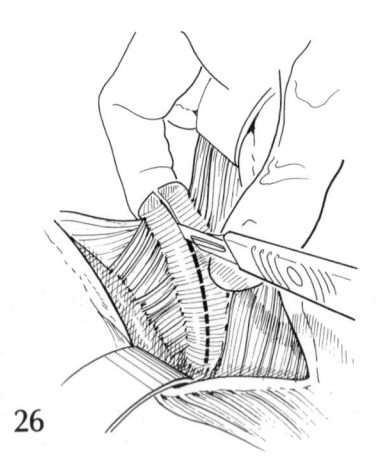

26

The soft tissue dissection is continued over the costal cartilage. The peritoneum is pushed off the deep surface of the costal cartilage and the cartilage split in its longitudinal axis. This serves as a useful marker when closing the wound.

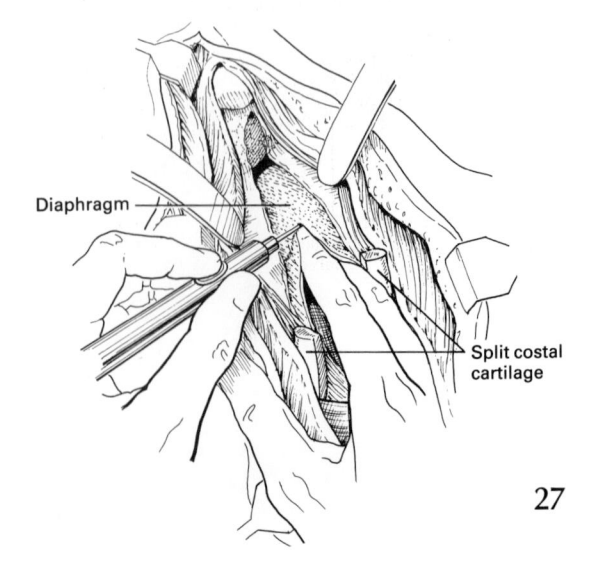

27

Using a gauze swab, a gap is developed between the peritoneum and diaphragm. When the diaphragm is cleared of peritoneum, it is divided 2 cm from the rib margin to the midline posteriorly.

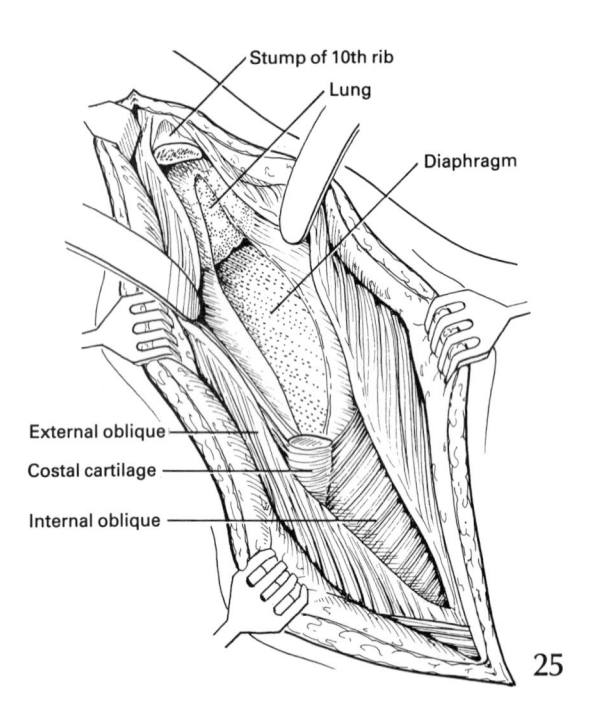

28

The plane is then developed medial to the psoas, reflecting the peritoneum with the ureter, to expose the underlying vertebral bodies between the psoas and the aorta. The sympathetic trunk is identified and protected in this interval.

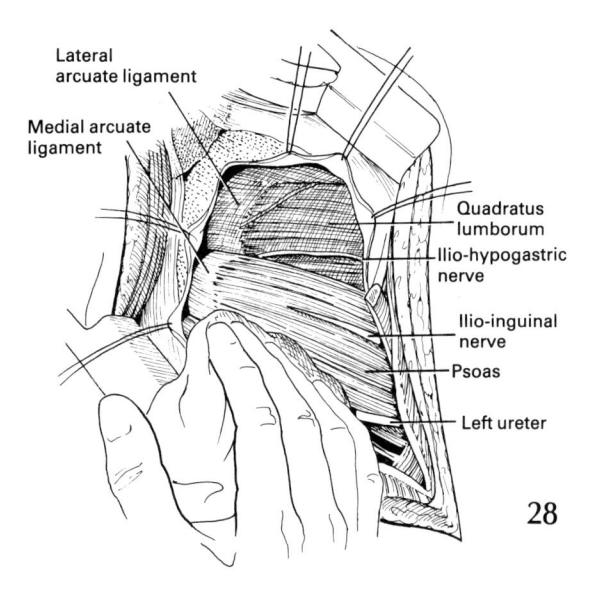

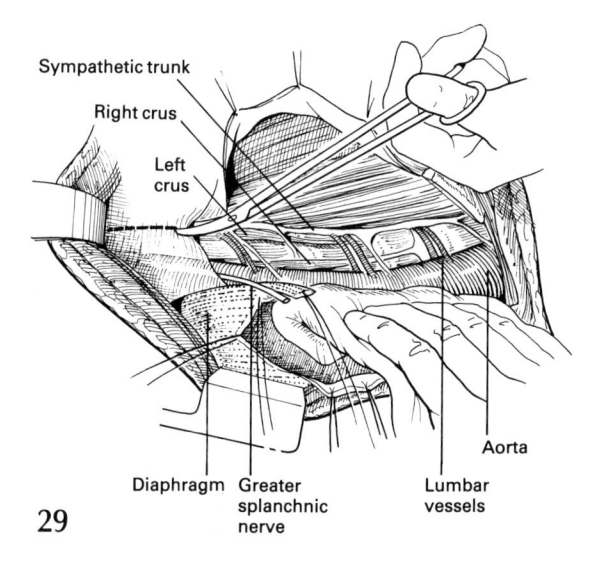

29

The parietal pleura is divided longitudinally over the vertebral bodies, and the segmental vessels ligated. Below the diaphragm, the left diaphragmatic crus (which arises from the anterior bodies and discs of L1 and L2) is divided and elevated. The greater splanchnic nerve on the crus superiorly is located and protected, and the sympathetic trunk caudally (which lies at the junction of the crus and psoas muscle).

Division of the right diaphragmatic crus extends the exposure to L3.

Closure

The left diaphragmatic crus is restored and the parietal pleura closed. The diaphragm is closed from posterior to anterior. Re-approximation of the split costal cartilage allows better definition of the abdominal layers for closure.

ANTERIOR RETROPERITONEAL APPROACH TO L2–5

Position of patient

30

The right semilateral position is preferred, with the right hip and knee slightly bent and the left leg extended. A slight tilt of the table in the lumbar region increases the costal margin to iliac crest distance.

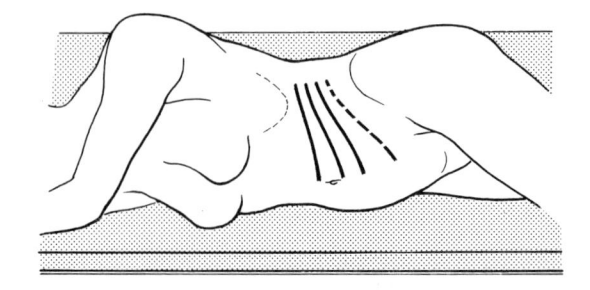

Incision

An oblique incision is made from the mid-axillary line to the edge of the rectus sheath. The level of incision depends on the vertebral level to be approached. L2–3 is above the umbilicus, L3–4 at the umbilicus, L4–5 in the upper half of a line between the umbilicus and symphysis pubis, and L5–S1 to the lower half of this line.

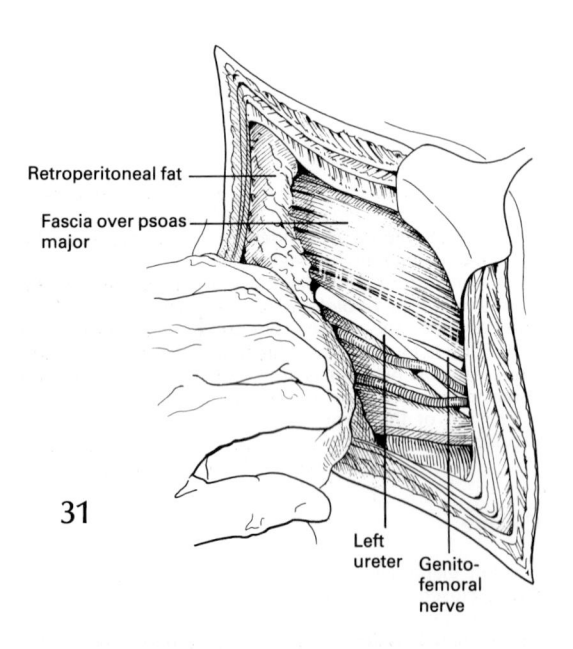

Dissection

31

The dissection is continued to the external oblique aponeurosis, which is divided in line with the skin incision, followed by internal oblique and transversus abdominis. Exposure of the retroperitoneal fat allows easy stripping of the peritoneum from the posterior abdominal wall. It is important to identify and protect both the genitofemoral nerve on the psoas and also the ureter which reflects forward with the peritoneum.

Approaches to the spine 611

32

Identification of the psoas muscle is the key to this approach. The sympathetic chain lies to the medial border of the psoas. The appropriate segmental artery and vein require ligation to develop the interval between the psoas and the great vessels (aorta, common iliac artery and vein). Exposure of the fourth lumbar vertebra often requires ligation of the iliolumbar vein.

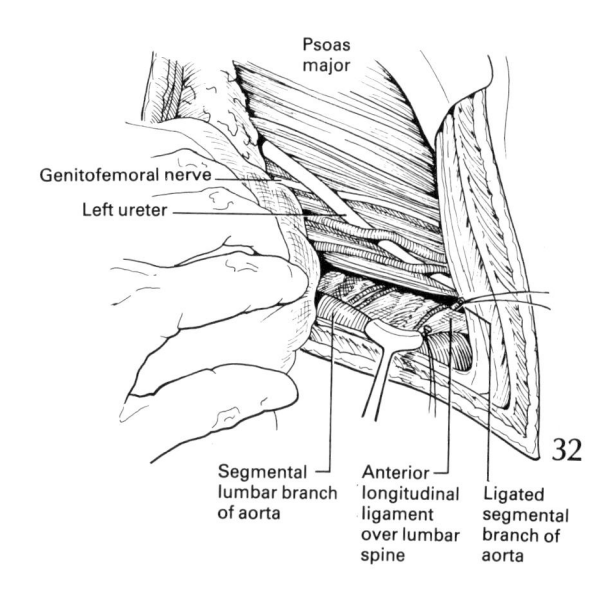

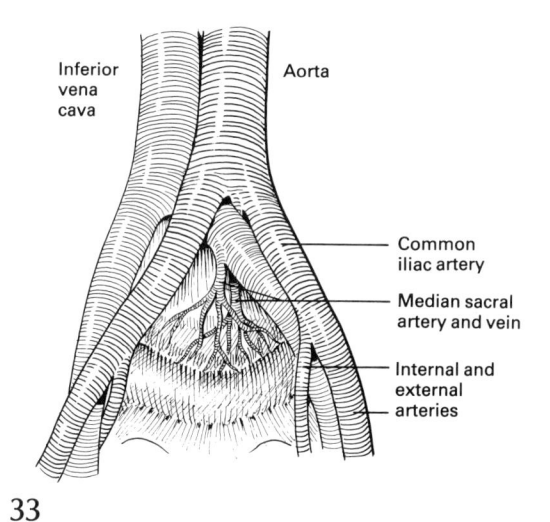

33

The approach to the L5–S1 disc depends on the level of bifurcation of the aorta (usually at the L4–5 disc level). Usually, the lumbosacral level is approached between the bifurcation of the great vessels.

Important structures to recognize and protect in the bifurcation are the middle sacral artery and veins, and the superior hypogastric plexus. The soft tissues are swept off the lumbosacral region to the right by blunt dissection only. To aid retraction, two Steinmann pins can be placed in the bifurcation into the L5 vertebral body.

Note: A low bifurcation of the iliac veins may require an approach to the lumbosacral disc from the left of the common iliac artery and vein, retracting both structures to the right.

Precautions

Care should be taken to protect the ureter, the sympathetic trunk, the great vessels, the iliolumbar vein, and the superior hypogastric plexus.

FRASER'S MUSCLE-SPLITTING APPROACH

34 & 35

An alternative anterior retroperitoneal approach is the muscle-splitting approach described by Fraser[5]. This involves splitting external oblique, internal oblique and transversus abdominis muscles in the line of their fibres, and dividing the rectus sheath vertically without dividing the rectus abdominis muscle.

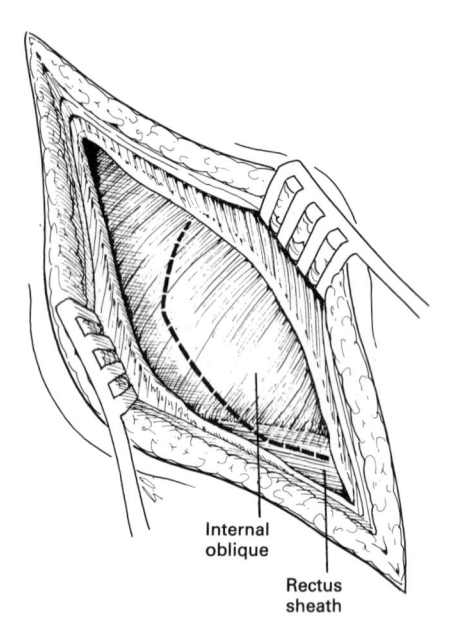

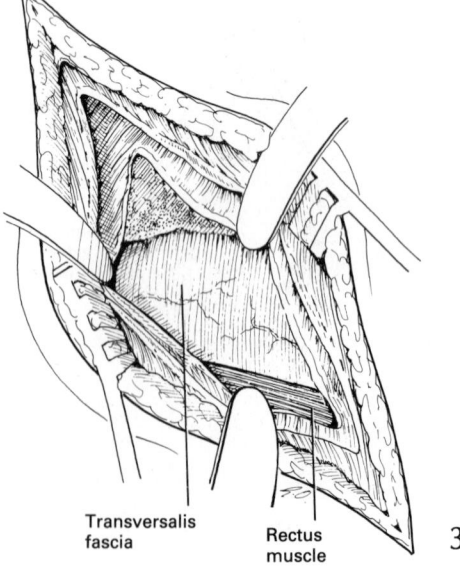

TRANSPERITONEAL MIDLINE APPROACH TO L4–S1

Preoperative procedures

Both a urinary catheter and a nasogastric tube should be passed.

Position of patient

The patient is placed on a table which is angled to produce slight hyperlordosis.

Incision

36

A longitudinal midline incision is made from the symphysis pubis, curving around the umbilicus.

A more cosmetic alternative is the Pfannenstiel incision but this requires transection of the rectus abdominis muscle.

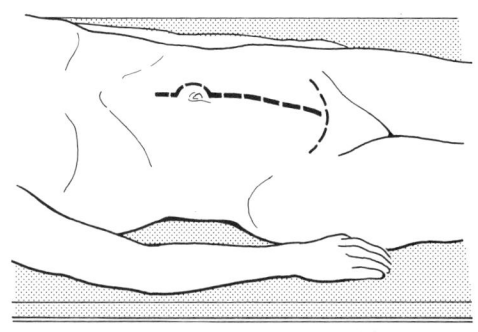

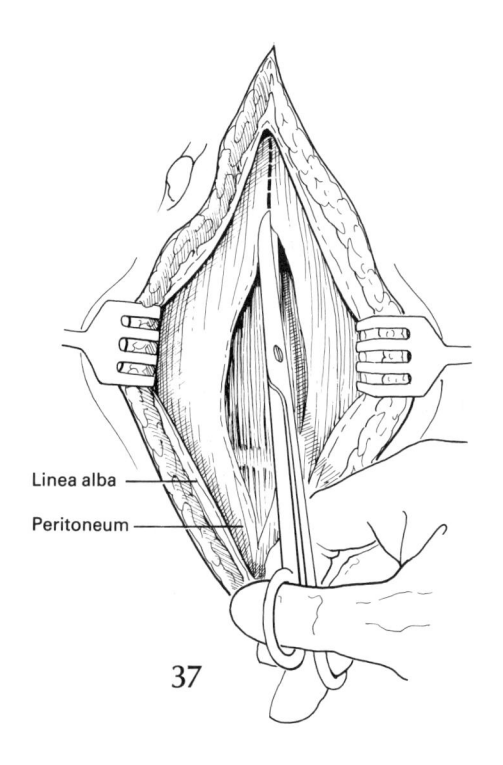

Dissection

37

The linea alba is incised longitudinally, and the rectus abdominis muscles are separated to expose the peritoneum. The peritoneum is picked up with forceps and incised in line with the incision, taking care to avoid the bladder inferiorly.

38

With the patient in a 30° Trendelenburg posture and the abdominal contents packed in a cephalad position, it is then necessary to identify the great vessel bifurcation, common iliac vessels, and soft prominence of the lumbosacral disc.

The retroperitoneal space over the sacral promontory is injected with saline to separate the peritoneum from the vessels and superior hypogastric plexus. The median sacral vessels may be ligated but the superior hypogastric plexus must be protected by avoiding sharp dissection or diathermy in this area, and sweeping the structures off the disc space from left to right.

Approaching the L4–5 disc from within the bifurcation depends on the level of bifurcation. Ligation of the iliolumbar vein is always required for L4–5 exposure.

Precautions

Retraction of the great vessels may cause vascular damage, particularly to the left common iliac vein. Damage to the superior hypogastric plexus must be carefully avoided to prevent retrograde ejaculation and sterility.

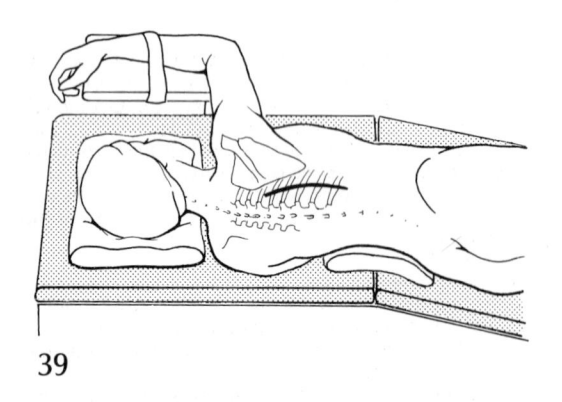

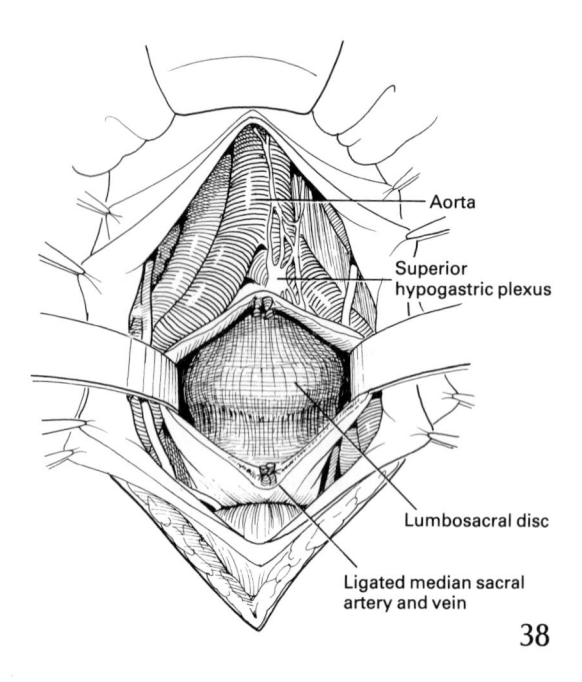

COSTOTRANSVERSECTOMY

First described by Menard in 1894, this approach is mainly used for evacuation of abscesses of the thoracic spine. It has, however, been described for decompression following trauma and tumours and for biopsy[6].

The main advantage of this approach is that it does not enter the thoracic cavity, and should be reserved for limited exposures in high-risk patients.

Position of patient

39

Either the prone position or a lateral decubitus, with 20° anterior tilt can be used.

Incision

A curved linear incision centred over the involved rib 8 cm lateral to the spinous process is commonly used, but an alternative is a midline incision.

Dissection

40

The dissection is continued through the trapezius and paraspinal muscles to reach the the appropriate rib. The muscle attachments are separated from the rib, costo-vertebral joint and transverse process. The transverse process is divided at its base, and the rib divided 6–8 cm from the midline.

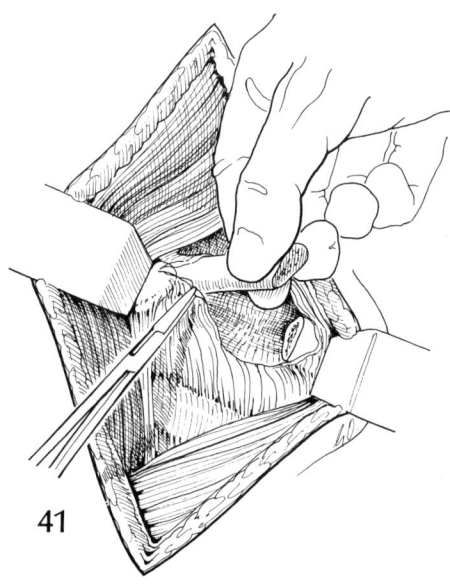

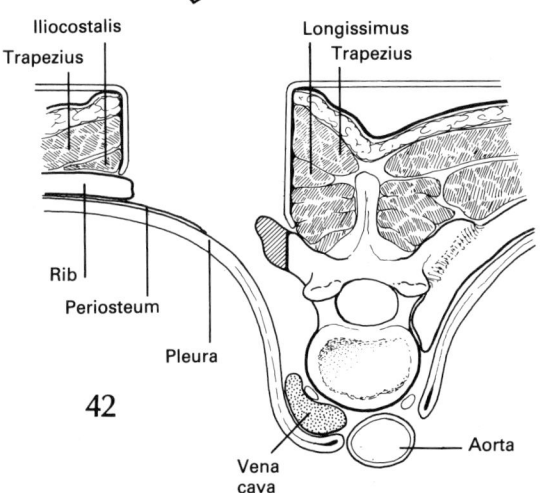

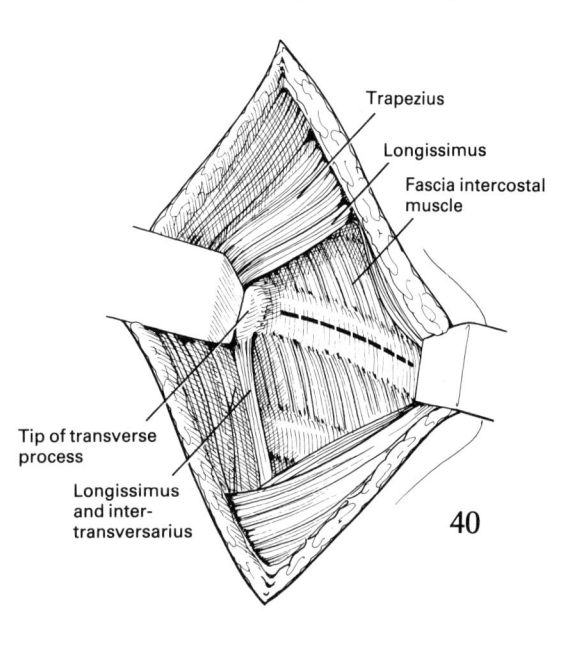

41 & 42

The costovertebral joint is removed with the adjacent transverse process and rib to expose the pleura and neurovascular structures below. Abscesses can be drained by resecting a portion of rib only, while exposing the vertebral body and disc requires removal of the transverse process, often over more than one level.

Precautions

1. Care must be taken with the neurovascular bundle, which leaves the intervertebral foramen caudal to the base of the transverse process, and courses on the inferior edge of the rib.
2. The pleura, which may be thickened by infection, should be carefully stripped by blunt dissection off the anterolateral vertebral body.

616 Thoracic and lumbar spine

Posterior approaches

POSTERIOR APPROACH TO C1–7

Position of patient

43

The patient is placed prone, is anaesthetized, and to control an unstable fracture, a halo traction is applied.

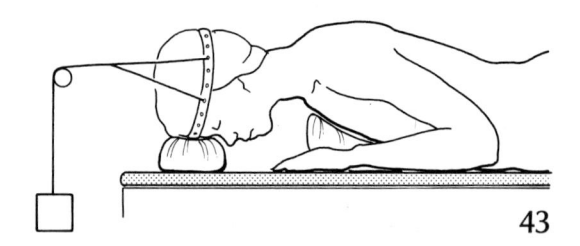

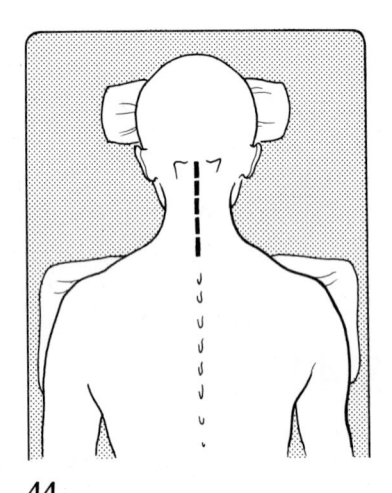

Incision

44

A midline incision is made extending two spinous processes above and below the level to be approached. The median raphe is identified and divided down to the spinous processes using cutting diathermy.

45 & 46

Cobb elevators are used to strip the paraspinal muscles off the spinous processes and laminae.

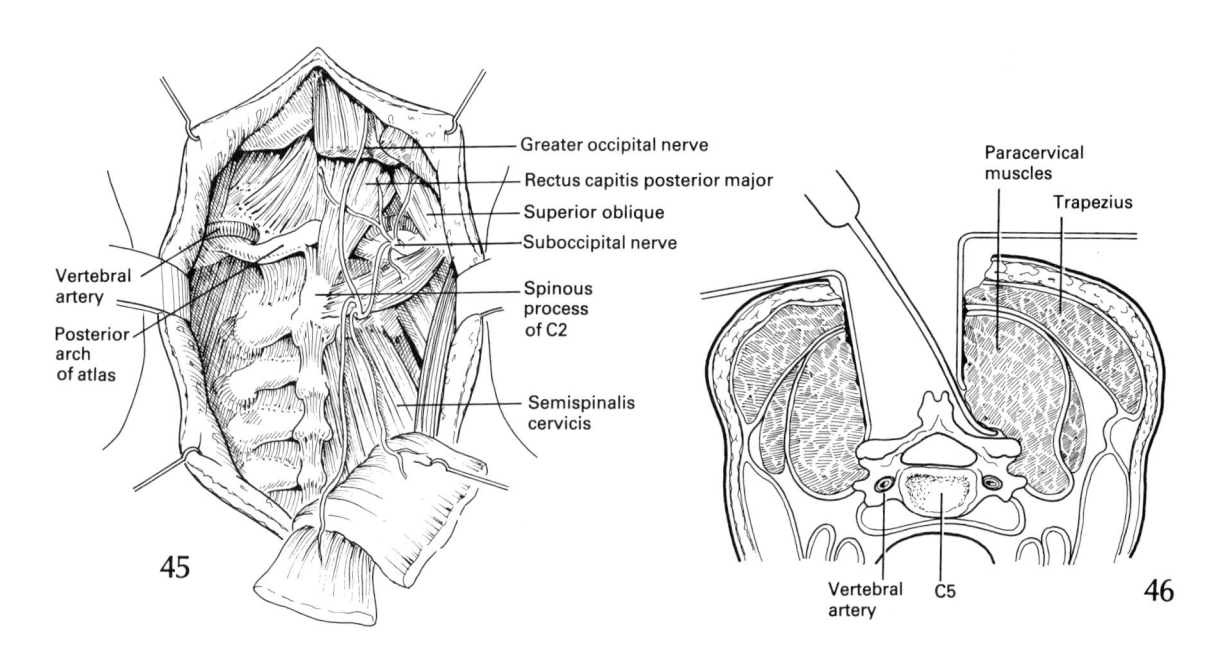

Figure 45: Labels: Vertebral artery; Posterior arch of atlas; Greater occipital nerve; Rectus capitis posterior major; Superior oblique; Suboccipital nerve; Spinous process of C2; Semispinalis cervicis.

Figure 46: Labels: Paracervical muscles; Trapezius; Vertebral artery; C5.

Dissection

47

The dissection is carried as far laterally as necessary to expose the lamina, facet joints and transverse processes. To expose the cervical canal, the ligamentum flavum is incised and removed with as much lamina as necessary for adequate visualization. Care must be taken to preserve the facet joints if possible to reduce the risk of producing instability.

Precautions

1. The vertebral artery must be protected by avoiding too lateral a dissection at C1, no more than 1.5 cm laterally in each direction, and penetration of the atlanto-occipital membrane superior to C1.
2. Care must be taken with the greater occipital nerve which ascends medially and superiorly after emerging from beneath the inferior oblique.
3. The suboccipital nerve is at risk as it emerges between rectus capitis posterior major and inferior oblique.

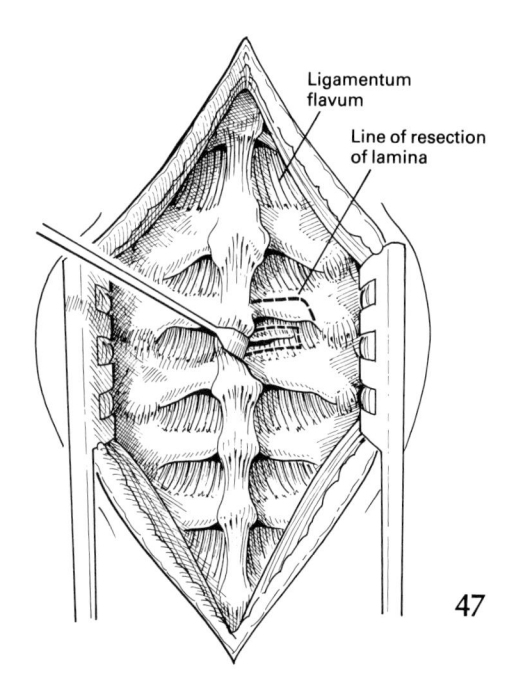

Figure 47: Labels: Ligamentum flavum; Line of resection of lamina.

POSTERIOR APPROACH TO THORACIC SPINE

Incision

48a

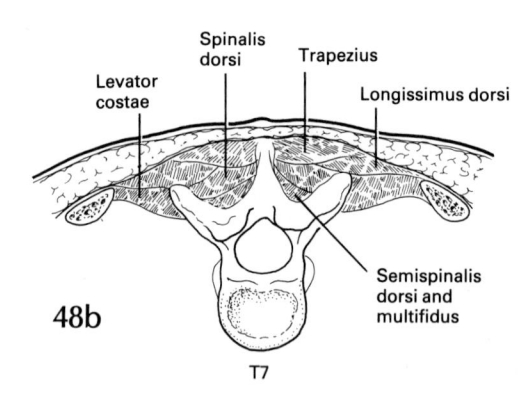

A posterior longitudinal midline incision is centred on the appropriate spinous process.

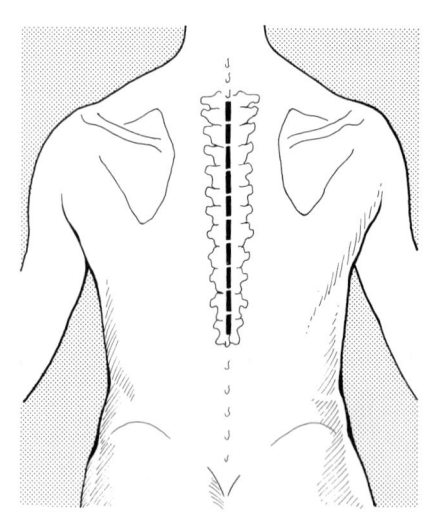

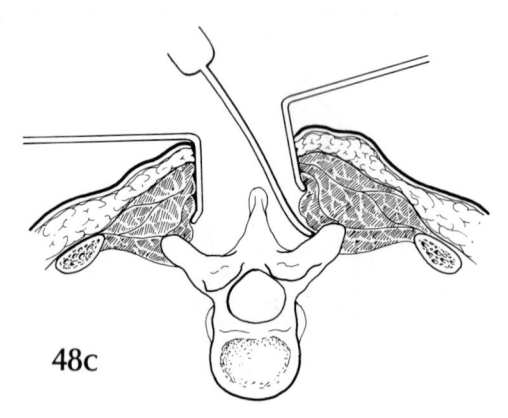

Dissection

48b & c

The deep fascia is divided in the midline and around the spinous processes with cutting diathermy. Cobb periosteal elevators are used to reflect the paraspinal muscles as far as the transverse processes if necessary. The vessels between the transverse processes should be coagulated but care taken to avoid penetration of the intertransverse ligament.

Precautions

1. The muscles should be stripped subperiosteally to preserve their blood supply.
2. Bleeding from the posterior external venous plexus should be controlled with coagulation or tamponade.

Approaches to the spine 619

POSTERIOR APPROACH TO LUMBAR SPINE

Position of patient

49

The position of the patient is important to prevent pressure on the abdomen which increases venous congestion. Lateral or prone positions are described, but variations of the knee–elbow position are popular.

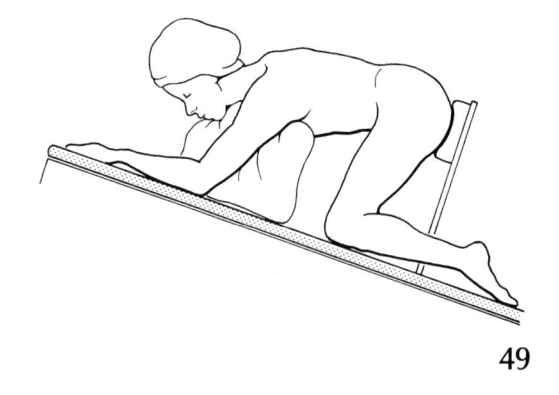

49

Incision

50

A midline incision is made, using cutting diathermy, to open the thoracolumbar fascia.

50

Exposure

51 & 52

The paraspinal muscles are subperiosteally reflected with Cobb elevators as far as the facet joints, and a deep self-retaining retractor used. If intertransverse exposure is required, the soft tissue is cleared from the pars interarticularis and lateral aspect of facet joints with cutting diathermy and Cobb elevators. A blood vessel inferior to the transverse process should be coagulated, and the intertransverse fascia identified.

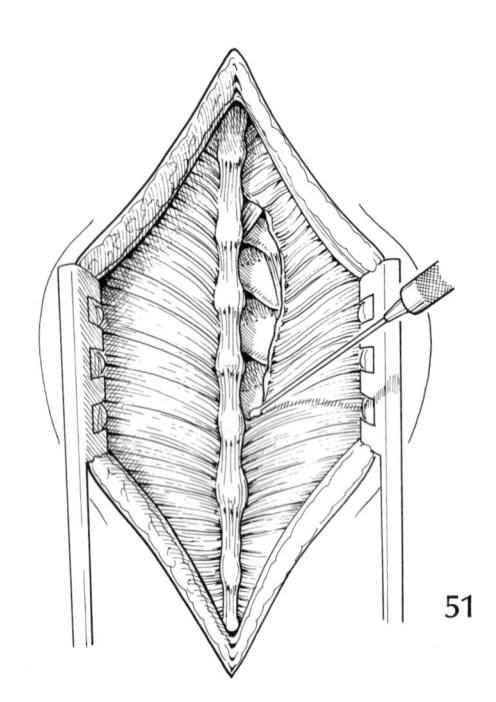

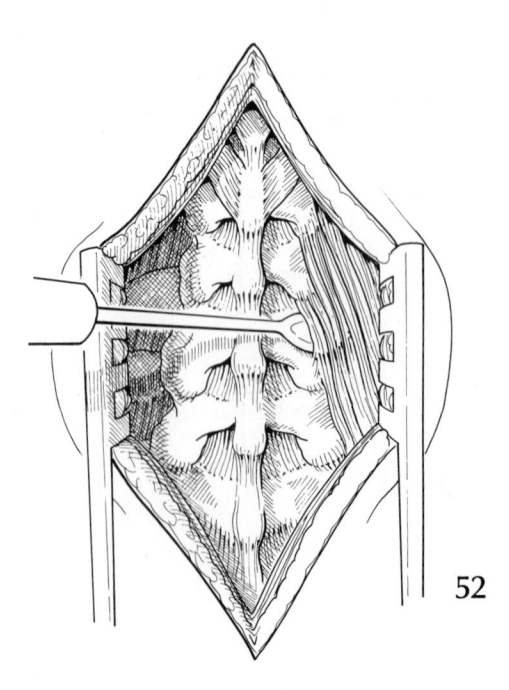

53 & 54

Exposure of the dura and nerve roots requires incision or removal of the ligamentum flavum. This is incised near the inferior lamina and away from the midline. It may be reflected medially, as a flap, or removed with a Kerrison rongeur. It should be remembered that the ligamentum flavum extends cephalad approximately 50 per cent under the superior lamina.

The pedicle should be identified with a probe. The nerve root exits caudally around the pedicle, while the intervertebral disc is 1 cm cephalad to the pedicle.

Precautions

1. In the intertransverse area, the vessels inferior to the transverse process are at risk and penetration should be avoided anterior to the intertransverse ligament.
2. Care should be taken with the vertebral venous plexus surrounding the nerve roots and posterior aspect of vertebral body.
3. The iliac vessels anterior to the vertebral bodies may be injured if instruments pass through the anterior annulus fibrosis.

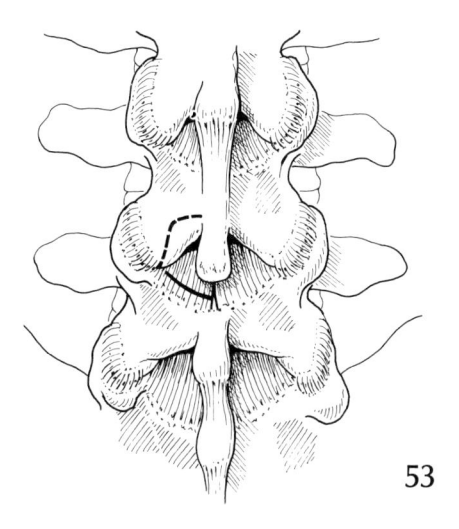

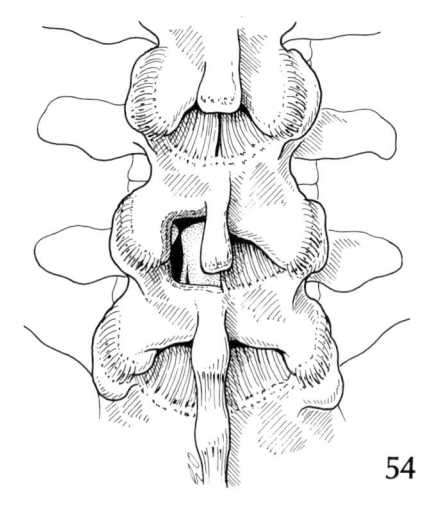

PARASPINAL APPROACH TO LUMBAR SPINE

Several lateral approaches to the lumbar spine have been described[7], most of which are lateral to the three muscles of the sacrospinalis group. Wiltse[8] described a paraspinal approach in 1968, primarily used for lumbosacral fusions, but later extended its use to central canal discectomy, decompression lateral to the pedicle ('far out syndrome'), and even decompression of the opposite side[9].

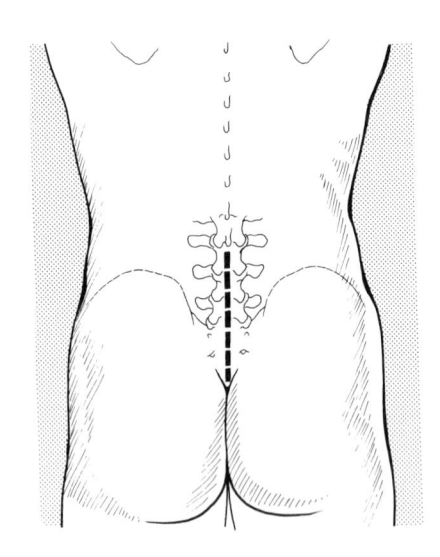

Position of patient

The position is as for the midline posterior approach (see Illustration 49).

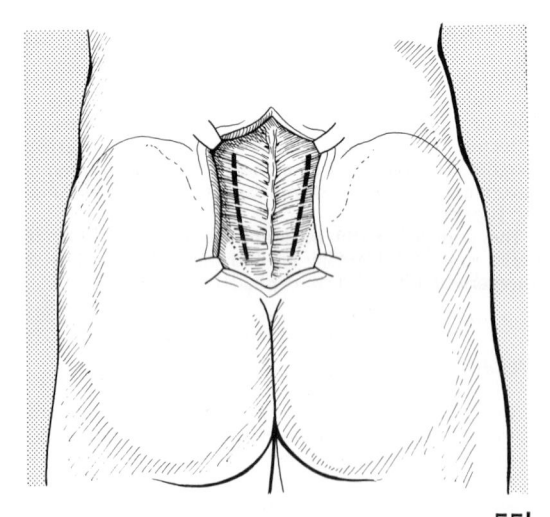

Incision

55a, b & c

Previously, two vertical incisions, three finger's-breadth from the midline, were described, but a midline skin incision with lateral fascial incisions is more cosmetic.

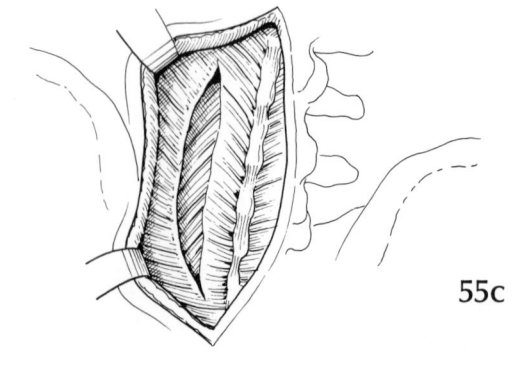

Exposure

56

A finger is passed at the L4–5 level between the multifidus and longissimus muscles of the sacrospinalis group. The transverse fibres of multifidus need to be separated by cutting diathermy from the heavy fascial extension of the combined longissimus and iliocostalis muscles below the L5 level.

Precautions

1. Dissection anterior to the transverse processes should be avoided for the spinal nerves may be injured.
2. Care should be taken with the lumbar arteries and veins just above the bases of the transverse processes.

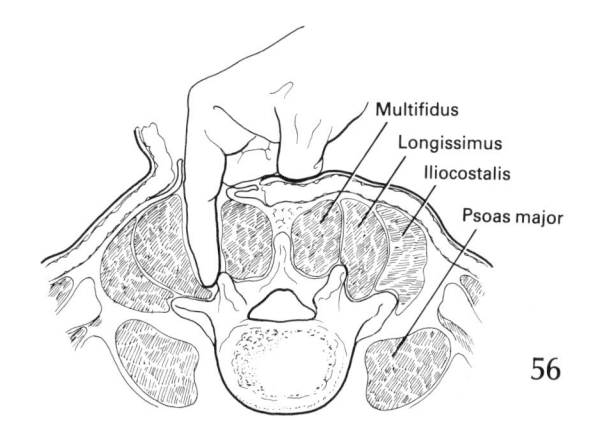

References

1. Kocher ET. *Textbook of operative surgery*, 3rd ed. London: Adam & Charles Black, 1911.
2. Hall JE, Denis F, Murray J. Exposure of the upper cervical spine for spinal decompression by a mandible and tongue-splitting approach. *J Bone Joint Surg [Am]* 1977; 59-A: 121–3.
3. Fang HSY, Ong GB, Hodgson AR. Anterior spinal fusion: the operative approaches. *Clin Orthop* 1964; 35: 16–33.
4. Turner PL, Webb JK. A surgical approach to the upper thoracic spine. *J Bone Joint Surg [Br]* 1987; 69-B: 542–4.
5. Fraser RD. A wide muscle-splitting approach to the lumbar spine. *J Bone Joint Surg [Br]* 1982; 64-B: 44–6.
6. Bohlman HH, Eismont FJ. Surgical techniques of anterior decompression and fusion for spinal cord injuries. *Clin Orthop* 1981; 154: 57–67.
7. Mathieu P, Demirleau J. Traitement chirurgical du spondylolisthésis douloureux. *Rev Orthop* 1936; 23: 352–63.
8. Wiltse LL. The paraspinal sacrospinalis-splitting approach to the lumbar spine. *J Bone Joint Surg [Am]* 1968; 50-A: 919–26.
9. Wiltse LL, Spencer CW. New uses and refinements of the paraspinal approach to the lumbar spine. *Spine* 1988; 13: 696–706.

Illustrations by Peter Cox

Spinal injuries

Sir George Bedbrook OBE, OStJ, MS(Melb), HonMD(WA), HonFRCS(Ed), HonDTech(WAIT), FRCS, FRACS, DPRM(Syd), FCRM(Hon)
Emeritus Consultant Orthopaedic Surgeon and Spinal Surgeon, Royal Perth Hospital and Spinal Unit, Royal Perth Rehabilitation Hospital, Western Australia

Philip H. Hardcastle FRCS(Ed), FRACS
Consultant Surgeon, Spinal Unit, Royal Perth Rehabilitation Hospital, Western Australia

Introduction

Spinal injuries cause a spectrum of different fractures and/or dislocations which may result in a neurological loss of different degrees. Management decisions will depend on the neurological state, fracture or dislocation type, age and associated injuries.

APPLICATION OF SKULL CALIPER OR HALO

Indications

1. To assist in surgical reduction of fractures, dislocations and fracture-dislocations of the cervical spine. The calipers or halo may be left in position for periods of up to 10 weeks and optimally for not less than 6 weeks.
2. To maintain reduction obtained by closed manipulative reduction. The calipers or halo remain in position for the same period as above.
3. To assist postural nursing of some stable fractures and cervical spinal injuries (usually for short periods only).

Contraindications

All stable injuries involving a fracture and/or some subluxations. These include compression and extension injuries. (Stability can be determined by flexion–extension lateral X-rays taken under sedation if necessary.) The spine should be positioned by the surgeon. Stability can frequently be decided by the pathological type of injury. Over 60 per cent of all fractures and dislocations of the human spine are pathologically and clinically stable immediately after the injury.

Preparation of scalp

Adequate hair must be removed in all cases and the scalp thoroughly cleaned. All associated lacerations must be carefully cleaned and sutured, if necessary under local anaesthetic.

1

Towelling must be arranged so that the naso-occipital line is visible. The lines, nasion to occiput and between the pinnae, are then marked with Bonney's blue or suitable marking ink. If a halo is being applied, the hair should be cut short over the halo area at least. The hair and scalp should be carefully cleaned.

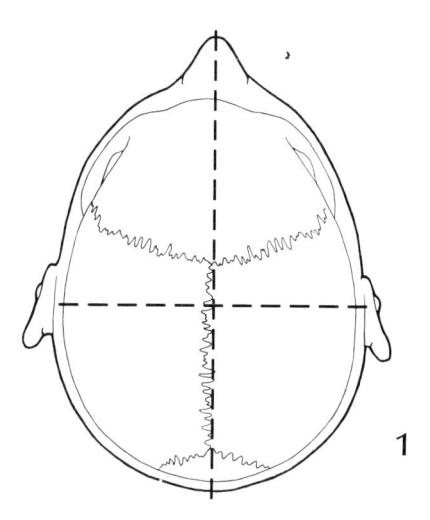

Preparation for calipers or halo

2a

The calipers (Crutchfield, Bennett, Vinke) are opened to the maximum width and a suitable size selected so that the pins will be vertical to the calvarium and the points are either: in front of the coronal line if extension is to be assisted; on the coronal line if neutral traction is required; or behind the coronal line if flexion is required.

The points on the skin should be marked clearly.

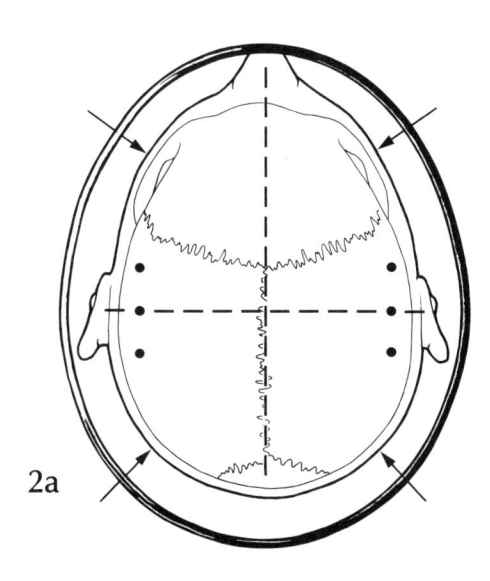

2b

The halo must be carefully positioned to allow 1–1.5 cm clearance of the skull and to be horizontal to the skull 1–2 cm above the pinnae and the supraorbital ridges. Four screws should be positioned and the skin marked (hair is not usually fully removed).

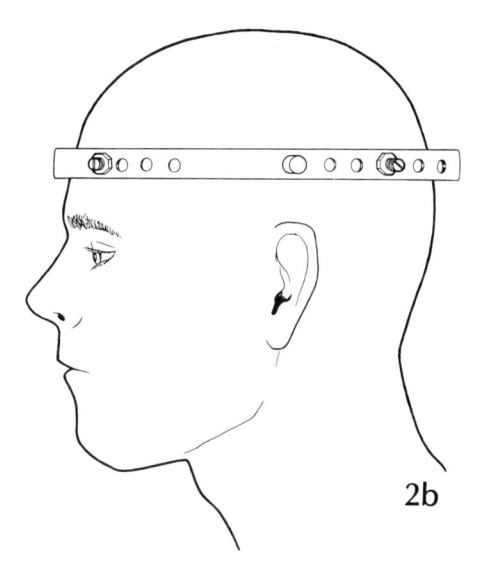

Anaesthesia

3

Intradermal local anaesthesia using 1 ml 2 per cent lignocaine with bilateral subcutaneous local anaesthesia 1–2 ml over the marked spots is used. A maximum of 5 ml on each side deep to the scalp in the pericranial space for caliper insertion is used, and 3–5 minutes should be allowed to elapse for adequate effect.

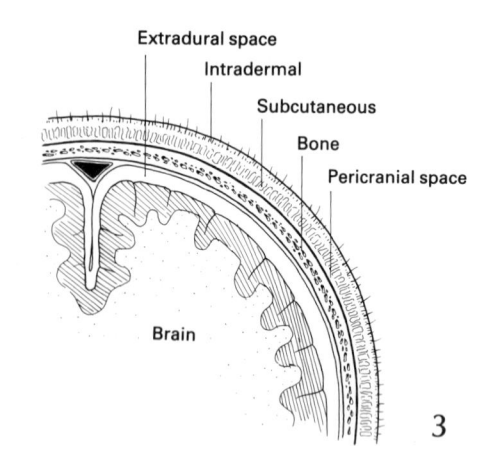

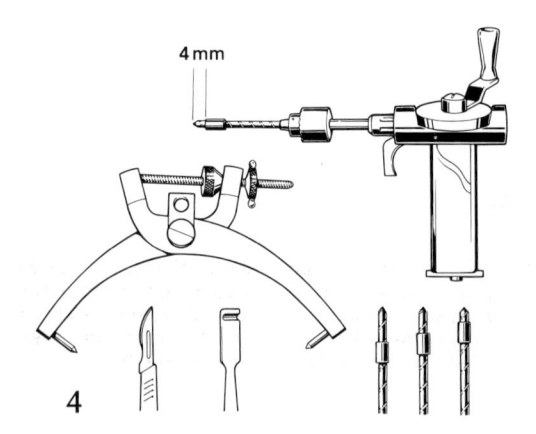

Instruments

4

A No. 15 scalpel, Howarth dissector, guarded twist drills with guard at 2, 3 and 4 mm from distal end of 3 mm drill (the caliper ends must only go through the outer table of the skull, the average depth being 4 mm), hand drill, head caliper or halo (select right size), and screws for halo and spanners are used.

Incision

5

Caliper

Compressing the marked spot on the first side (right or left) with two fingers, a short incision is made in the coronal plane. This is usually 5 mm long, but is never longer than 1 cm.

Halo

No incision is needed for the halo screws but stab wounds to the skull will be more comfortable for the patient.

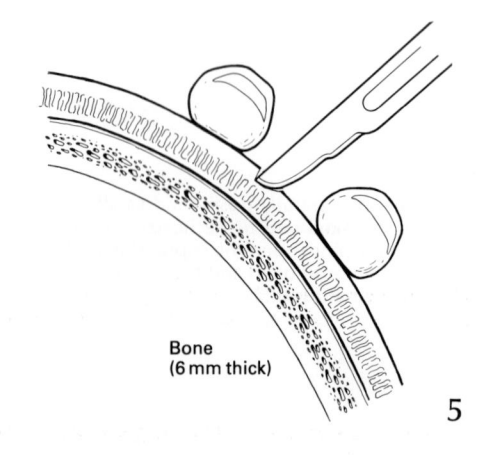

Spinal injuries 627

Caliper

6a

Bleeding is not usually excessive. A Howarth periosteal resector is used to bare the bone. A hole is then drilled in the outer table using a guarded drill to a depth of only 4 mm (maximum 5 mm).

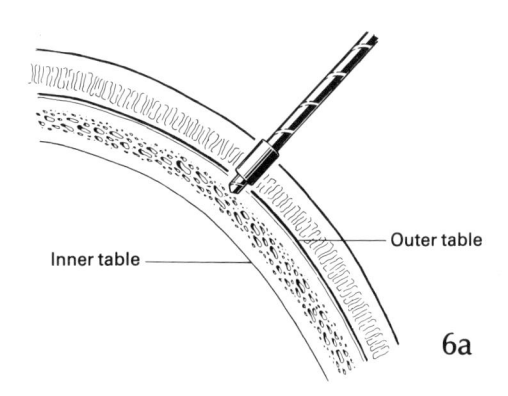

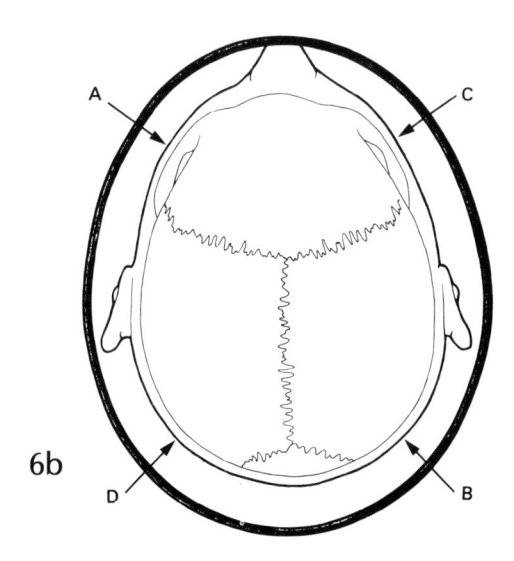

Inner table — Outer table

6a

Halo

6b

No drill is needed for application of the halo. With an assistant holding the halo level, screws are inserted via the skin to the depth of outer table. The position of the screws is checked and they are then tightened in order A–B–C–D. The assistant must hold the halo level.

6b

Caliper

7

The drill is removed; using the open caliper point the hole is found and the surgeon ascertains that it will locate well.

Halo

Each screw must be checked and the surgeon may need to alter the alignment.

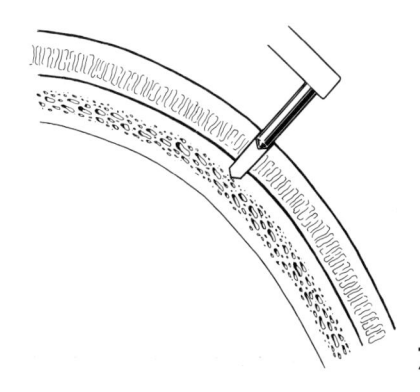

7

Second incision for caliper

When the caliper point has been positioned in the first hole (right or left), the position of the second incision should be checked. The caliper is removed and a second incision is made. Drilling should be as for the first procedure with the assistant maintaining pressure over the scalp at the first incision if necessary to control any haemorrhage.

Locating the caliper

8

When the second hole is finished, the caliper is located first in one drill hole and then in the second. The caliper is tightened in a manner appropriate to the type used.

The area surrounding each pin is anointed with either a sealed dressing with Friars' balsam (or a similar compound) or silver sulphadiazine cream which is changed daily as for burns.

The halo must be carefully checked and dressings applied if needed. The halo must finally be horizontal in the erect posture or vertical in the supine posture.

Complications

Complications include penetration of the inner table. If this occurs, the halo or caliper should be reinserted properly. Infection such as soft tissue cellulitis or osteomyelitis may occur. However, this is rare, the incidence being 1 in 500. To remedy infection, it should be treated with the appropriate drug to prevent recurrence. The caliper may work loose, but can be tightened with the finger daily. The halo may not be horizontal – this must be checked and repositioned if necessary. The caliper or halo must be kept firm by daily checks.

POSTURAL REDUCTION PLUS MAINTENANCE

Indications

All fractures and dislocations of the spine, either with or without operative treatment.

Advantages

1. Will effect total or partial reduction in all except 11 per cent of thoracolumbar fracture-dislocations which have locked facets and approximately 25 per cent of cervicothoracic fracture-dislocations which have locked facets
2. Allows muscle recovery
3. Prevents further neuromuscular damage
4. Encourages postural reflexes in extension
5. Prevents flexion-contractures
6. Creates a physiological position for neurological injury to recover.

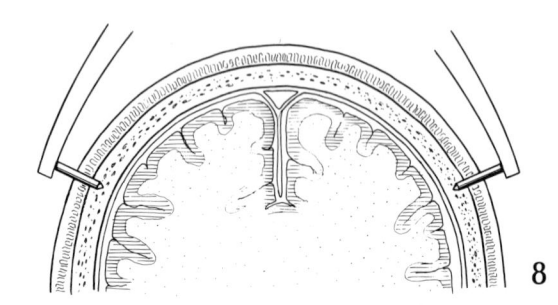

Duration

For the first 6–8 weeks reduction should be maintained as strictly as possible. The 'danger' period for redislocation is the third week, usually because posture is not carefully maintained.

Method

9–12

The patient is maintained in either a supine, prone or lateral position on a normal hospital bed using pillows in the lordotic areas of the spine. The patient is turned by a special team every 2 hours.

On special beds such as the Stoke Mandeville Egerton bed, turning is carried out by automatic electrical devices with only one attendant. Bed blocks of various heights made of blocked rubber or pillows are used.

Special points

13 & 14

The level of sensory loss and the level of the fracture must be marked on the skin so that posturing can be accurate. When cervicothoracic fracture-dislocations are being postured, a pillow is needed at the level of T1–T2 to achieve good extension. At the thoracolumbar junction the pillow must not be too large at first or adynamic ileus will be aggravated. The height of the pillows can be increased slowly until the maximum is obtained. Reduction can be achieved by cautious introduction of flexion in the postural care management, initially combined with traction if needed.

Cleft cleavage compression fractures may be stable or unstable, the latter with flexion or extension translational forces as well as compression. CT scans may reveal canal encroachment which can resolve spontaneously. Surgery is indicated for neurological deterioration.

All posture must be checked clinically and by X-ray in bed.

While perfect reduction is always the goal, multiple fractures at two or more levels are frequent pathologically so that the surgeon must judge the alignment and displacement remembering that, only in cases with displacement on lateral X-rays greater than one half of the anteroposterior diameter of a vertebra, is canal alignment grossly reduced.

Increasing accuracy with tomography, including oblique and axial views, has demonstrated the morbid anatomy as multifactorial in most flexion-rotation injuries.

Fracture-dislocations greater than half width on lateral plates can readily redisplace. As mentioned previously, reduction can be achieved by cautious introduction of flexion in the postural care management, initially combined with traction if needed before applying extension.

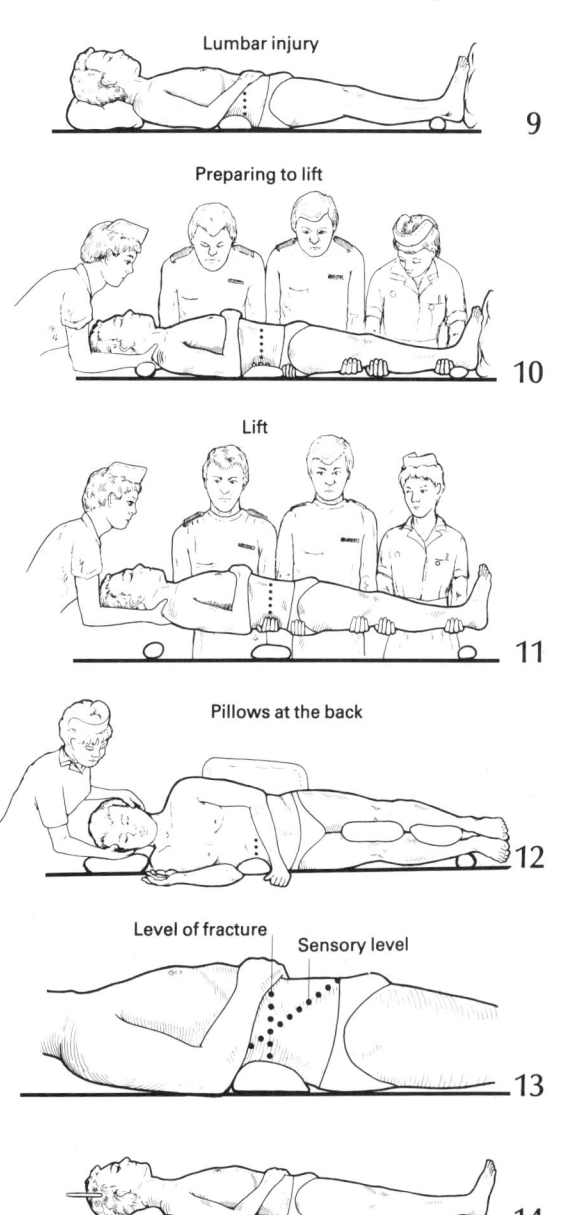

Contraindications

There are no contraindications to postural care.

This is the universal method required in all cases. Rarely in thoracolumbar injuries (1–2 per cent), more commonly in cervicothoracic injuries (26 per cent), extension forces have caused the injury, usually with displacement greater than the first X-rays reveal. Reduction can be achieved by cautious introduction of flexion in the postural care management, initially combined with traction if needed.

CERVICAL SPINE

Fracture-dislocation with or without tetraparesis or tetraplegia

CLOSED REDUCTION

Indication

Flexion-rotation dislocations of the cervical spine with single facet fracture-dislocation and with bilateral fracture-dislocation.

Timing

Reduction should be performed as soon as possible after injury, and by the right surgeon in the right place.

Methods

1. Slow 'manipulation' and reduction without general anaesthesia if over 24 hours since the accident
2. Rapid instantaneous manipulation and reduction with general anaesthesia if under 24 hours
3. Open reduction using either the anterior method or the posterior method (in first few days after injury).

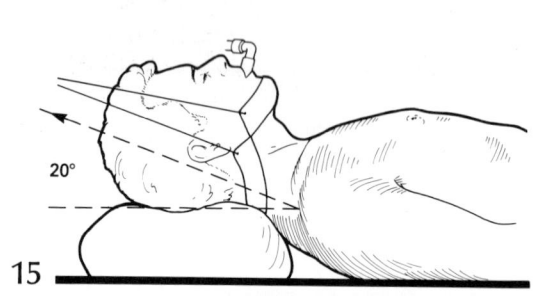

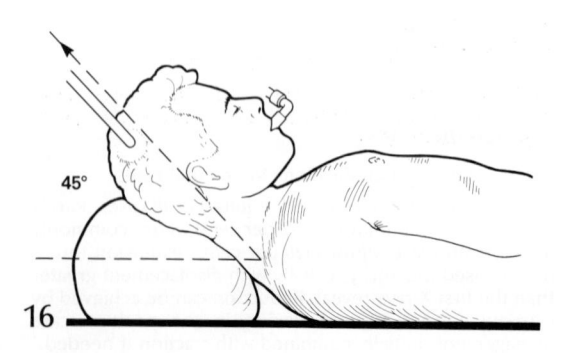

Decision on method

All cervical fracture-dislocations with 'locked' facets seen within 24 hours of injury, with or without spinal cord damage, should be treated under general anaesthesia by closed manipulative reduction by experienced surgeons, providing that there is no contraindication (e.g. pulmonary, cerebral or other injury) to general anaesthesia.

After 24 hours those without cord damage can be so treated, but the surgeon should first consider a closed method without general anaesthesia for those with cord damage or spinal cord oedema.

In bilateral facetal dislocations with (or without) fracture, occasionally open reduction is needed early (within the first week).

Selection of either an anterior or posterior method will depend on the place and the surgeon. There is *no* haste in complete lesions. In incomplete lesions, reduction time depends on patient fitness.

Method with general anaesthesia

15

Manual traction is applied by a halter, caliper or halo, and general anaesthesia is commenced, including intubation and relaxant.

Bilateral dislocation

16

The head is flexed to 45°, applying manual traction to unlock, with a pillow or sandbag under the cervical spine.

17a, b, c & 18

Maintaining traction, the head is slowly extended to unlock completely. A soft 'click' usually indicates reduction. The head should be extended 30–40°.

A lateral X-ray film is taken to confirm reduction.

Crutchfield calipers or halo are applied as described.

If reduction is not achieved, the process is repeated once.

If reduction has still not been achieved, then one further attempt can be made by a more experienced operator or the surgeon should progress to the slow reduction method (*see below*).

If not already applied, a halo or head traction calipers are then applied as described, with the head held in the reduced position.

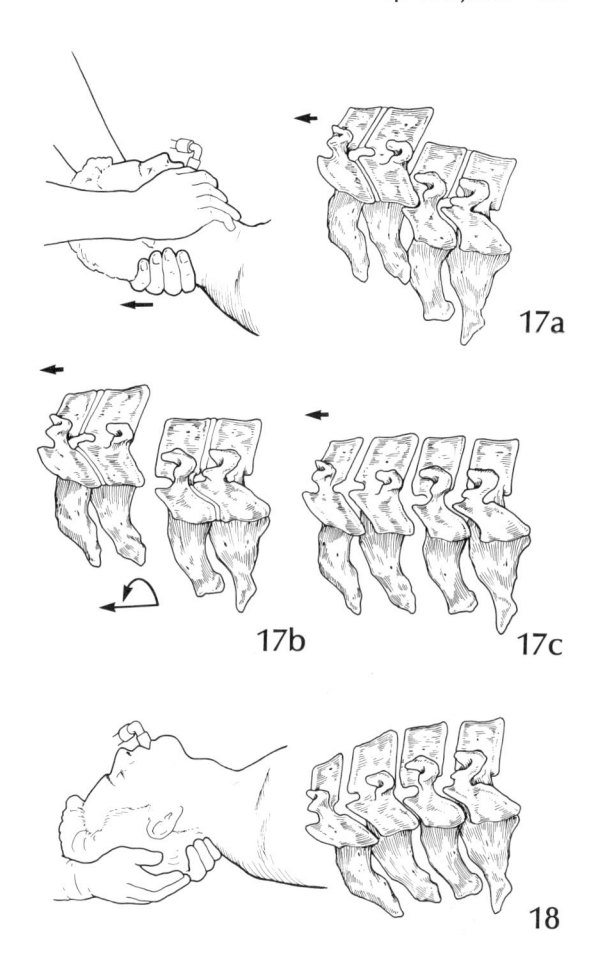

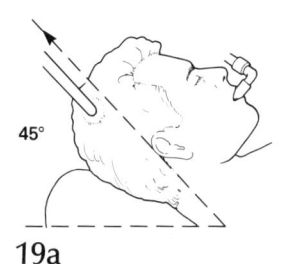

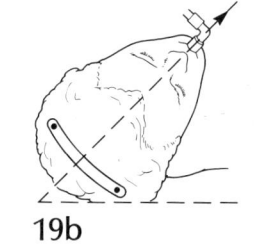

Unilateral dislocation (Walton manoeuvre)

19a & b

The head is flexed to 45° in the coronal and sagittal axes, and to the opposite side from the facet dislocation, with traction maintained.

632 Thoracic and lumbar spine

20 & 21

Traction is maintained while the head is rotated away from the side of dislocation around the intact side, thus unlocking the dislocation as the head is returned to neutral.

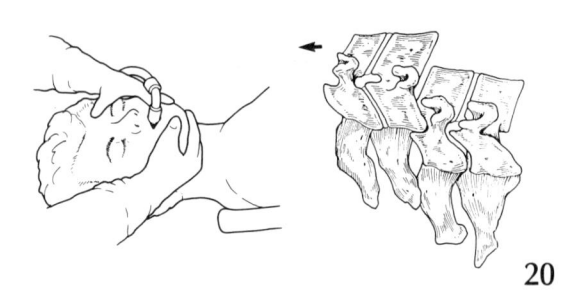

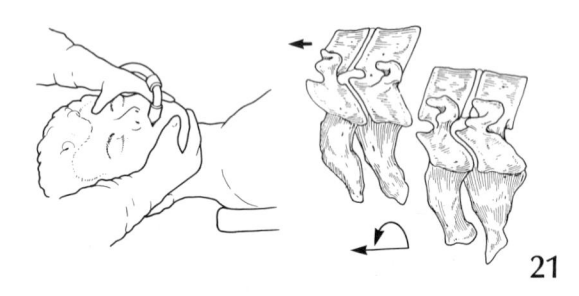

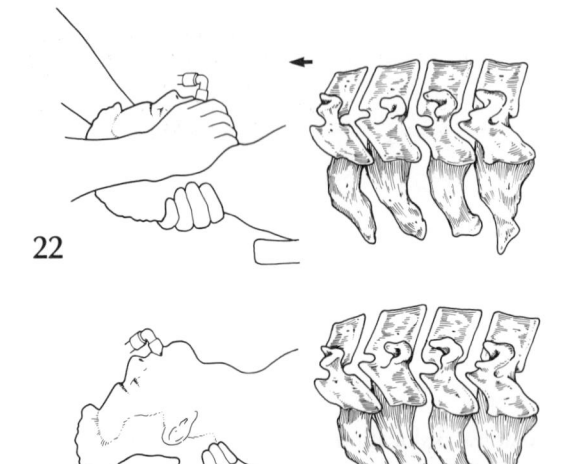

20

21

22

22 & 23

The head is then rotated back to neutral as extension is increased. As this procedure is carried out, the head is then finally extended to maintain the reduction.

An X-ray is taken to check reduction.

The procedure is repeated if, after careful study of oblique and the original anteroposterior and lateral plates to see that the sides are correctly identified, reduction has not been accomplished.

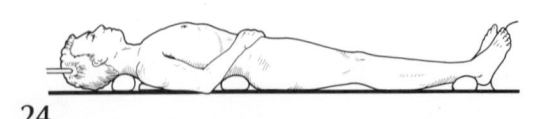

23

24

After reduction, head calipers or halo are applied and postural care commenced to maintain reduction.

24

Method without general anaesthesia

Bilateral fracture-dislocation

25

Head calipers or halo are positioned under local anaesthesia and, using pillows to posture, traction is applied in flexion (30°–40°) with a 7 kg weight.

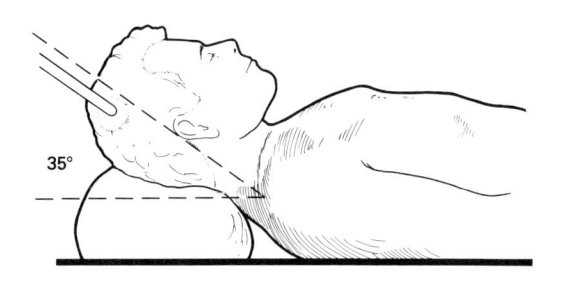

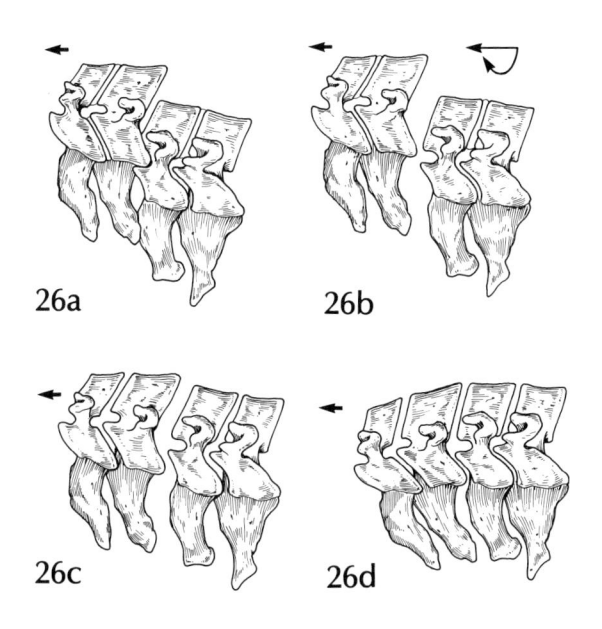

26a–d

The X-ray is checked and, if the fracture-dislocation is not distracted and unlocked, the weights are increased by 2 kg every 30–45 minutes, the X-ray (lateral only) being checked each time. The patient is sedated until 'unlocking' occurs; flexion is adjusted as necessary.

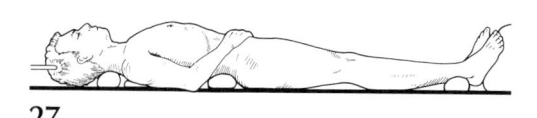

27

Traction is maintained while a pillow is inserted under the cervicothoracic area and the head lowered into the extended position. Unlocking is checked by X-ray.

634 Thoracic and lumbar spine

Unilateral dislocation

28a–d

Traction is applied slowly in two planes, coronal and sagittal. The traction is increased on both axes as for bilateral dislocation. Unlocking is checked by X-ray. The head is brought to neutral and then extended.

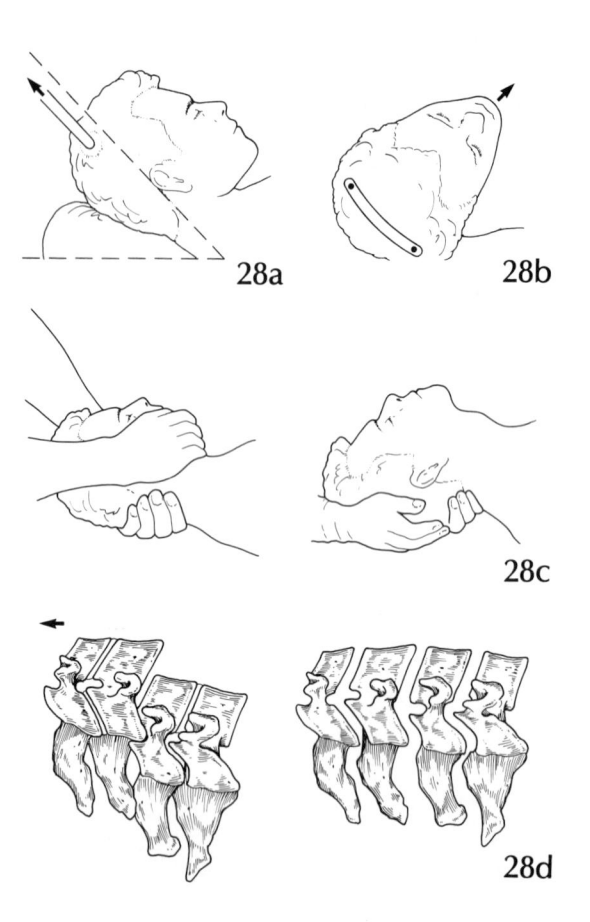

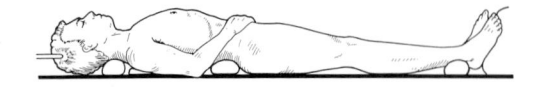

28a

28b

28c

28d

29

The reduction is maintained very carefully with posture and traction. Sufficient extension may be maintained for 6–8 weeks or the surgeon may use a halo and then halo vest to maintain position. The position is *not* always easy to maintain.

29

OPEN POSTERIOR REDUCTION

Indications (generally agreed)

1. Failed conservative method slow or rapid (bilateral dislocation)
2. Locked facets (bilateral)
3. Neural deterioration in either facetal dislocation or gross compression subluxation injuries.

Note: A locked unilateral facet dislocation is not regularly an indication for open reduction.

Contraindications

1. Multiple injuries
2. Gross respiratory difficulties
3. Any infection.

Note: Procedures (anterior or posterior) do not regularly give neural improvement.

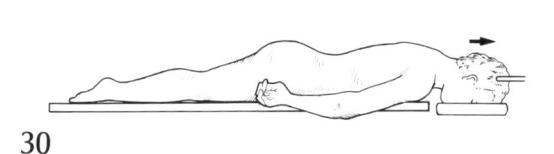

Procedure

30

The patient is carefully postured prone on a neurosurgical table, maintaining traction of 25–30 kg. The head must be comfortable, the eyes protected, and the head-piece must be adjustable.

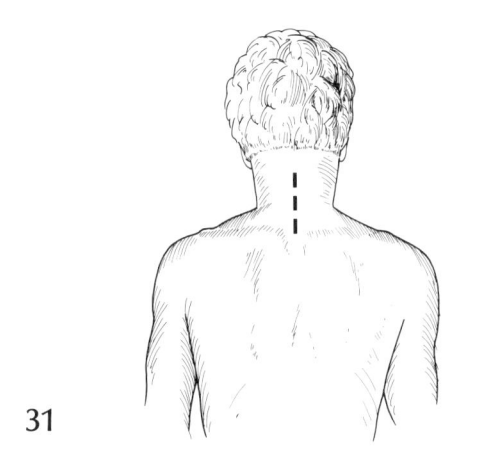

Incision

31

An incision is made along the spinal processes, from two above the level of dislocation to two below. The wound is deepened to clean the laminae carefully; these are usually partly cleared by the accident. After retraction, the facets are exposed as in the lumbar approach (*see Illustrations 67a & b*).

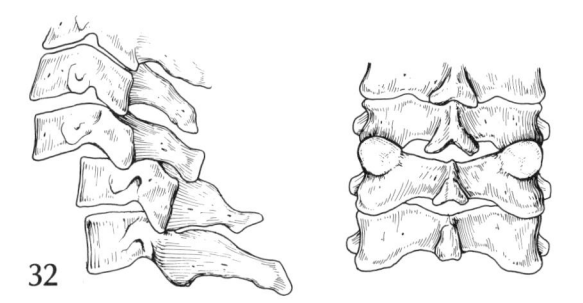

Reduction of dislocation

32

After intact spinous processes are identified above and below the injury site any laminal fracture must be treated by excision or elevation – caudocephalic traction force is applied in 25°–30° flexion to gently reduce – altering head posture as necessary.

Partial or complete facet excision may be required to unlock the dislocation. The facet is then reduced by extension.

Fixation

33 & 34

Most surgeons rely on wire splintage suitably laced through the spinous processes above and below. Some use plates or clamps which, because of the sheaving or overlapping of laminae, may be difficult to apply. Laminal wiring such as in the Gallie procedure (see p. 644) is also used with quadrilateral fixation devices. Bone grafting of the two segments, as in Gallie fusion, is also used (see Illustrations 59, 60, 61).

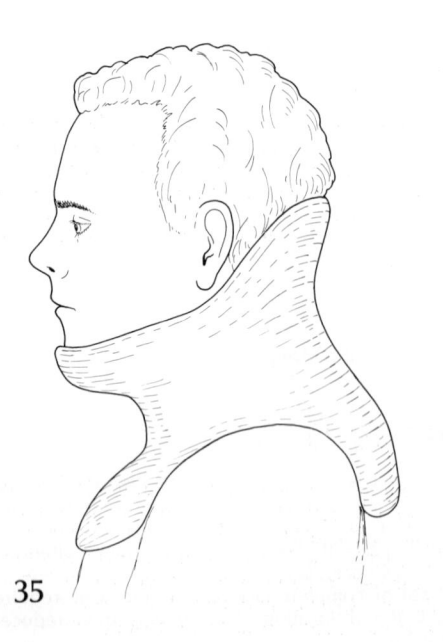

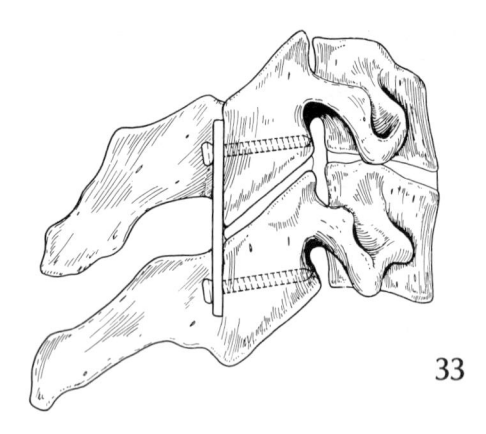

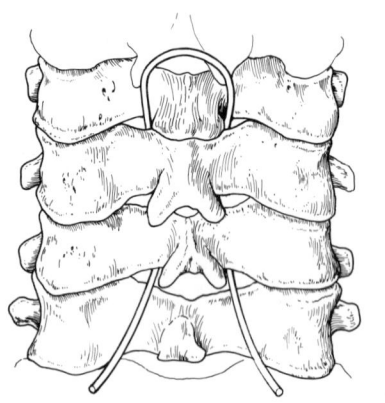

Wound closure

35

The wound is closed using the usual physiological closure.
After the wound is closed, a suitable moulded collar is applied in extension, and traction of 10–15 kg is maintained for a period until the patient is conscious. A halo vest can then be applied within a few days to allow mobilization.

Fractures requiring fusion

ANTERIOR STABILIZATION

This section describes anterior surgery in treatment of spinal fractures with spinal fusion and reduction of bilateral fracture-dislocation after injury.

Indications

Generally agreed:

1. To treat non-union at all levels
2. To stabilize the spine in fractures of the cervicothoracic area proven to be unstable 6–8 weeks after accident. These are usually of the flexion-rotation type
3. To fuse and stabilize after extensive laminectomies. Such an indication is very small, with the proven lack of usefulness of laminectomy in the management of spinal fractures with paraplegia
4. To correct spinal deformity.

Not generally agreed:

1. To reduce acute fracture-dislocations (this is rarely needed pathologically)
2. To remove intracanal fragments occupying 30 per cent or more of the spinal canal in incomplete neural lesions where neurological recovery has plateaued.

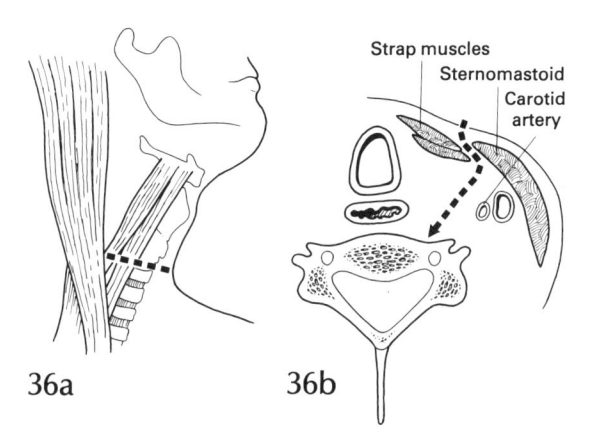

Anterior cervical approach

36a & b

A transverse incision is made at the level of the cricoid or above and below this level, depending on the vertebrae to be approached, through the platysma down to the anterior border of the sternomastoid. The incision is continued along this anterior border and between the strap muscles and carotid sheath onto the prevertebral fascia.

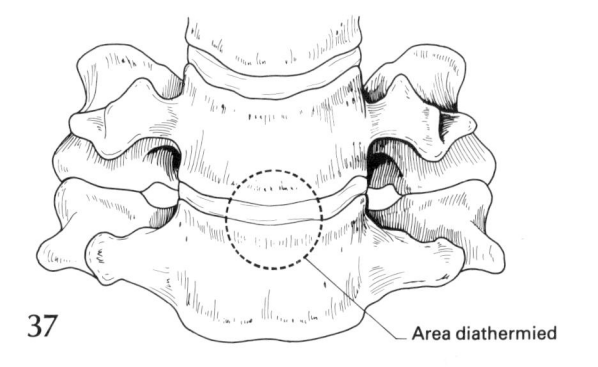

37

The prevertebral fascia is thus exposed. The disc spaces of C4–5, C5–6, C6–7 and even C7–T1 can be exposed.

Identification with lateral X-ray is usually important when a dowel is to be used. The disc space is exposed and prepared using diathermy in the shape of a circle, approximately 1–5 cm in the midline, to prevent excessive bleeding.

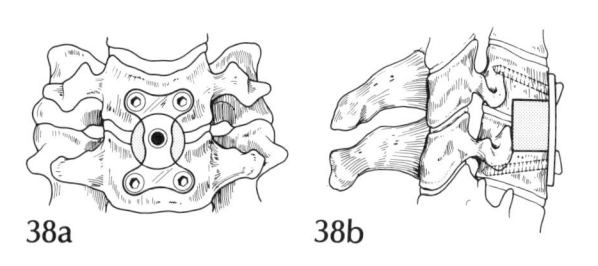

38a & b

In acute injuries, preservation of the anterior longitudinal ligament is important. The surgeon may decide to use a key graft or a small plate with cancellous screws. A 2.0 mm drill should be used, and the posterior cortex should not be breached. If the bone is osteoporotic, it is better to stabilize the spine posteriorly if fixation is necessary or to use external fixation (halo or Minerva plaster jacket).

Dowel method

39

A serrated dowel drill is then used to cut a circular hole of suitable depth to leave the posterior cortex intact. A drill is then inserted inside the dowel cylinder, and disc and bone are removed.

The possibility of multiple techniques means that an experienced surgeon with availability of other methods such as key graft or plates should perform the procedure. Cases where there is intracanal intrusion needing removal should be decompressed anteriorly. In acute cases the fragments can be removed with rongeurs and curettes. In late cases these fragments have to be drilled out with a diamond burr.

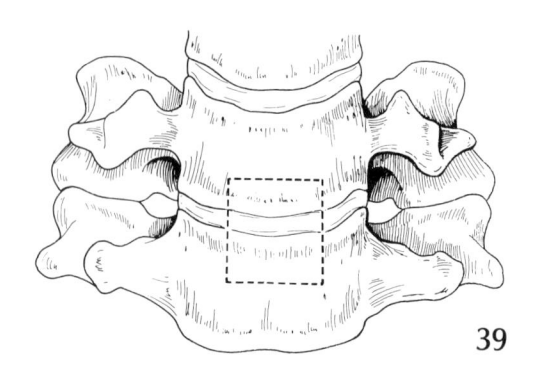

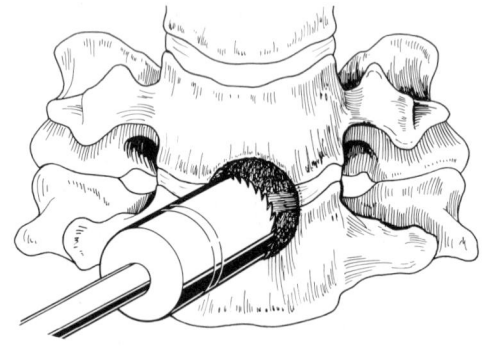

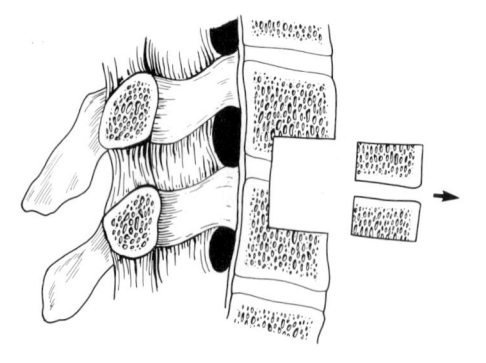

40 & 41

The cylindrical hole is cleared carefully and then, with the anaesthetist effectively inducing traction, a dowel is inserted firmly to give a tight fit.

The body of the vertebra needs careful assessment if a plate and screws are to be used so that cancellous screws give firm fixation.

42

If a key graft is used, a bicortical block of the required size must be removed and carefully fashioned.

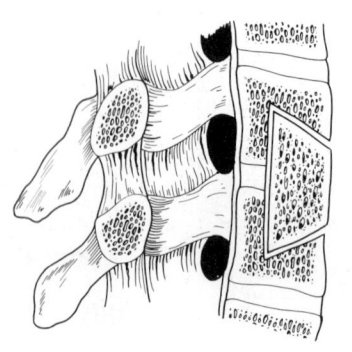

Spinal injuries 639

Taking a dowel graft

43 & 44

Using the dowel set illustrated, dowels are cut from the iliac crest behind the anterior superior iliac spine at the gluteal tubercle.

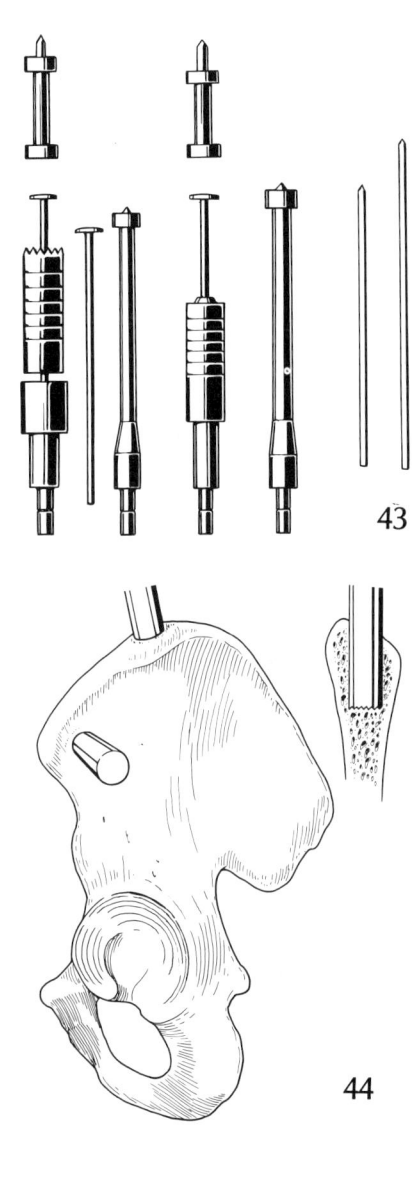

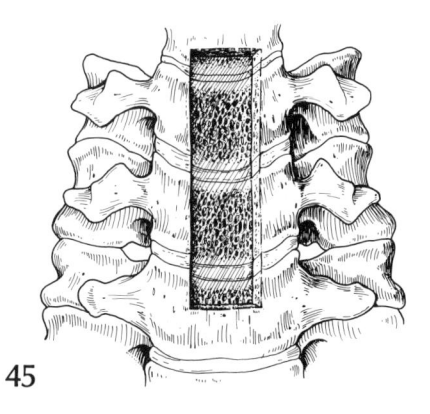

45

If an iliac or fibular strut is to be used to bridge two or three discs, a trench is fashioned with chisels.

The graft is fractionally longer than the trench or is fashioned with pegs or angles to lock. By maintaining traction as the graft is inserted, a tight fit is achieved. With the increased availability of cortical plates and cancellous screws, some surgeons will use these. They call for extra surgical expertise and the surgeon must be ready to remove them after use. Biological methods such as grafts are superior techniques.

Thoracic and lumbar spine

POSTERIOR FUSION WITH PLATES OR WIRES

Indications

1. Bifacetal dislocation unreduced by conservative methods
2. Redisplacement after reduction
3. Correction of kyphotic deformity after anterior release and fusion
4. Segmental instability.

Technique

46 *(see also Illustration 32)*

Midline incision and subperiosteal dissection out to the lateral aspect of the facet joint is performed. Dislocation is reduced. If a fracture of the superior articular process is present it is removed with rongeurs.

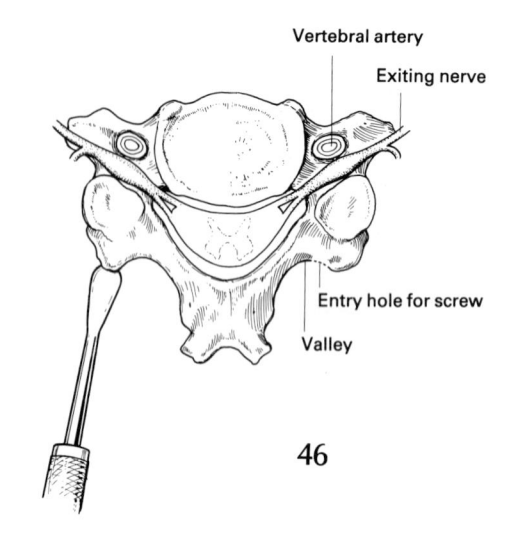

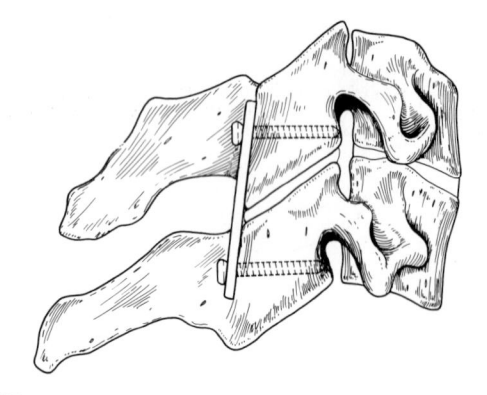

47

A two-hole spinal plate is inserted across the facet joint with one screw above and one below. For kyphotic deformity longer plates may be used. Cortex screws (3.5 mm) are used after pre-drilling with a 2.0 mm drill. In small articular processes 2.7 mm screws can be used.

48

Screws are placed above and below the level of the facet joint in the sagittal plane and angled 10° laterally. The entry point for the screw is 3 mm below the midpoint of the superior facet joint. The latter is approximately 5 mm from the lateral articular border. This avoids damage to the vertebral artery and the exiting spinal nerve which is under the pedicle. (The pedicle is too small for screw fixation.) Screw lengths range from 14 to 19 mm. No fusion is performed and the plates are not removed.

Wire 'fixation' can be used, encircling the laminae as in the Gallie fusion, or by drill holes through the spinous processes.

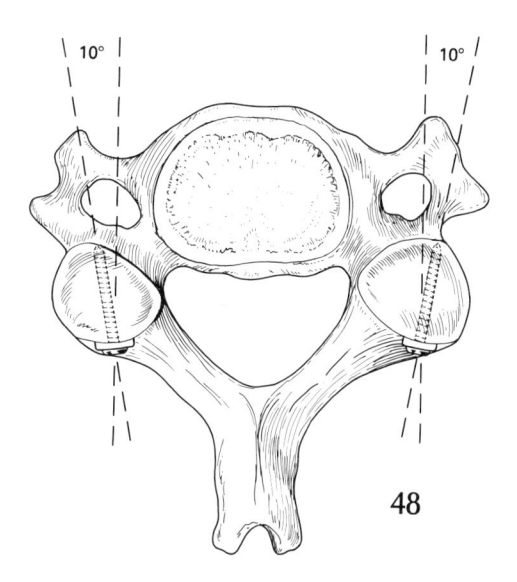

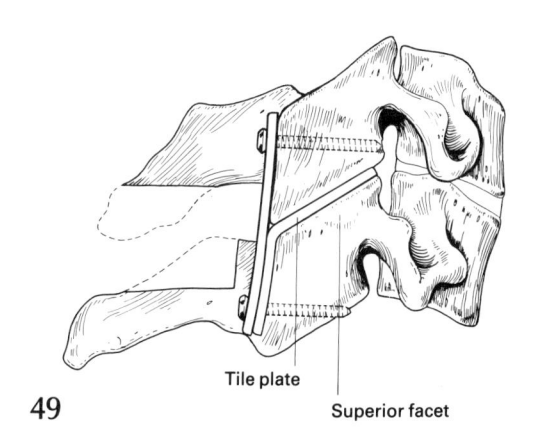

49

A Tile plate (Roy Camille) can be used to replace the superior articular facet if it is fractured. A two-hole plate is inserted adjacent to this.

Atlanto-axial fractures and dislocations

INTERNAL FIXATION OF ODONTOID FRACTURES

Indication

Unstable fracture through the base of the odontoid which does not unite after 8–12 weeks of adequate immobilization[1].

Technique

50

The patient is positioned as for a cervical fusion with the neck extended and turned slightly to the left. A sandbag is placed under the cervical spine.

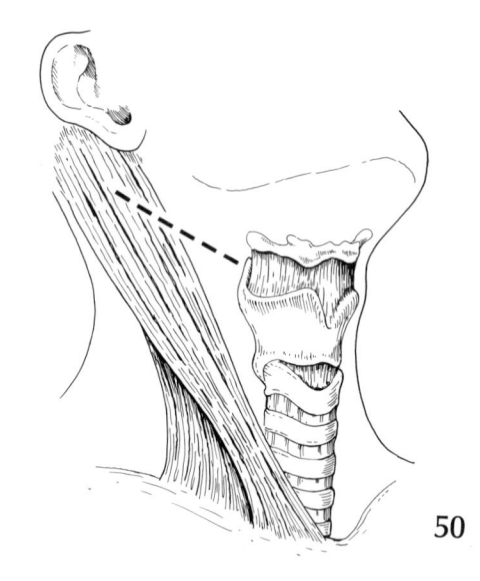

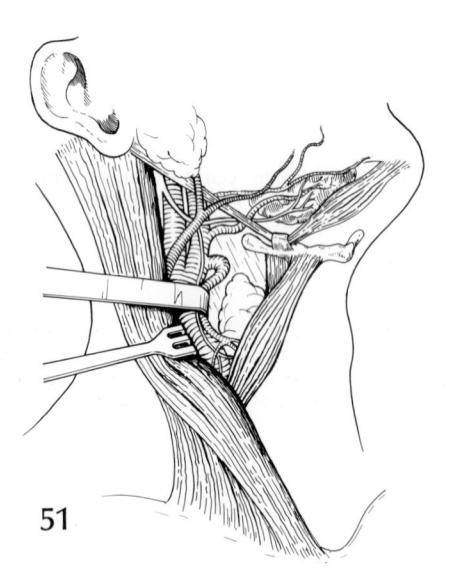

51

A right oblique incision is made at the C3–4 level. Platysma is incised in the line of the skin incision. Vessels are retracted laterally and the prevertebral fascia is exposed. The superior thyroid artery and vein are retracted inferiorly and the hypoglossal nerve superiorly.

Spinal injuries 643

52a & b

The inferior margin of the C2 vertebral body is confirmed by the image intensifier. A K-wire is inserted using a drill across the fracture site.

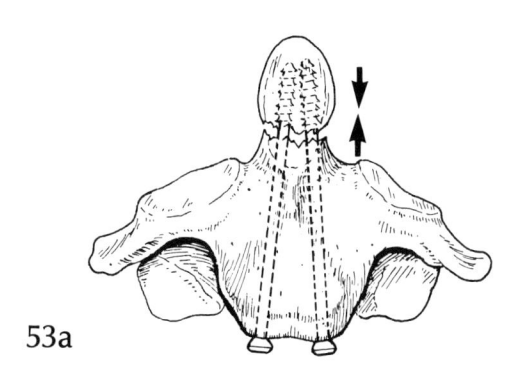

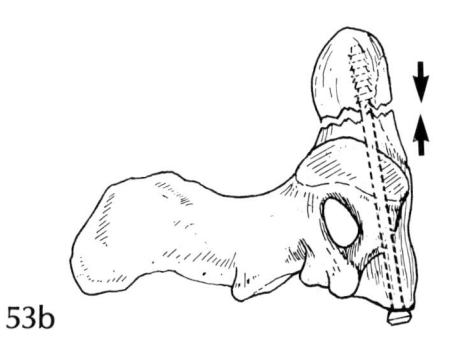

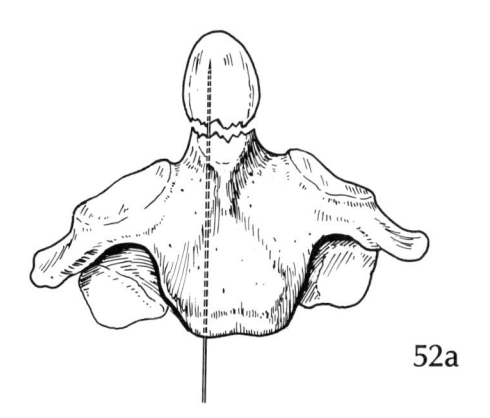

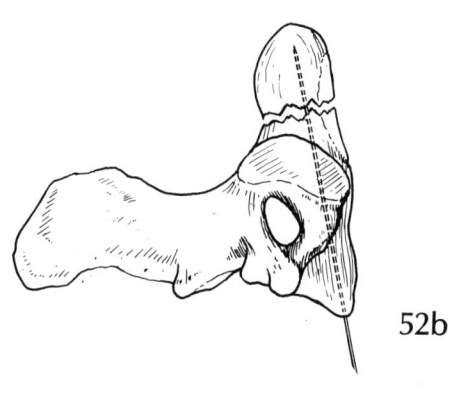

52a

52b

53a

53b

53a & b

Two AO 4.5 mm cancellous screws are inserted after pre-drilling with a 2.0 mm drill just past the fracture site.
   External immobilization is necessary for 3 months using either a halo or moulded Philadelphia collar.

644 Thoracic and lumbar spine

SPINAL FUSION OF GALLIE TYPE

Indications

1. Ununited fracture of the dens
2. Subluxations of the atlanto-axial joint.

The type of person must be carefully assessed; those at great risk need to be particularly considered. The pathology is multifactorial.

Method

54 & 55

A midline incision is made from the occiput to C5. Incised skin and deep fascia are tough and need sharp dissection. The incision is made in the midline between the trapezii and the right and left splenius capitis to expose the spinous processes. Muscle is dissected off the spinous processes with a sharp cutting and coagulating diathermy. Careful haemostasis is essential.

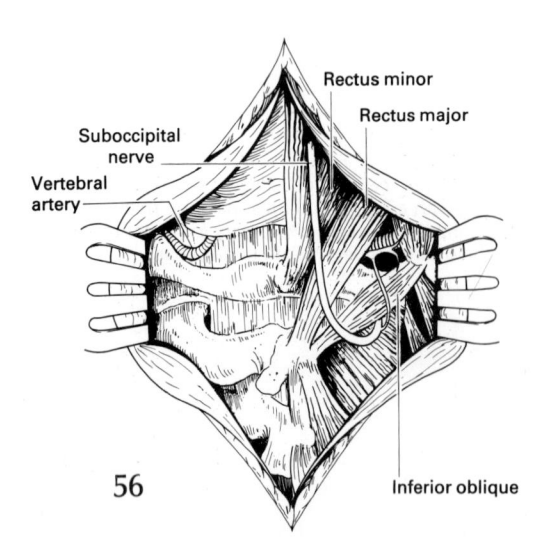

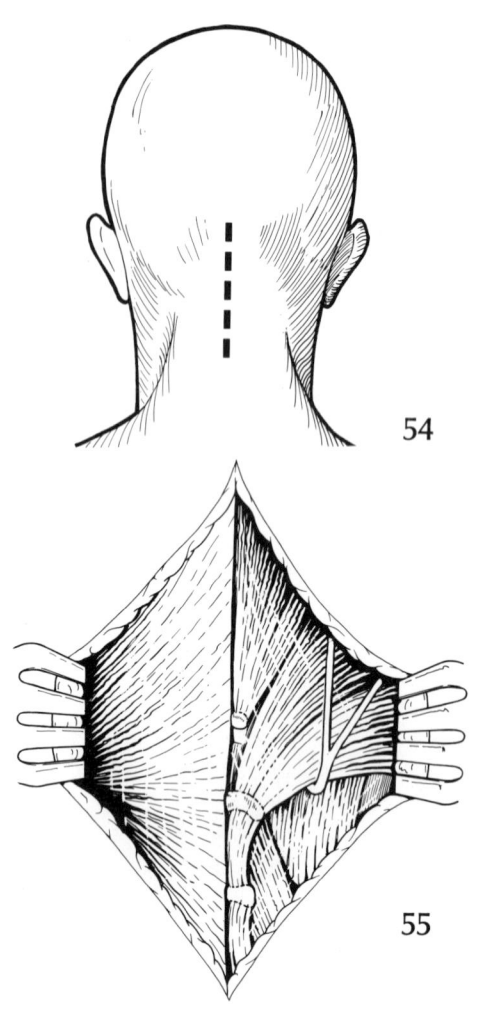

56

The laminae of C1, C2, C3 and the occiput are cleared by subperiosteal dissection. Using a Cobb elevator sharp dissection is carried laterally at each level. The surgeon should watch for venous bleeding laterally.

The muscle masses are retracted using Gelpis' retractors first, and, as dissection proceeds, a laminectomy retractor.

The arch of the atlas is exposed.

With great care subperiosteal dissection is carried laterally. The vertebral artery at the junction of the lateral one-third and medial two-thirds should be carefully avoided. Wide lateral dissection of the laminae of C1, C2 and C3 will thus be obtained. The venous channels are sealed off with cautery, gauze swabs or felt squares. Decortication of the laminae can be effected using nibblers and Capener chisels. Nibbler exposure of the cancellous bone in the C1 laminae can be performed gently.

Spinal injuries 645

57

The graft is removed from the ilium and cut in the shape of an inverted 'U' to fit the laminae of C1 and spinous processes of C2.

A long skin incision is made vertical to and deepening to the iliac crest. The bony–fascial incision is then made at right angles.

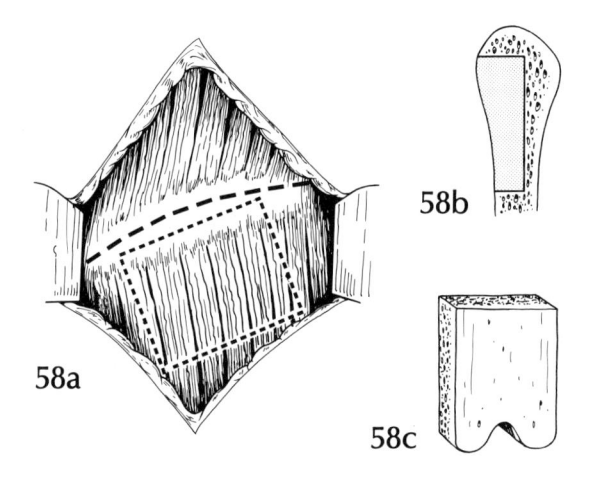

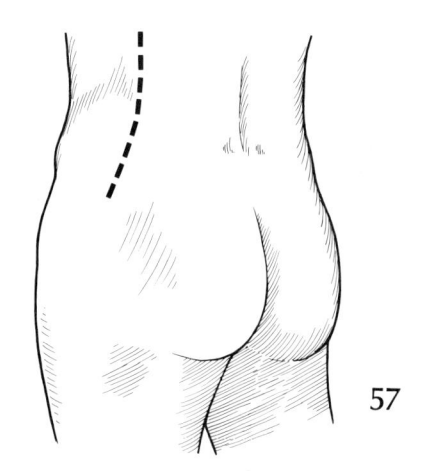

57

58a, b & c

The gluteal muscles are cleared from the iliac wing by subperiosteal dissection.

Using adequate retraction, a quadrilateral area of about 5 cm in diameter is marked out and then the outer table only is removed, using sharp chisel dissection. This gives a graft about 1 cm thick, curved in the line that will take the cervical spine and can then be cut into the inverted 'U'.

58a
58b
58c

59

Suitable curved dissectors (McCormack and aneurysm dissectors) between the dura and laminae are used to pass a wire loop under the arch of C1 and C2.

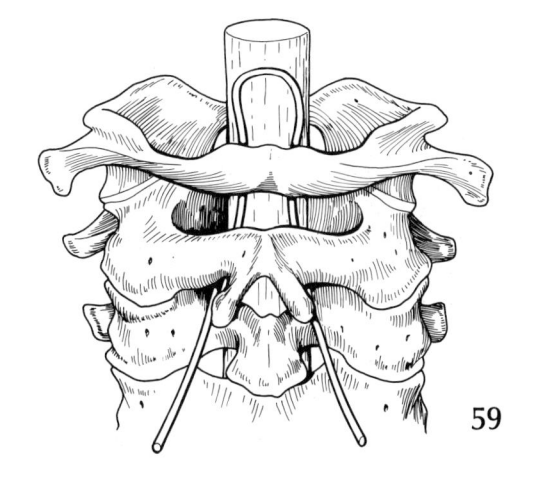

59

646 Thoracic and lumbar spine

60a, b & c

The graft is placed, cancellous surface down, onto the laminae after a cancellous bed has been prepared and laid well laterally. If a laminectomy has been performed at C1 then the graft is placed more lateral on both sides and fixation of C1–2 is achieved by screws across the C1–2 facet joints. The AO malleolar screw is inserted through the lamina of C2 and directed laterally and cranially across the joints.

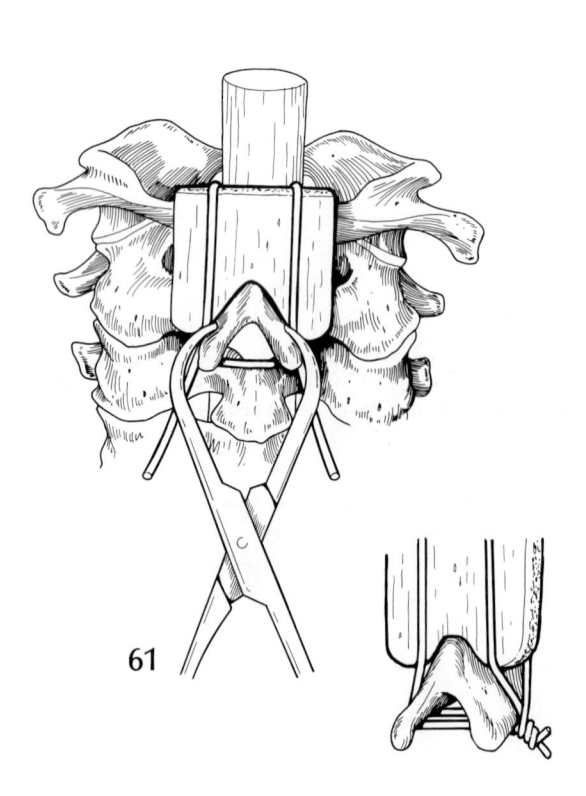

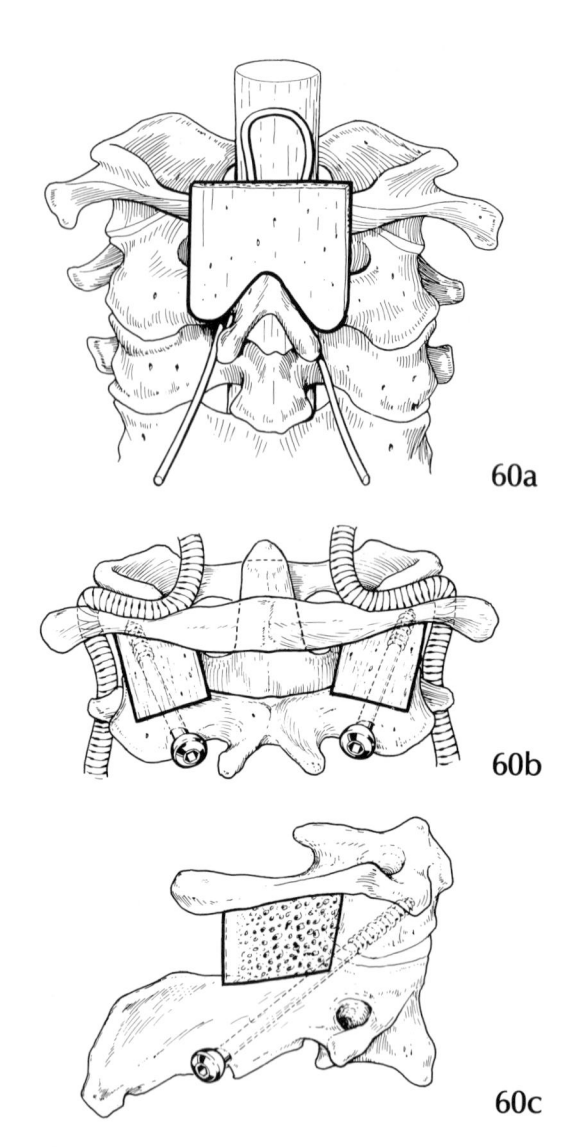

60a

60b

60c

61

The wires are tightened to fix the graft securely in position.
 The wound is closed in layers, sewing the splenius muscles together, the trapezius muscles together, the subcutaneous fascia and the skin using drainage.

Postoperative management

The patient sits up in bed as soon after the operation as possible. Traction is discontinued if used prior to operation; a polythene collar is applied postoperatively and an immediate soft collar is usually used for support.
 Fusion usually takes about 3 months.

THORACOLUMBAR SPINE

Fracture-dislocation with locked facets with or without paraplegia

CLOSED REDUCTION

Indications

1. Failure of postural reduction
2. When open reduction is contraindicated by infection, multiple injuries, other complications such as pulmonary, or psychological or religious reasons
3. Before open reduction.

Reduction under general anaesthesia

62

The patient is placed supine with relaxation ensuring that the fracture site is at the break in the table so that the spine can be flexed or extended.

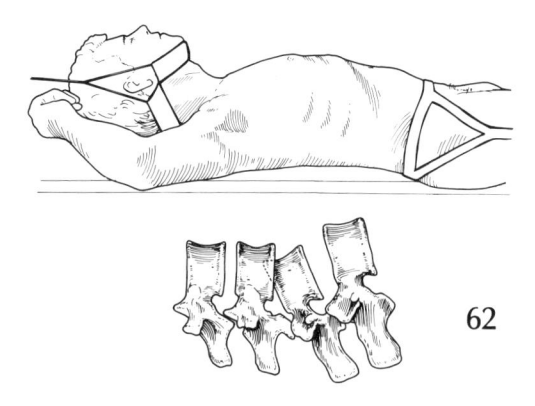

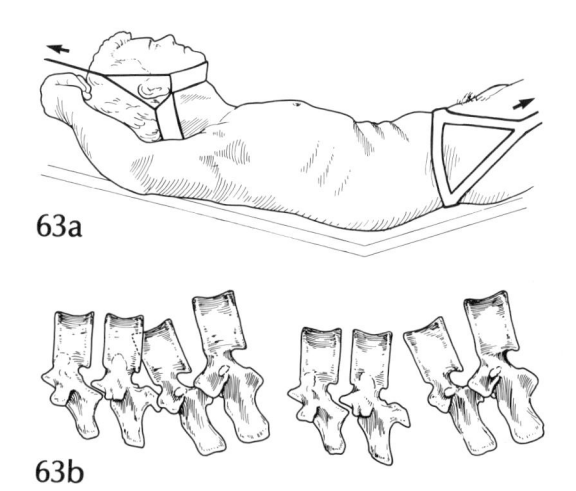

63a & b

Traction is applied manually and usually *via* a harness to the head or thorax and pelvis to distract the fracture in the flexed position by 'breaking' the table.

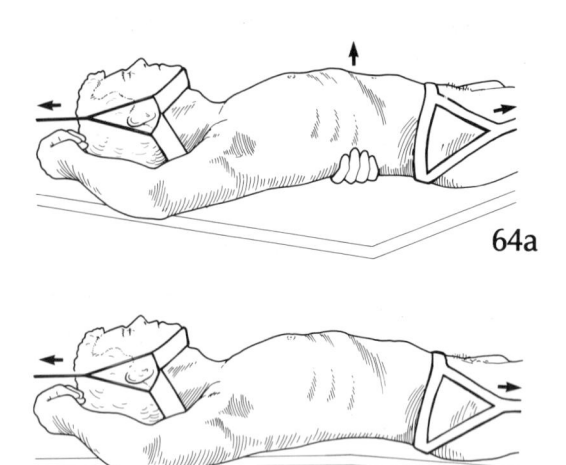

648 Thoracic and lumbar spine

64a, b & c

Traction is applied continuously while the operator exerts a forward thrust to the prominent spinous process, thus lifting (patient supine) the thoracolumbar spine into lordosis. The lumbar column below the fracture-dislocation can usually be felt to move forward and be locked by the anterior longitudinal ligament which is rarely injured. Reduction can be checked by a lateral X-ray at this point.

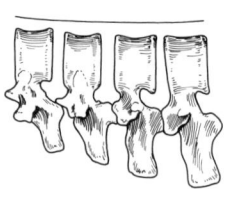

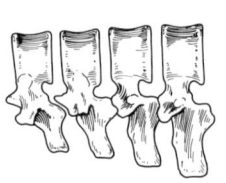

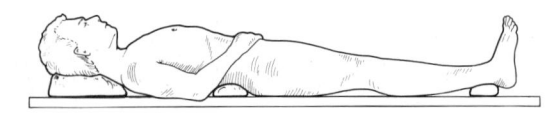

65a & b

Traction and extension are maintained. The table is reversed, a gallbladder rest is raised under a pillow to give hyperextension, thus 'fixing' the intact anterior longitudinal ligament. Traction is released but postural reduction is maintained.

The X-ray is checked. The above process is repeated if necessary, and the patient is allowed to recover from relaxant anaesthesia so that the muscle tone assists.

The patient is taken off the operating table by a sliding method onto a rigid surface to hold reduction. The rigid surface is removed in the ward when the patient is fully conscious.

Postural reduction is maintained.

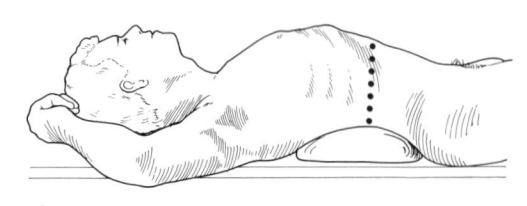

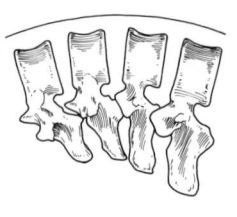

OPEN REDUCTION AND INTERNAL FIXATION

Indications

1. Deformity, e.g. kyphosis greater than 35°, kyphoscoliosis, lateral shift, lateral flexion injuries with pars interarticularis fracture
2. Bilateral locked facets
3. Central nervous system deterioration. Intracanal fragments associated with cleft cleavage injuries will resorb gradually over 1–2 years and are not regularly an indication for immediate surgery. However, in incomplete neural lesions where neurological recovery has plateaued and the fragments occupy more than 30 per cent of the canal, it is worthwhile considering removal of these fragments, particularly if the spinal canal is of small dimensions.

Contraindications

1. Local skin infection
2. Medical complications.

Relative contraindications are:

1. Age
2. Complete neural lesion without significant displacement or deformity.

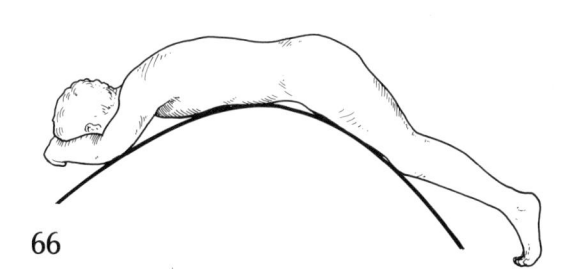

66

Procedure

X-rays and a CT scan should be available.

Partial postural reduction is maintained while the patient is taken to the operating theatre and anaesthetized with general anaesthesia.

The patient is turned with a 'log roll' by staff and placed carefully on a suitable frame to prevent abdominal compression. This will usually flex the spine at the fracture site, but will not reproduce the original deformity at the time of the accident. Adjustable frames are preferred to allow the spine to be extended.

650 Thoracic and lumbar spine

Exposure

67a & b

A midline incision is made centred over the site of the fracture-dislocation, extending two or three segments above and below the fracture site. The fascia is then carefully cleared of soft tissue (except muscle) by cutting and coagulation diathermy: the muscle from the spinous processes and laminae are cleared with a Cobb elevator.

It is usual for the erector spinae muscles to have been stripped and lacerated by the accident.

Retractors are inserted. The extent of laminar clearance depends on the type of fixation to be used. *Instrumentation over as few segments as possible is advisable depending on the mechanism of the vertebral body fracture.*

The dislocated locked facets, if present, will be thus exposed.

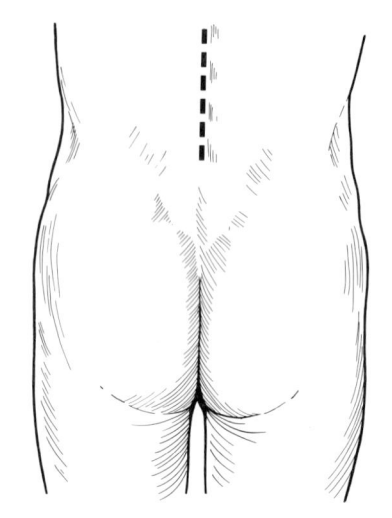

67a

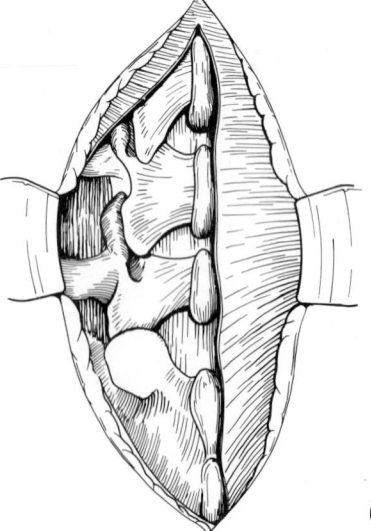

67b

Spinal injuries 651

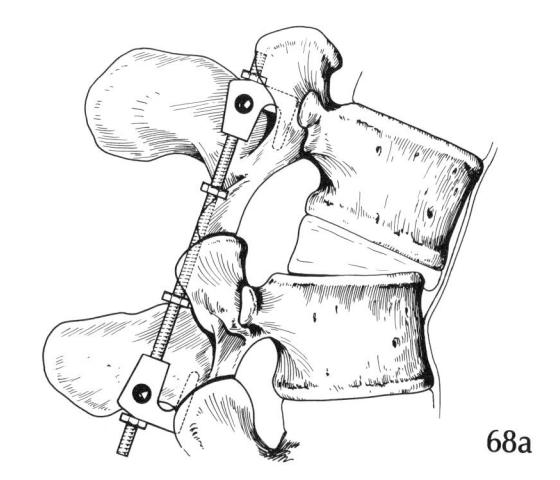

Reduction of dislocation

68a, b & 69

Using the intact spinous processes and suitable bone-holding forceps, the dislocation is reduced first by caudocephalic traction and then by suitably lifting the upper over the lower facet. If this is not possible, laminotomy and partial removal of the superior facet will help. Harrington compression clamps are applied to the laminae above and below the dislocation and are gradually tightened (by a tension band) until dislocation is reduced. Alternatively, a plate or Hartshill rectangle can be used to stabilize the dislocation.

Indications for surgery (compression fractures)

1. Deteriorating neurology
2. Severe compression anteriorly with height loss of more than half a vertebra
3. Intracanal fragments encroaching on greater than one-third of canal diameter in the cervical or thoracic region and half or more in the lumbar region in incomplete neural lesions.

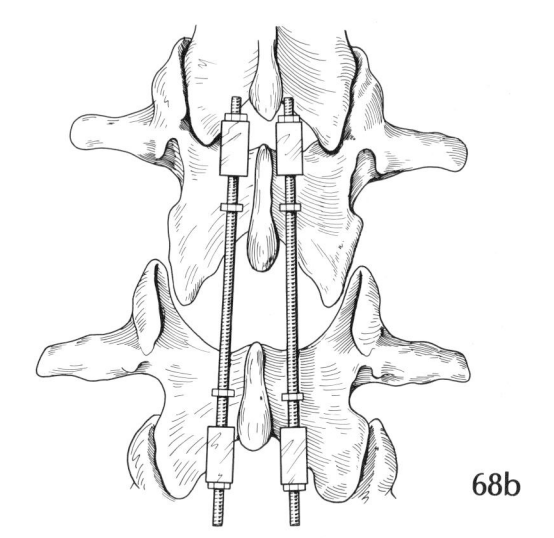

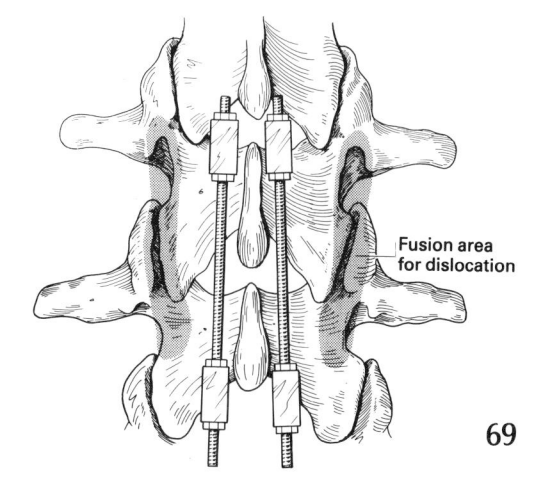

Cleft cleavage fractures

70

Intracanal fragments may displace and cause increased neural compression during reduction of compression fractures. These are therefore visualized using a hemilaminotomy if necessary or, in the unusual case where this is not possible, intraoperative ultrasound or myelography can be used. Care should be taken with intracanal fragments that have rotated through 180° as these can displace during the reduction if the posterior longitudinal ligament is torn.

The method of fixation will depend on the type and site of fracture. Short segment fixations are preferred. Multisegment stabilizations using distraction rods or spinal plates are used when there is significant kyphosis or scoliosis. Spinal fusion should be limited to less than two movement segments.

Fractures with considerable intracanal involvement can be managed by the anterior approach initially and certain fractures may require a combined approach.

It should be remembered, however, that such fractures may be treated regularly by conservative methods as the intracanal fragment can be naturally absorbed if the posterior longitudinal ligament is intact. The posterior longitudinal ligament is likely to be torn if there is more than 50 per cent intracanal involvement or the fragment is abnormally rotated[2].

Application of distraction rods and sublaminar wires

71a–d

The upper hook site is prepared by exposing the facet joint two levels above the fracture site. The capsule is removed and a small piece of the inferior facet is removed. Bifid upper hooks allow better control of rotation and are preferred.

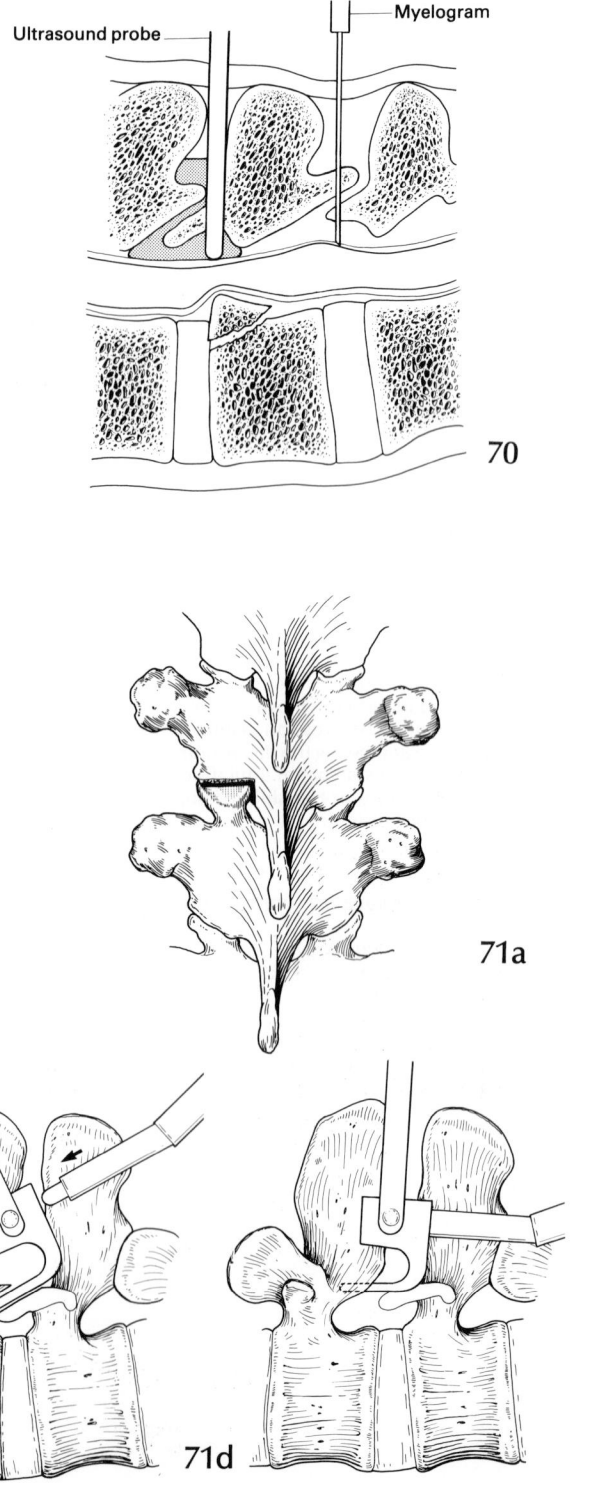

Spinal injuries 653

72a & b

The lower hook site is prepared by removing lamina from the lamina two segments below the fracture. Care should be taken not to remove bone from the pars interarticularis as this may fracture when distraction is applied. It may be necessary to remove bone from the inferior aspect of the lamina above to allow entry of the hook into the spinal canal. Long flanged hooks or square-holed hooks are preferred.

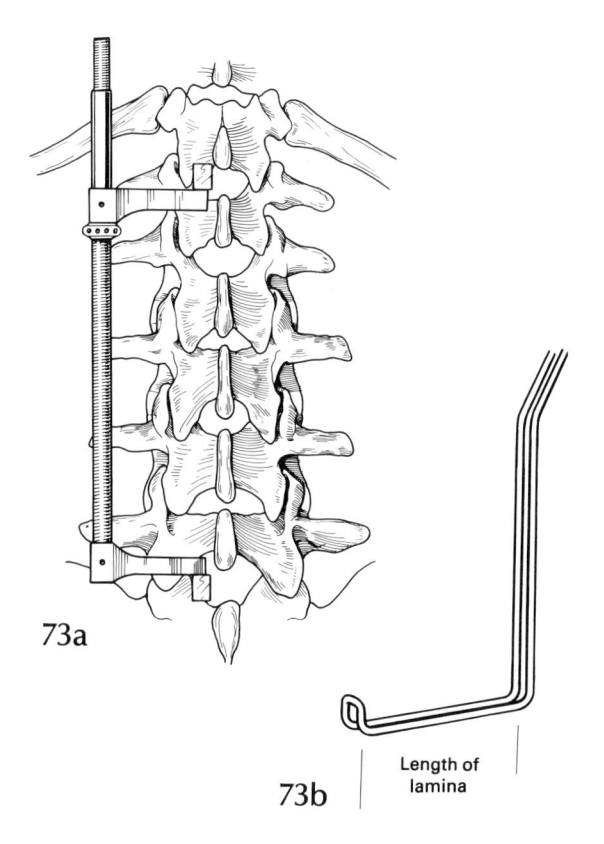

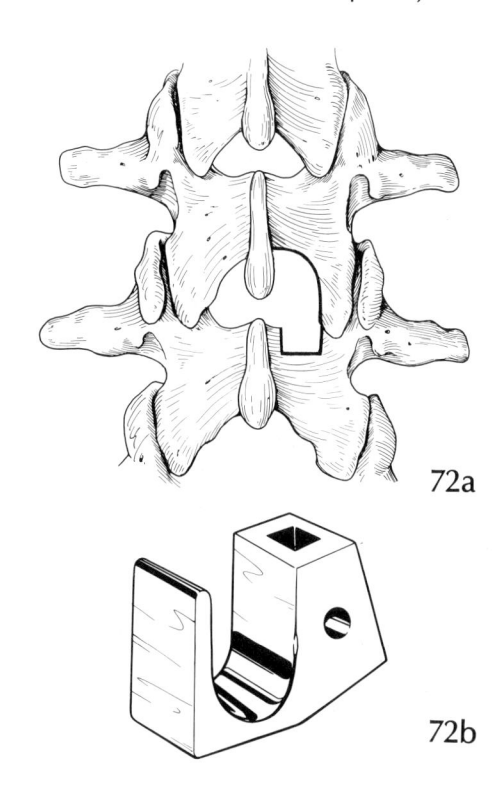

72a

72b

73a & b

The ligamentum flavum is removed at each level and sublaminar wires are passed around the intact lamina. An outrigger is inserted and reduction of the fracture performed.

73a

73b   Length of lamina

74a & b

A Moe rod of appropriate size is pre-bent into a small amount of lordosis or kyphosis, depending on the region. The rod is inserted through the upper hook and then, using a rod pusher or sequestrum forceps, the rod is manipulated into the lower hook while it is held with hook holders. It is sometimes necessary to remove some lamina from the dorsal aspect of the adjacent cranial vertebrae to allow the pre-bent rod to enter the lower hook. Sublaminar wires are then used to help fixation.

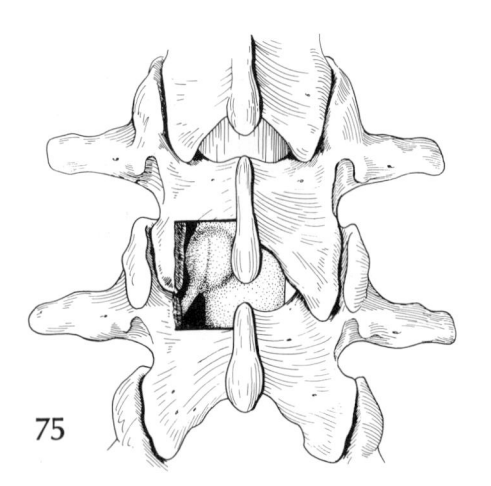

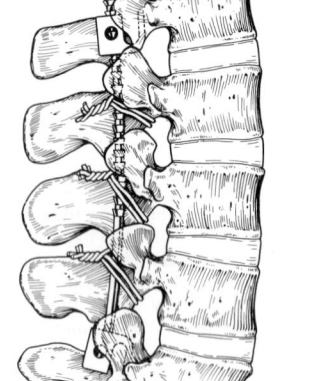

75

Distraction is applied and the spinal canal inspected by direct vision, ultrasound or intraoperative myelography to confirm reduction of the intracanal fragment. The outrigger is removed.

The spinal cord should not be retracted when visualizing intracanal fragments.

76

A second distraction rod is inserted or, in cases of kyphoscoliosis, a short segment compression system can be applied to the convex side. The sublaminar wires are tightened. *Sublaminar wires are not used around compression systems as the hooks may protrude into the spinal canal.* Postoperative external supports are not necessary. The rods are routinely removed 12 months after surgery.

It may be better in cases of severe compression fractures at this stage to replace the bone rods with a short segment system (Harrington compression clamps, spinal plate or Hartshill rectangle) to supplement the fusion area to prevent late kyphosis which can occur after removal of the implants.

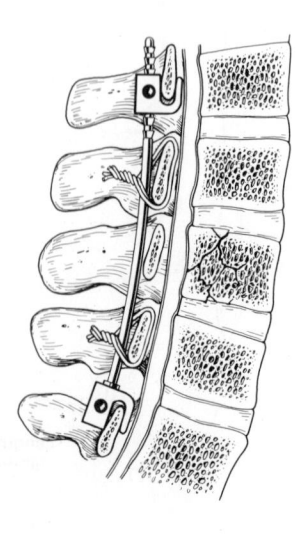

AO internal fixators

77

The apophyseal joints are exposed one segment above and below the fracture. K-wires are inserted into the pedicles at a point 1 mm below and lateral to the apophyseal joint. The pedicle lies directly medial to the transverse process and is an excellent landmark. The K-wires should converge towards the midline by 10° in the lower thoracic spine and 15° in the lumbar spine. The image intensifier is used to confirm that the wires are within the pedicle. It should be remembered that the exiting nerve root at each intervertebral segment is directly below the pedicle.

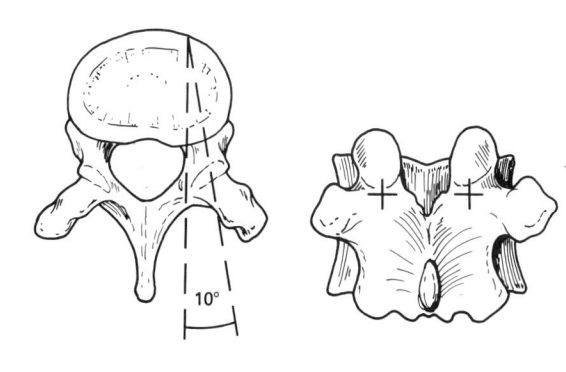

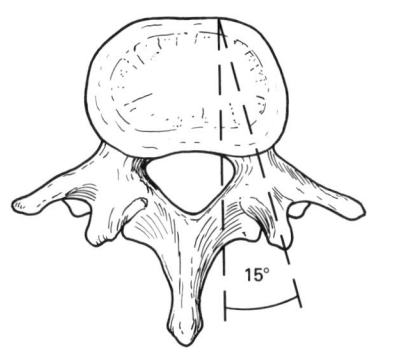

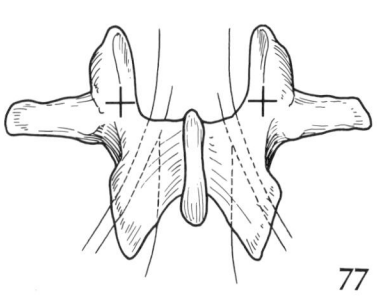

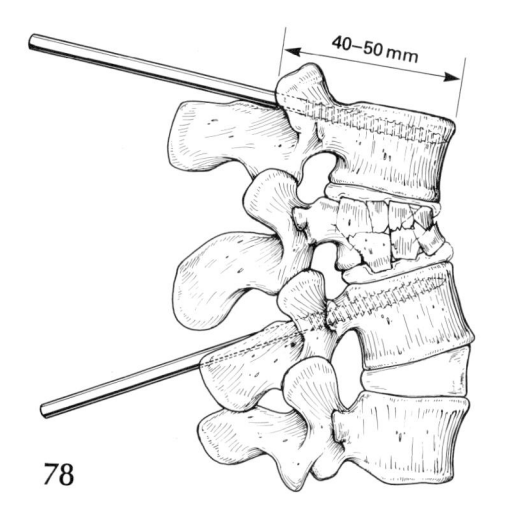

78

A 3.5 mm drill is used to breach the posterior cortex only. The Schanz screws are then inserted using the contralateral K-wire as a guide to a distance of about 40 mm.

The Schanz screws are advanced towards the anterior cortex of the vertebral body using the image intensifier. The screws are inserted to a distance of approximately 40–50 mm.

656 Thoracic and lumbar spine

79a & b
Sacral screws are inserted through the middle of the base of the sacral facet and angled downwards and outwards for a distance of 30 mm.

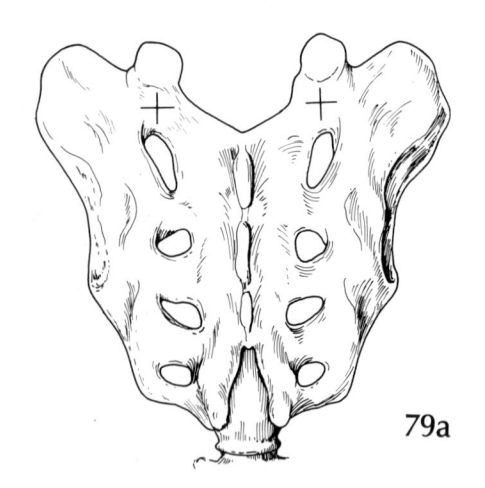

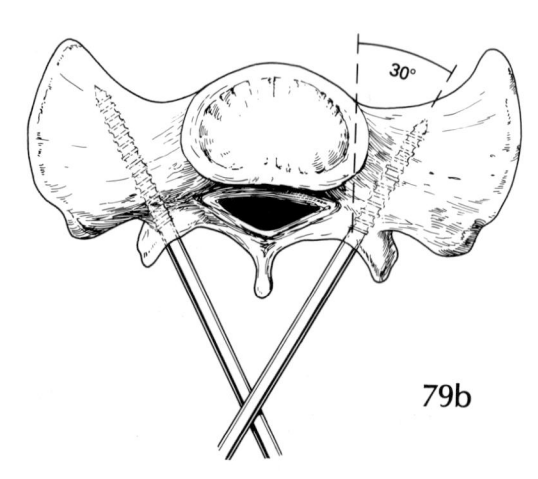

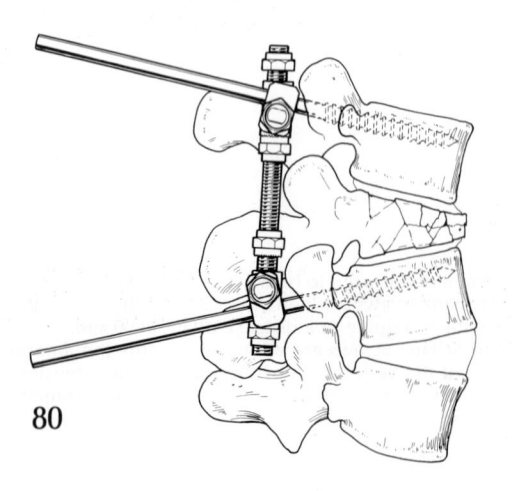

79a

79b

80
Reduction is achieved by manipulating the Schanz screws. The rods are placed over the Schanz screws with the nuts loosened on the medial side of the pins. The toothed clamps must interlock with the washer. Care should be taken if there is a fracture of the posterior vertebral body. To prevent further posterior displacement of such fragments, the nuts must be placed on the clamps as shown.

80

81

The kyphosis and/or scoliosis is corrected by approximating the posterior ends of the Schanz screws. To apply a greater compressive force during reduction, a cerclage wire is tightened around the dorsal ends of the Schanz screws to provide a longer lever arm. Distraction or compression of the vertebral body can be performed by loosening one nut and tightening its counterpart so the Schanz screws move downwards or away from each other depending what force is necessary. With compression injuries the more cranial and caudal nuts are loosened and the two middle nuts tightened to apply distraction.

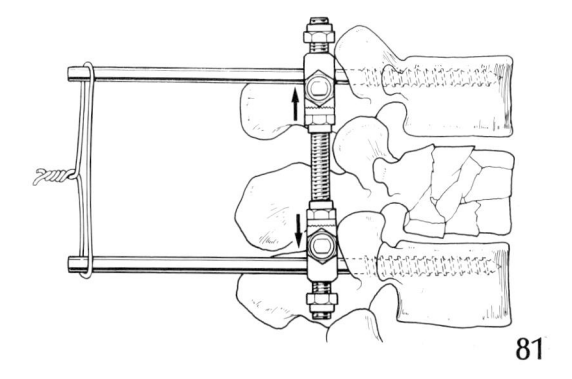

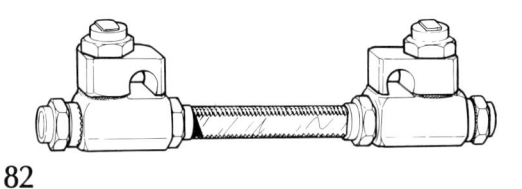

81

82

82

The Schanz screws are secured by tightening the lateral nuts and the wire is removed.

83

The final compression of the nut collar is achieved by tightening the inferior nut on the cranial Schanz screw and the superior nut on the caudal Schanz screw. The counter nuts are then tightened.

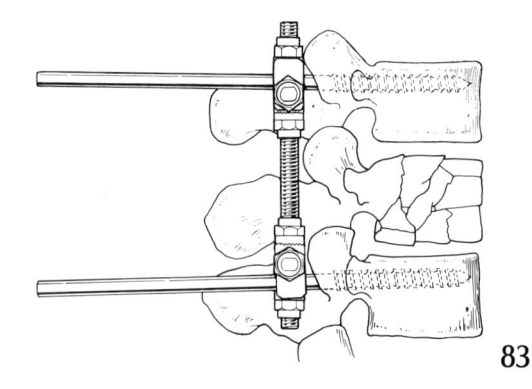

83

84

The rods can be further stabilized by twisting two diagonally crossed cerclage wires around the ends of the fixator to help control lateral forces. This provides a closed system.

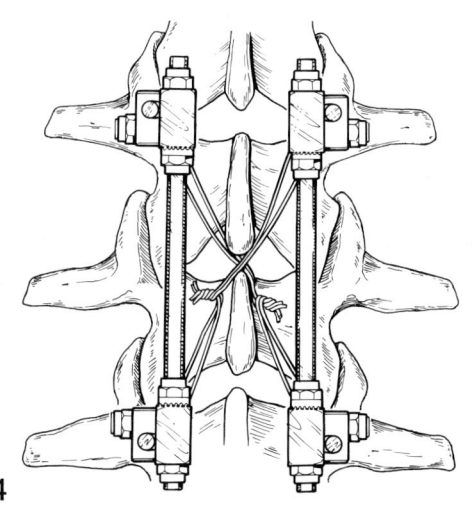

84

85

Bone grafting of major defects in the vertebral body is recommended. A 6 mm hole is drilled into one or both pedicles of the fractured vertebra. In cases where the pedicle is mobile, it can be retracted laterally, although it may be necessary to remove the medial aspect at its base and to allow access to the vertebral body. As much bone graft as possible is inserted into the vertebral bone. Autogenous corticocancellous bone from the iliac crest is recommended.

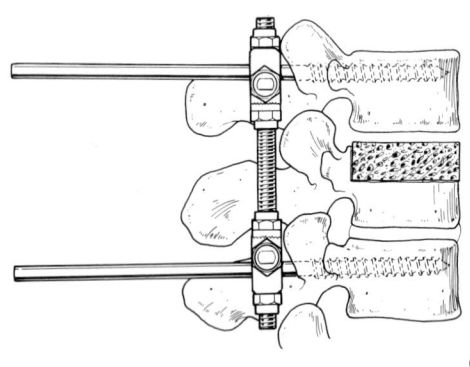

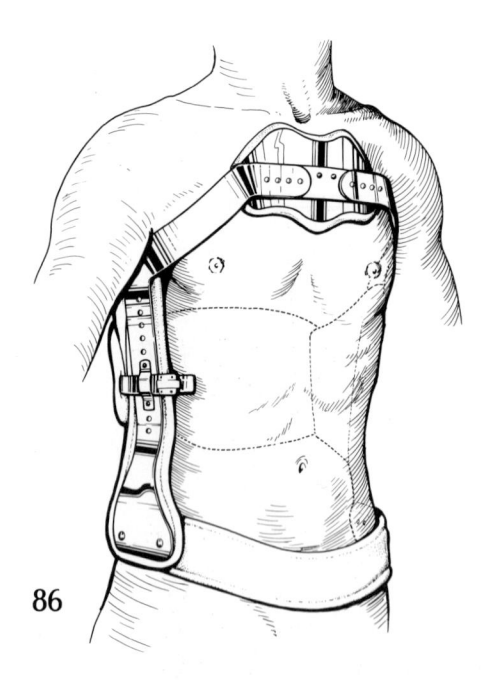

86

Mobilization can begin within the first week using a Jewett-type brace, depending on the neural status. Protection with this brace is for 6 to 12 weeks depending on the nature of the injury. The implant is removed 12–18 months after surgery.

Spinal injuries 659

Spinal plates

87a, b & c

Spinal plates provide good stability and can be used for short-segment stabilization where there is dislocation without significant vertebral compression, or for long stabilization between two or three segments above and below the vertebral fracture. The technique of insertion of the pedicle screws is the same as the Schanz screws, except they only need to enter the vertebral body and do not need to be advanced as far anteriorly. If a long segment fixation is used, the plates should be bent to allow a small degree of lordosis.

Roy Camille plates allow up to two screws to be inserted in any one pedicle if it is large enough.

When a scoliosis is present, the screws are tightened segmentally on the convex side first. Local posterolateral fusion is performed over no more than two segments. Spinal plates can be removed 12–18 months after insertion.

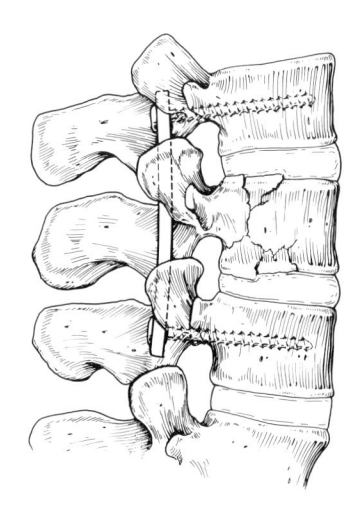

87a

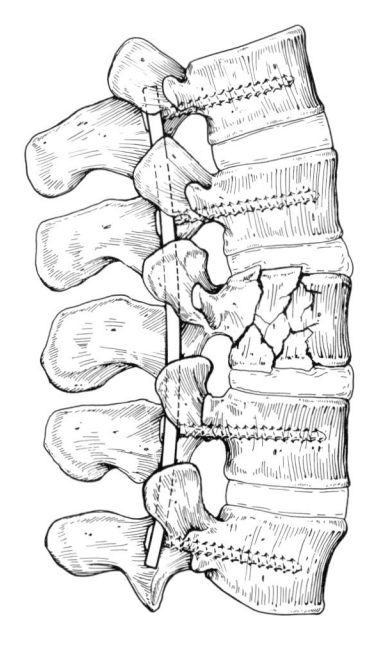

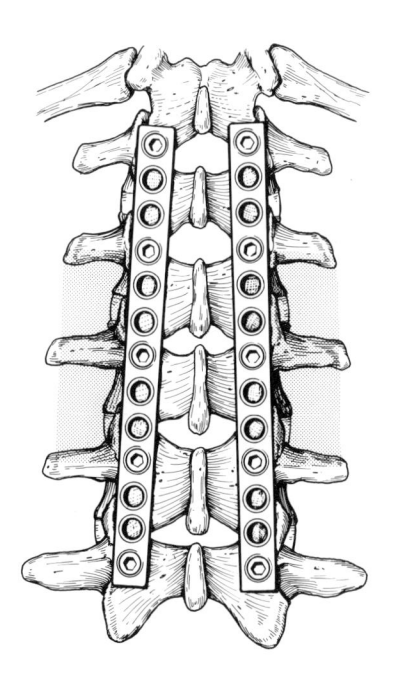

87b

87c

POSTERIOR FUSION

88a

Dislocation without anterior wedging requires only an interfacet fusion by denuding the articular cartilage on the surface of the facet joint.

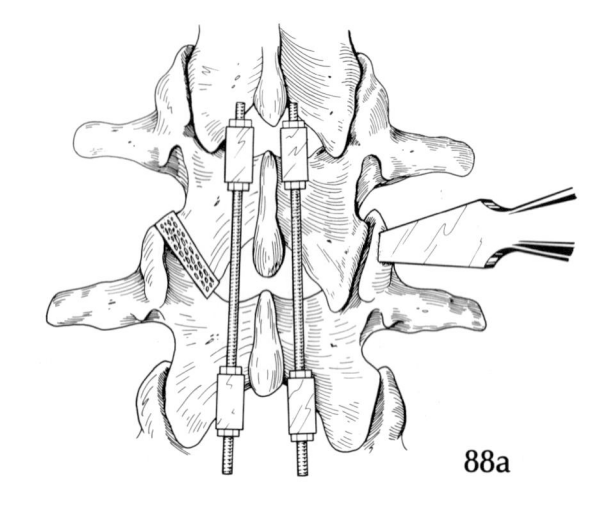

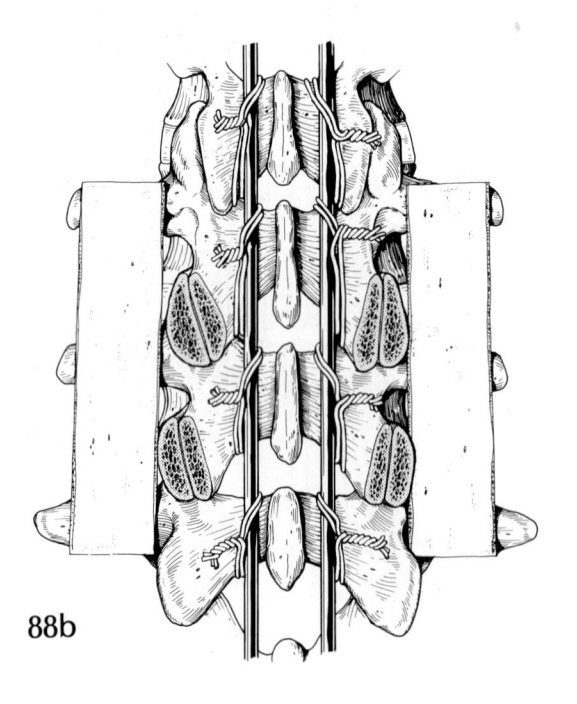

88b

When there is considerable vertebral body wedging, the fusion should be posterolateral using either an intertransverse process or Moe-type fusion. Only two intervertebral levels need to be fused. The resultant disability from multilevel fusion is not warranted, and the small residual kyphosis or loss of correction, occurring with short-segment stabilization, that may occur after removal of the implant causes little disability. Bone graft can be taken from the spinous processes, lamina or iliac crest. Bank bone or Ceros 80/82 are satisfactory alternatives.

Hartshill rectangle

89

A closed spinal rod system can be a good method of segmental fixation. The Hartshill rectangle (Surgicraft Hartshill, Redditch, UK) must be pre-bent into lordosis to allow reduction of compressive fractures, and fixation should be two to three segments above and two segments below the level of the fracture. For dislocation without vertebral body comminution, only one level above and one below will need to be stabilized.

The length of the rectangle should be from the top half of the lamina of the cranial level to the lower half of the caudal lamina to be instrumented.

The Hartshill bridge can be put over the rectangle to provide partial screw stabilization where the lamina is deformed. The bridge can be moved up or down the rectangle so that the lateral hole lies directly over the pedicle.

It is important that the upper and lower sublaminar wires are secured into the corners of the rectangle adjacent to the roof. The 20 gauge (UK) wires are turned in a clockwise direction and tightened until there is no movement with normal pressure in a caudal–cranial direction between the wires and the rectangle. Then the knot is cut at least four turns from the rectangle and embedded by turning in a clockwise direction. The sharp ends are then carefully punched so that no sharp ends are palpable.

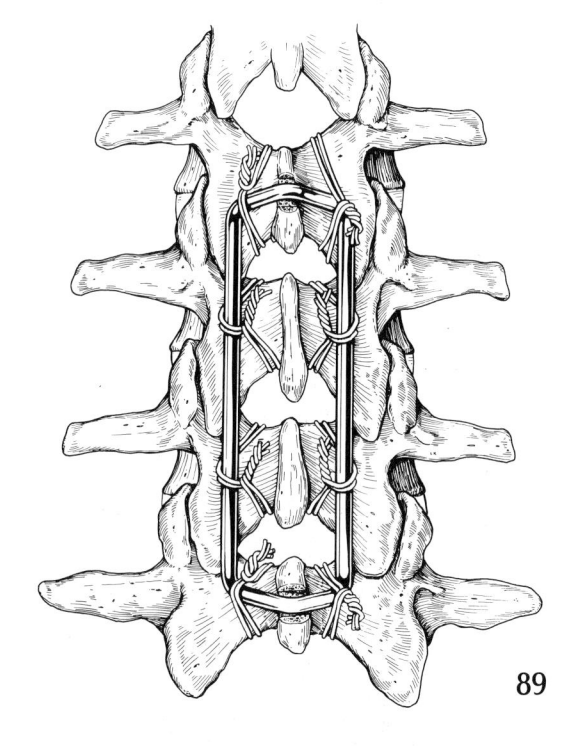

Kyphotic deformities and intracanal fragments

ANTERIOR DECOMPRESSION AND FIXATION

Indications

1. Correction of late kyphotic deformities
2. Intracanal fragments occupying greater than 30 per cent of the spine in the cervical and thoracic region and 50 per cent in the lumbar spine in the presence of incomplete paralysis
3. Traumatic incomplete paraplegia which has plateaued in its recovery with the presence of intracanal fragments
4. Pathological fractures.

Thoracic approach

90a & b

This entails a thoracotomy using the usual techniques (see 'Anterior procedures for spinal deformity' pp. 504–511). The rib can be removed for bone graft or osteotomized to improve access. The approach is made in line with the rib two segments above the kyphotic vertebrae. In cases of severe kyphosis it may be necessary to use the rib three segments above, particularly if the angle of the ribs is increased in the horizontal plane. Dividing the diaphragm 1 cm from its insertion into the rib and extending the incision down onto the rectus allows excellent access to the upper lumbar spine (thoracoabdominal approach).

The transverse process and the rib head are identified, the latter being removed if necessary. The vertebral body is cleared of soft tissue and the segmental vessels are divided at about the mid-vertebral level.

91 & 92

The nerve root is retracted but is then used as a guide to follow into the neural canal. The pedicle may be removed and the dura is thus exposed from the lateral side.

The posterior two-thirds of the vertebral body is then excised using chisel cuts, maintaining the posterior cortex and the posterior longitudinal ligament. A powered diamond drill can be used to help removal of bone. The anterior third of the body is preserved to provide a blood supply for the graft. If kyphosis is being corrected in the late stage, division of the anterior longitudinal ligament and even anterior bone resection may be necessary.

After the vertebral body has been removed, the vertebral cortex and posterior longitudinal ligament remain intact. It is then possible to remove the bone at the apex of the curve, opening the extradural space through the posterior longitudinal ligament if necessary.

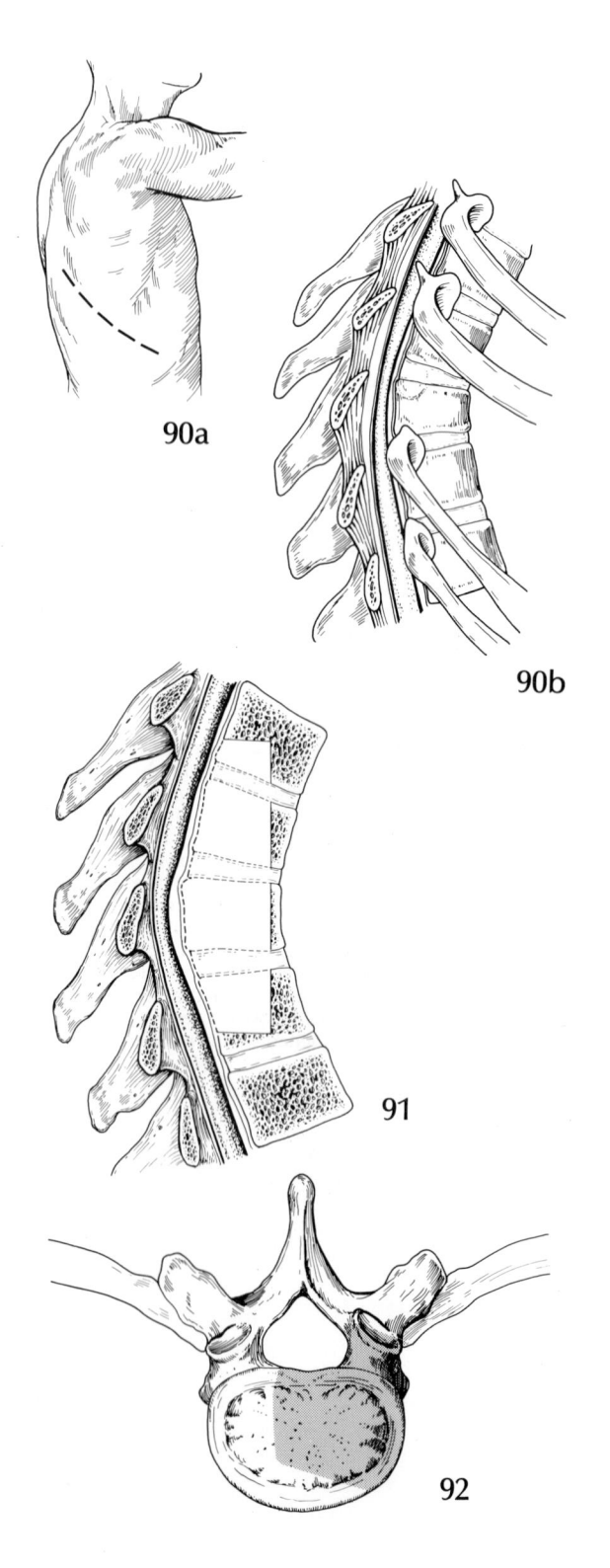

Spinal injuries 663

93

The surgeon continues cranially or caudally until the whole of the hump has been removed or, in the case of an intracanal fragment, the restoration of the spinal canal. It is important to move right across the midline to the opposite side and to ensure that all of the posterior vertebral body is thus excised. The cord will move forward.

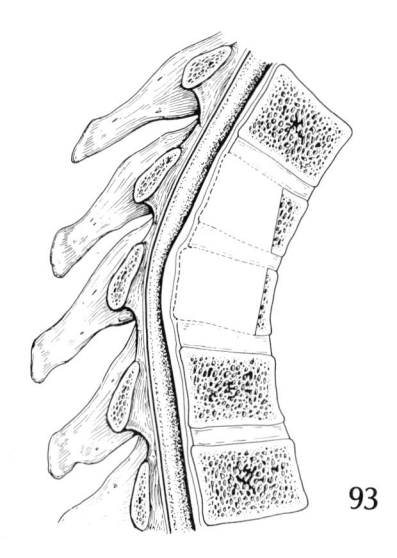

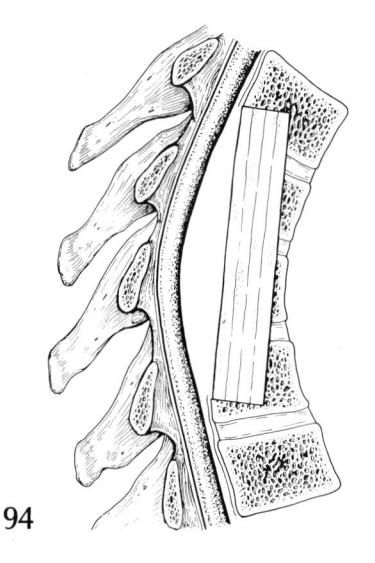

94

Autogenous corticocancellous graft can be obtained by removing a tricortical block of no more than 2 cm in width from the iliac crest to fit the defect. The cranial side of the rib can be cut out and used to form an osteoblastic reconstruction of the iliac crest defect.

The bone removed during vertebrectomy is replaced. The fibula, bank bone or bone graft substitute (ceramic or stainless steel) may also be used.

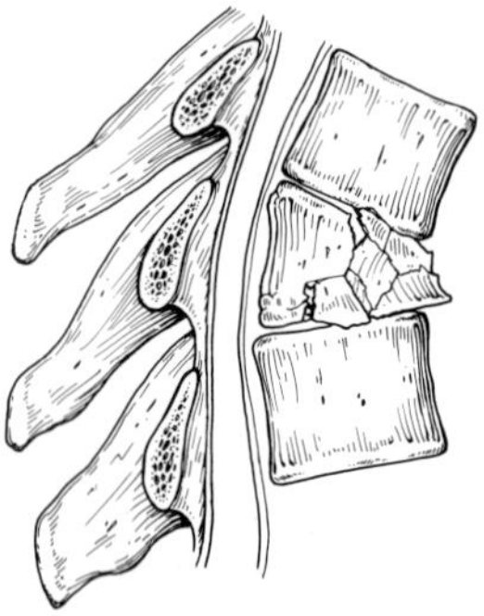

664 Thoracic and lumbar spine

CORRECTION OF KYPHOSIS

95a–d

Modified Dwyer screws (Kostuik[3]) of appropriate length are inserted as close to the vertebral end-plate as possible and a Harrington rod inserted with distraction. Graft from either the iliac crest or rib is inserted. A Hall rod is then inserted posterior to the Harrington rod. It is fixed by Dwyer screws which are crimpled after the rod has been inserted.

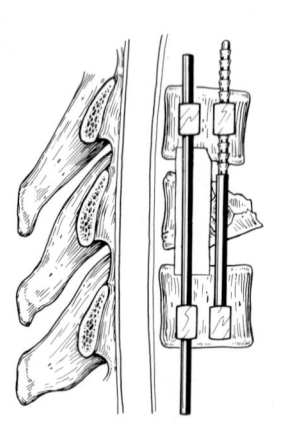

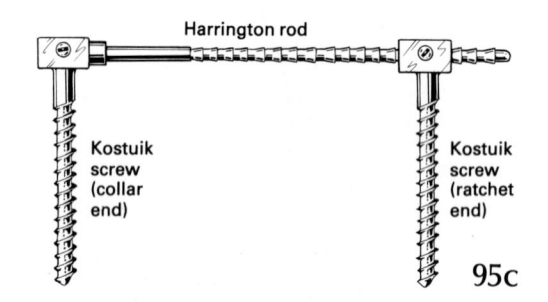

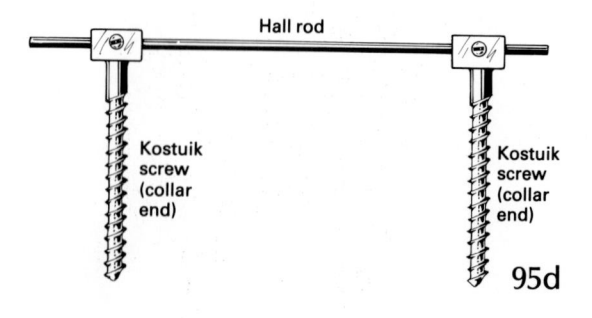

Spinal injuries 665

96a & b

The author has used the Dunn[4] device which also provides a system for stabilization of anterior defects. It consists of two rods linked by vertebral body bridges. The bridges are fixed to each vertebral body by a screw and a staple. They must be used on the right-hand side of the spine and can be used from the mid-thoracic level to L4. If the vena cava is in direct contact with the implant, a 6 cm Teflon felt pad is placed between the implant and the vessels.

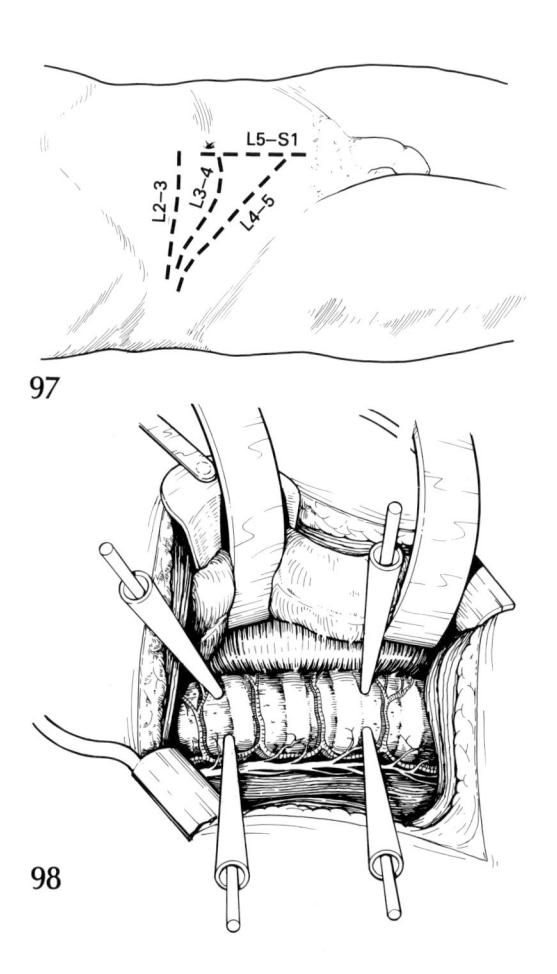

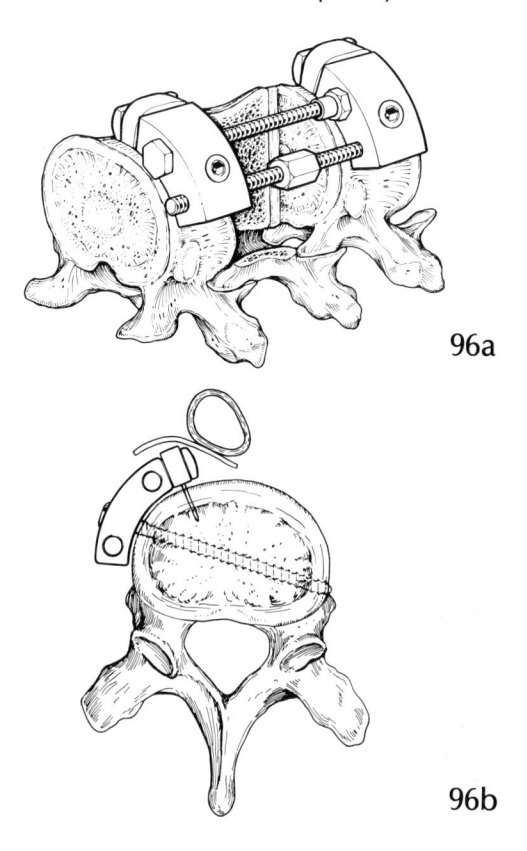

96a

96b

97

Lumbar approach

97 & 98

A lumbar incision as for a nephrectomy is used, exposing the spine by sweeping the peritoneal structures towards the medial side, making certain that the ureter is swept forwards. The disc spaces of L2–3 to L5–S1 can be exposed.

98

666 Thoracic and lumbar spine

99a & b

At the thoracolumbar junction, a more extensive approach (thoracoabdominal) is usually used along the tenth or eleventh rib and extending into the rectus abdominis. The retroperitoneal space is entered by carefully incising the costal cartilage in the line of the skin incision. L2 can be exposed by a subdiaphragmatic approach along the twelfth rib. It is necessary to divide both crura just proximal to their insertion to allow adequate retraction of the vessels. Steinmann pins with plastic covers are inserted into the vertebral bodies to provide retraction of major vessels, psoas muscle and sympathetic chain. L3 and L4 are best approached by a standard retroperitoneal approach.

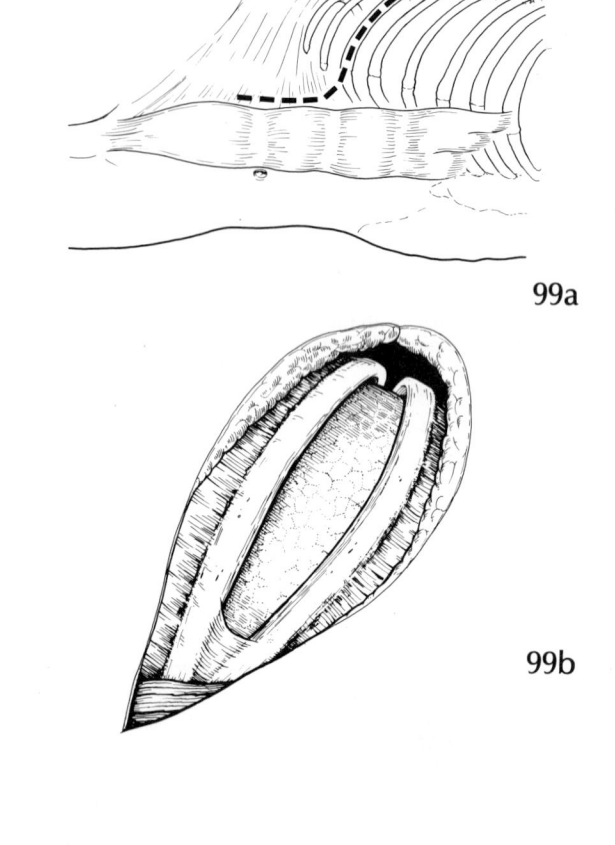

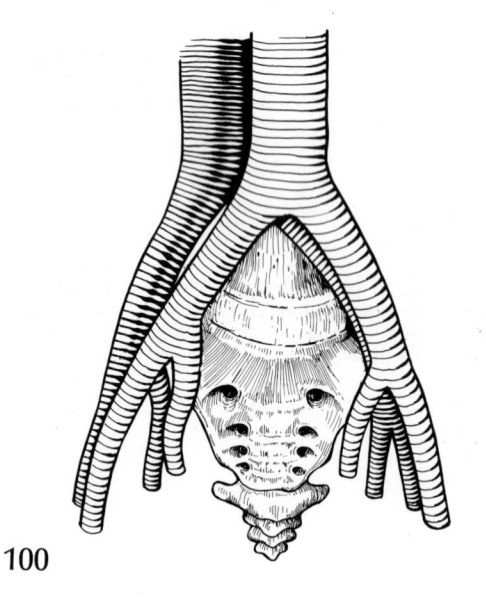

99a

99b

100

L5 can be exposed via an extraperitoneal approach either between the vessels or by ligating the iliolumbar vein to allow the common iliac vessels to displace towards the other side. Alternatively, a transperitoneal approach (Freebody) will provide excellent access to L5 and the sacrum.

100

Application of plaster of Paris spinal jacket

Indications

1. Unstable cervical fracture with deformity
2. Spinal fractures unsuitable for prolonged traction or a halo vest
3. Lumbar fractures treated conservatively.

Requirements

101

The following instruments and materials are required: Risser table, two canvas slings 10 × 25 cm (for derotation strap), head halter (disposable), stockinette (two sewn jackets, one with sleeves), orthopaedic felt (non-adhesive 25 × 40 cm), orthopaedic felt (non-adhesive 25 × 25 cm), two straps 5 cm × 4 m, two dozen plaster of Paris 15 cm, four plaster of Paris 10 cm, plaster knife, plaster saw, plaster scissors and a bucket of water (lukewarm).

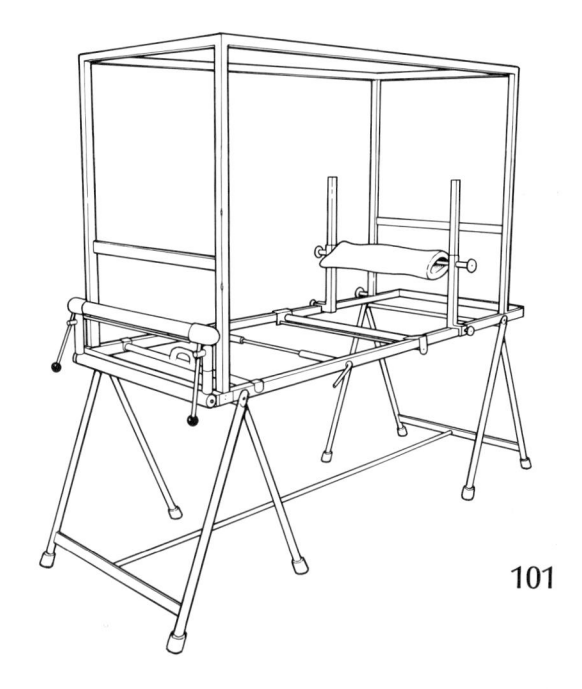

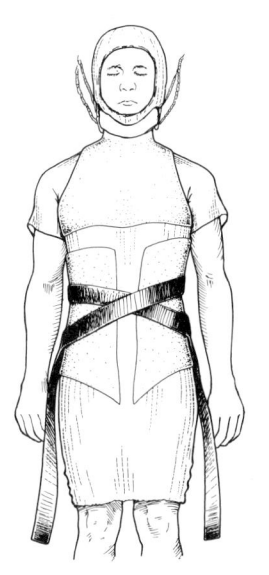

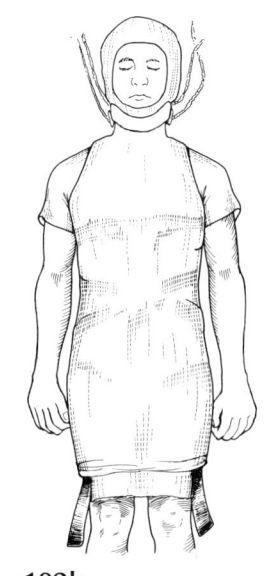

101

Method

Plaster slabs are prepared for the back, shoulders, neck (front and back) and side. Fifteen-centimetre plaster is used. The length of the slabs will depend on the patient's size and should be six thicknesses.

102a & b

Two stockinette jackets are applied, one with sleeves. Between the jackets, felt padding is applied around the pelvis and over the iliac crests to meet at the front. Felt may be placed over the stomach and/or chest to give an edge to any windows which may be cut.

Two straps are crossed over between the stockinette jackets around the pelvis with the ends left free to use for pelvic traction.

102a   102b

668 Thoracic and lumbar spine

103

A Glisson sling is applied over the two jackets to apply cervical traction.

The patient is placed on the Risser table, ensuring that the lower cross support is below the coccyx and the top support is across the mid-shoulder. The head is put on the rest as high as possible. Three people should be present.

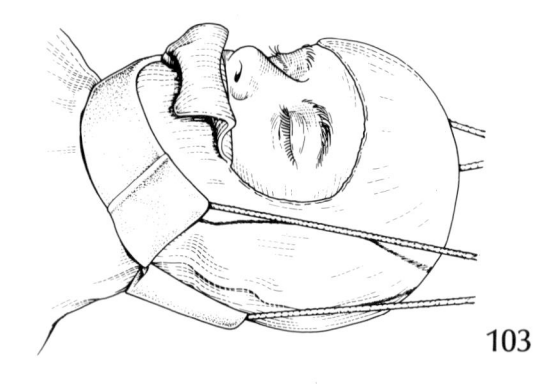

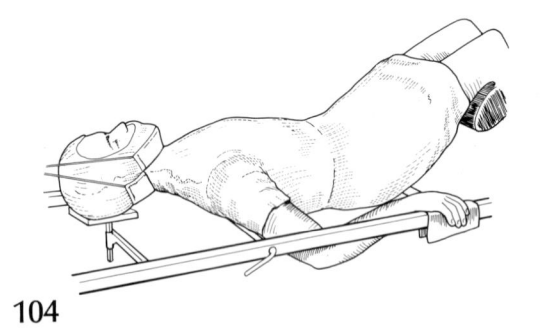

104

Traction is now applied, making sure that stockinette and any padding is kept smooth. When sufficient traction has been reached, the plastering is commenced. It is important that the plaster is applied quickly and evenly by at least three people. An extra person is helpful to steady the head. Two or three 15 cm plaster rolls are applied to the patient, covering as much as possible.

105

Slabs are applied to the body, pelvis, shoulders, back, front and sides of the neck, and are bound in by 15 cm plasters. Care is taken in moulding the plaster, particularly the neck and pelvic areas which are prone to pressure. The neck is moulded well under the occiput and mandible, and forward up over the larynx to create a hump to facilitate easy swallowing.

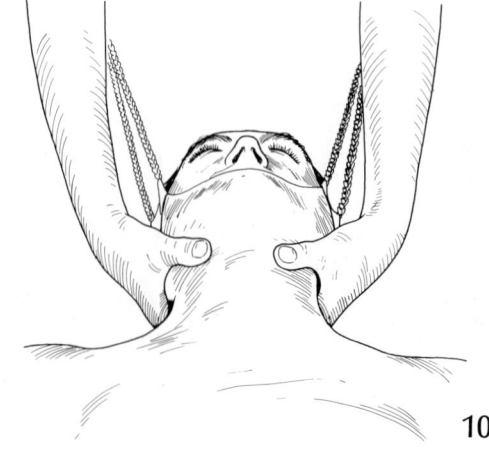

106

Two derotation straps are applied around the thoracolumbar area to achieve normal spinal curves while the plaster is drying. These are used only if a deformity is to be corrected.

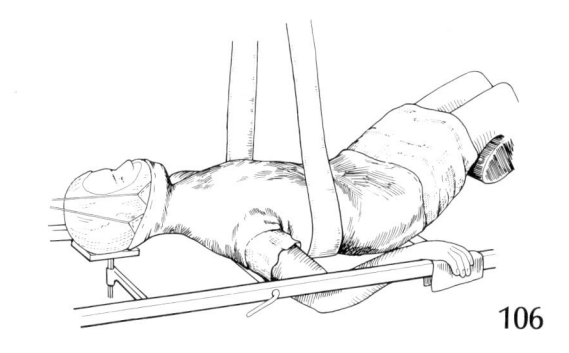

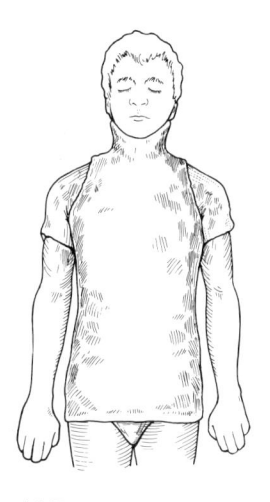

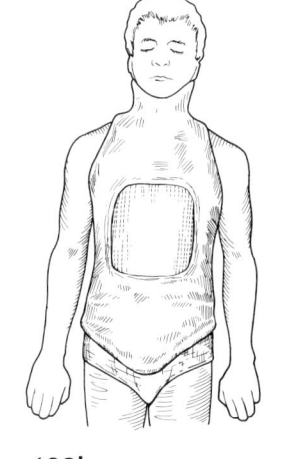

107a & b

The straps and Glisson sling are removed and the patient is placed on the bed for trimming when the plaster is almost dry.

107a   108b

References

1. Anderson LD, D'Alonzo RT. Fractures of the odontoid process of the axis. *J Bone Joint Surg [Am]* 1974; 56-A: 1663–74.

2. Willen JAG, Gaekwad UH, Kakulas BA. Burst fractures in the thoracic and lumbar spine: a clinico-neuropathologic analysis. *Spine* 1989; 14: 1316–23.

3. Kostuik JP. Anterior fixation for fractures of the thoracic and lumbar spine with or without neurologic involvement. *Clin Orthop* 1984; 189: 103–15.

4. Dunn HK. Anterior stabilisation of thoracolumbar injuries. *Clin Orthop* 1984; 189: 116–24.

Acknowledgements

The section on 'Application of Plaster of Paris Spinal Jacket' was kindly contributed by R. Lukey of the Royal Perth Rehabilitation Hospital, Western Australia.

Illustration 89 is reproduced courtesy of John Dove, Surgicraft Hartshill spinal fixation, A W Showell (Surgicraft) Ltd, Britten Street, Redditch, Worcestershire B97 6HF, UK.

Illustrations by Peter Cox

Recurrent anterior dislocation of the shoulder

William Angus Wallace FRCS Ed, FRCS Ed(Orth)
Professor of Orthopaedic and Accident Surgery, University of Nottingham, UK

Introduction

Aetiology

Dislocations of the glenohumeral joint are common injuries and are frequently associated with a tendency to recurrence, particularly in the young. The initial episode may involve minor or major trauma, depending on the susceptibility of the individual. An indirect injury to the shoulder, with a forcible abduction and lateral rotation strain to the arm, is the most common mechanism. The risk of recurrence after an anterior dislocation depends on the initial mechanism of injury and the age of the patient.

Simonet and Cofield[1] have shown from a review of 116 cases, followed up 5 years after injury, that patients aged under 20 years at the time of their first anterior dislocation have a 66 per cent incidence of recurrent dislocation and, in addition, an 18 per cent incidence of subluxation symptoms. Patients from 20 to 40 years had a 40 per cent incidence of recurrence with a further 9 per cent having subluxation symptoms, while in their series there were *no* recurrences in those aged over 40 but 10 per cent had subluxation symptoms. If the initial dislocation had been the result of an athletic or sporting injury and the patient was aged under 30 years the prognosis was worse, with the incidence of recurrence rising to 77 per cent.

Management of the initial dislocation

The first dislocation may reduce spontaneously, but if the patient attends hospital with the shoulder still dislocated an anteroposterior and modified axial radiograph[2] is recommended. Once dislocation is confirmed, reduction may be attempted by suspension of a weight from the patient's wrist while he lies prone on a table or trolley with the arm hanging over the edge. If this fails, in dislocations treated within the first 12 hours an attempt at reduction using sedation is recommended, but only if the proximal humerus has been shown to be free of fracture lines on plain radiographs. In all other circumstances the patient should be given a full general anaesthesia with muscle relaxation before the shoulder is reduced. For manipulative reduction the Hippocratic method is the safest: the operator's unshod foot is placed in the patient's axilla and firm sustained traction applied to the arm until the humeral head suddenly jumps back into joint. Kocher's manoeuvre, which involves a forcible rotation, is no longer recommended as it has been the cause of a significant number of iatrogenic humeral neck fractures.

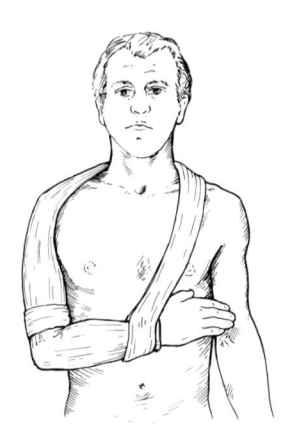

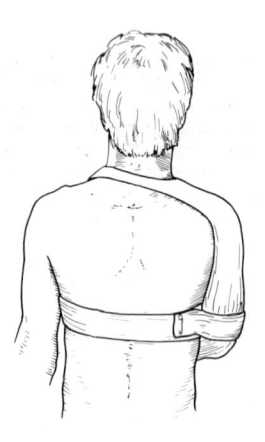

1

In those who spontaneously reduce and in patients who require manipulative reduction, further immobilization of the shoulder is recommended using a Gilchrist sling[3] made from a 3 metre length of stockinette. Alternatively, a broad arm sling and body bandage, or a commercially available shoulder immobilizer may be used.

The period of immobilization is currently a source of contention. Kiviluoto *et al.*[4] (1980) have shown, in patients under the age of 30, that there is an increased incidence of recurrence if only 1 week of immobilization is used compared with 3 weeks. However, Hovelius[5,6] has shown no difference between those mobilized early and those immobilized for 3–4 weeks. The lowest recurrence rate has been reported by Yoneda, Welsh and MacIntosh[7] who treated young university students with 5 weeks' absolute immobilization in a sling and body bandage and found their recurrence rate was reduced to only 17 per cent.

A sensible management policy would be that patients under 35 at the time of their first dislocation should be treated with strict immobilization for 5 weeks if they wish to return to active sport or for 3 weeks if they are likely to lead a less active life. In those over 35 years recurrence is rare irrespective of treatment, therefore only 1 week of immobilization is required, but no sporting activities for 6 weeks.

Preoperative

Assessment of patients with recurrent anterior dislocations

Four questions should be asked if a patient seeks help for a recurrent anterior dislocation of the shoulder.

1. Are the symptoms severe enough to warrant surgical treatment? Normally surgery is only considered if dislocation has recurred on at least two occasions or when subluxation symptoms are significantly interfering with everyday life.
2. Is there documentary evidence of the initial dislocation and if so in which direction did the humeral head displace?
3. Is it absolutely sure that the direction of the recurrent dislocation is anterior?
4. Does the patient have a 'loose' shoulder or multi-directional instability?

If radiographs are available from the first episode then the diagnosis will be supported *but* the patient could also have a 'loose' shoulder. The direction of instability is established clinically by carrying out two tests – the anterior apprehension test and the posterior stress test.

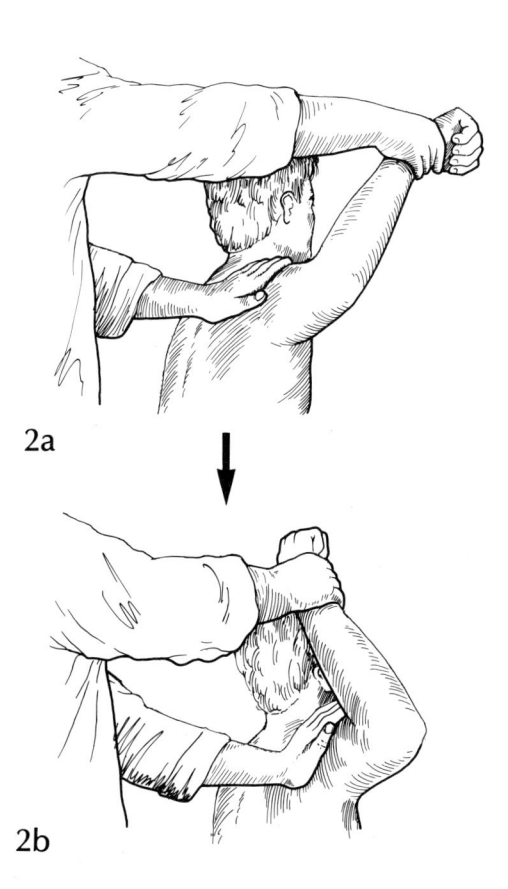

Anterior apprehension test[8]

2a & b

The affected arm is abducted to 90° in neutral rotation and the examiner gently rotates the arm laterally while controlling the scapula with his other hand as shown. If the shoulder is unstable anteriorly the patient will develop apprehension and the anterior third of deltoid or the subscapularis will develop spasm to protect the shoulder from dislocating.

Posterior stress test[9]

3a & b

The patient lies in the supine position. The examiner stabilizes the scapula by resting his hand between the scapula and the examination table. He places his fingers behind the neck of the scapula and the humeral head and moves the arm to 90° abduction in neutral rotation. The elbow is kept at 90° and the arm is brought forwards into flexion with the examiner applying firm axial pressure through the humeral shaft in order to attempt to displace the humeral head posteriorly. The examining hand will feel the humeral head sublux or dislocate in a posterior direction and this will be confirmed by then reversing the manoeuvre and extending the shoulder again when the head will be felt to 'clunk' back into joint.

Sulcus sign[10]

4

The 'loose' shoulder is identified by eliciting the sulcus sign. The patient is seated and asked to relax. The surgeon applies downward traction to the arm while observing the contour of the shoulder he is examining. If a sulcus appears just below the acromion this indicates the humeral head has subluxed inferiorly and the shoulder is 'loose'.

If a 'loose' shoulder is diagnosed, referral to an orthopaedic surgeon with a special interest in shoulder problems is recommended; these patients are particularly difficult to treat, and there is a surgical failure rate in excess of 50 per cent.

Voluntary recurrent anterior dislocation

There are a group of patients who can anteriorly sublux or dislocate their shoulder at will. A number of these patients have psychological problems. They should be managed in the first instance by advice to stop dislocating the shoulder, to avoid any activities which are known to cause the shoulder to come out of joint and to build up the rotator cuff muscles with specific strengthening exercises. The majority of patients settle using this regime and surgery is rarely required.

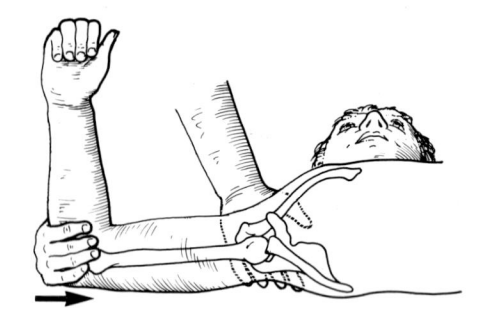

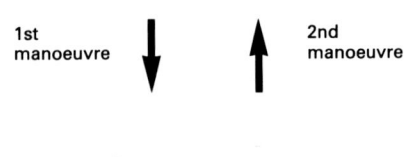

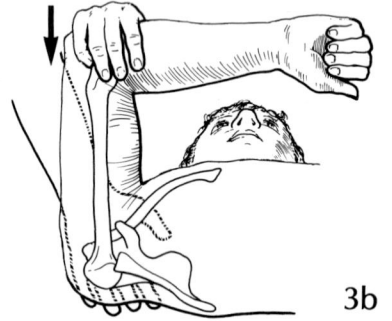

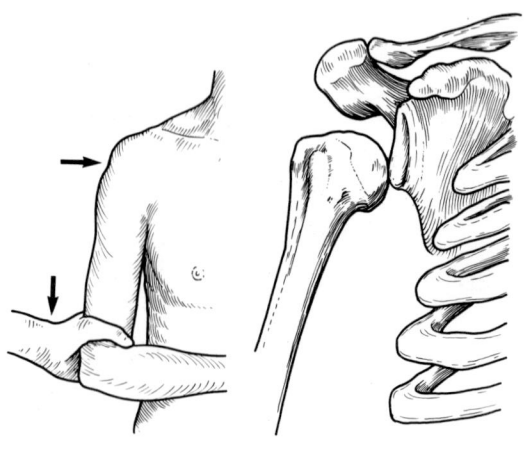

Pathological lesions

Carter Rowe[11] from Boston in 1978 reported his experience of surgical treatment of recurrent anterior dislocation over a period of 30 years. In 85 per cent of cases the capsule was completely avulsed or separated from the anterior glenoid rim. The glenoid labrum was absent or completely destroyed in 73 per cent, and intact but separated from the rim in a further 13 per cent of cases. Damage to the bony rim of the glenoid was present in 73 per cent of cases, with 44 per cent actually fractured. A Broca[12] or Hill–Sachs[13] lesion – a bony dent on the posterolateral aspect of the humeral head – was present in 77 per cent of cases. Rowe's failure rate using the Bankart operation was 3.5 per cent but increased to 5 per cent if a medium or large sized Broca lesion was present.

It has been shown by Pieper[14] that patients with recurrent anterior dislocation have a reduced humeral retroversion of $25° \pm 10°$ compared with the normal value of $40° \pm 6°$. This supports the concept of the Weber lateral rotation osteotomy[15] for the treatment of recurrent anterior dislocation. Unfortunately Pieper's findings have not been supported by Cyprien et al.[16] nor by Pfister and Gebauer[17] who have shown no difference in humeral torsion between normal controls and patients with anterior dislocation. Nor could they show a relationship between the glenoid version and recurrent dislocation.

Humeral rotation osteotomy will not be considered further.

Choice of operation

Table 1 shows the published success rates for different operations for recurrent anterior dislocation of the shoulder. The Putti–Platt operation is the traditional British operation but it suffers from two drawbacks – it has the highest recorded failure rate and it is usually associated with a marked loss of lateral rotation of the shoulder that limits its usefulness, particularly in sportsmen who require a good range of elevation and rotation.

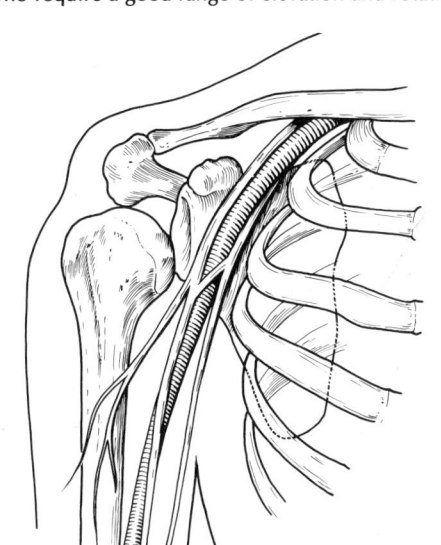

The best operation is usually the operation which the operator is most acquainted with and which he therefore does the best. My own preference is for the Bankart operation, particularly if the shoulder is only subluxing in an anterior direction, but it is difficult and may be tedious to carry out. The Boytchev procedure will produce a near-normal range of movement early after the operation (often within 4 months) but there is a 30 per cent incidence of temporary musculocutaneous nerve palsy.

Table 1 Results from recurrent dislocation operations

Operation	Dislocation plus subluxation recurrence rate (%)	Number of patients	Author
Putti–Platt	5	79	Quigley & Friedman (1974)[18]
	14	132	Morrey & Janes (1976)[19]
	19	68	Hovelius (1979)[20]
Bankart	5	18	Adams (1948)[21]
	4	145	Rowe et al. (1978)[11]
	4	45	Zinnecker (1984)[22]
Bristow–Helfet	7	30	Helfet (1958)[23]
	16	31	Albrektsson et al. (1982)[24]
	13	112	Hovelius (1984)[25]
Magnuson–Stack	3	75	DePalma et al. (1967)[26]
	2	154	Karadimas et al. (1980)[27]
	3	38	Ahmadain (1987)[28]
Boytchev	0	17	Conforty (1980)[29]
	0	26	Ha'Eri (1986)[30]
	12*	17	Sugimoto et al. (1987)[31]

* 2 patients had one minor subluxation each in the early postoperative period

Structures to protect in anterior shoulder surgery

5

Operations on the front of the shoulder are carried out close to the distal part of the brachial plexus. The illustration shows the close proximity of these nerves. The nerve which is most vulnerable is the musculocutaneous nerve which lies behind the conjoined tendons of biceps and coracobrachialis and passes into the posterior aspect of the coracobrachialis muscle. This nerve is usually well protected when the conjoined tendon is attached but as soon as a coracoid osteotomy is performed it becomes vulnerable; great care must be taken to avoid a traction injury to the nerve. The nerve usually enters the coracobrachialis muscle at least 5 cm distal to the coracoid but its anatomy is very variable.

676 Shoulder

Operations

The approach to the front of the shoulder is similar for most of the operations. It is therefore appropriate to describe the standard approach and then the different techniques for each operation will be described in detail. The closure technique and postoperative management will finally be presented.

Position of patient

6

The patient is placed supine on the operating table with the trunk at a 45° head-up tilt. A sandbag or 500 ml infusion bag is placed behind the medial border of the scapula to throw the shoulder forward for easier surgical access. The head is supported either with a head ring or, as shown, with a neurosurgical head support. A surgical preparation of almost half the trunk and the *whole* of the affected arm is recommended. A thyroid-type double head-drape is used to isolate the patient's head and the anaesthetic equipment from the surgical field. The arm is draped separately to facilitate manoeuvrability.

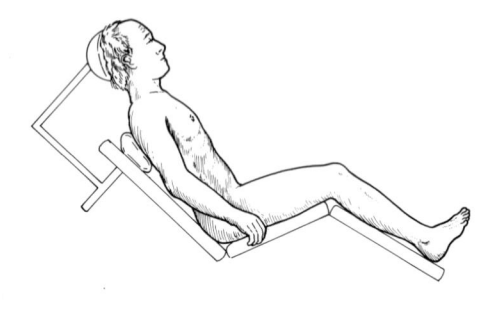

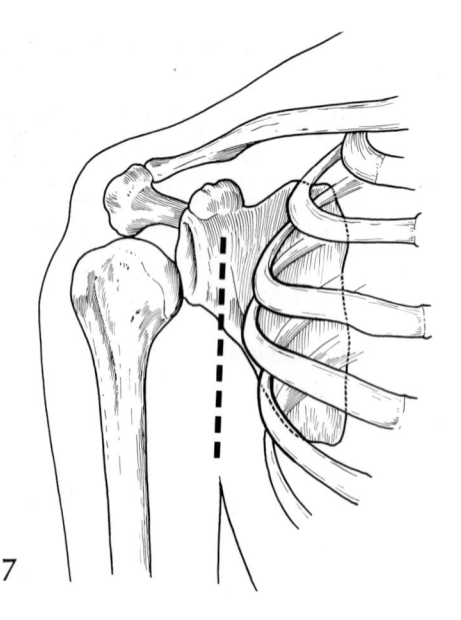

Skin incision

The incision varies depending on whether the patient is male or female.

7

In men the standard incision is from the tip of the coracoid vertically downwards towards the anterior axillary fold for a distance of 8 cm. This allows easy access through a large incision and provides an excellent exposure of the deeper anatomy.

8

In women cosmesis is exceptionally important. Two alternative cosmetic incisions can be used – the 'bra-strap' incision or the axillary approach. In the former, the incision is hidden behind the patient's bra strap, and in order to site it correctly it is essential to mark the position of the bra strap before operation.

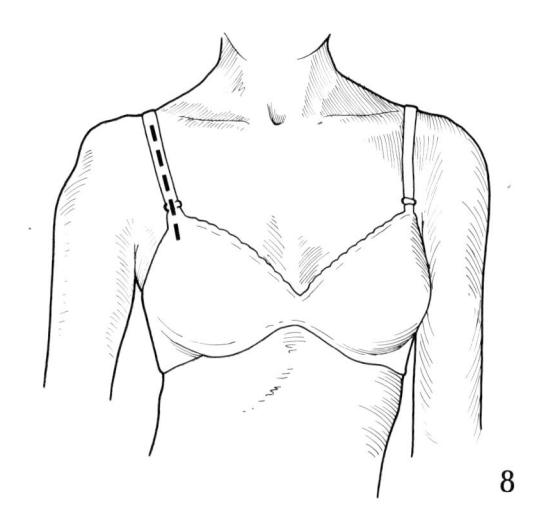

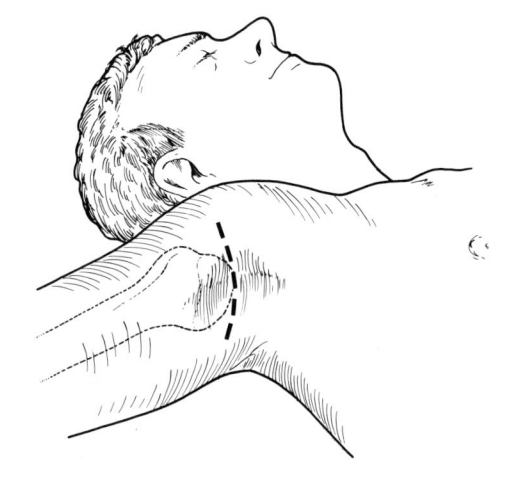

9

The axillary incision is made in the anterior half of the apex of the axilla and is extended forward as far as the anterior axillary fold formed by the pectoralis major tendon. The skin edges are then widely undermined and the lowest centimetre of the musculotendinous junction of the pectoralis major is divided. Abduction of the arm and retraction upwards of the pectoralis major tendon reveal the subscapularis tendon and conjoined tendon, and the coracoid may also be exposed. The pectoralis major should be repaired during closure. The disadvantages of the axillary approach are the more limited access and the occasional development of a thickened scar causing axillary discomfort.

678 Shoulder

Approach through the first muscle layer

10

The subcutaneous fat is divided and the deltopectoral groove is sought. This is located by identifying the cephalic vein distally and dissecting it proximally. As it passes upwards in the deltopectoral groove it dives down between the deltoid and pectoralis major. The vein is preserved but its lateral tributaries are either cauterized, or ligated between sutures, and then divided. If the main vein is damaged it may be tied off with no ill effect. The groove is then opened widely and held open with one pair of self-retaining retractors.

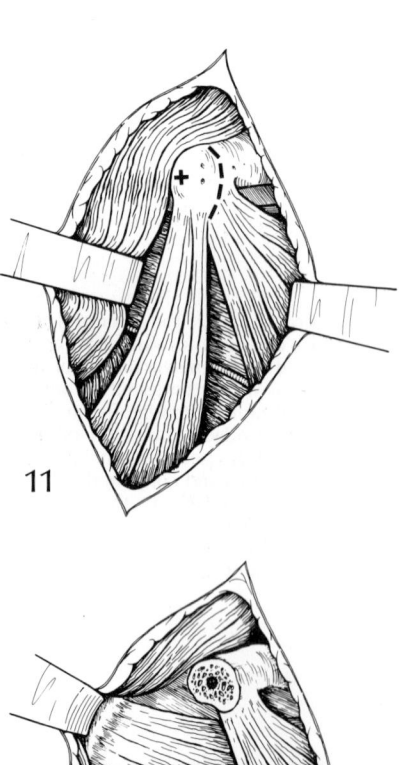

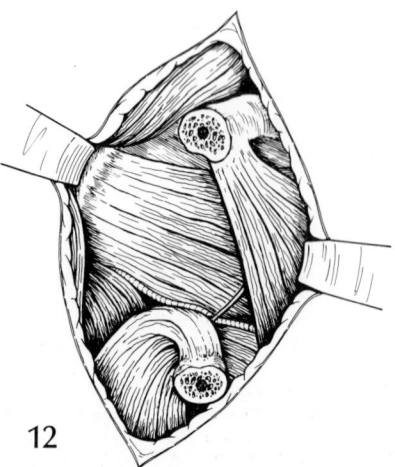

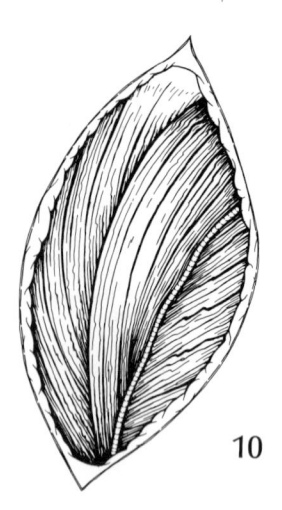

Approach through the second muscle layer

11 & 12

The coracoid process is now exposed in the upper part of the wound. The conjoined tendon of origin of coracobrachialis and the short head of biceps constitute the second layer. A cruciate stab incision is made on the tip of the coracoid, and the coracoid is predrilled using a 2.5 mm drill and tapped with a 3.5 mm tap after measuring the depth of the drill hole. The periosteum approximately 1 cm from the tip of the coracoid is divided transversely and a coracoid osteotomy performed with either an osteotome or with an oscillating saw. A stay suture is then placed through the drill hole in the tip of the coracoid and the detached coracoid tip with the conjoined tendon attached is then reflected downwards. Care must be taken to avoid excessive traction on the conjoined tendon. The musculocutaneous nerve enters the deep surface of the coracobrachialis muscle and can be injured by injudicious traction. Once reflected downwards, the whole of the subscapularis muscle comes into view with the distal edge of the muscle identified by a leash of veins passing along its lower border.

PUTTI–PLATT OPERATION[32]

Approach through the third muscle layer

13

The inferior border of the subscapularis is indicated by the transverse leash of anterior circumflex humeral vessels and the dissection should go no lower than this point. The vessels are now cauterized or divided between ligatures. Lateral rotation of the humerus puts the subscapularis under tension. Two stay sutures are now inserted into the subscapularis muscle 4 cm medial to its humeral attachment. These sutures are essential before dividing the subscapularis because if allowed to retract the cut muscle will come to lie dangerously close to the main nerves arising from the brachial plexus and there is then a risk of nerve injury when the subscapularis is subsequently sought. Subscapularis is now divided transverse to its fibres and 2 cm medial to its humeral attachment. The deep surface of the subscapularis is usually adherent to the joint capsule, and although it is preferable to protect the anterior capsule of the shoulder joint as a separate layer during the division, this is not essential.

Entry into the shoulder joint

14

The anterior capsule of the shoulder is divided in the same line as the subscapularis tendon – 2 cm from the lateral insertion of the subscapularis. A Bankart retractor inserted into the joint will allow a good view of the anterior glenoid rim but there is no need to sublux the joint in order to demonstrate any Broca lesion.

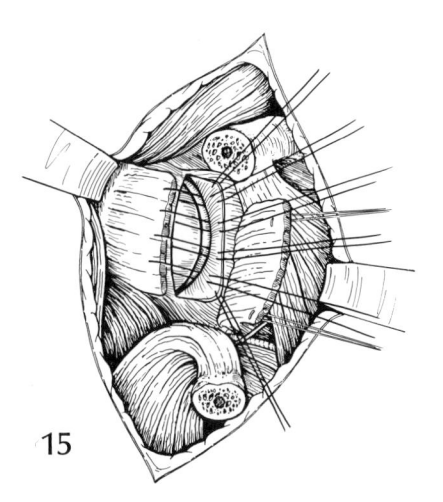

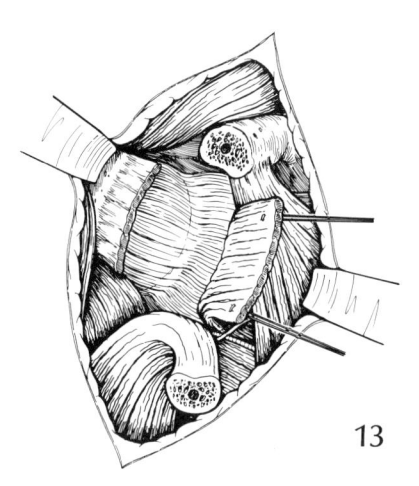

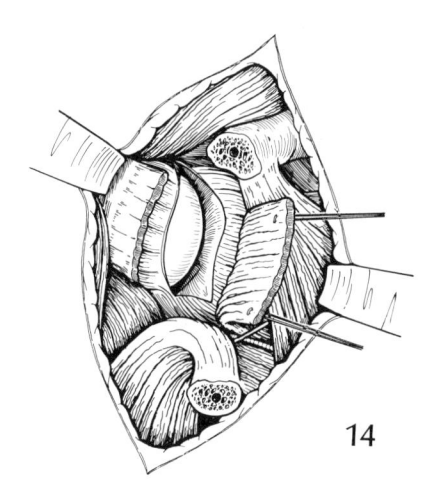

Attachment of subscapularis to the scapular neck

15

The lateral portion of subscapularis and the capsule are used as one flap in this operation. First the anterior scapular neck is roughened using a curette. The lateral flap is then sutured to the glenoid labrum and capsule so that it will adhere to the roughened area. Up to six braided non-absorbable mattress sutures are used and all should be inserted before they are tied as demonstrated. The humeral head should be levered backwards by the assistant as the sutures are tightened, but 45° of lateral rotation of the glenohumeral joint should still be possible at this stage.

Attachment of the medial capsular layer

16

The medial capsule is now double-breasted over the lateral subscapular layer and sutured using three braided non-absorbable sutures.

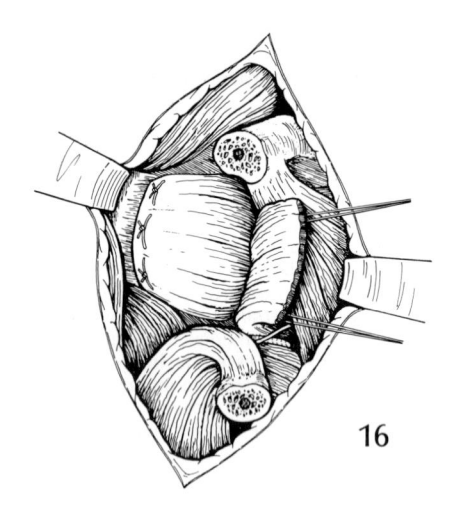

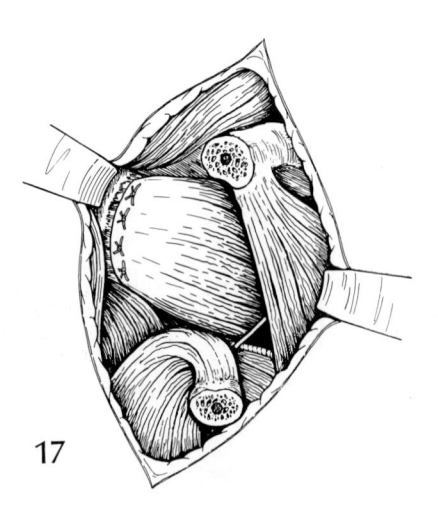

Attachment of the subscapularis layer

17

This is drawn across the deeper capsular layer and sutured with interrupted absorbable sutures to the deeper layers at a tension which will allow only 30°–45° of lateral rotation of the shoulder joint.

Reattachment of the coracoid

18

The coracoid is reattached with one 3.5 mm stainless steel screw of appropriate length. No washer is normally required as the screw usually settles nicely into the tip of the coracoid without cutting through.

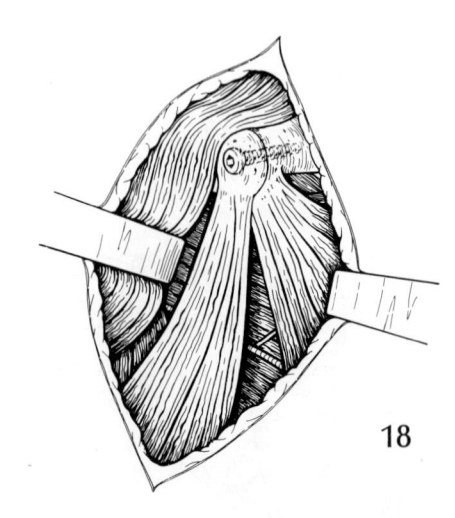

BANKART OPERATION[11]

Approach through the third muscle layer

19

This is very similar to the Putti–Platt except that the subscapularis is carefully dissected from the anterior capsule by sharp dissection as the subscapularis is divided and it is important *not* to divide the capsule at this stage. To avoid entering the joint a small amount of subscapularis tendon is often left on the anterior capsule.

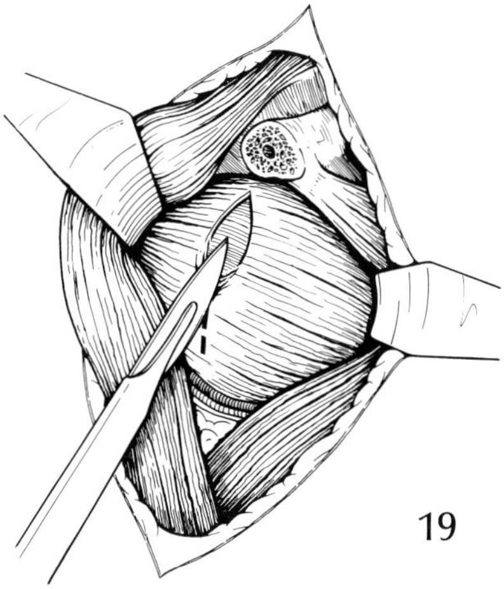

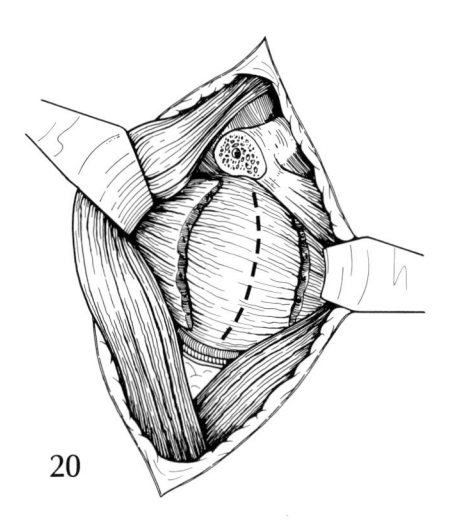

Entry into the shoulder joint

20

The arm is fully rotated laterally before a vertical incision is made into the joint just lateral to the rim of the glenoid. This ensures that the anterior flap will be of proper length to allow an adequate lateral rotation of the shoulder postoperatively.

Exposure of the anterior glenoid margin

21

The anterior glenoid rim is exposed more easily if a Bankart retractor is inserted into the joint. If the capsule is separated from the anterior glenoid rim, a Homan retractor is inserted into the glenoid neck and used to retract the medial part of the capsule. If the capsule and glenoid labrum are firmly attached to the anterior glenoid rim, these soft tissues can be used to reattach the anterior capsule and no drill holes are necessary.

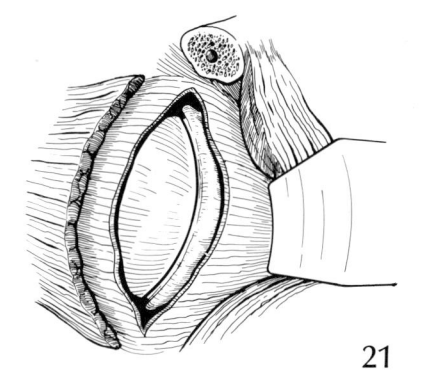

682 Shoulder

Preparing the anterior glenoid margin drill holes

22

The rim of the glenoid and the neck of the scapula can now be freshened with a curette or dental burr. Three or four holes are made through the rim using a right-angled dental drill and a strong, sharp-pointed towel clip. It is important that these holes are sufficiently deep to leave a solid anterior bridge after they have been drilled.

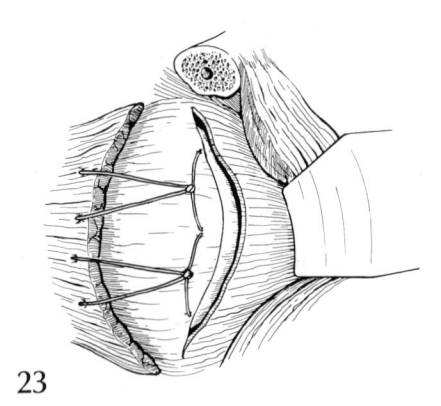

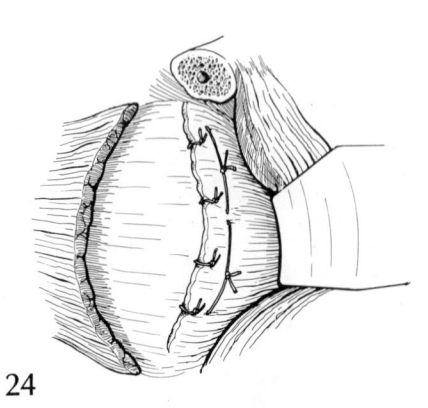

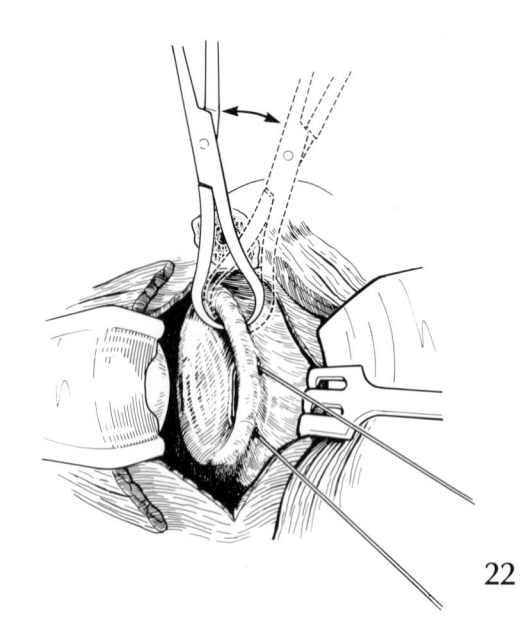

Attachment of the capsule to the glenoid

23 & 24

A No. 2, braided, non-absorbable suture is used. Using appropriate needles the sutures are placed through the holes as a mattress suture, with a small groove created in the articular cartilage, and then through the anterior capsular layer. *All* the sutures should be inserted before any are tied firmly with the arm in full medial rotation. The medial capsular flap is then sutured over the front of the repair using the ends of the same sutures, thus providing a solid reinforcement, and any free edge of medial capsule tacked down with interrupted absorbable sutures.

Repair of subscapularis

The subscapularis is repaired by end-to-end suture using three or four interrupted absorbable mattress sutures.

Reattachment of the coracoid

This is performed as in the Putti–Platt operation.

MODIFIED BRISTOW–HELFET PROCEDURE[25]

Technique

25

The subscapularis muscle and capsule of the shoulder are split longitudinally at a point between the middle third and the lower third of the muscle, and the gap held open with a self-retaining retractor. This gives access to the anteroinferior glenoid rim, which is roughened and drilled with a 3.2 mm drill to receive the attachment of the coracoid process. The coracoid is fixed using a 4.5 mm lag (malleolar) screw of sufficient length to engage the posterior cortex of the scapula. Hovelius[25] has clearly shown that the position of the coracoid is crucial to the success of this operation. It *must* be anchored on the inferior one third of the glenoid rim and its lateral edge should be flush with the articular surface of the glenoid with no palpable step. The conjoined tendon should be sutured to the subscapularis after removal of retractors to provide additional stability to the fixation.

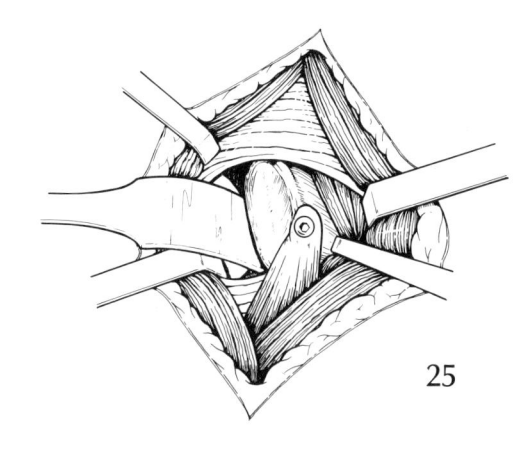

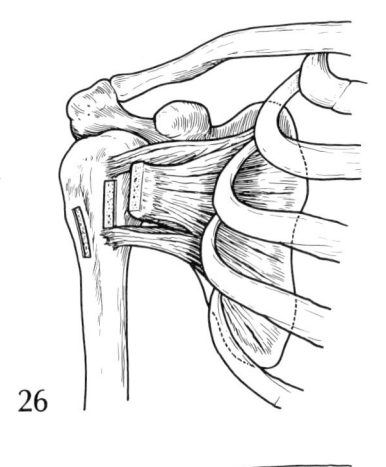

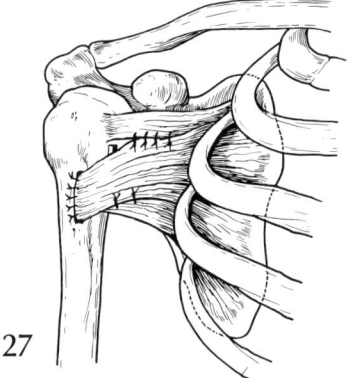

MODIFIED MAGNUSON–STACK PROCEDURE[26]

Technique

26 & 27

No osteotomy of the coracoid is required for this operation. The central four-fifths of the tendon of subscapularis is separated by incisions near its upper and lower margins. Its insertion is detached, taking a small wedge of bone and the capsulomuscular flap is dissected medially to allow inspection of the glenoid. The shoulder is then rotated medially and the subscapularis insertion is transplanted under reasonable tension lateral to the bicipital groove about 1 cm distal to the greater tuberosity. The bony wedge is placed in a shallow gutter and fixed either with staple or sutures. The upper and lower margins of the transferred tendon are sutured to local soft tissues.

MODIFIED BOYTCHEV PROCEDURE[30]

Technique

28 & 29

The conjoined tendons attached to the osteotomized coracoid process are retracted and freed downwards as far as the penetration of the coracobrachialis muscle by the musculocutaneous nerve. The musculocutaneous nerve must be identified either by careful dissection without undue traction or by palpation in view of the known occurrence of postoperative nerve palsies. The transverse leash of anterior circumflex humeral vessels at the lower border of subscapularis is identified and if necessary ligated. With the arm held in full medial rotation, a cholecystectomy forceps is passed between the subscapularis muscle and the capsule of the shoulder joint. A tunnel is created in this plane by opening the forceps and withdrawing the instrument. The tunnel is enlarged until the operator's little finger can be passed easily through the tunnel. The detached coracoid process with the conjoined tendons is passed through the tunnel and reattached to its original site with a 3.5 mm screw of appropriate length. It is important to check there is no tension on the musculocutaneous nerve at this stage. If there is, the lower fibres of subscapularis should be surgically divided to free the nerve.

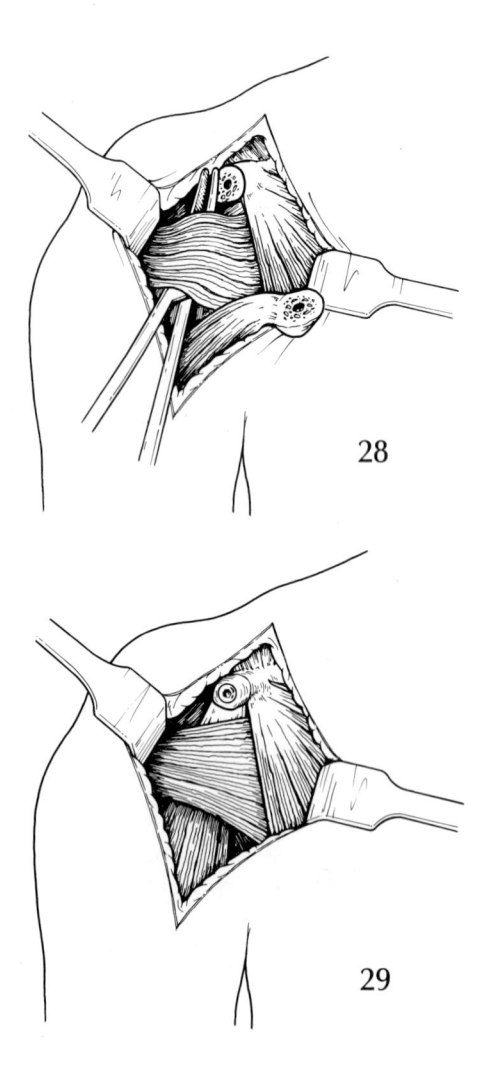

Closure

For all procedures the deltopectoral interval is loosely closed with two or three interrupted absorbable 0-gauge sutures over a suction drain. The subcutaneous fat is closed carefully with interrupted 2/0 absorbable sutures and the skin should be closed with 2/0 polypropylene continuous subcuticular suture reinforced with adhesive skin sutures. In the shoulder region there is no place for simple interrupted sutures because of the significant cosmetic deformity created by the suture holes which can be disfiguring. A simple absorbent, adhesive dressing is applied to the wound.

A Gilchrist sling (see *Illustration 1*) or a broad arm sling is applied in the operating theatre with a cotton wool axillary pad to absorb moisture.

Postoperative management

The patient remains in hospital for 24–72 hours, depending on the level of postoperative discomfort. The suction drain is removed at 24 hours after operation.

For the Putti–Platt, Bristow–Helfet and Magnuson–Stack procedures, a Gilchrist sling is recommended for 3–4 weeks. Alternatively, a broad arm sling under the clothes or a commercial shoulder immobilizer can be used for the same period. For the Bankart and Boytchev procedures a broad arm sling is required for only 10 days to 2 weeks.

No formal physiotherapy is required after any of these procedures. The patients are encouraged to 'use your arm as normally as possible'. Gentle swimming can be started from 6 weeks and a return to normal sports 3–4 months after operation.

References

1. Simonet WT, Cofield RH. Prognosis in anterior shoulder dislocation. *Am J Sports Med* 1984; 12: 19–24.

2. Wallace WA, Hellier M. Improving radiographs of the injured shoulder. *Radiography* 1983; 49: 229–33.

3. Gilchrist DK. A stockinette-Velpeau for immobilization of the shoulder girdle. *J Bone Joint Surg [Am]* 1967; 49-A: 750–1.

4. Kiviluoto O, Pasila M, Jaroma H, Sundholm A. Immobilization after primary dislocation of the shoulder. *Acta Orthop Scand* 1980; 51: 915–9.

5. Hovelius L, Eriksson K, Fredin H, et al. Recurrences after initial dislocation of the shoulder: results of a prospective study of treatment. *J Bone Joint Surg [Am]* 1983; 65-A: 343–9.

6. Hovelius L. Anterior dislocation of the shoulder in teenagers and young adults: a five year prognosis. *J Bone Joint Surg [Am]* 1987; 69-A: 393–9.

7. Yoneda B, Welsh PP, MacIntosh DL. Conservative treatment of shoulder dislocation in young males. In: Bayley I, Kessel L, eds. *Shoulder surgery*, Berlin: Springer Verlag, 1982; 76–9.

8. Gerber C, Ganz R. Clinical assessment of instability of the shoulder: with special reference to anterior and posterior drawer tests. *J Bone Joint Surg [Br]* 1984; 66-B: 551–6.

9. Norwood LA, Terry GC. Shoulder posterior subluxation. *Am J Sports Med* 1984; 12: 25–30.

10. Neer CS, Foster CR. Inferior capsular shift for involuntary inferior and multi-directional instability of the shoulder: a preliminary report. *J Bone Joint Surg [Am]* 1980; 62-A: 897–908.

11. Rowe CR, Patel D, Southmayd WW. The Bankart procedure: a long-term end result study. *J Bone Joint Surg [Am]* 1978; 60-A: 1–16.

12. Hartmann H, Broca A. Contribution a l'etude des luxations de l'epaule. *Bulletin de la Societe Anatomique de Paris*, 5Me Serie 1890; 4: 312.

13. Hill HA, Sachs MD. Grooved defect of the humeral head: frequently unrecognized complication of dislocations of the shoulder. *Radiology* 1940; 35: 690–700.

14. Pieper H-G. Correction of pathological amount of humeral retroversion in operative treatment of recurrent shoulder dislocation. In: Takagishi N, ed. *The shoulder*. Japan: PPS, 1987: 276–80.

15. Weber BG. Operative treatment for recurrent dislocation of the shoulder: preliminary report. *Injury* 1969; 1: 107–9.

16. Cyprien JM, Vasey HM, Burdet A, Bonvin JC, Kritsikis N, Vuagnat P. Humeral retrotorsion and glenohumeral relationship in the normal shoulder and in recurrent anterior dislocation (scapulometry). *Clin Orthop* 1983; 175: 8–17.

17. Pfister A, Gebauer D. The operative treatment of recurrent shoulder dislocation dependent of the retroversion angle: a computed tomography study. In: Takagishi N, ed. *The shoulder*. Japan: PPS, 1987; 270–5.

18. Quigley TB, Freedman PA. Recurrent dislocation of the shoulder: a preliminary report of personal experience with seven Bankart and 92 Putti–Platt operations in 99 cases over 25 years. *Am J Surg* 1974; 128: 595–9.

19. Morrey BF, Janes JM. Recurrent anterior dislocation of the shoulder. Long-term follow-up of the Putti–Platt and Bankart procedures. *J Bone Joint Surg [Am]* 1976; 58-A: 252–6.

20. Hovelius L, Thorling J, Fredin H. Recurrent anterior dislocation of the shoulder: results after the Bankart and Putti–Platt operations. *J Bone Joint Surg [Am]* 1979; 61-A: 566–9.

21. Adams JC. Recurrent dislocation of the shoulder. *J Bone Joint Surg [Br]* 1948; 30-B: 26–38.

22. Zinnecker HJ, Puhringer A, Bartalsky L. Experience in the treatment of recurrent anterior dislocation of the shoulder with a modified version of Bankart's procedure. In: Bateman JE, Welsh RP, eds. *Surgery of the shoulder*. Philadelphia: Decker. St Louis: CV Mosby, 1984: 91–3.

23. Helfet AJ. Coracoid transplantation for recurring dislocation of the shoulder. *J Bone Joint Surg [Br]* 1958; 40-B: 198–202.

24. Albrektsson BE, Herberts P, Korner L, Lamm CR, Zachrisson BE. Technical aspects of the Bristow repair for recurrent anterior shoulder instability. In: Bayley I, Kessel L, eds. *Shoulder surgery*. Berlin: Springer Verlag, 1982: 87–92.

25. Hovelius L. Operative treatment of recurrent anterior shoulder dislocation with the Bristow–Latarjet procedure. In: Bateman JE, Welsh RP, eds. *Surgery of the shoulder*. Philadelphia: Decker. St Louis: CV Mosby, 1984: 87–90.

26. DePalma AF, Cooke AJ, Prabhakar M. The role of the subscapularis in recurrent anterior dislocations of the shoulder. *Clin Orthop* 1967; 54: 35–49.

27. Karadimas J, Rentis GR, Varouchas G. Repair of recurrent anterior dislocation of the shoulder using transfer of the subscapularis tendon. *J Bone Joint Surg [Am]* 1980; 62-A: 1147–9.

28. Ahmadain AM. The Magnuson–Stack operation for recurrent anterior dislocation of the shoulder: a review of 38 cases. *J Bone Joint Surg [Br]* 1987; 69-B: 111–4.

29. Conforty B. The results of the Boytchev procedure for treatment of recurrent dislocation of the shoulder. *Int Orthop* 1980; 4: 127–32.

30. Ha'Eri GB. Boytchev procedure for the treatment of anterior shoulder instability. *Clin Orthop* 1986; 206: 196–201.

31. Sugimoto Y, Nakatsuchi Y, Saitoh S, Kutsuma T, Sugiura K. Boytchev procedure for recurrent dislocation of the shoulder. In: Takagishi N, ed. *The shoulder*. Japan: PPS, 1987: 261–5.

32. Osmond-Clarke H. Habitual dislocation of the shoulder. The Putti–Platt operation. *J Bone Joint Surg [Br]* 1948; 30-B: 19–25.

Illustrations by Peter Cox

Injuries of the acromioclavicular joint

William Angus Wallace FRCS Ed, FRCS Ed (Orth)
Professor of Orthopaedic and Accident Surgery, University of Nottingham, UK

Introduction

The acromioclavicular joint is one of the most commonly injured joints of the body. The injury is usually caused by a heavy fall onto the shoulder or a blow to the top of the shoulder as occurs in a rugby tackle. The patient experiences pain on the point of the shoulder immediately after the injury, with pain clearly localized to the acromioclavicular joint area, and often bruising appears 48 hours later.

The traditional management of this injury is conservative and this has been supported by recent reports by Bannister[1] and Dias[2]. Although there has been an eagerness in recent years to operate on these patients, work by Imatani[3] and by Glick[4] has clearly shown that the majority of sportsmen do well following non-operative management of their acromioclavicular joint dislocation. However, a small group of patients would appear to benefit from early surgery and an additional small group do require late surgical treatment after a poor result from non-operative treatment.

Classification

Three categories of injury are now widely recognized and were described by Allman[5].

Grade I injuries cause local damage, usually only to the superior acromioclavicular ligament with no joint disruption; there is no deformity – only local tenderness over the joint.

In Grade II injuries there is damage to both the superior and inferior acromioclavicular ligaments and stretching of the coracoclavicular ligaments, with a minor step (less than the height of the acromioclavicular joint) seen at the point of the shoulder.

In Grade III injuries the coracoclavicular ligaments are completely ruptured or avulsed; obvious deformity is present at the point of the shoulder with a high-riding clavicle and a weak shoulder. Bannister[6] has further divided Grade III injuries into Grade III-stable and Grade III-unstable injuries, with stability assessed on special stress radiographs taken with the elbow held at 90° while a weight of 5 kg is held in the hand. An additional indication of a Grade III-unstable injury is the clinical finding that the lateral end of the clavicle lies under the skin and is separated from its enveloping muscles – the trapezius above and the deltoid below.

Although all classifications concentrate on the vertical displacement on radiographs it is important also to examine clinically for anteroposterior displacement as it is usual for the lateral end of the clavicle to be displaced posteriorly after Grade III injuries. By gentle palpation, the lateral end of the clavicle and the acromion can be identified and their anteroposterior stability can be assessed by gentle pressure.

Indications for surgical intervention

Acute injuries

There is rarely an indication for surgical treatment for Grade I and Grade II injuries. Grade III injuries may be treated conservatively as recommended by Dias[2] who considered long-term disability was rare. There is merit in identifying the Grade III-unstable injury described by Bannister[6] and performing early open reduction and internal stabilization of this injury.

Late or chronic injuries (all grades)

In this situation the patient complains of either pain or deformity.

Pain If pain is the problem, this is usually due to mechanical pain either from muscle strain or from early arthritic change in the acromioclavicular joint. The degree of joint stability must first be assessed carefully. If the joint is stable, but arthritic, excellent results with a 90 per cent success rate will be obtained by resection of the lateral 1 cm of the clavicle[7] but with careful repair of the soft tissues. However, if the joint is unstable the joint surfaces must be assessed very carefully both before and at the time of operation. If the joint surfaces are in good condition the author recommends accurate open reduction and internal stabilization of the acromioclavicular joint. However, if the joint surfaces are badly damaged or cannot be accurately reduced a Weaver–Dunn procedure[8,9] is performed.

Deformity Patients with a chronic dislocation of the acromioclavicular joint have two deformities, an obvious 'bump' caused by the prominent lateral end of the clavicle together with the appearance of a dropped shoulder. In females the dropped shoulder may cause a problem with shoulder straps tending to fall off and apparent uneven hemlines of dresses. The 'bump' may be very obvious and can be fully corrected by operation as can the dropped shoulder, but in both cases one cosmetic problem will be replaced by another, the operation scar. Unfortunately scarring in the shoulder region is unpredictable and stretched and keloid scars may occur. The wise surgeon will counsel his patient carefully on the problem before operation and will take all appropriate steps to avoid unsightly postoperative scarring.

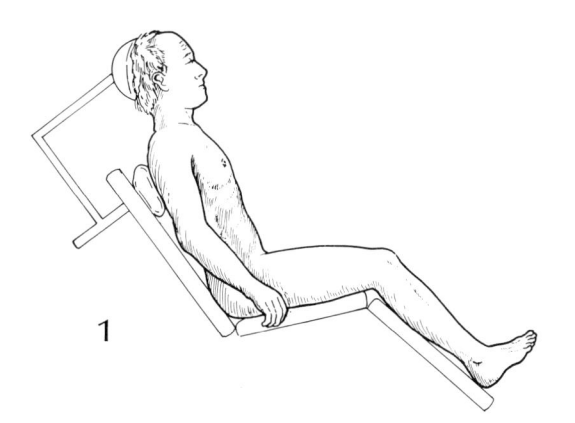

Operations

Position of patient

1

The patient lies supine with the operating table tilted upwards at an angle of around 40° (the deck-chair position). A sandbag is placed under the medial border of the scapula and the patient's head is supported either with a head ring or a neurosurgical head support but with the neck laterally flexed to the opposite side.

688   Shoulder

Incisions

2a, b & c

The author recommends one of two incisions – either (a) a vertical parasagittal incision which provides excellent access to the acromioclavicular joint and the deltoid muscle, or (b) a posterior coronally-directed incision which lies behind the acromioclavicular joint, provides less good access but is a very good cosmetic incision for females because it lies on the top of the shoulder and is usually not visible from in front or behind. Every attempt should be made to retain the continuity of the cloak of anterior muscles – the trapezius above and the deltoid below. The deeper approach to the acromioclavicular joint is through a vertical incision in the line of the muscle fibres and then through the joint.

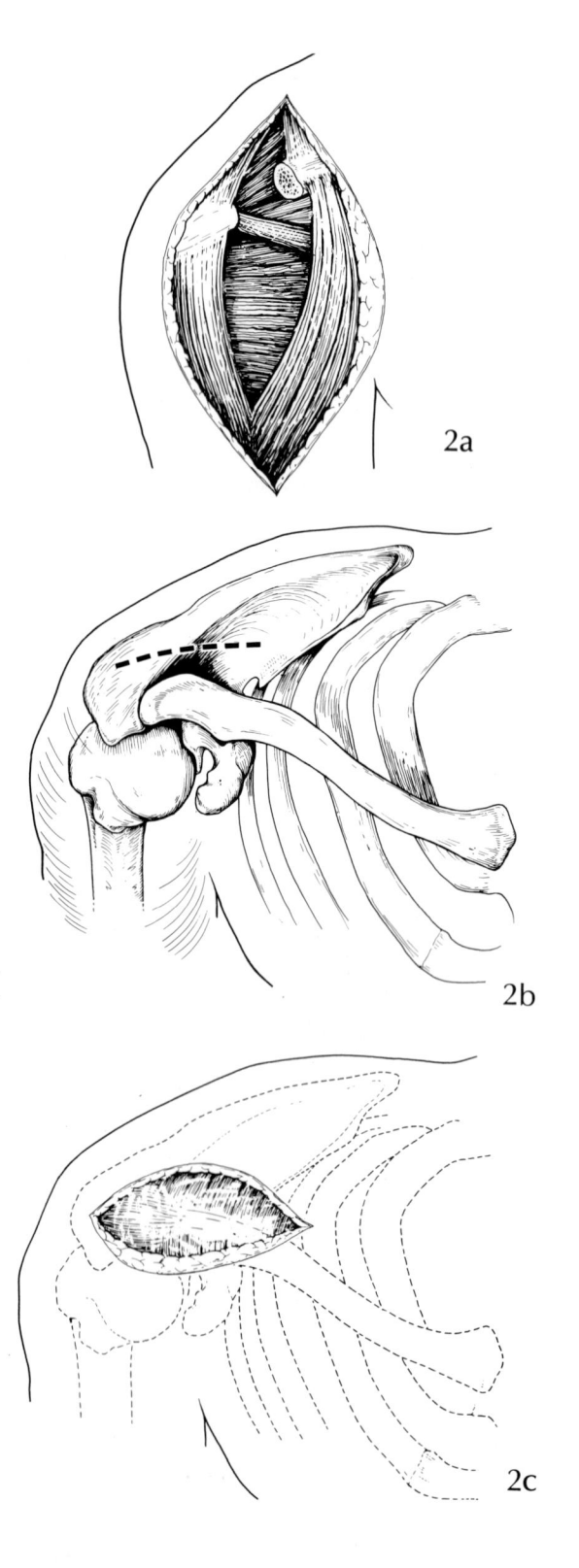

REDUCTION AND INTERNAL STABILIZATION

Open reduction

3

Under vision the acromioclavicular joint should be reduced after the necessary dissection and freeing-up of the soft tissues. Once the clavicle is fully reduced – with no step on inspection from the front and with the front edge of the clavicle matching the anterior edge of the acromion – the position should be held temporarily with one smooth K-wire inserted under power from the lateral end of the acromion, across the acromioclavicular joint into the clavicle.

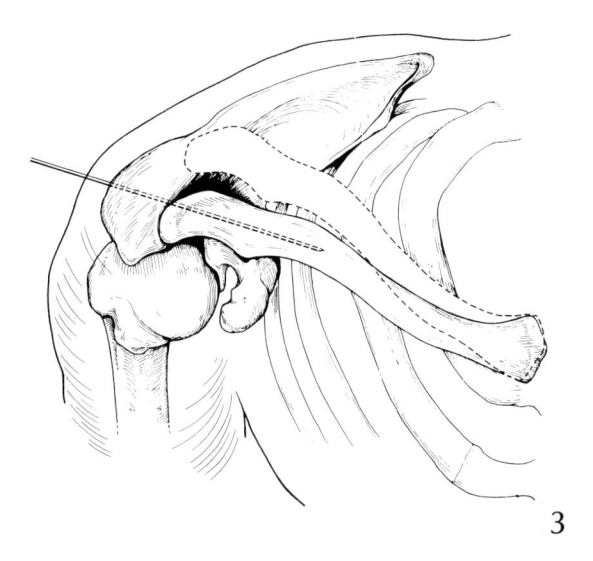

Stabilization with a coracoclavicular screw

4

This method is modified from the technique described originally by Bosworth[10]. The surgeon's index finger is passed through the vertical incision in the deltoid to palpate the coracoid and locate its position. The screw is to be positioned starting from the posterior part of the clavicle 4 cm from its lateral end and passing forward and downward to insert into the base of the coracoid. This is a difficult screw to position correctly and does require some experience. A 4.5 mm hole is first drilled in the clavicle and then a 3.2 mm drill is passed through this hole and the base of the coracoid is 'felt' with the tip of the drill while the surgeon's index finger again locates the tip of the coracoid manually. A 3.2 mm hole is now drilled into the base of the coracoid. A 4.5 mm AO screw of suitable length and with a large washer is now inserted through the hole and screwed into the coracoid until it starts to compress the clavicle onto the coracoid. The temporary K-wire fixation is now removed and the acromioclavicular joint inspected. The screw is adjusted and when stabilization appears satisfactory a check radiograph is taken to ensure the screw position is satisfactory and the radiological appearance is acceptable.

Soft tissue reconstruction should now be carried out around the joint, firmly repairing the superior acromioclavicular ligaments with the local soft tissues and finally ensuring a full repair of the deltoid and the trapezius with synthetic absorbable sutures.

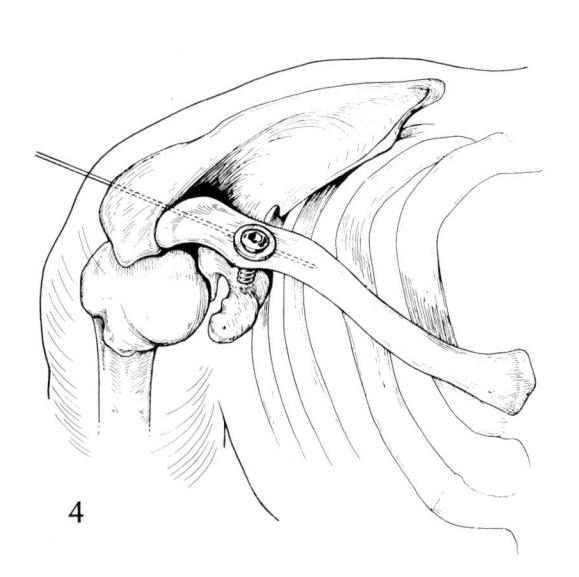

WEAVER–DUNN TECHNIQUE FOR CHRONIC DISLOCATIONS

5

The lateral end of the clavicle is exposed through a deep vertical incision and, after creating a soft tissue curtain of periosteum with trapezius above and deltoid below in continuity and with sharp dissection, that curtain is gradually pushed back medially from the lateral 2 cm of the clavicle. Using an oscillating saw, a bevelled cut is made, removing the lateral 2 cm of the clavicle and leaving the clavicle longer superiorly. A large (4.5 mm) drill hole is made in the lateral end of the clavicle to accommodate the coracoacromial ligament and two vertical 2 mm drill holes are inserted vertically through the superior cortex of the clavicle into the previously drilled hole. The freed acromial end of the coracoacromial ligament is now anchored with a No 2 non-absorbable suture using a Kessler or Bunnell tendon suture technique, and the suture ends passed through the 2 mm drill holes – thus opposing the coracoacromial ligament to the cut end of the clavicle. The suture is pulled tight, the lateral end of the clavicle is thus reduced and the suture tied. The deltoid and trapezius are now meticulously reconstructed using synthetic absorbable sutures.

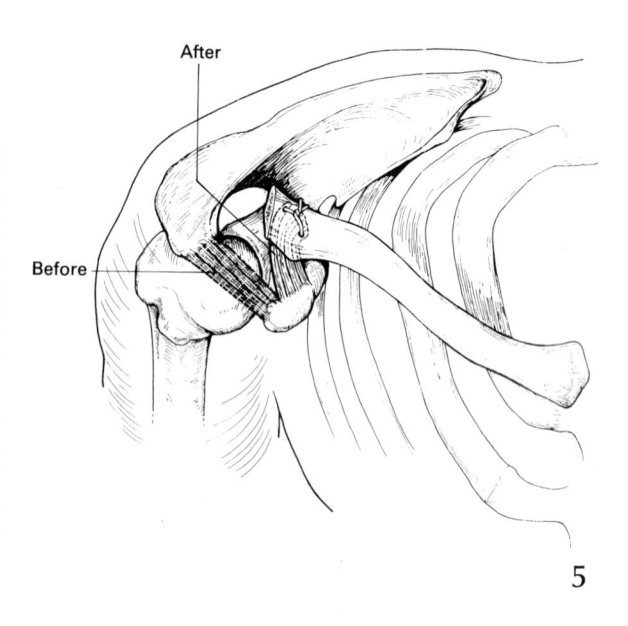

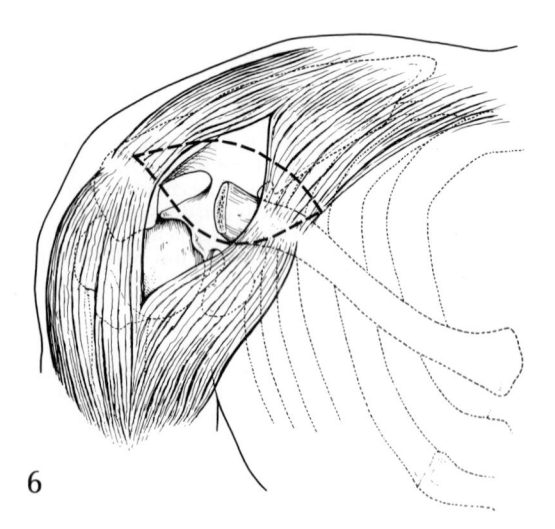

RESECTION OF THE LATERAL 1 CM OF THE CLAVICLE

6

The lateral end of the clavicle is exposed through a deep vertical incision and, after creating a soft tissue curtain of periosteum with trapezius above and deltoid below in continuity, the curtain is dissected back using sharp dissection to expose the lateral 1 cm of the clavicle. Using an oscillating saw with the blade parallel to the plane of the acromioclavicular joint an osteotomy is made which allows the lateral articular end of the clavicle to be removed.

Closure

For all procedures a careful and complete reattachment of the deltoid to the trapezius, with a resulting reinforcement of the repair of the new acromioclavicular joint, is essential. The subcutaneous tissues are approximated with interrupted absorbable sutures and the skin wound is closed with a subcuticular 2/0 polypropylene suture followed by adhesive wound closure strips to protect the healing wound from broadening. A broad arm sling (or Mastersling) is used for 2–3 weeks and mobilization of the shoulder carried out thereafter. For patients with a coracoclavicular screw in place, mobilization of the arm should be restricted to below shoulder level (i.e. 90° elevation) until after the screw is removed at 6–8 weeks after stabilization.

References

1. Bannister GC. The management of complete acromioclavicular dislocation: a randomised prospective controlled trial comparing early movement with coracoclavicular screw fixation. MCh Orth Thesis, University of Liverpool, 1983.

2. Dias JJ, Steingold RF, Richardson RA, Tesfayohannes B, Gregg PJ. The conservative treatment of acromioclavicular dislocation: review after five years. J Bone Joint Surg [Br] 1987; 69-B: 719–22.

3. Imatani RJ, Hanlon JJ, Cady GW. Acute, complete acromioclavicular separation. J Bone Joint Surg [Am] 1975; 57-A: 328–32.

4. Glick JM, Milburn LJ, Haggerty JF, Nishimoto D. Dislocated acromioclavicular joint: follow-up study of 35 unreduced acromioclavicular dislocations. Am J Sports Med 1977; 5: 264–70.

5. Allman FL. Fractures and ligamentous injuries of the clavicle and its articulation. J Bone Joint Surg [Am] 1967; 49-A: 774–84.

6. Bannister GC, Wallace WA, Stableforth PG, Hutson MA. The management of acute acromioclavicular dislocation. J Bone Joint Surg [Br] 1989; 71-B: 848–50.

7. Taylor GM, Tooke M. Degeneration of the acromioclavicular joint as a cause of shoulder pain. J Bone Joint Surg [Br] 1977; 59-B: 507.

8. Weaver JK, Dunn HK. Treatment of acromioclavicular injuries, especially complete acromioclavicular separation. J Bone Joint Surg [Am] 1972; 54-A: 1187–94.

9. Warren-Smith CD, Ward MW. Operation for acromioclavicular dislocation: a review of 29 cases treated by one method. J Bone Joint Surg [Br] 1987; 69-B: 715–8.

10. Bosworth BM. Acromioclavicular separation: a new method of repair. Surg Gynecol Obstet 1941; 73: 866–71.

Illustrations by Gillian Oliver

Arthroscopy of the shoulder

J. I. L. Bayley FRCS
Consultant Orthopaedic Surgeon, Royal National Orthopaedic Hospital, Stanmore, Middlesex, UK

Introduction

Shoulder arthroscopy is now established as a useful diagnostic and operative technique. In resistant shoulder pain and obscure instability, the clinical diagnosis may be altered in up to half the cases depending on the type and site of the pathology. In cases of shoulder pain in which no clinical diagnosis can be made with any confidence, arthroscopy reveals the diagnosis in two-thirds. The global results of anterior repair for unstable shoulders using arthroscopic techniques have been disappointing and the method is only applicable when there is a significant Bankart's labral detachment. On the other hand the results of anterior acromioplasty by arthroscopic techniques have been generally encouraging.

This chapter will only describe the technique of diagnostic arthroscopy of the shoulder, which deserves more general application.

Operation

Position

1

The patient is placed in the lateral position and the arm is draped free following skin preparation. For diagnostic arthroscopy the arm is not immobilized in traction but is held by an assistant so as to allow free movement. Preparation and draping are routine.

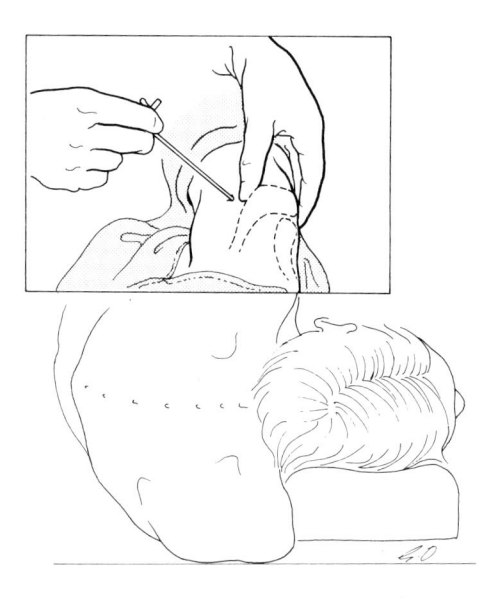

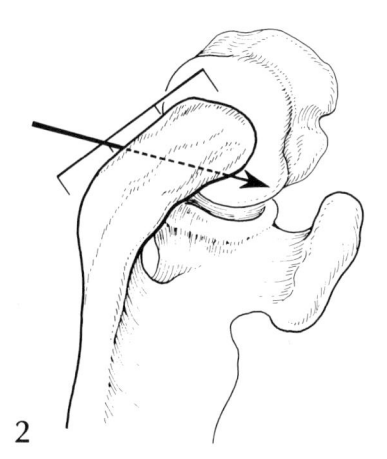

Approach to subacromial space

2

An attempt must be made in all cases to inspect the subacromial space. The arthroscope is introduced 'dry' just under the lateral border of the acromion at the junction of the posterior and middle thirds. Preinjection of irrigant should not be carried out since, if the needle does not enter the bursal space, injected fluid will collapse the walls of the bursa, making subsequent entry of the arthroscope difficult. The sharp trocar is used to penetrate the deltoid and then, using a blunt obturator, the arthroscope is advanced towards the acromioclavicular joint until a tell-tale 'give' in resistance is felt.

The telescope is introduced but irrigation is only begun under direct vision, since the arthroscope may be 'perched' at the bursal wall which can still be collapsed by fluid egress into surrounding areolar tissue. Under vision there is an opportunity to advance the arthroscope into the bursal space as irrigation begins. Using this technique it is possible, after suitable experience, to enter a defined bursal space in 80 per cent of cases. Separate irrigation for simple diagnosis is not usually required.

Arthroscopic appearances – subacromial space

The superficial surface of the supraspinatus tendon is easily seen and is usually smooth with no disruption of the bursal floor. The greater tuberosity, the deep surface of the anterior acromion and the coracoacromial ligament are all easily identified (Plate 1*). The deep surface of the acromioclavicular joint can only be seen when the bursal cavity extends sufficiently far medially.

The superficial surface of the supraspinatus tendon and the deep surface of the anterior acromion are visibly roughened in cases of 'impingement'. Sometimes flap tears may occur. They can be assessed by probing with a needle (Plate 2). Subtle changes can be appreciated which defy diagnosis by available imaging techniques.

Glenohumeral appearances

Glenohumeral joint arthroscopy should be preceded by examination under anaesthetic to assess laxity of the shoulder expressed as a percentage of the humeral head diameter. However, the technique is subjective and the presence of increased humeral head glide demonstrates laxity but does not imply symptomatic instability. The arthroscope is introduced via a posterior portal after preinjection of irrigant. The portal is placed a thumb's breadth below and a thumb's breadth medial to the posterior angle of the acromion. The arthroscope is introduced into the empty space between the humeral head and the glenoid, which can be appreciated by gliding the humeral head backwards and forwards on the glenoid by the thumb and forefinger placed astride the shoulder. The instrument is advanced down to the shoulder capsule with the sharp obturator, which is changed to the blunt obturator in order to penetrate the joint. A common mistake is to skid medially off the back of the scapular neck.

If there is some doubt as to the exact position of the glenohumeral joint line, the arthroscope with the blunt obturator can be used to 'palpate' the rim of the glenoid and the humeral head. It is then a simple matter to puncture the capsule in the space between the two. Having entered the joint, the obturator is changed for a standard 30° telescope. An outflow portal is only introduced for diagnostic arthroscopy if there is troublesome bleeding. Generally the field can be kept clear using hydrostatic distension with irrigant.

The origin of the biceps tendon from the supraglenoid tubercle provides the central reference point from which the inspection is begun (Plates 3 and 4). The tendon can be followed over the humeral head and into the bicipital sulcus, noting any degenerative, inflammatory or mechanical changes (Plates 5 and 6). The deep surface of the cuff can then be scanned when any deep surface disruption will be readily apparent.

The arthroscope is next advanced into the anterior compartment and the glenohumeral ligament complex inspected (Plate 7). The anterior glenoid rim is easily seen and any labral detachment is readily demonstrated. If necessary a hook or probe can be inserted through the 'quiet area' of the rotator interval just in front of and below the anterior acromion.

Next the arthroscope is swept around the glenoid rim into the inferior axillary recess. An assessment is made of any anteroinferior or inferior capsular pouch and the posteroinferior glenoid rim is inspected for signs of attrition which would indicate posterior instability (Plate 8). The instrument is then drawn through the posterior compartment, during which process an inspection of the posterior surface of the humeral head can be made (Plate 9). Subtle defects in the articular surface can be seen which would not be visible radiographically but which confirm the presence of anterior instability.

Finally, an assessment is made of the articular surfaces and the synovium. Early osteoarthritis causing shoulder stiffness can be differentiated from the frozen shoulder syndrome. Localized synovitis in the superior glenohumeral joint space, apparently a 'forme fruste' of the frozen shoulder syndrome, can be readily appreciated (Plate 10). It does not cause limitation of movement but can present with a typical subacromial painful arc syndrome which mimics supraspinatus impingement.

Postoperative management

After removing the arthroscope, sterile wound closure strips are applied to the skin portals and covered with a waterproof dressing. These are left in situ for 5 days. The shoulder is rested in a collar and cuff for 24 hours before allowing unrestricted activity.

*Colour plates 1–10 are on pages 695–696.

Arthroscopy of the shoulder

Plate 1. The superficial surface of the supraspinatus tendon can be seen in the lower part of the field. It is smooth and without bursal floor disruption.

Plate 2. The superficial surface of the supraspinatus tendon has clearly been disrupted by impingement on the undersurface of the anterior acromion, where there are also signs of wear. There is a partial thickness flap tear of the tendon which is being examined for size and mobility with a needle probe.

Plate 3. The right glenohumeral joint has been entered from the posterior aspect. The origin of the long head of biceps tendon can be seen from the supraglenoid tubercle. This is the reference point from which to begin inspection of the joint.

Plate 4. The biceps tendon has been followed through the superior glenohumeral space to the biceps sulcus, where it can be inspected in more detail by manoeuvring the draped arm.

Plate 5. The normal deep surface of the supraspinatus tendon of the left shoulder can be seen with its insertion into the greater tuberosity just behind the biceps sulcus.

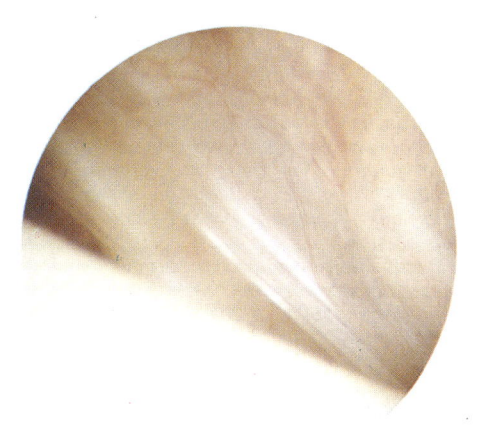

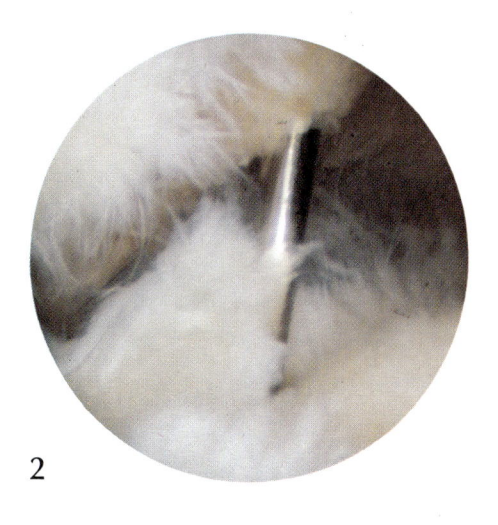

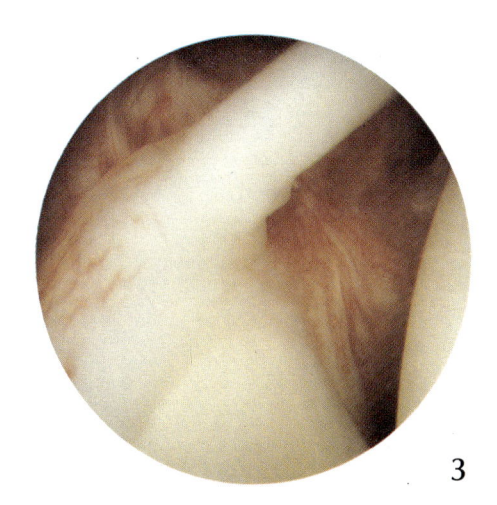

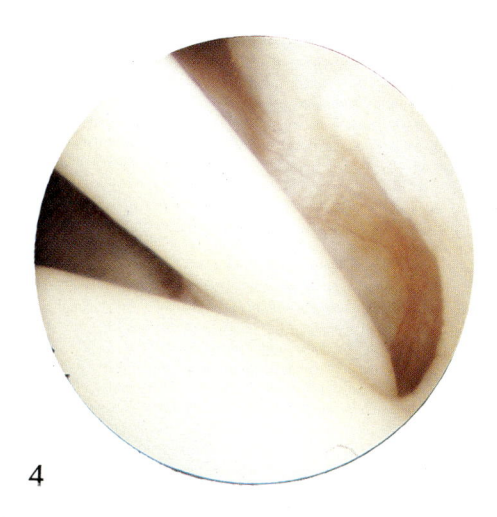

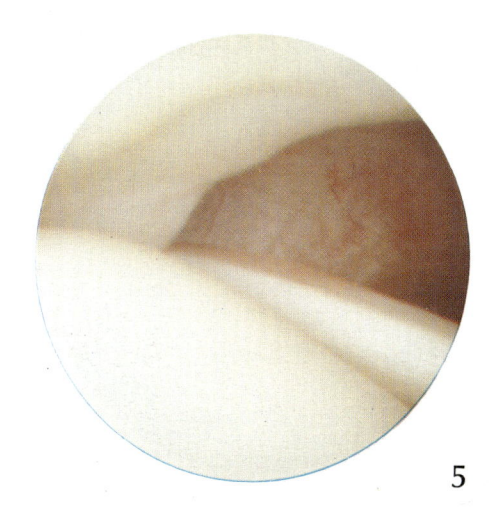

696   Shoulder

Plate 6. In this shoulder there is a deep surface cleft tear at the junction of supraspinatus and infraspinatus.

Plate 7. The right anteroinferior compartment of the glenohumeral joint is demonstrated from the posterior approach. The labrum has been detached from the rim of the glenoid and can be probed using a hook introduced through the 'quiet area' of the rotator interval.

Plate 8. The posteroinferior glenoid rim of the left shoulder has been disrupted as a result of recurrent posterior dislocation.

Plate 9. There is defect in the articular surface of the posterior aspect of the humeral head – a sure sign of post-traumatic anterior instability. In this case the defect was not seen with other imaging techniques because it is very shallow and does not broach the subchondral bone plate.

Plate 10. The superior compartment of the left glenohumeral joint is seen. There is a chronic low grade synovitis. The patient presented with a painful arc syndrome with no limitation of movement and elsewhere in the joint the synovium was not involved. Note the normal appearance of the humeral head and biceps tendon.

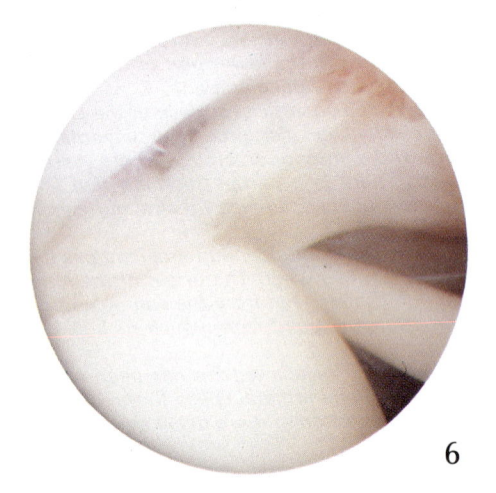

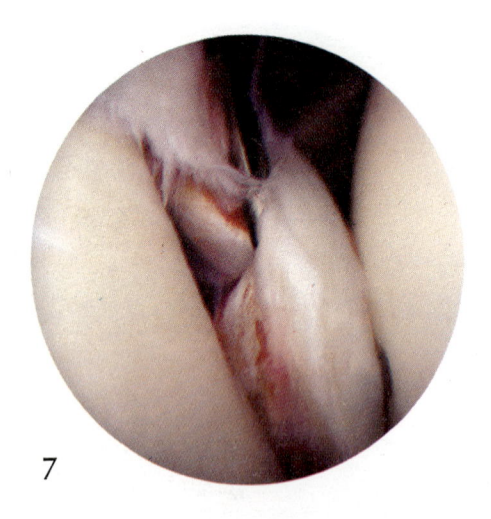

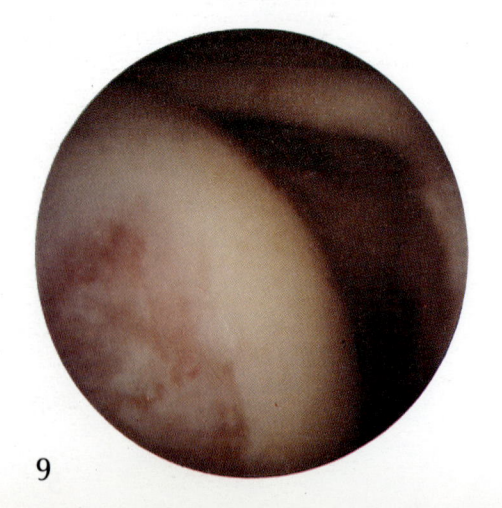

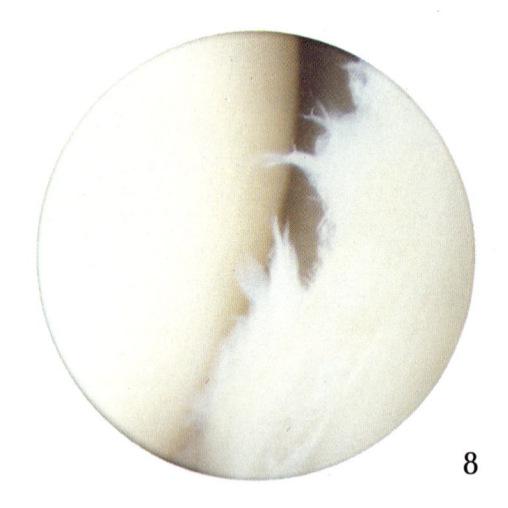

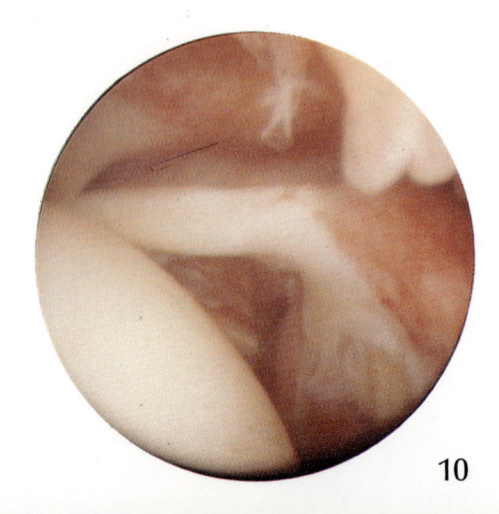

Illustrations by Gillian Oliver

Rotator cuff repair

J. I. L. Bayley FRCS
Consultant Orthopaedic Surgeon, Royal National Orthopaedic Hospital, Stanmore, Middlesex, UK

Introduction

The main aim of rotator cuff repair is to relieve pain, but operation may be indicated to restore a severe functional deficit or to preserve future function, particularly in a younger patient with an acute tear. Pain relief is generally good but restoration of function depends largely on the size and chronicity of the tear and the state of the tissues. Nevertheless, although global tears are the most taxing, repair can give surprisingly satisfactory results and is well worthwhile, provided pain and dysfunction are sufficient to justify the necessary prolonged rehabilitation.

The need for repair is determined by the extent and nature of the rupture. Longstanding attrition of the supraspinatus tendon beneath the anterior acromion may wear a small hole in the tendon with thickened margins such that rotator cuff function, though vitiated by pain, remains mechanically competent. In such cases it may suffice to decompress the tendon by anterior acromioplasty, particularly if the procedure is carried out arthroscopically. In large ruptures, however, where a substantial segment of tendon insertion has given way as a result of trauma in the young, or avascular degeneration in the older patient, the rotator cuff is rendered incompetent and repair is required. The outcome depends upon patient selection and surgical planning. The patient must be prepared to co-operate in a carefully controlled rehabilitation regime and to wait an average of 9 months before achieving full benefit from the surgery. Surgical planning involves the design and choice of an appropriate surgical approach to the subacromial region and selection of a suitable technique of repair.

Two surgical exposures are available to address the spectrum of pathology. Small or acute defects can be repaired through an anterior deltoid splitting incision such as might be used for a simple subacromial decompression. Large or chronic retracted defects are more easily dealt with via an approach which splits the acromion in the plane of the scapula. Preoperative assessment of the size of the rupture is therefore important; loss and weakness of active lateral rotation are useful clinical indicators of a significant cuff disruption.

Operation

Surgical exposure

1 & 2

The basic principle of any approach to the subacromial space is the preservation of trapeziodeltoid continuity. In the anterior approach, the skin is incised in a line which a bra-strap might occupy and deepened to the areolar tissue over the clavicle and deltoid epimysium. A full-thickness flap is developed as far lateral as the outer border of the acromion. The deltoid is now split in the line of its fibres for a distance of not more than 5 cm from the acromio-clavicular joint.

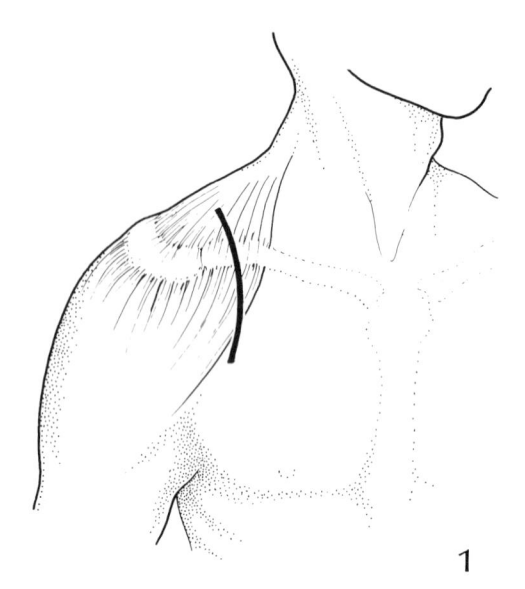

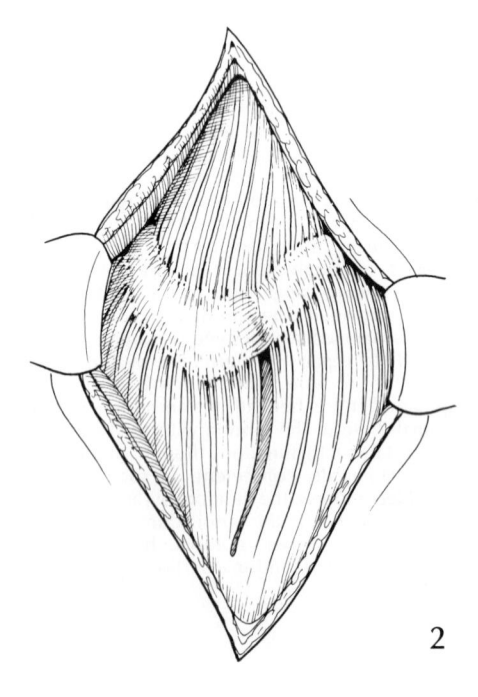

3

If it is intended to excise the acromioclavicular joint, the incision is extended proximally through the joint into trapezius. The acromial branch of the acromiothoracic artery requires coagulation where it runs anterior to the acromioclavicular joint deep to deltoid before exposing the coracoacromial ligament. An aponeurotic flap is now developed by sharp dissection over the acromion which carries deltoid with it and allows exposure of the anterior acromion part way along its lateral border. It is preferable to create an osteoperiosteal flap with an osteotome rather than risk compromising trapeziodeltoid continuity by tearing a thinning aponeurotic flap. A medial flap can be developed over the clavicle if excision of the acromio-clavicular joint is to be carried out either for access, cuff decompression, or treatment of an associated intrinsic acromioclavicular joint osteoarthritis.

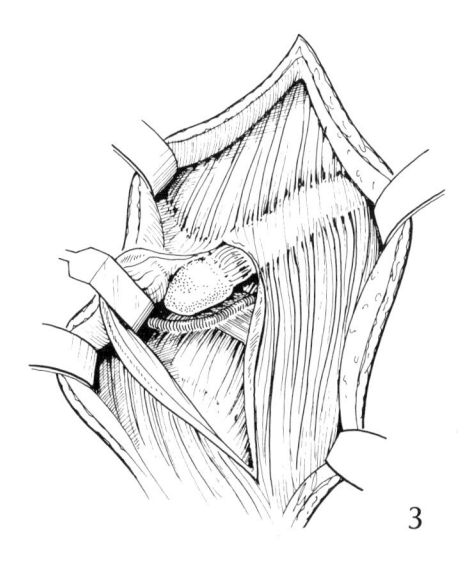

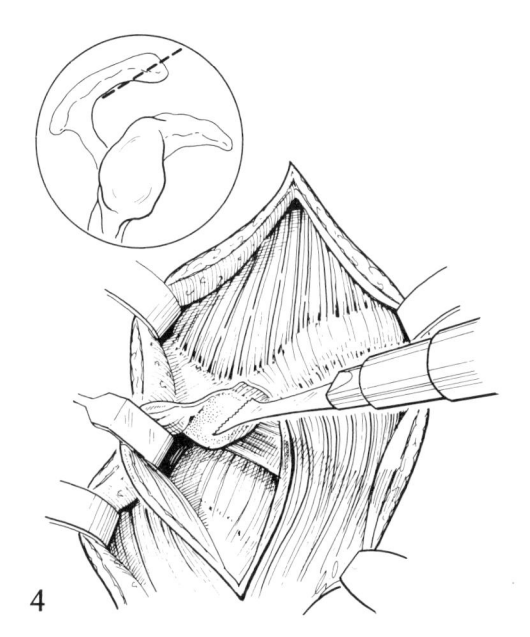

4

An anterior undercutting acromioplasty is now carried out with a reciprocating power saw, aiming to remove the hooked part of the anterior acromion and creating a flattened undersurface to the acromion with an upward slope from back to front.

700 Shoulder

5

If the outer end of the clavicle is to be excised it should be accomplished in a line running posteromedially – in order to avoid a prominent posterolateral corner to the residual stub of clavicle – and by undercutting to create deep space for the rotator cuff whilst preserving an acromioclavicular arch for deltoid purchase.

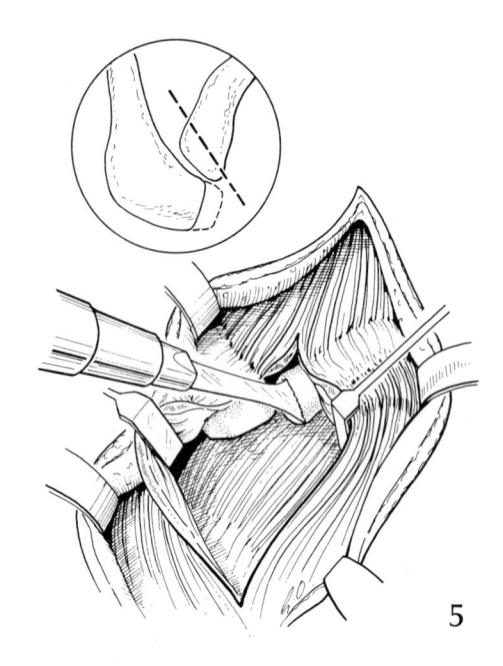

6

Large chronic cuff defects are better exposed through a more laterally disposed incision. The skin incision passes across the point of the shoulder in the line of the scapula and is developed to expose trapezius and deltoid.

7 & 8

After raising osteoperiosteal flaps the acromion is divided with a reciprocating saw in the line of the scapular blade, such that the osteotomy exits on the lateral border of the acromion at the point where it is intersected by a line extrapolated along the anterior border of the clavicle. By this technique, after enucleation of the anterior fragment of acromion and closure of the aponeurosis, the soft tissues bridge between the clavicle and acromion in such a way that the mechanical leverage of deltoid is reduced by no more than the distance the anterior acromion projected forwards beyond the line of the clavicle. After splitting trapezius and deltoid in the same line over no more than a 5 cm length distally to avoid the circumflex nerve and 3 cm proximally, division of the subacromial bursa will allow the cuff defect to be defined.

Having determined by preliminary inspection that repair is possible, the anterior fragment of acromion should be enucleated in the manner of a patellectomy from its aponeurosis by sharp dissection in order to improve access and to decompress the subsequent repair. Often the outer end of the clavicle also requires undercutting.

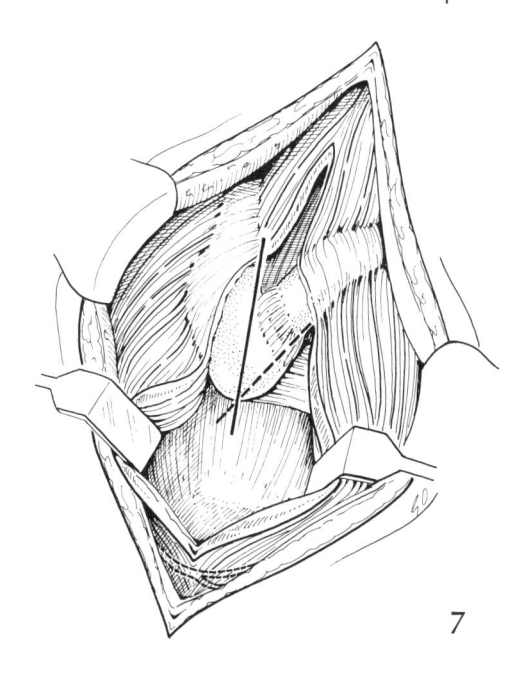

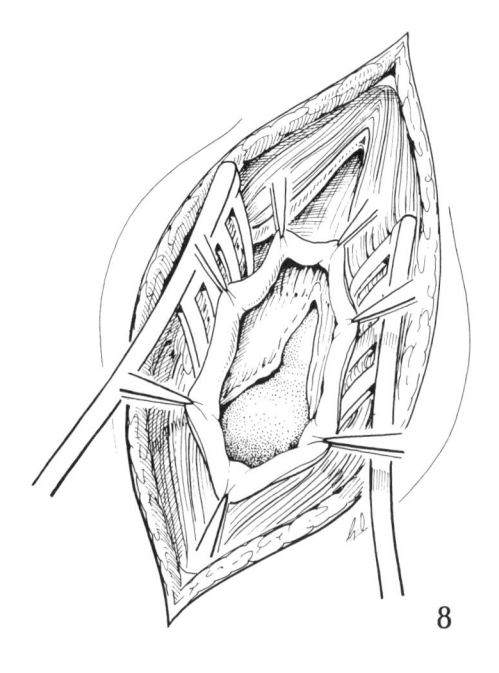

Repair

The principles of the repair are constant whichever approach is used. Firstly, a retracted cuff should be mobilized in order to bring it back towards its original insertion. Next, the fibrotic edges of the defect should be excised if possible to bleeding tissue, and finally the cuff should be resutured into a trough cut as close to the original insertion as possible and commensurate with allowing the arm to come close to the trunk without disrupting the repair. Associated splits are closed side-to-side.

Mobilization is usually not required in small or fresh tears but in chronic lesions there may be marked retraction. Bursal adhesions are first divided by sharp dissection whilst exerting traction on the cuff via stay sutures. Next, the coracohumeral ligament may require release from its coracoid attachment, and finally the transacromial approach allows a complete circumferential capsulotomy around the glenoid rim. Only in the presence of marked loss of cuff substance do these three manoeuvres fail to mobilize a retracted cuff sufficient to allow repair.

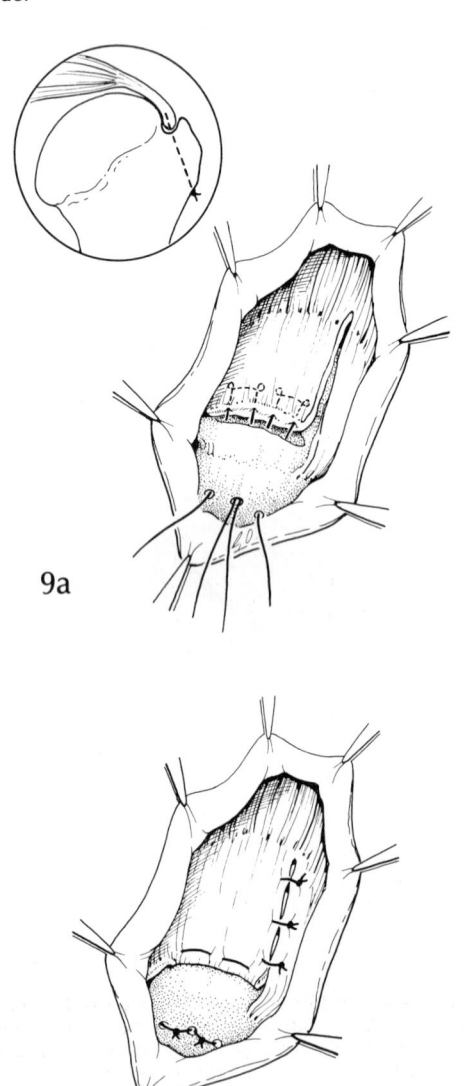

9a & b

Most tears are due to a combination of disinsertion and a longitudinal split. The pattern of each lesion should be studied to decide the correct method of repair. The disinserted segment is repaired into a trough cut into the greater tuberosity at the humeral articular margin, using a braided synthetic non-absorbable suture in a Kessler pattern stitch. The sutures are passed through drill holes in the base of the trough and tied over the outer cortex of the tuberosity. Any longitudinal component is sutured side-to-side. The repair does not need to be water-tight but should be secure when the arm is brought down to within 15° of the trunk.

In chronic tears, when loss of tendon substance and length may prevent direct reinsertion into the greater tuberosity, it is a mistake to cut the trough so far medial that it encroaches into the articular surface of the humerus. In the absence of proven artificial tendon substitutes, several reconstructive procedures have been described. None has proved to be markedly superior but in general it is better to use local tissue whenever possible. Two such procedures have stood the test of time.

BICEPS TENODESIS

The intra-articular tendon of the long head of biceps is sectioned at the level of the biceps sulcus. The distal portion is tenodesed to soft tissues within the sulcus and the proximal stump, still attached to the supraglenoid tubercle, is sutured into the trough and used as a spacer between supraspinatus and infraspinatus. The procedure sacrifices the humeral head depressing action of the biceps muscle, but in extreme cases the net gain is worthwhile.

SUBSCAPULARIS AND INFRASPINATUS TENDON TRANSPOSITION

10a & b

In a proportion of cases, despite marked retraction and loss of cuff tendon superiorly, the anterior and posterior tissues remain intact. Although it is important to preserve functioning cuff at the front and back, the upper half of these cuff remnants can be spared for transfer to the superior aspect of the humeral head to distribute cuff action equally around the articular circumference. The transposed tendons are sutured as earlier described into a trough cut in the greater tuberosity. The V-shaped defect between them can often be filled with the retracted stump of supraspinatus.

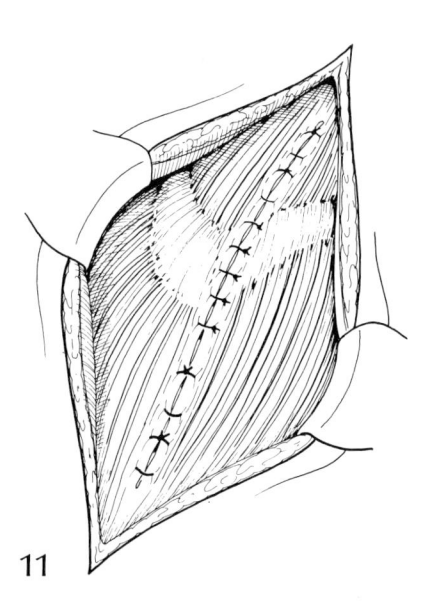

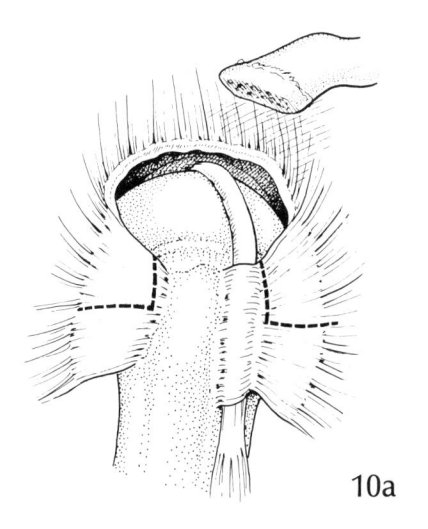

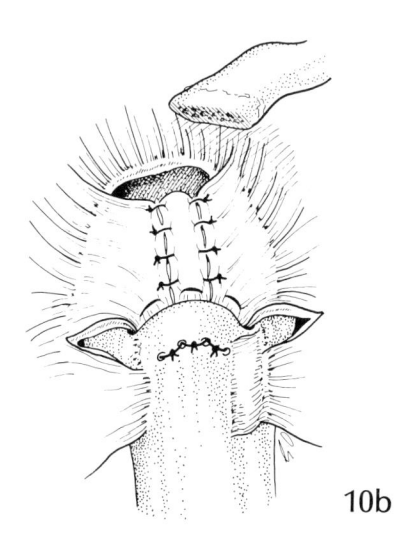

Wound closure

11

The trapeziodeltoid flaps are repaired side-to-side over a suction drain. The muscle layers should be apposed with horizontal – rather than vertical – mattress sutures through the epimysial layer to avoid muscle infarction.

704 Shoulder

Postoperative management

12 & 13

Pending tendon healing, no active use is allowed for 6 or 8 weeks but shoulder mobility is preserved by passive movement. The arm should be maintained in some elevation in order to protect the repair and to encourage blood flow to the tendon. Initially, therefore, the limb is supported in a roller towel whilst postoperative discomfort settles and, after 3–5 days is placed on a foam abduction wedge with which the patient is discharged home.

Passive mobilization into elevation is continued until 6 or 8 weeks from operation, when the abduction wedge is discarded and assisted active exercises are started. Thereafter shoulder control is progressively but gradually developed over the ensuing months. It is much better to aim for slow but steady progress rather than trying to push the shoulder beyond its limits.

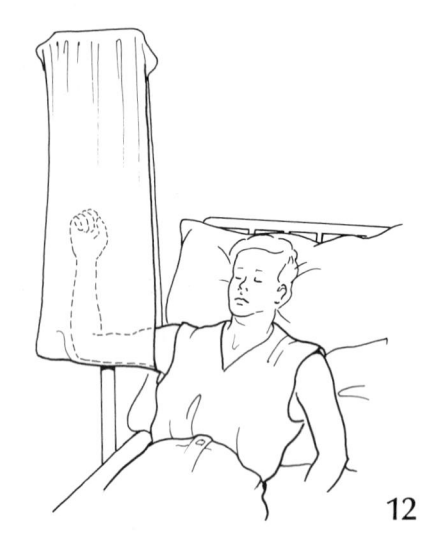

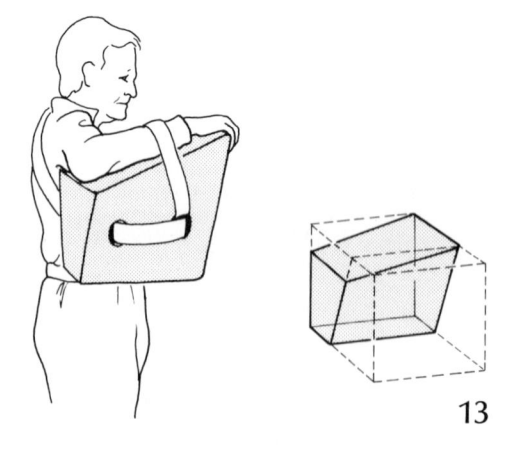

Illustrations by Gillian Oliver after B. Hyams

Operations for Erb's palsy

B. Helal MChOrth, FRCS
Honorary Consultant Orthopaedic Surgeon, The Royal London Hospital and The Royal National Orthopaedic Hospital, London, and Enfield Group of Hospitals, UK

S. C. Chen FRCS
Consultant Orthopaedic Surgeon, Enfield Group of Hospitals, UK

Introduction

Erb's palsy[1] is an upper brachial plexus birth palsy, in which the shoulder girdle muscles, especially the supraspinatus and infraspinatus muscles, are affected and a medial rotation and adduction deformity of the shoulder develops. The subscapularis muscle which functions normally becomes contracted as a result of its action being unopposed. There are several operations described for this condition, but the authors consider that Sever's modification[2,3] of Fairbank's operation[4] and the Bateman procedure[5] give satisfactory results.

Operations

SEVER'S MODIFICATION OF FAIRBANK'S OPERATION

Incision

1

An incision is made along the deltopectoral groove from the tip of the coracoid process to the insertion of the deltoid muscle.

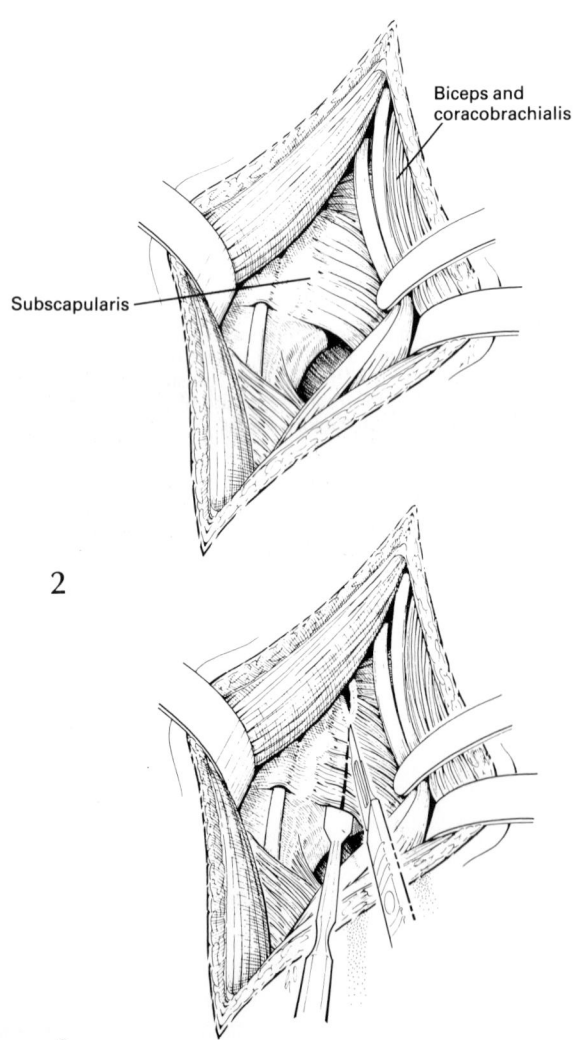

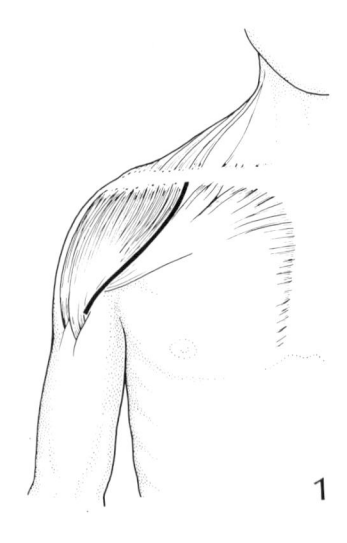

Exposure and release

2 & 3

The pectoralis major muscle is divided parallel to the humerus along the tendinous insertion. The coracobrachialis and short head of the biceps muscles are identified and retracted medially. This exposes the subscapularis muscle. The shoulder is laterally rotated and abducted and the subscapularis muscle cut without cutting the joint capsule by elevating the muscle from the capsule with a MacDonald dissector.

Postoperative management

A shoulder spica is applied with the shoulder abducted and laterally rotated, the elbow flexed to 90°, the forearm in supination and the wrist in a neutral position. The spica is removed after 2 weeks and physiotherapy started – both passive and active exercises.

MUSCLE TRANSFER FOR DELTOID PARALYSIS
(Bateman's operation)

Incision

4

The patient is placed prone. A T-shaped incision is made, the horizontal limb along the acromioclavicular arch and spine of the scapula.

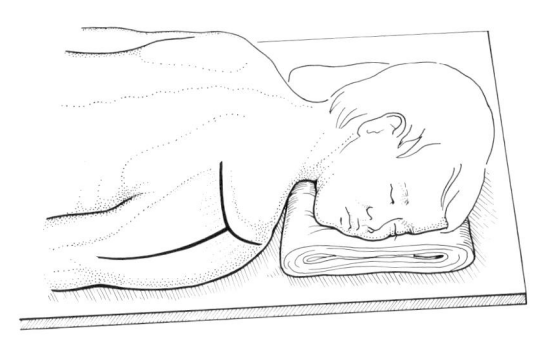

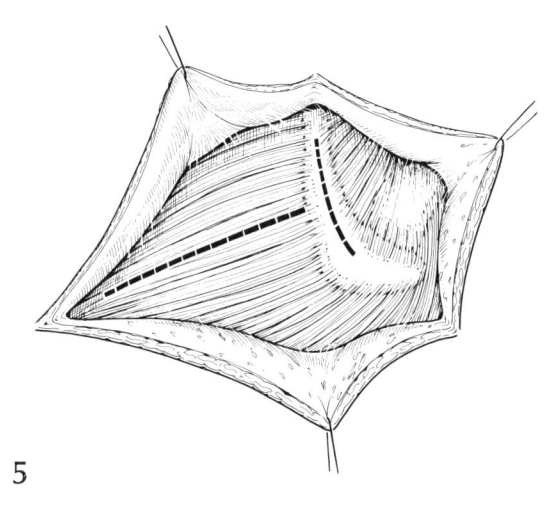

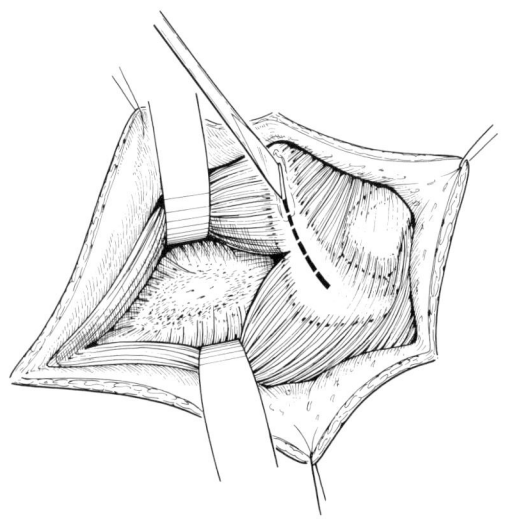

Osteotomy

5 & 6

The atrophied deltoid is exposed by retracting the flaps. The deltoid muscle is split longitudinally and the shoulder joint exposed. The spine of the scapula is osteotomied near its base, in a lateral direction, with the trapezius still attached to it.

The trapezius is detached from the lateral part of the clavicle avoiding damage to the coracoclavicular ligament. The shoulder is abducted to 90°. The lateral aspect of the humerus is freshened near the deltoid insertion.

7

The acromion with the trapezius is pulled over the humeral head and attached with screws to the humerus as close to the deltoid tuberosity as possible.

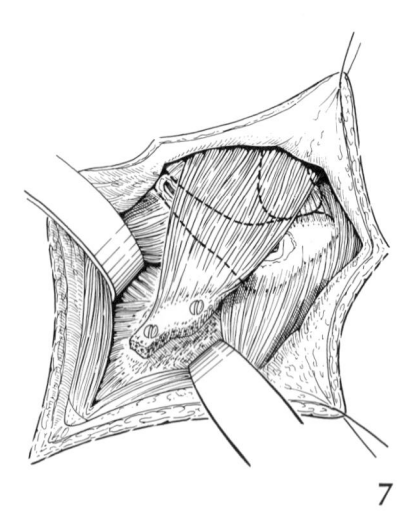

Postoperative management

The arm is immobilized with the shoulder abducted to 90° in a shoulder spica for 6 weeks. Gradually the arm is brought down to the side using an abduction splint. When the acromion has united with the humerus, passive and active exercises are started to re-educate the transferred muscle.

References

1. Erb WH. Ueber eine eigenthümliche Localisation von Lahmungen im Plexus brachialis. *Verh naturh-med Ver Heidelb* 1874–77; n.f., 2: 130–7.

2. Sever JW. Obstetric paralysis. *Am J Dis Child* 1916; 12: 541.

3. Sever JW. The results of a new operation for obstetrical paralysis. *Am J Orthop Surg* 1918; 16: 248–57.

4. Fairbank HAT. Birth palsy: subluxation of the shoulder joint in infants and young children. *Lancet* 1913; 1: 1217.

5. Bateman JE. *The shoulder and environs.* St Louis: Mosby, 1955.

Illustrations by Gillian Oliver after B. Hyams

Rupture of the biceps

B. Helal MChOrth, FRCS
Honorary Consultant Orthopaedic Surgeon, The Royal London Hospital and The Royal National Orthopaedic Hospital, London, and Enfield Group of Hospitals, UK

S. C. Chen FRCS
Consultant Orthopaedic Surgeon, Enfield Group of Hospitals, UK

Introduction

Rupture of the biceps occurs at one of two sites: rupture of the long head of biceps affects the elderly patient, while rupture of the distal tendon of biceps is a lesion of the young.

RUPTURE OF LONG HEAD

This usually causes very little disability in the elderly patient, as the short head of the biceps and the brachialis muscle are intact and can take over elbow flexion. The flexors of the forearm also contribute to this. However, there is some loss of muscle power, as about half the biceps muscle is made inactive by the rupture of the long head. There is, in addition, a slight cosmetic disfigurement as the biceps muscle becomes bunched up in the lower part of the upper arm. In patients who lead a robust life and need normal muscle power, it is necessary to reattach the long head, usually to the short head.

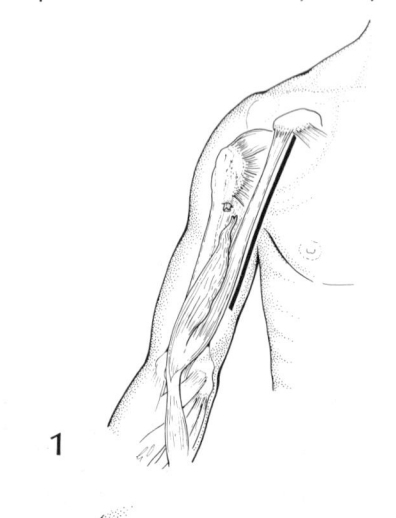

Operation

The elbow is kept flexed at 90° during the operation, to relax the long head of the biceps.

Incision

1

An incision is made along the medial border of the biceps muscle from the tip of the coracoid process to the middle of the upper arm.

Repair

2

The ruptured long head of the biceps is searched for and is usually found crumpled up in the lower and lateral part of the muscle belly of the biceps.

3

The short head of the biceps which is attached, with the coracobrachialis, to the tip of the coracoid process is identified. The long head is pulled proximally until the lateral belly feels the same in consistency as the medial belly of the biceps. The long head is anchored to the short head using three non-absorbable sutures.

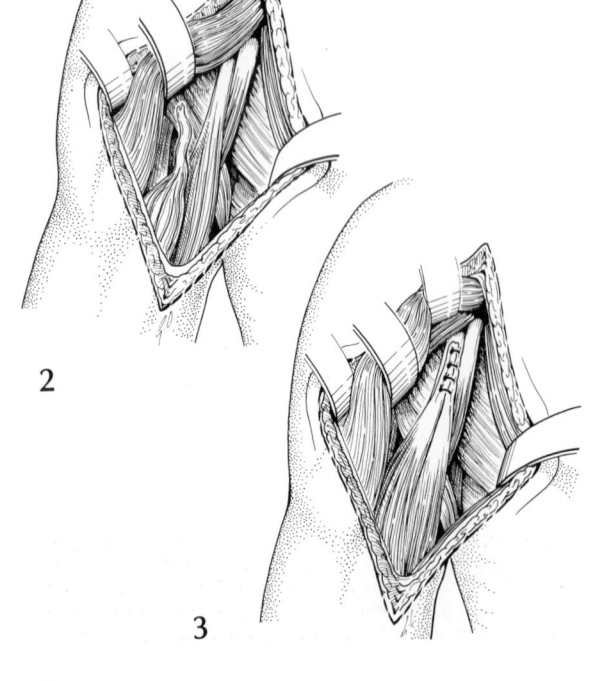

Postoperative management

4

The arm is nursed in a loop sling for 3 weeks. Passive exercise to the shoulder and elbow is started after 1 week.

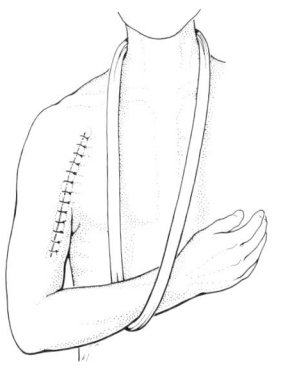

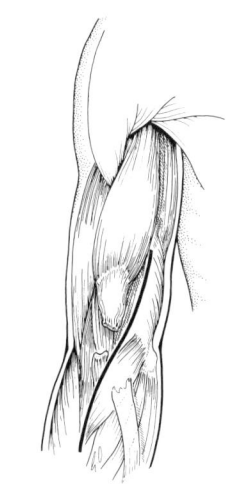

RUPTURE OF DISTAL TENDON

Unlike rupture of the long head, which usually occurs in the older patient and is due to some degeneration of the tendon, rupture of the distal tendon of the biceps occurs in the fit young man after strenuous activity. This lesion results in significant weakness and must therefore be repaired.

Operation

Incision

5

A lazy-S incision is made across the front of the elbow.

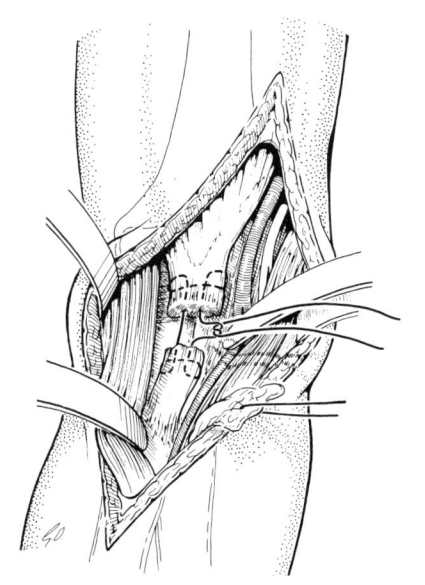

Repair

6

The median nerve and brachial artery must be identified. The ruptured ends of the distal tendon of the biceps are located. If these ends are not shredded, an end-to-end anastomosis of the tendons is performed with the forearm in supination to facilitate easier approximation.

7 & 8

If the tendon ends are frayed, a drill hole is made in the upper end of the radius as near as possible to the bicipital tuberosity. The tendon is threaded through the drill hole and sutured back on itself using non-absorbable sutures.

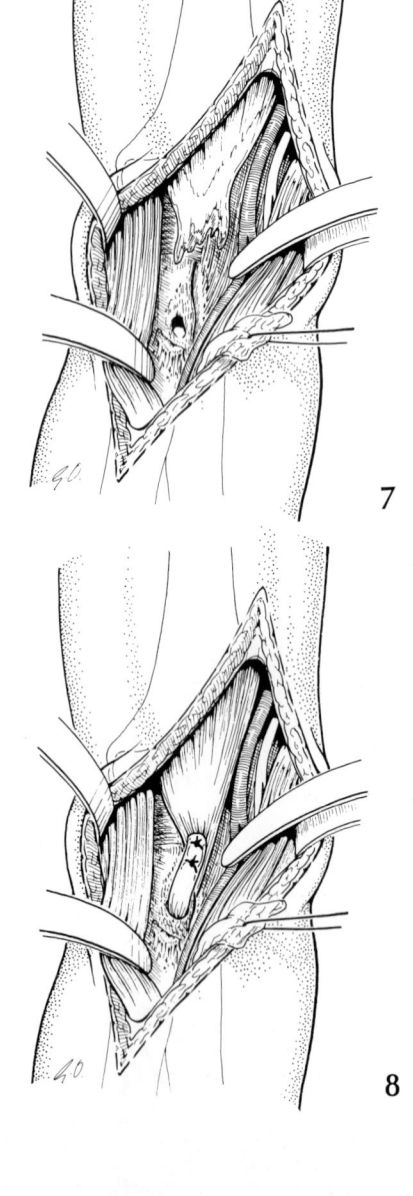

Postoperative management

9

An above-elbow plaster cast is applied to include the wrist and hand. This is removed at the end of 3 weeks and gentle mobilization exercises to the elbow are started.

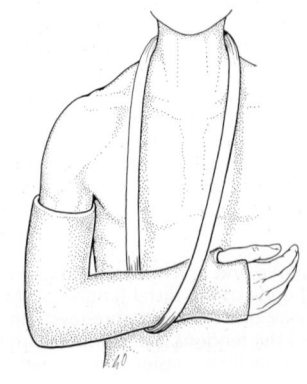

Illustrations by Peter Cox after P. G. Jack

Arthroplasty of the shoulder

Alan Lettin MS, FRCS
Consultant Orthopaedic Surgeon, St Bartholomew's Hospital and Royal National Orthopaedic Hospital, London, UK

Introduction

Indications

Arthroplasty of the shoulder is usually performed to relieve pain and restore a functional range of movement to patients suffering from pain and stiffness of the glenohumeral joint resulting from rheumatoid arthritis, post-traumatic arthritis or primary osteoarthritis. Arthroplasty may also be performed as a primary procedure for fractures and fracture-dislocations of the head of the humerus when they are unsuited to other methods of treatment.

The proximal part of the humerus may also be replaced using a special custom-made prosthesis for resectable tumours.

There are three types of arthroplasty: (1) excision arthroplasty, (2) hemiarthroplasty and (3) total replacement arthroplasty which is either constrained or unconstrained.

Excision arthroplasty

This is occasionally performed as a primary procedure following severe fractures and fracture-dislocations of the head of the humerus, when the rotator cuff is disrupted and the fragments of bone are too comminuted to allow satisfactory reduction and internal fixation. Although an excellent range of passive movement is frequently possible after the operation, active movement is usually poor because of the lack of a stable fulcrum, and movement is frequently painful.

Excision of the head of the humerus and the glenoid may occasionally be employed in the primary treatment of arthritic shoulders, but this has the same disadvantages.

Excision arthroplasty may be necessary when a replacement arthroplasty fails. As a secondary procedure it gives more satisfactory results because the stability of the false joint is improved by the excessive fibrous tissue which forms following the failure of the primary operation.

Hemiarthroplasty

Replacement of the head of the humerus (e.g. with a Neer prosthesis[1]) is best reserved for the early treatment of severe fractures and fracture-dislocations, when the rotator cuff is intact or capable of repair. Without the stability afforded by a functioning rotator cuff, the prosthesis subluxates superiorly on the glenoid and gives a poor result. It is usually unsatisfactory in rheumatoid arthritis.

Total replacement arthroplasty

Total replacement arthroplasty was introduced into modern surgical practice in 1969[2,3]. There are now several prostheses available but basically they fall into two groups, constrained and unconstrained.

In the first group, the glenoid may be replaced by a cup and the head of the humerus by a ball which articulates in the cup (e.g. Stanmore); or the ball is attached to the scapula and the cup is contained by the upper end of the humerus (e.g. Kessel).

The unconstrained replacements (e.g. Neer II) use an anatomically shaped humeral component of appropriate size to replace the head of the humerus and a shallow saucer-shaped ultra-high molecular weight polyethylene component to resurface the glenoid.

Because of their inherent stability, constrained replacements provide a stable fulcrum for muscle action and are not dependent on the rotator cuff for stability. They are therefore more suitable for the treatment of pain and limitation of movement resulting from severe rheumatoid and other forms of arthritis, when the rotator cuff is destroyed and cannot be repaired. When the rotator cuff is intact or repairable, an unconstrained replacement is more satisfactory and is less likely to become loose.

Even without an intact rotator cuff, the pain relief and movement resulting from total replacement arthroplasty are similar for the constrained and unconstrained replacements[4,5].

Preoperative

Position of patient and towelling

The patient lies supine with the affected side towards the edge of the operating table, and a firm oblong sandbag is placed between the shoulder blades. The head is towelled separately with double towels and the trunk and legs completely covered. A separate towel is firmly bandaged around the distal half of the upper arm, forearm and hand, leaving the limb free. The remaining uncovered skin may be conveniently sealed with two medium-sized adhesive drapes, which secure the towels in place.

Operation

Incision

1

The same approach to the shoulder may be used for each prosthesis. The skin and subcutaneous fat are incised from the clavicle to the anterior fold of the axilla, crossing the tip of the coracoid process of the scapula.

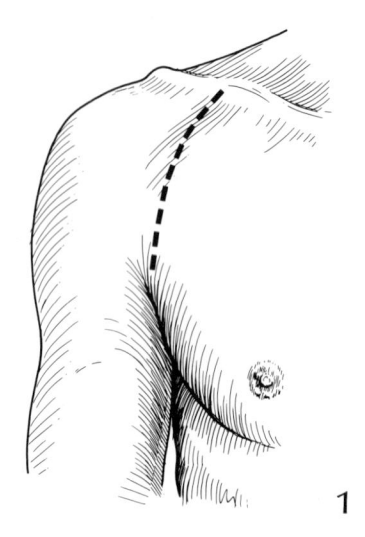

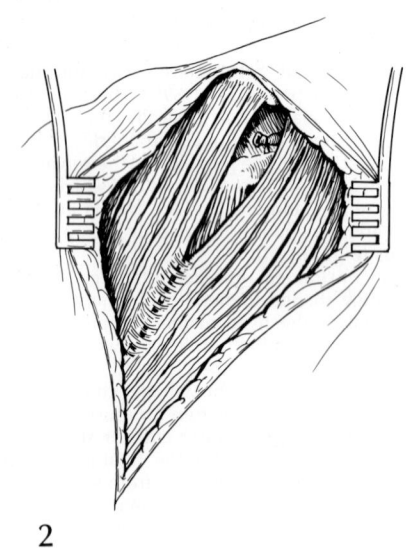

Exposure and development of deltopectoral groove

2

The subcutaneous fat is stripped from the underlying muscle by blunt dissection to expose the cephalic vein, which passes obliquely across the wound as it lies in the deltopectoral groove. This is ligated and divided at the lower margin of the wound and dissected proximally almost to the clavicle, and the tributaries are coagulated as they are divided. The proximal end of the vein is ligated and divided just below the clavicle before it disappears through the clavipectoral fascia. The free segment of the vein is removed to avoid troublesome bleeding later in the operation.

Exposure and division of coracoid process

3

The pectoralis major and deltoid muscles are separated with a self-retaining retractor. When absolutely necessary, exposure may be improved by detaching the clavicular portion of the deltoid from the clavicle as far laterally as the acromioclavicular joint, leaving sufficient muscle attached to the bone to hold sutures during closure. The coracoacromial ligament is divided. Then, after drilling a hole of 3 mm diameter along the centre of the coracoid process to facilitate later reattachment, it is resected with an osteotome or Gigli saw proximal to its muscle attachments.

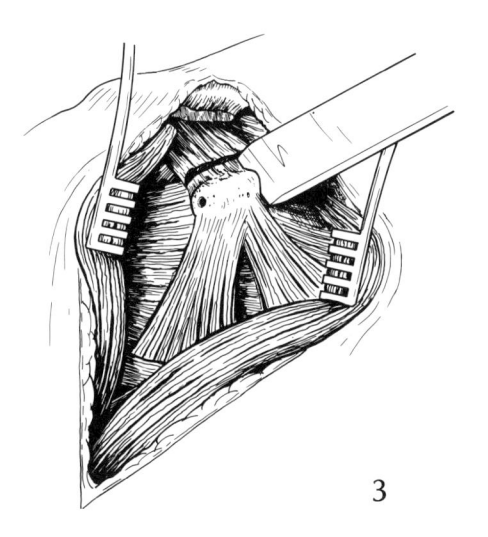

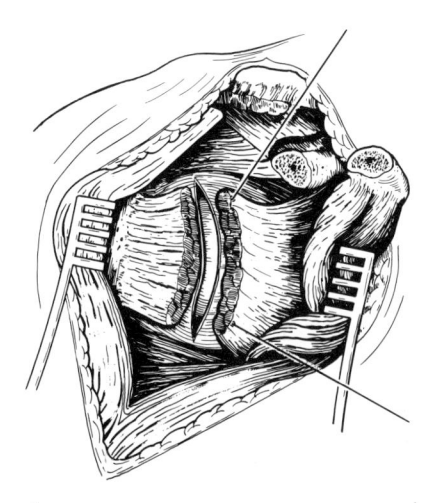

Division of subscapularis and exposure of joint

4

The upper and lower borders of the subscapularis muscle are identified and marked with stay sutures just lateral to the musculotendinous junction. The identification of the lower border is facilitated by the presence of one or more veins running parallel to it. These should be coagulated. The upper margin may be difficult to define. In rheumatoid arthritis, proliferating synovium frequently bulges over the upper border of the subscapularis. The subscapularis is divided through the tendinous part just lateral to the stay sutures and retracted medially. The underlying capsule cannot always be identified as a separate layer, but when it is a definite entity it is also divided and retracted with the muscle.

The supraspinatus or its remnants are identified. If present, they should be separated from the undersurface of the acromion by blunt dissection.

Resection of humeral head and exposure of glenoid

5

The head of the humerus is dislocated forward out of the wound and resected at the level of the articular margin with an osteotome or power saw. If the supraspinatus is intact, this leaves its attachment to the greater tuberosity undisturbed. When the head of the humerus is badly affected by disease then the articular margin may not be clear. When the Neer II prosthesis is used, the trial humeral component is laid alongside the humeral head to enable the level of resection to be marked; this lies at the maximum diameter of the bone. The bone is cut obliquely so the cut face is retroverted 30°–40° with respect to the plane of the humeral condyles and 45° to the long axis of the shaft (see *illustration 8b*). Care should be taken not to remove too much bone.

In the case of a severely comminuted fracture which cannot be reconstructed, the fragments are removed and the humerus trimmed as near as possible to the ideal plane of resection.

For excision arthroplasty no more need be done.

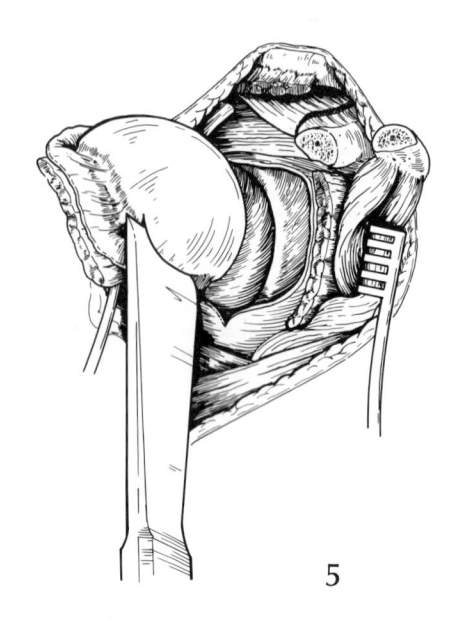

Preparation of the humerus and replacement of head of humerus alone

6

The medullary cavity at the centre of the cut surface is located and the loose cancellous bone removed with a curette from the upper end of the humerus; the debris is washed out. The prosthesis selected should have a medullary stem which fits the canal, and a head diameter equal to the diameter of the cut surface. After trial reduction, the prosthesis is cemented into place or left as a push-fit according to personal preference.

When a total replacement is to be used, excavation of the humerus is best left until after the glenoid has been prepared.

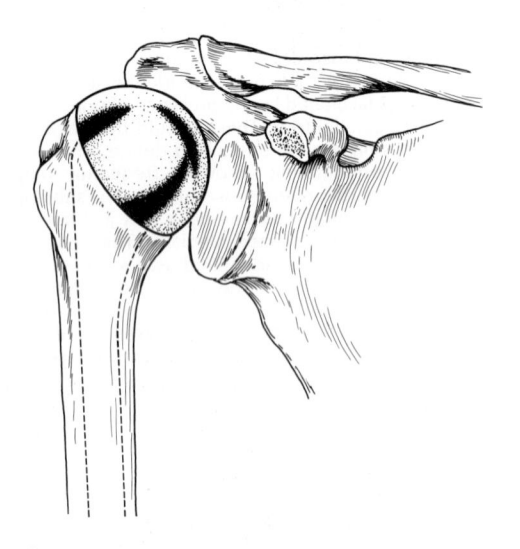

STANMORE PROSTHESIS

Preparation of glenoid

7

The resected humerus is returned to the wound and retracted laterally to expose the posterior capsule, which is divided along the margin of the glenoid. The tip of a Bankart retractor is slipped under the posterior lip of the glenoid to give access to the glenoid. This is much easier when the rotator cuff is degenerate or disrupted, but if intact it may be divided if exposure of the glenoid or the subsequent insertion of the prosthesis is unduly difficult.

The margins of the glenoid are defined carefully for the glenoid may appear to be much enlarged as a result of osteophyte formation. Any residual articular cartilage and the subchondral bone are carefully removed with a Capener gouge, leaving the rim of the glenoid intact. The underlying cancellous bone is removed carefully with a gouge and a sharp curette or powered burr to create as big a cavity as possible. The thick bar of bone in the lateral border of the scapula is excavated from within the inferior lip of the glenoid using Paton's burrs of increasing diameter and a small curette. The index finger of the non-dominant hand is placed on the costal surface of the lateral border of the scapula to give direction to the instrument. The cavity is made of sufficient size to take the inferior anchoring prong of the prosthesis.

The cancellous bone is removed from within the base of the coracoid process with a curette. Sometimes it is possible to create a shallow third hole in the spine of the scapula in the depth of the main cavity. These holes are to key the cement.

Trial reduction

8a & b

The inferior prong of the glenoid component of the prosthesis (right or left as appropriate) is inserted into the inferior keyhole and then the cup is tilted backwards into the cavity of the glenoid. The inferior lip of the cup should rest on the inferior margin of the glenoid, and the plane of the face of the cup should be in the line of the lateral border of the scapula. The cup cannot be completely contained by the glenoid but the upper prongs can be shortened if necessary to allow the cup to drop back into the cavity until it rests on the rim of the glenoid.

The humeral component of the prosthesis is inserted into the prepared cavity in the upper end of the humerus with the arm extended and laterally rotated. The plateau of the prosthesis rests on the cut surface of the humerus, and if the line of resection is correct, the head will be retroverted 30°–40° with respect to the humeral condyles. It is difficult to articulate the two components before they are cemented into place but it is possible to determine whether reduction will be possible without the need for resection of more bone from the upper end of the humerus.

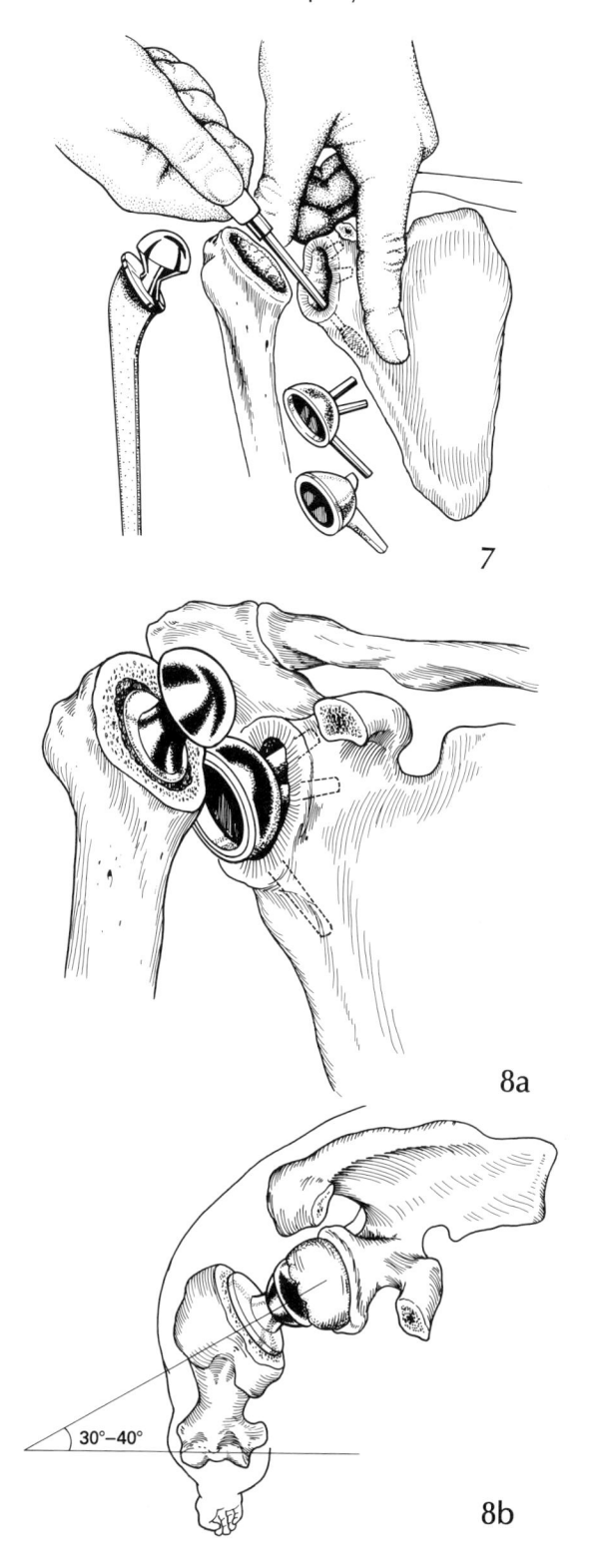

Insertion of the prosthesis

9

Debris is washed from the prepared glenoid cavity which should be made as dry as possible before being packed with acrylic cement. Care should be taken to ensure that the cement packs into the keyholes. The prosthesis is inserted as before, making sure that the inferior prong passes into the cavity in the lateral border of the scapula. While the prosthesis is held firmly in place with the tip of the index finger, excess cement is moulded around the cup to provide a smooth finish. The wound is flooded with cold saline until the cement is hard. Any excess cement is removed with bone nibblers. The medullary cavity of the humerus is packed with cement and the humeral component of the prosthesis is inserted; it may then be finally tapped home.

The two components can be articulated when the cement is hard by medial rotation of the arm and direct pressure on the upper end of the humerus. The components can be felt to snap together and resist distraction as the polythene retaining ring in the rim of the cup grips the head. If this is not the case it is usually due to a film of fluid or flap of soft tissue in the cup.

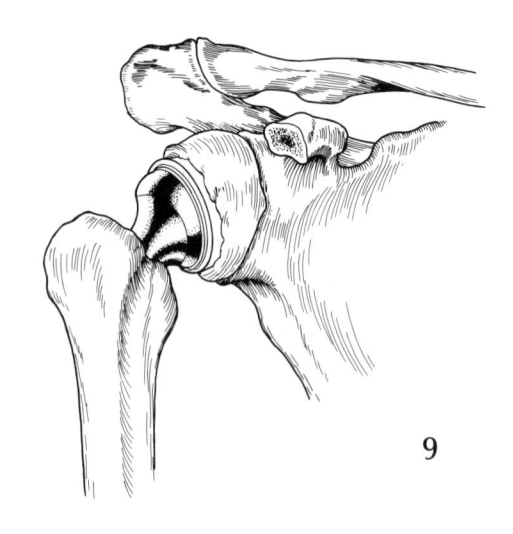

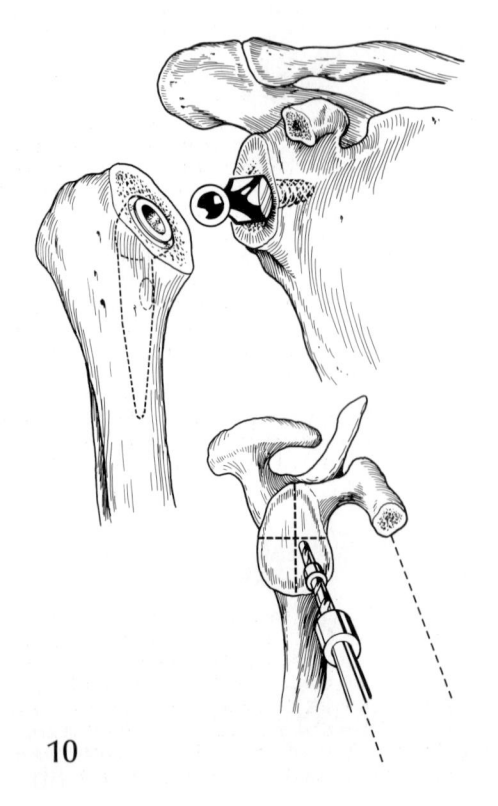

KESSEL PROSTHESIS

Preparation of glenoid and insertion of prosthesis

10

The glenoid is exposed as before. A hole is drilled into the scapula with a 6 mm twist drill, starting at a point just anterior and inferior to the centre of the glenoid. This starting point should be located with care after defining the true margin of the glenoid. The drill is directed in a line parallel to the axis of the coracoid process and so enters the thickest part of the scapula. The entrance of the hole is enlarged with the special countersinking tool. A trial reduction is carried out with the non-threaded glenoid component and the plastic humeral component as a prelude to any final adjustments to the resected humerus. It is impossible to alter the position of the glenoid component once the hole has been drilled because of the thin cross-section of the scapula. The threaded glenoid component is screwed into place with a special spanner and the humeral component cemented into the prepared cavity at the upper end of the humerus so that the rim of the socket lies flush with the resected surface. When the acrylic cement has set the components are articulated.

NEER PROSTHESIS

Preparation of glenoid and insertion of prosthesis

11a

The glenoid is exposed taking care to preserve the supraspinatus, when present. The template is placed on the glenoid so that the longitudinal slit is in line with the lateral border of the scapula. The subchondral bone is carefully perforated with a hand drill to create a series of holes the length of the slit. The template is removed and the holes joined together with bone nibblers or a powered burr.

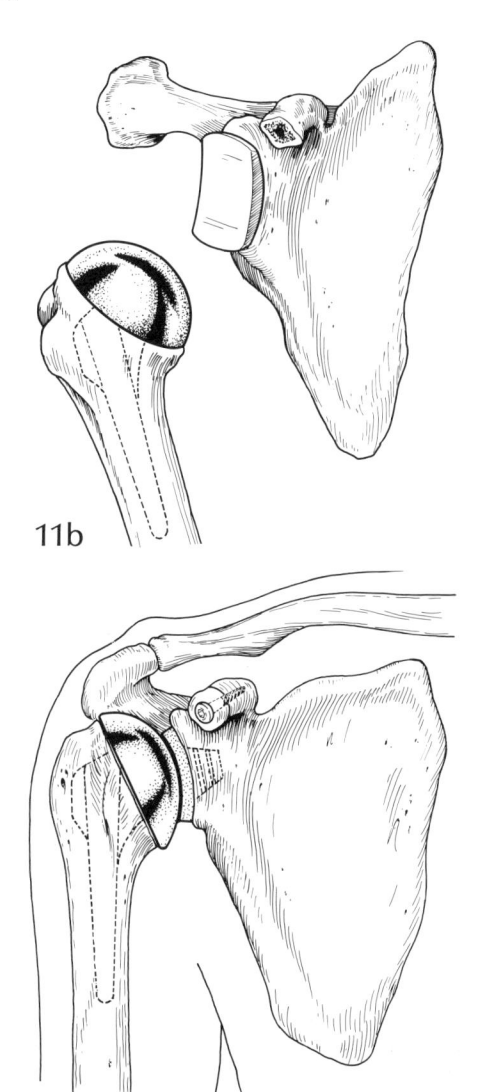

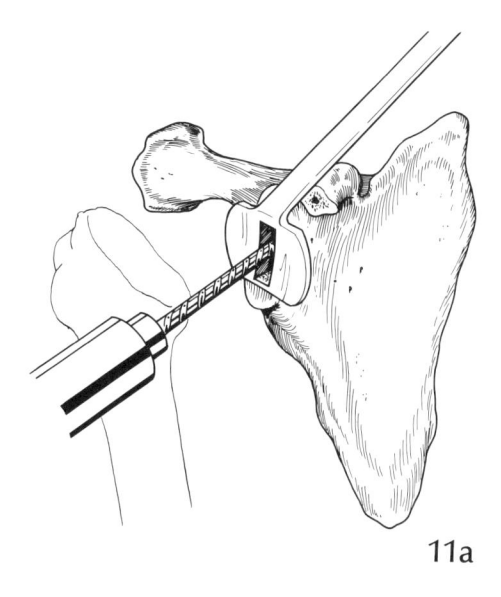

11b & c

The underlying bone from the glenoid is removed with a small curette or powered burr to create a cavity large enough to accommodate the keel of the glenoid component and the cement. The size of the cavity and the slit is checked with the trial prosthesis and progressively both the slit and the cavity are enlarged until the back of the trial prosthesis lies on the surface of the glenoid.

Any residual articular cartilage is carefully removed from the surface of the glenoid, leaving it roughened and irregular. The cavity is filled with cement and the real glenoid component inserted and held in place firmly until the cement sets. Surplus cement is then removed.

The upper end of the humerus is delivered from the wound and the arm is laterally rotated and extended to bring the prepared medullary cavity into view. A trial humeral component is selected with an intramedullary stem diameter which is easily accommodated and a head thickness which allows a trial reduction to be accomplished without tension on the soft tissues. The size of the prosthesis is adjusted as necessary using the larger intramedullary stems in large patients. When a satisfactory fit is achieved, the permanent prosthesis is cemented in place.

Closure

The subscapularis is repaired under slight tension with interrupted sutures. The tip of the coracoid process is reattached with a single screw or by sutures should it split. The clavicular portion of the deltoid is sutured to the clavicle if necessary and the deltopectoral groove closed before suture of the subcutaneous fat and skin. The arm is bandaged to the chest wall over a layer of cotton wool, with hand directed towards the opposite shoulder.

Postoperative management

After 24 hours the suction drains (if used) are removed. There is rarely any significant blood loss. A radiograph is taken of the shoulder through the dressing to confirm the satisfactory position of the prosthesis.

The bulky dressings are removed after 3–4 days and the arm supported in a sling. The sling is removed intermittently for pendulum exercises over the next 24–48 hours. Then passive flexion and extension exercises are begun, depending on the degree of discomfort, at first under supervision and later the patient is encouraged to use the unoperated arm to mobilize the operated shoulder. After 7–10 days isometric exercises against resistance are started to improve the tone of all muscle groups, the sling is discarded and the patient discharged from hospital. Stitches are removed after 10–14 days. Lateral rotation is avoided for 3–4 weeks. Movements slowly improve for 3–6 months after the operation with assiduous exercises, depending on the underlying condition and the state of the rotator cuff.

Complications

Dislocation

Dislocation may occur, especially whilst the muscles are atonic immediately after operation. Closed reduction is usually possible and in the case of late dislocation should be followed up by a further period of immobilization.

Loosening

If loosening of the prosthesis occurs it may be possible to replace it. The remaining bone adjacent to the glenoid usually proves inadequate for fixation, however, and coversion to an excision arthroplasty is preferable. Both components may be removed through the original incision, together with any loose cement or bone, leaving two flat surfaces. The soft tissues are carefully repaired and the abundant fibrous tissue, which is usually present, is left undisturbed. Postoperative management after excision arthroplasty is similar to that after replacement arthroplasty.

References

1. Neer CS. Articular replacement for the humeral head. *J Bone Joint Surg [Am]* 1955; 37-A: 215–28.

2. Lettin AWF, Scales JT. Total replacement of the shoulder joint. *Proc R Soc Med* 1972; 65: 373–4.

3. Lettin AWF, Scales JT. Total replacement arthroplasty of the shoulder in rheumatoid arthritis. *J Bone Joint Surg [Br]* 1973; 55-B: 217.

4. Lettin AWF. Total shoulder replacement in rheumatoid arthritis. In: Kölbel R, Helbig B, Blouth W, eds. *Shoulder replacement*. Berlin: Springer-Verlag, 1987: 103–11.

5. Kelly IG, Forster RS, Fisher WD. Neer total shoulder replacement in rheumatoid arthritis. *J Bone Joint Surg [Br]* 1987; 69-B: 723–6.

Illustrations by Peter Cox after C. M. Lamb

Arthrodesis of the shoulder

The late **Sir Henry Osmond-Clarke,** KCVO, CBE, FRCS(I), FRCS(Eng)
Former Orthopaedic Surgeon to Her Majesty Queen Elizabeth II; Consulting Orthopaedic Surgeon, The Royal London Hospital, London and Robert Jones and Agnes Hunt Orthopaedic Hospital, Oswestry, UK

Introduction

Indications

Arthrodesis of the shoulder is undertaken mainly for inflammatory conditions such as tuberculosis, much more rarely than formerly for paralytic lesions and rarely for osteoarthritis or rheumatoid arthritis of the shoulder, for gross injuries and after the resection of benign neoplasms.

The shoulder may be approached either from the front (or anterosuperiorly) or from behind.

Contraindications

Distraction at the shoulder joint The posterior operation should not be done for paralytic lesions of the shoulder unless it is combined with intra-articular ablation of the joint and fixation of the humeral head to the glenoid by pin or screw, otherwise the graft may act as a fulcrum about which the head of the humerus is levered out of the glenoid.

Preoperative

Position of patient

Anterior approach The patient lies on the back with a small sandbag under the scapula and buttock so that he is slightly tilted towards the opposite side.

Posterior approach The patient lies prone with the face turned towards the opposite side and the affected arm hanging over the edge of the table. The body part of a plaster of Paris shoulder spica should have been applied some days previously.

Anaesthesia

General anaesthesia with an endotracheal tube is satisfactory.

Operations

ANTERIOR OPERATION

Incision

1

The incision is like that used for recurrent dislocation of the shoulder (see p. 676) except that it is extended backwards to a point behind the posterior margin of the acromion.

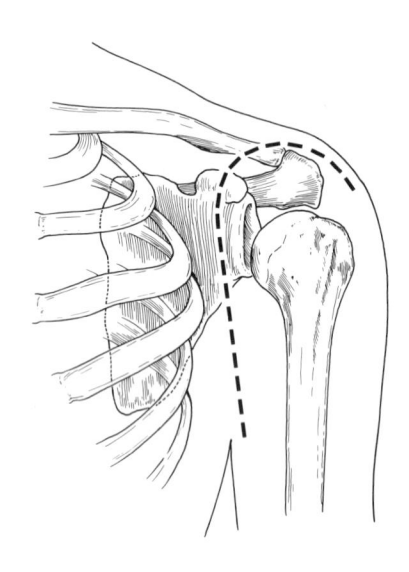

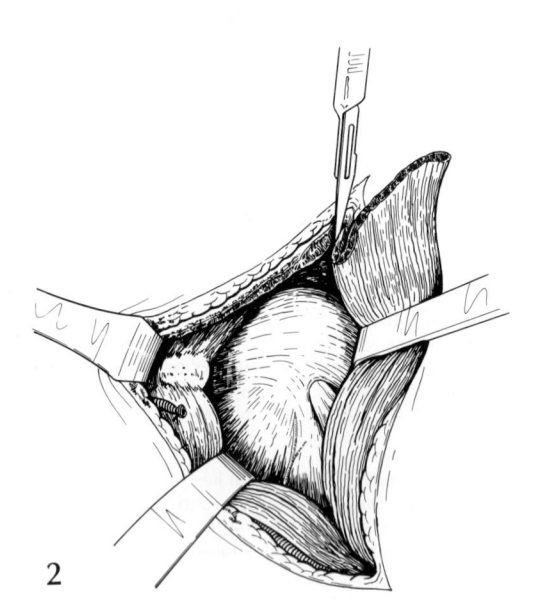

Exposure

2

The deltopectoral groove is identified and the same procedure carried out as in the similar stage of the Putti–Platt capsulorrhaphy (see p. 679). The cephalic vein is tied, and the deltoid muscle is detached from its clavicular attachment and from the anterior two-thirds of its acromial attachment. This exposes the coracoid process, the musculotendinous cuff and capsule and the long tendon of the biceps.

Division of capsule

3

The transverse humeral ligament and the capsule above it are divided longitudinally to free the tendon of the biceps.

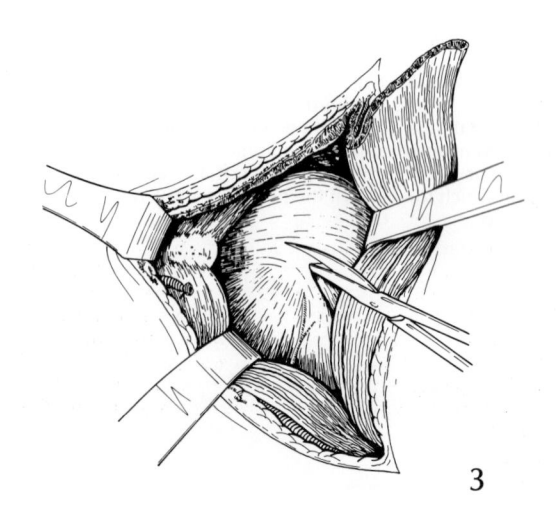

Entry into joint

4

The tendon of the biceps is retracted forwards and the musculotendinous cuff and capsule are divided transversely, opening up the shoulder joint.

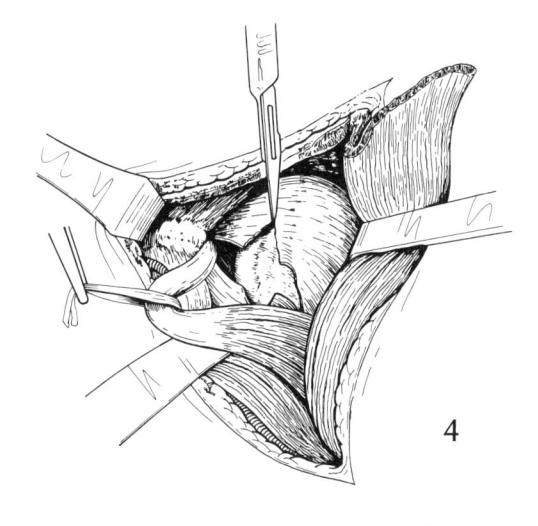

Preparation of bony surfaces

5

With a gouge the joint surfaces are thoroughly rawed, all the remains of the cartilage and sclerotic bone being removed to expose bleeding cancellous bone.

Positioning of arm

6

The humeral head is placed in contact with the glenoid and the arm is held in the position that will ensure optimum function. This is in fact the position which allows the patient to get his hand to his mouth and allows the arm to come to the side in repose. In an adult it amounts to 40° of abduction, 15°–25° of forward flexion and 25°–30° of medial rotation. An adolescent can be allowed about 50° of abduction because of the greater mobility of the scapula.

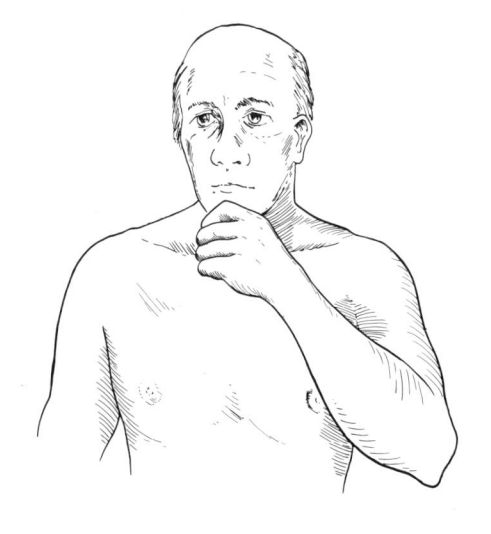

Insertion of guide wire

7

While the above position is carefully maintained by an assistant a guide wire is inserted from the outer aspect of the humerus at an angle of about 60° so that it penetrates the humeral head and the glenoid; it should be directed upwards and backwards. Its position is checked by radiographs.

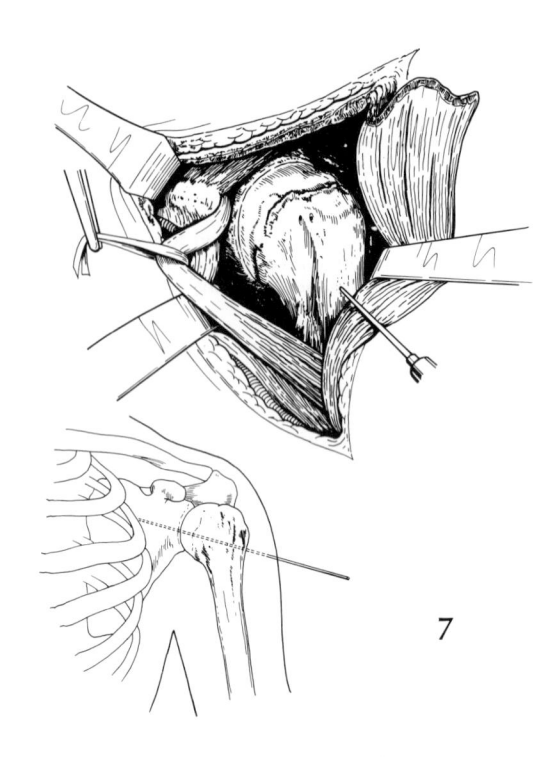

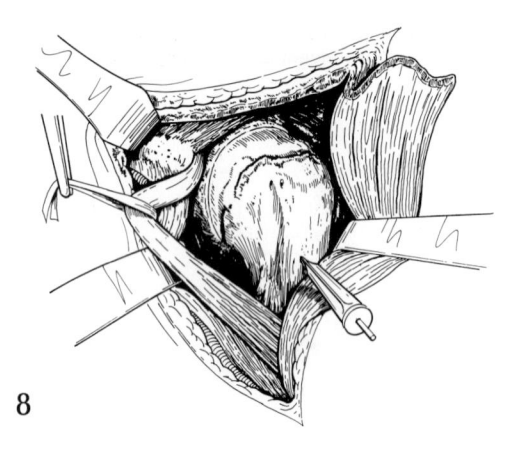

Insertion of Smith-Petersen nail

8

When a satisfactory position of the guide wire has been achieved a cannulated Smith-Petersen nail is driven over the wire and firmly impacted. Alternatively, one or two lag compression screws may be used. The wire is removed.

Arthrodesis of the shoulder

Reinforcement of arthrodesis

9

The arthrodesis is reinforced by bending the rawed acromion downwards and inserting it into a notch cut in the humerus.

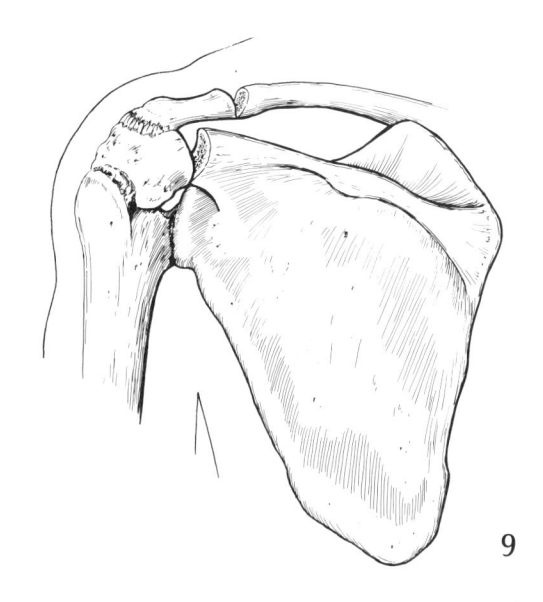

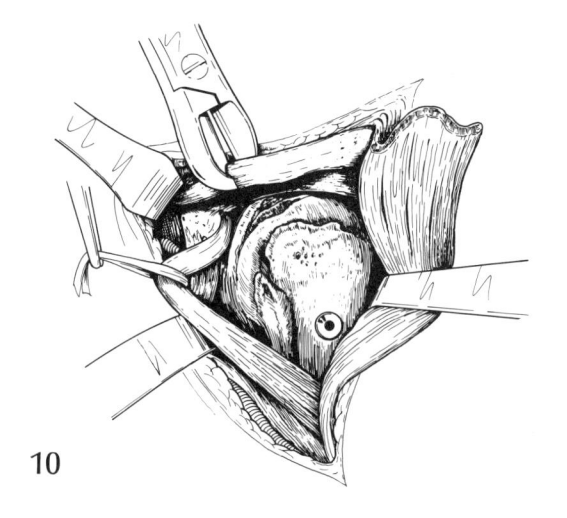

Mobilization of acromion

The above manoeuvre is facilitated by partly dividing the clavicle and the spine of the scapula. The soft tissue attachments should be left intact to ensure an adequate blood supply and to preserve a reasonably stable 'hinge'.

10

Part-division of clavicle The clavicle is partially divided by means of bone-cutting forceps.

11

Part-division of scapula The spine of the scapula is cut with bone-cutting forceps.

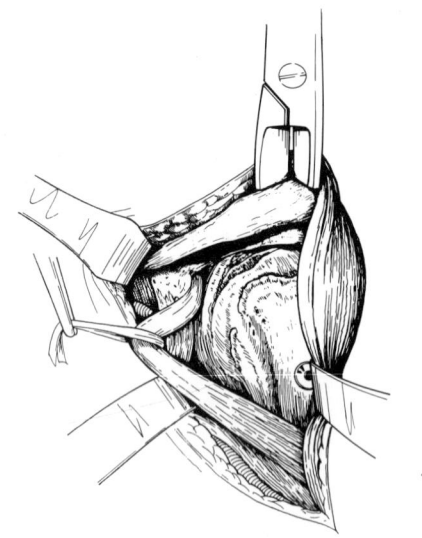

Formation of notch in humerus

12

The notch in the humerus is made by inserting a chisel from above downwards and fracturing the greater tuberosity outwards.

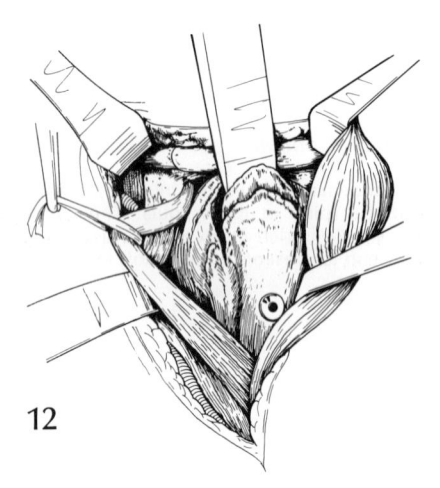

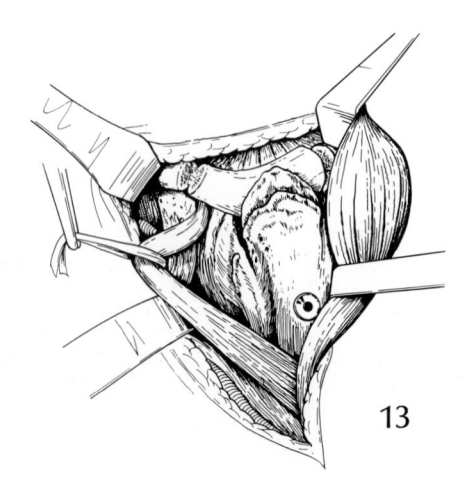

Completion

13

The outer parts of the clavicle and acromion are bent down into the gap formed by the outwardly levered tuberosity. One or two sutures keep them in snug contact. The wound is closed in layers.

Alternative techniques

Other techniques are in use. Some surgeons prefer to use a lag-screw rather than a Smith-Petersen triflanged nail. Others, notably Charnley and DePalma, describe the use of compression by Steinmann pins passed through the clavicle and acromion above and the neck of the humerus below.

THE POSTERIOR OPERATION

14

The aim of the operation is to insert a tibial graft, cut as illustrated, between the scapula and the humerus about 5 cm below the shoulder joint. It has been claimed by Brittain[1], the originator of this operation, that the compression force exerted by the arm constantly tending to adduct ensures more certain union than other methods.

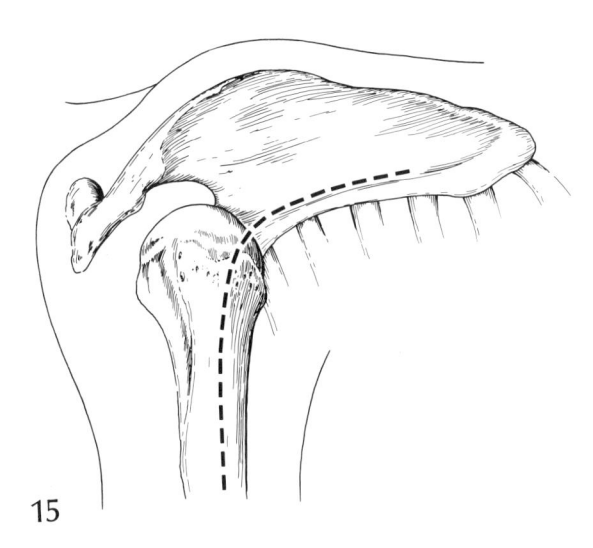

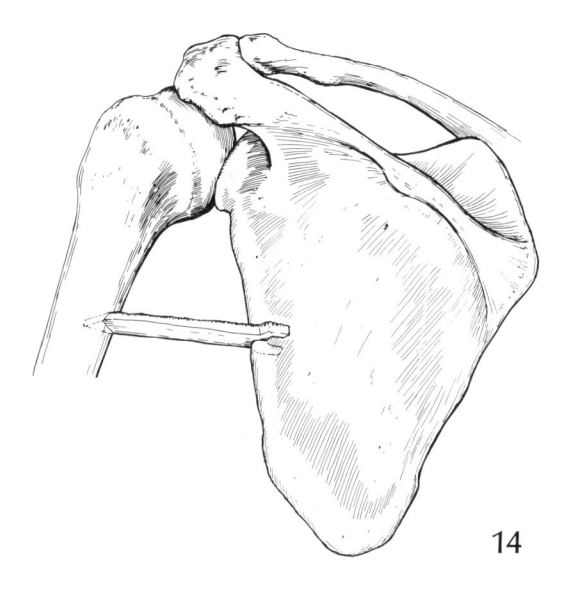

Incision

15

A curved incision is made, beginning near the lowest third of the scapula and extending along the axillary border and down the arm for about 10 cm.

Exposure

16

The incision is carried down through the teres minor muscle onto the axillary border of the scapula. If the circumflex scapular artery is in the way it is divided and ligated. The infraspinatus behind and the subscapularis in front are stripped from the scapula sufficiently to allow a notch to be made in the bone with nibbling forceps.

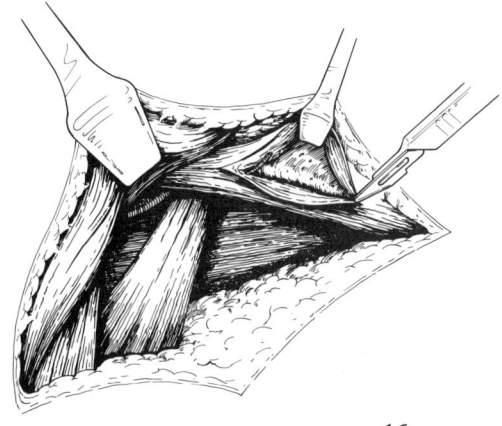

Notching of scapula and drilling of humerus

17

When the axillary border has been notched, the posterior border of the deltoid is retracted and the lateral and medial heads of the triceps are split to expose the shaft of the humerus just below its surgical neck. A suitable hole is drilled in the humerus; its position and direction are determined with due regard to the length of the graft (cut from the subcutaneous surface of the tibia at the beginning of the operation) and the correct positioning of the arm.

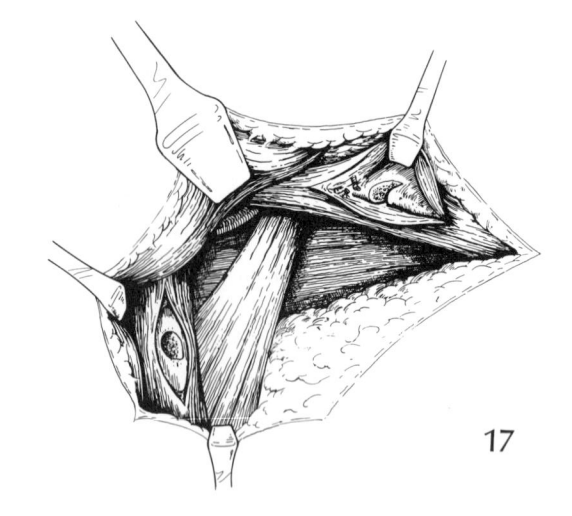

Insertion of graft

18

The graft is embedded firmly in both bones. It is usually easier to place it in the humerus first and then by manoeuvring the arm to coax the other end into the slot in the scapula. The wound is closed in layers.

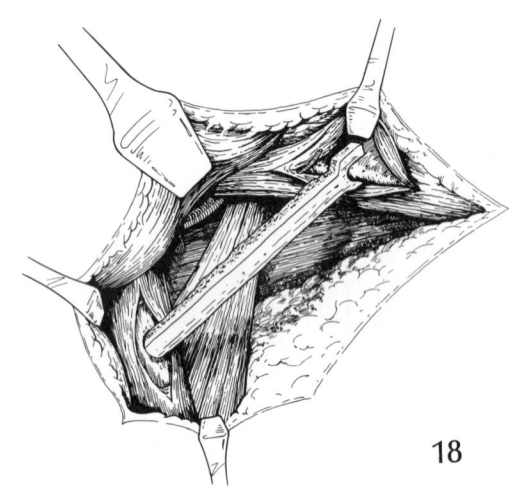

Postoperative management

ANTERIOR OPERATION

A plaster of Paris shoulder spica is applied; this is not easy on the anaesthetized patient, and it is therefore wise to remove the plaster and the sutures after about 2 weeks and to apply a fresh, snugly fitting spica which should be retained until union has occurred, usually in about 3–4 months. When the arthrodesis is firm the patient begins a course of exercises to mobilize the scapula on the chest wall and to restore the greatest possible function to the arm.

POSTERIOR OPERATION

The patient is carefully turned, and plaster of Paris is applied to the arm and connected with the previously applied body plaster to form a shoulder spica. Stitches are removed in about 2 weeks and a snugly fitting spica is applied; special care must be taken at this stage to avoid disturbing the attachments of the graft. The plaster must be worn for not less than 4 months because this graft takes a considerable time to revascularize.

Reference

1. Brittain HA. *Architectural principles in arthrodesis.* 2nd ed. Edinburgh and London: Livingstone, 1952: 168.

Illustrations by Peter Cox

Prosthetic replacement of the elbow

Thomas P. Sculco MD
Associate Director, Department of Orthopaedic Surgery, The Hospital for Special Surgery, New York, USA

Philip M. Faris MD
Clinical Associate Professor, Louisana State University Medical Center, USA

Introduction

The evolution of elbow arthroplasty has progressed from interposition arthroplasty to metal-to-metal uniaxial hinges to semiconstrained metal to polyethylene hinges and metal-to-polyethylene resurfacing arthroplasty[1]. Resection and interpositional arthroplasties, using organic and inorganic materials, have been attempted for degenerative disease of the elbow with varied success[2-6]. Because of this unpredictability, especially related to residual pain and instability, interposition arthroplasty has been virtually abandoned except for use in patients with haemophilia[7] and in the salvage of failed elbow prostheses.

In the mid 1950s, experimentation with hemiarthroplasty began[8-12]. The proximal olecranon, radial head, and distal humerus all were independently replaced using metal components with acrylic or metal stems. These were fixed to bone with screws, wires, or sleeves to attain mechanical fixation; results were mixed. With the introduction of methylmethacrylate, the problem of fixation to bone seemed lessened and further development ensued. In 1972, Dee[13] described a metal-to-metal hinge arthroplasty using methylmethacrylate and intramedullary fixation. Other similar hinges were developed by Scales, McKee, Shiers, and others during this period; their designs had varying success with short and intermediate follow-up[1].

As the understanding of the biomechanics of the elbow increased, prosthetic designs developed to give (1) the semiconstrained or sloppy hinge and (2) the unconstrained or resurfacing design. Examples of semiconstrained prostheses are the Coonrad, Mayo, Pritchard–Walker, Triaxial, and Volz. Examples of the unconstrained prostheses are the Ewald, London, Kudo, Liverpool, and Souter.

Biomechanics of the elbow joint

Analysis of elbow kinematics has developed slowly compared to data available on the knee and hip. Morrey and Chao[14] in 1976, presented a complex kinematic analysis of cadaveric elbows and confirmed Fisher's[15] observation that the axis of elbow flexion is fixed and localized to the centre of the trochlea. This axis must also be oriented in an oblique fashion relative to the humeral axis, allowing the carrying angle to change from approximately 10° of valgus in extension to 5° of varus in full elbow flexion. Axial rotation of the forearm occurred during elbow flexion and extension. In this study, the ulna was essentially fixed during axial rotation.

The variation in carrying angle from valgus in extension to varus in flexion was disputed by London[16] in 1981. He felt that this finding was erroneously based on an axis through the condyles at a right angle to the humeral shaft. When the axis of movement was defined as perpendicular to the plane of the trochlear sulcus, then flexion/extension of the humeroulnar and humeroradial joints is uniplanar. Instant centres were localized to the arc of the trochlear sulcus except in the last 5°–10° of extension when the instant centre moved toward the olecranon fossa, and in flexion when the instant centre moved toward the coronoid fossa. Similar variation was seen in the humeroradial joint.

The range of elbow movement required for activities of daily living has been elucidated by Morrey et al.[17] using a triaxial electrogoniometer. Ranges required varied from 15° of flexion for tying shoes to 140° for reaching the occiput. Total rotation required was 100° with 50° of supination needed for personal hygiene.

Although the elbow is not a weight-bearing joint as are the knee and hip, the forces acting across the joint are significant. Under physiological stress (i.e. lifting an 11 kg weight) forces of greater than body weight are predicted at 90° of flexion and increase to three times body weight at 20° of flexion[11]. Further increases in force occur as full extension is approached, as the forearm pronates, and as rapid acceleration is introduced. The direction of the forces applied is mostly shear at 90° of flexion and becomes more axial with increasing extension. Twisting moments about the humerus are also high, depending upon the activity for which the arm is used.

In summary, many factors must be considered in the design of an elbow prosthesis, including (1) adequate range of movement, (2) restoration of normal centres of rotation, and (3) twisting forces acting upon the joint.

Current design

The triaxial prosthesis, which has been used at The Hospital for Special Surgery since 1975, is a 'sloppy hinge' allowing 10°–12° of varus/valgus freedom and 4°–6° of rotational movement besides full flexion and extension. Some minor modifications in the original design have been made to improve its resistance to dislocation and fracture and to increase its component–bone–cement composite strength. Currently, the device consists of cobalt–chrome ulnar and humeral components with the humeral component having a built-in 7° valgus carrying angle. Articulation is via a polyethylene bearing interposed between the metallic humeral and ulnar components. The articulation, then, is a metal-to-polyethylene interaction which maintains its 'sloppiness' under a 65 newton compressive force. A distraction force of 49.5 newtons is required to disarticulate the components.

In a recent report, Inglis et al.[18] reported the 2–9 year results (mean 5 years) on 61 patients with 73 triaxial total elbow prostheses. The average arc of flexion was 28° to 125° with pronation of 68° and supination of 60°. Forty-six elbows were rated excellent, 18 good, 2 fair, and 7 were poor results. There were no cases of aseptic loosening, component migration, or circumferential progressive radiolucent lines. There were 16 major complications including infection in 3, persistent nerve palsies in 3, skin slough in 2, condylar fractures in 3, and dislocation in 5 elbow prostheses. The current design displayed a lower dislocation rate than the earlier axle design. Continuing design modifications are aimed at reducing the incidence of dislocations and improving load-transfer characteristics.

Indications

1. Pain is the chief indication for elbow arthroplasty.
2. Rheumatoid arthritis and juvenile rheumatoid arthritis are indications for which arthroplasty produces good results.
3. Degenerative, post-traumatic and ankylosed elbows give less satisfactory results.

Neither limitation of movement nor instability have shown marked improvement after arthroplasty.

Contraindications

Relative contraindications include previous elbow sepsis, severe bone loss, insufficient soft tissue coverage, absent triceps and/or biceps function, and poor wrist and hand function.

Operation

INSERTION OF THE TRIAXIAL PROSTHESIS

Position of patient

The patient is placed in a 45° lateral decubitus position with a sandbag placed beneath the ipsilateral shoulder.

Incision

1

A longitudinal incision, curved gently on the ulnar side of the olecranon, is begun approximately 7 cm proximal to the olecranon and carried 7 cm distal to the olecranon tip.

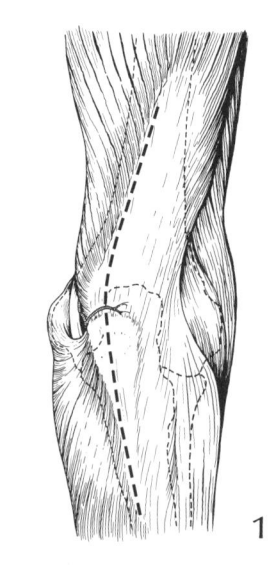

Dissection

The ulnar nerve is isolated near its exit from beneath the medial head of the triceps, dissected free from the cubital tunnel, and cleared distally to its first muscular branch. The ulnar nerve is isolated and retracted using a 6 mm Penrose drain held with a suture, not a haemostat, as this may produce undue traction on the nerve.

Exposure

2

The distal humerus is exposed subperiosteally through the medial intramuscular septum. The fascia of the flexor carpi ulnaris is incised longitudinally 1 cm medial to the ulnar crest. The fascial incision connects, in continuity, with the triceps incision. It is carried through the flexor carpi ulnaris directly to the ulna. The fascia and periosteum, along with the triceps insertion, are elevated sharply from the ulna and olecranon. Extreme care must be taken to keep the triceps muscle, triceps insertion, and ulnar periosteum in continuity. Elbow extension allows relaxation of these tissues. Further subperiosteal elevation of the anconeus provides access to the radial head, which is resected just proximal to the orbicular ligament. Because of the intrinsic stability of the triaxial prosthesis, the ulnar collateral ligament may be released from the medial humeral condyle, and the elbow will remain stable.

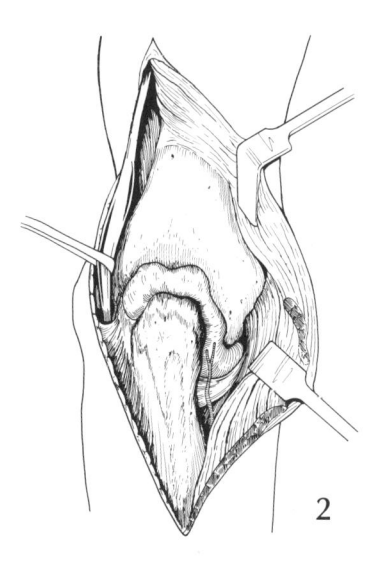

Complete capsulectomy is performed. The anterior ulna is cleared of soft tissue to the coronoid process or beyond if necessary for flexion contracture release. Commonly an osteophyte is present at the coronoid process and this is removed. It is particularly important to release soft tissue contractures from the coronoid to allow the ulna to be brought anterior to the humerus in full flexion. This is necessary to reduce the prosthetic components. The anterior humerus is likewise cleared of contracted soft tissue to allow complete elbow extension. All osteophytes are removed, especially along the medial and lateral olecranon.

Preparation for prosthesis

3a & b

Bone cuts are begun after adequate soft tissue release. The trial ulnar component is superimposed over the olecranon process and a rectangular cut is outlined using methylene blue. The ulnar intramedullary canal is located and the mouth of the canal is opened and shaped using the intramedullary broach and a high-speed burr. Trial placement of the ulnar component is performed and the olecranon is repetitively shaped until the ulnar component fit is snug and its centre of rotation corresponds with the anatomical centre.

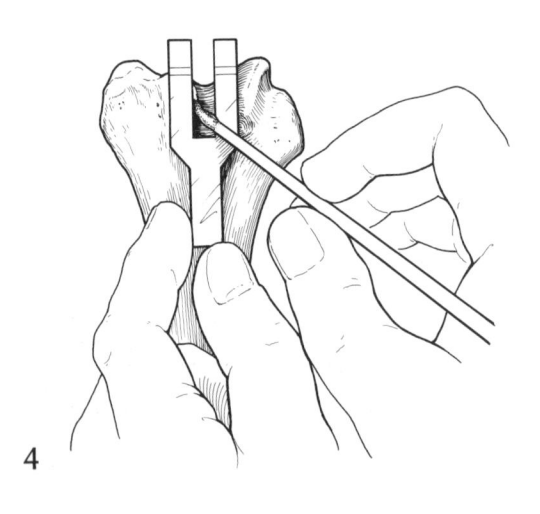

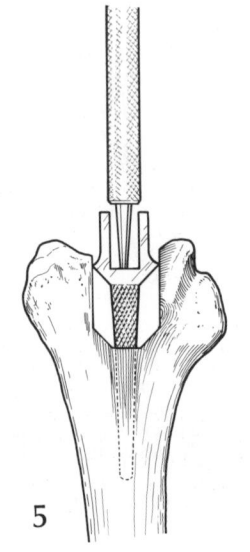

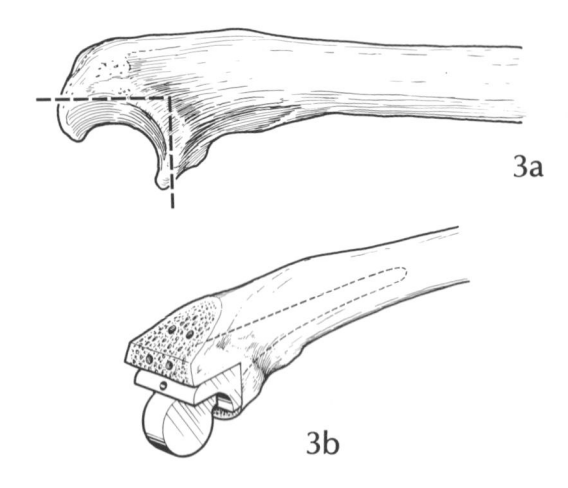

4

The humeral trial component is superimposed posteriorly over the humeral condyles. The posterior humeral surface must be adequately visualized. The cuts are outlined with methylene blue with the depth of cut fashioned to recreate the centre of rotation. It must be appreciated that the humeral medullary canal is slightly lateral to the centre of the trochlea and if the humeral cut is too far medial, fracture of the medial epicondyle may occur.

5

All cuts are made using a micro-oscillating saw. Broaches are provided for humeral and ulnar components. After all cuts are made and the trial components fit snugly, the trial humeral polyethylene is placed and the components are reduced in maximum flexion. Movement is tested. A full range of movement should be attained including full extension. If full extension is unobtainable, further soft tissue release anteriorly off the humerus and/or ulna is necessary. In extreme cases the humeral component may be seated more proximal in the humerus.

Insertion

The humeral and ulnar canals are plugged with bone plugs which are shaped and fitted for the canals. The canals are lavaged with pulsatile lavage and packed with methylmethacrylate. The final components are placed simultaneously and held in position. Excess methacrylate is removed and the cement is allowed to cure. The components are reduced in flexion. The elbow again is tested for stability and range of motion.

Closure

6

Three drill holes are placed in the olecranon in a medial to lateral direction and No. 1 non-absorbable sutures are placed through these holes. The triceps sleeve is reattached using the non-absorbable suture. The remainder of the fascial sleeve is then repaired over small vacuum drains. The ulnar nerve is allowed to lie in a position of least tension or compression, which may be anterior to the cubital tunnel.

Routine subcutaneous and skin closure follows and the arm is placed in 30° of flexion in a soft compressive dressing with medial and lateral plaster splints. No pressure should be allowed over the tip of the olecranon.

Postoperative management

Postoperatively, the drains are removed after 24–48 hours and prophylactic antibiotics are discontinued after 48 hours. On the fourth day, the dressing is changed and the arm is placed in a long-arm splint with a flexion-lock hinge. Movement is allowed from 30° to 90° of flexion for the first 3 weeks when the sutures are removed. The wound is watched closely and any evidence of wound inflammation, dehiscence, or necrosis requires cessation of exercises. The brace is removed at 3 weeks when strengthening and full range of movement exercises are begun.

Review of results

Semiconstrained resurfacing prostheses

To date there is a paucity of long-term clinical follow-up data available concerning resurfacing semiconstrained prostheses[19–25]. From the literature on resurfacing-type elbow replacements, the loosening rates are modest compared to hinges, pain relief is satisfactory, and restoration of function is good, but, unacceptable rates of instability, infection, and ulnar nerve palsy persist. A high proportion of these complications are soft tissue-related and, with adaptations of Bryan and Morrey's[26] triceps-sparing approach, may be diminishing.

Semiconstrained total elbow prosthesis

Beginning in 1974, several semiconstrained or 'sloppy' hinge-type prostheses were developed. Again, minimal long-term data is available concerning many of the designs currently being used (i.e. Volz, Schlein, Pritchard-Walker, Mayo, Coonrad, and Triaxial). Greater than two-year follow-up results in adequate numbers are available for the Mayo–Coonrad[27] and Triaxial[18].

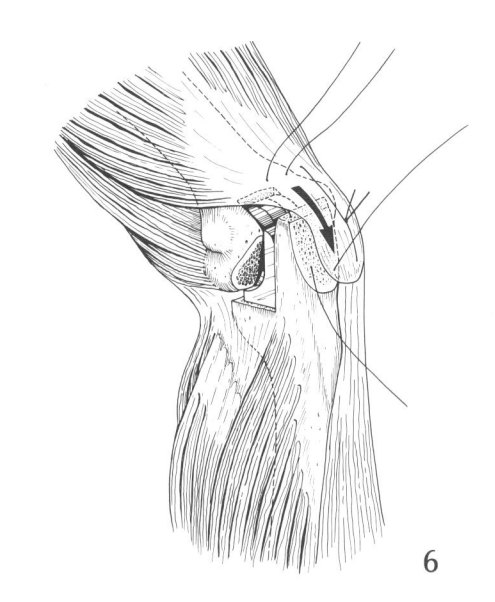

6

Complications and their treatment

Complications of elbow arthroplasty include most of those seen after other joint replacements (i.e. infection and loosening), but also include some that are more specific to elbow replacement (i.e. dislocation, skin slough, ulnar nerve neuropathy, and triceps disruption).

Infection

Overall, infections have been reported in 4–12 per cent of cases. This high rate may be due to the patient population, many of whom are steroid-dependent rheumatoid arthritics. Additionally, there is meager soft-tissue coverage at the elbow, and previously the use of the triceps tongue-type approach led to many wound problems. As in all arthroplasty surgery, deep infection carries a high morbidity. Our approach to this problem has been similar to our approach to all joint arthroplasties. We prefer implant removal, when this is possible, followed by thorough surgical debridement, 6 weeks of intravenous antibiotics (mean inhibitory concentration greater than 8:1) and reimplantation. Removal of ulnar and humeral components which are well fixed may be complex and if not performed with care may produce severe bone loss and fracture. In cases of inadequate soft tissue or bone stock, reimplantation is inadvisable and soft tissue interpositional arthroplasty is performed using external fixation. In an occasional, isolated case, when any surgical procedure might be contraindicated, *in situ* maintenance of the prosthesis using antibiotic suppression may be attempted, though is rarely successful.

Loosening

Loosening has not been a major problem with the triaxial prosthesis, occurring in only 2 per cent of cases to date. Primary revision of loose components is preferable, using custom-made long-stem prostheses. If bone stock is insufficient, then soft tissue interpositional arthroplasty is advisable. Arthrodesis is a reasonable alternative in young patients, but may be difficult to effect.

Dislocation

Dislocation of the ulnar component from the humeral polyethylene bearing may occur in two ways. It may be due to prosthetic uncoupling in extreme flexion (130°) which is rarely attained, and is treated by closed or open reduction and flexion-block orthosis. The other type of dislocation occurs later postoperatively in those very active individuals who place extreme varus/valgus rotational loads on the elbow at 90° of flexion. In this case, cold flow deformation of the polyethylene bearing progresses until the ulnar component is no longer 'captured' by the bearing and disarticulates. This complication is also uncommon and is treated by replacement of the polyethylene bearing. A yoke may be a useful addition to prevent recurrence.

Skin problems

Skin problems of major proportions have diminished significantly since development of the triceps sleeve approach. Simple areas of delayed wound healing or small eschars may be treated with changes in sterile dressing. If delay in healing persists or if skin slough is greater than 1–2 cm then skin grafting and/or muscle pedicle flap coverage may be required. Skin problems must be treated aggressively and with care as involvement deep to the prosthesis can be catastrophic and jeopardize the survival of the implant.

Neuropathy

Ulnar nerve neuropathy has been reported in 5–15 per cent of cases and most frequently is a sensory paraesthesia which resolves spontaneously. This complication is best prevented at the time of surgery by protection and gentle handling of the nerve. Anterior transposition at the time of arthroplasty is indicated if the nerve does not lie untethered in the cubital tunnel. Neurolysis and anterior transposition may be required postoperatively if symptomatic improvement does not occur over a 12-month period.

Triceps disruption

Triceps disruption, if discovered early, may be treated by extension splinting or casting for 4 weeks. When disruption is appreciated later (after 2 weeks) then reattachment or reconstruction is necessary.

Summary

Total elbow arthroplasty is an appropriate surgical procedure with good clinical results when restricted to those disease entities for which it is most successful, i.e. those patients with juvenile and adult-onset rheumatoid arthritis and osteoarthritis. All other arthropathies should be approached with caution. Current designs and techniques are improving as are the long-term results; however, the complication rate remains high. The surgical technique is demanding and attention to detail is imperative. The triceps sleeve approach, use of a prosthesis which allows the use of a soft tissue sleeve for stress distribution, recreation of the anatomical centre of rotation, and intensive postoperative rehabilitation are recommended to maximize results and minimize complications.

References

1. Coonrad RW. History of total elbow arthroplasty. In: Inglis AE, ed. *Symposium on total joint replacement of the upper extremity, New York 1979.* St Louis: Mosby, 1982: 75–90.
2. Knight RA, Van Zandt LL. Arthroplasty of the elbow: an end-result study. *J Bone Joint Surg [Am]* 1952; 34-A: 610–78.
3. Dee R, Reis M. Non-prosthetic elbow reconstruction. *Contemp Orthop*, 1987; 14(2): 37–48.
4. Murphy JB. Arthroplasty. *Ann Surg* 1913; 57: 593–647.
5. Putti V. Arthroplasty. *J Orthop Surg* 1921; 19 (old series): 419.
6. Shahriaree H, Sajadi K, Silver CM, Sheikholeslamzadeh S. Excisional arthroplasty of the elbow. *J Bone Joint Surg [Am]* 1979; 61-A: 922–7.
7. Smith MA, Savidge GF, Fountain EJ. Interposition arthroplasty in the management of advanced haemophilic arthropathy of the elbow. *J Bone Joint Surg [Br]* 1983; 65-B: 436–40.
8. Barr JS, Eaton RG. Elbow reconstruction with a new prosthesis to replace the distal end of the humerus: a case report. *J Bone Joint Surg [Am]* 1965; 47-A: 1408–13.
9. MacAusland AR. Replacement of the lower end of the humerus with a prosthesis: a report of four cases. *West J Surg* 1954; 62: 557–66.
10. Mellen RH, Phalen GS. Arthroplasty of the elbow by replacement of the distal portion of the humerus with an acrylic prosthesis. *J Bone Joint Surg* 1947; 29: 348–53.
11. Street DM, Stevens PS. A humeral replacement for the elbow: results in 10 elbows. *J Bone Joint Surg [Am]* 1974; 56-A: 1147.
12. Torzilli PA. Biomechanics of the elbow. In: Inglis AE, ed. *Symposium on total joint replacement of the upper extremity, New York 1979.* St Louis: Mosby, 1982: 150–68.
13. Dee R. Total replacement arthroplasty of the elbow for rheumatoid arthritis. *J Bone Joint Surg [Br]* 1972; 54-B: 88–95.
14. Morrey BF, Chao EYS. Passive motion of the elbow joint: a biomechanical analysis. *J Bone Joint Surg [Am]* 1976; 58-A: 501–8.
15. Fisher G, cited by Fick R. *Handbuch der Anatomie und Mechanik der Gelenke, unter Bericksichtigung der Bewegenden Muskeln.* 1911; 2: 299.
16. London JT. Kinematics of the elbow. *J Bone Joint Surg [Am]* 1981; 63-A: 529–35.
17. Morrey BF, Askew LJ, An KN, Chao EY. A biomechanical study of normal functional elbow motion. *J Bone Joint Surg [Am]* 1981; 63-A: 872–7.
18. Figgie HE III, Inglis AE. Current concepts in total elbow arthroplasty. *Adv Orthop Surg* 1986; 9: 195–212.
19. Ewald FC, Scheinberg RD, Poss R, Thomas WH, Scott RD, Sledge CB. Capitello-condylar total elbow arthroplasty: two to five year follow-up in rheumatoid arthritis. *J Bone Joint Surg [Am]* 1980; 62-A: 1259–63.
20. Davis RF, Weiland AJ, Hungerford DS, Moore JR, Volenec-Dowling S. Non-constrained total elbow arthroplasty. *Clin Orthop* 1982; 171: 156–60.
21. Rosenberg GM, Turner RH. Non-constrained total elbow arthroplasty. *Clin Orthop* 1984; 187: 154–62.
22. Kudo H, Iwano K, Watanabe S. Total replacement of the rheumatoid elbow with a hingeless prosthesis. *J Bone Joint Surg [Am]* 1980; 62-A: 277–85.
23. Soni RK, Cavendish ME. A review of the Liverpool elbow prosthesis from 1974 to 1982. *J Bone Joint Surg [Br]* 1984; 66-B: 248–53.
24. Pritchard RW. Anatomic surface elbow arthroplasty: a preliminary report. *Clin Orthop* 1983; 179: 223–30.
25. Roper BA, Tuke M, O'Riordan SM, Buestrode CJ. A new unconstrained elbow: a prospective review of 60 replacements. *J Bone Joint Surg [Br]* 1986; 68-B: 566–9.
26. Bryan RA, Morrey BF. Extensive posterior exposure of the elbow: a triceps sparing approach. *Clin Orthop* 1982; 166: 188–92.
27. Morrey BF, Bryan RS, Dobyns JH, Linscheid RL. Total elbow arthroplasty: a five year experience at the Mayo Clinic. *J Bone Joint Surg [Am]* 1981; 63-A: 1050–63.

Illustrations by Gillian Oliver after B. Hyams

Tendon replacement to restore elbow flexion

B. Helal MChOrth, FRCS
Honorary Consultant Orthopaedic Surgeon, The Royal London Hospital and The Royal National Orthopaedic Hospital, London, and Enfield Group of Hospitals, UK

S. C. Chen FRCS
Consultant Orthopaedic Surgeon, Enfield Group of Hospitals, UK

Introduction

Before any operation to restore elbow flexion is carried out, it is important to ensure that the hand and fingers are capable of normal function and that the muscles to be transferred have normal power. If the forearm flexor muscles are normal they can be used to restore elbow flexion. However, if they are paralysed or weak then the pectoralis major or minor, the sternomastoid, the latissimus dorsi or the triceps muscle may be used.

Operations

STEINDLER FLEXORPLASTY[1,2]

1

To assess whether the forearm flexor muscles are capable of flexing the elbow, the shoulder is abducted to 90° and with the forearm supinated the patient attempts to flex the extended elbow. If this can be performed the muscles are strong enough for transfer.

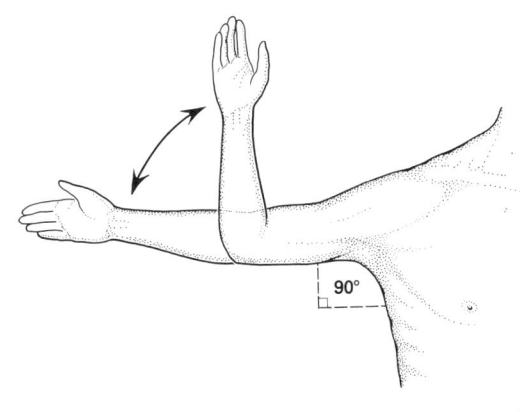

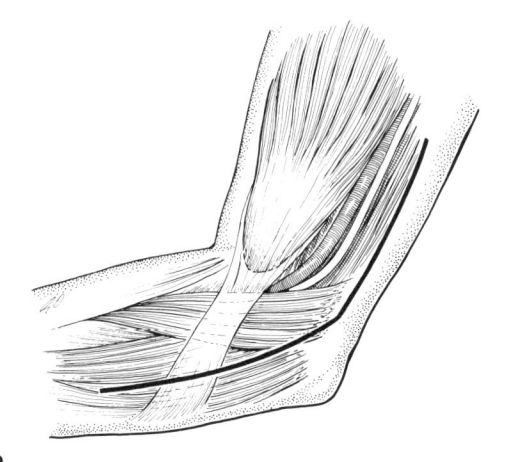

Incision

2

A curved incision is made over the medial side of the elbow starting from about 7.5 cm above the medial epicondyle and ending on the anterior surface of the forearm.

Mobilization of flexor muscles

3

The ulnar nerve is identified behind the medial epicondyle and it is retracted backwards. The medial epicondyle is osteotomized with the common flexor origin.

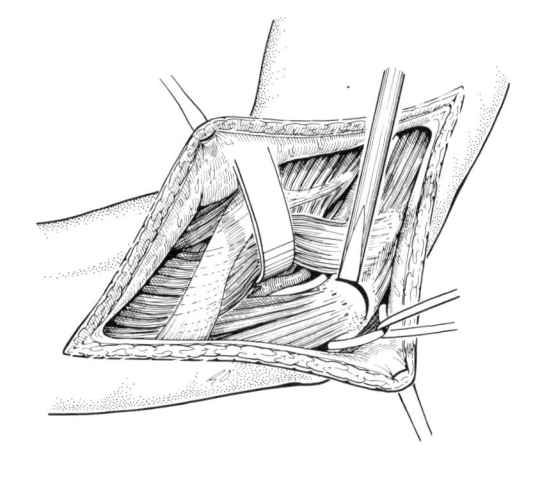

4

The humeral head of pronator teres, flexor carpi radialis, palmaris longus, flexor digitorum sublimis and flexor carpi ulnaris are freed for about 5 cm distally. An area of the humerus is freshened with an osteotome about 5–7.5 cm proximal to the medial epicondyle.

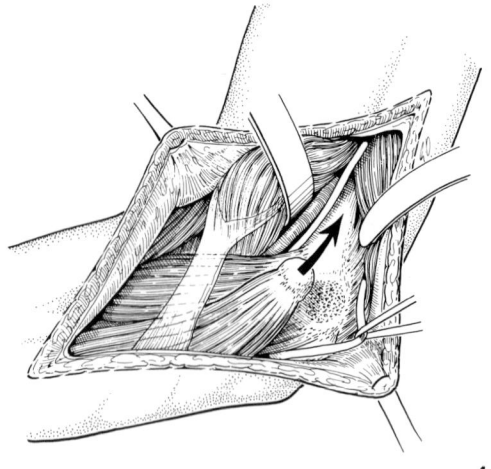

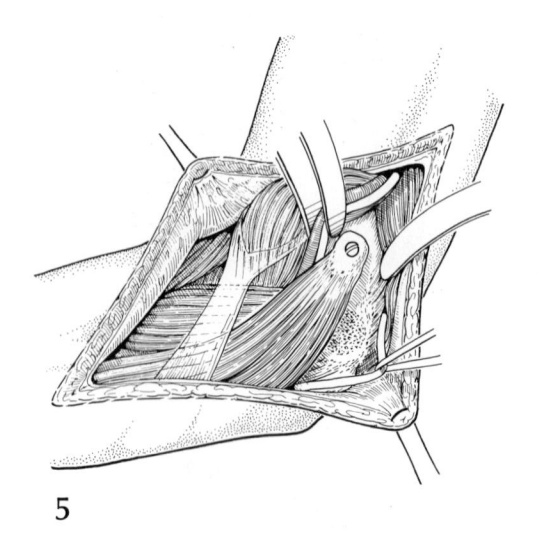

Reattachment of common flexor origin

5

A point on the medial side of the humerus is chosen such that, when the common flexor origin is brought up to it, the elbow will be flexed about 45°. A screw is used to fix the detached medial epicondyle onto this area of the humerus.

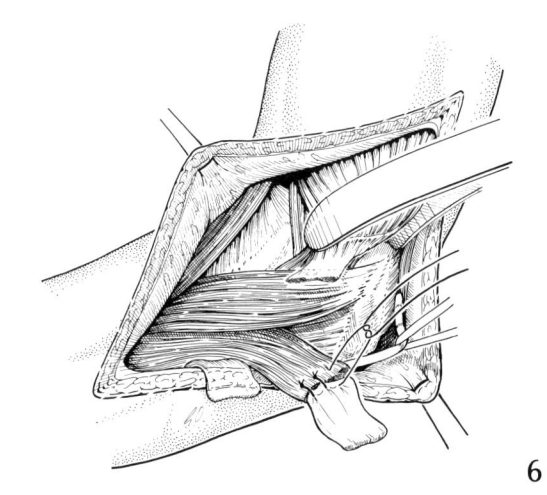

Bunnell's modification of Steindler flexorplasty[3]

6, 7 & 8

The main disadvantage of the Steindler flexorplasty is that the forearm becomes pronated during elbow flexion and the patient may even develop a pronation contracture of the forearm. Bunnell's modification eliminates this problem. Instead of fixing the detached medial epicondyle on the medial side of the humerus, the common flexor origin is detached without osteotomizing the medial epicondyle. The common flexor origin is lengthened with a graft of fascia lata. This is advanced 5 cm up the lateral side of the humerus. It is attached by raising an osteoplastic flap and suturing the fascia lata graft under the flap. The point of attachment should be the same as for the Steindler flexorplasty.

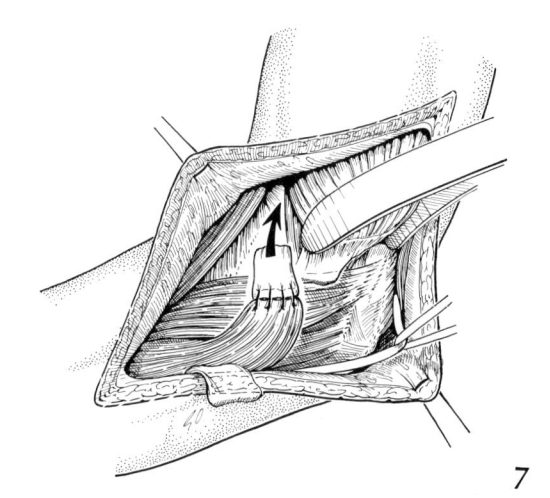

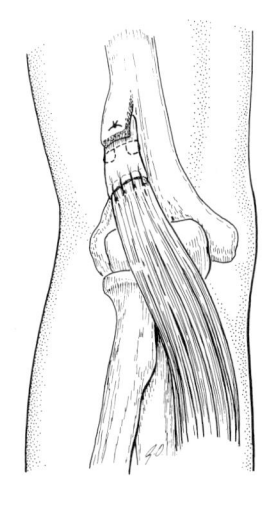

740 Elbow

Postoperative management

9

An above-elbow cast is applied with the elbow in 80° of flexion and the forearm in mid-pronation. At the end of 6 weeks, the plaster cast is removed and gradual mobilizing exercises are started – both passive and active.

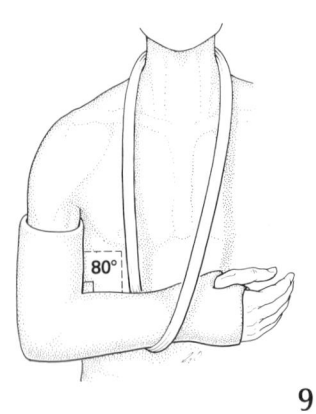

ANTERIOR TRANSFER OF THE TRICEPS TENDON (Bunnell[4] and Carroll[5])

Posterior incision

10

An incision is made along the posterolateral aspect of the upper arm, and the triceps tendon exposed.

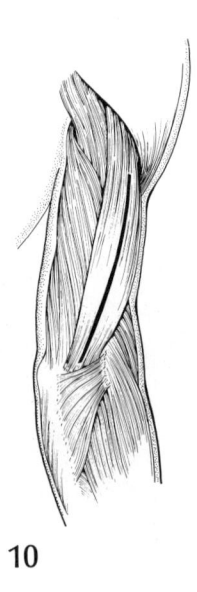

Mobilization and lengthening of triceps

11

The triceps tendon is detached at its insertion to the olecranon process of the ulna and dissected from the lower fourth of the shaft of the humerus. The tendon of the triceps is lengthened with a free graft of fascia lata.

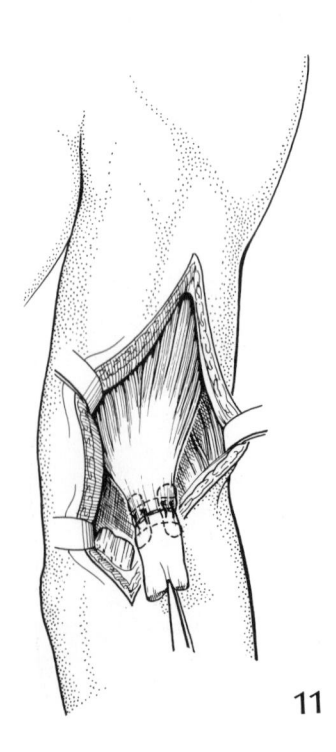

Anterior incision and tendon transfer

12 & 13

Another incision is made on the anterolateral aspect of the arm and forearm, and the lengthened tendon of the triceps brought round the lateral aspect of the humerus. The brachioradialis muscle and the radial nerve are retracted laterally and the pronator teres medially. The forearm is supinated and the biceps tendon is identified.

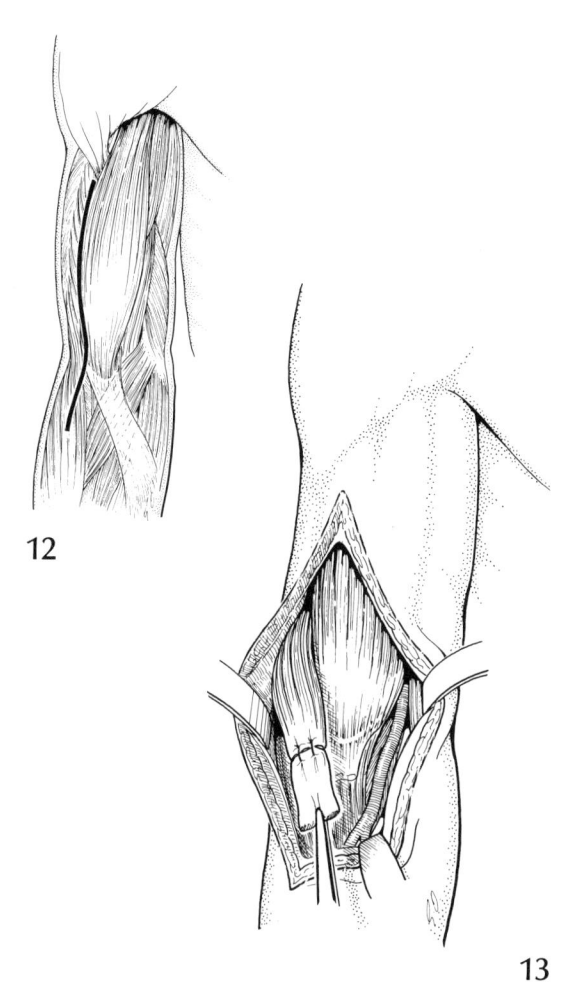

Attachment

14

The biceps tendon is split as near to its insertion to the radial tuberosity as possible and the lengthened triceps tendon passed through this. It is sutured to the biceps tendon using non-absorbable sutures with the elbow at 90° of flexion and the forearm fully supinated.

Postoperative management

An above-elbow plaster cast is applied for 6 weeks with the elbow acutely flexed at 80° and the forearm in mid-pronation. Passive and active exercises are started at the end of the 6 weeks.

742 Elbow

TRANSFER OF THE PECTORALIS MAJOR TENDON
(Brooks and Seddon[6])

This operation to restore elbow flexion is carried out if a Steindler flexorplasty is not feasible and if the biceps muscle is completely paralysed. For the operation to be successful muscles controlling the shoulder joint must be normal; otherwise the shoulder must be stabilized by fusion.

Incision

15

An incision is made along the deltopectoral groove starting from the level of the coracoid process and extending along the upper third of the upper arm.

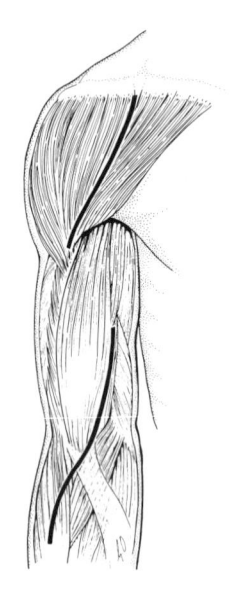

Dissection of pectoralis major

16

The tendon of the pectoralis major is cut as close to the bony insertion as possible. The pectoralis muscle is mobilized by finger dissection towards the clavicle, taking care not to damage the blood vessels and nerves supplying this muscle.

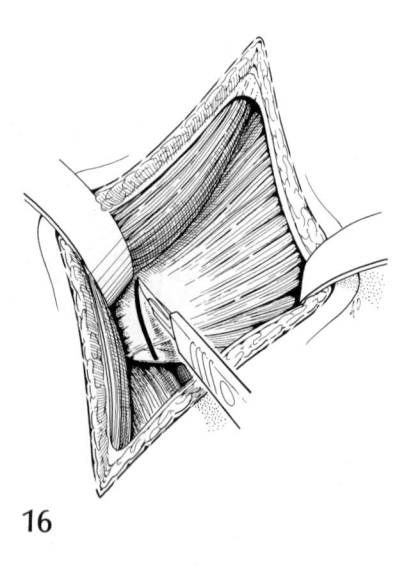

Mobilization of biceps

17

The long head of the biceps is exposed by retracting the deltoid laterally. This is cut as near as possible to the supraglenoid insertion without opening the shoulder joint.

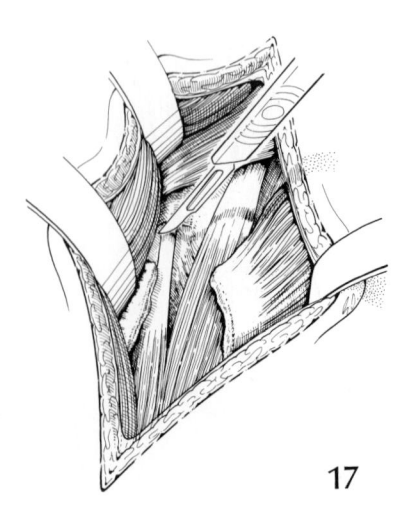

18

The muscle belly of the long head of the biceps is mobilized and separated from the short head. The blood vessels supplying the long head of the biceps muscle are ligated and divided.

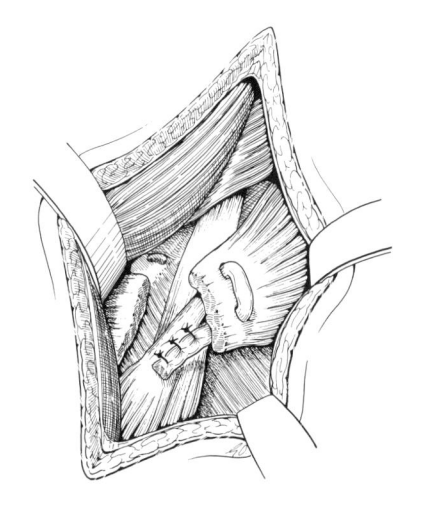

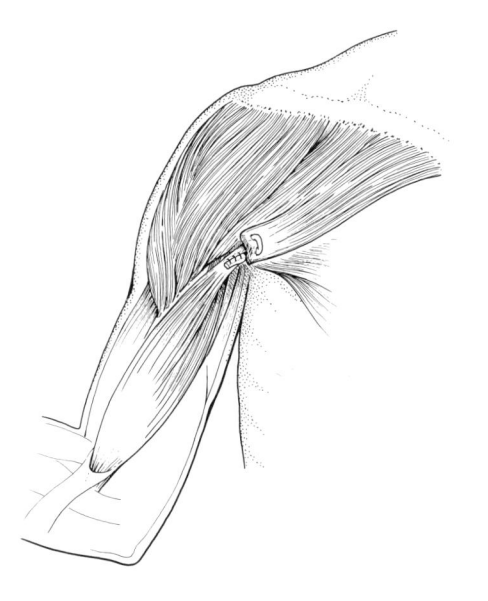

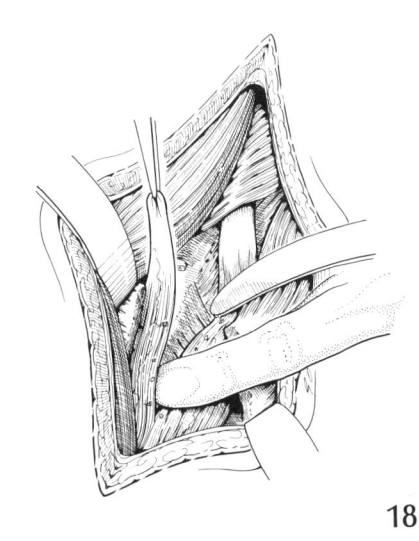

Transfer through anterior incision

A lazy-S incision is made on the anterior aspect of the elbow starting from the medial border of the biceps muscle to the lateral side of the forearm (see *Illustration 15*). The muscle belly of the long head is separated from the short head. Any additional nerves or blood vessels are divided and the muscle belly is freed right down to the radial tuberosity. The surgeon should ensure that the muscle belly of the long head of the biceps is completely freed by bringing it out through the elbow incision.

The muscle belly is replaced in the wound in the original position and the tendon of the long head is replaced into the proximal incision.

19 & 20

Two button-hole incisions are made in the pectoralis major tendon and the long head of the biceps is threaded through these so that it doubles back on itself. With the elbow flexed to 90° the biceps tendon is tautened and sutured to itself using non-absorbable sutures. This is further augmented by sutures placed between the pectoralis major and biceps tendons.

Postoperative management

A well-padded plaster backslab is applied with the elbow flexed to 90°. The backslab is removed at the end of 3 weeks and gradually the elbow is extended. The extension should not be too rapid, otherwise the tendon replacement will over-stretch. It usually takes about 3 months for extension to return.

References

1. Steindler A. Muscle and tendon transplantation at the elbow. *Am Acad Orthop Surg Instr Course Lect* 1944; 276–83.

2. Steindler A. Reconstruction of the poliomyelitic upper extremity. *Bull Hosp Joint Dis* 1954; 15: 21–34.

3. Bunnell S. Restoring flexion to the paralytic elbow. *J Bone Joint Surg [Am]* 1951; 33-A: 566–71.

4. Bunnell S. Tendon transfers in the hand and forearm. *Am Acad Orthop Surg Instr Course Lect* 1949; 6: 106–12.

5. Carroll R. E. Restoration of flexor power to the flail elbow by transplantation of the triceps tendon. *Surg Gynecol Obstet* 1952; 95: 685–8.

6. Brooks DM, Seddon HJ. Pectoral transplantation for paralysis of the flexors of the elbow. A new technique. *J Bone Joint Surg [Br]* 1959; 41-B: 36–43.

Illustrations by Gillian Oliver

Tendon reconstruction in the forearm

B. Helal MChOrth, FRCS
Honorary Consultant Orthopaedic Surgeon, The Royal London Hospital and The Royal National Orthopaedic Hospital, London, and Enfield Group of Hospitals, UK

S. C. Chen FRCS
Consultant Orthopaedic Surgeon, Enfield Group of Hospitals, UK

Introduction

Tendon reconstruction may be necessary in the forearm for either spasticity or paralysis. Spasticity of a muscle may be due to cerebral palsy, or could follow a cerebrovascular accident. The more usual indication is for paralysis of a muscle due to irreversible nerve injury, or a neuromuscular disease, e.g. poliomyelitis, multiple sclerosis or muscular dystrophies. It is important to determine whether the neuromuscular disorder is progressive, because the transferred tendon may later be involved in a progressive lesion.

Before surgery is undertaken, it is advisable to give the patient a course of physiotherapy or splintage in order to correct any fixed deformities and to assess the state of the affected muscles over a period of 2–3 months. In spastic paralysis it may be necessary to produce a temporary paralysis of the overactive muscles by nerve block in order to assess the strength of their antagonists. It is also important to observe the psychological make-up of the patient to assess whether he or she is well-motivated.

It is only after a period of conservative therapy that surgical treatment should be advised.

SPASTIC CONDITIONS

Pronation deformity of the forearm

Pronation deformity of the forearm is not very disabling, and is preferable to a supination deformity, as most actions of the hand are carried out with the forearm in some degree of pronation. However, a pronation deformity associated with a flexed and ulnar-deviated wrist, usually seen in cerebral palsy, is disabling.

There are two surgical procedures which are equally satisfactory.

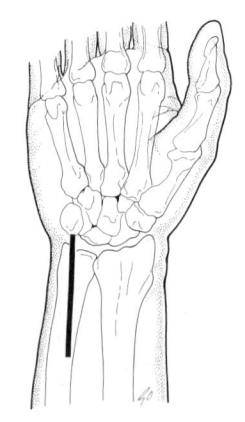

TRANSFER OF FLEXOR CARPI ULNARIS (Green and Banks[1])

1

A longitudinal incision is made on the anterior aspect of the wrist, extending 4 cm proximally from the pisiform bone.

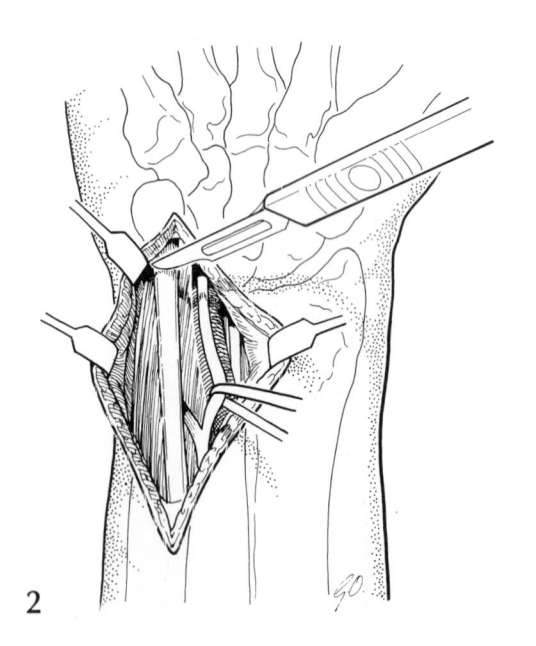

2

The ulnar nerve is identified and protected. The tendon of the flexor carpi ulnaris is detached from the pisiform bone and freed by sharp dissection from the ulna. A strong suture is attached to the end of the tendon.

3a & b

A second longitudinal incision is made over the muscle belly of the flexor carpi ulnaris, starting 4 cm from the medial epicondyle and extending about 8 cm distally. The tendon of the flexor carpi ulnaris is brought out through this incision. The muscle belly is dissected from the ulna and the deep fascia, taking care to protect the ulnar nerve and its branches.

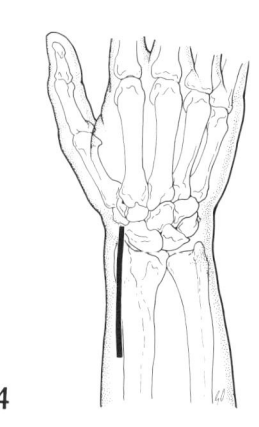

4

A third longitudinal incision is made on the dorsum of the wrist over the tendon of the extensor carpi radialis longus, extending from the wrist joint line proximally for about 5 cm. The tendon of the extensor carpi radialis longus is identified.

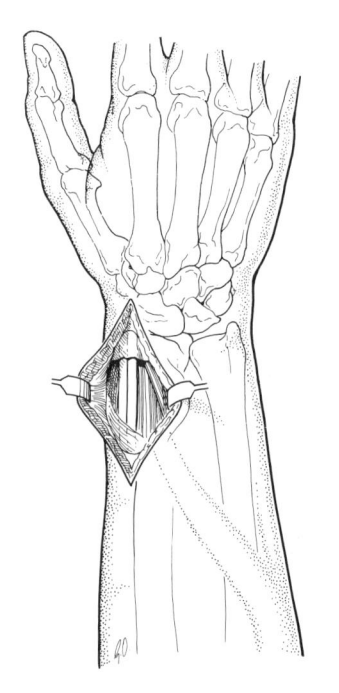

5

A check is made that the muscle belly and tendon of the flexor carpi ulnaris are freed along its course from its origin, and can be brought across the dorsum of the wrist. A tunnel is made from the proximal anterior incision, around the ulnar side of the forearm, to the dorsal incision.

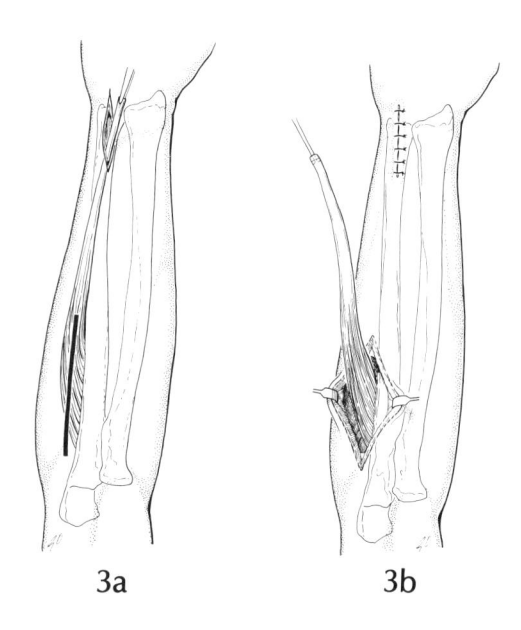

6

The tendon of the flexor carpi ulnaris is brought out of the dorsal incision through this tunnel. The strong suture attached to the end of the tendon greatly facilitates this manoeuvre. A check is made to ensure that the muscle belly and tendon of the flexor carpi ulnaris are in a direct line of action for attachment to the extensor carpi radialis longus.

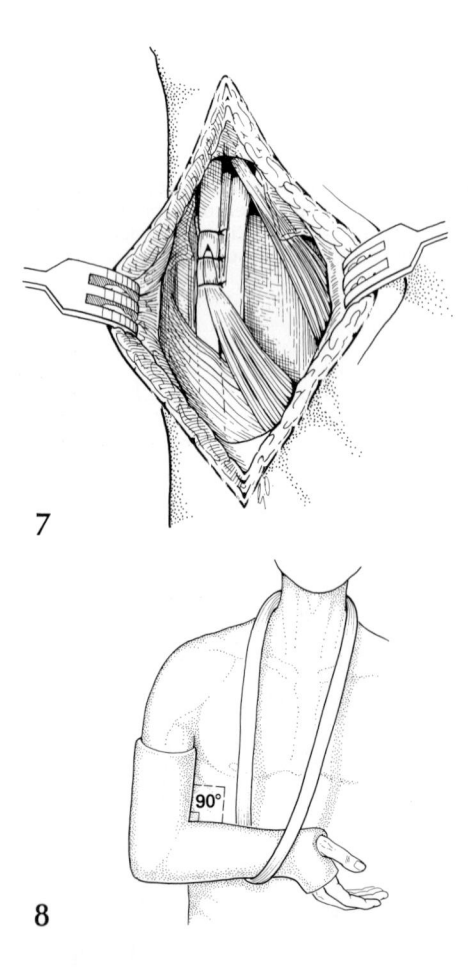

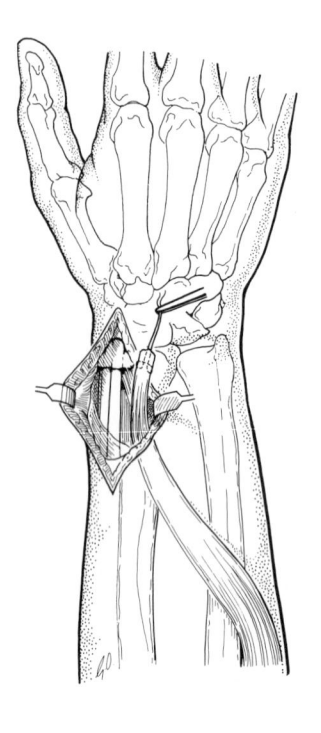

7

A small incision is made in the tendon of the extensor carpi radialis longus, and then the tendon of the flexor carpi ulnaris is passed through it. With the wrist in full dorsiflexion, and the forearm in supination, the tendons are sutured together.

If less supination and radial deviation are required, the tendon of the extensor carpi radialis brevis is chosen for attachment to the tendon of the flexor carpi ulnaris.

The wounds are sutured.

8

An above-elbow plaster cast is applied with the elbow flexed at 90°, the forearm in full supination and the wrist in dorsiflexion.

Postoperative management

Passive and active exercises of the fingers and thumb are carried out to maintain mobility of their joints. The plaster cast is bivalved at the end of 3 weeks and converted into a night splint. Elbow, forearm and wrist exercises are added to the finger exercises. The night splint is worn for a further 6 weeks.

REDIRECTION OF PRONATOR TERES TENDON
(Sakellarides, Mital and Lenzi[2])

9

A ventral longitudinal incision is made over the radius in the mid-forearm. The lateral cutaneous nerve of the forearm and the superficial branch of the radial nerve are identified and protected from injury. The brachioradialis muscle is identified and retracted medially.

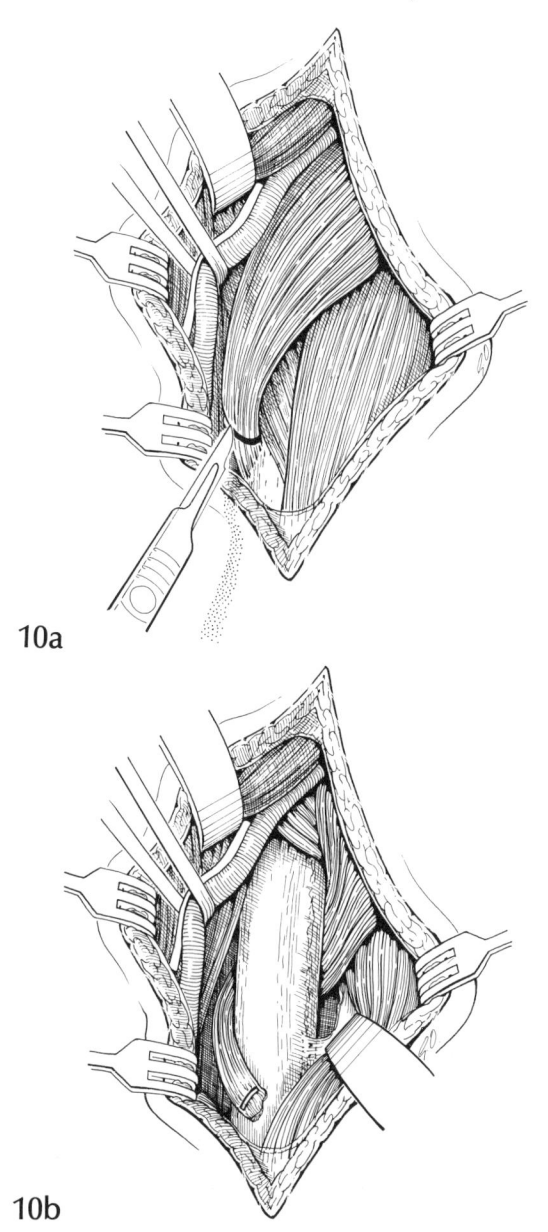

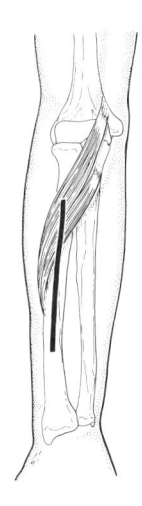

10a & b

Next, the tendon of the pronator teres is identified and detached from its insertion to the radius. A non-absorbable suture is passed through the end of the tendon using a Kessler stitch.

The interosseous membrane is detached from the radius. The tendon of the pronator teres is passed through the interosseous space and around the lateral side of the radius. Using a large drill, a hole is made in the radius at the same level as the original insertion of the pronator teres. The tendon of the pronator teres is passed through the hole in the radius. With the forearm in full supination and the elbow flexed at 90°, the tendon of the pronator teres is tied to the radius. The wound is closed.

Postoperative management

An above-elbow plaster cast is applied. At the end of 3 weeks the plaster cast is converted into a night splint, and mobilizing exercises to the elbow and wrist are carried out. The night splint is used for 8 weeks.

750 Forearm, wrist and hand

Supination deformity of the forearm

In paralytic disorders, active pronation of the forearm may be lost. This can be disabling to the patient, as satisfactory hand function relies on the ability of the forearm to be actively pronated. However, the biceps muscle may be functioning normally, and active supination is possible. In the early stages, passive pronation is present; but in longstanding supination deformities of the forearm there may be contractures of the inferior radio-ulnar joint and the interosseous membrane, and even passive pronation may be lost.

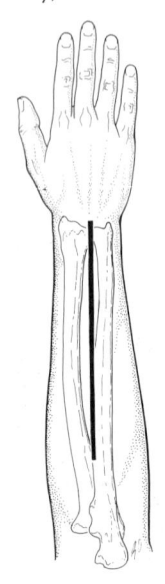

CAPSULOTOMY OF THE INFERIOR RADIO-ULNAR JOINT AND RELEASE OF THE INTEROSSEOUS MEMBRANE OF THE FOREARM (Zancolli[3])

11

A long dorsal incision is made in the forearm, starting from the inferior radio-ulnar joint and extending proximally three-quarters of the length of the forearm.

12

The extensor muscles are retracted medially and the interosseous membrane exposed by careful dissection. The posterior interosseous nerve is in the substance of these muscles and is therefore fairly well protected from damage. The interosseous membrane is incised at its attachment to the ulna. The inferior radio-ulnar joint is exposed and a dorsal capsulotomy is carried out. A check is made that passive pronation is possible at this stage. If not, the supinator muscle may have to be released. The wound is sutured.

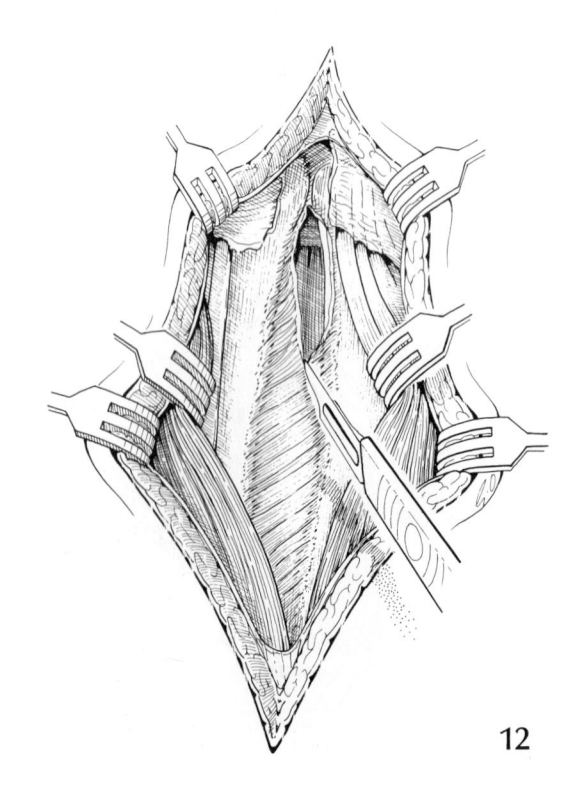

REDIRECTION OF BICEPS TENDON

13a & b

An S-shaped incision is made on the front of the elbow starting medially above the joint and ending over the radial head. The brachial artery and median nerve are identified and protected from injury. The biceps tendon is next identified.

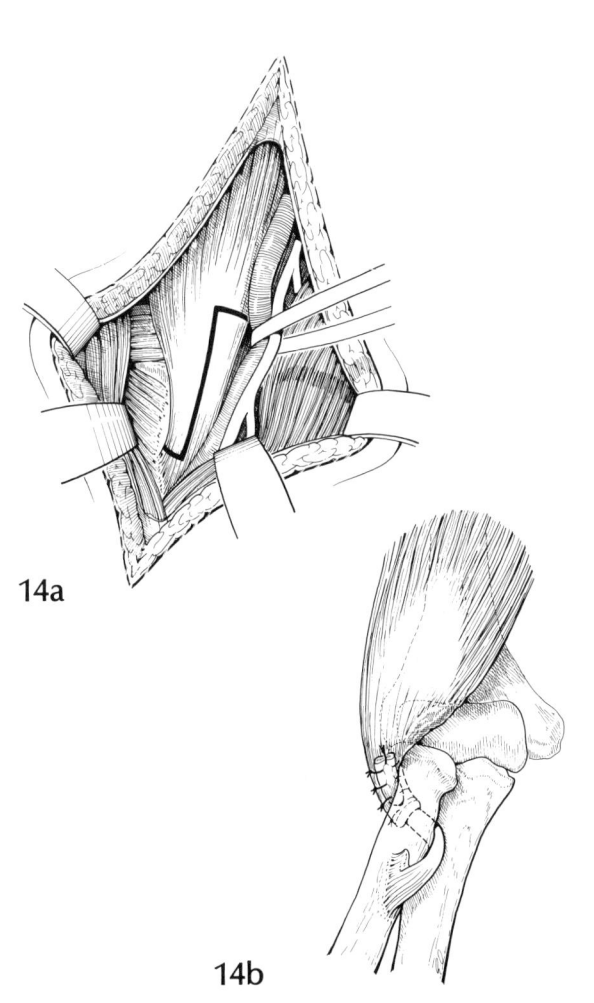

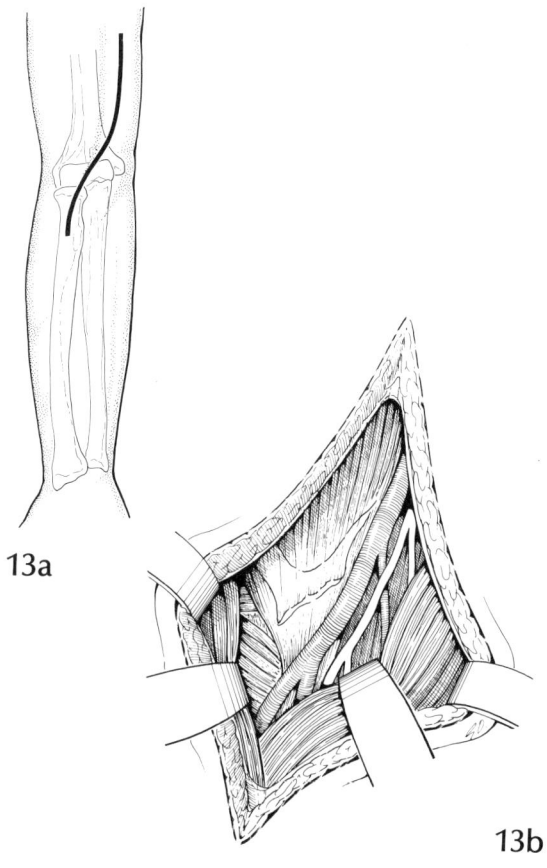

14a & b

A long Z-shaped incision is made in the tendon near its insertion to the radial tuberosity. The distal part of the tendon is then passed medially and posteriorly to the radius and brought out onto the lateral side of the radius. With the elbow flexed at 90°, the tendon is reattached to its proximal end under tension. The wound is closed.

Postoperative management

An above-elbow plaster cast is applied with the elbow flexed at 90°, and the forearm pronated. At the end of 3 weeks, the plaster cast is converted to a night splint, and pronation exercises are commenced. The night splint is worn for 8 weeks and then discarded.

752 Forearm, wrist and hand

Flexion deformity

In cerebral palsy, there may be severe flexion deformities of the wrist and fingers, which cannot be corrected passively, due to overactivity or contracture of the flexor muscles of the forearm.

By releasing these flexor muscles from their origins it may be possible to extend not only the wrist but also the fingers.

RELEASE OF THE FLEXOR MUSCLES OF THE FOREARM

15

An S-shaped incision is made, starting proximally behind the medial epicondyle and crossing the front of the elbow joint into the middle of the forearm over the ulna. The medial cutaneous nerve of the forearm is identified and protected.

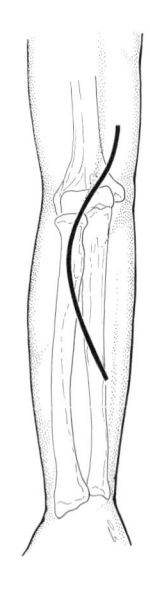

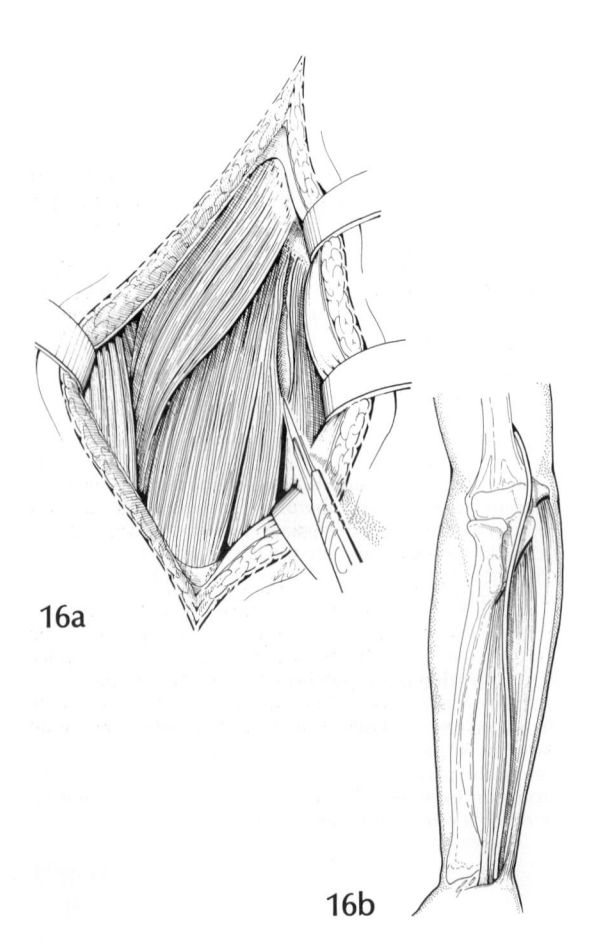

16a & b

The ulnar nerve is identified and dissected from its groove behind the medial epicondyle. The medial intermuscular septum is excised at this stage, to facilitate anterior transposition of this nerve at a later stage.

The fibrous arch of the flexor carpi ulnaris is incised and the branches of the ulnar nerve to the flexor carpi ulnaris and flexor digitorum profundus are identified. The origins of these two muscles are then detached and freed distally down to the middle of the ulna.

17

Next, the origins of the pronator teres, flexor carpi radialis, flexor digitorum sublimis, palmaris longus and flexor carpi ulnaris are detached from the medial epicondyle. The median nerve is now seen passing between the two heads of pronator teres. The ulnar nerve is transposed anterior to the elbow joint. The subcutaneous tissue and skin are sutured.

Postoperative management

A below-elbow plaster cast is applied with the forearm in supination, and the wrist and fingers in the extended neutral position. Flexion and extension exercises for the elbow are started early. At 3 weeks the plaster cast is converted into a night splint, and active and passive movements of the wrist and fingers are carried out. The night splint is discarded at the end of 8 weeks.

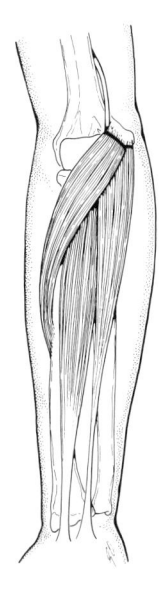

PARALYTIC CONDITIONS

One or a combination of the three nerves to the hand may be irreversibly damaged, by injury.

Radial nerve palsy

When the radial nerve is damaged in the upper arm, usually in the radial groove of the humerus, all the muscles in the limb supplied by it are paralysed. They are the brachioradialis and the extensor carpi radialis longus supplied by the main radial nerve; and the extensor carpi radialis brevis, supinator, extensor digitorum communis, extensor digiti minimi, extensor carpi ulnaris, abductor pollicis longus, extensor pollicis brevis, extensor pollicis longus and extensor indicis supplied by the posterior interosseous nerve. In addition, the sensory branches of the radial nerve are also damaged, and there is loss of sensation of the dorsal and radial border of the hand.

When the posterior interosseous nerve alone is damaged, the brachioradialis and the extensor carpi radialis longus are spared, and there is no sensory loss as the posterior interosseous nerve is a pure motor nerve.

In a radial nerve palsy, there is loss of dorsiflexion of the wrist, thumb and fingers, and abduction of the thumb. Three tendon transfers can provide these movements.

1. The pronator teres is transferred to the extensor carpi radialis brevis to provide wrist extension.
2. The flexor carpi ulnaris is transferred to the extensor digitorum communis to provide extension of the fingers.
3. The palmaris longus, if present, is transferred to the extensor pollicis longus to provide thumb extension; if the palmaris longus is absent, the flexor carpi ulnaris is transferred to the extensor pollicis longus (in addition to the extensor digitorum communis).

Extension of the fingers will also extend the wrist.

In a posterior interosseous nerve palsy, the pronator teres is transferred to the abductor pollicis longus, the flexor carpi ulnaris to the extensor digitorum communis, and the palmaris longus to the extensor pollicis longus (brachioradialis if palmaris longus is absent). The extensor carpi radialis longus is active, and reinforces wrist extension.

TRIPLE TRANSFER

Mobilization of flexor carpi ulnaris and palmaris longus

18

An L-shaped ventral incision is made along the lower half of the forearm on the ulnar side, with the transverse limb along the flexor crease of the wrist and its junction with the vertical limb centred on the pisiform bone.

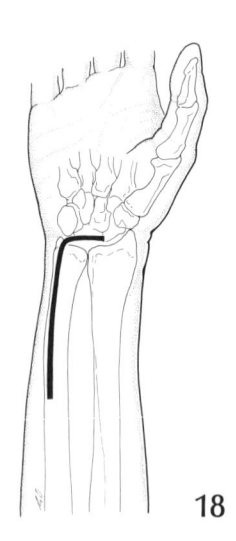

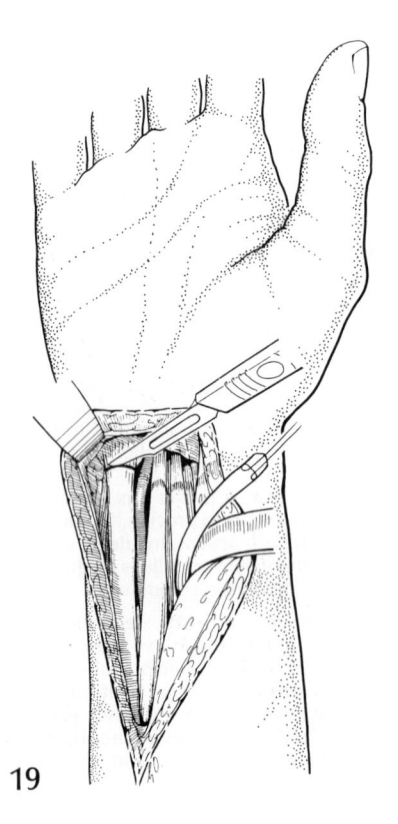

19

The tendon of the flexor carpi ulnaris is identified and detached from the pisiform bone, taking care not to damage the superficial and deep branches of the ulnar nerve. The muscle belly is freed from the ulna and mobilized proximally to the upper third of the forearm. If present, the tendon of the palmaris longus is also detached from the palmar fascia and mobilized.

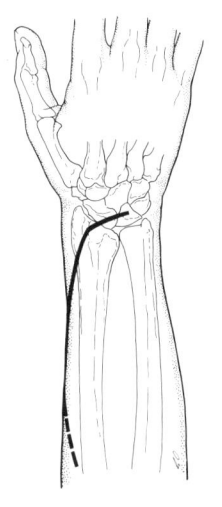

Mobilization of pronator teres

20a & b

A second L-shaped incision is made on the dorsum of the forearm with the transverse limb along the dorsal crease of the wrist and the vertical limb along the distal half of the radial side of the forearm. The proximal edge of the extensor retinaculum is identified, incised across and a flap based proximally is made in the deep fascia.

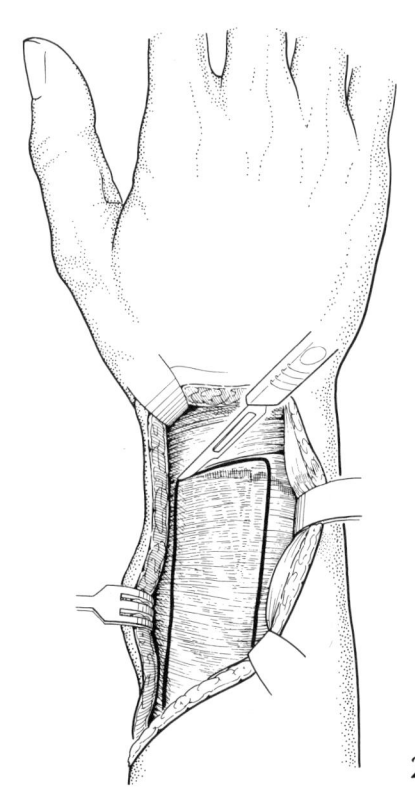

756 Forearm, wrist and hand

21a & b

The flap is turned back and the extensor tendons are exposed. The tendons of the abductor pollicis longus, the extensor pollicis longus, the extensor digitorum communis and the pronator teres (PT) are identified. The extensor pollicis longus is freed and brought out of its groove to lie in the same plane as the tendons of the extensor digitorum communis. The pronator teres is detached from the radius and held with an end-suture.

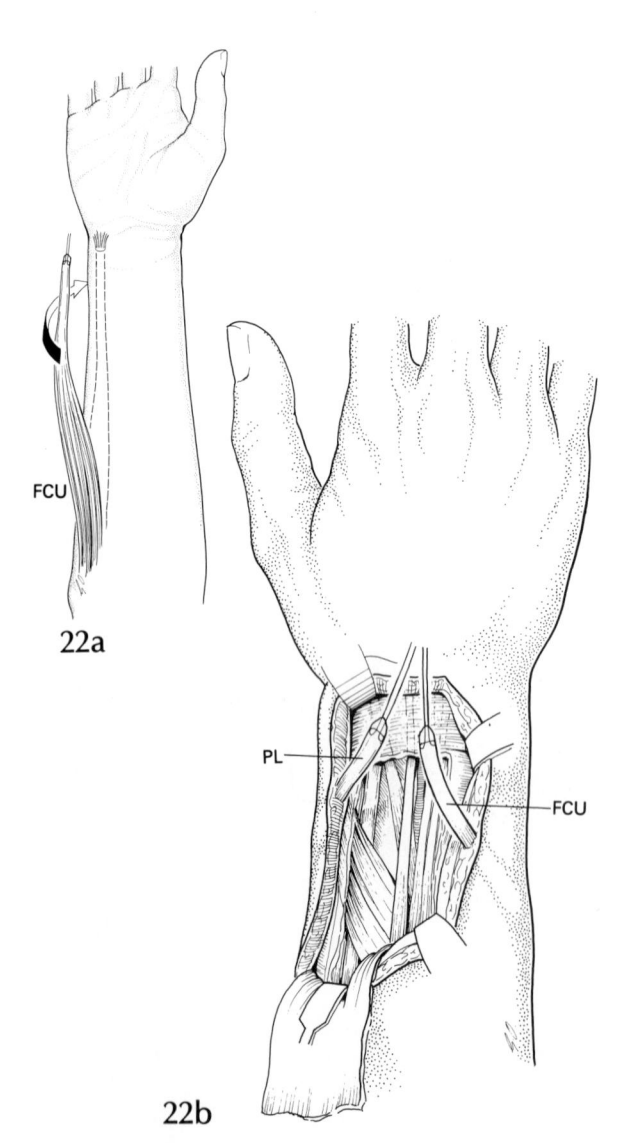

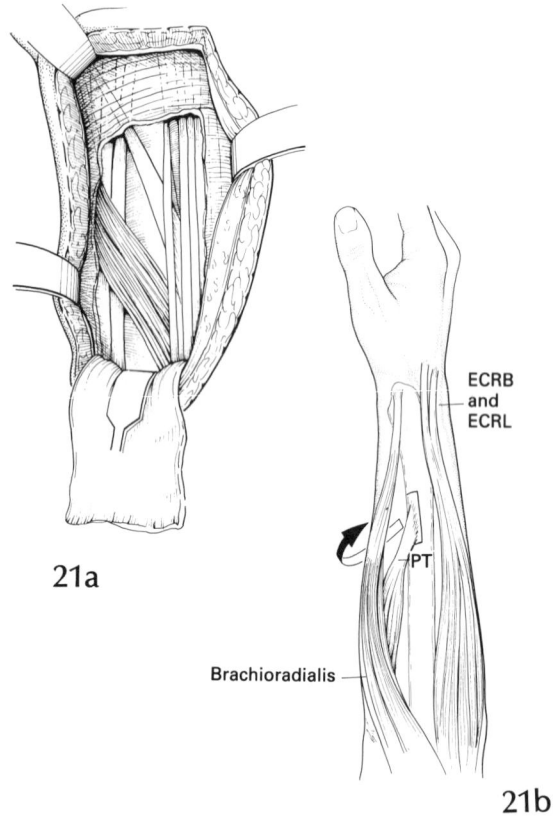

Transfer of flexor carpi ulnaris

22a & b

Oblique subcutaneous tunnels are made on the radial and ulnar sides of the forearm extending distally from the dorsum to the ventral sides proximally. The tendon of the flexor carpi ulnaris (FCU) is passed along the ulnar side of the forearm to emerge on the dorsum. Similarly, the tendon of the palmaris longus (PL) is passed along the radial side. The positions of these two tendons are checked to make sure that their lines of pull are as near to the direction of pull of the extensor digitorum communis, extensor pollicis longus and extensor carpi radialis brevis (ECRB).

23

The wrist is held in full dorsiflexion. The fingers are held with the metacarpophalangeal joints in full extension, the proximal and distal interphalangeal joints in full flexion. The thumb is held fully extended and abducted. A thin Kirschner wire is passed through the tendons of the extensor digitorum communis and the extensor pollicis longus. The tension of each tendon is checked to make sure that the correct tension is applied to each. This is checked by extending the wrist, when full passive flexion of the fingers should be possible; and by flexing the wrist, when full extension of the fingers should occur.

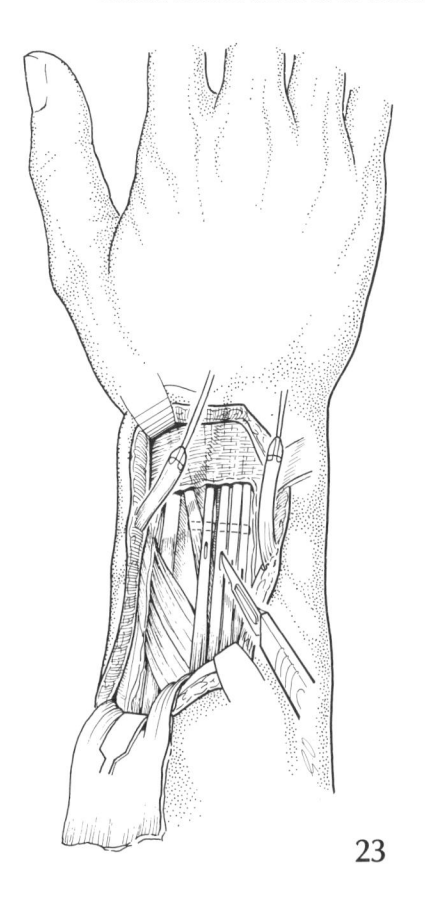

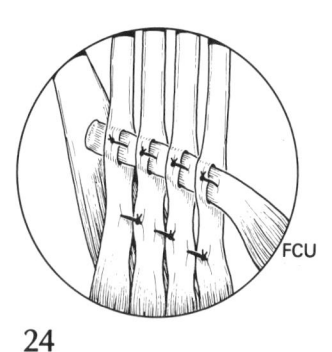

24

A No. 15 blade is passed through each tendon in an oblique direction, and along the line of pull of the flexor carpi ulnaris tendon. Sufficient muscle fibres are dissected away from the end of the flexor carpi ulnaris tendon to enable it to be passed through and to be sutured to each tendon with non-absorbable sutures. The Kirschner wire is now removed.

Transfer of pronator teres and palmaris longus

25a, b & c

The tendon of the extensor carpi radialis brevis is split near its insertion, and the pronator teres (PT) is passed through and sutured to it with non-absorbable sutures.

The tendon of the extensor pollicis longus is split, and the palmaris longus (PL) tendon is passed through and sutured to it with non-absorbable sutures.

If the palmaris longus is absent, the brachioradialis is used.

Closure

The flap in the deep fascia on the dorsum of the forearm is sutured back into place. The subcutaneous tissue and skin are sutured.

The L-shaped incision on the ventral surface of the forearm is then sutured in layers.

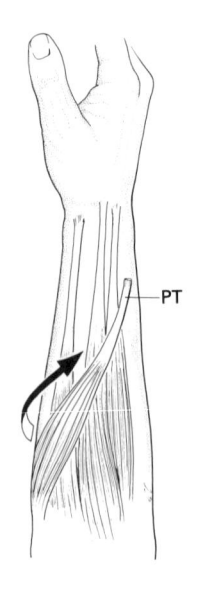

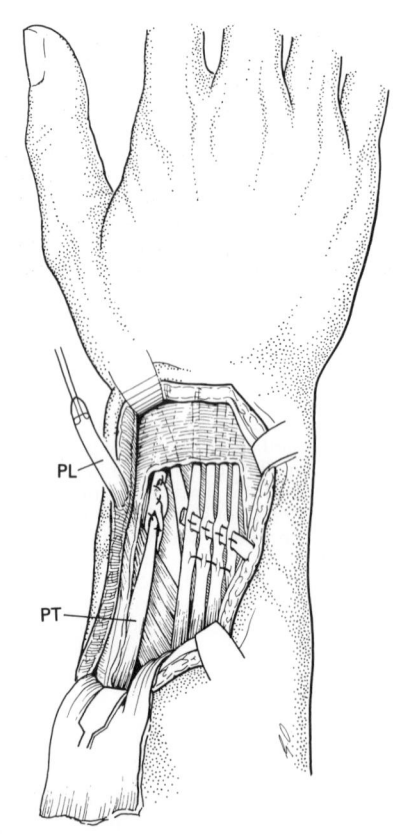

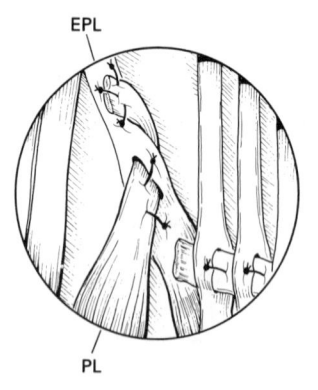

Postoperative management

26

A well-padded below-elbow plaster backslab is applied with the wrist in full dorsiflexion, the metacarpophalangeal joints flexed at 90°, and the interphalangeal joints fully extended. At the end of 3 weeks the plaster backslab is removed and converted into a night splint. Active thumb, finger and wrist exercises are started. The night splint is discarded at the end of 2 weeks.

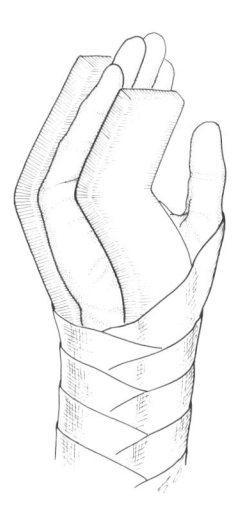

26

Median nerve palsy

When the median nerve is damaged in the arm above the elbow, the flexor group of muscles, i.e. pronator teres, flexor carpi radialis, flexor digitorum sublimis, palmaris longus, flexor carpi ulnaris, radial part of the flexor digitorum profundus, flexor pollicis longus and pronator quadratus, are paralysed leading to loss of forearm pronation, wrist flexion, index and middle finger flexion, and thumb flexion and opposition. There is also sensory loss in the median nerve distribution.

The thumb movements are restored by two reconstructions: the extensor indicis is used to provide thumb opposition; and the extensor carpi radialis longus is transferred to the flexor pollicis longus to provide thumb flexion. The muscle bellies of the flexor digitorum profundus to the ring and little fingers are innervated by the ulnar nerve which is undamaged, so they are sutured to the flexor digitorum profundus tendons of the index and middle fingers to provide a mass action in flexion. In addition, the brachioradialis is transferred to the conjoined tendons to reinforce the mass action.

Protective sensation may be restored to the thumb and index finger by transferring island flaps from the ring and little fingers.

Forearm, wrist and hand

TRANSFER OF EXTENSOR INDICIS TO THE THUMB
(Burkhalter, Christensen and Brown[4])

27

A small transverse incision is made on the dorsum of the metacarpophalangeal joint of the index finger.

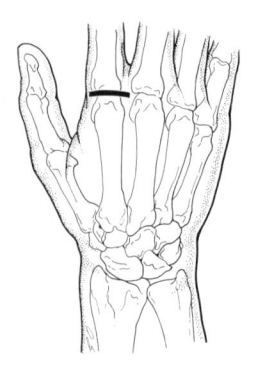

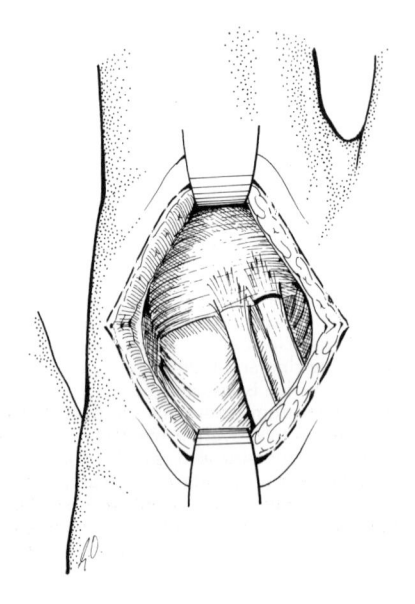

28a & b

The tendon of the extensor indicis proprius is identified lying on the ulnar side of the extensor digitorum communis tendon. It is divided and the distal stump is sutured onto this tendon. The proximal end of the extensor indicis proprius is freed as much as possible with blunt dissection.

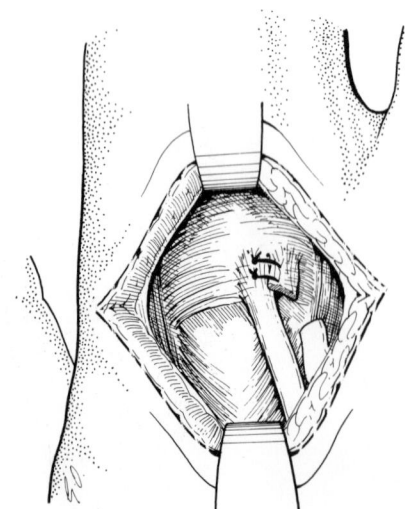

29

A longitudinal incision about 3 cm long is made on the ulnar side of the forearm just proximal to the flexor crease of the wrist. The muscle belly of the extensor indicis is identified by tugging on its tendon in the distal wound. The proximal part of the tendon is freed by blunt dissection. Using a blunt hook, the tendon is brought out of the proximal wound. The distal wound is now sutured.

A tunnel is made in the subcutaneous tissue towards the pisiform bone, making sure that the tunnel is always kept in the superficial tissues, so as not to damage the ulnar nerve and its branches in this area.

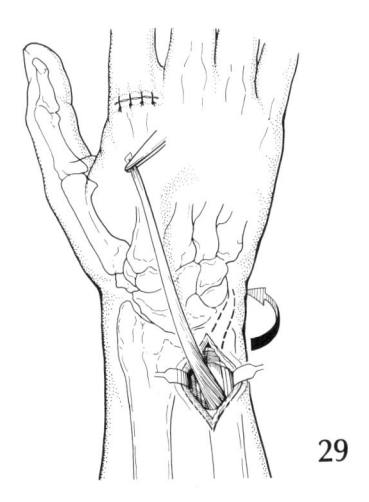

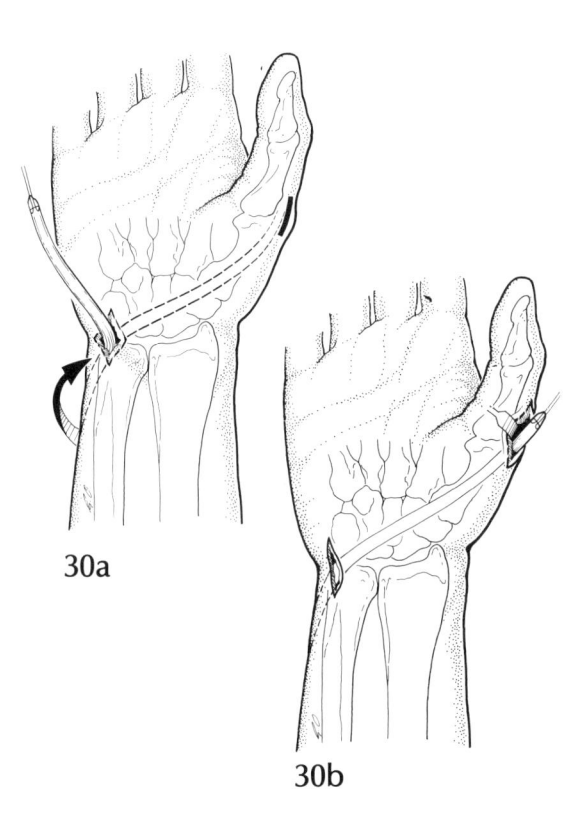

30a & b

A small incision 1 cm long is made just distal to the pisiform. The tunnelling is continued towards the radial side of the metacarpophalangeal joint of the thumb, where a small incision 2 cm long is made. The extensor indicis tendon is now brought out through the incision just distal to the pisiform. It is then re-routed towards the thumb, and brought through the wound on its radial side.

31

A button-hole is made in the abductor pollicis brevis tendon, and the extensor indicis tendon is passed through and sutured to it, with the thumb held in full abduction, and the wrist in 10° of palmarflexion.

Correct tension is important. If it is too tight, an abduction contracture of the thumb can occur. If it is too loose, satisfactory opposition is not possible.

The wounds are now sutured.

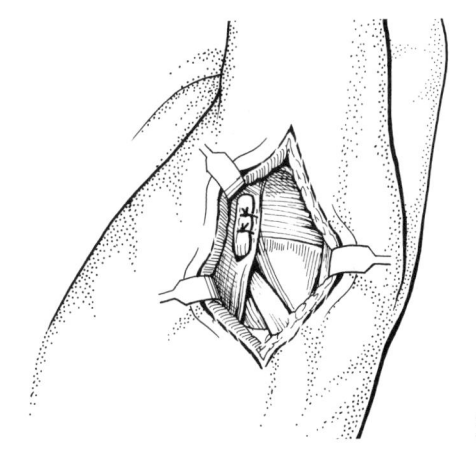

762 Forearm, wrist and hand

TRANSFER OF BRACHIORADIALIS TO FLEXOR DIGITORUM PROFUNDUS

32

An L-shaped incision is made on the flexor surface of the forearm with the transverse limb across the crease of the wrist, and the vertical limb 5 cm long on the radial side. The radial nerve and its branches are identified and protected.

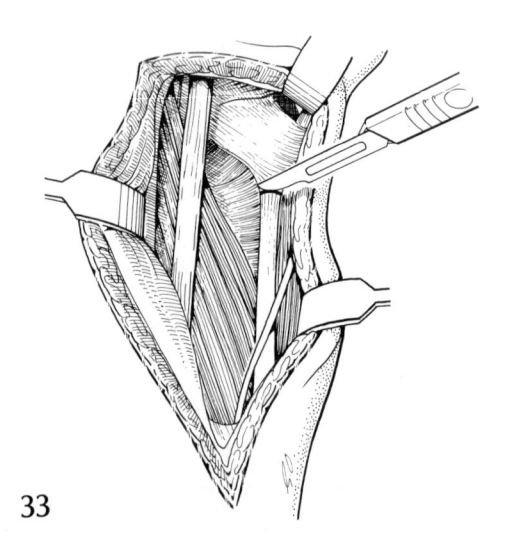

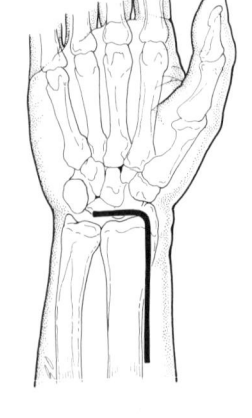

33

The brachioradialis is detached from its insertion to the lateral side of the lower end of the radius and freed, so that its direction of pull is in line with the flexor digitorum profundus tendons.

34

The four tendons of the flexor digitorum profundus are identified and sutured together with non-absorbable sutures. The flexor digitorum profundus tendons to the index and middle fingers are then cut proximally to free them from their paralysed muscle bellies. The brachioradialis tendon is sutured under tension to the conjoined flexor digitorum profundus tendons on the radial side.

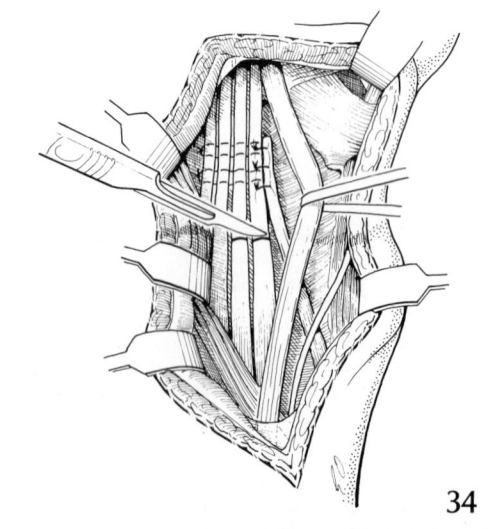

TRANSFER OF EXTENSOR CARPI RADIALIS LONGUS TO FLEXOR POLLICIS LONGUS

35

A transverse incision is made over the insertion of the extensor carpi radialis longus and extended to the base of the second metacarpal. The tendon is detached and freed by blunt dissection. It is brought out on the radial side onto the flexor surface of the forearm.

36

The flexor pollicis longus tendon is identified, and the extensor carpi radialis longus tendon is attached to it by interweaving the two tendons together, with the wrist in neutral position, the thumb in 20° of flexion at the interphalangeal joint, full extension at the metacarpophalangeal joint, and full abduction at the carpometacarpal joint.

The L-shaped wound on the flexor surface of the forearm and the small transverse wound on the dorsum of the wrist are now sutured.

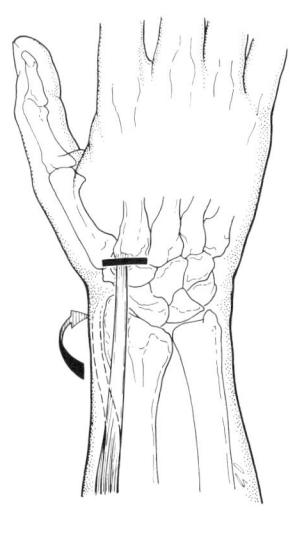

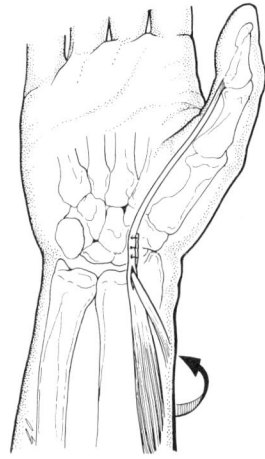

Postoperative management

A plaster backslab is applied with the wrist in a neutral position, the metacarpophalangeal joints of the fingers in 90° flexion, and the proximal and distal interphalangeal joints in full extension. The thumb is immobilized in full abduction at the carpometacarpal joint, in neutral position at the metacarpophalangeal joint, and in 20° of flexion at the interphalangeal joint. The Kleinert technique of early mobilization is not used, as the extensor carpi radialis longus and extensor indicis are extensors and may pull off in the immediate postoperative phase. The plaster backslab is removed at the end of 3 weeks, and passive and active thumb and finger exercises are started.

Ulnar nerve palsy

When the ulnar nerve is damaged in the arm, above the elbow, the ulnar part of the flexor digitorum profundus is paralysed, leading to loss of flexion of the distal interphalangeal joints of the ring and little fingers; the flexor carpi ulnaris is also paralysed, leading to loss of ulnar deviation of a palmarflexed wrist. In addition, the ulnar nerve supplies most of the intrinsic muscles in the hand, and paralysis of these muscles results in a weak grip. Paralysis of the adductor pollicis and the first dorsal interosseus results in a weak pinch.

Tendon reconstruction of the hand is dealt with elsewhere, but it is important to realize that combined nerve lesions can occur, and will influence tendon reconstruction in the forearm.

Combined median and radial nerve paralysis

In this situation the ulnar nerve is the only functioning nerve, and the muscles which it innervates, namely flexor carpi ulnaris and the medial part of the flexor digitorum profundus, are those available for transfer.

The flexor carpi ulnaris is transferred around the ulnar side of the forearm to the extensor digitorum communis and extensor pollicis longus, and the four tendons of the flexor digitorum profundus are joined together by non-absorbable sutures.

It is necessary to carry out an arthrodesis of the wrist as there are no functioning prime movers of this joint. The arthrodesis is always carried out after the tendon transfers.

The thumb can be flexed at the metacarpophalangeal joint by the flexor pollicis brevis which is supplied by the ulnar nerve, but it may be necessary to arthrodese the interphalangeal joint to provide a good pinch grip.

Combined median and ulnar nerve paralysis

In this situation, only the radial nerve is functioning. The palmar surface of the hand, including the finger tips, is anaesthetic. Only the extensor muscles in the forearm, namely brachioradialis, extensor carpi radialis longus, extensor carpi radialis brevis, extensor indicis, extensor digitorum communis and extensor carpi ulnaris, are active.

The extensor carpi radialis longus is transferred to the flexor digitorum profundus, and the brachioradialis to the flexor pollicis longus, to provide flexion of the fingers and thumb. A closed fist is usually associated with an extended wrist and therefore these transferred tendons are synergistic in their actions. Therefore, the wrist should never be arthrodesed.

It may be necessary to carry out metacarpophalangeal arthrodesis of the thumb, and Zancolli capsulodesis[5] of the metacarpophalangeal joints of the fingers.

Combined radial and ulnar nerve paralysis

In this situation, only the median nerve is functioning in the forearm. The muscles innervated by it, namely pronator teres, flexor carpi radialis, flexor digitorum sublimis, palmaris longus, flexor carpi ulnaris, the radial two tendons of the flexor digitorum profundus and flexor pollicis longus, are available for transfer.

Flexor carpi radialis longus is transferred around the radial side of the forearm into the extensor digitorum communis and extensor pollicis longus. If the palmaris longus is present it is transferred to the abductor pollicis longus. Clawing of the ring and little fingers is corrected by Zancolli capsulodesis[5].

It is usually necessary to arthrodese the wrist joint, but this is done only as the final stage in the treatment, after the tendon transfers have been carried out.

References

1. Green WT, Banks HH. Flexor carpi ulnaris transplant and its use in cerebral palsy. *J Bone Joint Surg [Am]* 1962; 44-A: 1343–52.

2. Sakellarides HT, Mital MA, Lenzi, WD. Treatment of pronation contractures of the forearm in cerebral palsy by changing the insertion of the pronator radii teres. *J Bone Joint Surg [Am]* 1981; 63-A: 645–52.

3. Zancolli EA. Paralytic supination contracture of the forearm. *J Bone Joint Surg [Am]* 1967; 49-A: 1275–84.

4. Burkhalter W, Christensen RC, Brown P. Extensor indicis proprius opponensplasty. *J Bone Joint Surg [Am]* 1973; 55-A: 725–32.

5. Zancolli EA. Clawhand caused by paralysis of the intrinsic muscles: a simple surgical procedure for its correction. *J Bone Joint Surg [Am]* 1957; 39-A: 1076–80.

Illustrations by Peter Cox

Surgery of the wrist

I. J. Leslie MChOrth, FRCS
Department of Orthopaedic and Traumatic Surgery, Bristol Royal Infirmary, Bristol, UK

RHEUMATOID ARTHRITIS

General considerations

Surgery of the rheumatoid hand and wrist requires careful preoperative evaluation. It must be remembered that rheumatoid arthritis is a systemic disease, and that surgery of the peripheral part of the upper limb is a single event in the long-term management of the systemic disease as well as other treatment that may be necessary in other joints of the upper and lower limbs. Careful patient selection is crucial and the decision for surgery should be taken in conjunction with the rheumatologist. Therefore, ideally, combined clinics with rheumatologists should be held and the timing of surgery, as well as the operative procedure, should be carefully evaluated at these clinics. The therapist is an extremely important member of the evaluating team and should have a particular interest in both rheumatoid disease and hand therapy.

Indications and principles in planning surgery

While there are specific indications for individual operations, it is uncommon for there to be only one particular problem which requires one operation. Surgery needs to be planned as multiple operations may well be required. Certain general principles must be taken into consideration when planning such surgery. These are detailed below.

1. An assessment of *shoulder and elbow function* is important. It is pointless reconstructing a hand when it cannot be put to any good use because of painful restriction of elbow and shoulder joint function.

2. The mere presence of a *deformity of the hand* does not necessarily mean an operation is required. Rheumatoid disease has a slow progression and patients adapt very well to a slowly progressive deformity. Surprisingly, good function can be maintained without pain in a very deformed hand. A careful functional assessment of the hand must be performed and this is best done by the therapist who will have the time and facilities available to sit down with the patient and discuss the problems and requirements. The therapist should be included in the discussion when surgery is being considered.

The cosmetic appearance of the hand is not an important indication for surgery; however, in young people with rheumatoid arthritis this may be an important factor to the patient. Considerable psychological problems may result from a deformity and the surgeon should be prepared to undertake surgery for this reason, provided that function is not compromised, and a careful discussion of this aspect should be undertaken with the patient.

3. While surgery for arthritic joints is usually undertaken because of *pain*, this may not necessarily be so in the hand and wrist. It is important to discuss with the patient the reason for operating, i.e. relief of pain, improvement of function, or both.

4. The patient with rheumatoid disease may well have significant problems with the lower limbs and for that reason may have to use walking aids. Therefore *the need to use crutches* or a walking stick may alter the type of surgery which is considered in the upper limb, i.e. a wrist arthrodesis versus a wrist arthroplasty.

5. When planning surgery of the rheumatoid hand and wrist, the general principle should be to *start reconstruction proximally and work distally*, leaving the thumb until last, e.g. metacarpophalangeal joint replacement will not work well if the patient has an unstable, painful wrist. The order of surgery should be considered along the following guidelines.

(a) Wrist joint
(b) Metacarpophalangeal joints of the fingers
(c) Proximal interphalangeal joints of the fingers
(d) Thumb (if the thumb is done last it can then be put into the best position of function to correspond to the position achieved in the fingers).

6. It is important that the surgeon gains the confidence of the patient when multiple surgical procedures may well be necessary. For this reason it is usually better to *start with a simple procedure* which has a high success rate. The more difficult procedures can then be performed at a later date when the patient understands what is required in the postoperative programme and the surgeon can assess how the patient will respond to the more complicated procedures. While the simple procedures can be performed by any competent orthopaedic surgeon, those that require more intricate work on the joints and tendons and thus carry a high risk of loss of function should be left to a surgeon who is more skilled in the atraumatic techniques that are required and who has access to the expertise available from a skilled hand therapist.

7. It is important that the *patient's expectations* of the operations are not higher than those of the surgeon. The patient must be aware of why the operation is being performed and also be prepared to undergo an extensive rehabilitation programme postoperatively.

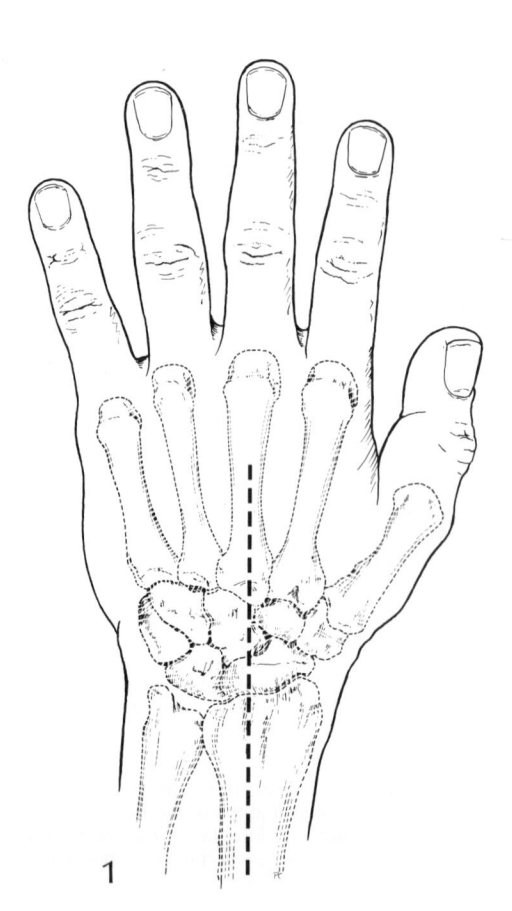

8. It is advisable to *operate on only one hand at a time* as the patient will be extremely incapacitated if both hands are in splints or bandages. The amount of surgery performed on one hand at any one time must also be restricted as extensive operations, especially on the dorsal and palmar aspect, may result in significant swelling and subsequent stiffness.

9. *Prophylactic surgery* may be necessary and this mainly involves the preservation of tendon function, i.e. synovectomy and decompression of synovial compartments.

Operations

DORSAL SYNOVECTOMY

Synovitis of the extensor tendons, especially when tense and painful, may result in rupture of one or more of the extensor tendons. The extensor retinaculum remains intact and allows an increased pressure to develop within the dorsal compartments. Synovium will bulge at each end of the retinaculum, producing an 'hour glass' effect. Decompression is necessary to prevent tendon rupture.

Indications

Indications for dorsal synovectomy are persistent swelling of the dorsal compartments despite medical treatment and ruptured extensor tendons.

Incision

1

A straight longitudinal incision is made in line with the shaft of the third metacarpal. It extends from a point approximately 6 cm proximal to the wrist joint to the level of the mid-shaft of the metacarpal.

Approach

The incision is taken directly down to the extensor retinaculum. Veins and cutaneous nerves should be preserved. The delicate skin should be lifted by the assistant using skin hooks to avoid grasping with forceps. A scalpel is used to develop the plane between the subcutaneous tissue and the extensor retinaculum. Excessive retraction on the skin should be avoided and the skin flaps should be kept as thick as possible. On the radial side some terminal branches of the radial nerve may be seen and these should be preserved and lifted with the subcutaneous tissue.

2

The extensor retinaculum is incised as shown and is lifted from the ulnar side towards the radial side. The extended Flap A will be used as a sling for extensor carpi ulnaris. Flap C is left attached on the ulnar side and Flap B is left attached on the radial side. Segment D is left in place to stop the tendons bow-stringing on wrist dorsiflexion. It is necessary to dissect the vertical septa off the dorsal surface of the radius, taking care not to buttonhole the retinaculum.

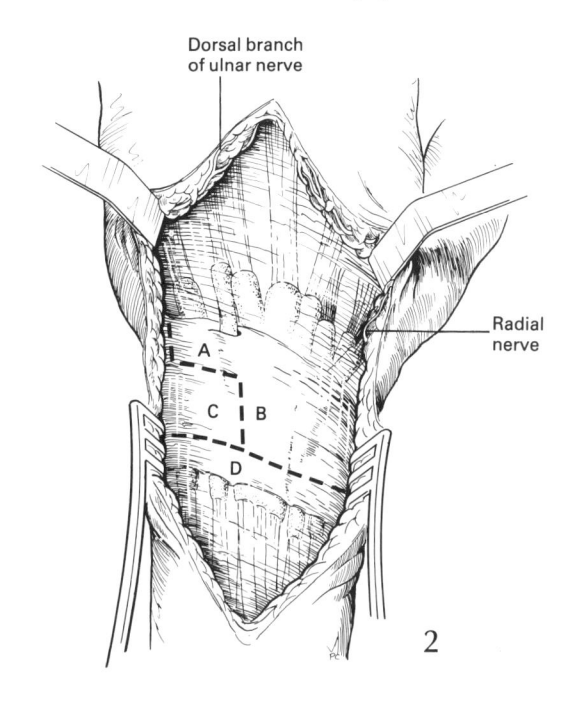

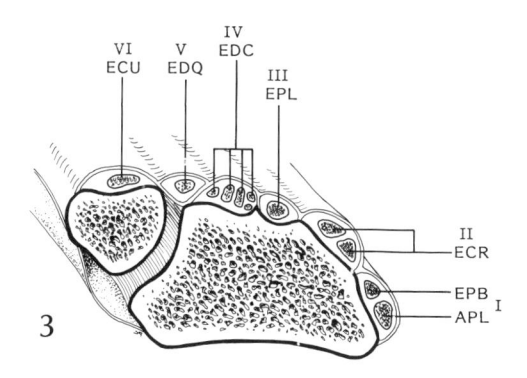

3

The compartments of the extensor mechanism at the wrist joint are shown. The dissection can be carried radially to expose extensor pollicis longus unless there is significant synovial involvement of the extensor carpi radialis tendons, in which case the retinaculum should be lifted to expose the next compartment.

768 Forearm, wrist and hand

Synovectomy and reconstruction

4a & b

The synovium is dissected off the tendons by sharp dissection with a scalpel or scissors. It can also be pulled off using a pair of curved artery forceps. A blunt hook is used to lift the tendons clear of the wrist joint. Any sharp spicules on the underlying bone should be removed. At this stage the following procedures can be carried out if necessary.

1. Synovectomy of the wrist
2. Excision of the distal end of the ulna
3. Synovectomy of the distal radio-ulnar joint
4. Repair of extensor tendons.

The terminal branch of the posterior interosseous nerve can be found on the distal radius underlying the extensor tendon to the middle finger. It is often worth dividing this with bipolar coagulation as it helps to relieve pain on the dorsum of the wrist.

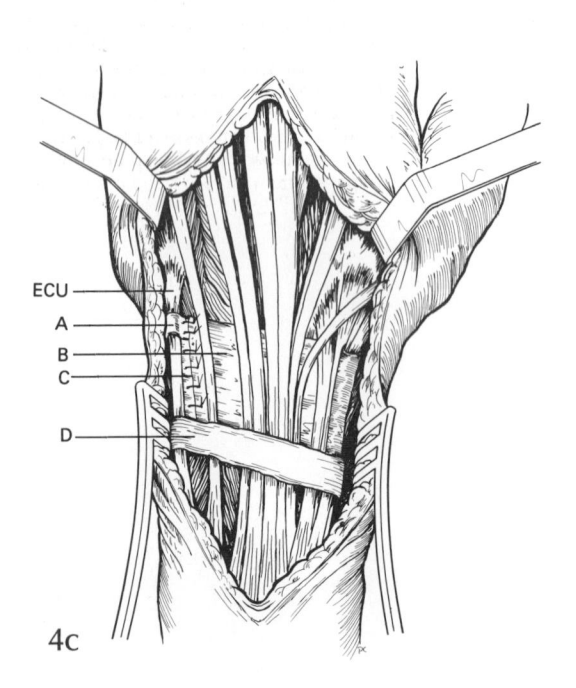

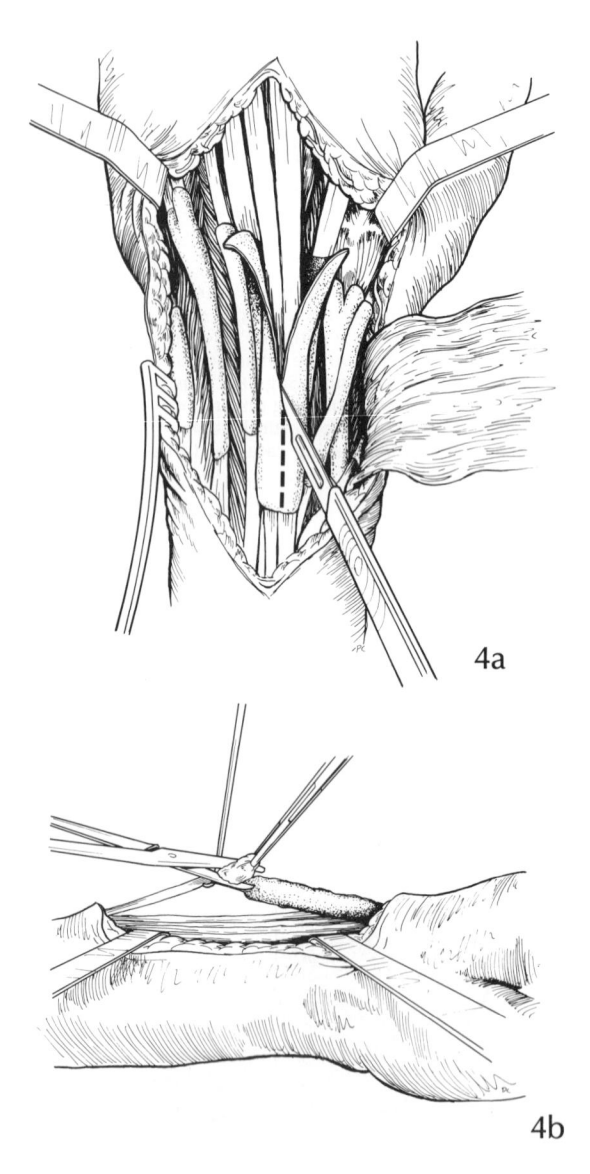

4c

Following synovectomy, the extensor retinaculum is passed beneath the extensor tendons of the thumb and fingers and is sutured back to the ulnar flap using an absorbable suture material. Flap A of the retinaculum is passed beneath the tendon of the extensor carpi ulnaris and brought back over the top of it to create a pulley. It is sutured to Flap B using a braided polyester suture material. This reconstruction places the extensor carpi ulnaris tendon over the distal end of the ulna, reduces the ulnar deviation forces and helps to elevate the carpus.

Skin closure and postoperative management

A small suction drain is placed beneath the skin which is sutured in one layer with interrupted 4/0 nylon. A soft gauze dressing is applied followed by a soft wool dressing. A plaster slab is placed on the palmar aspect for 10 days until the wound is healed. Mobilization of the wrist and fingers is then commenced unless extensor tendon repair has been performed, in which case the fingers and wrist are immobilized for 3 weeks followed by dynamic extension splinting to the fingers.

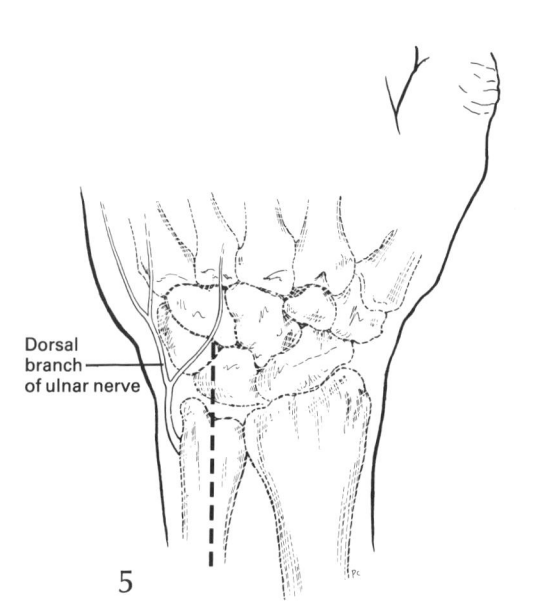

DARRACH'S PROCEDURE (excision of the distal end of the ulna)[1]

Rheumatoid arthritis at the wrist joint level usually also involves the radio-ulnar joint. It may produce a painful synovitis, arthritis or subluxation of the distal ulna.

Indications for operation

Indications are painful subluxation of the distal radio-ulnar joint secondary to rheumatoid arthritis, osteoarthritis or old wrist fractures, and painful supination/pronation of the forearm with tenderness of the distal radio-ulnar joint.

In patients with rheumatoid arthritis, this operation is usually done in association with other wrist procedures such as a synovectomy, arthrodesis or arthroplasty. In the patient with osteoarthritis it will usually be performed as an isolated procedure.

Incision

5

When the procedure is performed in isolation, a longitudinal incision is made on the dorso-ulnar side of the distal ulna. Care is taken to preserve the dorsal branch of the ulnar nerve which crosses the ulnar border of the hand between the ulnar styloid and the pisiform. However, its position can be variable. The extensor retinaculum is incised longitudinally, leaving a flap on the ulnar side which will enable the retinaculum to be repaired at the end of the procedure. The capsule of the distal radio-ulnar joint is now exposed.

770 Forearm, wrist and hand

Approach

6a & b

When this procedure is performed in association with other operations on the dorsum of the wrist joint, exposure through the retinaculum will be similar. The tendons of extensor carpi ulnaris and extensor digiti minimi are mobilized and retracted. A longitudinal incision is then made in the capsule from the ulnar styloid for about 3 cm proximally. The periosteum is incised and the neck of the ulna is exposed subperiosteally. The soft tissues are retracted by placing two small bone levers around the palmar side of the neck, ensuring that the tips of the retractors remain in close contact with the bone.

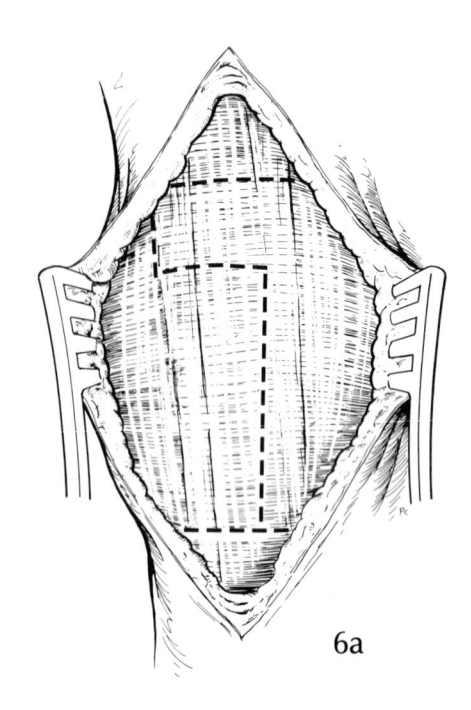

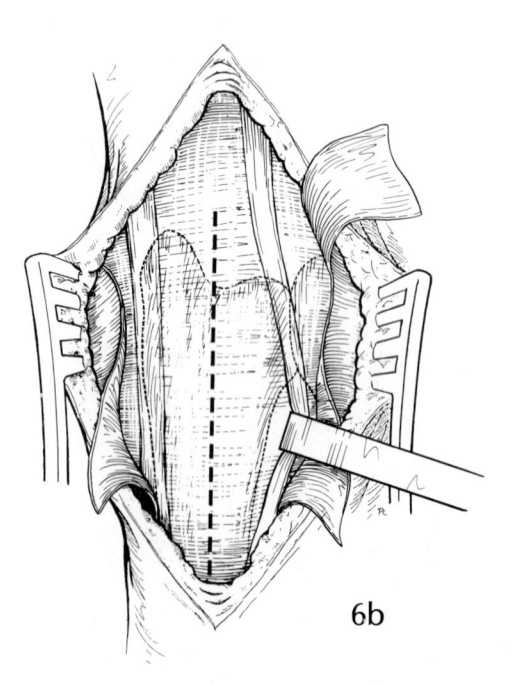

6a

6b

7

A sagittal power saw is used to divide the bone at the level of the proximal limb of the sigmoid cavity of the radius. This is usually about 1.25–2 cm from the ulnar styloid. If more than 2 cm of ulna are resected, then the proximal end tends to sublux, creating an unpleasant prominence beneath the skin, and the tendon of extensor carpi ulnaris may click over the end. An alternative method of division of the ulna is to drill multiple holes at the level of resection and then complete the procedure with bone cutters. The distal fragment of ulna is grasped with pointed bone-holding forceps and, after rotation and elevation, sharp dissection is used to release it from its soft tissue attachments. The fragment is extracted. Excess synovium is then removed from the radio-ulnar joint.

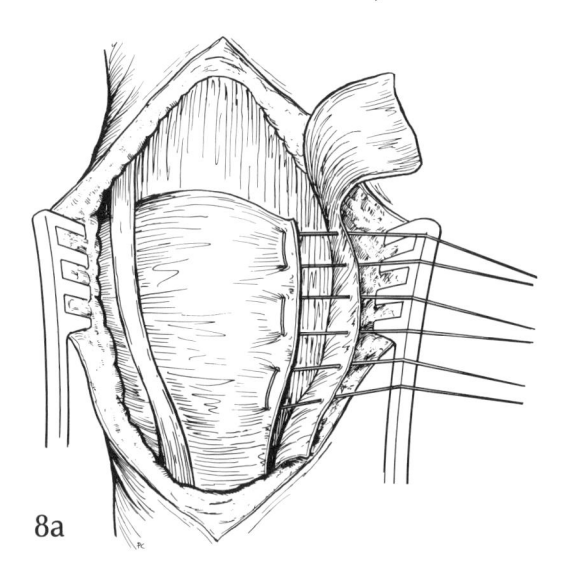

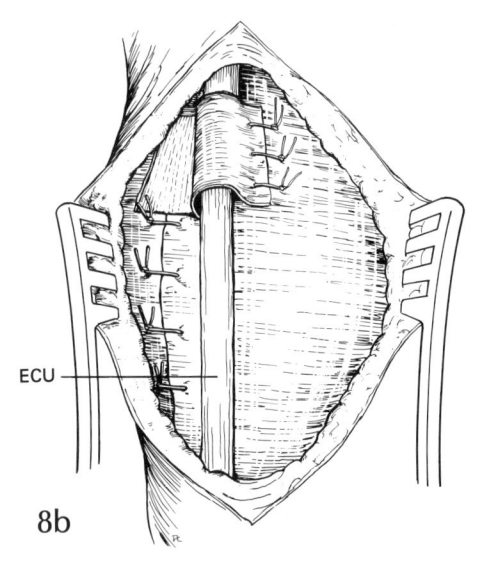

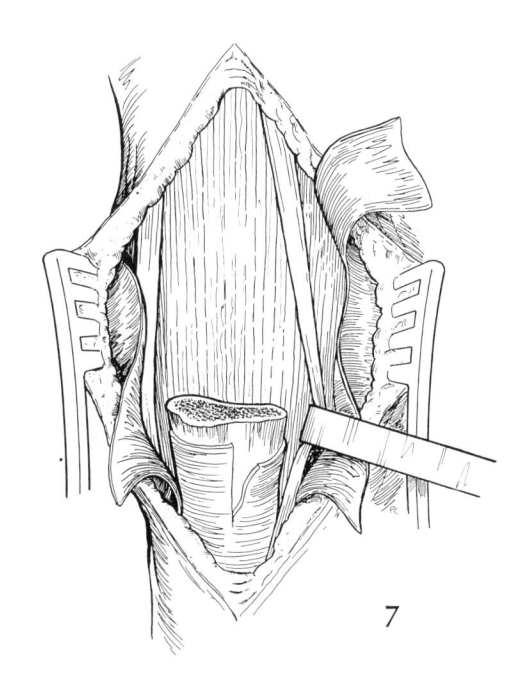

Closure

8a & b

An assistant depresses the distal end of the ulna while the dorsal capsule is repaired with absorbable 2/0 suture material. The retinaculum is sutured firmly over the stump of the ulna and the flap of retinaculum is used to create a pulley for the extensor carpi ulnaris. The skin is closed with interrupted 4/0 nylon.

9a & b

If the distal end of the ulna tends to sublux dorsally, a flap of palmar capsule can be raised on a distally based flap and sutured to the dorsal surface of the ulna via drill holes. The flap is sutured in place with the forearm supinated and an assistant depressing the ulna. The wound is dressed with cotton gauze and wrapped in wool. The forearm is supinated and a plaster slab is applied to the palmar surface of the wrist.

Postoperative management

The hand is elevated for 48 hours and then maintained in a sling, allowing movement of the shoulder, elbow and fingers, but no forearm rotation. The slab is removed at 3 weeks and a full mobilization programme followed.

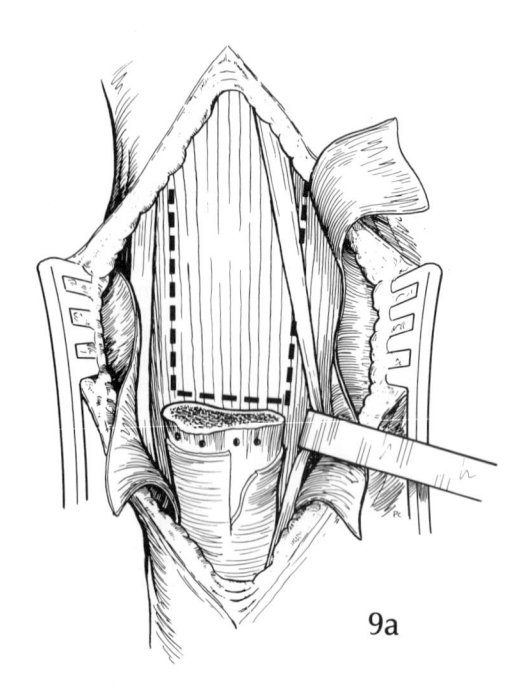

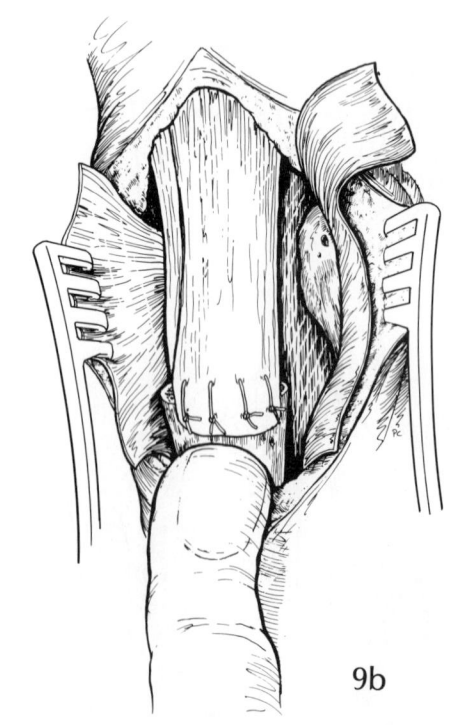

THE LAUENSTEIN PROCEDURE

The potential complications of the Darrach procedure are progressive ulnar translocation of the carpus, ulnar deviation and subsequent painful instability of the wrist. The Lauenstein procedure leaves the distal end of the ulna as an articular surface for the carpus and allows mobility by creating a pseudarthrosis proximal to the head of the ulna[2].

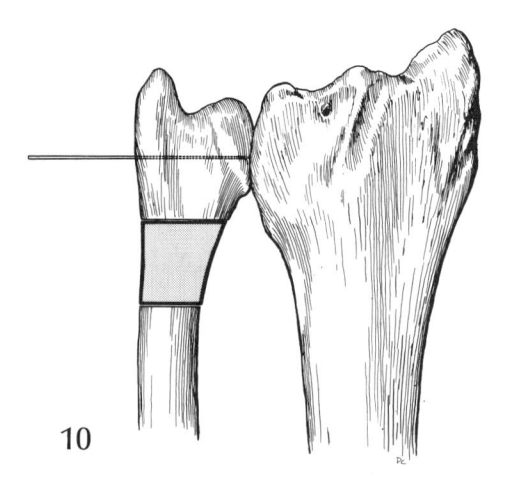

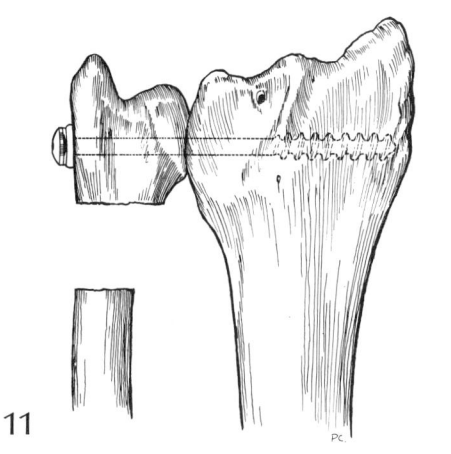

Indications

The indication for this procedure is painful subluxation of the distal radio-ulnar joint associated with arthritic changes in those who are young, and in those who show a potential for ulnar translocation of the carpus, e.g. those in whom ulnar translocation is already present or where the 'slope' of the radius is steep towards the ulnar side.

Incision

This is the same as for excision of the distal end of the ulna as an isolated procedure.

Procedure

10

After the ulna has been exposed subperiosteally, a 2 mm Kirschner wire is drilled into the head of the ulna in the coronal plane with the wrist in neutral rotation. It will be used to manipulate the bone.

11

Osteotomy of the neck is performed with a sagittal power saw at a level just proximal to the radial articular surface of the distal radio-ulnar joint. A second osteotomy is made about 12–15 mm proximal to this and a segment of ulna is removed. The radio-ulnar joint is exposed by manipulating the distal fragment with the Kirschner wire. Articular cartilage is removed from the surfaces of both the distal ulna and the radio-ulnar articulation of the radius. The head of the ulna is then apposed to the distal radius and a Kirschner wire is driven across this joint. Pointed bone reduction forceps hold the position while the Kirschner wire is removed and replaced with a small-fragment AO cancellous screw.

12

Alternatively, a 1.6 mm Kirschner wire can be driven through the opposite cortex of the radius and left protruding so that it is just palpable beneath the skin. A second Kirschner wire is inserted obliquely to the first. Both are cut off flush with the ulna and will later be removed from the radial side. Bone graft taken from the excised piece of ulna can be used to augment the fusion.

The edges of the proximal ulna stump are rounded off and the dorsal capsule is sutured over this distal stump while the forearm is supinated and an assistant depresses the bone. If the shaft of the ulna tends to protrude despite this, then a palmar flap of capsule can be elevated leaving its hinge distally, as in the Darrach procedure. This is then sutured through drill holes to the distal stump.

Closure and postoperative management

These are the same as for the Darrach procedure, except that splinting should be continued for 4 weeks.

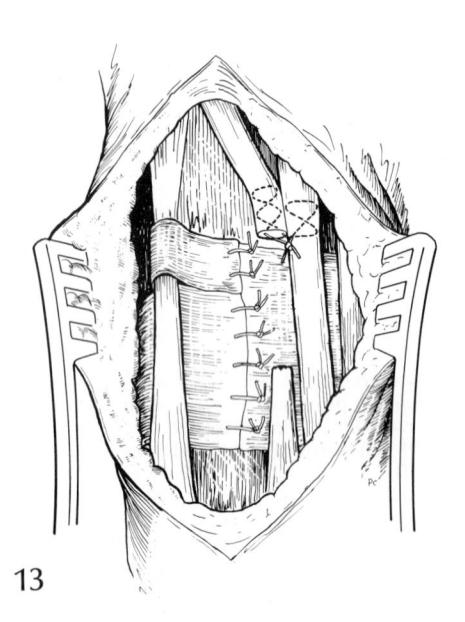

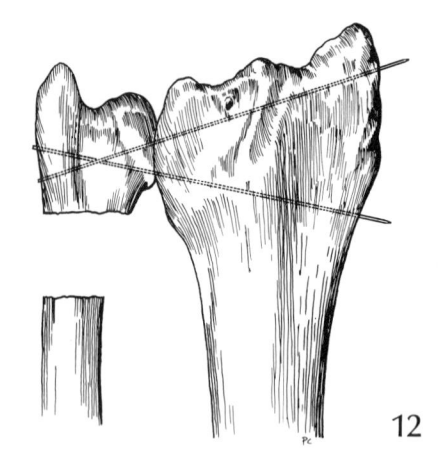

RECONSTRUCTION OF RUPTURED EXTENSOR TENDONS

Reconstruction of one or several ruptured extensor tendons, excision of the head of the ulna or fusion of the wrist joint may be necessary during dorsal synovectomy for rheumatoid arthritis.

13

Rupture of a single tendon If only one tendon is ruptured, and this is usually the extensor digiti quinti, then a side-to-side anastomosis can be made with the adjacent extensor tendon using 4/0 non-absorbable braided suture material. Tension should be applied to the distal stump of the ruptured tendon at the time of the anastomosis. The correct tension is always difficult to achieve. However, after the anastomosis, when the wrist is fully flexed, the finger should come into full extension; and when the wrist is fully dorsiflexed, the finger should adopt a position of flexion similar to the others. With the wrist in neutral, full passive flexion should be achieved without pulling the anastomosis apart.

Rupture of two tendons The tendons to the ring and little finger are usually the two that are found ruptured. Both of these can be anastomosed to the intact tendon of the middle finger; however, it is then more difficult to gauge the correct tension. The above criteria apply in determining the correct tension.

Transfer of extensor indicis proprius

If the extensor indicis is available then this can be used to provide active extension to the ring and little fingers.

Procedure

14 & 15

The extensor tendons at the wrist joint will already be exposed for a dorsal synovectomy. A separate transverse incision is made over the head of the second metacarpal.

The extensor indicis proprius lies on the ulnar side of the extensor digitorum communis. Prior to distal division of the extensor indicis proprius, an anastomosis with 4/0 absorbable suture is made between the indicis proprius and the communis while slight traction is applied to the proprius. This reduces the extensor lag which occurs after this procedure. The extensor indicis proprius is then divided just proximal to the anastomosis. It is pulled proximally into the wrist incision and then anastomosed to the conjoint distal ends of the ruptured extensor tendons. Anastomosis may be made end-to-end or by weaving the proprius through the other two tendons.

Postoperative management

A palmar plaster slab is applied holding the wrist in 20° of dorsiflexion and the proximal phalanx of the fingers in full extension.

At 10 days the sutures are removed and dynamic extension traction is applied to the proximal phalanges while the wrist is maintained in dorsiflexion. Active flexion against the resistance of the elastic bands is then allowed for the subsequent 3 weeks, at which time the splintage is removed. A night splint is applied for 6 weeks holding the fingers extended.

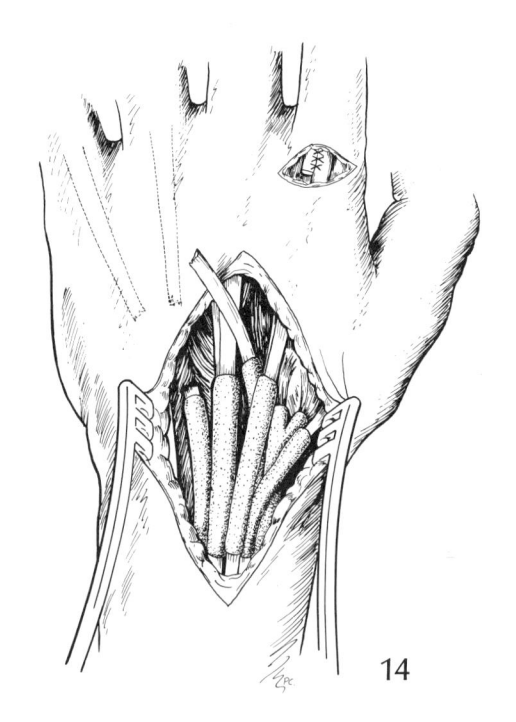

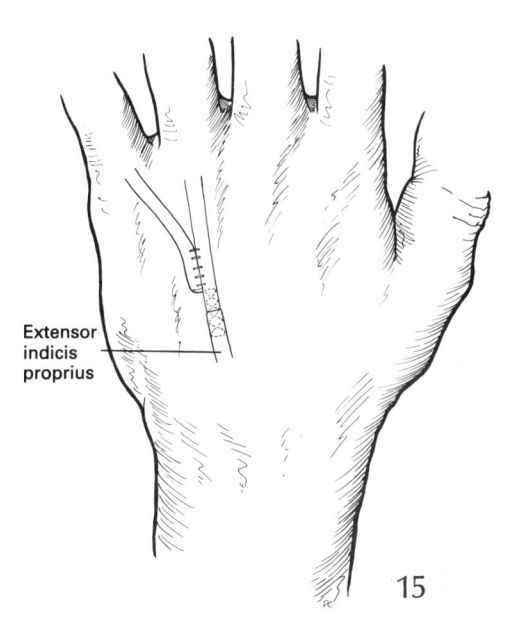

Rupture of all extensor tendons

If all the extensor tendons to the fingers are ruptured, then it is necessary to transfer the flexor digitorum superficialis from the ring finger or from the ring and middle fingers. The tendons of extensor carpi radialis longus or extensor carpi ulnaris may be used but often require a bridging graft.

Procedure

16a & b

A transverse incision is made at the distal palmar crease at the base of the ring finger. The flexor digitorum sublimis (FDS) is isolated by a small incision in the distal palmar crease just proximal to the A1 pulley. The finger is flexed and the FDS is divided as distally as possible. After the tendon has been withdrawn above the wrist the wound is closed with interrupted nylon. FDS to the middle finger may be taken then if two tendons are to be used.

A zigzag incision is made over the palmar aspect of the forearm commencing approximately 2–3 cm proximal to the flexor wrist crease. Flexor digitorum superficialis from the ring finger is then withdrawn into the wound. Tendon-passing forceps are then placed subcutaneously around the radial border of the forearm to emerge in the volar incision. The tendon is grasped and delivered into the wound over the dorsal aspect. An anastomosis is made to the four extensor tendons to the fingers. If FDS from the middle finger is used as well then it is sutured to extensor digitorum communis (EDC) of index and middle fingers, while FDS from the ring finger is sutured to EDC of ring and little fingers.

If extensor pollicis longus is also ruptured, then one of the following tendons may be transferred into the distal stump: extensor carpi radialis longus, extensor pollicis brevis, flexor digitorum superficialis to the middle finger, or palmaris longus.

Postoperative management

A bulky dressing is applied with a palmar plaster slab holding the wrist in 20° of dorsiflexion and supporting the proximal phalanges. The arm is elevated for 48 hours. When the patient is comfortable at 3 to 5 days, dressings are reduced and a new splint applied. At 3 weeks dynamic extension splinting is applied to the proximal phalanx of each of the fingers. A static night splint is also used. Active flexion against resistance is encouraged for a further period of 3 weeks and then the patient is allowed free of the splints for periods during the day. The resting night splintage is continued for a total of 8 weeks.

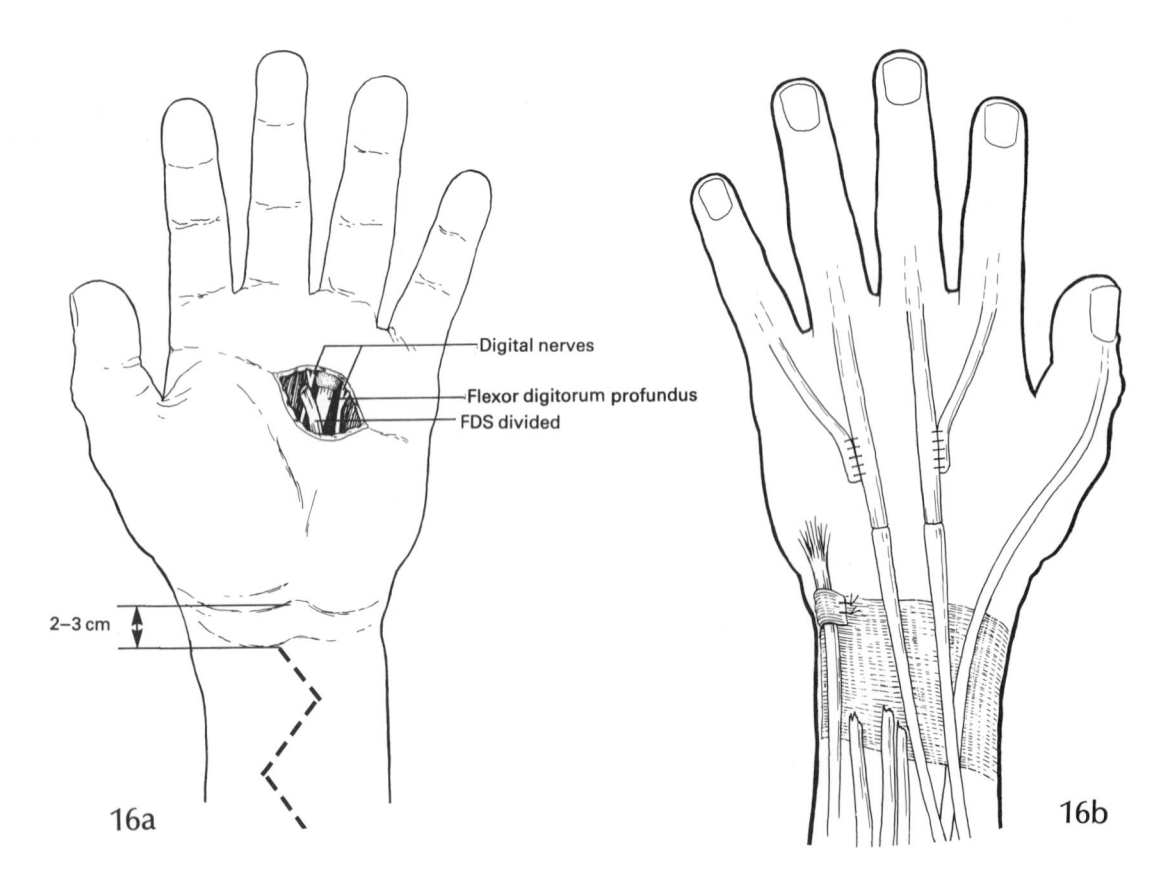

FLEXOR SYNOVECTOMY

Proliferative synovium around the flexor tendons at the level of the wrist joint may produce an hour-glass deformity on the palmar aspect. Swelling will appear in the palm of the hand as well as proximal to the wrist crease. Hydrocortisone injections are usually given in the early stages.

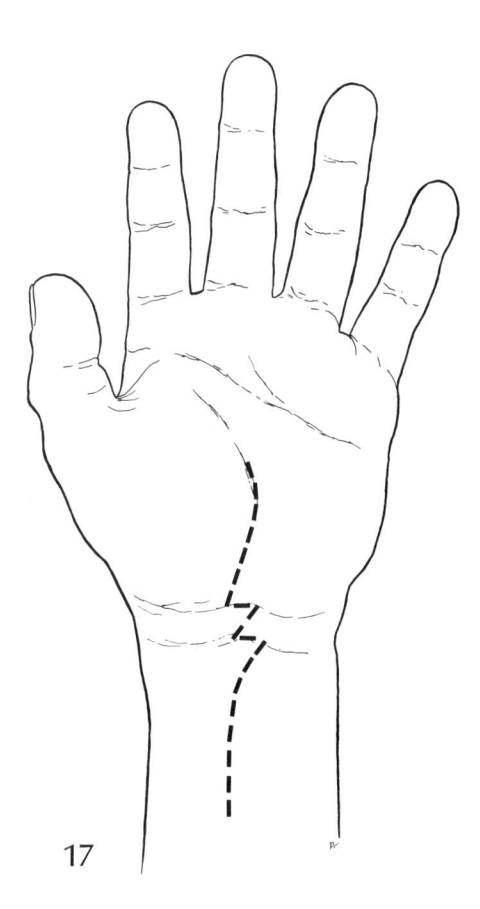

Indications

There are three indications for operation: symptomatic compression of the median nerve; rupture of flexor pollicis longus and/or other flexor tendons; and persistent swelling and pain despite medical treatment.

Incision

17

A longitudinal incision is made in the mid-palmar line which extends proximally across the wrist joint in a zigzag fashion.

Approach

18a & b

The subcutaneous fat and the palmar aponeurosis are divided by sharp dissection, maintaining traction on the skin with skin hooks. Vessels are coagulated with bipolar diathermy. A midline incision is made in the deep fascia of the forearm and the median nerve identified. A vessel loop is placed around the nerve and all subsequent dissection is performed on its ulnar side. The flexor retinaculum is divided under direct vision to expose the carpal tunnel. Care must always be taken to ensure that the motor branch of the median nerve is not divided. The median nerve is retracted to the radial side and the synovium is removed from round the flexor tendons by sharp dissection. The floor of the carpal tunnel is palpated and any sharp spicules of bone are removed with nibblers.

Closure

The tourniquet is released and the wound is packed with swabs soaked in saline while the arm is elevated for 3 minutes. Obvious bleeding points are coagulated with bipolar diathermy. A small vacuum drain is inserted. The skin is closed with interrupted 4/0 nylon. A well-padded palmar plaster slab is applied holding the wrist in approximately 20° of dorsiflexion.

Postoperative management

The arm is elevated for 48 hours and the drain is removed at 24 hours. The patient is discharged with the hand resting in a high arm sling for 3–4 days. Active finger movements are encouraged as soon as the patient is comfortable. The plaster slab and the sutures are removed at 10 days and full mobilization of the wrist is allowed.

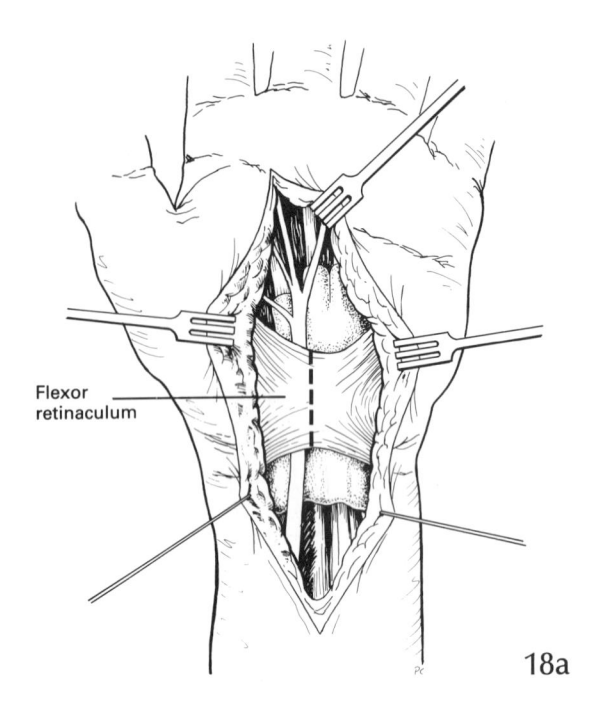

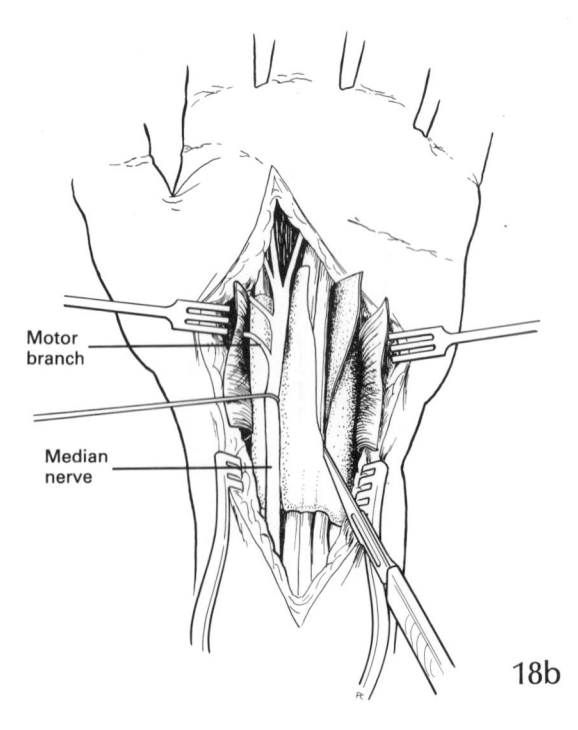

ARTHRODESIS OF THE WRIST

Indications

Indications are severe pain in the wrist on flexion/extension combined with radiological changes of Grade III or IV; loss of hand function owing to volar subluxation of the carpus (volar translocation); bone destruction with ulnar translocation and loss of hand function. This may occur after a previous excision of the head of the ulna.

Before proceeding to surgery, the patient should be given a wrist splint which will provide the opportunity to see what the wrist is like after an arthrodesis. However, the splint will reduce rotation of the forearm whereas fusion will not. The splint will also give the surgeon some help in deciding if a fusion will improve the pain and/or function of the wrist joint. Careful consideration should be given before arthrodesing the second wrist in bilateral cases as an arthroplasty may give better function.

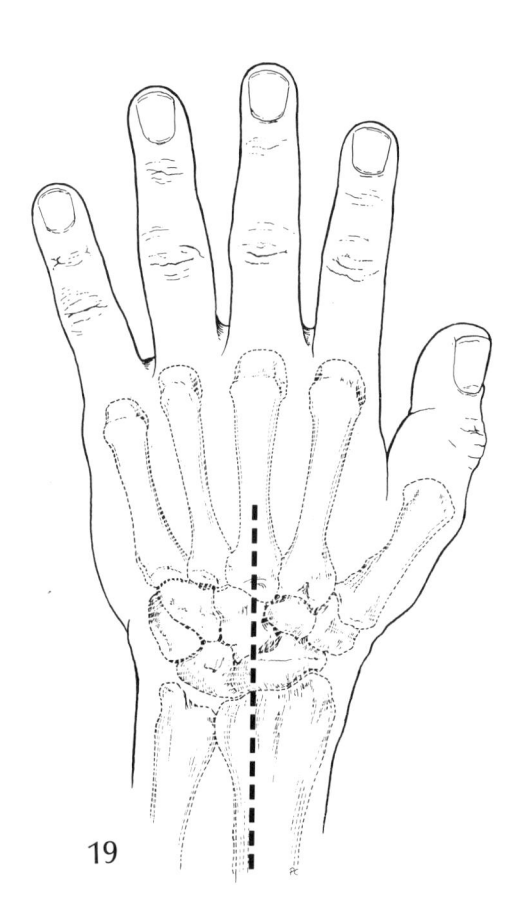

Incision

19

A straight dorsal incision is centred over the wrist joint and extends from a point 4 cm proximal to the wrist to the proximal third of the third metacarpal. It is important to make the incision of adequate length so that excessive traction on the skin edges is avoided during the operation.

Exposure

20

A dorsal synovectomy is usually performed as previously described. The retinacular flaps are made as before, but it is unnecessary to leave a proximal retinacular band. The dorsal capsule of the radiocarpal joint is incised transversely at the distal end of the radius. It is elevated, leaving the capsule attached distally. The distal end of the ulna is excised and the articular surface of the radiocarpal joint is exposed by flexing the wrist. Bone nibblers are used to remove synovium and remnants of articular cartilage. If the joint alignment is satisfactory, then the third metacarpal will lie in line with the radius and it is not necessary to perform an extensive dissection.

If there has been palmar or ulnar translocation of the wrist joint, then it may be necessary to release further sections of capsule on the ulnar, palmar and radial sides. When dissecting on the radial side it is essential to take care not to damage the abductor pollicis longus or the extensor pollicis brevis tendons which lie in very close apposition to the distal end of the radius. After further capsular dissection the wrist can be fully flexed to display the entire distal end of the radius as well as the carpal bones. It may be necessary to resect some bone from the dorsum of the distal radius to expose a reasonable area of cancellous bone and enable the carpus to sit on the end of the radius. The carpus and the distal end of the radius are shaped so that one fits into the other. Sometimes it is necessary to make a transverse cut with the power saw in order to achieve two flat surfaces if there has been gross erosion on the palmar aspect of the radius.

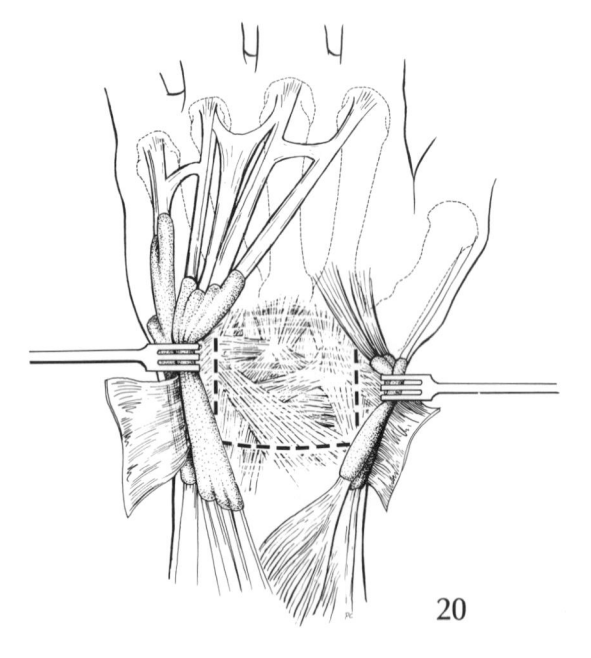

Internal fixation

21a & b

This is achieved by passing a Steinmann pin down the shaft of the third metacarpal, through the carpal bones and across the wrist joint into the medulla of the radius[3].

A longitudinal incision is made over the metacarpophalangeal joint of the third metacarpal. The extensor hood is divided on the ulnar side and the extensor tendon is retracted to the radial side. The capsule and synovium are divided in the midline. A Steinmann pin approximately 15–20 cm in length is mounted on a T-handle and introduced through the head of the metacarpal. It is passed along the shaft, across the carpus until the point is seen to emerge. It is then lined up with the medullary cavity of the distal radius and driven longitudinally along it. Care must be taken not to miss the shaft of the radius completely or to penetrate its soft cortex. Bone graft taken from the head of the ulna is packed into any available space and the hand is manually impacted against the radius. The Steinmann pin is countersunk deep into the articular surface of the metacarpal using a punch or a specially designed threaded introducer. If rotation of the carpus on the radius is a problem, then an oblique 2 mm Kirschner wire can be inserted through the radial styloid and across into the carpus. Alternatively, a bone staple can be placed across the dorsum.

If the metacarpophalangeal joint of the middle finger is not involved in the disease, then a Steinmann pin can be passed in a retrograde direction from the carpus to emerge between the second and third metacarpal heads[4]. This is then driven back down the centre of the radius.

This type of arthrodesis produces a wrist in neutral position, which would seem to be quite satisfactory for the patient with rheumatoid disease, even if both wrists are fused[5].

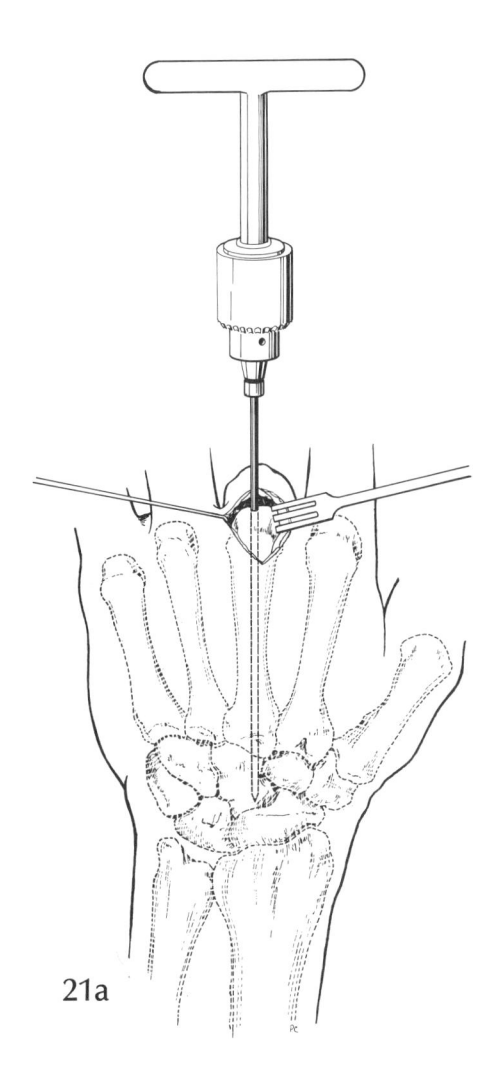

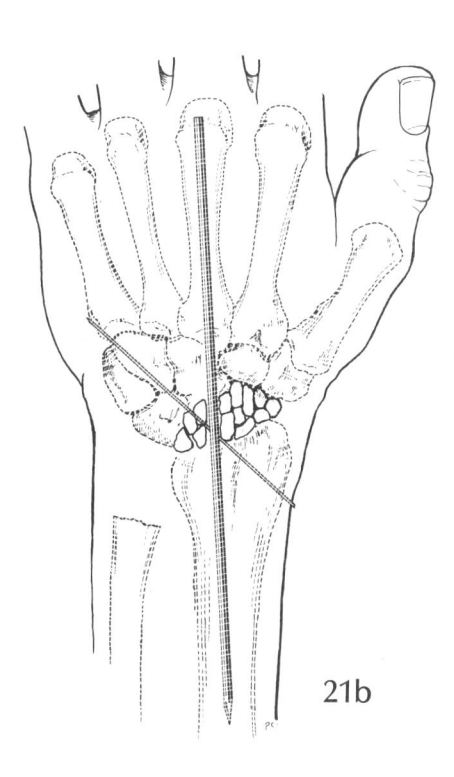

Closure

The distally based flap of dorsal capsule is sutured back to the distal radius with absorbable suture material and this covers the bone graft. The extensor retinaculum is then placed beneath the extensor tendons and sutured to itself on the ulnar side, depressing the shaft of the ulna at the same time. A small vacuum drain is inserted and the skin is closed with interrupted nylon.

Postoperative management

Gauze dressings are applied to the wound and a well-padded palmar plaster slab is applied. The arm is elevated for 48 hours and the drain is then removed. At 2 weeks the sutures are removed and a complete short-arm plaster is applied supporting the wrist. This is kept in place for 8–10 weeks or until fusion is sound.

Limited wrist arthrodesis (Chamay)

If the mid-carpal joint is reasonably well-preserved the lunate and the proximal carpal row may be fused to the radius and some wrist movement will be maintained[6]. This technique should always be considered before undertaking complete arthrodesis of the wrist in rheumatoid arthritis.

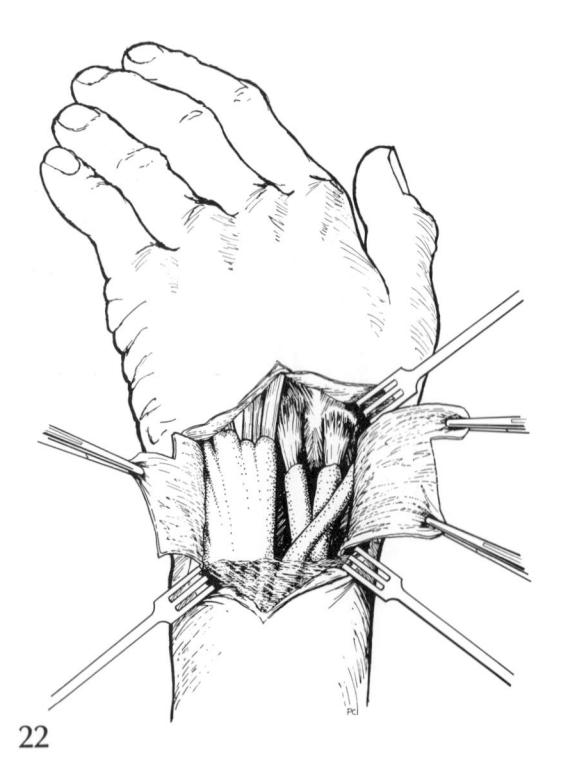

ARTHROPLASTY OF THE WRIST

Arthroplasty of the wrist in rheumatoid arthritis has gained popularity in recent years and the Swanson Silastic (Dow Corning, UK) prosthesis[7] is perhaps the most widely used. Since arthrodesis is such a successful operation, the role of arthroplasty is still controversial. However, when a patient requires an operation on both wrists, it is useful if one hand is fused to give good power grip and the other has a replacement arthroplasty to maintain some movement which is helpful for toilet purposes.

Contraindications

Contraindications to arthroplasty are extensive extensor tendon rupture, especially if the wrist extensors are compromised; insufficient bone stock, especially in the distal radius; a history of previous infection; and poor skin cover. An anteroposterior and a true lateral radiograph are essential in the planning of the operation.

Incision

A straight longitudinal incision is made in the line of the third metacarpal. It should extend for approximately 6–8 cm proximal to the wrist joint. Care is taken to preserve cutaneous nerves and veins.

Procedure

22

The extensor retinaculum is divided longitudinally on the ulnar side over the line of the extensor digiti minimi, leaving a longer flap on the distal edge. The retinaculum is reflected towards the radial side with its base between the first and second dorsal compartments. The retinaculum on the ulnar side is elevated to expose extensor carpi ulnaris. A narrow strip of retinaculum is left proximally to prevent bow-stringing of the extensor tendons. A synovectomy of the extensor tendons is performed.

23 & 24

A transverse incision is made across the capsule of the wrist joint just proximal to the articular surface. This flap of capsule is reflected distally leaving it attached to the dorsum of the carpal bones. The head of the ulna is resected. The capsular attachment to the radial styloid is reflected distally, taking care not to injure the tendons in the first two dorsal compartments. The wrist is palmarflexed to expose the distal end of the radius and the carpal bones. A power saw is used to make a transverse cut across the distal end of the radius leaving, if possible, some of the subchondral bone to give support to the prosthesis. The lunate and the proximal pole of the scaphoid are removed either with a rongeur or a sagittal power saw.

The medullary cavity of the distal radius is reamed, using a broach, curette or a Swanson burr mounted on a power driver. It is reamed to take the appropriate trial prosthesis. The medullary cavity of the third metacarpal is identified. This can be done by passing a Kirschner wire through the head of the capitate and out through the head of the third metacarpal. The wire is then removed and this track is opened up, using initially a hand burr followed by a Swanson burr mounted on a power reamer.

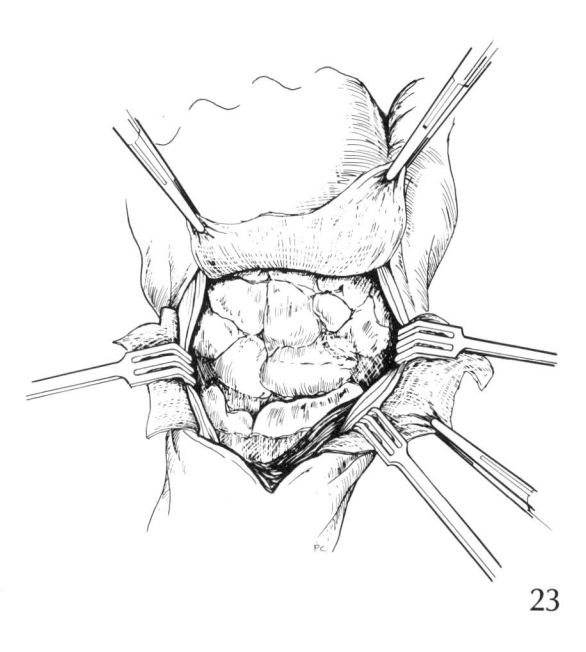

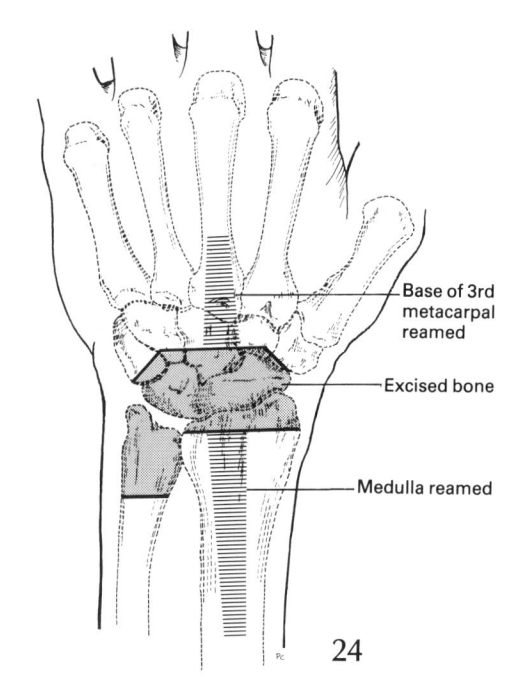

25a & b

The cavity is shaped to accommodate the distal end of the trial prosthesis which should not extend beyond the metaphysis of the third metacarpal. The trial prosthesis is then inserted into the distal radius and then the distal stem is introduced into the palmarflexed carpus as the wrist is dorsiflexed. The range of movement is tested and 30° of dorsiflexion and palmarflexion should be possible. If there is impingement on dorsiflexion, then it may be necessary to resect more of the distal end of the radius.

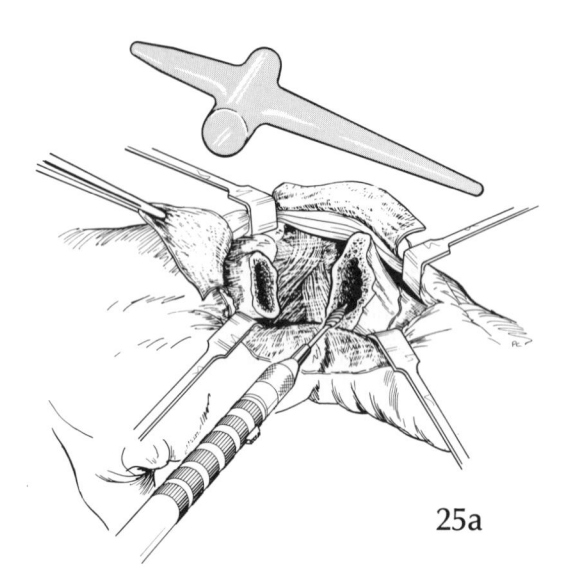

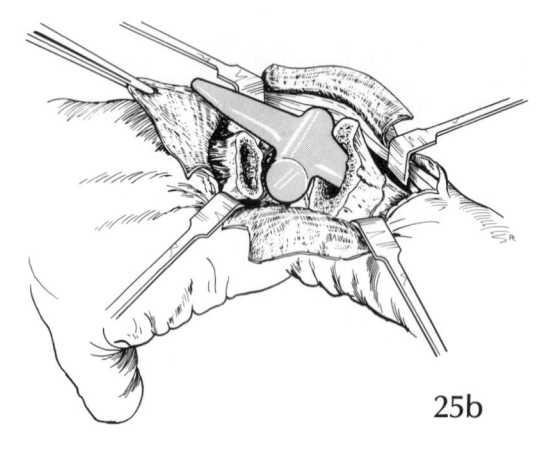

25a

25b

26a & b

If grommets (titanium protective sleeves) are to be used then the appropriate size is inserted into the prepared cavities and further reaming may be necessary to allow these to fit well into the bone. The distal grommet is normally used on the dorsal surface and the proximal grommet on the palmar surface. The size of the grommet corresponds to the prosthesis.

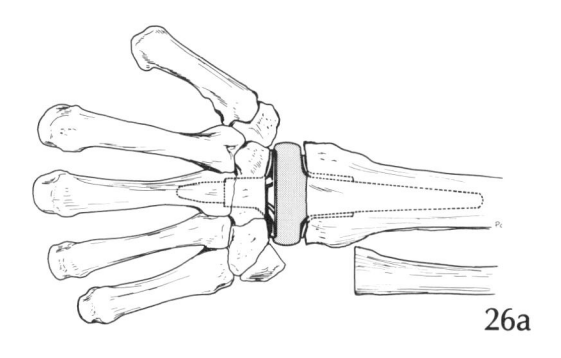

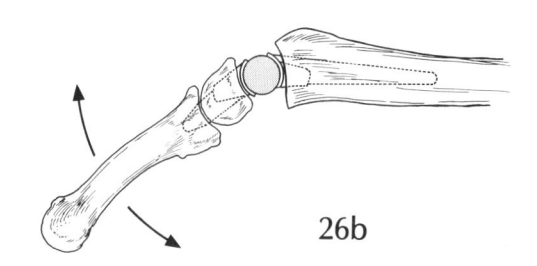

27

The trial prosthesis and grommets are removed. A 1 mm round burr is used to make two holes on the palmar aspect of the distal radius, and 2/0 braided non-absorbable sutures are used to reattach the palmar capsule to the distal end of the radius. Three further holes are drilled on the dorsal surface of the distal radius and the suture material passed through the holes, leaving the needles attached to each of the three threads.

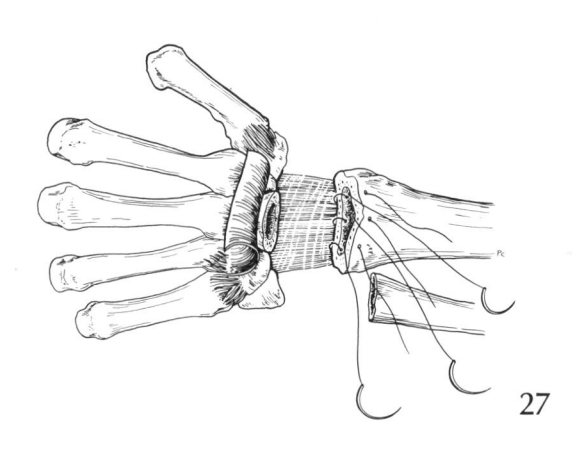

The bone cavities are washed out thoroughly with saline. Titanium grommets of the appropriate size are inserted into the distal end of the radius and into the carpal cavity. The definitive prosthesis of correct size is now removed from the packet and care is taken not to touch it with the gloves nor to rest it on any surface. The electrostatic charge on the Silastic material will attract foreign material and it should be handled with non-toothed forceps. The long proximal stem is inserted into the distal end of the radius, the wrist is palmarflexed and the distal stem inserted into the carpal cavity. The wrist is dorsiflexed and a stable reduction should be achieved.

Closure

28a & b

The distally based dorsal capsular flap is sutured to the distal end of the radius using the suture material previously inserted through the bone. The extensor retinaculum is passed beneath the extensor tendons and sutured as described for a dorsal synovectomy, holding extensor carpi ulnaris on the dorsum. A suction drain is inserted and the skin is closed with 4/0 monofilament sutures. A bulky dressing is applied with a palmar plaster slab holding the wrist in neutral.

Postoperative management

The arm is elevated for 7–10 days. The drain is removed at 48 hours. At 10 days the dressing is reduced and sutures are removed. A below-elbow cast is then applied to the arm for a further 4 weeks. On its removal mobilization is commenced. Sometimes it may be helpful to use a dynamic extension splint.

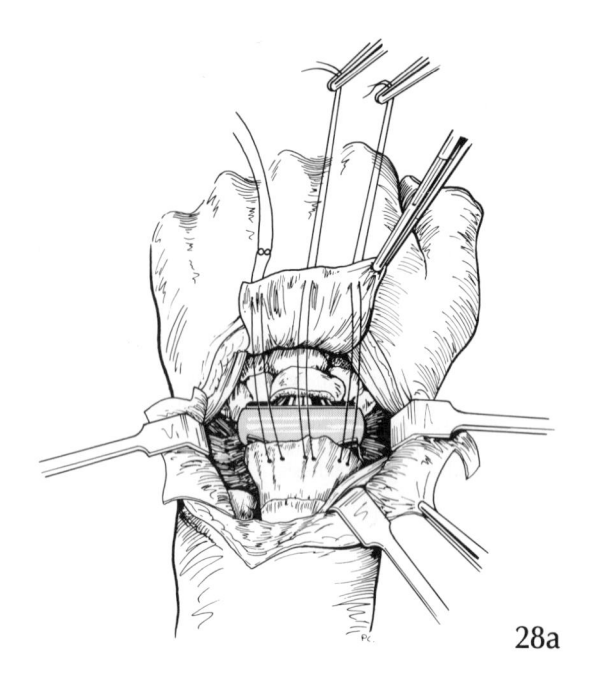

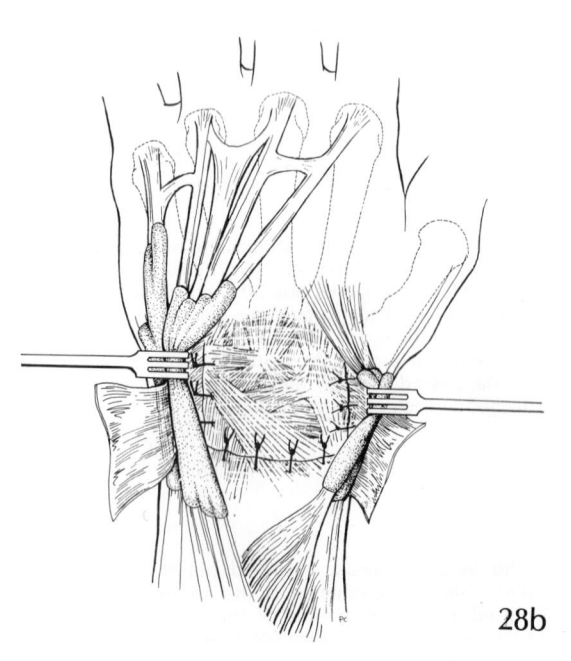

DECOMPRESSIVE PROCEDURES

DE QUERVAIN'S DISEASE

This condition is an aseptic inflammation of the synovium lining the abductor pollicis longus tendon and the extensor pollicis brevis tendons as they pass over the lower end of the radius and under the extensor retinaculum. The condition is more common in women and is characterized by pain over the distal end of the radius aggravated by thumb movement. There is often local swelling and tenderness over the radial styloid area which radiates proximally along the line of the two tendons. Adduction of thumb with ulnar deviation of the wrist may produce pain (Finkelstein's test). Occasionally there is crepitus in the tendon sheath when the thumb is moved. The diagnosis can be confused with osteoarthritis of the carpometacarpal joint of the thumb.

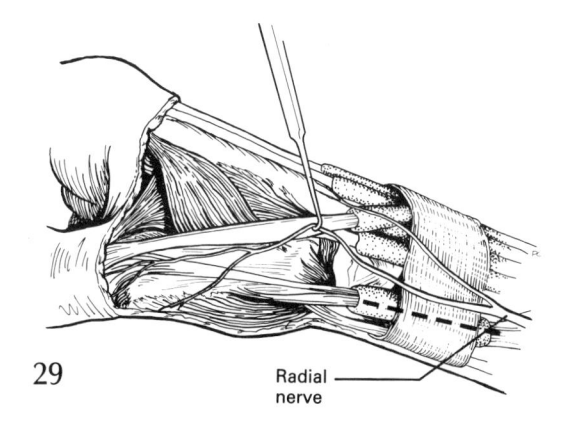

Conservative treatment Conservative measures should be tried before surgical intervention. Repetitive use of the thumb should be avoided if it is possible and this may require a change in occupation. The thumb may be supported in a crêpe or elastic bandage and longer relief may be achieved by the application of a moulded lightweight splint which should immobilize the wrist and the thumb up to the proximal phalanx. The injection of a local steroid agent into the tendon sheath is often quite beneficial and may have a long-lasting effect. Care must be taken not to inject into the substance of the tendon.

Indications for operation

If the conservative measures fail and the patient's housework and/or occupation is being limited, then exploration is indicated.

Procedure

29

It is preferable to carry out the operation using a tourniquet on the upper arm and with regional or general anaesthesia. The local injection of an anaesthetic agent may distort the anatomy.

A longitudinal or zigzag incision is made over the tendon of extensor pollicis brevis or slightly to the dorsal side. It is possible to use a transverse incision which has a better cosmetic result but places the terminal branches of the radial nerve at greater risk.

The skin edges are elevated using skin hooks and the extensor retinaculum is exposed, taking great care to avoid damage to the terminal branches of the radial nerve. The thickened extensor tendon sheath is incised along its dorsal border and the tendons of abductor pollicis longus and extensor pollicis brevis are identified. Abductor pollicis longus may exist as more than one tendon, but this may lead the surgeon to believe that both tendons have been decompressed. It is important to identify extensor pollicis brevis separately and release it from its own subcompartment. Traction on the tendon will help to identify it. Some surgeons excise a segment of the tendon sheath to prevent recurrence.

The tourniquet is released, haemostasis secured and the skin closed with a subcuticular suture. A bulky wool and crêpe bandage is applied to restrict movement of the thumb. This is removed when the suture is taken out at 7–10 days.

29

Radial nerve

Complications

Damage to the terminal branches of the radial nerve can result in a painful neuroma at the site of the operation. This may be more of a problem to the patient than the original tenovaginitis. Careful dissection in the longitudinal line is essential.

CARPAL TUNNEL DECOMPRESSION

Compression of the median nerve in the carpal tunnel produces the classic symptoms of paraesthesia in the median nerve distribution, waking the patients at night and often causing them to shake the hand in order to gain relief. The symptoms may persist during the day, causing clumsiness owing to alteration of sensation in the tips of the fingers and there may be weakness of thumb abduction. The condition occurs most commonly in women and often there is no clear aetiology. However, it is known to be associated with pregnancy, rheumatoid arthritis, myxoedema, and following a Colles' fracture.

The clinical picture can be confusing as pain can radiate proximally up the forearm and care must be taken to differentiate it from more proximal nerve lesions, especially those in the cervical spine region. Phalen's test is useful: this involves maintaining the wrist in full palmar-flexion for 1–2 minutes and, if positive, the symptoms will be reproduced. Tinel's sign may be positive over the carpal tunnel. If any doubt exists, then motor and sensory electrical studies are essential. If any skeletal abnormality is suspected, a radiograph, showing a skyline view of the tunnel, may be helpful.

Conservative treatment A splint holding the wrist in slight dorsiflexion may relieve nocturnal symptoms, and can be used as a diagnostic test. Steroids are sometimes injected into the carpal tunnel, and often produce a good response but repeated injections should not be given. Also, great care must be taken to avoid injection of the steroid into the substance of the median nerve.

Anaesthesia

The operation is generally carried out under regional or general anaesthesia using a tourniquet on the upper arm. However, it can also be performed by local infiltration of 0.5 per cent bupivacaine into the area of the incision. A high arm tourniquet can still be used as long as it is inflated just before the skin incision is made; the patient can usually tolerate the discomfort of the tourniquet for 10–20 minutes, which is sufficient time for the surgeon to expose the nerve. The tourniquet can then be released.

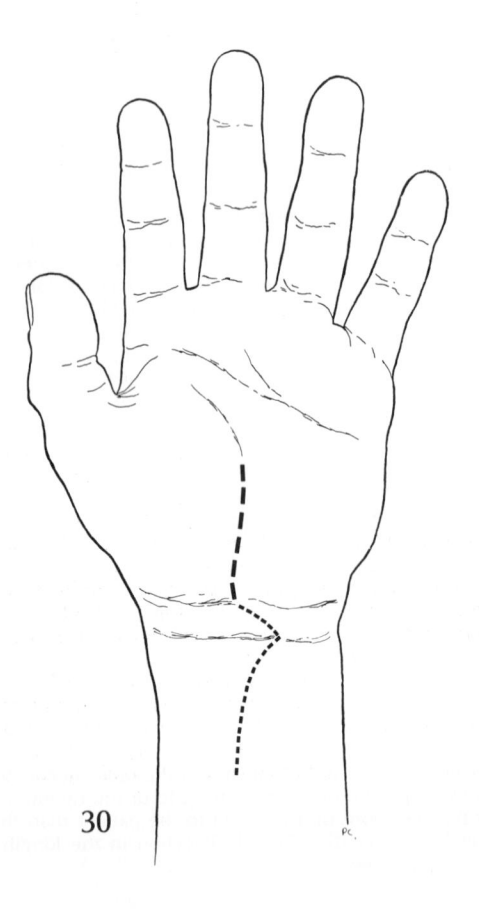

Incision

30

A longitudinal incision is made to the ulnar side of the midline of the palm. It commences at the distal wrist crease and extends distally for about 5 cm or to a line level with the ulnar side of the extended thumb. If it is necessary to extend the incision proximally, then the skin should be incised in a zigzag or curvilinear fashion across the wrist creases.

Exposure

31

The skin edges are elevated and retracted with skin hooks to put the underlying tissue under tension. Using sharp dissection, the palmar aponeurosis is divided longitudinally taking care not to damage the superficial palmar arterial arch which will appear at the distal end of the wound. The transverse carpal ligament is divided on the ulnar side of the midline; once an entry point has been made, a MacDonald dissector is passed proximally and distally in the carpal tunnel to clear any adhesions.

The transverse carpal ligament is then divided completely from the distal edge proximally to expose the carpal tunnel. Great care must be taken to avoid damage to the motor branch of the median nerve which in some hands may arise from the palmar aspect of the nerve and enter the transverse carpal ligament close to the midline. The edges of the ligament should be retracted; then, using a blunt dissection technique, the median nerve should be identified and, in particular, the motor branch should be sought to confirm its position and to clear it from surrounding tissue. The other terminal branches of the median nerve are carefully released.

The remainder of the carpal tunnel is inspected to exclude other space-occupying lesions, e.g. lipoma, ganglion or osteophyte. The tunnel proximal to the distal wrist crease can be inspected by elevating the skin with a retractor and, with the median nerve identified, any remaining restriction produced by the deep fascia can also be incised without extending the skin incision above the wrist. The author does not perform an internal neurolysis of the nerve at a primary operation. The tourniquet is released, the vascular flow to the median nerve is observed and haemostasis is secured.

The subcutaneous fat layer is sutured with a fine absorbable material and subcuticular polypropylene is used for the skin.

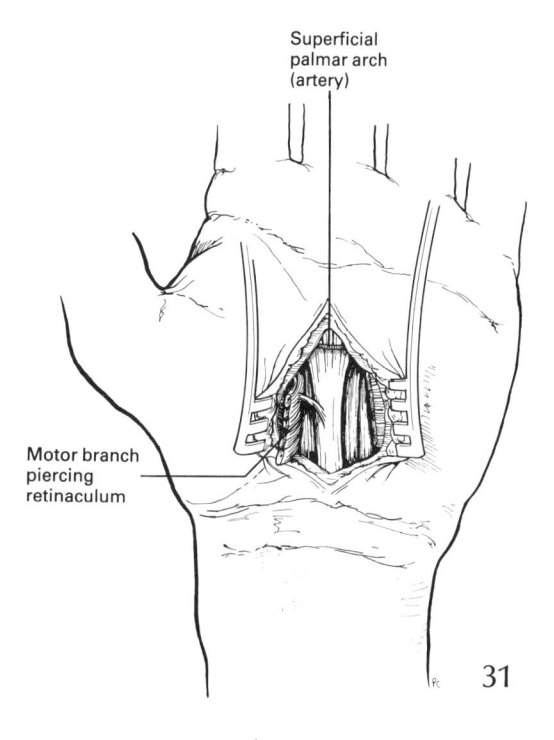

Postoperative management

A gauze dressing is applied to the wound, followed by a bulky wool and crêpe bandage with the wrist held in slight dorsiflexion. This is kept in place for 10 days until the sutures are removed.

Complications

Damage to the motor branch of the median nerve can produce a significant disability. It is important to identify this nerve and it is surprising how often it is seen emerging from the palmar aspect of the median nerve and penetrating the flexor retinaculum close to the longitudinal incision. If it has been divided it is important to recognize it and perform a primary repair. If the incision is continued above the wrist crease, it is important to preserve the superficial palmar branch of the median nerve. Damage to this can produce a painful neuroma.

The scar following a carpal tunnel release can be quite tender. This may be due to the formation of small neuromata in the line of the scar but can usually be well treated by desensitization exercises.

It is important to hold the wrist slightly dorsiflexed postoperatively as the tendons and nerve can bowstring across the divided flexor tunnel. This dorsiflexed position can usually be maintained by a bulky bandage, but a small plaster slab on the palmar aspect is used by some surgeons.

GANGLION AT THE WRIST

The commonest site for a ganglion at the wrist joint is on the dorsal aspect on the radial side of the common extensor tendons. It is usually more obvious on palmarflexion of the wrist and may disappear on dorsiflexion. It may be tender, cause an ache when using the wrist or just be a cosmetic nuisance. If a ganglion is not annoying a patient in any of the above ways, it is probably best left alone as many will resolve spontaneously, particularly in children.

The next most common site is on the palmar aspect of the wrist on the radial side, in relationship to the flexor carpi radialis tendon. The radial artery is often stretched over the palmar surface of this ganglion.

EXCISION OF A DORSAL GANGLION

Procedure

32a & b

The operation should be performed using a high arm tourniquet with either general or regional anaesthesia. Local infiltration of anaesthetic usually distorts the anatomy and may make the dissection difficult.

On the dorsum of the wrist, a transverse incision is made over the ganglion. The skin edges are retracted; then, using blunt longitudinal dissection, and taking care to avoid the terminal branches of the radial nerve, the extensor retinaculum is exposed. It will be necessary to incise the extensor retinaculum, and then the ganglion with its investing fascia layers will be apparent. It is important to establish the correct plane of dissection, which is more easily done if the ganglion remains intact. The extensor tendons should be retracted to each side and care taken to avoid damage to them. The ganglion can usually be traced down to the dorsal capsule of the wrist joint. Some surgeons prefer to excise a small piece of the dorsal capsule with the ganglion while others try to ligate the neck of the ganglion and sew the dorsal capsule of the wrist joint over the top.

The tourniquet is then released and haemostasis secured. The extensor retinaculum is repaired with an absorbable suture and the skin closed with a subcuticular polypropylene suture.

Postoperative management

The wound is covered with a gauze dressing and wrapped in a bulky wool and crêpe bandage which helps to immobilize the wrist joint for the first 10 days until the suture is removed.

Complications

On the dorsal surface it is possible to damage the terminal branches of the radial nerve which may produce an area of numbness distal to the wound or may produce a painful neuroma.

The ganglion recurs in approximately 5 per cent of cases. The patient should be informed of both these possible complications before surgery.

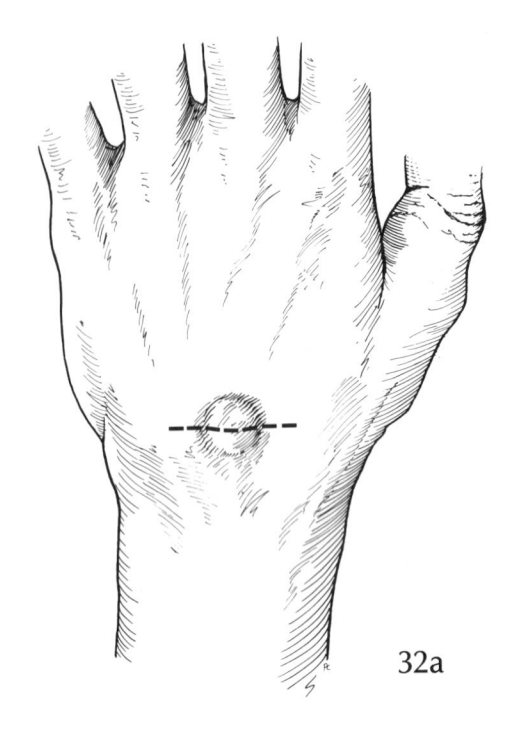

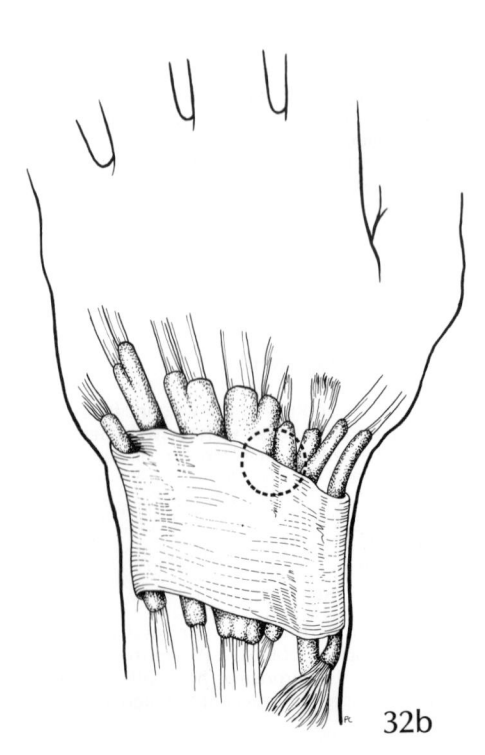

EXCISION OF A PALMAR GANGLION

A longitudinal lazy-S incision is made over the ganglion. Since the radial artery often overlies the ganglion, it is important to identify this vessel proximally and dissect it free from the ganglionic tissue. Having retracted the artery, the dissection of the ganglion is carried down to the wrist joint where it is amputated and the capsule oversewn. It is important in this procedure to release the tourniquet to establish the continuity of the radial artery prior to skin closure.

The wound is closed with a subcuticular suture. Postoperative management is the same as for the dorsal ganglion, and recurrence is as frequent.

OSTEOARTHRITIS

Osteoarthritis of the wrist joint usually results from previous trauma or from Kienböck's disease of the lunate. If the osteoarthritis only involves two or even three carpal joints then a limited arthrodesis may be performed. However, if the radiocarpal and mid-carpal joints are involved then it will be necessary to perform an arthroplasty or an arthrodesis of the wrist joint. Arthroplasty of the wrist joint has not been popular in post-traumatic arthritis because such patients usually put significant forces through the wrist joint once the pain has been relieved. This is in contrast to the patient with rheumatoid arthritis who has multiple joint involvement above and below the wrist joint and therefore the forces applied are minimal.

Arthrodesis of the wrist joint allows a patient to perform most manual tasks and is therefore preferable to arthroplasty, especially in the manual worker. If mobility of the wrist joint is of utmost importance, then arthroplasty or limited arthrodesis could be considered.

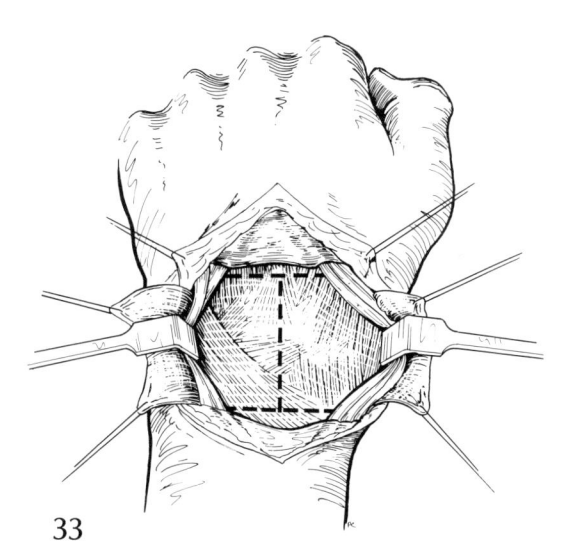

In osteoarthritis advantage can be taken of the good bone stock on each side of the wrist joint which enables internal fixation to be more rigid than that which can be obtained from the osteoporotic bone of rheumatoid arthritis.

PANARTHRODESIS OF THE WRIST

While it is usual for the wrist to be fused in approximately 20° of dorsiflexion in order to aid power grip, it can be fused in a straight position with little disability. The arthrodesis can be performed using a bone graft for internal fixation, or a plate can be applied to the dorsal surface together with the bone graft in order to provide the fixation. The approach is the same for each operation.

Position of the patient

The patient lies supine with the forearm resting on a table. The tourniquet is applied to the upper arm. The patient can be slightly tilted towards the side of the operation by a sandbag placed under the opposite buttock, which will elevate the pelvis to enable a bone graft to be obtained.

Incision

A lazy-S longitudinal dorsal incision is made extending from the proximal third of the third metacarpal to 3 cm proximal to the wrist joint.

Exposure

33

The skin edges are lifted with skin hooks and the dorsal veins ligated if they are an obstruction. The extensor retinaculum is divided on its ulnar side and reflected towards the radial side. The extensor tendons are retracted to expose the distal end of the radius and the dorsal area of the carpus up to the base of the third metacarpal. If necessary, the extensor carpi radialis tendons may be detached from their insertion and reflected proximally.

The dorsal capsule of the wrist joint is incised in the shape of an I. Flaps are retracted medially and laterally. The wrist is flexed and the articular cartilage is removed from the carpal bones and from the distal radius with gouges and bone nibblers. The distal end of the ulna can be excised if it is involved in the arthritic process and can be used as a bone graft.

Bone graft fixation

34a

The proposed graft will be placed on the dorsum of the carpus extending from the base of the third metacarpal proximally to a point 2 cm proximal to the distal end of the radius. A trough approximately 2 cm wide should be made over the radius, carpus and the base of the third metacarpal. After cutting the edges of the trough the bone can be excavated using a chisel or a gouge.

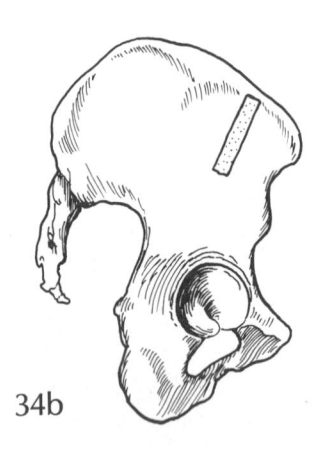

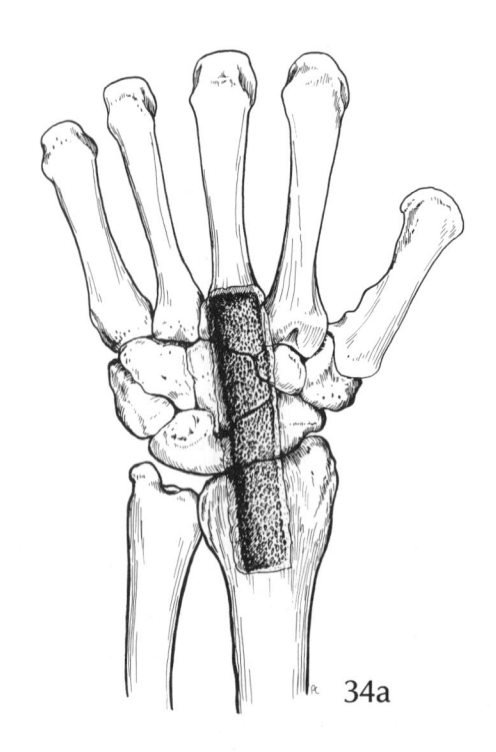

34a

34b

Bone graft is taken from the opposite ilium. The outer surface of the ilium is exposed below the iliac crest. The graft required is approximately 8 cm long and 2 cm wide and is taken in a caudo-cranial direction from the outer table of the iliac bone. The site of the graft is marked using an osteotome: the outer table and cancellous bone are penetrated but the inner table is not. A curved osteotome is then used to lift this graft, together with underlying cancellous bone, away from the inner table. It is important to take the graft from this area as it has a slight concavity which, when applied to the dorsum of the wrist, produces a slightly dorsiflexed position.

34b

Seating of the graft

35

Prior to fixation of this graft the wrist joint is opened while in palmarflexion, articular cartilage is removed, and cancellous bone taken from the iliac crest is impacted into the joint. The wrist is dorsiflexed and the bone graft strut is placed in the trough and shaped to lie flush with the surface of the carpus. It is held in place by a lag screw which passes through the radius and a second one which passes through the base of the third metacarpal. This produces quite firm fixation of the wrist.

Plate fixation

36

The articular cartilage is removed from the joint and a trough is cut on the dorsum of the distal radius and carpus. Cancellous bone graft is packed into the joint space. The required position of the wrist is determined and fixed with Kirschner wires. A 3.5 mm cancellous screw is passed through the radial styloid to the capitate and the position is checked. A corticocancellous bone graft is placed in the trough and an 8-hole, 3.5 mm AO dynamic compression plate is then applied from the base of the third metacarpal to the distal radius. It should be contoured to produce about 20° of dorsiflexion.

Closure

It may be possible to suture the dorsal capsule of the wrist joint over the plate or the graft, but this is not essential. The extensor retinaculum is passed deep to the tendons and sutured in place over the graft or the plate. It is helpful to leave one strip of the extensor retinaculum on the dorsal surface of the tendons to limit the bowstringing, especially if there has been any degree of dorsiflexion left in the wrist.

A small suction drain is left in the wound and the skin is closed with interrupted sutures. A well-padded dressing is applied with a plaster slab on the palmar aspect of the wrist.

Postoperative management

Bone graft fixation It is advisable to leave the wrist supported in a below-elbow plaster cast for a period of 12 weeks or until fusion has been established.

Plate fixation A well-padded volar plaster slab should be left in place until the sutures are removed at 14 days. A heat-moulded splint is then applied for a period of 12 weeks. This can be a removable splint but must be left in place except for essential toilet of the skin until fusion is complete.

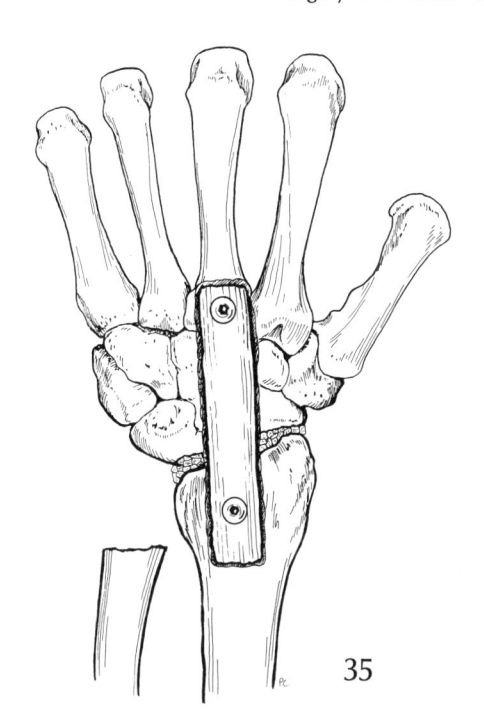

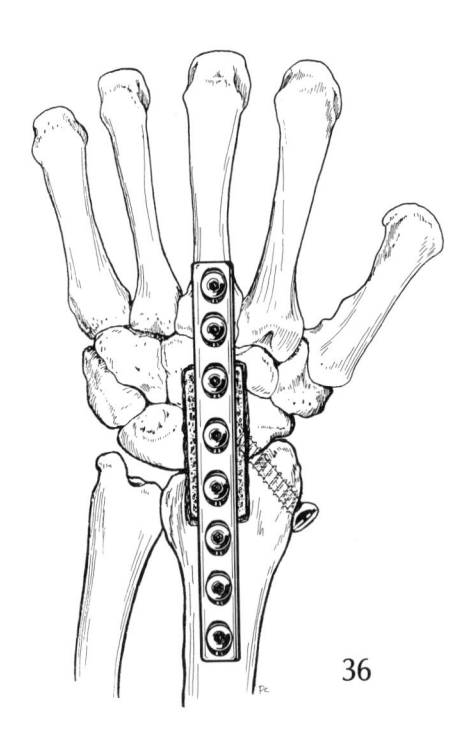

FRACTURES OF THE CARPAL SCAPHOID

37

Fractures of the carpal scaphoid not associated with dislocations should be treated conservatively in a plaster cast. There is considerable controversy concerning the extent of the plaster and the position of the wrist. However, a short-arm cast which encloses the proximal phalanx of the thumb in a position of function achieves a union rate of 95 per cent, and more extensive immobilization would appear unnecessary[8,9].

The duration of immobilization that is required varies with the site of the fracture. Fractures of the tuberosity and distal third require 6 weeks of immobilization. Fractures of the waist and the proximal third require 12 weeks of immobilization[8]. The plaster cast is removed after these intervals and further radiographs in four planes are necessary. It may be difficult at this stage to tell if union is complete but the patient should be allowed to mobilize the wrist and be reviewed in 4 weeks with further radiographic and clinical assessment.

Operative intervention may be necessary at this stage if radiographically there is established non-union, especially if there has been a change in position of the scaphoid since the original radiograph. Non-union occurs predominantly in fractures of the waist and the proximal pole. If, after 4 weeks of mobilization, the fracture is clinically and radiographically un-united then operative intervention is recommended. If the patient is asymptomatic yet the radiograph shows that the fracture has not yet united, then the treatment is open to controversy. London[10] recommends that the non-union be treated only if it is symptomatic, suggesting that there is a state of asymptomatic fibrous union which may never cause problems. However, other authors[11,12] suggest that osteoarthritis is the eventual outcome of an asymptomatic non-union and that operative intervention should be performed even in the absence of clinical symptoms.

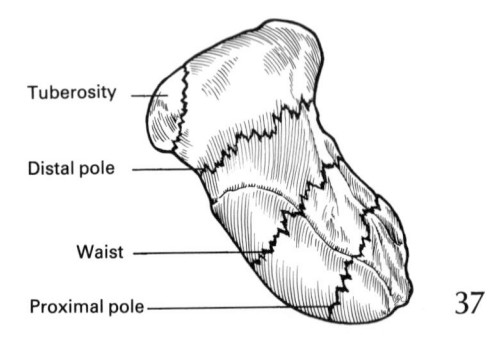

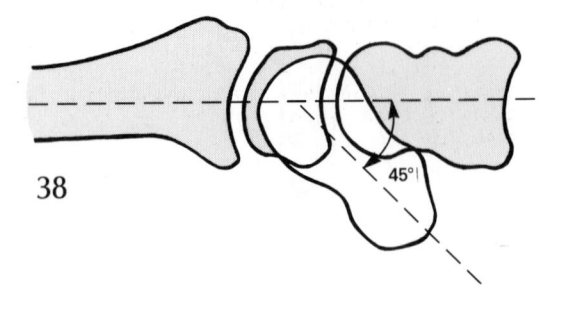

38

It is important to scrutinize the lateral view of the wrist carefully to detect evidence of carpal instability[13]. The normal scapholunate angle is 45°.

39a & b

A fracture of the waist of the scaphoid may cause the distal pole to tilt anteriorly, thus creating dorsiflexion of the lunate (dorsal intercalated segmental instability pattern). Disruption of the ligamentous structures may allow abnormal movement at the fracture site and therefore increase the risk of non-union. Those patients with gross instability should have a primary internal fixation of the scaphoid. In late cases it is important to recognize this anterior collapse of the carpal scaphoid which effectively reduces the overall length of the bone. The anterior collapse should be corrected by the insertion of a wedge graft which restores the scaphoid to the correct length.

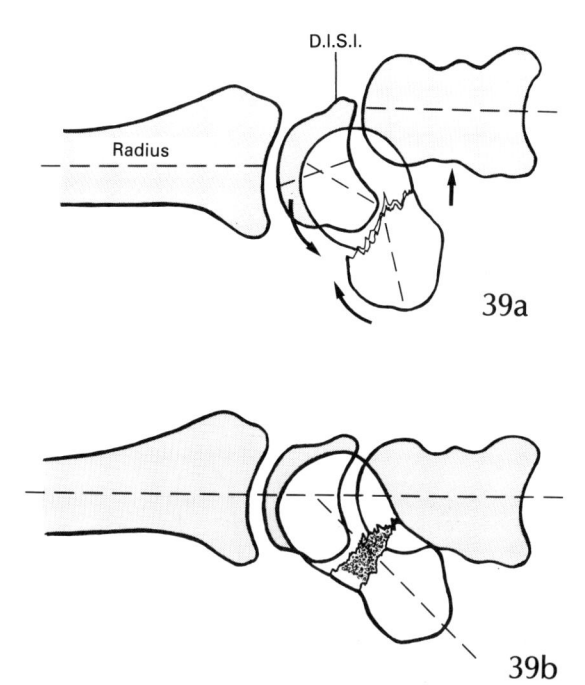

Indications for operation

Early

1. Acute trans-scaphoid perilunate dislocations of the wrist or any other dislocation of the wrist joint in which the scaphoid is fractured.
2. Displacement of the scaphoid fracture greater than 2 mm.

Late

1. If, after removal of plaster at 12 weeks, the fracture shows established non-union and early cyst formation on each side of the fracture line.
2. If, after 4 weeks of mobilization following the plaster removal at 12 weeks, the fracture remains un-united and the patient is symptomatic.
3. If, after 4 weeks of mobilization following removal of the plaster, the fracture remains un-united but the patient is asymptomatic (this indication is controversial at the present time).
4. An un-united fracture of the carpal scaphoid which presents late (often due to a further injury) and there is a carpal instability pattern.
5. If, after a fresh injury the symptoms of an old un-united scaphoid fracture are brought to light and do not settle down after a 4-week period of plaster immobilization. There is a relative indication for internal fixation if there is an instability pattern, as there would appear to be a risk of late degenerative change.
6. An established non-union of the scaphoid associated with symptomatic degenerative change of the wrist joint which may require excision of the radial styloid, limited carpal arthrodesis or a panarthrodesis of the carpus from the radius to the base of the third metacarpal.

Operations

Internal fixation of the scaphoid with or without bone graft and the Matte–Russe bone grafting procedure[14] are the two most commonly performed operations. The success rate for established non-union is similar for each procedure although the Matte–Russe bone graft procedure requires a longer period of plaster immobilization. In the acute injury internal fixation is the treatment of choice.

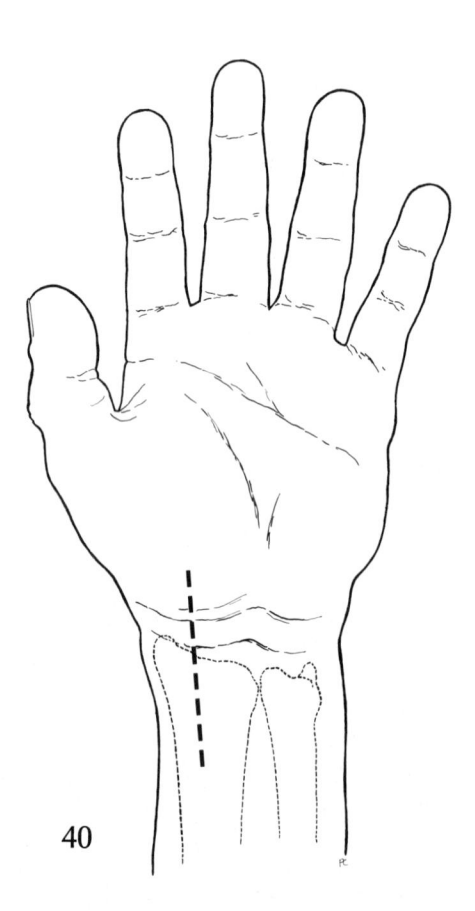

MATTE–RUSSE BONE GRAFT OF THE CARPAL SCAPHOID

Position of patient

After induction of general anaesthesia, the patient is placed supine and a tourniquet applied to the upper arm. A sandbag is placed under the opposite buttock to enable a bone graft to be taken from the iliac crest, and this site is then prepared.

Incision

40

An anterior approach is made to the wrist joint. A 5 cm longitudinal incision is made over the tendon of flexor carpi radialis and it is centred at the level of the tip of the styloid process. Care should be taken to identify the superficial palmar branch of the radial artery, which should be ligated.

Approach

41

The tendon sheath of flexor carpi radialis is opened and the tendon is retracted, releasing it from its tunnel distally. A longitudinal incision is made in the base of the tendon sheath, dividing the capsule longitudinally; the joint may then be entered. The deep volar radiocarpal ligaments will need to be reconstructed at the end of the procedure.

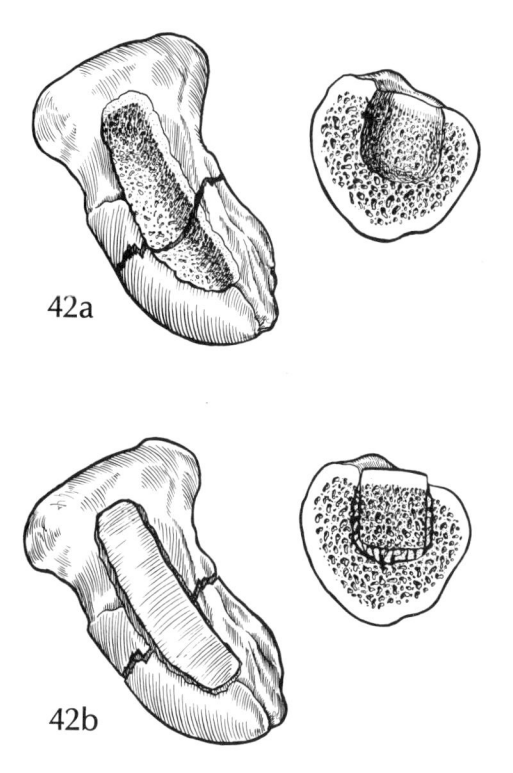

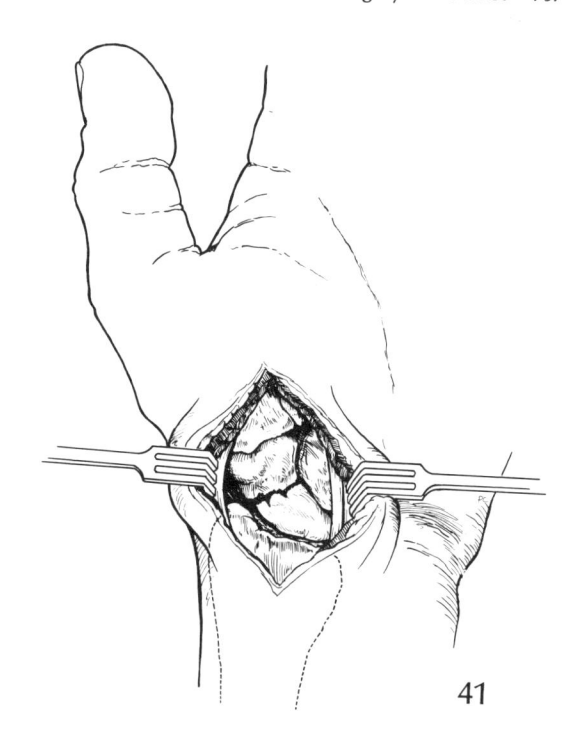

Procedure

42a & b

The fracture is identified and an egg-shaped cavity is created in both fragments using a small osteotome and curette. The anterior cortex is undermined distally and proximally. This creates an anterior trough in the bone.

A small corticocancellous graft is taken from the iliac crest through a small transverse incision. A small amount of cancellous bone is taken at the same time. The bone graft is trimmed to fit into the cavity. The cortex of the graft lies superficially and the fragments are distracted while the graft is pressed into the cavity. Release of the fragments should create a stable graft. The cavity around the graft is packed with small fragments of cancellous bone. If the graft is not stable then two longitudinal Kirschner wires can be used to maintain stability.

43

A modification of this technique is to use two small corticocancellous grafts, placing the cancellous surfaces face-to-face and inserting the graft on its side[15].

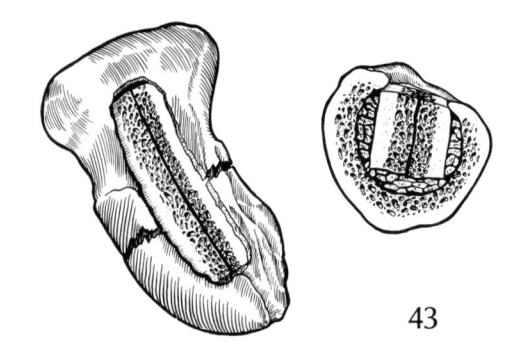

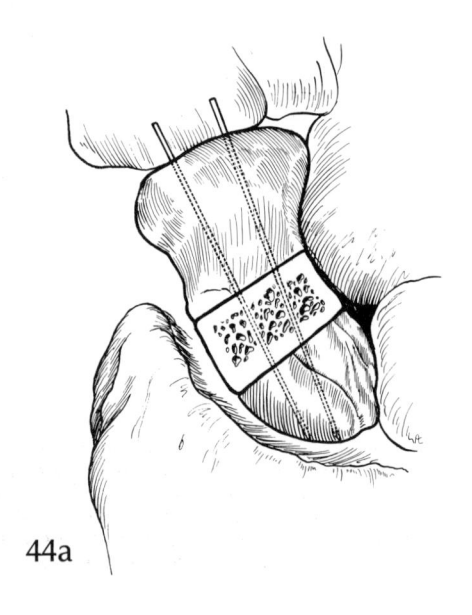

43

44a & b

If there is a collapse of the scaphoid bone on the lateral view then it is important to open out the volar aspect with the bone graft. The lateral view of the fractured side should be compared with the unfractured side in order to establish the correct length of the scaphoid bone. It is possible to plan the size of the wedge with preoperative drawings[16]. It is usually necessary to fix these grafts with Kirschner wires or even a screw.

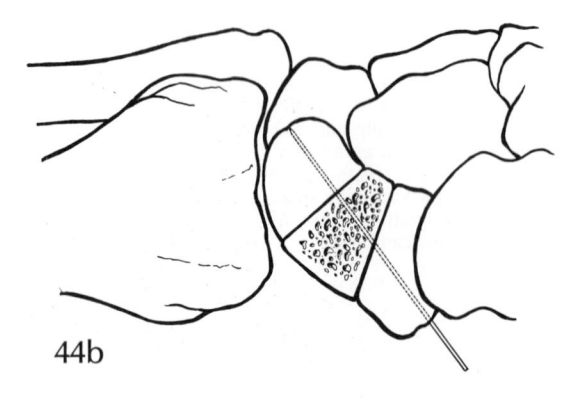

44a

44b

Closure

The volar radiocarpal ligaments are repaired using interrupted sutures. It is easier to place all the sutures before tying any of them. The synovium is closed over the tendon of flexor carpi radialis and the skin sutured. A well-padded bandage is applied followed by a volar plaster slab with a gutter on the ulnar side.

Postoperative management

The dressing is reduced after 10 days and a below-elbow plaster applied, including the proximal phalanx of the thumb. This is left in place for 12 weeks.

Surgery of the wrist 799

INTERNAL FIXATION OF THE SCAPHOID

AO scaphoid lag screw

Position of patient

A tourniquet is applied to the upper arm and the patient's hand rests pronated on a hand table. It is necessary to have X-ray facilities peroperatively.

Incision

45

A straight incision is made over the dorsoradial side of the carpus extending from the base of the thumb to the radial styloid and then curving slightly across the back of the wrist.

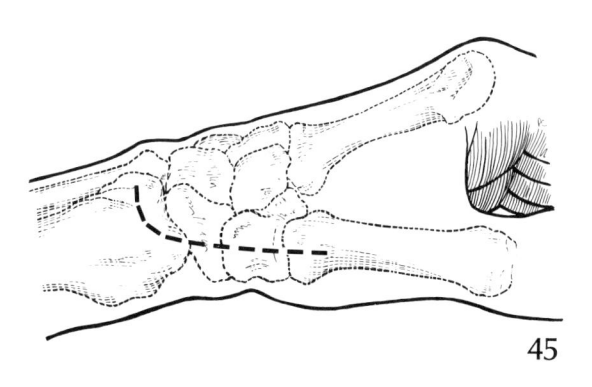

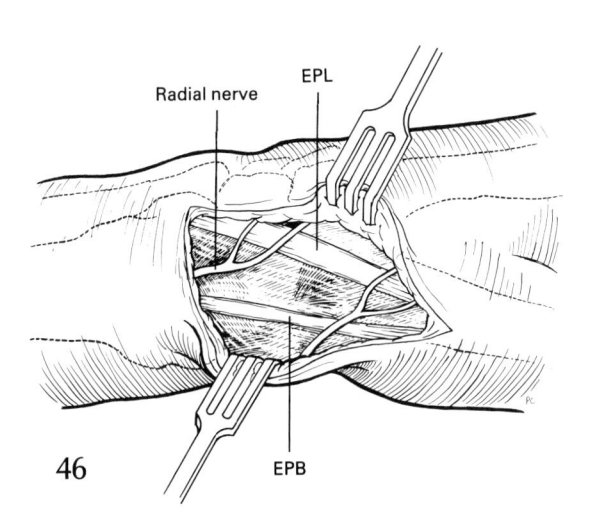

Exposure

46

Superficial veins may be ligated. It is important to preserve the terminal branches of the radial nerve and also the radial artery as it crosses the floor of the fossa. The tendons of extensor pollicis longus and extensor pollicis brevis are retracted. The capsule of the wrist is exposed and an oblique incision is made in line with the scaphoid.

47

The fracture is identified and a small bone hook is inserted around the proximal pole. Care should be taken not to dissect the capsule of the dorsal ridge of the scaphoid as this will influence the blood supply.

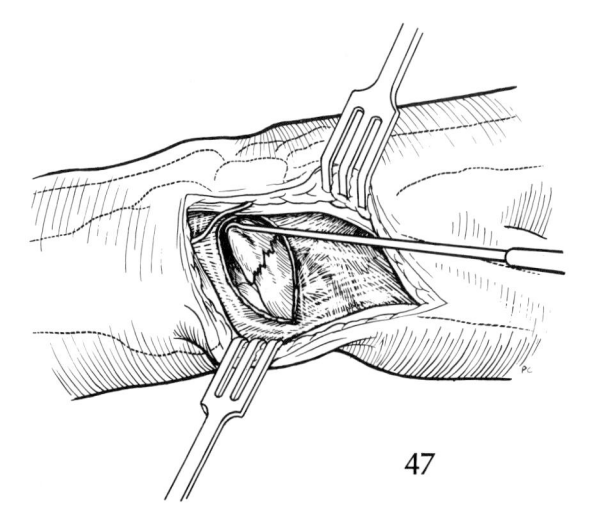

48a & b

Using the drill guide, the surgeon inserts a Kirschner wire along the long axis of the scaphoid. A check radiograph is taken in the posteroanterior and lateral directions. The length of the screw required is determined by measuring the length of Kirschner wire protruding from the scaphoid and subtracting that length from the total length of another similar Kirschner wire. A 2 mm drill hole is made parallel to the Kirschner wire using the drill guide. The proximal cortex is tapped using the 3.5 mm tap and an appropriate length of 3.5 mm cancellous screw is inserted into the scaphoid.

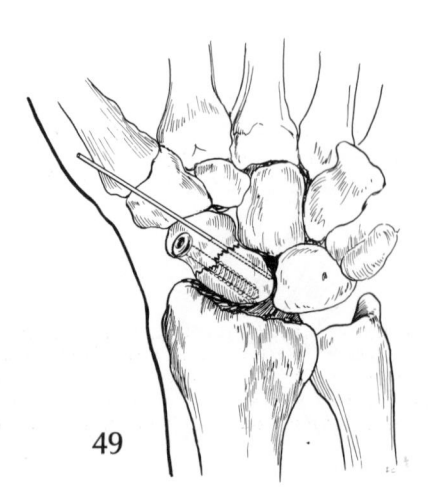

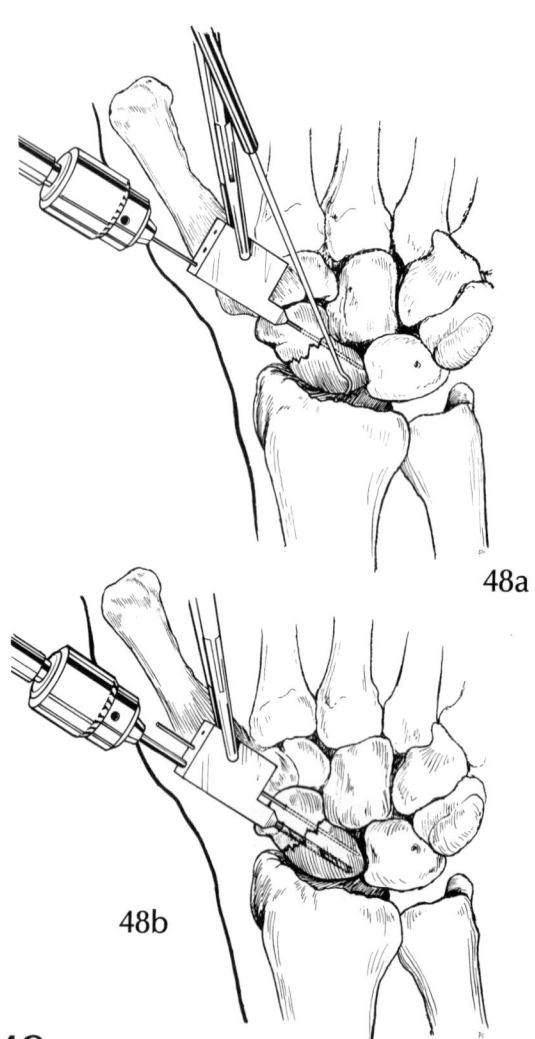

49

Compression should be observed at the fracture site. Check radiographs should be taken to ascertain the position of the screw. The Kirschner wire is removed. The capsule is closed with interrupted sutures. The skin is closed with interrupted nylon. A padded bandage is wrapped round the hand and a plaster volar slab applied with a gutter around the ulnar side.

Postoperative management

The plaster slab and bandages should be reduced at 10 days and sutures can be removed. A lightweight splint is applied for a further 2 weeks and if check X-ray films are satisfactory at that stage, total mobilization can be commenced. Full force should not be taken through the wrist for 3 months.

The Herbert bone screw

50 & 51

The insertion of a screw into the scaphoid is a difficult procedure as there is little margin for error in the alignment. A screw has been designed which overcomes some of the difficulties encountered previously. The screw does not have a head, but in its place is another thread which has a different pitch to that of the distal end of the screw[17]. Therefore the head of the screw does not protrude from the bone and compression is achieved by the differential pitch of the threads at each end of the screw. Both ends of the screw remain buried in the bone and the screw does not have to be removed. A jig is necessary for its insertion and it is essential, before commencing the operation, to make sure that all the necessary instruments and the complete range of screws are available in the set

This procedure is technically demanding and Herbert's precise instructions should be studied carefully. The jig is difficult to place in the correct position and concern about ligamentous and vascular damage to the distal end of the scaphoid has been expressed[18].

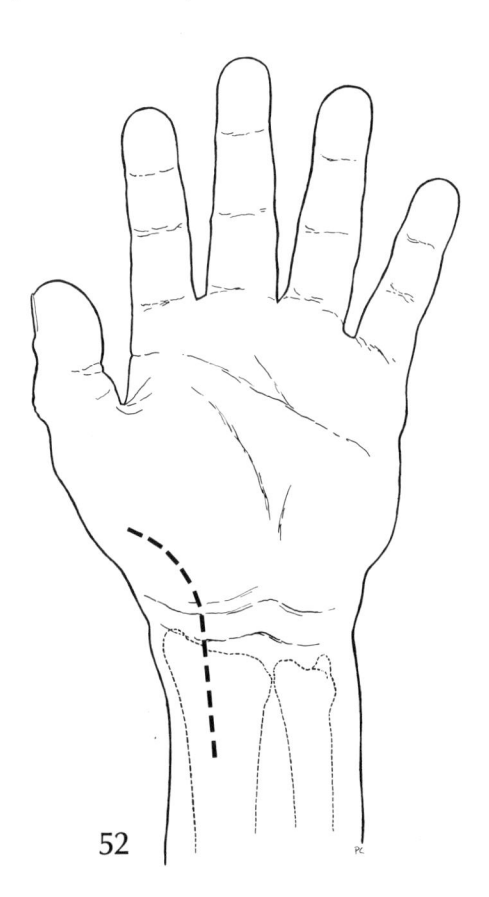

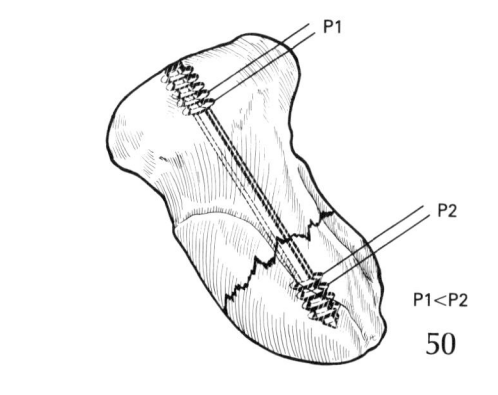

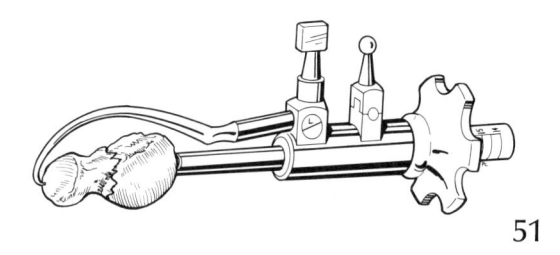

Preparation of the patient

The patient is placed supine on the operating table with a tourniquet applied to the upper arm and the hand resting on the table. If the screw is being inserted for an established non–union it may be necessary to take a bone graft and therefore the contralateral iliac crest should be prepared.

Incision

52

An anterior approach is made to the wrist joint. A longitudinal incision is made along the line of the flexor carpi radialis; distally it curves radially along the thenar eminence.

Approach

The superficial branch of the radial artery is ligated. The flexor sheath of flexor carpi radialis is divided longitudinally and the tendon retracted. The tendon is released from its tunnel distally. The bed of the tendon is then incised longitudinally to expose the wrist joint and the scaphoid.

802 Forearm, wrist and hand

Procedure

53

In the acute situation the fracture is reduced and the Herbert jig is applied. The hook of the jig must be inserted into the proximal pole. It will be necessary to dissect the ligaments between the scaphoid and the trapezium to lift the scaphoid forward so that the jig can be applied distally. The guide is then clamped to the distal pole and it should be seen to compress the fracture line.

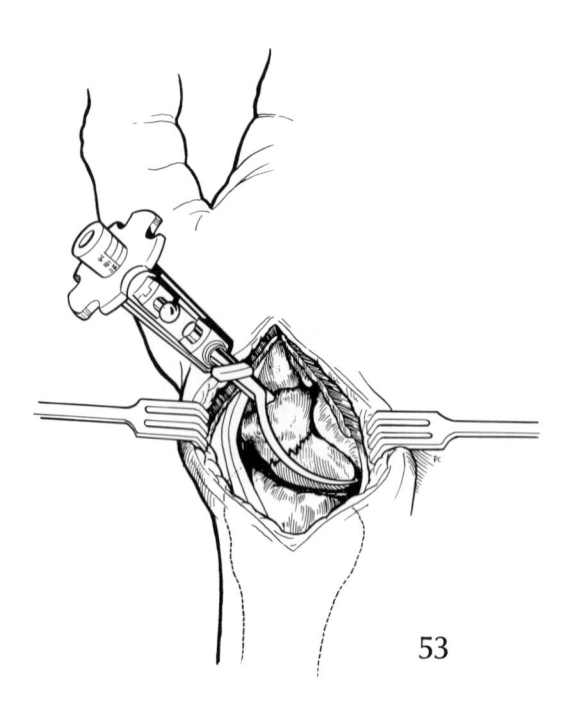

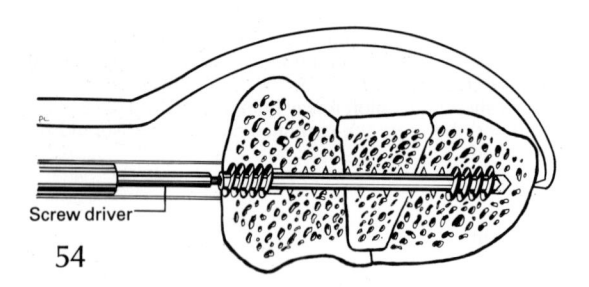

54

If the screw is being inserted into an established non-union then the fibrous tissue is removed from the fracture site and the cavity so created is packed with cancellous bone. It may be necessary to insert an anterior wedge of bone taken from the iliac crest. This should be a corticocancellous graft. The fracture is opened up, the wedge inserted and it is then held there by the compression of the jig.

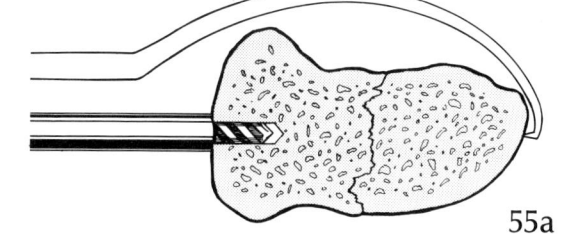

55a, b, c & d

With the jig in place, a pilot drill is inserted into the proximal end for the trailing edge of the screw (a). A long drill is then inserted for the leading edge of the screw (b), the bone is then tapped and the length of the screw is measured directly from a scale on the jig (c). Insertion of all instruments is done through the jig and the instruments are so designed that the correct length of drilling and tapping is always achieved.

A screw of appropriate length is then inserted through the jig and tightened. Compression should be seen at the fracture line (d). The jig is removed and the stability of the fracture tested.

Closure

The anterior volar capsule is closed with interrupted non-absorbable sutures as described above for the Matte–Russe graft procedure.

Postoperative management

A radiograph is taken to check the position of the screw. The hand is wrapped in a well-padded bandage with a plaster cast on the volar aspect. At 10 days the cast and the sutures are removed and a light heat-moulded wrist splint is applied for a total period of 4 weeks. During this time the patient removes it for gentle mobilization.

Precautions

Care must be taken not to dissect the scaphoid too extensively from its distal pole. The jig must be applied accurately if the screw is to achieve its aim of producing compression across the fracture.

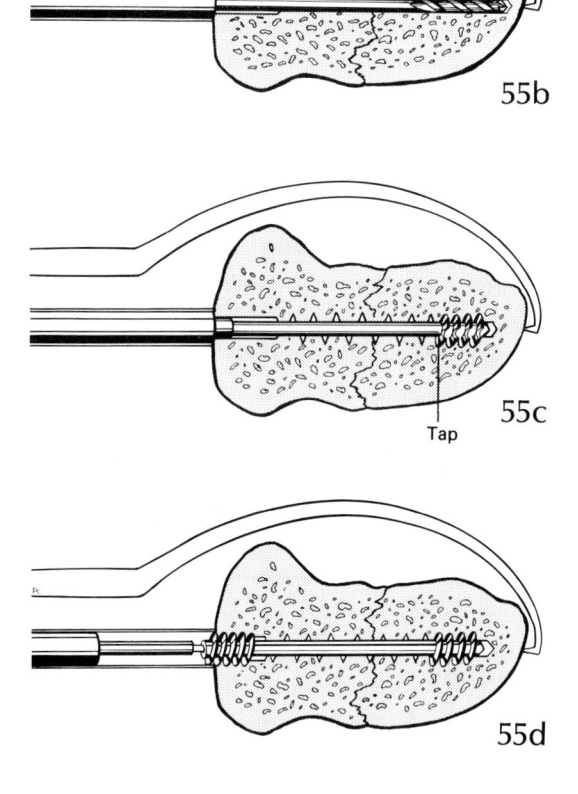

FRACTURES OF THE PROXIMAL POLE WITH A SMALL FRAGMENT

56

If at operation the proximal pole is found to be too small or completely avascular then bone grafting procedures and fixation will not be possible. Excision of the small proximal fragment leaves a space into which the capitate may migrate and it is therefore advised that a small piece of Silastic be carved and used as a spacer. Some surgeons use the moulded Silastic scaphoid and cut off the proximal end, while others use a block of Silastic and cut it to the necessary shape at the time of the operation[19].

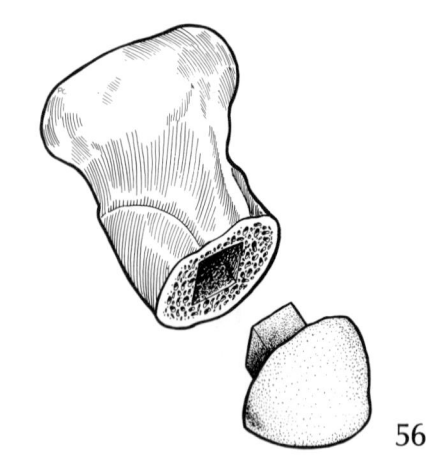

56

References

1. Darrach W. Anterior dislocation of the head of the ulna. *Ann Surg* 1912; 56: 802–3.

2. Gonçalves D. Correction of disorders of the distal radio-ulnar joint by artificial pseudoarthrosis of the ulna. *J Bone Joint Surg [Br]* 1974; 56-B: 462–4.

3. Clayton ML. Surgical treatment at the wrist in rheumatoid arthritis: a review of 37 patients. *J Bone Joint Surg [Am]* 1965; 47-A: 741–50.

4. Millender LH, Nalebuff EA. Arthrodesis of the rheumatoid wrist: an evaluation of 60 patients and a description of a different surgical technique. *J Bone Joint Surg [Am]* 1973; 55-A: 1026–34.

5. Papaioannou T, Dickson RA. Arthrodesis of the wrist in rheumatoid disease. *Hand* 1982; 14: 12–6.

6. Chamay A, Della Santa D, Vilaseca A. Radiolunate arthrodesis: factor of stability for the rheumatoid wrist. *Ann Chir Main* 1983; 2: 5.

7. Swanson AB, Swanson G de G, Maupin, BK. Flexible implant arthroplasty of the radiocarpal joint: surgical technique and long-term study. *Clin Orthop* 1984; 187: 94–106.

8. Leslie IJ, Dickson RA. The fractures carpal scaphoid: natural history and factors influencing outcome. *J Bone Joint Surg [Br]* 1981; 63-B: 225–30.

9. Taleisnik J. *The wrist*. New York: Churchill Livingstone, 1985.

10. London PS. The broken scaphoid bone: the case against pessimism. *J Bone Joint Surg [Br]* 1961; 43-B: 237–44.

11. Ruby LK, Stinson J, Belsky MR. The natural history of scaphoid non-union: a review of 55 cases. *J Bone Joint Surg [Am]* 1985; 67-A: 428–32.

12. Mack GR, Bosse MJ, Gelberman RH. The natural history of scaphoid non-union. *J Bone Joint Surg [Am]* 1984; 66-A: 504–9.

13. Fisk GR. Carpal instability and the fractured scaphoid. *Ann R Coll Surg Engl* 1970; 46: 63–76.

14. Russe O. Fracture of the carpal navicular: diagnosis, non-operative treatment and operative treatment. *J Bone Joint Surg [Am]* 1960; 42-A: 759–68.

15. Green DP. The effect of avascular necrosis on Russe bone grafting for scaphoid non-union. *J Hand Surg [Am]* 1985; 10A: 597–605.

16. Fernandez DL. A technique for anterior wedge-shaped grafts for scaphoid non-union with carpal instability. *J Hand Surg [Am]* 1984; 9A: 733–7.

17. Herbert TJ, Fisher WE. Management of the fractured scaphoid using a new bone screw. *J Bone Joint Surg [Br]* 1984; 66-B: 114–123.

18. Botte MJ, Mortensen WW, Gelberman RH, Rhoads CE, Gellman H. Internal vascularity of the scaphoid in cadavers after insertion of the Herbert screw. *J Hand Surg [Am]* 1988; 13A: 216–20.

19. Zemel NP, Stark HH, Ashworth CR, Rickard TA, Anderson DR. Treatment of selected patients with an ununited fracture of the proximal part of the scaphoid by excision of the fragment and insertion of a carved silicone-rubber spacer. *J Bone Joint Surg [Am]*; 66-A: 510–7.

Illustrations by Gillian Oliver

Tendon transfer for mobile radial deviation of the wrist

B. Helal MChOrth, FRCS
Honorary Consultant Orthopaedic Surgeon, The Royal London Hospital and The Royal National Orthopaedic Hospital, London, and Enfield Group of Hospitals, UK

S. C. Chen FRCS
Consultant Orthopaedic Surgeon, Enfield Group of Hospitals, UK

Introduction

In rheumatoid disease the inferior radio-ulnar joint is often involved early. The synovitis around the ulnar head results in inhibition of the ulnar carpal muscles. This, in turn, encourages ulnar deviation at the metacarpophalangeal joints[1]. While there is passive mobility in an ulnar direction this can be corrected by tendon transfer. Ferlic and Clayton[2] have carried out tendon transfer of the extensor carpi radialis longus to the extensor carpi ulnaris. In our experience much of the power is dissipated in extending the wrist. Helal[3] modified this transfer by splitting the transferred extensor carpi radialis longus and implanting half into the flexor carpi ulnaris and half into the extensor carpi ulnaris. This transfer has proved an effective ulnar deviator of the wrist. There is an added bonus, as the limb passing to the flexor carpi ulnaris stabilizes the ulnar shaft as the procedure is usually combined with ulnar head excision.

Operation

Incisions

1

Three skin incisions are made on the dorsum of the forearm and wrist:

1. Over the insertion of extensor carpi radialis longus
2. In line with this tendon in the lower third of the forearm
3. On the ulnar side, over the distal end of he ulna.

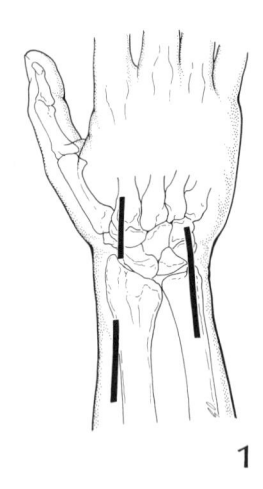

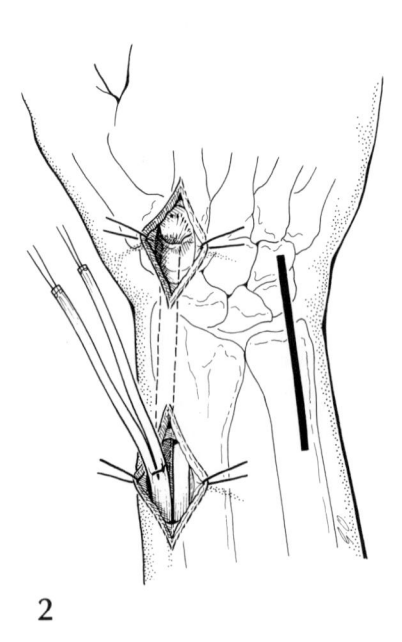

Transfer

2

The tendon of extensor carpi radialis longus is detached from its insertion and brought out through the proximal incision. It is split and a suture placed through the bifurcation to prevent further separation.

3

The split tendon is tunnelled through subcutaneous tissue to the ulnar side.

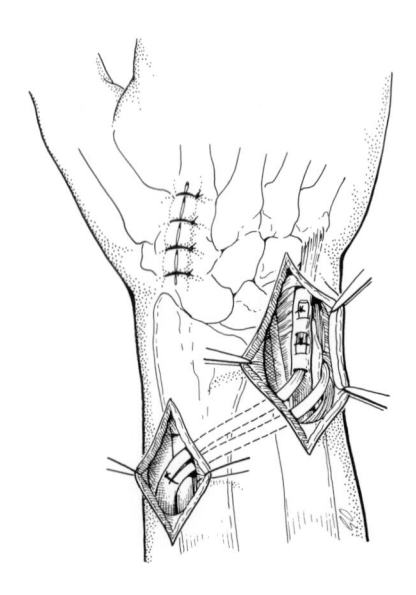

Exposure of ulnar tendons

4

The tendons of extensor carpi ulnaris and flexor carpi ulnaris are identified. In isolating the flexor carpi ulnaris care must be taken to protect the ulnar nerve which is close by.

Attachment

One limb of the split transferred tendon is woven into each of the ulnar carpal tendons with the wrist held in full ulnar deviation.

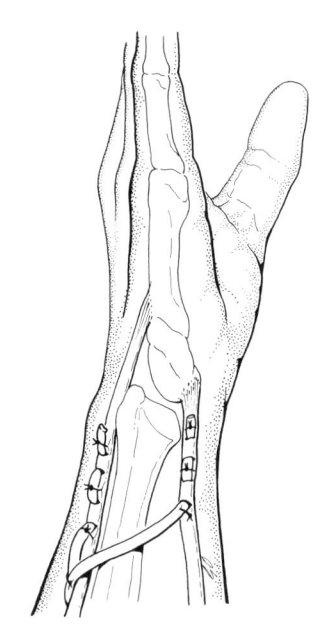

Postoperative management

A below-elbow plaster cast is applied with the wrist in ulnar deviation for a period of 4 weeks.

References

1. Stack HE, Vaughan Jackson OJ, The zig-zag deformity in the rheumatoid hand. *Hand* 1971; 3: 62.

2. Ferlic DC, Clayton ML. Tendon transfer for radial rotation in the rheumatoid wrist. *J Bone Joint Surg [Am]* 1973; 55-A: 880–1.

3. Helal B. The flexor tendon apparatus in the rheumatoid hand. *Clin Rheum Dis* 1984; 10: 479–500.

Illustrations by R. C. Pearson and Gillian Oliver

Tendon injuries in the hand

John P. W. Varian FRCS, FRACS(Orth)
Consultant Hand Surgeon, Blackrock Clinic, Dublin, Ireland

Much of the text in this chapter remains unchanged from the previous edition and is the work of the late Mr. R. Guy Pulvertaft. The present author has amended and expanded it in the light of his experience and some of the changing trends in tendon surgery.

Introduction

The problems set by tendon divisions in the hand are complex and their treatment varies with the site of injury, but the following observations have a general application.

1. A tendon heals readily when held in apposition and the union is sufficiently strong at 3–4 weeks to withstand slight strain.
2. Damaged tendons have a marked tendency to become adherent to the surrounding tissues, limiting their gliding movement.
3. A gentle and precise technique is essential and necessitates the use of the finest instruments and a suture material which does not provoke a tissue reaction.
4. A bloodless field, using a tourniquet, is necessary. Most surgeons remove the tourniquet and secure haemostasis prior to closure. Others, including the author, prefer to use meticulous haemostasis throughout the operation, especially during the early dissection, and then close prior to tourniquet release. The essential objective is the prevention of postoperative haematoma and the surgeon should use the technique which suits him best in attaining this objective.

Indications for operation

EXTENSOR TENDONS

Distal interphalangeal joint (mallet deformity)

1

Rupture or division of the extensor attachment to the distal phalanx is best treated by splintage in extension for 6–8 weeks or longer if the treatment has been delayed. The splint needs to be tolerable to the patient and effectively maintained. Several patterns of splint have been described; the one illustrated (devised independently by Parker and by Stack) is suitable and preferred to plaster or internal fixation.

Operative treatment is reserved for those cases in which conservative treatment has failed or which are seen late. The choice lies between arthrodesis of the distal joint or repair of the tendon. The former is often difficult to achieve and the latter tends to give poor results. Most patients are therefore advised against secondary surgery. Where tendon repair is undertaken there must be a full passive range of movement in the terminal joint.

Secondary repair is possible where there has been open severance of the tendon. In closed rupture the tendon ends are difficult or impossible to identify and tendon plication as described by Vilain[1] is preferable. Iselin[2] has reported satisfactory results excising a wedge of skin and tendon, and including both tissues in the repair suture. Operative treatment is also advisable when a considerable fragment of bone has been avulsed with the tendon and especially when this is accompanied by subluxation of the main fragment. In these circumstances the operation becomes very difficult if there is delay after injury and should not be attempted if the delay exceeds 3 weeks.

Proximal interphalangeal joint (boutonnière deformity)

The extensor tendon divides over the proximal phalanx into a central band which is attached to the base of the middle phalanx and into two lateral bands which bypass the proximal interphalangeal joint and join to be inserted into the base of the distal phalanx. Division of the central band allows the proximal joint to flex and the distal joint is drawn into hyperextension. The lateral bands migrate forwards and act as flexors of the proximal joint. Secondary ligamentous contractures lead to a fixed deformity of both joints.

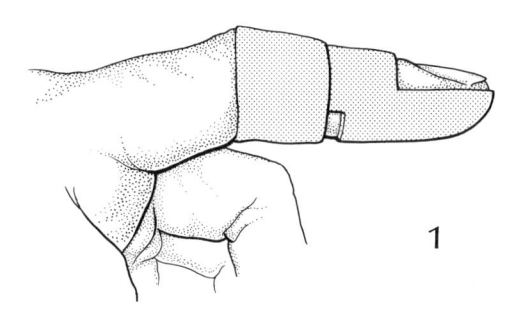

2, 3a & b

When a rupture or division of the central band is seen within 5 or 6 weeks after injury, a good result can usually be obtained by splintage in extension for a period of 4–6 weeks, followed by protective mobilization in a dynamic splint. A suitable static type is the Bunnell splint which is fitted as illustrated to permit flexion of the distal joint. The Capener dynamic splint is recommended for the mobilization phase. It may also be used to correct a moderate flexion contracture.

Operative treatment is reserved for those cases which fail to respond to conservative measures and for those that are manifestly unlikely to do so. Secondary repair by simple scar excision and end-to-end suture is usually possible up to 3 months after injury but once secondary contractures develop it may not be possible to reconstitute the normal anatomy. Matev[3] corrects the deformity by transposing one of the lateral bands to the base of the middle phalanx and lengthens the other band to overcome the hyperextension of the distal phalanx. Littler and Eaton[4] centralize the lateral bands over the proximal joint, relying on the oblique retinacular ligament of Landsmeer and the lumbrical muscle to extend the distal joint.

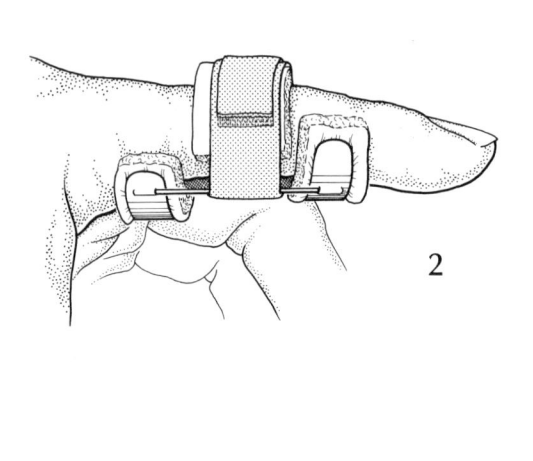

Hand and wrist

Tendon retraction after division over the metacarpophalangeal joint is usually slight and an early case may be treated successfully by splintage in extension. If there is any doubt, and always in later cases, surgical repair is advisable. Tendons divided in the central and proximal parts of the hand and over the wrist joint always require repair. In late cases it may not be possible to obtain apposition of the tendon ends and a tendon graft or a tendon transfer may be needed.

FLEXOR TENDONS

Flexor digitorum profundus in the finger

When the profundus tendon alone is divided beyond the superficialis attachment, good results can be obtained by immediate suture. Delayed suture is possible if the vincula are intact and retraction has been prevented. This is likely if the laceration occurred when the profundus muscle was relaxed. (Remember that this is the case in the finger during strong pulp-to-pulp pinch against the thumb.) In these circumstances end-to-end repair is often possible up to 6 weeks after the injury, bypassing the distal pulley.

If the tendon retracted into the palm, as commonly occurs in tendon avulsion, direct repair becomes impossible after only a few days as the tendon becomes too swollen to be threaded back through the pulleys and superficialis decussation. Consideration should then be given to tendon grafting which should be delayed for 4–6 months to allow the hand to settle after the original injury. A thin tendon, preferably plantaris, is used and reaches from the proximal palm to the distal phalanx. The undamaged superficialis tendon is not disturbed. This operation is justified for someone whose occupation demands fingertip action and for children. The purpose is to achieve perfection and, as the possibility of disturbing superficialis function exists, the operation should only be undertaken when the indications are clear and the surgeon is experienced in tendon grafting[5].

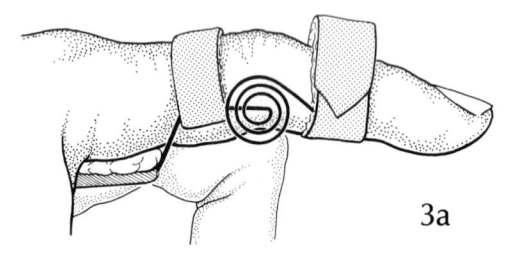

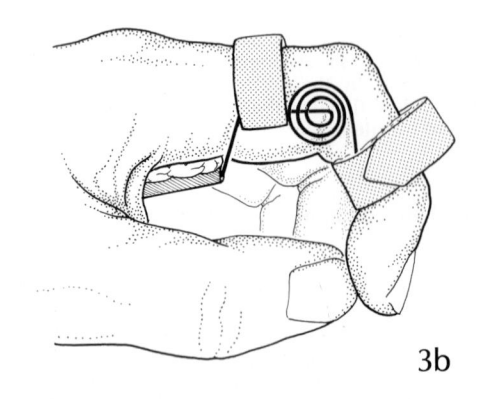

The alternative procedure is fixation in suitable flexion of the distal joint by arthrodesis or tenodesis. This should be postponed for at least 6 months as in the author's experience most patients become accustomed to the loss of flexion in the terminal joint and do not want surgery.

Flexor digitorum profundus and superficialis in the finger

During recent years there has been a movement towards the wider use of primary suture of flexor tendons divided within the digital theca, the technique of which is described in the chapter on 'Primary repair of the divided digital flexor tendon' (see pp. 828–835). *It must be stressed that the results are likely to be disappointing unless the facilities and the technique are of the highest order; failure will foul the ground for subsequent tendon grafting.* Neither primary suture nor tendon grafting are recommended unless the surgeon has studied the subject fully and has had adequate training in the exacting technique. When these conditions are not satisfied, it is wiser to do no more than clean and suture the wound and refer the case for tendon grafting later. The tendons are replaced by a graft when the digit has recovered from the initial trauma and all reaction has resolved, which may take 4–6 months. Apart from the inconvenience to the patient there is no inherent harm in the delay for excellent results can be achieved even after a lapse of years, provided that the digit is in good overall condition[6]. It is useless to expect tendon grafting to succeed in the presence of severe scarring, contracture or complete sensory loss. If these conditions prevail, consideration should be given to the two-stage operation described on pp. 836–854.

Flexor pollicis longus

Division of flexor pollicis longus in the distal part of the thumb should be treated by immediate suture. In the region between the metacarpophalangeal joint and the wrist the tendon is in close relationship to the sensory nerves of the thumb and the motor branch to the thenar muscles. These structures are at risk during a tendon repair and, if injured, lead to a worse disability than the lack of distal joint flexion. If the surgeon is inexperienced, it is better to perform skin suture only, with a view to tendon grafting later. However, in experienced hands, primary repair produces better results than in the finger because there is only one flexor tendon to the digit and less risk of adhesion.

In general, function can be restored in all late cases by tendon grafting. However, it must be remembered that a thumb lacking flexion at the interphalangeal joint produces little disability in many individuals, whereas a severe flexion contracture in this joint which may result from a tendon graft, can be disabling. It is advisable therefore to avoid splinting the interphalangeal joint in full flexion in the postoperative period.

Palm

Suture of the superficialis and profundus tendons divided at the same level in the palm is apt to be followed by cross-union which limits the flexion action to superficialis. Meticulous suture of sharp-cut tendons will avoid this complication, but when the tendon ends are ragged it is advisable to cut back superficialis and restrict the repair to profundus. Superficialis to the ring and little fingers should always be sacrificed in the palm. Superficialis to the index and middle fingers has an important action in strong pulp-to-pulp pinch and should be repaired if possible. Appropriate posturing of the finger in the postoperative period will separate the two tendon repairs and reduce the risk of cross-union. Secondary suture may be practicable if the proximal end is held by the lumbricalis muscle but in late cases end-to-end contact may not be obtainable and the gap should be closed with a free graft taken from superficialis.

Wrist

Tendons divided at the wrist level retract severely and their muscles shorten and prevent apposition even in a fairly recent case, which necessitates the use of multiple bridge grafts for reconstruction. It is imperative, therefore, to perform immediate suture of tendons in this region if the wound conditions permit. End-to-end suture of all the tendons is performed, using the more rapidly applied Bunnell double right-angle stitch[7] which saves time especially when repair of associated nerve injury is carried out at the same operation.

ANAESTHESIA

In Great Britain general anaesthesia is used unless there is some special indication for plexus or local nerve block anaesthesia. However, regional anaesthesia is the more common choice in many countries where general anaesthesia is not so readily available. With the advent of neurotracers and longer acting anaesthetics the techniques are becoming easier. Many would consider it an advantage to have the limb paralysed in the immediate postoperative period, avoiding the uncontrolled movements often seen during the recovery from general anaesthesia, which increase the risk of haematoma formation and the risk of dehiscence of the repair[8].

812 Forearm, wrist and hand

Operations for individual tendon injuries

TENDON JUNCTIONS

Suture material

Stainless steel wire causes no tissue reaction and has proved a most satisfactory suture material. Care must be taken to avoid kinking; a reef knot is tied and the wire may be cut off flush with the knot leaving no protruding ends. Monofilament wire (British wire gauge 40) can be obtained swaged to 2.5 cm bayonet-ended malleable needles which were specifically developed for tendon surgery. Synthetic fibres (4/0) are also widely used. Material should always be non-absorbable. The two junctions most commonly used in primary repair are shown in *Illustrations 4* and *5*. Other techniques have been described[9, 10, 11].

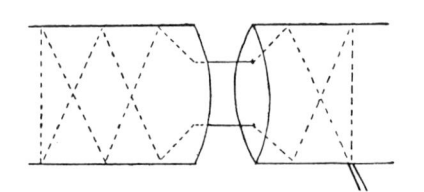

Bunnell criss-cross stitch

4

This stitch used to be the commonest method used in end-to-end tendon repair. As the result of claims that it causes ischaemia of tendon ends it has now become less popular than the Kessler stitch[12] (*see below*).

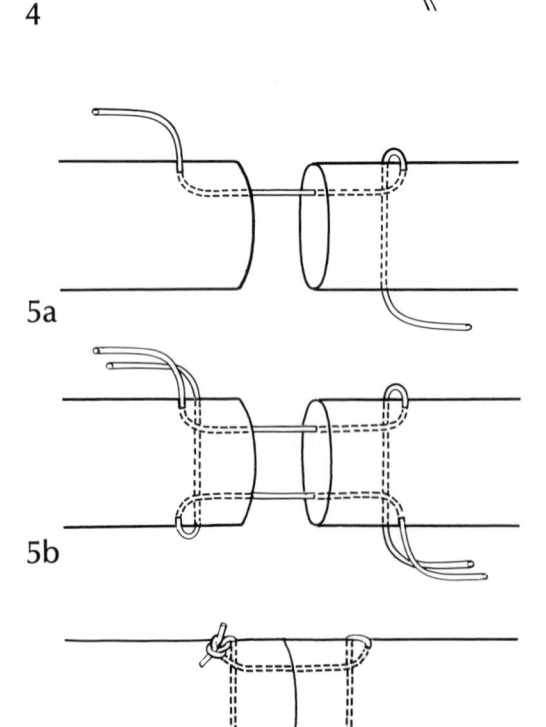

4

Kessler grasping stitch

5a, b & c

This stitch has the advantage of requiring fewer penetrations of the tendon and it is claimed that is has less tendency to compress the tendon ends and embarrass the blood supply. It has been modified by many surgeons who now no longer tie a half-knot at each corner as described by Kessler but insert the suture as shown. It is also easier to insert the suture into each tendon end in turn and tie the knots at the tendon junction, especially during primary repair when flexor sheath is being preserved.

5a

5b

5c

Bunnell double right-angle stitch

6

This stitch can be inserted rapidly and is a convenient and adequate technique to use when many tendons are divided at the wrist level, especially when time is of the essence, as during a replantation.

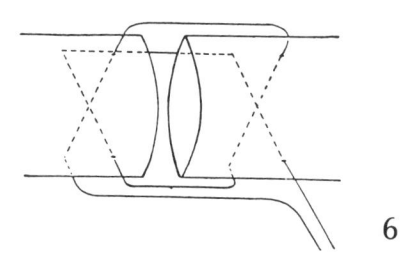

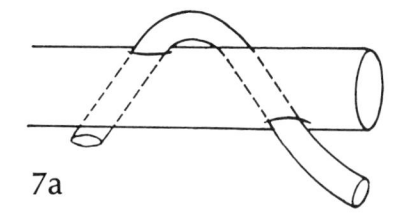

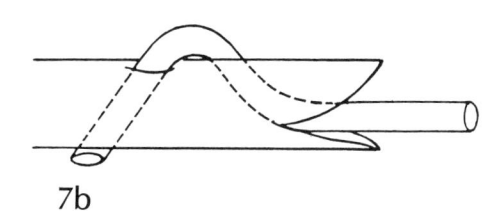

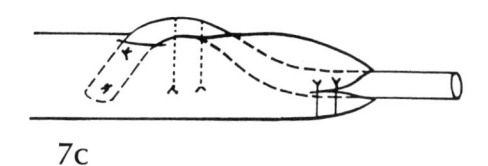

6

7a

Pulvertaft interlacing method

7a, b & c

The interlacing and fishmouth technique[13] is recommended when a slender tendon needs to be joined to a larger tendon and is suitable for the proximal attachment of a graft. It combines the neatness of an end-to-end junction with the strength of an interlacing suture.

7b

7c

Attachment of graft to distal tendon stump

8a-d

Several methods of attachment of the distal end of a tendon graft have been described but a simple one is as follows. The graft is taken through the fingertip with a Reverdin needle (Downs Surgical, Mitcham, UK) as described by Pulvertaft[13]. This gives good control of the graft beyond the tendon stump leaving the wound clear of instruments to facilitate suturing. It also allows tension adjustment at the distal junction. Sutures of 6/0 material are then inserted at three points as shown (*b* and *c*). The stump is then turned back and a further three sutures are inserted (*d*). Finally the stump is tacked down to the volar surface of the graft with a single suture. It is important to ensure that this tendon stump is short enough to lie distal to the distal interphalangeal joint.

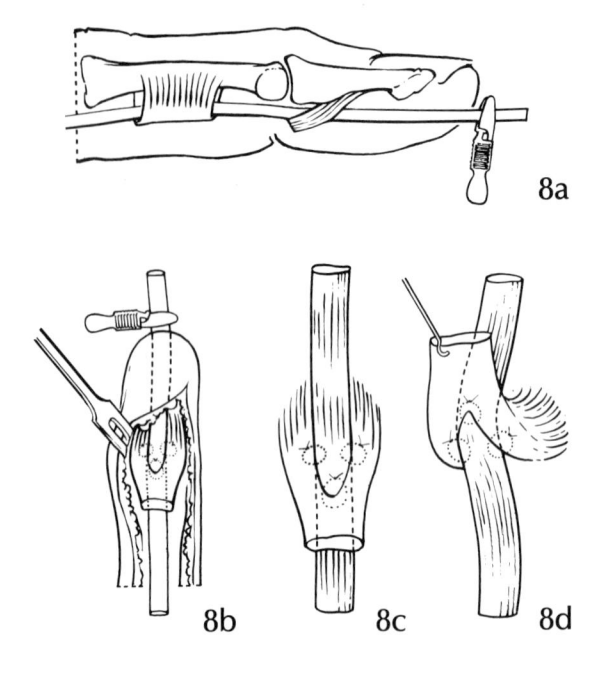

Bunnell withdrawal stitch

9

The Bunnell withdrawal stitch[7] is a neat method of attaching the distal end of the tendon or tendon graft, where there is inadequate profundus stump. The wire is passed through the phalanx to emerge on the nail where it is tied over a dental wool roll. The tendon end is snugged into a drill hole made in the volar cortex of the base of the distal phalanx. The accurate passage of each wire can be facilitated by the use of hollow needles, through which the wire is passed (*see Illustrations 13* and *14* and accompanying text). A simple wire loop is left around the proximal end of the suture and taken through the volar skin. This is then used to pull out the suture after division of the suture at the dental roll.

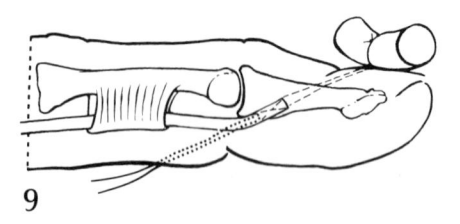

REPAIR OF MALLET FRACTURE

(Repair of tendon rupture is as that for boutonnière deformity – see *Illustrations 16–19*).

Incision

10

The incision is angled. The transverse arm is placed midway between the distal interphalangeal joint and the nail fold. The longitudinal arm follows the midlateral line to midway between the interphalangeal joints.

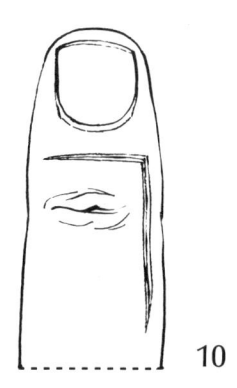

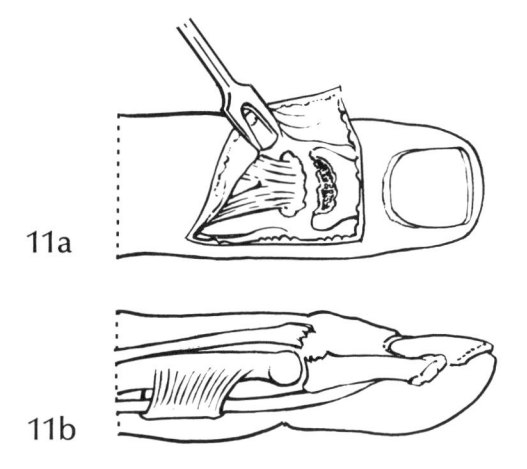

Exposure of extensor tendon

11a & b

The flap is raised exposing the extensor tendon. The two lateral bands are seen joining to form the single tendon which is inserted into the dorsal surface of the base of the distal phalanx. The fracture with haematoma around it is seen here.

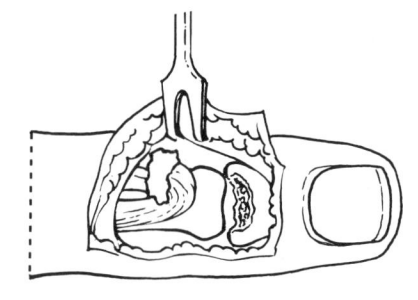

Display of fracture surfaces

12a & b

The avulsed fragment of distal phalanx is reflected proximally with the insertion of the extensor tendon. The bone surfaces are cleared of haematoma but no bone is excised. At this stage the joint is open and the articulation clearly visible.

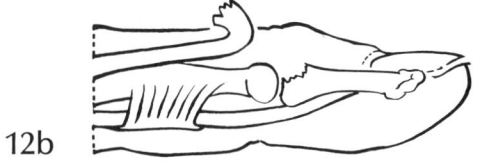

Passage of needles

13a, b &c

A large needle (18 gauge) is passed through the fracture surface in the main fragment and on through the fingertip to appear on the volar surface of the skin. This is used to railroad (c) a small hypodermic needle (25 gauge) back so that the point appears at the fracture site. This is repeated with a second pair of needles.

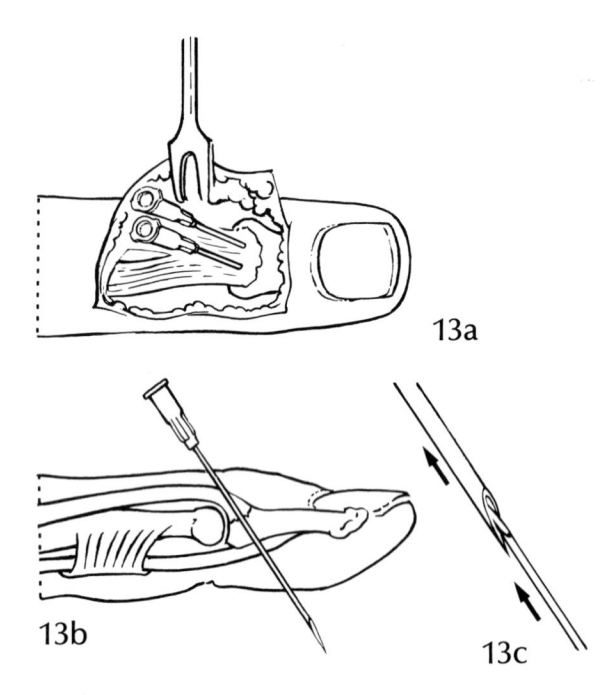

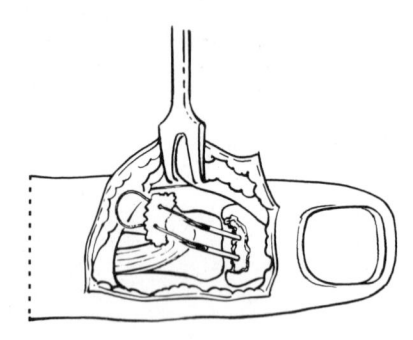

13a

13b

13c

14a

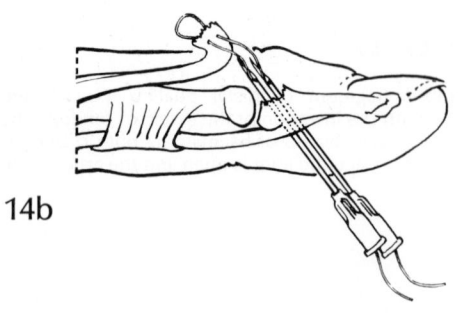

Insertion of suture

14a & b

A stainless steel wire suture is passed through the small bone fragment or around it if the fragment is too small or comminuted. The suture should pass through the extensor tendon at its insertion. Each end of the wire is then passed down one of the needles. Stainless steel 4/0 wire is adequate for simple avulsion but where there is subluxation of the joint 2/0 wire should be used.

14b

Tendon injuries in the hand 817

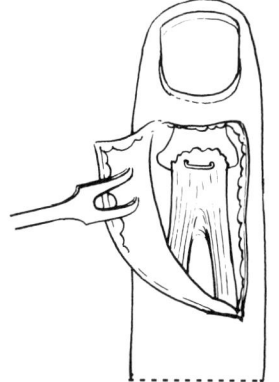

Reduction of fracture and tying of suture

15a–e

The suture is pulled tight to approximate the fragments and can be tied over a dental roll on the volar surface of the finger. A pull-out suture is unnecessary as simple removal is possible as for a skin suture (b). Alternatively the dissection can be carried around the side of the distal phalanx to the flexor aspect and the suture tied over the bone (c). This is more difficult but ensures a tighter, more secure repair. Where there has been subluxation a fine Kirschner wire may be passed across the joint for added security after the suture has been tied (d and e).

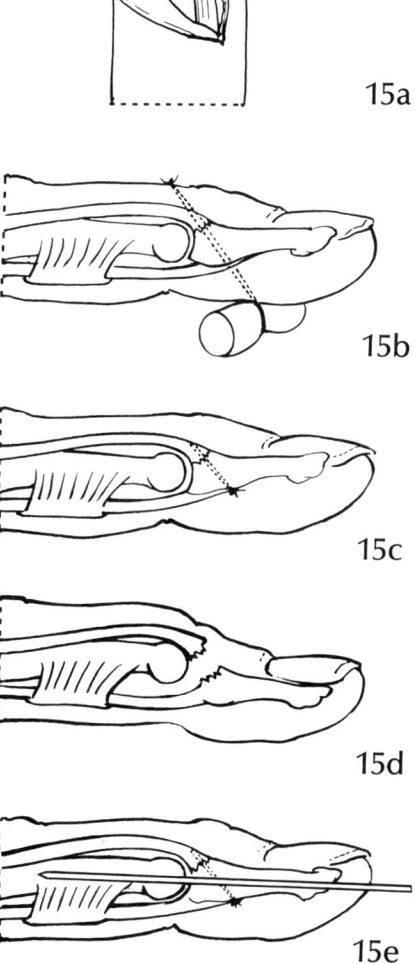

SECONDARY REPAIR OF BOUTONNIÈRE DEFORMITY

Incision

16

A curved incision is used which passes anteriorly almost as far as the midlateral line of the joint. The transverse crease lines over the dorsal surface of the joint are avoided.

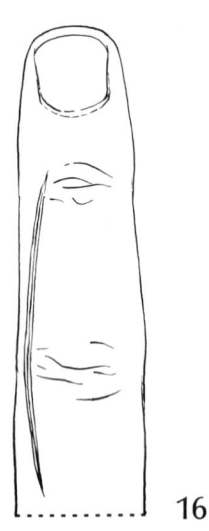

Exposure of extensor tendon

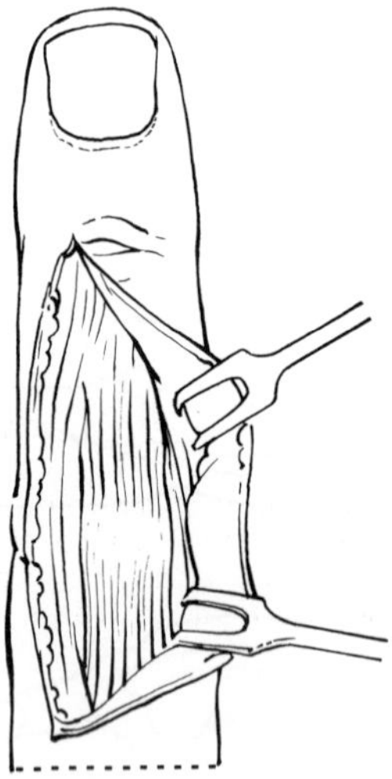

17

The skin and subcutaneous tissue are turned back revealing the extensor tendon. Here is seen the severed central band which is white and the scar tissue in the gap which is opalescent. The two lateral bands pass by the side of the joint to become one tendon over the middle phalanx. In a longstanding case they will have slipped forwards and release of the transverse retinacular ligaments on their flexor aspect will be necessary. It may also be necessary to release the oblique retinacular ligament (Landsmeer) to permit recovery of flexion at the terminal joint.

Removal of scar tissue

18

The scar tissue is removed and the joint opened. At this stage it is advisable to separate the central band completely from the lateral components. The central band is usually found to be adherent to the neck of the proximal phalanx. These adhesions must be freed so that the tendon moves easily when drawn in the distal direction.

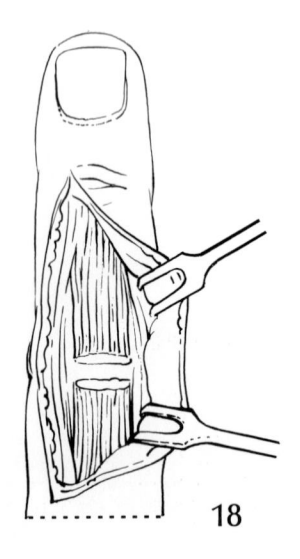

Suture of central band to distal remnant

19

The central band is sutured to the distal remnant with a Kessler stitch combined with a few small approximating stitches or, if the distal stump is very short, several small horizontal mattress sutures may be used. The lateral bands are held in contact with the sides of the central band with a few fine stitches (not illustrated). The final tension should allow the finger to lie in the correct position relative to the other fingers.

A similar technique may be used in the secondary repair of mallet deformity, using the incision shown in *Illustration 10*. Where there is an evulsion fracture causing the boutonnière deformity, the technique described for mallet fracture should be used (*see illustration 10–15*).

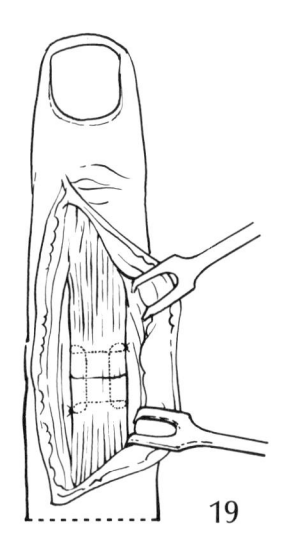

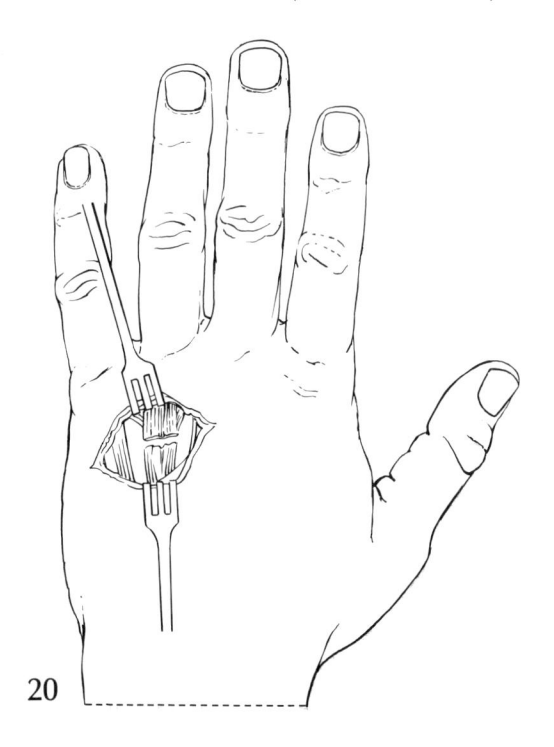

REPAIR OF TENDONS ON THE BACK OF THE HAND

Incision

20

Often the existing laceration allows adequate visualization of the tendon ends as shown but if necessary one end of the wound may be extended proximally to permit retrieval of the retracted proximal tendon stump. Dorsal digital veins should be preserved where possible. Division of cutaneous nerve branches may lead to painful neuroma formation.

21

Suture of the tendon

Where it is ragged the tendon is tidied up by excising the tags. A clean severance (as with glass) requires no further excision of tendon tissue. The Kessler stitch is used and the tendon ends drawn together. This stitch is ideally suited to this situation as it grips the tendon fibres, which tend to be easily frayed at the ends, and it does not bunch up the flat tendon.

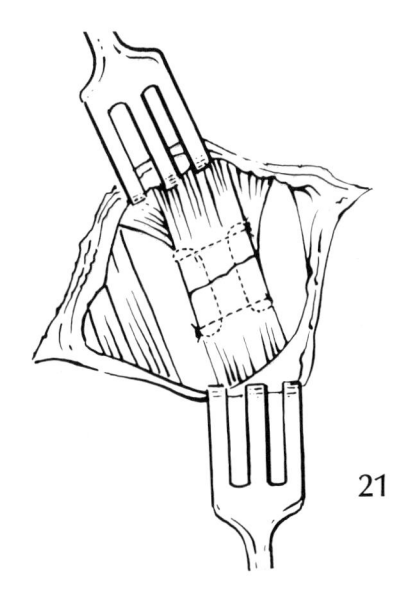

Flexor tendon divisions showing suitable method of repair

22

Zone 1: beyond superficialis

Primary suture should be performed if wound conditions are satisfactory; otherwise the skin is sutured and secondary suture or a tendon graft is performed later.

Zone 2: 'no man's land'

Primary suture or secondary graft depending upon the circumstances.

Zone 3: the palm

Primary suture should be performed if wound conditions are satisfactory; otherwise the skin is sutured and secondary suture or bridge graft performed later.

Zones 4 and 5: carpal tunnel and wrist

Primary suture is highly desirable. Delay necessitates bridge grafting (see *Illustration 31*).

In Zones 2 and 4, superficialis to the ring and little fingers should not be repaired, in order to avoid cross-union to the profundus repair, except where, in Zone 2, the laceration is distal to the intact vinculum longum. In these circumstances, the pull of the unrepaired superficialis puts tension on the vincular artery and compromises the blood supply to the profundus tendon. Both tendons should therefore be repaired in spite of the increased risk of cross-union.

PRIMARY REPAIR IN THE FINGER

This is often the procedure of choice and is fully described in the chapter on 'Primary repair of the divided digital flexor tendon' (pp. 828–835).

TENDON GRAFT OPERATION

Graft source

Palmaris longus, plantaris and extensor digitorum longus are suitable. Flexor digitorum superficialis is ideal for a short bridge graft but is less suitable to use as a full-length graft. Palmaris muscle occasionally extends down the tendon too far to leave sufficient length of pure tendon. It is exposed through a short transverse incision above the wrist and a similar incision in the mid-forearm and drawn out. Plantaris is sufficiently long to serve as two grafts and is of appropriate size; occasionally it is very thin and should not be used. Its presence cannot be determined until the first incision is made on the medial border of the tendo Achillis. A second incision is made in the midcalf, three fingers'-breadth behind the medial border of the tibia. The gastrocnemius muscle is retracted and the plantaris is seen on its deep surface; it is divided in the distal wound and drawn out of the proximal wound. Although a tendon stripper is commonly used, it has been found more satisfactory to remove these tendons in the manner described. A toe extensor tendon is best removed through a full exposure and is of ample length if divided above the extensor retinaculum. A leash of four tendons may be taken if required, but it must be remembered that the fifth toe does not possess a short extensor muscle and will drop into flexion if its sole extensor tendon is removed.

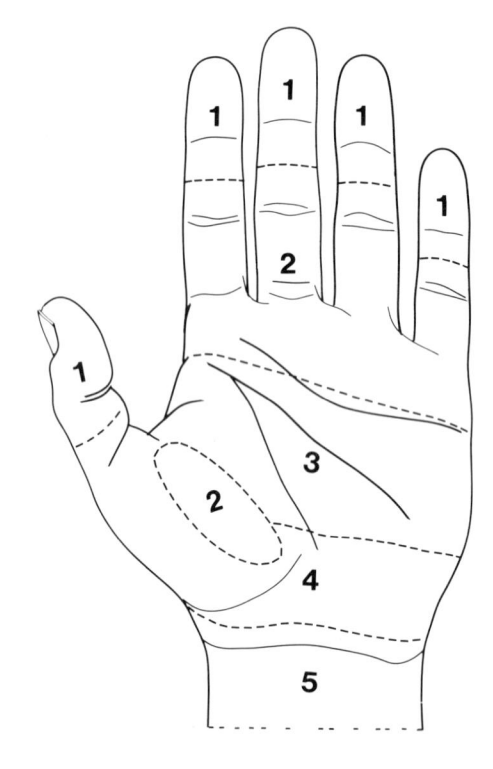

Incisions

23

In the case of the index finger, the incision (A) is made in the exact midaxial line from the nail root to the thenar crease, which it then follows to the proximal part of the palm. A similar incision is used for the little finger, but the palmar incision follows the distal crease for about 3 cm and then is continued into the proximal palm parallel to the thenar crease. For the middle and ring fingers, separate palmar incisions (B) are made in the appropriate crease lines; these may be joined to the finger incision if it is found necessary to expose the base of the finger.

The thumb requires three separate incisions: midaxial in the thumb, the thenar crease and above the wrist just medial to the tendon of flexor carpi radialis.

The Bruner zig-zag incision[14] is commonly used for the finger and gives an excellent exposure but the midaxial approach is more suitable for the operative technique to be described. The latter approach is also preferable when performing a tenolysis which may be indicated later. It cannot be used for a tenolysis once a Bruner approach has been used for the first operation without incurring the risk of delayed skin healing.

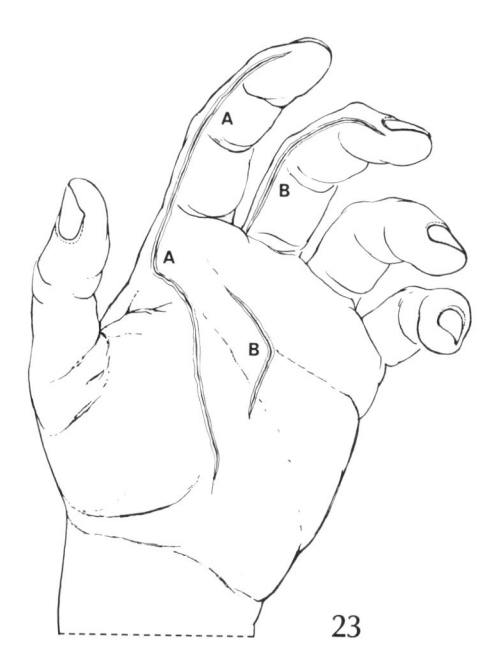

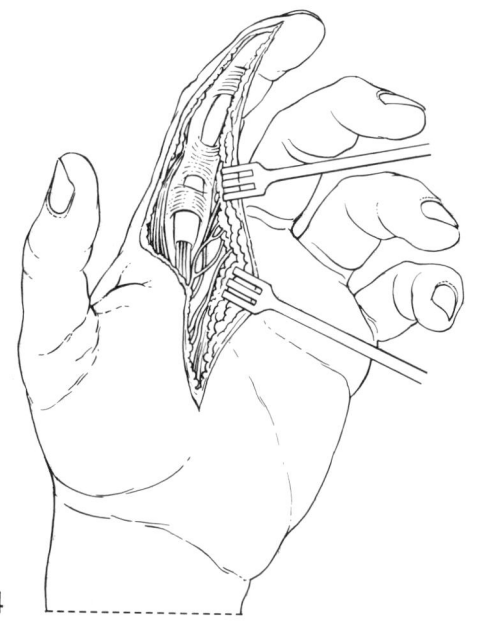

Exposure of the digital theca

24

The incision is deepened, passing posterior to the digital vessels and the digital nerve which are carried forwards in the flap. Care must be taken not to injure these structures which are shown crossing the operative field. The dorsal branch of the digital nerve arises just beyond the base of the proximal phalanx (not illustrated). It is not always possible to preserve this small nerve, but it should be looked for and retained if it does not unduly embarrass the exposure. This sensory branch assumes particular significance when the digital nerve has been injured more distally. The digital theca containing the tendons is fully exposed. The lumbrical muscle is seen on the radial side of the finger.

Selective excision of the digital theca and insertion of the graft

25

The theca is cut away leaving three bands to serve as pulleys. These are situated in front of the metacarpophalangeal joint and the midparts of the proximal and middle phalanges. The two proximal pulleys are essential to prevent bowstringing and should be reconstructed if adequate pulleys cannot be fashioned from a damaged and fibrosed theca. The profundus tendon and the proximal part of the superficialis tendon are completely removed. The distal part of the superficialis tendon is not removed if it is firmly adherent and its excision would leave raw tissue along the course of the graft.

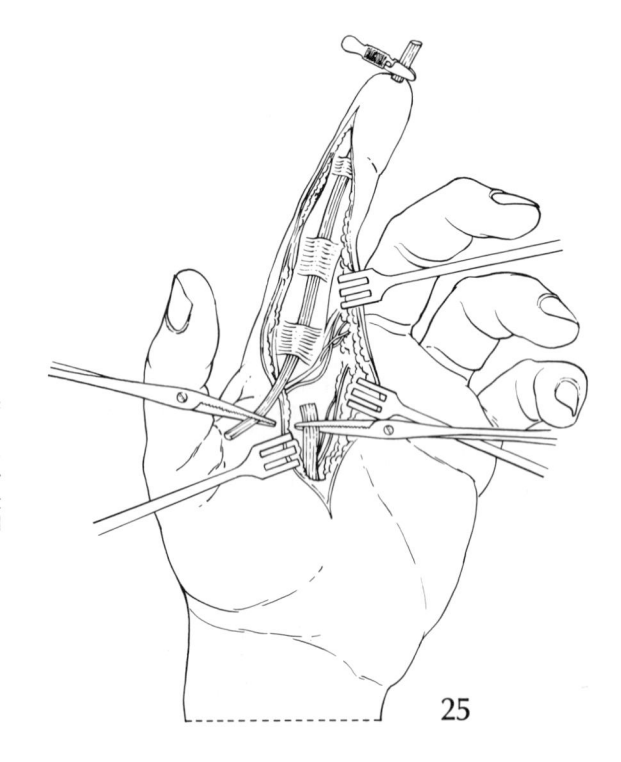

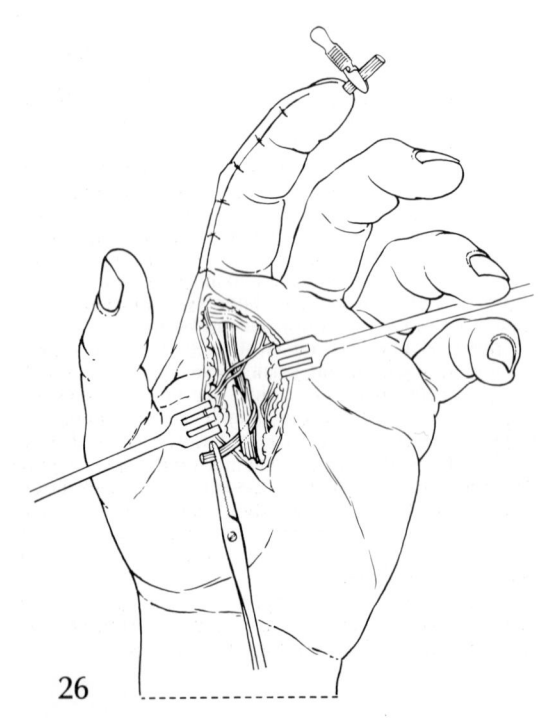

26

The graft is inserted and its proximal end attached to the profundus or the superficialis tendon, whichever is found to possess the better amplitude of movement. The fishmouth technique (see *Illustration 7*) is used. When the graft is attached to profundus, the junction is covered by the lumbricalis muscle provided that this muscle is not fibrosed resulting in a 'lumbrical plus' syndrome. The superficialis of the little finger is a weak muscle and is not suitable to use as a motor tendon. It is helpful to hold the proximal part of the motor tendon by a transfixation needle during this stage of the operation. Note the illustration shows the proximal junction being performed after the distal junction and closure of the finger. This is the author's preference.

Distal attachment of the graft

The graft is attached to the stub of the profundus tendon by the technique described (see *Illustration 8*) or by the Bunnell method (see *Illustration 9*).

Tension of the graft

27

The tension must be carefully adjusted until the finger lies in a slightly more flexed position than would appear correct in relation to the other fingers. The finger posture should be observed while moving the wrist through its full passive range. The patient has had tendon grafts for the middle and ring fingers. Tension can be adjusted at either junction. The author prefers to use the proximal junction for this as it is easier to suture the distal junction with the finger straight before tension is adjusted.

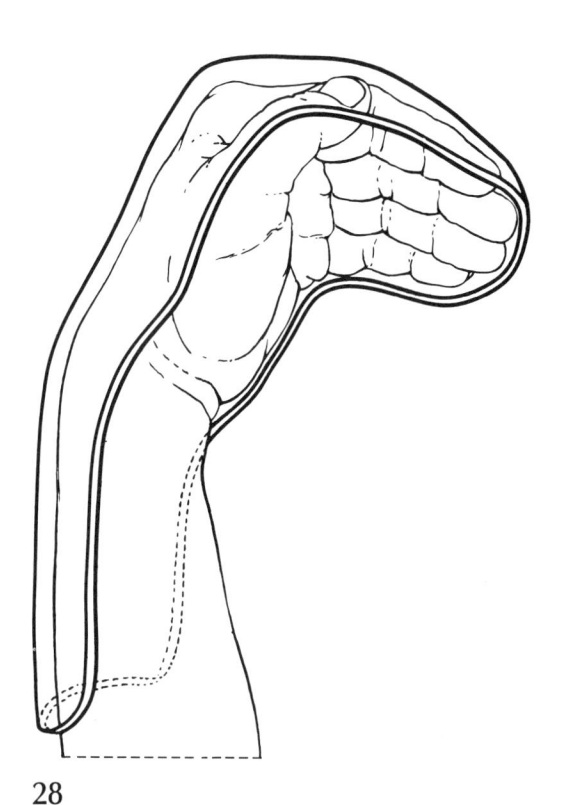

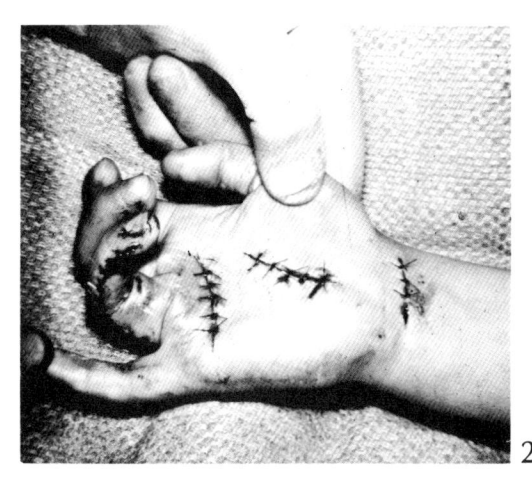

(*Reproduced from* Hand Surgery, *Figure 13, p. 305, by courtesy of J. E. Flynn and Williams and Wilkins Co, 1975*)

Completion of the operation

28

If it is felt necessary to secure haemostasis, the hand is covered with a moist dressing and held well elevated, combined with tilting of the table, and the tourniquet is removed from the arm. This position is maintained for 8–10 minutes by which time it is not unusual to find that bleeding has ceased. Any persistent haemorrhage is controlled by bipolar coagulation or ligation. Perfect haemostasis is essential and the wound is washed clear of blood before being closed.

The wound is dressed with tulle gras. A little fluffed dry gauze is placed between the fingers and the palm is filled with cotton gauze. Other materials can be used such as polyurethane foam, wire wool or real wool. Wool substitutes which are made from paper become moistened by sweat and wound exudate in the palm and rapidly lose their resilience. They should not be used. It should be noted that the palmar concavity is triangular and the dressing should be shaped accordingly. Rolls of bandage or wool should not be used as they tend to hold the metacarpophalangeal joints straight and allow the fingers to flex at the interphalangeal joints. The optimal position of wrist in half flexion, metacarpophalangeal joints fully flexed, and interphalangeal joints slightly flexed is held most easily by a dorsal plaster of Paris hood, which should be extended above the elbow in young children. Other surgeons splint the interphalangeal joints in flexion arguing that it is easier to recover extension with splints than to recover flexion. The author finds that splinting the interphalangeal joints in flexion produces an unacceptable number of uncorrectable flexion contractures. The limb is held elevated for 48 hours.

TENDON GRAFT FOR FLEXOR POLLICIS LONGUS

29a & b

The three incisions are: midaxial in the thumb reaching from the base of the nail to just proximal to the metacarpophalangeal joint; almost the full length of the thenar crease; and above the wrist medial to the flexor carpi radialis tendon. Through the thenar crease incision, the palmar aponeurosis is incised to expose the first lumbrical muscle, the digital nerve to the radial side of the index finger, both digital nerves to the thumb and the flexor pollicis longus tendon lying between these two nerves. The distal tendon junction is performed as in the fingers. The proximal junction is a fishmouth at the wrist proximal to the carpal tunnel.

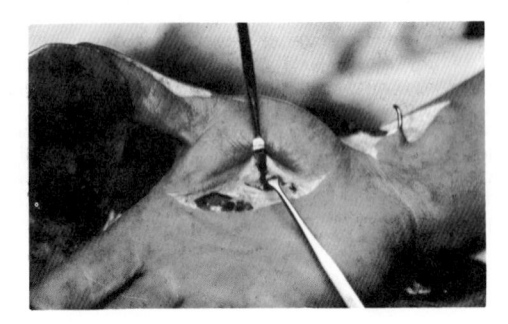

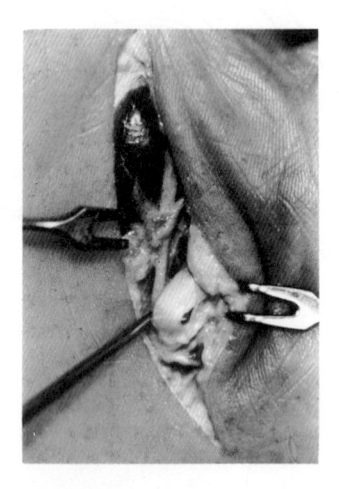

(Reproduced from the American Journal of Surgery 1965; 109: 350, Figure 18 by permission of Dunn-Donnelly Publishing Co.)

TENDON DIVISIONS IN THE PALM

Suture

30

The incision is determined by the position of the existing wound or scar, bearing in mind that a wide exposure is needed to repair nerves in addition to the tendons and that the tendon is likely to be divided at a more distal level than the wound would suggest. In a secondary repair one can expect to find considerable scar tissue which demands a painstaking dissection. The superficialis and profundus tendons are both sutured when conditions are suitable, but if there is a risk of cross-union it is wiser to cut back superficialis and suture only the profundus tendon as illustrated (*see* Introduction). Tendons severed in the distal part of the palm are considered to be in Zone 2 (*see* Illustration 22) and treated accordingly.

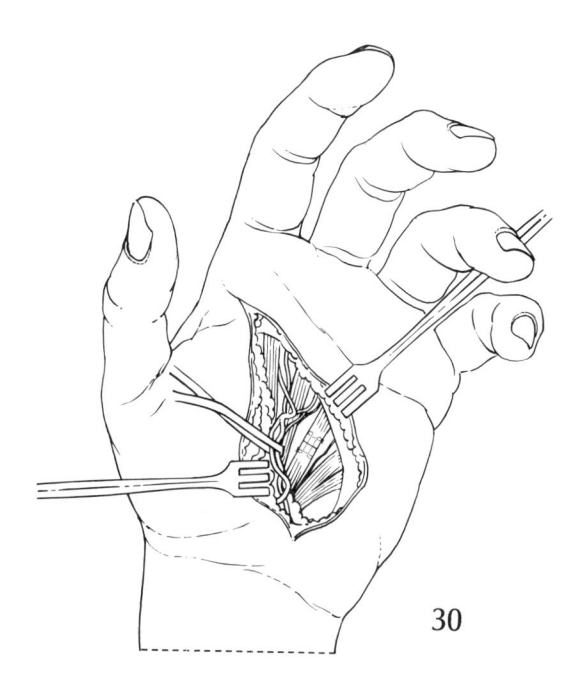

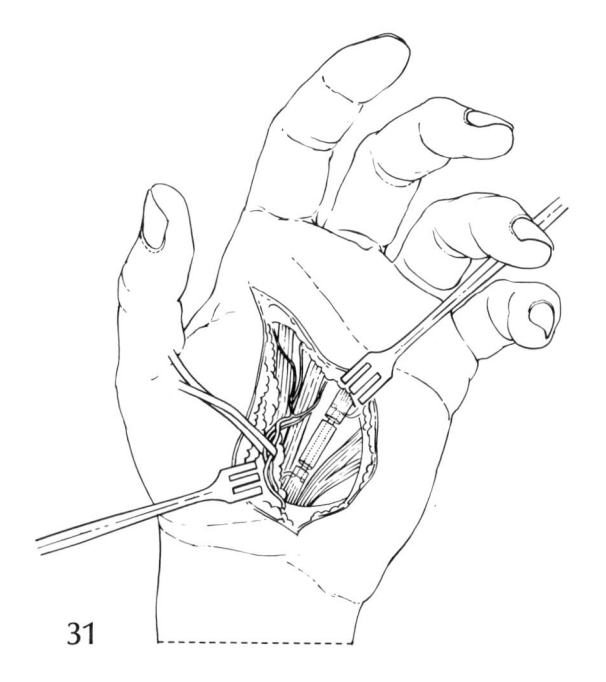

Bridge graft

31

In cases where there has been a delay of some months it may be difficult or impossible to bring the tendon ends into apposition. An effective repair may be performed by using a short superficialis graft to bridge the gap in the profundus tendon. The suture passes through the graft in the manner shown; in this illustration the wire has not yet been drawn tight and knotted.

826 Forearm, wrist and hand

TENDON DIVISIONS AT THE WRIST

32

The first step in dealing with a major injury of this kind is to enlarge the wound in distal and proximal directions and indentify the structures. Respect should be paid to the angles of the flaps which should if possible be greater than 90°.

There are 12 tendons, two main nerves and two main arteries on the flexor aspect of the wrist and two tendons – abductor pollicis longus and extensor pollicis brevis – on the radial aspect. All may be divided and it is not surprising that confusion arises when searching for the corresponding ends. Once the anatomy is clearly seen, the surgeon can proceed confidently with the repair work which may take several hours to complete. Although many hands have survived the loss of both main arteries, this cannot be taken for granted, particularly in older persons, and in any case problems associated with vascular insufficiency may arise later. Both arteries should be anastomosed. All tendons, with the possible exception of palmaris longus, should be sutured when they are divided proximal to the carpal tunnel. It is probably wiser to ignore the superficialis tendons when they are divided within the tunnel.

Opinion differs about the wisdom of primary or secondary suture of nerves divided under these circumstances; if a formal suture is not performed the nerves should be held together to prevent shortening and to preserve the orientation.

In a later reconstructive operation it is not possible to bring the tendon ends together without excessive positioning of the joints. Continuity can be restored to the essential tendons by the interposition of bridge grafts taken from superficialis when the conditions are favourable. The alternative procedure is tendon transference.

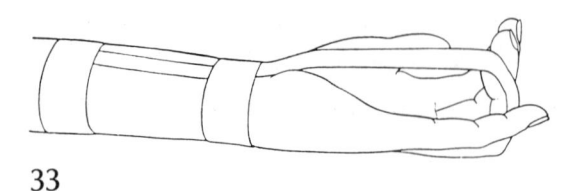

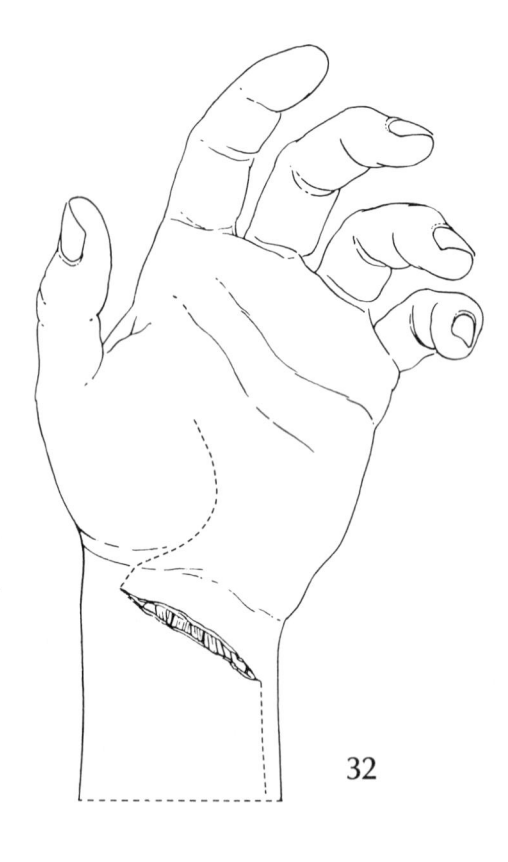

Postoperative management

33

At this stage – some 3–5 weeks after tendon suture – when it is customary to permit movements, there is a special risk of the tendon junction giving way for two reasons: the union is immature and adhesions limit the free gliding of the tendon which in a normal hand allows the strain to be taken up gradually. It is therefore unwise to allow complete freedom immediately after the primary splintage has been removed. Some form of protective splintage is advisable such as a check-rein strap or elastic, or a spring device.

Movements return slowly and the patient requires constant encouragement. He should be kept under personal supervision until the final state is reached which may not be for 6–9 months after operation. Occasionally, the operation of tenolysis is indicated for cases in which the active range fails to attain the passive range of movement. The temptation to try early tenolysis should be resisted. The operation is best carried out about 12 months after repair.

EXTENSOR TENDONS

Mallet deformity

The finger is splinted with the distal interphalangeal joint extended, leaving the proximal interphalangeal joint free for 5 weeks followed by 3 weeks of spring splintage (long Capener splint).

Boutonnière deformity

The finger is splinted with the proximal interphalangeal joint extended for 4 weeks followed by 3 weeks of spring splintage (short Capener splint). The distal joint may be left free.

Back of the hand

The forearm, wrist and fingers are splinted with the wrist in extension and the metacarpophalangeal and interphalangeal joints in slight flexion for 3 weeks. The fully extended position of the fingers is unnecessary and can lead to joint stiffness. During the following 2 weeks, flexion of the fingers is limited by a pad of steel wire or a volar slab bandaged into the palm against which the fingers can squeeze.

FLEXOR TENDONS

Fingers, palm and wrist

The wrist and hand are held in a plaster hood in the position described (*see Illustration 28* and accompanying text) for 3 weeks. After the removal of splintage, digit extension is limited for the further week (2 weeks in children, for whom a plaster cast is used in the first stage) by the use of an elastic check-rein strap. This strap allows flexion exercises to be practised but prevents excessive extension. Passive extension by the patient or physiotherapist should be discouraged until 6 weeks after the operation.

Physiotherapy

There can be no denying that a good physiotherapist markedly increases the quality of the results. It is important for the therapist to know how much to strain a tendon repair with passive exercises during the early stages of rehabilitation. Later, tenodesis can be cleared especially on the extensor aspect of the hand by skilled deep friction massage and ultrasonics. Many patients are afraid to attempt active exercises for fear of 'doing damage' and it is in these cases that supervised active exercises are useful, particularly in young children.

However, the patient's own intelligent cooperation is the most important factor in the aftercare and if this is lacking a good result is rarely achieved. It is for this reason that flexor tendon surgery in children under 5 years frequently gives disappointing results. As tendon union becomes stronger more active work in the occupational therapy department is given and in most hospitals this department is responsible for producing the vast range of heat-malleable plastic splints that can be so useful in rehabilitating the injured hand.

References

1. Vilain R. Repair of the extensor of the finger at its distal end. In: Stack HG, Bolton H, eds. *Proceedings of the Second Hand Club, 1956–1967*. London: The British Society for Surgery of the Hand, 1975: 155–6.

2. Iselin F, Levame J, Godoy J. A simplified technique for treating mallet fingers; tenodermodesis. *J Hand Surg* 1977; 2: 118–21.

3. Matev I. Transposition of the lateral slips of the aponeurosis in treatment of longstanding 'boutonnière deformity' of the fingers. *Br J Plast Surg* 1964; 17: 281–6.

4. Littler JW, Eaton RG. Redistribution of forces in the correction of the boutonnière deformity. *J Bone Joint Surg [Am]* 1967; 49-A: 1267–74.

5. Pulvertaft RG. The treatment of profundus division by free tendon graft. *J Bone Joint Surg [Am]* 1960; 42-A: 1363–71, 1380.

6. Pulvertaft RG. Flexor tendon grafting after long delay. In: Tubiana R, ed. *The hand*. Vol 3. Philadelphia: W. B. Saunders, 1988: 244–54.

7. Bunnell S. Tendons. In: *Bunnell's surgery of the hand*. 5th ed. Rev. by J. H. Boyes. Philadelphia: Lippincott, 1970: 393–409.

8. Rank BK, Wakefield AR, Hueston JT. *Surgery of repair as applied to hand injuries*. 4th ed. Edinburgh: Churchill Livingstone, 1973: 84.

9. Shaw PC. A method of flexor tendon suture. *J Bone Joint Surg [Br]* 1968; 50-B: 578–87.

10. Tsuge K, Ikuta Y, Matsuishi Y. Intra-tendinous tendon suture in the hand: a new technique. *Hand* 1975; 7: 250–5.

11. Becker H, Orak F, Duponselle E. Early active motion following a beveled technique of flexor tendon repair: report on fifty cases. *J Hand Surg* 1979; 4: 454–60.

12. Kessler I. The grasping technique for tendon repair. *Hand* 1973; 5: 253–5.

13. Pulvertaft RG. Tendon grafts for flexor tendon injuries in the fingers and thumb. *J Bone Joint Surg [Br]* 1956; 38-B: 175–94.

14. Bruner JM. The zig-zag volar digital incision for flexor tendon surgery. In: Stack HG, Bolton H. eds. *Proceedings of the Second Hand Club, 1956–1967*. London: The British Society for Surgery of the Hand, 1975: 423–4.

Illustrations by Adrian Shaw

Primary repair of the divided digital flexor tendon

Harold J. Richards FRCS
Formerly Consultant in the Surgery of Orthopaedics and Trauma, University Hospital of Wales and Prince of Wales Orthopaedic Hospital, Cardiff, UK

Blood supply of flexor tendon

The maintenance of a good blood supply to the divided and repaired digital flexor tendon is the single most important factor in obtaining good healing and return of function in the repaired tendon.

Blood is supplied to the digital flexor tendon via fragile vincula, which run to the dorsal surface of the tendon from the adjacent underlying phalanges.

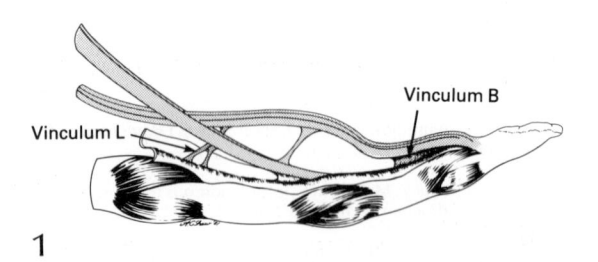

1

The vincula are of two types: the short (VB) and the long (VL). The short runs to the flexor tendon near its insertion and is only occasionally ruptured or damaged as when a spontaneous rupture of the long flexor occurs.

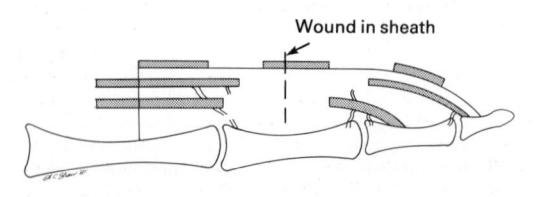

2

The vinculum longus, however, ruptures easily if it is attached to the proximal divided end of the tendon, which then retracts towards the palm.

3

The vinculum carries not only the blood supply (B) to the tendon but also the nerve supply (N) as shown in a section of the vinculum 6 hours after division of the flexor tendon.

When the blood supply is adequate the digital flexor tendons have the ability to heal by means of their own cells[1-6].

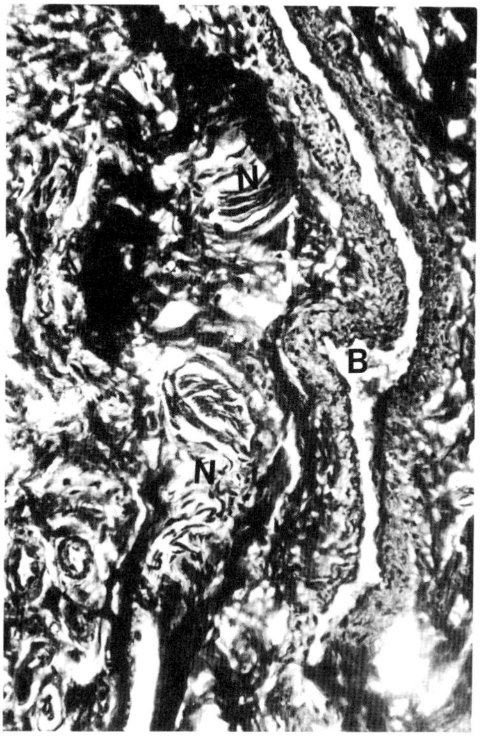

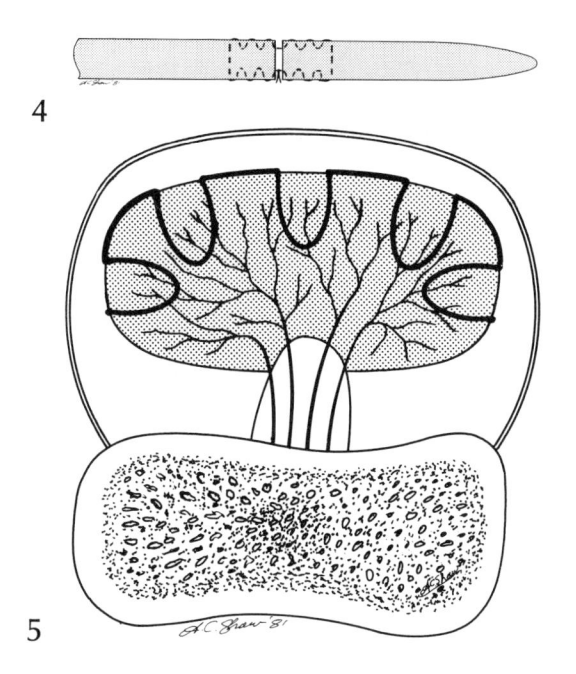

4 & 5

Within the flexor tendon the blood vessels run longitudinally at various depths, but they intercommunicate[7,8]. The richest blood supply is near the point of entry of the vinculum and in the central area of the tendon whilst the peripheral areas, particularly the volar aspect, have the poorest blood supply. It is essential that the suture used for repairing the tendon should interfere with the blood supply as little as possible.

The suture should, therefore, take hold of the tendon along its periphery and when running across the tendon should go through the volar half of the tendon only. The worst type of suture is a constricting one going through the full thickness of the tendon, such as a figure of eight.

Impairment of blood supply which occurs when the proximal end of the divided tendon retracts, rupturing the vinculum and its blood vessels and nerves, leads after suture of the tendon to considerable adhesion formation during healing, particularly if a constricting suture is also used. The adhesions result from connective tissue penetrating the healing tendon carrying an essential new blood supply, but the penalty for this assistance is the formation of massive adhesions which result in loss of function of the tendon after healing has taken place.

830   Forearm, wrist and hand

Preoperative

Indications for operation

Primary repair of the divided digital flexor tendon should be undertaken when the following conditions are met.

1. There is no extensive loss of soft tissue.
2. There is no gross contamination of the wound.
3. There are no fractures which cannot be immobilized.
4. The divided tendon ends can be approximated.
5. Adequate skill and facilities are available. These are difficult operative procedures and experience in tendon surgery is necessary. A bad result from primary repair makes any further salvage operation more difficult and impairs the final level of function of the hand.

Initial treatment

The wound should be cleaned, dressed or closed.

6

The wrist should be put in a position of full flexion and maintained in this position by splintage, usually a plaster of Paris cast or slab, supported by a non-elastic bandage. This will prevent or limit the retraction of the cut proximal end of the divided flexor tendon and protect its blood supply.

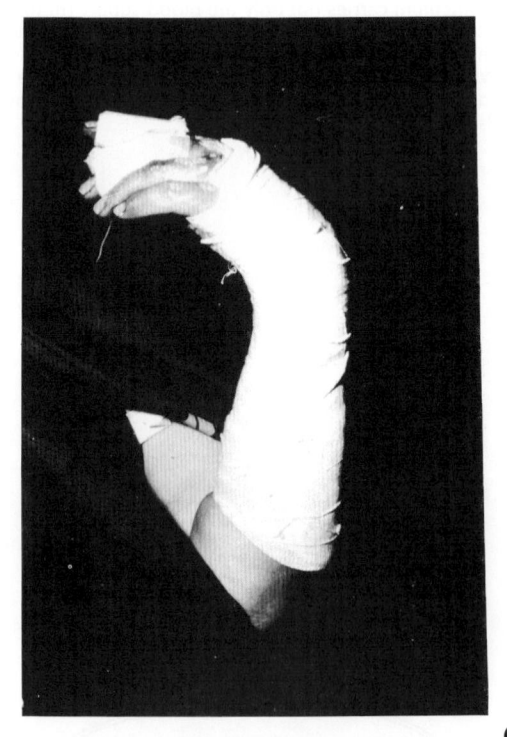

Technique of repair

Under general anaesthesia, without the application of a tourniquet and with the wrist held in full flexion, the original wound is explored. Flexing the finger usually brings the distal cut end of the tendon into the wound. Full flexion of the wrist usually does not bring the proximal cut end into the wound, but in most cases this can be achieved by massaging the digit from the palm distally. If the latter manoeuvre fails a delicate artery forceps can be passed proximally along the fibrosynovial sheath and the tendon grasped and pulled distally.

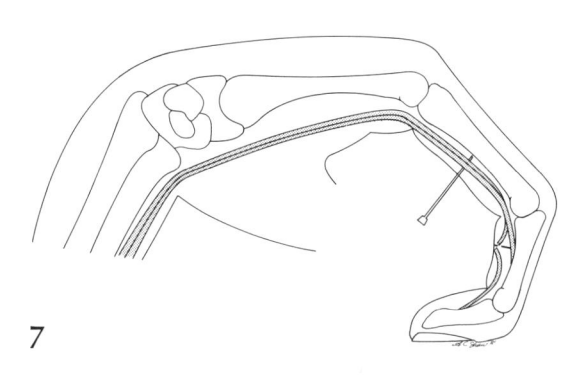

7

Once in the wound it can be maintained in this position by passing a hypodermic needle through the skin, fibrosynovial sheath and tendon. A non-reactive suture (3/0) can then be inserted as shown in *Illustrations 4* and *5*. The suture should run at least 1 cm along the length of the tendon before running transversely. At this point and beyond there is less softening of the tendon during healing than at the area around the site of the tendon division. The suture should be securely tied and cutting out is prevented by positioning of the wrist, hand and fingers in flexion after repair. If the tendon ends are poorly coapted, a running suture through the epitenon and outer margin of the tendon may be used (6/0 or 7/0 nylon is suitable).

8

Where there is difficulty in approximating the cut ends, or bringing them into the original wound, the latter will have to be extended as shown. The wound in the fibrosynovial sheath will have to be enlarged in a similar fashion. Where both tendons have been divided, both should be sutured, as the long vinculum runs to both tendons and the repair of one only would allow the other to retract proximally with rupture of the vinculum, blood and nerve supply. It may not be possible fully to close the fibrosynovial sheath when both tendons have been sutured.

After repair of the tendon or tendons, the fibrosynovial sheath is repaired using a non-reactive suture (5/0). Divided digital nerves, and at least one artery, are also sutured (see Chapter on 'Microsurgical techniques', *The Hand*, pp. 242–247). Where there is difficulty in getting the cut tendon into the wound and the latter has to be extended, it may be necessary to apply a tourniquet to control bleeding, but once the ends have been isolated the tourniquet should be removed as this makes it much easier to get the proximal cut end into the wound. If a pneumatic cuff type of tourniquet is applied to the upper arm following elevation of the limb and without preliminary use of an Esmarch bandage, the tourniquet can be retained, as this method does not lead to difficulty in getting the proximal cut tendon end into the wound.

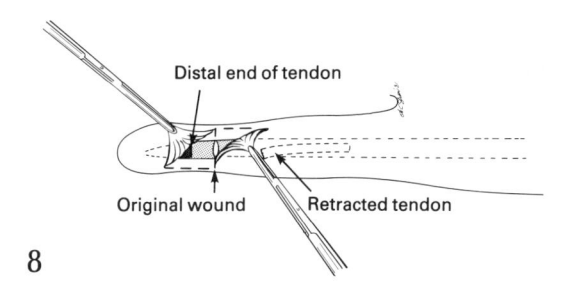

Delay in primary repair

Usually it is possible to approximate the divided cut ends of the flexor tendon at up to 2 weeks in an adult and 4 weeks in a child after the date of the injury. However, the following problems are encountered.

1. The proximal end of the divided tendon will have retracted with rupture of the vinculum and impairment of blood supply.
2. Adhesions form, making it difficult to get the distal end into the wound.

These difficulties can be overcome as far as isolation of the tendon ends is concerned by using a radiological investigation known as a tenogram[9]. A tenogram is obtained by injecting a radiopaque material (25 per cent Hypaque, Stirling Research, Guildford, UK) into the fibrosynovial sheath.

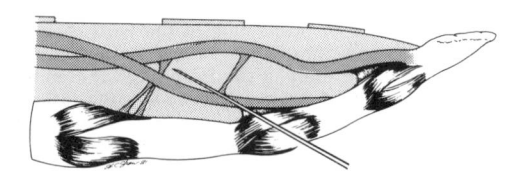

9

10

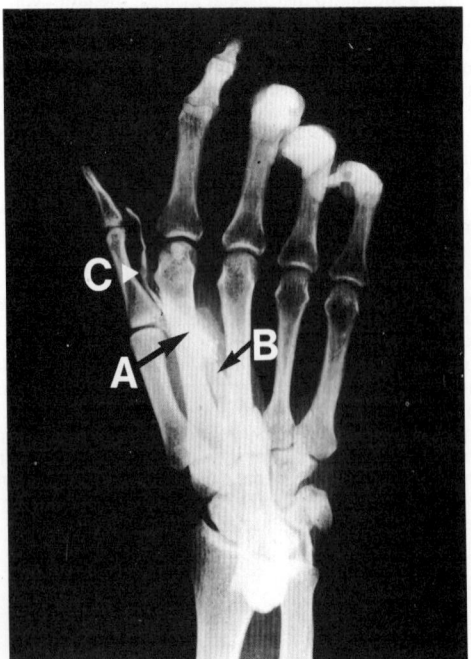

TENOGRAPHY TECHNIQUE

Any non-irritable opaque medium can be used for outlining the digital flexor tendon sheath but 25 per cent Hypaque is suitable. The normal closed digital flexor tendon sheath will accommodate 2 ml of this fluid, but if the sheath is connected to the common sheath (see *Illustration 10*) then more fluid can be injected as it will travel up and fill the compound flexor sheath. Five millilitres of Hypaque are drawn up into the syringe to which a fine hypodermic needle is attached.

9

The needle is then inserted obliquely into the lateral aspect of the finger and directed towards the proximal end of the digit. When the needle strikes the fibrosynovial sheath some resistance is felt but with a little firm pressure the needle passes through the sheath. The opaque medium is injected and if the needle is within the sheath, then the fluid passes easily out of the syringe. The patient can usually feel the fluid passing into the sheath and frequently will indicate accurately in which direction the fluid is flowing. A finger placed on the sheath will also detect the flow of the opaque medium along the fibrosynovial sheath. If no adhesions are present then the sheath will accommodate approximately 2 ml, but if there are adhesions, then only a limited amount of fluid will pass into the sheath, the amount depending on the degree of adhesion formation. The needle is passed into the lateral aspect of the finger so that it will slip between the tendons; if pushed into the sheath from the front of the finger, the needle is likely to penetrate the flexor tendon and prevent the opaque fluid from passing into the sheath[9].

TECHNIQUE OF DELAYED REPAIR

10

The finger is then opened at the site of the original wound (A) and over the proximal (B) and distal (C) ends of the tendon. The latter (B and C) are then threaded along the fibrosynovial sheath into the original wound and sutured. In order to approximate the cut tendon ends, both the wrist and finger may have to be flexed and postoperatively held in this position for 3 weeks. If the blood supply has been impaired then the tendon will heal with adhesions and the finger will be in a fixed flexion position. The patient should be warned of this before operation and also told that a further operation, a tenolysis, will be necessary in a year's time to restore function.

The long flexor tendon is most difficult to repair between its insertion and the insertion of the short flexor, particularly if repair is attempted 48 hours or more after injury. The distal fibrosynovial sheath is flat and small and the cut tendon tends to swell; if the sheath has been widely opened it is almost impossible to resuture it. An alternative technique of inserting a suture using a 3/0 non-reactive suture with a straight needle at either end is employed.

11

The needle is introduced as previously described into the proximal end of the divided long flexor tendon. It is then inserted into the cut distal end of the tendon and passed throughout its length and out through the pulp at the tip of the finger.

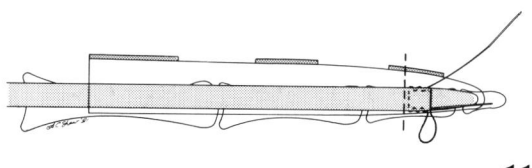

12

The other straight needle is passed in a similar direction.

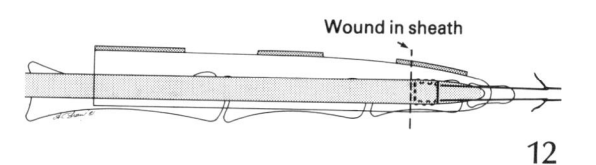

13

An incision is then made into the pulp tissue along one of the natural creases and the insertion of the long flexor tendon is exposed. The two sutures passing out through this insertion are isolated. The straight needles are then cut off and the sutures are drawn back into the pulp area.

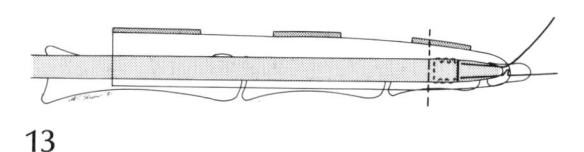

14

The retracted suture ends are then threaded on to a curved needle and passed through the insertion of the long tendon to take a firm hold of it. The sutures are then tied.

Alternatively the sutures are tied at the tip of the finger over a button. This procedure has the disadvantage that the suture will probably have to be removed by a further operation.

Division or spontaneous rupture of the long flexor tendon, where the vinculum is intact, presents no difficulties as the tendon does not retract and can be repaired without difficulty, generally with an excellent functional result, as the blood supply is good. It may, however, be necessary to use a tenogram to isolate the proximal cut end.

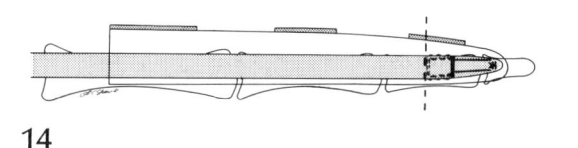

Postoperative management

The wrist is immobilized in full flexion using a plaster of Paris cast and the finger is allowed to take up its physiological position. The plaster cast extends from below the elbow to the tips of the fingers, except in a young child up to the age of 6, where the plaster extends above the elbow joint. The forearm is held in supination, with the elbow flexed to 100°, as this gives the best position for venous drainage from the fingers and minimizes swelling of the digit. The plaster cast is removed after 3 weeks and active exercises started. Each individual joint is mobilized separately, as well as in conjunction with the other joints. Maximum recovery of movement usually occurs within 3 months of the operation.

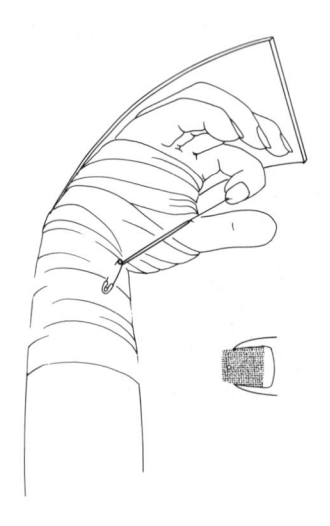

15

Kleinert[10] has advocated guarded extension exercises using rubber bands which hold the finger in flexion for the first few weeks after operation.

An elastic band is secured to the nail by adhesive or to a nylon loop passed through the nail tip. The insert shows the method favoured by the author: a strip of ordinary zinc oxide strapping is folded onto itself, sticky sides together, and shaped as shown; a hole is cut in the distal end for attaching the traction apparatus and the strapping is then stuck onto the nail using one of the superglues.

The band is secured to the splint so that the tension on the digit maintains it in greater flexion than its fellows. It is important that the proximal interphalangeal joint is not flexed to over 70° or fixed flexion deformity may occur, impairing the result. The patient is encouraged to extend actively the digit from the first postoperative day. The flexor muscles are inhibited by active extension, effectively reducing tension across the suture line. Close supervision is necessary if this technique is adopted.

TENOLYSIS

16

Where, after a flexor tendon repair, function is very limited or the finger is in a position of fixed flexion deformity, tenolysis should be undertaken, but not until 1 year after the operation and the tendon has had time to re-establish a normal blood supply. A tenogram may be helpful in outlining the area of adhesion.

A lateral incision is made in the finger over the area of adhesion and the skin, subcutaneous tissue and fibro-synovial sheath are raised in one flap. The adhesions are all divided so that the tendon moves freely and the skin only is sutured. As soon as the patient recovers from the anaesthetic active movements are commenced.

Where the adhesions involve the tendon sheath in its proximal end the incision has to be extended into the palm so that this part of the sheath can be explored and the adhesion divided.

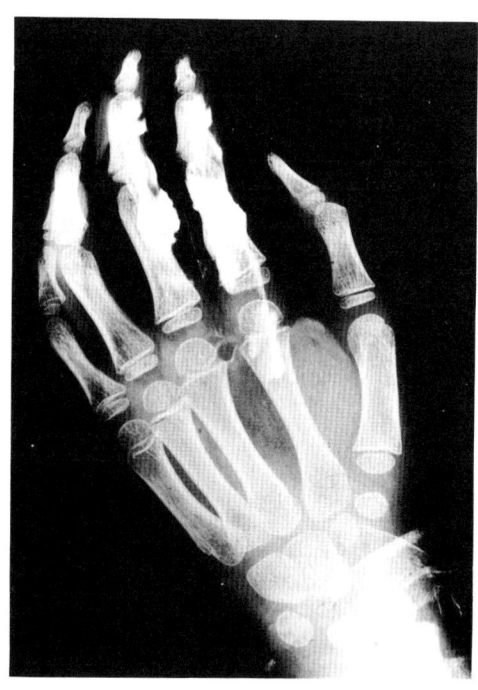

References

1. Matthews P, Richards H. The repair potential of digital flexor tendon: an experimental study. *J Bone Joint Surg [Br]* 1974; 56-B: 618–25.

2. Matthews P, Richards H. Factors in the adherence of flexor tendon after repair: an experimental study in the rabbit. *J Bone Joint Surg [Br]* 1976; 58-B: 230–6.

3. Richards HJ. Primary and delayed repair of flexor tendons in the fingers. *J Bone Joint Surg [Br]* 1964; 46-B: 571.

4. Richards HJ. Digital flexor tendon repair and return of function. *Ann R Coll Surg Engl* 1977; 59: 25–32.

5. Richards HJ. Factors affecting the healing and return of function in the repaired digital flexor tendon. *Aust NZ J Surg* 1980; 50(3): 258–63.

6. Richards HJ. Repair and healing of the divided digital flexor tendon. *Injury* 1980; 12: 1–12.

7. Edwards DAW. The blood supply and lymphatic drainage of tendons. *J Anat* 1946; 80: 147–52.

8. Brockis JG. The blood supply of the flexor and extensor tendons of the fingers in man. *J Bone Joint Surg [Br]* 1953; 35-B: 131–8.

9. Richards HJ. Radiographic localization of severed tendons and of adhesions within a synovial sheath. *J Bone Joint Surg [Br]* 1962; 44-B: 744.

10. Kleinert HE, Meares A. The quest of the solution to severed flexor tendons. *Clin Orthop* 1974; 104: 23–9.

Illustrations by Michael J. Courtney

Two-stage tendon reconstruction using gliding tendon implants

James M. Hunter MD
Clinical Professor of Orthopedic Surgery, Thomas Jefferson University, Philadelphia, Pennsylvania, USA;
Chief, Hand Surgery Service, Department of Orthopedics, Thomas Jefferson University Hospital

Peter C. Amadio MD
Assistant Professor of Clinical Orthopedics, SUNY, Stony Brook, New York, USA;
Active Staff, St John's Episcopal Hospital, Smithtown, New York

Introduction

Following mutilating trauma to the hand, the early priorities of treatment should emphasize the maintenance of good circulation, protective skin coverage, proper alignment of the bones and joints and the restoration of a soft bed for tendon gliding. Damaged tendons may be taught to glide again by supervised exercises. Often, however, in spite of careful primary treatment, the tendon and tendon gliding bed have been so damaged that a healing complex of scar develops and function is lost. It is the purpose of this chapter to outline the techniques of two-stage tendon reconstruction using a gliding tendon implant to assist organization of a new tendon bed prior to tendon grafting.

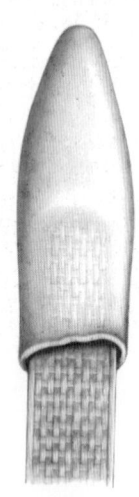

Implants

1

Twenty-five years of experimental and clinical research have resulted in the evolution of both a passive and an active implant gliding programme for two-stage tendon reconstruction. The implants are designed to provide firmness and flexibility to permit secure distal fixation and minimize buckling during the passive push phase of gliding. This is achieved by combining an inner woven Dacron (du Pont, USA) core for strength and an outer sheath of silicone rubber for inertness and low-friction gliding.

Passive gliding programme and implant

2

This programme implies that the distal end of the implant is fixed securely to bone or tendon while the proximal end glides free in the proximal palm or forearm. Movement of the implant is produced by active extension and passive flexion of the digit.

The passive implant is available commercially as a silicone-coated woven Dacron tape in widths of 3, 4, 5 and 6 mm with two different distal fixation possibilities. The blunt tip passive implant can be fixed by suture. A passive implant with a metal plate for distal screw fixation is also available.

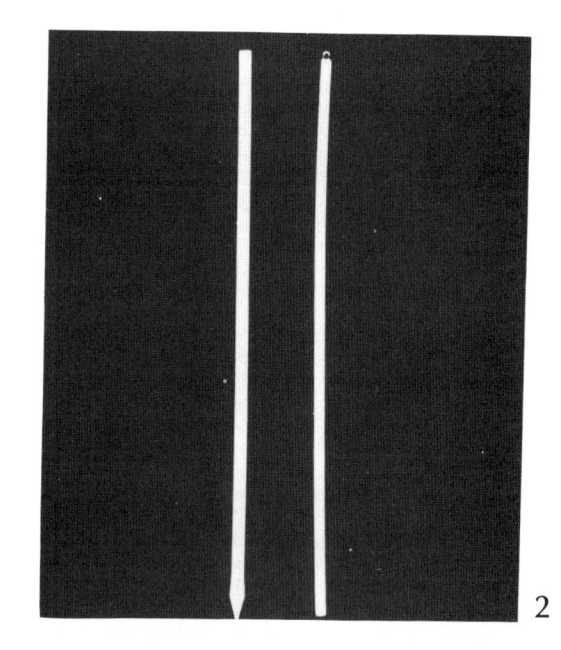

Active gliding programme and implant

3

The active tendon implants are fixed at the distal end to the distal phalanx or middle phalanx of the finger by either a screw twist wire or a Dacron weave through bone. Implants are fixed proximally in the forearm to the motor tendon by either a loop-to-loop technique or by suturing the Dacron weave into the motor tendon in the forearm. These methods permit the Stage I period to be extended indefinitely. The patient could have function for months or years before implant replacement by a tendon graft or another implant.

The active tendon implants that are currently available are constructed with special porous weaves of Dacron that will permit tissue ingrowth as well as permit enhanced flexibility of the constructed tendon. The length of the tendons may be changed by peeling the silicone from the Dacron and gently opening the two woven Dacron cords with a scalpel.

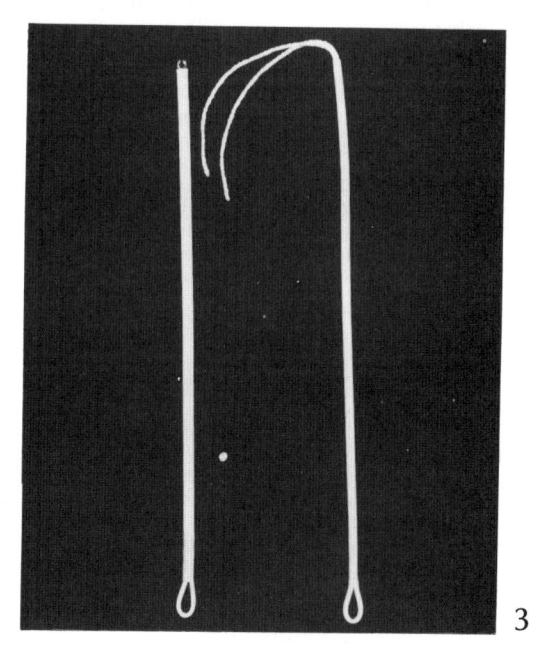

Care of tendon implants

Silicone rubber is highly electrostatic and, as a result, attracts airborne particles and surface contaminants. For this reason, once the implants have been removed from their sterile packets, they should be kept moist at all times. Gloves and instruments which contact the implants should always be wet. Attention to these details will minimize the risk of synovitis postoperatively.

Indications for surgery

More than 25 years of surgical experience have shown the two-stage technique of tendon reconstruction to be useful in cases of both chronic and acute tendon injuries. The basic indication is a scarred soft tissue bed which could compromise gliding after tendon graft or transfer. It has been shown experimentally that a fine, glistening, fluid-secreting sheath is formed about the gliding tendon implant, which, after removal of the implant, provides a more suitable bed for gliding of a tendon graft or transfer than the scarred tissue initially present at the time of Stage I.

By improving the quality of the tendon bed, the surgeon capable of achieving a good result with flexor tendon grafting in a finger with minimal scarring may now see similar results in initially poorer grade cases when using the two-stage method. Candidates for tenolysis and tendon grafting should also be considered candidates for two-stage reconstruction since only at the time of surgery can the surgeon truly assess the extent of tendon-bed injury.

A second indication for two-stage tendon reconstruction would be the necessity for concurrent surgery which might compromise the usual rehabilitation pattern for one-stage tendon reconstruction, repair or transfer. Simultaneous pulley reconstruction makes rehabilitation after tenolysis or one-stage tendon grafting difficult; combining pulley reconstruction with two-stage grafting allows the active movement to be deferred until pulley healing is completed. Similarly, after tendon repair, nerve injuries or concomitant fractures, particularly those of the proximal phalanx which violate the fibro-osseous canal, may require immobilization to the detriment of tendon rehabilitation. In these predictably poor situations, the use of a tendon implant can again maintain a gliding bed until later tendon reconstruction is possible. Earlier use of a tendon implant on the flexor surface may simplify replantation surgery by allowing, for example, concentration on active movement of repaired extensors in a Zone II level amputation.

Contraindications to two-stage reconstruction

Acute infection is the only absolute contraindication, as with all reconstructive surgery involving implants. Some relative contraindications should also be considered. Formation of a good gliding bed for tendon function following finger injury is a dynamic metabolic process which requires a certain minimal level of tissue viability for support. The stiff, scarred finger with destroyed joints, damaged nerves and vessels cannot be expected to support the necessary nutritional requirements for successful healing following extensive reconstruction of any kind and will usually be served best by amputation.

Even more important to consider preoperatively is the level of patient cooperation and motivation available. Considerable therapy will usually be required to convert the potential gains made at Stage I surgery into actual ones after Stage II. If the patient is unable or unwilling to cooperate or to attend frequently enough for the surgeon to detect trouble spots early, complex reconstructions should not be undertaken. Prior to surgery, all patients should have hand therapy designed to mobilize stiff joints and to improve to the maximum the condition of the soft tissues. The timing of surgery should finally combine the judgment of surgeon, hand therapist and patient. Again, patient input and motivation are the keys to a successful result.

Antibiotic therapy

As with other orthopaedic implants, preoperative broad-spectrum intravenous antibiotics are recommended, beginning just prior to surgery and continuing for 48 hours postoperatively. The use of antibiotics containing irrigation solution is also advised.

Anaesthesia

If a passive implant reconstruction is definitely to be performed, either general or axillary block anaesthesia is recommended to control operative and tourniquet pain, as dissection and reconstruction may be extensive. If consideration is being given to tenolysis versus staged grafting or if the active implant programme is elected, local anaesthesia (1 per cent lidocaine infiltration) is recommended, to be supplemented with intravenous fentanyl and droperidol (Innovar) or meperidine and diazepam to control tourniquet pain and patient restlessness. This technique allows the surgeon to assess completeness of the tenolysis and also is helpful both in checking active amplitude of potential donor motor units and in setting proper tension to either the active implant or tendon graft. The anaesthetist should be experienced with the technique as often a very fine balance must be struck to provide sufficient sedation on the one hand, and a patient awake enough to cooperate when active movement is required, on the other. With the local sedation technique, the tourniquet is intermittently deflated at roughly half-hour intervals to prevent tourniquet paralysis and to evaluate function if appropriate. This anaesthetic technique is well tolerated by most patients and can be used for procedures lasting as long as 4 or 5 hours.

PASSIVE PROGRAMME

Stage I

Preoperative assessment of active and passive range of movement

4

The angular movement of each joint in degrees and the distance that the finger pulp fails to touch at the distal palmar crease are recorded and made a part of the permanent record of each patient for progress comparison and follow-up, typically: (*1*) before Stage I; (*2*) 6 weeks after Stage I; (*3*) preferably active movement during Stage II surgery after graft juncture with appropriate tension; and (*4*) monthly after Stage II.

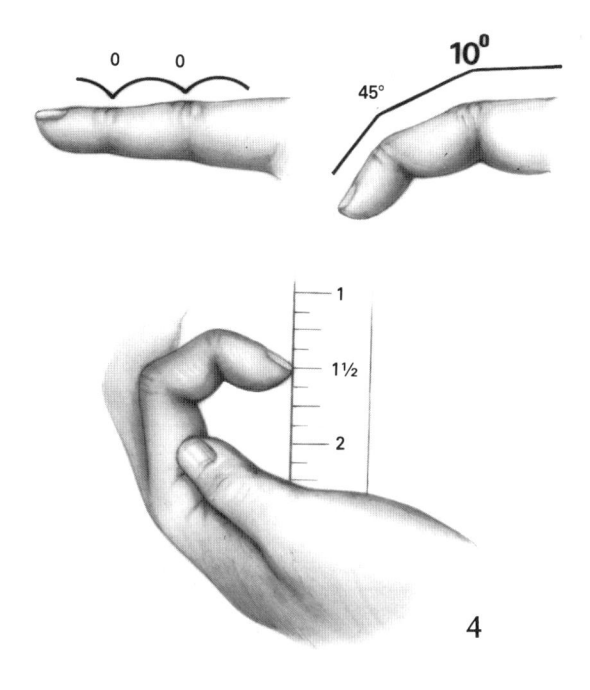

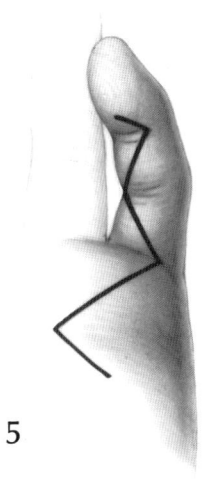

THE OPERATION

Incisions for flexor tendon reconstruction

5

The damaged flexor tendons and scarred sheaths are exposed through the volar zig-zag incisions popularized by Julian Bruner. The skin flap should be full-thickness, with the apices overlying the neurovascular bundles. Longer flaps may develop marginal necrosis. The neurovascular bundles must be carefully protected.

6

A separate curved incision is made in the distal forearm to expose the finger flexors and the plane between the profundus and superficialis where the implant will lie.

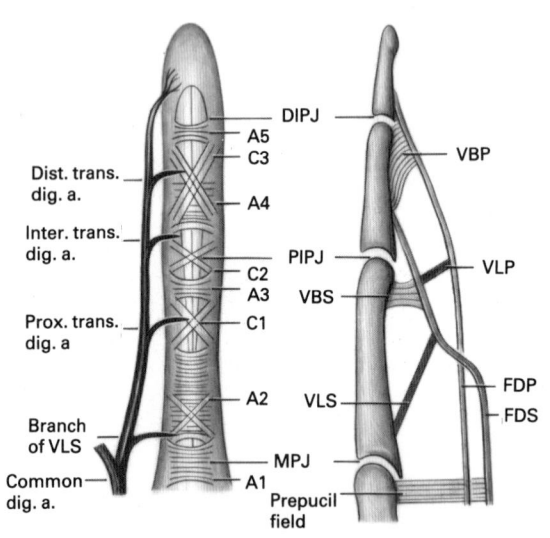

7

DIPJ, distal interphalangeal joint
PIPJ, proximal interphalangeal joint
MPJ, metacarpophalangeal joint
VPB, vincula brevia profunda
VLP, vincula longa profunda
FDP, flexor digitorum profundus
FDS, flexor digitorum superficialis
VBS, vincula brevia superficialis
VLS, vincula longa superficialis
A1-5, annular pulleys 1–5
C1–3, cruciform pulleys 1–3
VF, variable fibre

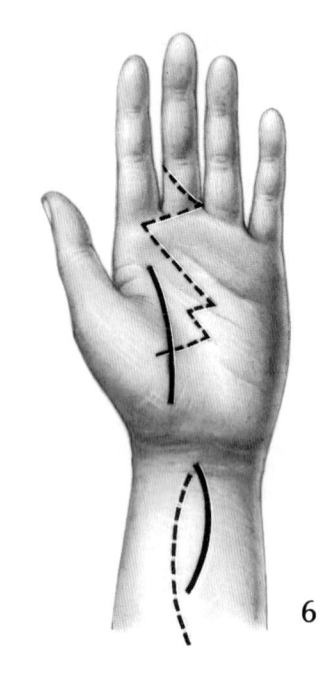

At the level of the cruciate pulleys, the digital arteries give four transverse tributaries which supply the synovial bed and vincular system. If possible, these should be preserved.

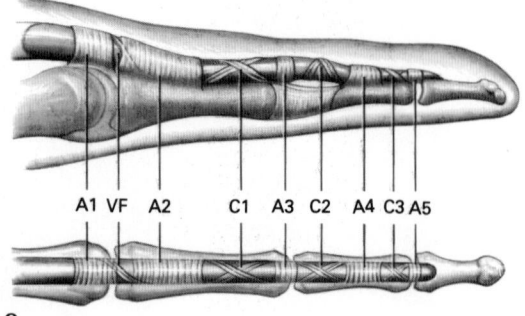

8

All undamaged segments of the pulley system should be preserved. Typically, transverse window incisions are made to expose the damaged tendons:

1. between A1 and A2 in the variable fibre (VF) area;
2. at the mid A2 level;
3. at the level of the cruciate pulleys C1, C2 and C3.

Excision of damaged tendons

9

This portion of the operation must be done carefully to avoid further injury to the tendon bed and will often be very time-consuming. A generous stump of profundus tendon, at least 1 cm, should be left attached to the distal phalanx. It is usually necessary to sacrifice the A5 pulley to perform this adequately.

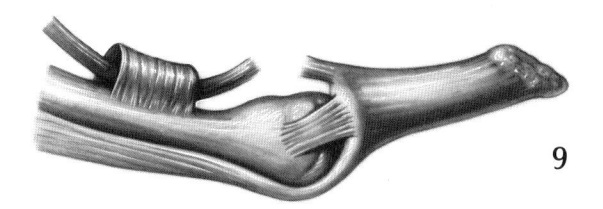

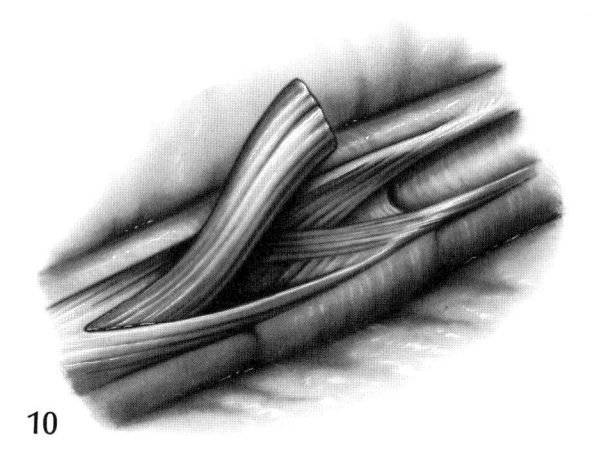

10

If the superficialis tendon bed has not been injured, it is left intact over the proximal interphalangeal joint. Scarring of the tendons at the proximal interphalangeal joint level is often responsible for flexion contracture. Meticulous dissection of mature scar here will permit increased range of movement later. Care must be taken to preserve the volar proximal interphalangeal joint capsule.

11

Severely scarred segments of sheath should be removed and later replaced with new pulleys. Collapsed annuli may be dilated with fine haemostats.

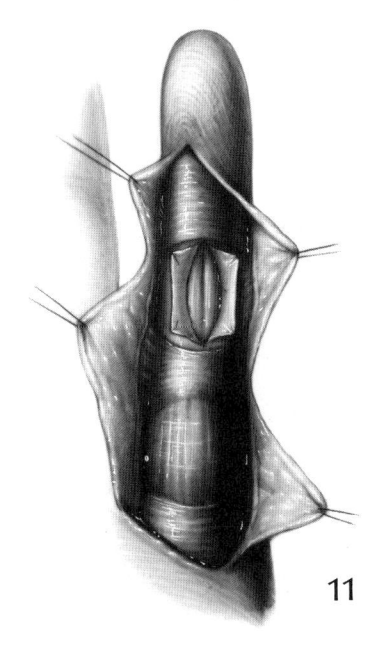

Division of flexor tendons in palm and excision of lumbrical muscle in palm

12

After the scarred tendons have been pulled proximally through the A1 pulley, they are transected in the palm. Scarred lumbrical muscle is resected. If the palm is uninjured, the lumbrical and profundus complex with surrounding mesotendon is carefully preserved for Stage II juncture. Usually, however, when staged tendon reconstruction is planned, scarring is present at this level and proximal juncture is planned in the distal forearm.

If more than one implant is to be used and crowding is noted in the carpal canal, the sublimi may be pulled through the carpal canal and excised in the forearm.

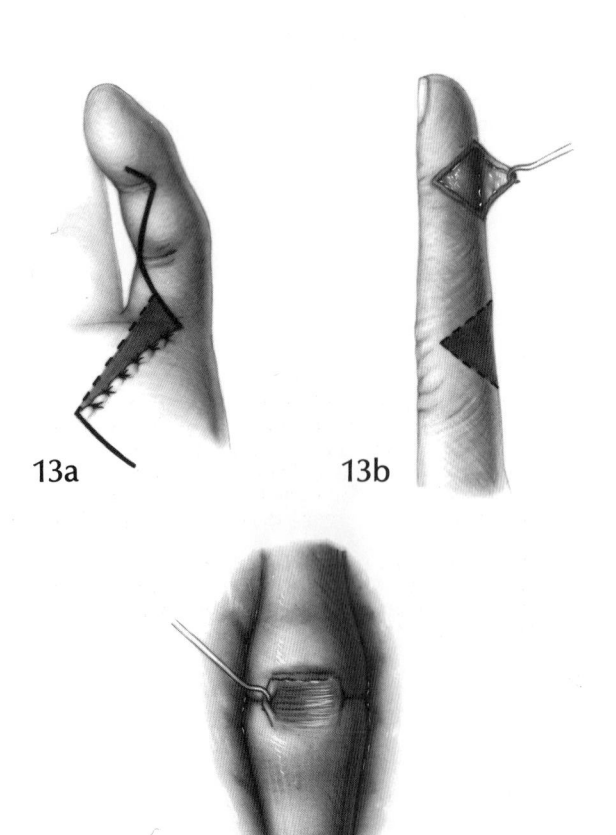

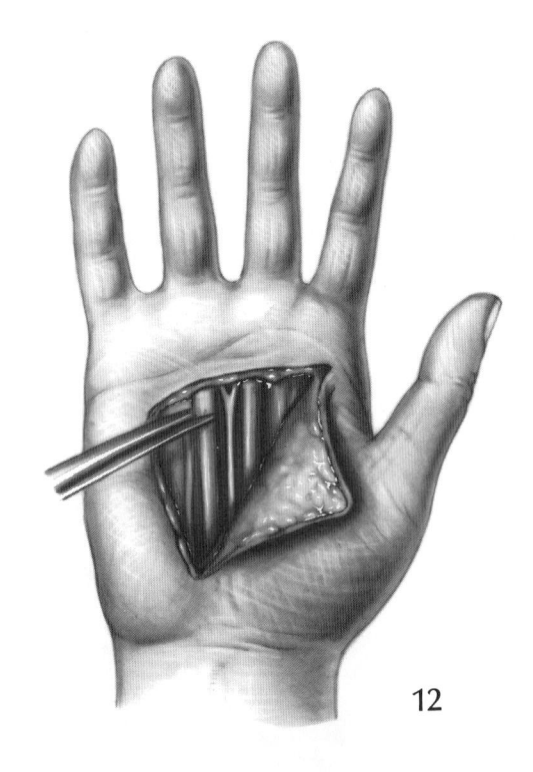

Release of skin and joint contractures

13a–c

Finger joints should be left undisturbed if all contractures can be released by tendon removal and incision of contracted cutaneous ligaments of Cleland or the oblique retinacular ligament of Landsmeer. Shifting or advancement of skin flaps may be necessary (a). The Y-V advancement technique may be applied to release skin tension (b).

Persistent joint contracture can be released by capsulotomy of the accessory collateral ligaments and volar plate (c). If volar capsulotomy is performed, the proximal interphalangeal joint should be immobilized postoperatively by a transarticular smooth Kirschner wire for approximately 10 days, then splinted in between therapy sessions afterwards. These procedures will be most effective when the vascular status of the finger is unimpaired. In all instances of contracture release, the tourniquet should be deflated and the vascularity of the finger inspected frequently. In poor situations, arthrodesis or amputation may be indicated.

Contractures which are not fully released at the time of surgery cannot be expected to resolve during postoperative therapy. The goal of therapy should be to maintain the movement obtained at surgery.

Pulley reconstruction

14

Normal active flexion cannot be expected with a deficient pulley system. Mechanically, the pulleys serve to hold the tendons close to the axis of movement of the joint. This produces a maximum angular movement for each unit of tendon excursion. Thus, bowing must lead to diminished active range, regardless of the passive potential of the joint. In the already injured finger, scarring may form below the bowed tendon, further limiting function.

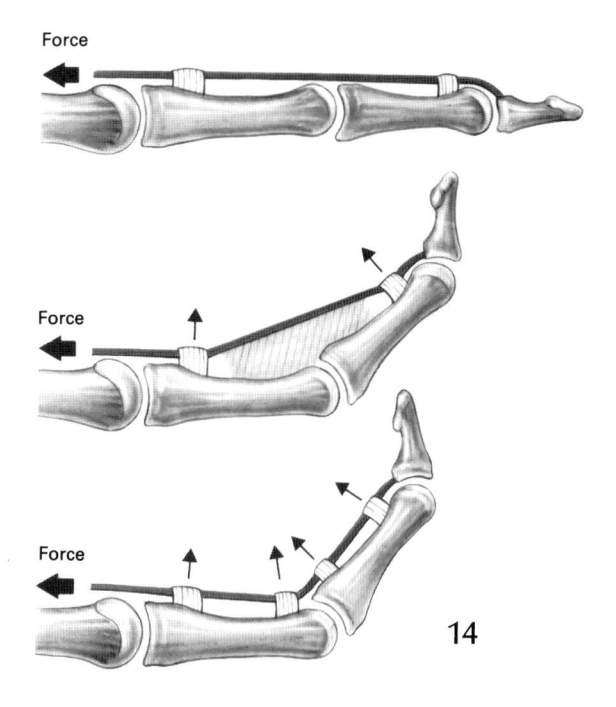

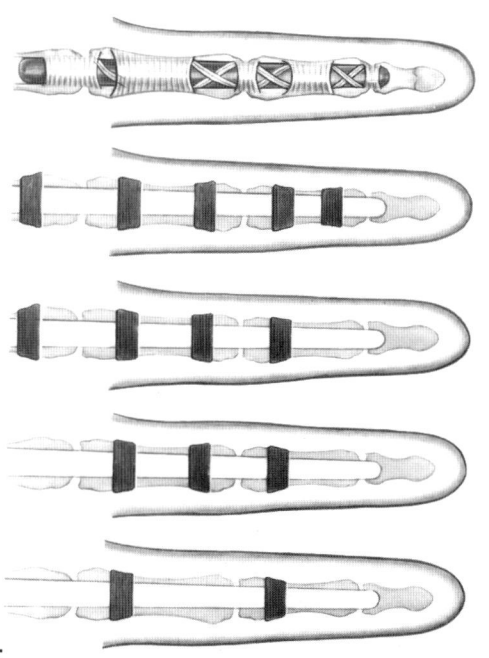

15

In order to preserve normal movement, therefore, it is imperative to conserve or reconstruct as many functional pulleys as possible. For purposes of reconstruction, it may be better to think of the long A2 pulley as performing two separate functions: a distal restraint for the metacarpophalangeal joint and a proximal one at the proximal interphalangeal joint.

In reconstruction, a four-pulley system is preferred. The diagram shows the anatomical situation (top) and, in decreasing preference from top to bottom, four experimentally tested pulley reconstruction possibilities.

16

Portions of excised sublimis and profundus tendons are excellent for pulley building. Several basic principles should be kept in mind. As stated above, the closer the reconstruction comes to the anatomical situation, the greater the potential for excellent active movement after the tendon grafting. Pulleys should be wide and sturdy. We prefer passing the pulley graft completely around the bone extraperiosteally but beneath the extensor tendon on the proximal phalanx and around the extensor tendon on the middle phalanx. The pulley graft should be passed around the bone twice, then sutured to itself at the remaining rim of fibro-osseous canal. We have found a Mixter haemostat helpful in passing the graft around the phalanx. Care must be exercised to retract the neurovascular bundle on each side of the finger so the graft may be passed close to bone without compromising the bundles.

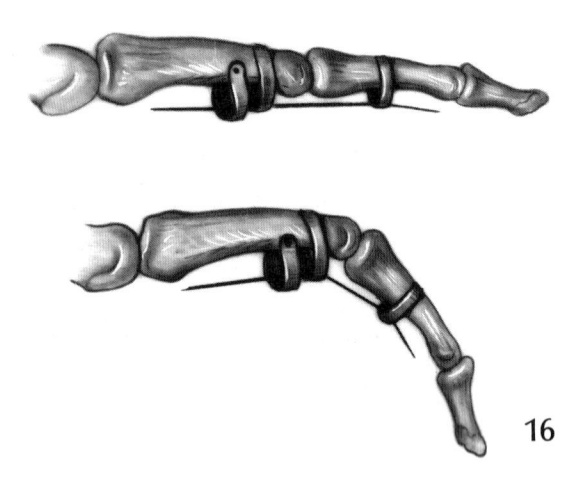

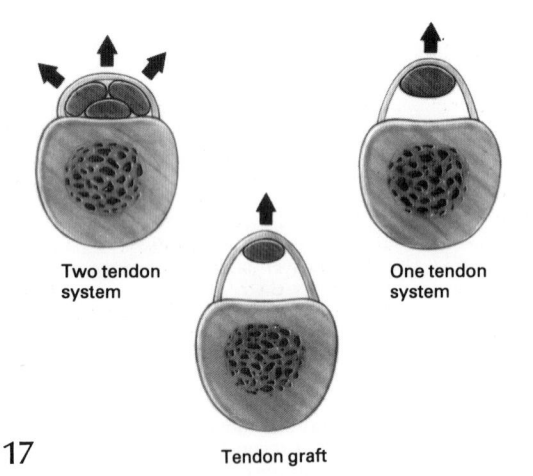

17

The pulleys should conform to the implant but not bind it. In this regard it is important to remember that the eventual tendon graft will be much smaller than the two-tendon system it replaces; reconstructed pulleys do not need to be as roomy as normal ones. Indeed, there may be an element of bowing in even normal pulleys after grafting, as shown in the diagram. For this reason, we currently recommend using the smaller implants, 3–4 mm in women and 4–5 mm in men, when reconstructing the pulley system.

The reconstructed pulley should be close to the joint for the reasons mentioned above but must not be so close or so bulky as to be a mechanical impediment to flexion.

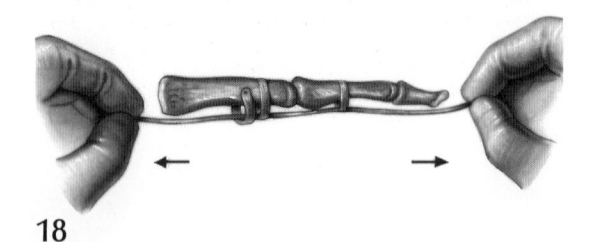

18

Tendon implant sizers are placed through the pulley system. With the finger held extended, the moistened implant is pulled gently back and forth to check for binding. Overly tight pulleys may lead to buckling and synovitis later.

19

Through the forearm incision, the superficial and deep flexors are identified and a preliminary selection of a Stage II motor tendon unit is made. A malleable blunt tendon carrier is passed from distally through the carpal canal to present in the forearm, between the superficialis and the profundus. The instrument is passed gently, seeking the soft mesotendon spaces. The proximal end of the implant is pulled into the forearm through the eye of the passer. The distal end is threaded through the pulley system to the fingertip. The implant should be long enough to extend proximal to the carpal canal in full finger extension. Excess length can be trimmed sharply at this time.

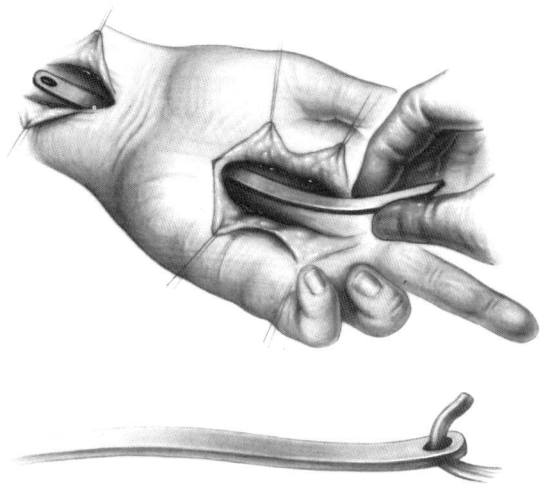

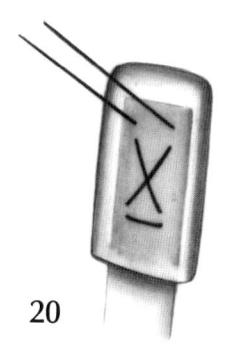

20

Distal end fixation will depend on the type of passive implant chosen. In any case, the flexor profundus stump should be freed to its distal attachment fibres in the distal phalanx. For the blunt tip implant, sutures should be placed in the implant as shown, being careful to keep the suture in the more central area to gain purchase in the Dacron tape. Suture placed only in the silicone rubber will not hold – the implant will loosen postoperatively and synovitis will develop. We prefer a 4/0 monofilament wire suture with a taper cut needle to minimize damage to the implant.

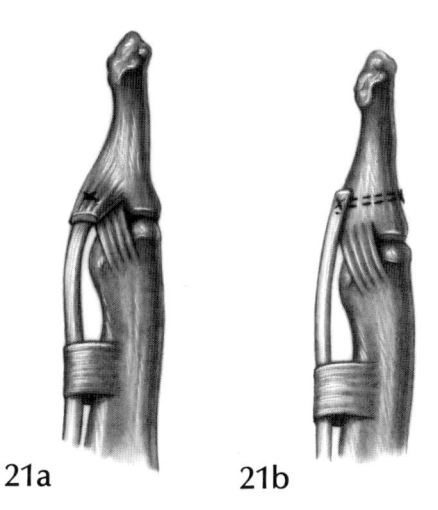

21a & b

Depending on the quality of the profundus stump, the blunt tip implant may be sutured directly to the profundus or fixed to the distal phalanx by passing the implant wire suture through two drill holes in the base of the phalanx. The implant is snugged against bone and the sutures tied on the dorsum of the distal phalanx through a separate incision. With either fixation technique, laterally reinforcing sutures of 5/0 monofilament wire are recommended as well.

22

If the screw-fixation passive implant is chosen, the implant must be threaded from distal to proximal through the pulley system and palm as the metal end-plate is bulkier than the implant itself and has sharp seating spikes which could damage the tendon bed. The plate is placed on the distal phalanx and a guide hole is made with a 11 mm (0.45 inch) Kirschner wire proximal to the nailbed. A self-tapping 2 mm Woodruff screw is then inserted to fix the plate securely to the phalanx. The screw should just penetrate the distal cortex of the phalanx. If too distal on the phalanx, it may damage the germinal matrix of the fingernail. Usually, the 6, 8 or 10 mm screw is used.

The alternative technique for fixing the metal plate to bone is by twist-fixing metal wire around the plate through drill holes in the bone.

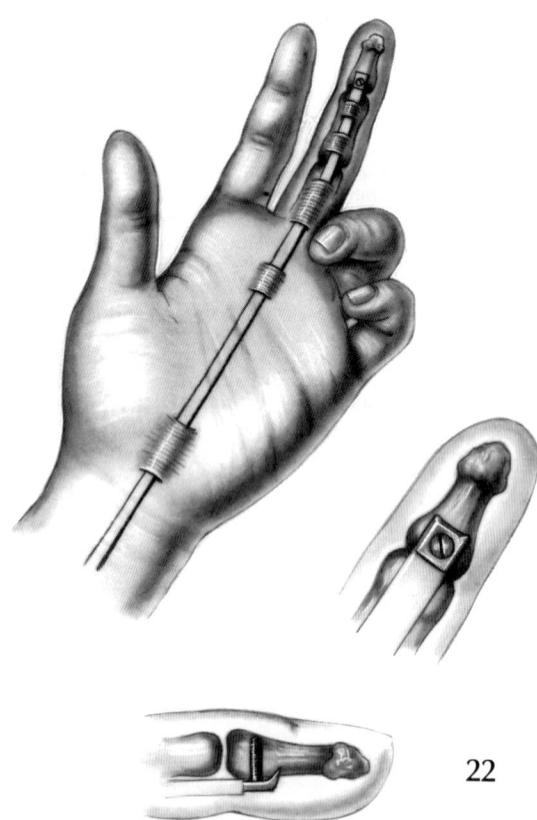

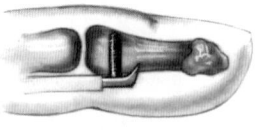

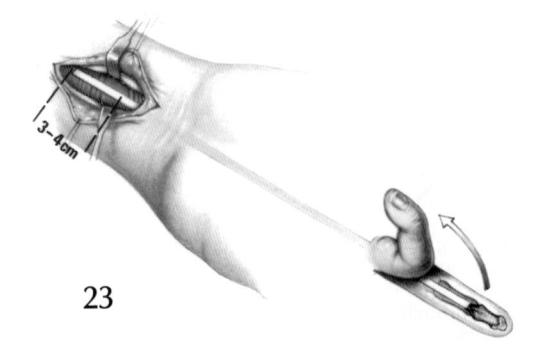

23

Passive gliding of the implant is tested by moistening the implant bed with saline, and holding the wrist and finger in neutral while passively flexing and extending the finger. Movement should be free, with a measured amplitude of implant movement between 3 and 4 cm at the proximal end. Any buckling must be corrected before closure or synovitis will develop between Stage I and Stage II.

Testing pulley system and recording range of movement

24

This is the important last manoeuvre of Stage I before wound closure. The free proximal end of the implant is grasped and pulled, bringing the finger from extension to maximum flexion. The following are recorded.

1. The predicted active range of movement versus the passive range of movement.
2. The measured distance of the proximal end necessary to produce the active function. This will assist in selection of the Stage II motor tendon.
3. The attitude of the finger in relation to the pulley system. Is another pulley necessary to improve function? Should a sagging pulley be snugged down closer to the bone? A pulley may rupture during this manoeuvre, requiring resuture or a tendon graft.
4. Finally, after these forceful manoeuvres the security of the distal end attachment of the tendon implant should be carefully checked.

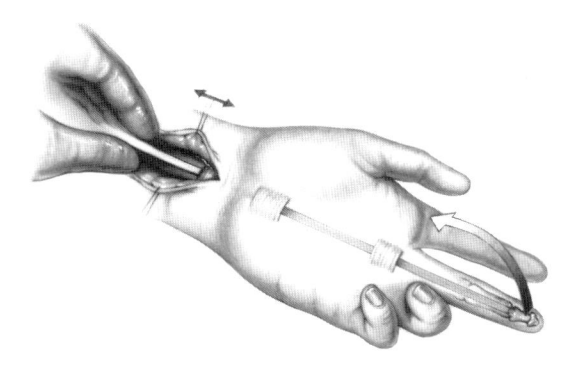

24

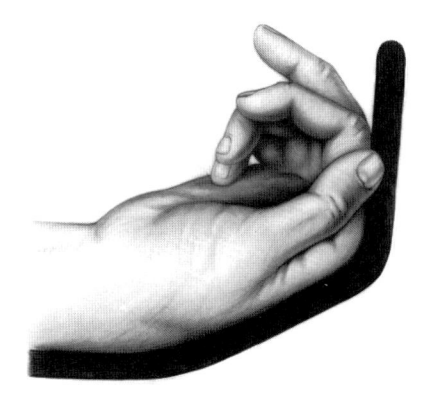

25

The wound is closed from distal to proximal and finally the soft tissue recess for the implant in the forearm is checked with a moistened gloved finger and passive gliding is reviewed. The hand is positioned with the wrist and metacarpophalangeal joints in flexion for closure and final dressing. This position after Stage I permits the proximal sheath to form in the long position.

25

POSTOPERATIVE MANAGEMENT

During the first 3 weeks, the patient is kept in the dorsal splint between therapy sessions. All therapy should be initially performed under the supervision of a hand therapist and the patient closely monitored for the development of synovitis. During the first week, gentle passive movement is started. If a flexion contracture was present preoperatively, extension splinting of the affected joint may also begin at this time. Regular passive stretching under the supervision of the hand therapist is begun during the third week and the patient is taught to flex the finger passively both with the opposite hand and by trapping or taping with an adjacent finger. Joint movement should be recorded regularly. When the patient has a soft supple finger with movement equal to that obtained in the operating room at the time of Stage I surgery, he is ready for the second stage.

26a & b

Between Stage I and Stage II, the movement and position of the implant should be checked radiographically in extension and flexion – at 6 weeks and on the day prior to Stage II are suggested.

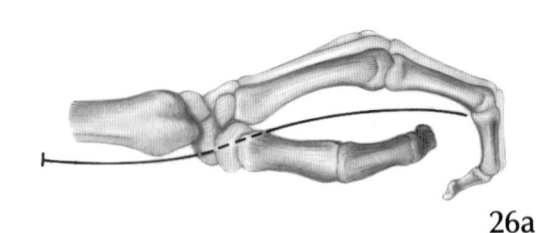

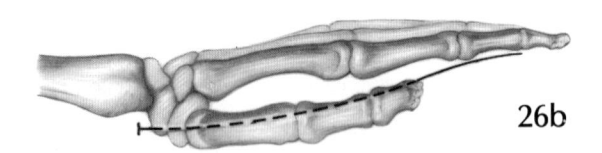

Complications

If good judgement in patient selection and exact surgical techniques have been followed, complications after Stage I surgery should be rare. A complication that may occur is synovitis about the implant, which may be of two types. The most common situation is an aseptic synovitis secondary to mechanical irritation about the implant, which is characterized by pain, swelling and perhaps erythema but no signs of systemic illness. This problem is best treated by prevention. Synovitis can be minimized by careful handling of the implant to minimize accumulation of foreign particles by electrostatic attraction. Careful construction of the pulley system to avoid bowing and buckling will also do much to eliminate this problem. Distal juncture disruption is the most common cause of synovitis; again, careful attention to the details of the implant fixation are the best prevention. Finally, over-vigorous therapy may also result in synovitis.

Purulent synovitis is almost always due to contamination of the implant secondary to postoperative wound breakdown. Typically, this occurs over the distal phalanx in the region of initial injury in Zone II. Such fingers may be better treated initially by special salvage procedures, discussed below. If purulent synovitis does occur, early drainage and antibiotic irrigation may save the situation; if not, the implant should be removed and after adequate healing, the patient re-evaluated for repeat Stage I surgery.

Whatever the cause, aseptic synovitis once diagnosed is treated first by rest. If the symptoms do not resolve within 1 week, consideration should be given to early Stage II surgery. By 3 weeks after Stage I, sufficient neosheath is usually present to support Stage II surgery. Continued mobilization of the finger in the face of synovitis will result in a thickened sheath which will not support gliding or nutrition of the Stage II graft.

Stage II

THE OPERATION

Replacement of implant with a tendon graft

27

On the operating table, the passive range of movement is recorded to be compared with the Stage I range of movement. Improvements are frequently noted after Stage I hand therapy. Distal and proximal incisions are made to identify the sheath and implant. Distally, the implant is left attached to the tendon stump. Proximally, the implant is identified and the sheath at the site of the juncture is carefully examined. Portions of soft sheath may be retained at the surgeon's discretion; however, if synovitis has been present, any thickened sheath must be completely removed from the area extending from the proximal juncture site as far as the wrist flexion crease. The potential active range of movement is recorded starting with the hand and finger flat on the table. The measured rule is held by the proximal end of the implant. The implant is pulled firmly and the surgeon should note: (1) the excursion of the implant to produce the range of movement from maximum extension to maximum flexion; (2) the distance the finger pulp rests from the distal palmar crease; (3) joints with restricted movement; (4) the gliding of the implant and the fluid lubrication system of the tendon bed.

28

The motor tendon is selected and grasped with a small haemostat. The hand is elevated and the tourniquet is released while the lower leg is prepared to remove a long plantaris tendon graft. The technique is that described by Paul Brand.

A long toe extensor tendon may be used when the plantaris is absent. This technique uses the Brand type stripper and two incisions; (1) distally over the metatarsal joint of toe 3 or 4 and; (2) proximally at the retinacular level of the ankle. The fifth toe often has only one extensor tendon and should not be used as a donor for tendon grafting.

The graft is freed in the distal segment, passed through the proximal incision and stripped to the muscle attachment. Excellent long grafts have been removed by these techniques. Shorter tendon grafts such as palmaris longus, extensor indicis, extensor digiti minimi and segments of superficialis are removed by a standard technique and may be used for: (1) thumb, little finger and superficialis fingers with the juncture in the forearm; or (2) index, long and ring fingers to a tendon junction in the uninjured palm.

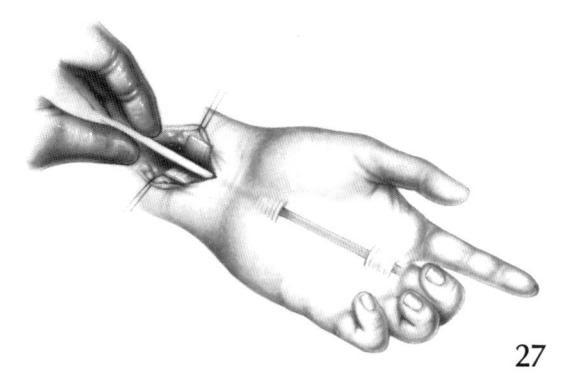

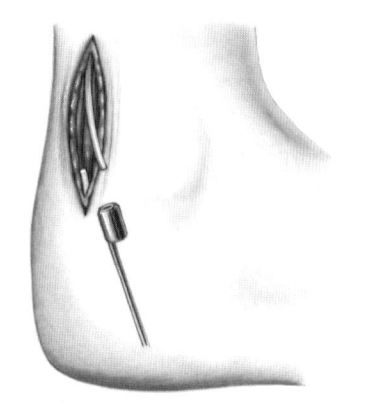

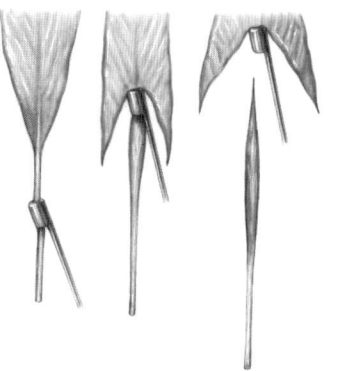

850 Forearm, wrist and hand

Removal of tendon implant and insertion of tendon graft

29

The tendon graft, carefully stripped of peritenon, is sutured to the proximal end of the implant and pulled through the new tendon bed. The implant is detached from the distal phalanx and discarded.

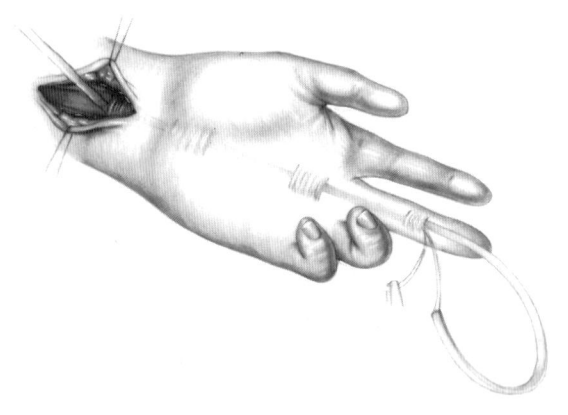

29

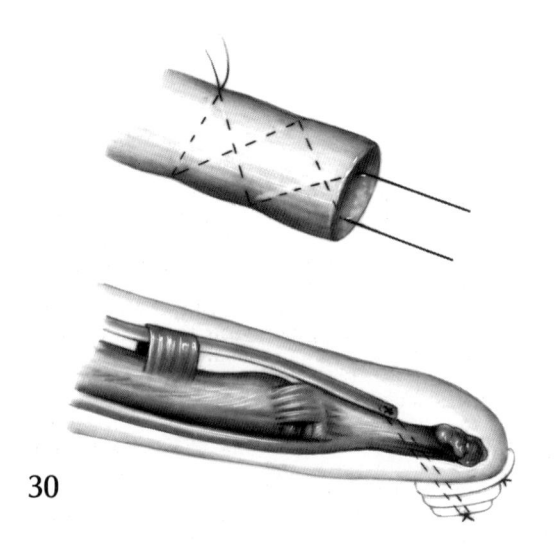

30

The tendon graft is secured distally by a Bunnell type suture technique to bone with monofilament 4/0 wire using a button dorsally on the fingernail. A pull-out wire is no longer used; if only one or two weaves are used in the tendon, the wire suture can be easily removed later by traction distally after the knot over the button has been cut.

The distal juncture should be carefully prepared to minimize the risk of rupture. The drill hole at the base of the phalanx should be enlarged so that the distal portion of the graft seats within the bone. Lateral reinforcing sutures of 3/0 braided polyester complete the juncture. An ophthalmic S-1 needle has been found helpful in placing these sutures in the confined space of the fingertip.

After the distal juncture is completed, the skin there should be closed since closure will be awkward after graft tension has been set.

30

Selection of a tendon motor

31

The tendon motor must supply the same excursion as that required to flex the finger fully with traction on the tendon graft. Selection of an appropriate motor unit, particularly in the previously traumatized extremity, is greatly facilitated by having the patient sedated but awake and cooperative at the time of Stage II surgery, as previously described.

Patient cooperation also eliminates the guesswork inherent in setting proper graft tension.

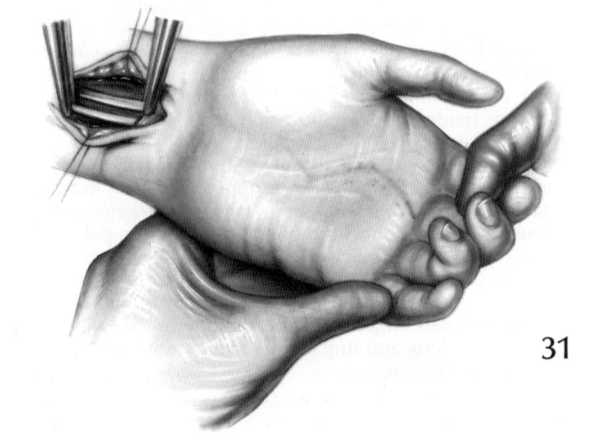

31

32a & b

When the tension is correct, the graft tendon is sutured to the motor tendon using the Pulvertaft end-weave technique. Interrupted monofilament 35 gauge wire is our suture of choice. It is extremely important to be sure that the suture passes through both the motor and graft tendon to prevent subsequent slipping of the proximal juncture. The juncture is more bulky than the implant so that proximal sheath may need to be excised at this point to permit free excursion of the juncture region.

After wound closure, a dorsal plaster splint is applied with the wrist flexed 30°, the metacarpophalangeal joints 70° and the proximal interphalangeal joints slightly flexed. A suture of 2/0 nylon may be placed through the fingernail at this time and fashioned into a loop for attachment of postoperative elastic band control.

POSTOPERATIVE MANAGEMENT

Postoperative tendon gliding requires close supervision of the patient by the therapist. Rubber band elastic flexion used early helps to protect the new tendon junctures and is applied either in the operating room or the next day. The patient is instructed to extend the finger actively against the rubber band and to allow the band to flex the finger passively, in a scheme similar to that recommended by Kleinert and others for rehabilitation after acute flexor tendon repair. It is important that the tension on the rubber band be minimal when the finger is flexed; otherwise, early proximal interphalangeal joint contractures may develop. The hand therapist should begin instructing the patient in passive movement of the interphalangeal joints during the first week. Passive flexion beyond the degree created by the rubber band is encouraged and active extension with the metacarpophalangeal joints flexed is allowed. The extension block splint is discontinued during the fourth week and a wrist cuff to which the rubber band is attached is substituted. This allows the patient to spend more time on wrist and metacarpophalangeal joint extension. The dorsal splint can be eliminated sooner if there has been difficulty in obtaining good graft sliding and active movement or if there has been a flexion contracture; later, if active movement has returned quickly. The rationale for the latter recommendation is the assumption that easy early movement implies fewer adhesions to the graft and, consequently, slow vascular ingrowth and presumably slower juncture healing. Conversely, stiffness and poor gliding would imply a greater vascular contribution to the healing process and more rapid healing.

During the sixth week, the button and distal wire suture are removed and light passive stretching may begin. Active flexion is encouraged with use of the Bunnell wood block and similar training techniques to develop supple gliding planes of connective tissue around the graft. At 8 weeks light resistive activities are begun and at 12 weeks heavy resistance and work therapy can be introduced.

Complications

The most common complications after Stage II are adhesions and rupture of the tendon graft junctures. Restrictive adhesions are most common at the proximal juncture site but may occur anywhere. They are particularly likely to develop where tight pulleys bind the graft, where inadequate pulleys allow the graft to bowstring and scar to deposit beneath the bowed graft, or in areas with poor overall tissue nutrition with consequent inadequate fluid nutrition to the graft.

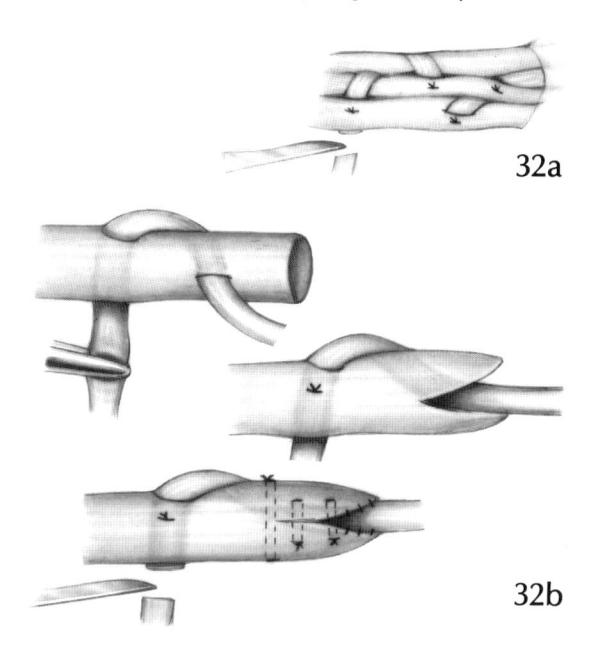

If at the completion of Stage II rehabilitation adhesions are significantly restricting movement, tenolysis should be performed. Sedation combined with local anaesthesia is preferred for tenolysis since only by observing active tendon movement can all the restricting adhesions be identified. Adhesions which do not limit movement should be looked upon as providing nutrition to the graft and should not be disturbed.

Tenolysis should begin at the region of the proximal juncture; extensions may be necessary proximally as well as distally, as intermuscular scar may also limit active movement. Early movement after tenolysis is essential if the gains achieved at surgery are to be maintained. An indwelling silicone rubber catheter through which 0.5 per cent bupivacaine hydrochloride (Marcain) can be injected prior to therapy sessions has been found to be extremely helpful in controlling pain during the first postoperative week. The patient should be encouraged to take the finger through a full range of active movement several times each hour. Careful supervision by a hand therapist is required.

Rupture of the tendon graft is usually due to faulty technique in preparing junctures initially. So-called 'stretching' of the graft is probably an incomplete manifestation of this problem.

Occasionally late rupture may be due to a combination of increased activity level and incomplete juncture healing. Typically, these patients have regained movement quickly after Stage II, presumably having fewer vascular adhesions as mentioned previously. The best treatment is prevention through awareness of the situation; however, often these grafts may be salvaged by early exploration and graft reattachment.

Special indications

THE SUPERFICIALIS FINGER

33

The two-stage technique may be indicated in special circumstances to reconstruct severely damaged fingers with poor distal skin. The implant may be carried distally to the superficialis and fixed by any of the techniques described above. The distal joint can be amputated, fused or tenodesed as necessary. Stage II techniques for superficialis finger reconstruction are identical to those for standard Stage II surgery.

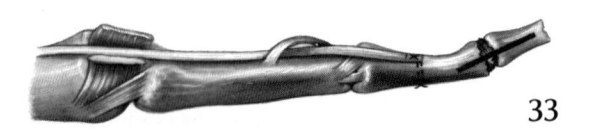

THE SUPERFICIALIS FINGER BY TENDON GRAFT RECESSION

34

After Stage II tendon grafting, a pulley rupture, distal or proximal to the proximal interphalangeal joint, may result in a bowed finger. A useful result may be salvaged by detaching the tendon graft distally and attaching the graft to the base of the middle phalanx. Tenodesis or arthrodesis of the dorsal interphalangeal joint completes the procedure.

EXTENSOR TENDON RECONSTRUCTION

35

In some cases of extensor tendon injury, a dorsal scar may restrict the movement of a primary graft or transfer. The two-stage technique may be used to good advantage in these patients, suturing the implant distally to the dorsum of bone of either the proximal or middle phalanx and extending it proximally into the forearm.

A pulley to help centralize the implant is essential and may be made from available extensor tendon or free graft material. The lateral band system should be functional on at least one side.

Requirements for tendon excursion on the extensor side are considerably less than for flexors, particularly when intrinsics are available to extend the interphalangeal joints, and the reconstruction need only extend to the metacarpophalangeal joint. Often sufficient action is provided by the neosheath between the forearm musculature and the phalanx so that active movement is possible through this connection even prior to Stage II grafting. If the implant is then removed and no graft inserted, the sheath will collapse and form a strong fibrous band – a sort of neotendon which eliminates the necessity for grafting. This is particularly helpful in a hand which otherwise could require multiple tendon grafts, such as a replanted hand.

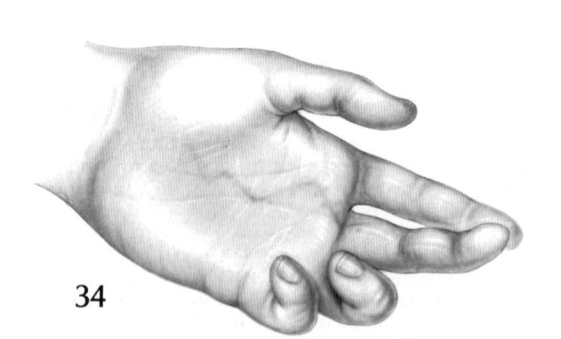

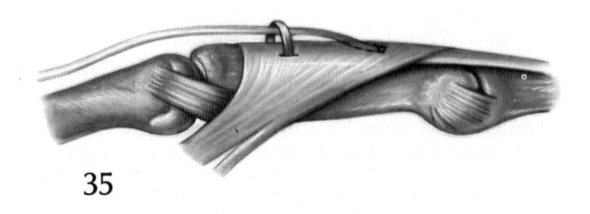

ACTIVE PROGRAMME

Stage I

The surgical principles of Stage I surgery for the passive programme apply equally to the active programme. Local anaesthesia should be used to facilitate selection and testing of the motor unit. Specific technical points which will be covered here relate to implant fixation and selection of a motor unit.

The active programme generally shares the same indications as the passive programme. Situations in which poor finger nutrition might limit neosheath formation and healing after Stage II may be better candidates for the active than the passive programme, for example, the older patient. Factors which would weigh against the active programme include: necessity for tenolysis in adjacent digits, since the splinting necessary to protect the active implant junctures would compromise rehabilitation for the tenolysis; and simultaneous multiple pulley reconstructions, since the immobilization required to protect the pulleys would compromise early active movement of the implant.

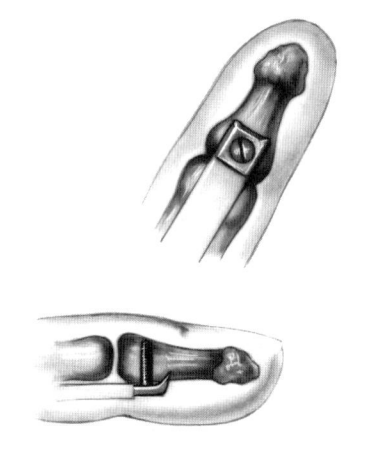

Stage I

THE OPERATION

Distal fixation

36

The implant* should be threaded from distal to proximal through the reconstructed tendon bed. With the finger extended, the proximal loop should be just proximal to the carpal canal so that the fixation can be to the tendon rather than to the muscle belly of the motor unit. The distal screw-fixation device is similar to that in the passive implant. If the braided cord implant is used, the cords can be separated distally until the implant is of the desired length. The braided cord may be sutured into tendon or bone.

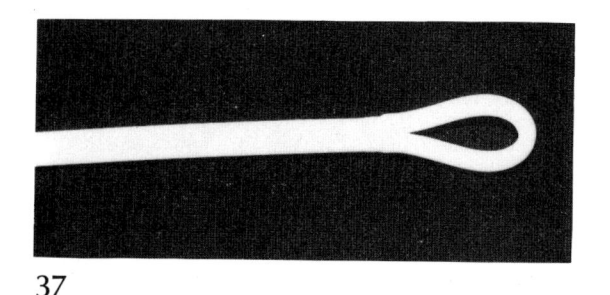

Proximal juncture

37

The motor unit is selected from those available as in Stage II of the passive programme, attempting to make the best possible match between required excursion of the implant and available amplitude of the motor. The motor unit tendon is passed through the implant loop and sutured to itself with a Pulvertaft weave technique. Free ends of Dacron braid may be woven into the tendon for suture fixation as an alternative technique.

---

* Active Tendon Implant for Total Tendon Replacement – The Holter Housner International Co., Bridgeport, PA, USA

POSTOPERATIVE MANAGEMENT

Rehabilitation after the Stage I active implant is similar to that after Stage II in the passive programme, except that it may progress more quickly, as the healing which must occur is from well-vascularized tendon to itself rather than from well-vascularized tendon to avascular graft and from avascular graft to bone. The wrist cuff is usually employed after the third week and light resistive exercises begun after the sixth week.

Complications

In addition to the complications of the passive implant, both proximal and distal implant juncture rupture is a potential hazard of the active programme. Unlike the passive programme, however, in which juncture separation is detected only indirectly – by fortuitous radiography or with the development of synovitis – active implant rupture is immediately evident by sudden loss of active flexion. If the distal juncture fails, Stage II tendon grafting should be considered, since the implant will retract and the distal sheath will close. If the proximal juncture fails, however, the active programme can be simply converted to the passive programme and rehabilitation continued, with elective Stage II grafting at the appropriate time.

Stage II

THE OPERATION

If the active implant is functioning well, Stage II surgery may be delayed indefinitely. When, either electively or because of juncture separation, State II grafting is indicated, the technique is similar to that for Stage II of the passive programme. Since the motor has already been selected and prepared, the proximal end of the tendon graft is passed through the loop in the motor unit and woven to itself by the Pulvertaft technique (*see Illustration 32*) or the graft may be woven into the tendon and sutured. Again, the proximal juncture is bulky so that sheath may need to be excised in the forearm to allow for maximal amplitude of the juncture region.

POSTOPERATIVE MANAGEMENT

Stage II postoperative therapy and complications are identical for the active and the passive programmes with the exception that in Stage II gliding movement occurs rapidly and special precautions are necessary.

Summary

Flexor tendon reconstruction through the two-stage programme is a proven, useful method to restore function to the injured hand. The active implant, currently in the clinical experimental stages, has the potential to incorporate the benefits of active movement even earlier in the rehabilitation course. As research makes the tension interface between living tissue and synthetic materials more durable, a true artificial tendon will also be developed.

Illustrations by Paul Richardson

Dupuytren's contracture

W. M. Steel FRCS (Ed)
Consultant Orthopaedic Surgeon, Department of Postgraduate Medicine, University of Keele, Hartshill, Stoke-on-Trent, UK

Introduction

Aetiology

Dupuytren's disease is inherited as a dominant gene. It becomes increasingly prevalent in the older population and is much commoner in men than women. Epileptics have a 15 times higher incidence of the disease than the normal population, suggesting a genetic linkage but many of these also have a history of treatment with drugs such as phenytoin. Chronic alcoholics and patients whose hands are immobilized are also prone to the disease. Dupuytren's contracture has been called 'the Viking's curse', since its geographical incidence corresponds to the Viking homelands and the spread of Viking invaders at the beginning of the second millennium. However, studies in Japan from old people's homes have shown an incidence not dissimilar from that noted in Caucasian surveys. There have been numerous studies on the relationship to manual labour, but although the disease can follow a single traumatic incident, there seems no definite linkage with repetitive hand trauma.

Pathology

Despite interesting microscopic studies and detailed collagen analysis, the pathological mechanism is still unknown. What stimulates fibroblasts to hyperplasia and new collagen production is uncertain. The presence of an increased amount of Type III collagen in Dupuytren's tissue is probably a reflection of the production of new relatively immature collagen by active fibroblasts. The formation of the nodule seems to be the primary process whilst the development of cords is a secondary phenomenon resembling work hypertrophy. There have been several elegant studies of the anatomy of the diseased fascia which help in the understanding of the pattern of the contracture and provide an essential anatomical basis for surgical dissection.

Dupuytren's diathesis

Several factors are known to have an adverse influence on the prognosis of the disease and, if they are present, the patient should be warned of the possible gloomy outlook. These are a definite inheritance, bilateral involvement, the presence of ectopic lesions (knuckle pads, plantar nodules, penile lesions of fibrosis of the corpus cavernosum – Peyronie's disease), associated diseases (epilepsy, alcoholism), and an early onset. In patients with such a diathesis, surgery may well have to be repeated frequently as the condition progresses to involve the palm and digits of both hands. Recurrence, as well as extension of the disease, will be common.

Clinical features and natural history

Nodules are often seen in the earlier stage of the condition and are sometimes painful and tender when they first appear. They generally occur in the line of the finger rays. Skin pits are usually found in the palm, often at the distal palmar crease. They are said to arise when adhesions develop between the longitudinal and vertical fibre systems. The most frequently observed feature is the cord, extending across a joint and producing a flexion contracture. The cords may be entirely palmar, causing a metacarpophalangeal contracture, entirely digital or, more usually, involving both areas. Although most often seen in the little and ring rays, cords are not uncommon in the radial fingers and thumb. Even the terminal interphalangeal joints are occasionally involved. The progression of contracture is extremely variable and is not linear.

In a study of a series of patients with very early Dupuytren's contracture, after only one year 9 per cent had progressed, after 3 years 22 per cent had deteriorated and at 6 years 48 per cent. In the patients with a diathesis, contractures develop with great rapidity, whilst in the elderly patient with involvement of a single ray the process may take many years. Prolonged contracture leads to permanent joint stiffness causing considerable disability.

Prognosis

The overall risk of recurrence and/or extension is 34 per cent but this figure rises to 78 per cent in the patient with a diathesis and falls to 17 per cent in the elderly, slowly progressive case. The ability to correct a contracture is to some degree unpredictable. It can generally be said that metacarpophalangeal flexion deformities can always be corrected. Interphalangeal contractures may be fully correctable, partially correctable or quite incorrigible. A short history of contracture of less than 6 months is a favourable factor, whereas dense skin involvement is not. The patient should be warned that correction is unlikely to be complete but an attempt is always worthwhile.

Preoperative

Timing of surgery

With general practitioners and the lay public becoming increasingly aware of the condition, patients are presenting more frequently with early disease. The presence of a palmar nodule, skin pit or simple cord without any joint contracture does not usually warrant surgery but occasionally nodules require removal for pain. The patient should be given an explanation of the disease and advised to return at the first sign of deformity. A simple test is the inability to place the hand flat on the table, palm down. When contractures are present, surgery should be considered and the appropriate operation selected. There is seldom extreme urgency to operate for Dupuytren's disease, but the patients should be seen every 3 to 4 months and surgery brought forward if there is progression of the deformity. The exception is the patient with an occupation involving manual skills who should be treated at the first sign of contracture. In some elderly patients with very mild contractures, it may be reasonable to observe the condition without resorting to immediate surgery. Where two hands are involved, it is not always appropriate to operate first on the worst hand. If the contracture on the most seriously affected side seems irremediable, the best choice is often to correct the other hand which is still salvageable. Dominance and the patient's requirements for work and recreations influence the choices. Clinical photographs should be taken.

Selection of operation

In the absence of deformity, or in an elderly patient well-adjusted to a virtually static flexion deformity, no operation is necessary.

Fasciotomy

This is a good procedure for the elderly patient with a single, well-defined band, deep to mobile skin, and causing only a metacarpophalangeal contracture. The morbidity is trivial but there is a risk of recurrence. It is also a useful preliminary operation in very severe Dupuytren's contracture, where skin toilet is impossible, prior to the major operation. Fasciotomy plus skin graft has been suggested as an option, but it is not necessary to close skin in the palm and an 'open-palm' fasciotomy is quite satisfactory.

Limited fasciectomy

There is no longer any place for the extensive fasciectomy which was once preferred, in which attempts were made to excise all the palmar aponeurosis in an effort to prevent extension of the disease. The morbidity from this procedure was unjustified and there is no evidence that prophylactic excision of the palmar fascia prevents extension or recurrence. The current practice is to limit fasciectomy to the area of diseased tissue in the palm and digits. Moreover, it is now felt that as little normal tissue as possible should be removed, the diseased fascia should be painstakingly dissected out, preserving not only the neurovascular bundles but also as much as possible of the palmar and digital fat.

Dermofasciectomy

Replacement of involved skin is the only known method of preventing local recurrence of Dupuytren's disease. It is used in the treatment of recurrence, almost entirely in the digits, but there have been advocates for its use in the anticipation and prevention of recurrence in those patients with a diathesis where extensive skin involvement is noted at the primary operation.

Amputation

There is a definite place for the removal of digits with troublesome interphalangeal contractures which have proved incorrigible at primary or secondary operation. Often the patient will suggest amputation rather than have a useless protruding finger.

Other measures

Very occasionally proximal interphalangeal contractures, which do not correct during fasciectomy, may be relieved by careful and judicious capsulotomy, but the surgeon should be wary of embarking on heroic release of the collateral ligaments and volar plate as not infrequently this results in an even more vicious contracture. Surgical trauma to the flexor mechanism and to the interphalangeal joints should be kept to an absolute minimum during surgery if rapid return of function is to be achieved. Arthrodesis of the proximal interphalangeal joints in semi-flexion may be employed but is seldom an appropriate choice in the ulnar two digits. The success rate of interphalangeal joint arthroplasty in arthritis is so poor that its use in Dupuytren's disease should be discouraged.

Operative principles

Whether general or regional anaesthesia is used is a matter for the preference of individual surgeons and anaesthetists; either is appropriate. As in all hand surgery, certain requirements are essential, namely good lighting, a comfortable seat with arm support, good position of the hand, quiet, unhurried conditions, fine instruments, a bloodless field and adequate assistance. Incisions are planned to permit maximum exposure of the fascia to be dissected, but with the minimum risk of skin flap ischaemia and necrosis. They are placed so as to reduce the possibility of scar contracture across joints. Delicacy in handling the tissues and the avoidance of clumsy blunt dissection reduce postoperative oedema and fibrosis. Ideally the tourniquet should be released at the end of the dissection in order to achieve good haemostasis. This can be rather time-consuming and equally satisfactory prevention of haematoma can be obtained by elevation of the limb for 24 hours immediately after surgery or by using the 'open-palm' technique.

DISEASE INVOLVING ONE RAY

1 & 2

A longitudinal approach to the digit offers the most satisfactory exposure for fasciectomy and avoids the problem of dissecting the difficult area at the base of the finger through transverse incisions. Various techniques are used to prevent skin contracture and marginal wound necrosis. The most widely used is a longitudinal incision over the diseased cord, broken up by appropriate Z-plasties at the transverse skin creases. Its advantage is the direct exposure of the diseased tissue with excellent access. The disadvantage is that quite often the skin flaps are of poor quality and may slough.

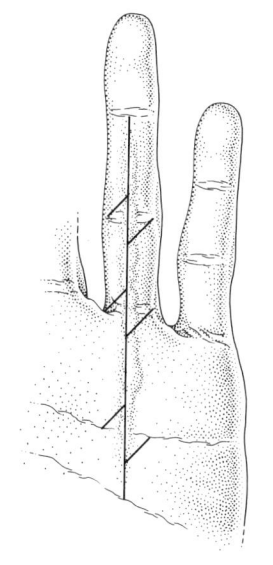

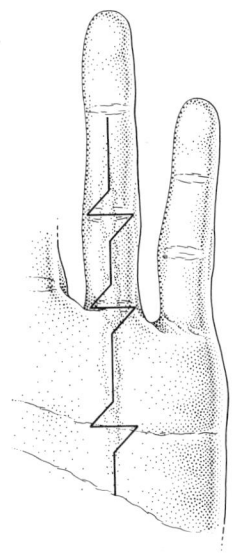

3

The Bruner zigzag approach avoids the need for Z-plasty but affords no skin lengthening at closure. Large flaps raised across densely involved dermal areas may be at risk.

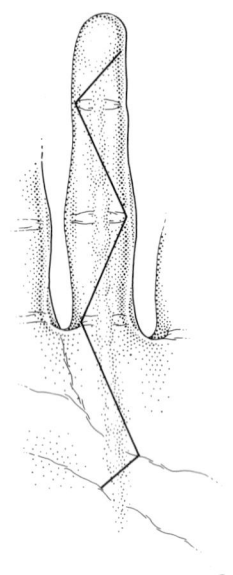

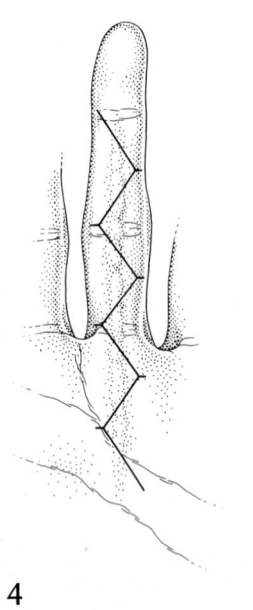

4

A third compromise is the multiple V–Y technique. Some skin lengthening is achieved and Z-plasty planning and manipulation is avoided.

5

In occasional circumstances, particularly the ulnar border of the little finger, a sinuous digito-palmar incision can be used.

The incision should be planned so that it extends to the interphalangeal crease beyond the last flexed joint, thus permitting access to the distal attachments of the cord. The first and often most difficult step is the dissection of the skin from the diseased nodule or cord. The dermis is often very adherent to the involved tissue and separation is tedious. Damage to the dermal circulation at this stage will carry the risk of skin necrosis. Sharp scalpel dissection is essential and magnification can be helpful. As the band is defined, the skin flaps become more secure. Frequent changing of the scalpel blade is necessary. Once the skin has been completely isolated from the diseased tissue, resection can then commence. It is wise to work from proximal to distal. After careful transverse incision of the fascial cord in the proximal palm, the involved tissue is separated from the transverse palmar ligament and paratendinous fibres. At the level of the mid-palm, the nerves and vessels are much more deeply situated than the cord and need not be disturbed. At the level of the metacarpophalangeal joint the deep vertical fibres are seen and can be divided without deeper dissection. At this stage the neurovascular bundles must be isolated and preserved. The cords are then traced to the finger and the neurovascular bundles carefully protected.

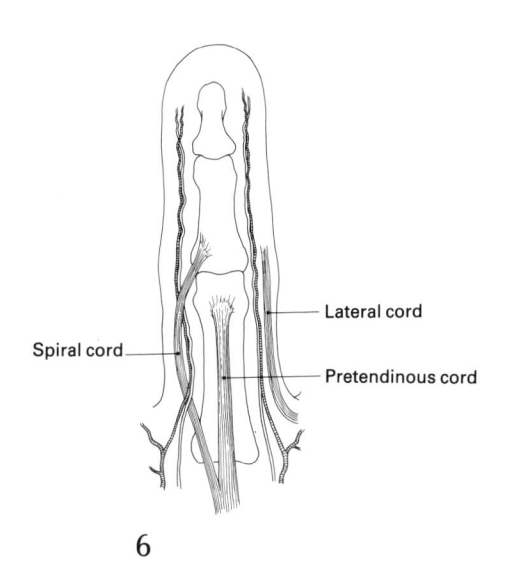

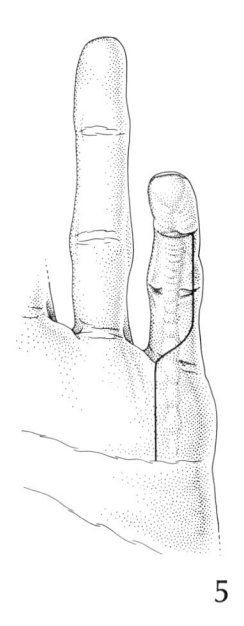

6

Detailed anatomical studies have increased our understanding of the pattern of involvement in the digit. The three types of cord, which should be recognized, are the central pretendinous cord, the spiral cord and the lateral cord. The central cord is comparatively easily dissected away from the flexor tendon sheath and the neurovascular bundles. The lateral cord usually lies lateral and deep to these structures, the fibres are attached to skin and seldom distort the neurovascular bundle; they are often continuous with the natatory ligament which may also be involved in the Dupuytren's process. This cord seldom contributes much to the proximal interphalangeal contracture. The most troublesome cord is the spiral, which as its name implies spirals around the neurovascular bundles, lying first deep and then superficial to these structures.

Knowledge of the anatomy is the key to safe dissection. The cord is never attached to nerves and vessels which pass through a tunnel on their way to a lateral and more superficial position. By defining the tunnel and dividing the cord carefully, the neurovascular bundle can be isolated and the cord removed in two parts. The cord's distal attachment is to the base of the middle phalanx and it is often necessary to retract the nerves and vessels to reach the distal insertion. On the ulnar side of the little finger, the spiral cord usually emanates from the tendon of abductor digiti minimi, and is continuous with that structure.

DISEASE INVOLVING MORE THEN ONE RAY

7

The advantages of a longitudinal approach to digital dissection can be combined with Skoog's approach to palmar disease and the 'open-palm' technique. This combination has an advantage over a strictly longitudinal approach in allowing good access for the removal of widespread disease. The use of the 'open-palm' technique reduces the risk of haematoma following palmar dissection, permits early mobilization of the hand and reduces tension in the longitudinal digital incisions. The digital approach may be a midline vertical incision broken by Z-plasty, particularly when the band is central, or by the Bruner incision, which can be so planned as to give good access to laterally placed disease.

Skoog technique

Skoog emphasized the need to separate and preserve intact the transverse palmar ligament which is never involved by Dupuytren's disease. The transverse incision is made over the extent of the palmar disease, a vertical extension is made proximally, and distal longitudinal incisions fashioned over the cords extending to the digits. These incisions can be parallel or Y-shaped. The triangular skin flaps over the proximal palm need only be developed to expose the borders of the involved aponeurosis. Distally, the flaps are raised only as far as the limits of the disease. The fatty tissue in the web space outlined by the quadrilateral or triangular flap is not disturbed and there should be no problem in the blood supply of the skin. Skoog emphasized a conservative excision in the palm; the longitudinal diseased fascia is separated from the transverse palmar ligament and removed. The paratendinous septa are not disturbed and it is quite unnecessary to dissect out and isolate the neurovascular structures. By leaving the delicate connective and fatty tissues, bleeding in the palm is reduced and swelling is minimal. Function is rapidly restored.

Having isolated the involved palmar tissue, the base of the triangle which it forms is divided carefully and, working distally, is dissected away by scalpel from the underlying flexor tendon, paratendinous fibres and transverse palmar ligament. There is no need to isolate the neurovascular bundles in the mid-palm. As the dissection proceeds into the distal palm, the deep connections will be seen and must be carefully isolated from the neurovascular structures. The vertical septa are divided just deep to the plane of the fascia. There is no need to remove them at a deeper level as they are not diseased nor do they lead to recurrence. Further dissection in the finger proceeds as outlined earlier.

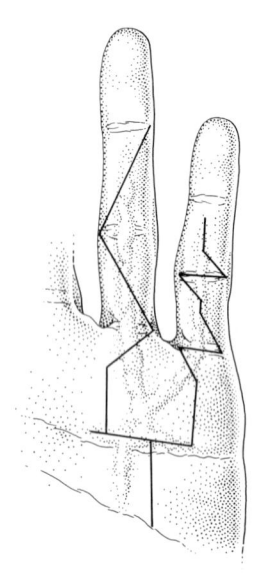

7

'Open-palm' technique (McCash)

8 & 9

The 'open-palm' technique recognizes that the blood supply of the palmar skin is so good that healing will occur regardless of wound suture. The technique can readily be combined with the Skoog approach. All the longitudinal wounds are closed but the transverse palmar wound is left open. Since there has been only a selective aponeurectomy in the palm, the dead space is minimal. A single layer of paraffin gauze is applied to the open wound, followed by fluffed gauze, wool padding and a crêpe bandage. At 5–7 days, the wound is examined and the patient instructed in active flexion and extension exercises. If necessary, the hand therapist can assist. Since there is no tension of the wound, the patient need not fear disrupting the sutures. The open wounds are remarkably pain-free and comfortable. Dressings thereafter are changed once or twice a week and the patient seen weekly in the hand clinic. No haematoma ever develops and no wound has ever failed to heal within 4 weeks. Infection is unknown. The postoperative regime is not tedious and is amply rewarded by the freedom from complications.

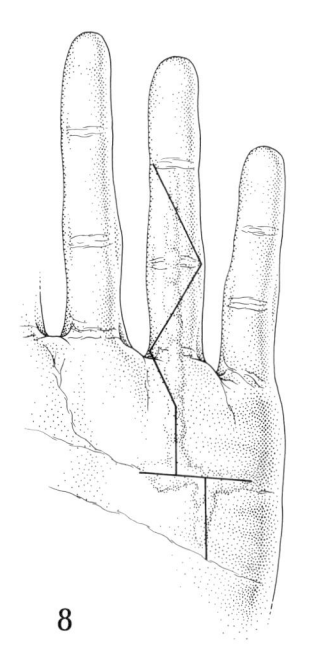

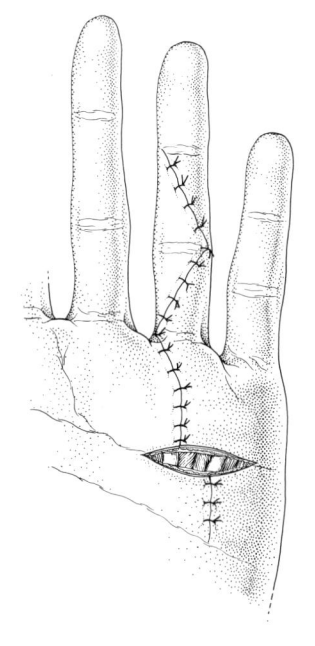

Joint contractures

At the end of the dissection the skin flaps are carefully palpated between finger and thumb to detect any residual nodules or Dupuytren's tissue. Palpation is the most sensitive method of detecting residual cords in the finger which may lie undetected. If there has been incomplete correction of a proximal interphalangeal contracture, it is permissible to divide the fibrous flexor sheath and the check-rein ligaments. Open capsulotomy, though favoured by some, carries a definite risk of loss of flexion, a more serious handicap than loss of extension. Accurate recording of the preoperative and residual flexion contracture is essential.

Haemostasis

Haematoma formation has been greatly reduced since the demise of extensive radical fasciectomy. The use of longitudinal incisions minimizes the risk of a palmar dead space, whilst the 'open-palm' technique completely eliminates the possibility of palmar haematoma. Bleeding can be reduced further by the use of bipolar diathermy during the operation, facilitated by allowing a little blood to remain in the vessels. Release of the tourniquet is widely practised and allows inspection of skin flaps as well as good haemostasis. A firm pad of wire wool or fluffed gauze is packed into the palm and bandaged firmly but not tightly. Forcible extension of the whole hand is to be avoided. Elevation of the limb from the moment of tourniquet release can be extremely effective in preventing haematoma and should be continued for at least 24 hours. Suction drainage is used if extensive palmar dissection has been necessary.

Skin closure

The wounds are closed with 4/0 nylon interrupted sutures, tension must be avoided and it is preferable to leave small gaps rather than to suture tightly. The 'open-palm' technique helps to reduce tension in the longitudinal finger wounds. Where Z-plasties are used, the skin is rearranged with regard to the principles of that technique.

DERMOFASCIECTOMY

Fasciectomy combined with excision and grafting of skin is frequently used in recurrent Dupuytren's contracture, and by some surgeons as a primary procedure in severe Dupuytren's disease. In patients with a strong diathesis in whom there is obvious skin involvement, it may be appropriate to anticipate recurrence by dermofasciectomy as a primary procedure. Skin proximal to the distal palmar crease need not be excised since it will not cause contracture.

The fasciectomy is carried out in the usual way through a midline incision. Particular care must be taken to avoid opening the fibrous flexor sheath, since leakage of synovial fluid will float off the graft. If the sheath is just slightly nicked it may be closed. Similarly, the proximal interphalangeal joint must not be opened. These strictures are easily met in primary fasciectomy but more difficult in recurrent disease. The area to be grafted must extend to the mid-axial line of the digit at the finger creases, but need not necessarily at points between. After fasciectomy and skin excision, a graft is cut to a pattern and sutured in place with a tie-over dressing. It is preferable for cosmetic reasons to take a full-thickness graft, using the inner arm or groin as the donor site.

RECURRENT DISEASE

When previous surgery has been carried out, dissection is considerably more difficult. The planes between normal and diseased tissue are lost and there is no longer separation between the cords and the neurovascular bundle. Careful exposure of the nerves and vessels is essential. The fibrous flexor sheaths may well be transgressed and, if joint contracture is not relieved by fasciectomy, then further capsular dissection will be necessary. If there is a need to replace involved skin there must be no synovial leakage from flexor sheath or proximal interphalangeal joint. That may limit the extent of the correction or, if synovial leakage does occur, skin grafting is precluded.

FASCIOTOMY

10

This procedure is often appropriate in elderly patients with metacarpophalangeal contractures, caused by single cords under mobile skin. The closed technique is easily perfomed under local anaesthesia. The skin overlying the cord and the tissues deep to the cord are infiltrated with 1 per cent local anaesthetic. A number 15 scalpel blade is inserted between skin and cord and, whilst tension is applied, the blade is rotated so that its cutting edge is applied to the cord. Without pressing on the knife, the cord is forced against the blade until the cord is fully divided. Fasciectomy at two levels in the palm is advisable to prevent recurrence.

Fasciotomy in the finger carries a considerable risk of damage to digital nerves and vessels. It should never be done closed but a small open fasciotomy is permissible, provided the neurovascular bundle can be seen and isolated. Following operation a simple dressing is applied but it is advisable to splint the hand and fingers in the corrected position to prevent relapse and recurrence.

AMPUTATION

The general principles of digital amputation are followed with one addition, the dorsal skin of the amputated digit should be filleted and used to replace involved skin in the palm or proximal finger. Thus, scarred adherent skin can be replaced by supple uninvolved dorsal skin. The only disadvantage is the appearance of hair in the palm of hirsute individuals.

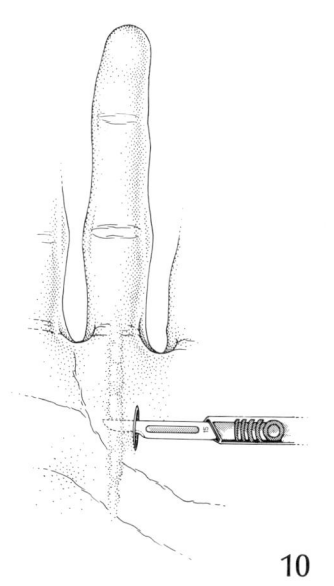

10

Postoperative management

Careful postoperative care and close supervision are the keys to the avoidance of complications. The limb is elevated for at least 24 hours after operation. The patient may then mobilize with the arm in a high sling and be discharged from hospital. At the first postoperative visit 5 to 7 days after operation, the wound should be inspected. At this stage haematoma can be recognized and released; infection, which should be extremely rare, can be treated; marginal skin necrosis, if less than one centimetre in extent, will usually heal without difficulty but larger areas should be excised and grafted before scarring and contracture spoil the operative result. When no complications have occurred the patient is encouraged to commence active flexion of the fingers. If there is any difficulty or reluctance, the aid of a hand therapist is enlisted.

Swelling of the hand should be minimal, provided the surgery has been gentle, the dressings properly applied and haematoma prevented. If there is evidence of swelling or oedema this must be treated vigorously as it is often the first sign of impending reflex sympathetic dystrophy. If the swelling is serious, the patient should be readmitted for elevation of the limb, ice packs and hand therapy. Lesser degrees may be supervised as an outpatient with similar treatment.

Open wounds are dressed at the first visit and at weekly intervals thereafter. The patient is instructed to ignore the wound and move the fingers freely. By the second week there should be sufficient wound healing to permit more vigorous exercises by the patient and, where necessary, with the help of the therapist. Sutures should be left for at least 14 days before removal. Once sound wound healing has occurred, paraffin wax may be used as a preliminary to exercise periods. Bouncing putty and other aids can be introduced to assist in building up hand strength. Occupational tasks and a programme of home activities are used at this time.

The use of splintage following Dupuytren's surgery is not universally accepted but it certainly has a place in the maintenance of the operative correction and the prevention of relapse. Splints must be individually designed, changed regularly as the contracture improves, and supervised daily by the therapists. They may be introduced as early as 1 week or as soon as the wound permits. Splintage must be intermittent and interspersed with an active exercise programme. Night splintage for several months after operation is often useful.

Recurrence

The development of further Dupuytren's disease in the area of operation is termed recurrence. It may occur within a few weeks of surgery or be delayed for years. Patients with a diathesis and those with dense skin involvement are most prone to this complication. Recurrence and/or extension has been noted in 78 per cent of patients with a strong diathesis, compared with 17 per cent in the unilateral late-onset case with no family history. Further contracture will take place if the recurrence affects the digital tissues. Second operations should be delayed until scars are mature, and revisions should be accompanied by skin excision and replacement whenever it is involved. The prospect of correction diminishes in these patients.

Extension

The development of further Dupuytren's disease outside the area of primary operation is termed extension and is not infrequent, particularly in those with a diathesis. Patients should be warned of this possibility. The treatment of the extension follows the lines of primary disease and offers no special difficulties.

Further reading

Egawa T, Horiki A, Senrui H. Dupuytren's contracture in Japan. In: Hueston JT, Tubiana R, eds. *Dupuytren's disease*, 2nd ed. Edinburgh: Churchill Livingstone, 1985: 100–3.

Hueston JT, Tubiana R. *Dupuytren's disease*, 2nd ed. Churchill Livingstone, 1985.

Hueston JT. The control of recurrent Dupuytren's contracture by skin replacement. *Br J Plast Surg* 1969; 22: 152–6.

Hueston JT. *Dupuytren's contracture*. Edinburgh: Livingstone, 1963.

King EW, Bass DM, Watson HK. Treatment of Dupuytren's contracture by extensive fasciectomy through multiple Y-V-plasty incision: short-term evaluation of 170 consecutive operations. *J Hand Surg* 1979; 4: 234.

Ling RS. The genetic factor in Dupuytren's disease. *J Bone Joint Surg [Br]* 1963; 45–B: 709–18.

Lubahn JD, Lister GD, Wolfe T. Fasciectomy in Dupuytren's disease: a comparison between the open palm technique and wound closure. *J Hand Surg [Am]* 1984; 9–A: 53–8.

Luck, JV. Dupuytren's contracture: a new concept of the pathogenesis correlated with surgical management. *J Bone Joint Surg [Am]* 1959; 41-A: 635–64.

McCash CR. The open palm technique in Dupuytren's contracture. *Br J Plast Surg* 1964 17: 271–80.

McFarlane RM. Patterns of the diseased fascia in the fingers in Dupuytren's contracture: displacement of the neurovascular bundle. *Plastic Reconstr Surg* 1974; 54: 31–44.

McGrouther DA. The microanatomy of Dupuytren's contracture. *Hand* 1982; 14: 215–36.

Mikkelsen OA. Dupuytren's disease: the influence of occupation and previous hand injuries. *Hand* 1978; 10: 1–8.

Millesi H. The clinical and morphological course of Dupuytren's disease. In: Hueston JT, Tubiana R, eds. *Dupuytren's disease*, 2nd ed. Edinburgh: Churchill Livingstone, 1985: 114–21.

Skoog T. The transverse elements of the palmar aponeurosis in Dupuytren's contracture: their pathological and surgical significance. *Scand J Plast Reconstr Surg* 1967; 1: 51–63.

Illustrations by Robert Lane

Trigger finger and thumb

Neil Citron MChir, FRCS
Consultant Orthopaedic Surgeon, St Helier's Hospital, Carshalton, Surrey, UK

Introduction

This common condition usually occurs in middle age and affects women more often than men. The patient complains of a digit which intermittently 'snaps', 'locks', or 'dislocates' on active movement. Closer questioning elicits a history of pain over the volar aspect of the metacarpophalangeal joint and on examination a nodule may be felt on the flexor tendon, especially in the thumb. Most cases are due to stenosis of the entrance to the fibrous flexor tendon sheath at the level of the A1 pulley, due to a chronic inflammatory tenosynovitis of unknown aetiology. This narrowing causes the development of a localized thickening of the flexor tendon, and as this passes to and fro beneath the pulley it gives rise to a momentary pain and feeling of resistance.

As the condition progresses, the tendon nodule size increases and triggering becomes constant. In severe cases the nodule can occasionally jam distal to the constriction in the sheath and the patient is unable to flex the digit. More often, in severe cases, there is limitation of extension as the nodule cannot pass distally. If this is prolonged, secondary flexion contracture of the proximal interphalangeal joint may ensue.

It is common to have more than one finger involved in the condition, often sequentially. This is especially so in diabetic patients and those with renal failure.

Rheumatoid tenosynovitis of the flexor tendons can cause triggering owing to masses of synovial proliferation on the tendon. Diagnosis of the condition is important as surgical treatment is different and more extensive than the idiopathic type[1] and will not be discussed here.

Conservative treatment

If triggering is of relatively short duration, the tendon sheath can be injected from proximal distally with local anaesthetic and steroid. A wide (21-gauge) needle should be used to obtain a good 'feedback' of the fluid pressure in the synovial sheath: injection should be without resistance, whereas if the needle has been advanced into the tendon itself a greater resistance is felt. Injection of steroid into tendons causes damage and predisposes to their rupture.

Preoperative

Rheumatoid disease should be excluded by clinical examination. Local sepsis is an absolute contraindication.

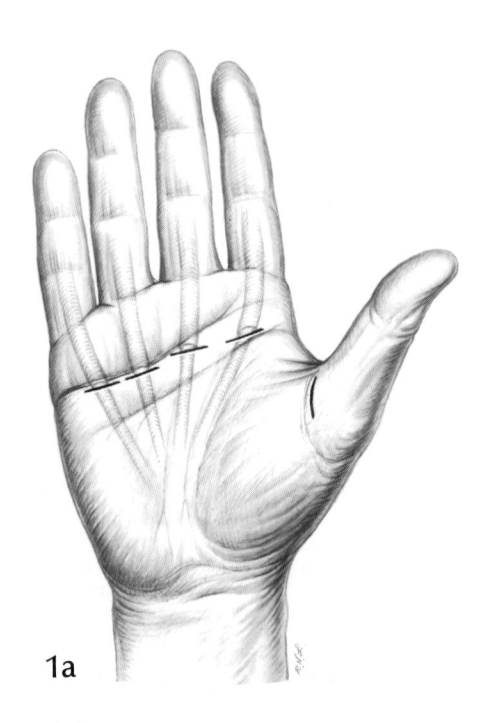

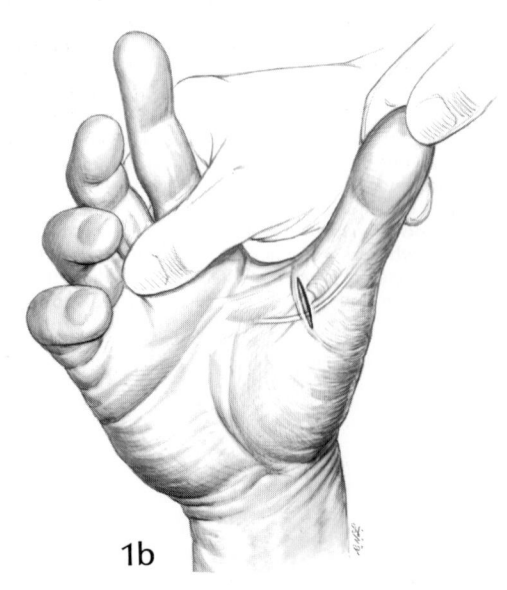

1a

1b

Anaesthesia

The operation may be performed under local or general anaesthesia. Where local anaesthesia is chosen, the skin in the web spaces around the finger is cleaned with 70 per cent ethanol. This is then allowed to evaporate. A 5 ml syringe filled with 1 per cent lignocaine without adrenaline is used with a 23-gauge needle. This is introduced deep into the web space parallel to the palm of the hand and aspiration attempted to avoid inadvertent intravascular injection. Then 2.5 ml of 1 per cent lignocaine without adrenaline is slowly injected deep into the web space on either side of the finger concerned. While waiting for the anaesthetic to take effect, the preparations for surgery continue.

A padded pneumatic tourniquet is placed around the forearm at its point of maximal circumference just distal to the elbow. This is more comfortable for the patient than an upper arm tourniquet. The hand and distal forearm are cleaned and draped in the usual manner. The hand is exsanguinated by elevation for 3 minutes. The patient then clenches his fist, including the thumb, and the tourniquet is rapidly inflated before he releases again.

Operation

Incision

1a

A small transverse incision using a No. 15 blade is made at the base of the finger just proximal to the distal transverse palmar crease for the ulnar three fingers and just distal to the proximal palmar crease for the index finger. Placing the incision next to a skin crease has two advantages.

1. Sweat and dirt do not collect in the wound as they do in the crease.
2. The effect of the crease is to evert the edge of an incision adjacent and parallel to it, so facilitating skin closure.

One way of checking the correct site of the skin incision is by the fact that the skin crease of the proximal interphalangeal joint is equidistant from the centre of the finger pulp and the proximal edge of the A1 pulley.

1b

For surgery on the thumb, an assistant holds the hand with the wrist flexed 90° so the surgeon can be face-on to the true volar surface of the digit. The incision is on this surface, just distal to the metacarpophalangeal joint crease. This avoids danger to the radial digital nerve which is very superficial at this point. Care should be taken here to ensure that the incision is through skin only, as both digital nerves are very superficial at this level.

Trigger finger and thumb 867

Dissection

2

A path is cleared down to the tendon sheath by blunt dissection and the sheath then defined on its volar aspect and the lateral sides.

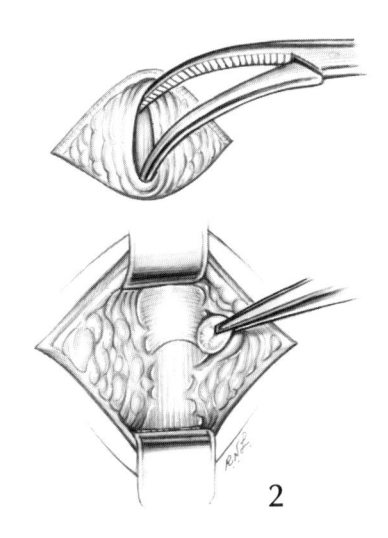

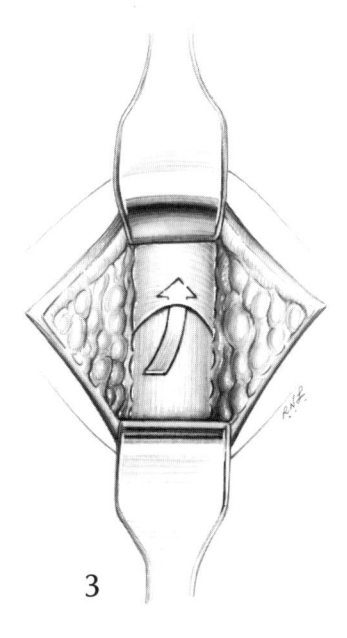

3

There is no need formally to dissect the digital nerves and vessels as they lie in a fibrofatty sheath and are pushed away *en bloc* during the dissection. The edge of the tendon sheath, the A1 pulley, will now be visible as a whitish crescentic edge whose position can be confirmed by moving the finger to and fro and seeing that it does not move, unlike the tendons. The position of the edge can be confirmed by introducing the flat edge of a MacDonald dissector between the sheath and the tendon. A local tenosynovitic reaction may be evident.

Release

4

Using a No. 15 blade with the sharp edge always turned *towards* the tendon, a 0.5 cm strip of the pulley is resected. Alternatively, the tendon sheath is divided longitudinally for 1 to 1.5 cm. The running of the flexor tendons is again checked and if the nodule is still snagging on the edge of the pulley a little more tendon pulley can be resected to enlarge the aperture further or the central slit extended by 0.5 cm. Care is taken to ensure that the tendon nodule does not impinge on the intact edge of the pulley when the finger is in full extension at all joints simultaneously, otherwise there is a risk of a contracture developing of the proximal interphalangeal joint.

In the index finger, special care should be taken to ensure that only a minimum of pulley is removed, or else a bow-stringing effect of the long flexor tendons can occur across the palm, rotating the finger into ulnar deviation. On no account should the nodule in the tendon be touched. Surgery is confined to the sheath! The patient is then asked to straighten the finger *fully,* maximally extending all the joints simultaneously, and confirm the free movement of the digit. A local synovectomy may be undertaken and is said to reduce the amount of postoperative tenderness.

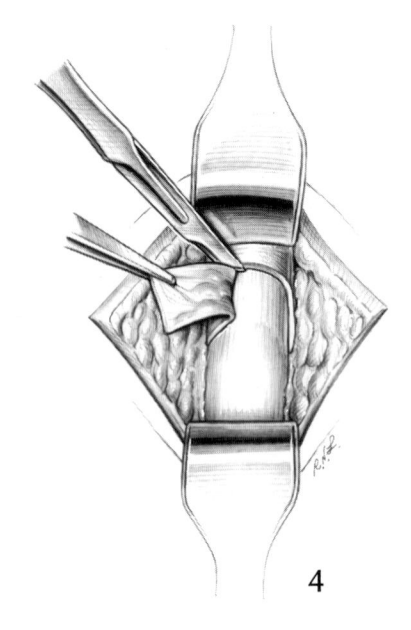

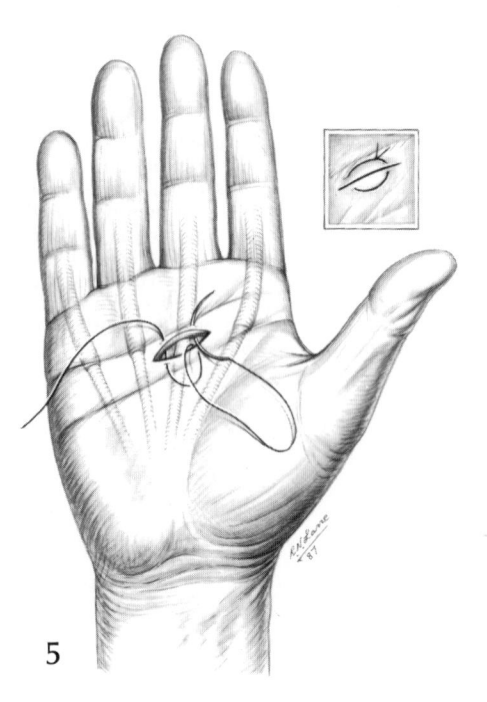

Closure

5

The skin is closed with one or two sutures, taking care to evert the wound edges. A single horizontal mattress suture is often all that is required. No subcutaneous sutures are used. An airstrip dressing is applied to the wound followed by an elasticated, gently compressive bandage. The tourniquet is now released and removed completely from the arm and the patient rests with his hand elevated for at least half an hour before going home in a high sling.

Postoperative management

The compressive dressing is removed on the next day by the patient himself. He is instructed to move his finger normally, beginning on the day after the operation, in order to maintain a full range of movements. After 10 days the sutures can be removed and any residual flexion deformity of the proximal interphalangeal joint corrected by dynamic extension splinting.

TRIGGER THUMB IN INFANCY AND CHILDHOOD

In infancy the thumb is usually locked in flexion because the nodule cannot pass into the narrowed sheath. The condition should be distinguished from other conditions presenting as a thumb flexion deformity.

Thirty per cent of cases presenting at birth will recover spontaneously and so operation can be deferred. Twelve per cent of those presenting at 6–24 months will have spontaneous recovery so that operation can be deferred for them also.

Operation should be undertaken if the condition persists until the child is 2 years old or else irreversible contracture of the interphalangeal joint will occur. Those cases presenting over the age of 2 years require immediate surgery.

Details of operative technique are similar to that in adults except that some form of magnification is usually used. General anaesthesia is required. Special care should be taken to avoid cutting the digital nerves to the thumb. Care should be taken to make the initial incision through the skin only and no deeper: the digital nerves should be positively identified.

Acknowledgements

I would like to thank Dr G. Foucher MD, of Strasbourg, France, for his valued instruction and comments.

Reference

1. Ferlic DC, Clayton, ML. Flexor tenosynovectomy in the rheumatoid finger. *J Hand Surg* 1978; 3: 364–7.

Further reading

Clark DD, Ricker JH, MacCallum MS. The efficacy of local steroid injection in the treatment of stenosing tenosynovitis. *Plast Reconstr Surg* 1973; 51: 179–80.

DeHaan MR, Wong LB, Petersen DP. Congenital anomaly of the thumb: aplasia of the flexor pollicis longus. *J Hand Surg* 1982; 12A: 108–9.

Dinham JM, Meggitt BF. Trigger thumb in children: a review of the natural history and indications for treatment in 105 patients. *J Bone Joint Surg [Br]* 1974; 56-B: 153–5.

Fahey JJ, Bollinger JA. Trigger fingers in adults and children. *J Bone Joint Surg [Am]* 1954; 36-A: 1200–18.

Froimson AI. Trigger thumb and fingers. In: Green DP, ed. *Operative hand surgery*. Vol. 2. Edinburgh: Churchill Livingstone 1982: 1510–3.

Uchida M, Kojima T, Sakurai N. Congenital absence of flexor pollicis longus without hypoplasia of thenar muscles. *Plast Reconstr Surg* 1985; 75: 413–6.

Illustrations by Philip Wilson

Operations for congenital dislocation of the hip

A. Catterall MChir, FRCS
Consultant Orthopaedic Surgeon, Royal National Orthopaedic Hospital, Stanmore, UK

Introduction

A decision to operate on a child with congenital dislocation of the hip is not taken in isolation but within the framework of a protocol of management in which the aim of treatment is to produce a congruous concentric reduction of the femoral head within the acetabulum by conservative means if possible.

There are four stages in this protocol:

1. Correction of any soft tissue contracture.
2. Reduction of the femoral head into the acetabulum.
3. Maintenance of the reduction until the hip is stable.
4. Follow-up to assess the subsequent development of the hip joint.

In the management of this protocol it must be emphasized that it is not wise to proceed from one stage to the next without radiological confirmation that the previous stage has been achieved.

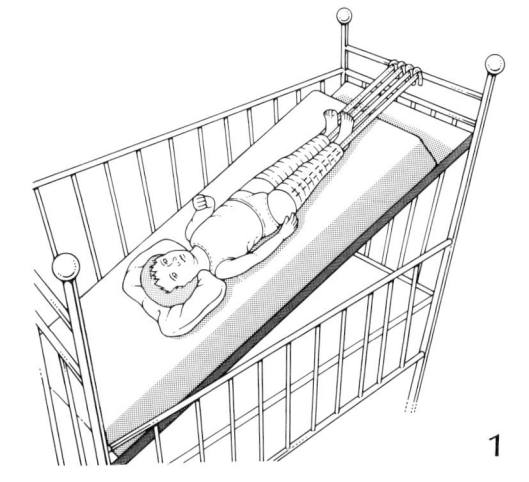

1 & 2

In the younger child it is usually possible to overcome the soft tissue contracture by traction of the Pugh's type for a child under the age of 1 year or by using an overhead frame between the ages of 1 and 3 years. Over the age of 3 years the incidence of avascular necrosis increases the risks of conservative treatment and makes open reduction a better option. Where the soft tissue contracture is being corrected by the use of gallows traction, skin traction is applied to the leg and allowed to set for 1 to 2 hours before the legs are suspended by fixed traction to the overhead loop. The legs are progressively abducted over 2 weeks and the child encouraged to move actively within the bed.

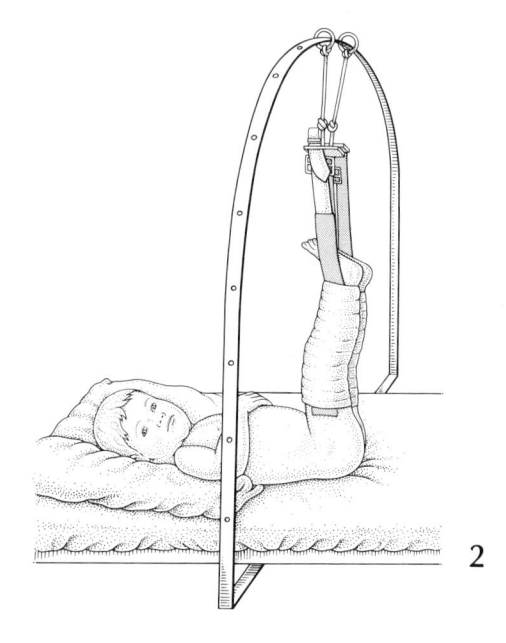

3

When approximately 60° of abduction has been obtained on each side, usually at 2 weeks, radiographs are taken to see if the femoral head remains high; if this is confirmed, cross-traction is applied. If during the course of this progressive abduction the adductors become unduly tight, an adductor tenotomy is performed under general anaesthesia (see below).

Once the femoral head has been brought opposite the acetabulum and this has been confirmed radiologically, the hip is examined under anaesthesia. The object of this examination is to decide whether the femoral head will engage the acetabulum, and determine the position in which it is most stable. A plaster is now applied with the leg in this position (usually 90° of flexion, 40°–60° abduction). The knees are allowed free. This plaster is retained for a total of 6 weeks and during this time the child is encouraged to mobilize. This period may be thought of as the 'trial of closed reduction', as reduction of the dislocation is not a sudden incident as it is in traumatic dislocation but an evolving process.

At the end of the 'trial of reduction' the child is readmitted and again examined under anaesthesia. If the hip is now stable and the radiographs show a concentric reduction then the trial is regarded as successful and the conservative treatment in plaster continued for a further 6 months. If there is doubt about the congruity of the hip joint an arthrogram is performed.

On occasions the adductors remain very tight and unyielding after 2 weeks of traction. In these circumstances a subcutaneous tenotomy may allow conservative treatment to continue.

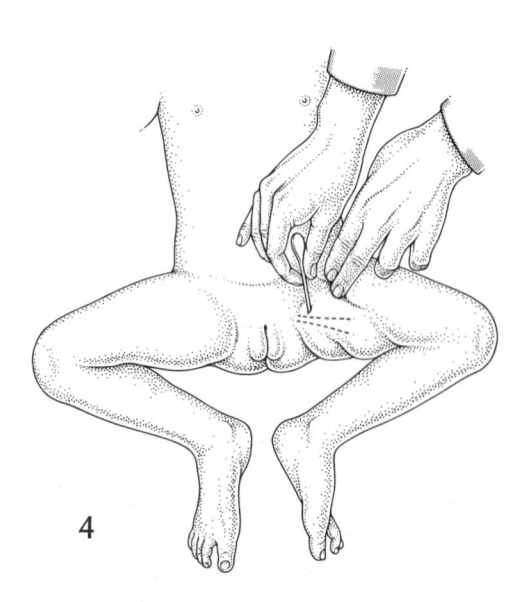

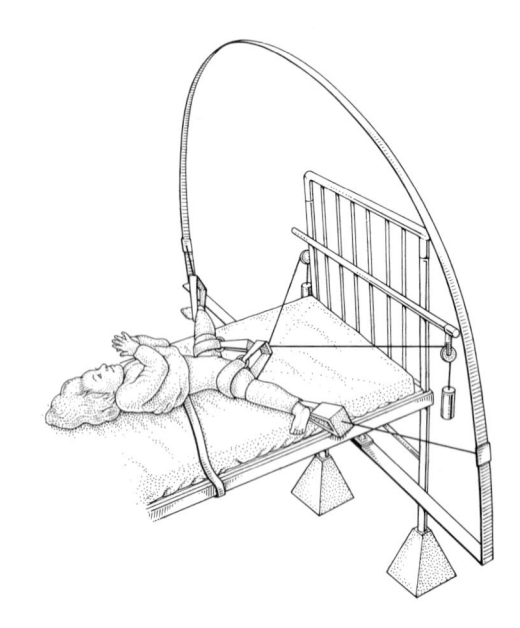

CLOSED ADDUCTOR TENOTOMY

4

This operation is performed under general anaesthesia with the child temporarily removed from the frame but with the traction maintained in position. The legs are placed with the hip in 90° of flexion and in abduction without undue tension. The tendon of the adductor longus is palpated and its attachment to the tibial pubic tubercle identified. The femoral artery is now palpated and a finger placed medial to this to protect the femoral vein. A tenotome is now inserted percutaneously 1 cm from the attachment of the adductor longus and medial to the finger protecting the femoral vein. The tendon is divided. A full release of all the adductors is not performed as this may produce unnecessary bleeding.

OPEN REDUCTION

Indications

Within this protocol of management the indications for open reduction of the hip are relatively simple.

1. Failure to correct the soft tissue contracture.
2. Failure of the hip to engage at the time of the examination under anaesthetic.
3. Failure of the 'trial of reduction' to produce a concentric reduction.
4. A child over the age of 3 years at presentation. There is an increased risk of avascular necrosis in these children.

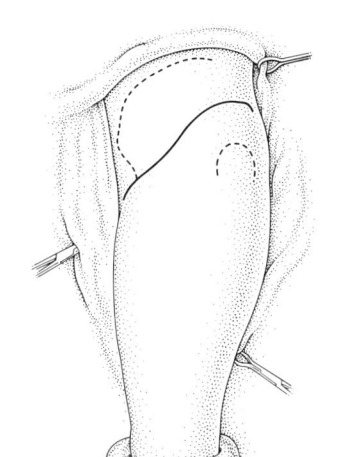

Position of patient

For open reduction, Pemberton acetabuloplasty or the lateral shelf acetabuloplasty the patient is placed on the operating table with the affected hip and buttock supported on a sandbag so that a half-lateral position is achieved.

Incision

5

The same incision and approach is used for all operations on the hip joint. Whereas in the younger child the iliac apophysis is split in order to obtain access to both sides of the wing of the ilium, in the adult the muscles are detached from the iliac crest for the same purpose.

The incision is made half-way between the greater trochanter and the iliac crest, parallel to the iliac crest and curved downwards at its distal medial end. It is deepened through the superficial fascia and the bleeding controlled. The proximal flap is now retracted over the iliac crest and the remaining fat and fascia incised in the line of the iliac crest.

Fascia lata and iliac crest

6

The interval between the sartorius and the tensor fasciae latae is identified by a dense white area starting from the anterior superior iliac spine. As this is incised care must be taken to identify and preserve the lateral cutaneous nerve of the thigh on the medial side of the incision. The interval is deepened and extended up to the anterior superior iliac spine. Small bleeding vessels from the transverse circumflex iliac vessels must be controlled. The iliac apophysis is now split in the line of the crest and detached from it. The bulbous end of this apophysis passes deeply downwards towards the anterior inferior iliac spine. The apophysis will not detach from the bone until this bulb has been divided. The wing of the ilium is now exposed subperiosteally.

874 Pelvis and hip

Detachment of the rectus femoris and dissection of the psoas

7 & 8

The rectus femoris is now identified and its straight and reflected head dissected from the underlying capsule. The straight head is divided at its attachment at the anterior inferior iliac spine and the reflected head from its distal attachment of the capsule. There is always bleeding from the superior gluteal artery at this point and this must be controlled. The rectus femoris is turned down distally and held with a stay suture. The psoas muscle covering the medial capsule is identified and dissected down to its attachment at the lesser trochanter. As the dissection proceeds medially the tendon of the psoas will be demonstrated and it is detached as near to the lesser trochanter as possible. This is facilitated by flexing and laterally rotating the leg.

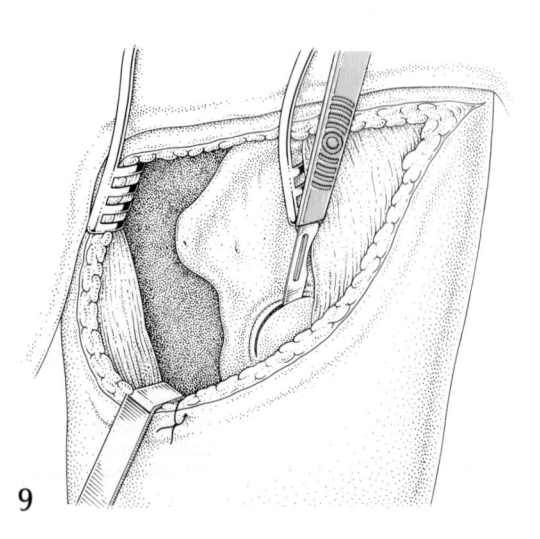

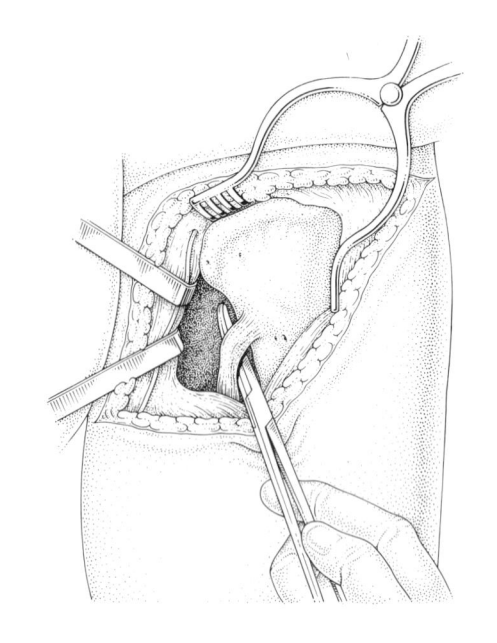

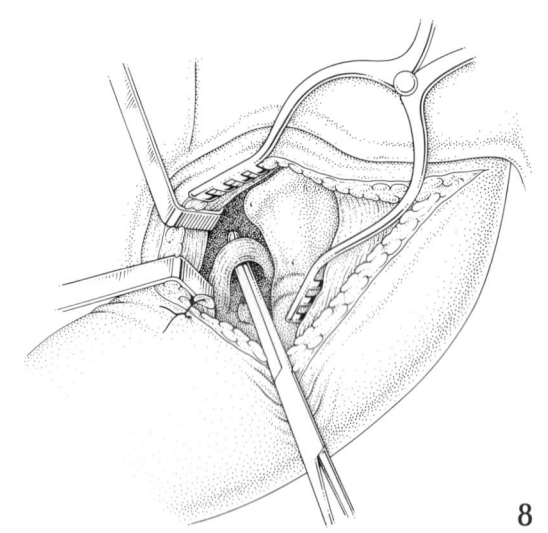

Dissection and incision of the capsule

9

The remaining portions of the capsule are now dissected cleanly superiorly, inferiorly and laterally so that the true and false acetabula are identified. The capsule is now opened by an incision parallel to its capsular attachment to the pubes and 1 cm distal to it.

Assessment of stability

When the capsule is opened the hip joint is inspected and this is facilitated by extending the capsular incision medially towards the transverse ligament and laterally by a vertical incision in the false capsule. The possible intracapsular obstructions to reduction are:

1. The ligamentum teres.
2. The inturned acetabular labrum or limbus.
3. The capsule.
4. The transverse ligament of the acetabulum.
5. Fatty tissues on the medial wall of the acetabulum or pulvina.
6. The shape of the acetabulum.

10a, b & c

In true congenital dislocation the shape of the acetabulum is relatively normal with the labrum inverted, while in acetabular dysplasia with subluxation the anterolateral aspect is deformed and the labrum everted producing the double-diameter acetabulum. In the older child and those with a neurological defect this may be an indication for a Pemberton acetabuloplasty.

All these structures must be inspected. If possible the lateral acetabular labrum should be preserved as it represents the lateral growing point of the acetabulum margin. Its obstructing value to reduction may be overcome by full release of the inferior capsule and division of the transverse ligament which converts the cavity of the acetabulum from a cone to a cup-shape.

The open reduction may be considered adequate when on returning the femoral head to the acetabulum it appears fully contained or covered and is stable to axial pressure with the leg in flexion, abduction and medial rotation. If this degree of stability cannot be achieved an acetabuloplasty of the Pemberton type is required.

On occasions the soft tissues are excessively tight on attempted reduction of the femoral head. Forced reduction at this stage will result in avascular necrosis of the femoral head. This may be prevented by shortening the femur by 1–2 cm. The operation should be performed through a separate incision (see femoral osteotomy p. 884).

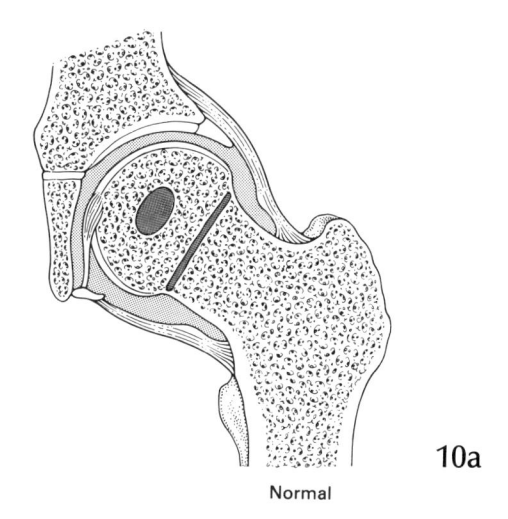

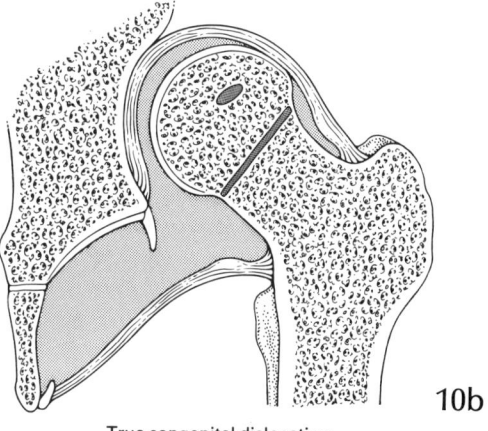

10a
Normal

10b
True congenital dislocation

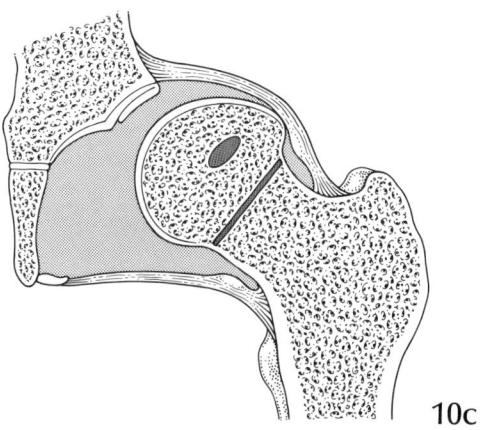

10c
Acetabular dysplasia and subluxation

Test of stability

11a, b & c

The stability of the joint to axial loading is now assessed in (a) flexion, abduction and medial rotation; (b) abduction and medial rotation; and (c) medial rotation alone. If flexion is required for stability, an innominate osteotomy is indicated and may be performed at the same time as the open reduction (see chapter on 'Innominate osteotomy' pp. 893–899). Where abduction and medial rotation alone are required the realignment is more conveniently obtained by a femoral osteotomy which will also correct the persisting femoral anteversion. This is best undertaken at a later stage because of the risk of avascular necrosis.

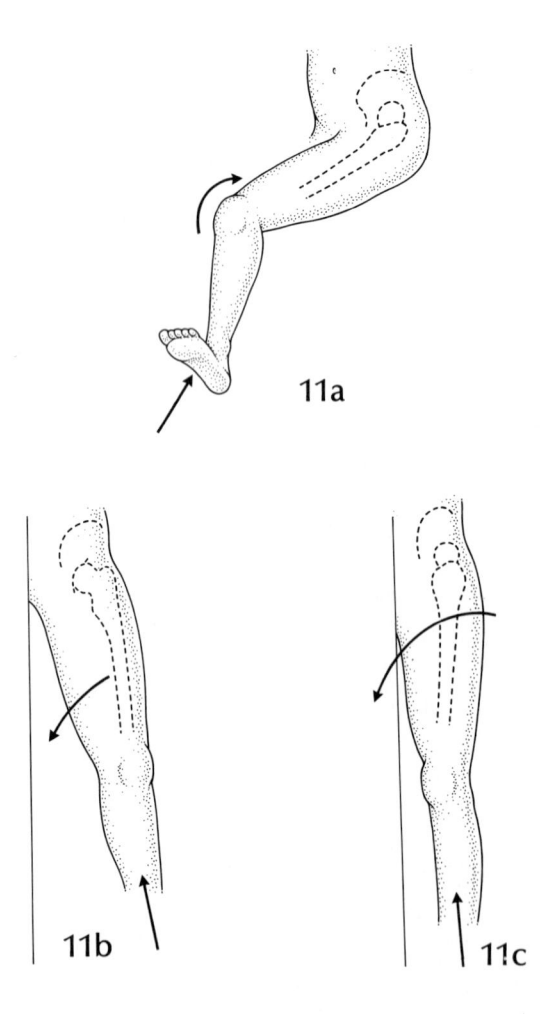

Reduction of the femoral head and repair of the capsule

12a & b

The vertical incision made in the capsule of the false acetabulum is now extended down to the base of the femoral neck at its superior point. This creates a flap of anterior capsule which may be advanced medially providing good cover for the femoral head as it is reduced and also a factor preventing redislocation. In repairing the capsule three sutures are usually used. The first is placed from the region of the anterior inferior iliac spine and passes to the base of the flap at the lateral border of the femoral neck. The remaining two sutures are placed in the capsule medial to this and what was previously the anterior capsule is plicated over them. The leg is placed in the position of maximal stability while this repair is being performed. The rectus femoris is reattached to the anterior inferior iliac spine. If after the repair of the capsule there is no lateral rotation of the hip, a realignment osteotomy of the femur will be required. This is ideally performed 2 weeks after operation.

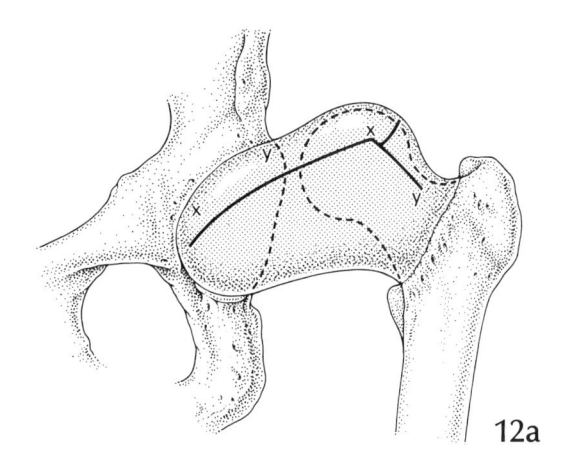

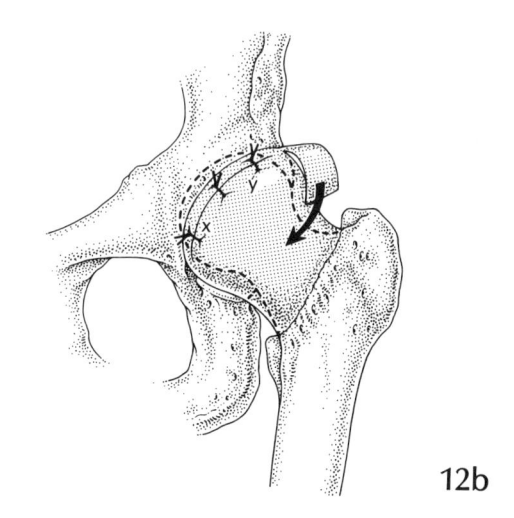

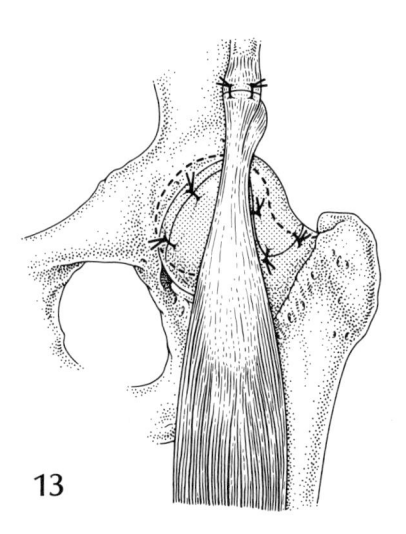

Closure

13

Once the capsule has been repaired and the rectus femoris reattached, the iliac apophysis is then repaired with three sutures. The incision in the fascia lata is closed. The subcutaneous tissues and skin are closed. Where possible a subcuticular stitch should be used as this produces a neater scar than interrupted sutures.

878   Pelvis and hip

THE PEMBERTON ACETABULOPLASTY

The object of this procedure is to improve the stability of the femoral head at the time of open reduction when it can be shown that the anterosuperior part of the acetabulum is deficient, and there is a 'double-diameter acetabulum'. The acetabular labrum is usually found everted and adherent to this portion of the acetabulum. These circumstances are found in acetabular dysplasia with subluxation, either primary or secondary to previous surgery or neurological disease such as cerebral palsy. The hip is approached as for an open reduction.

Technique

14a, b & c

Once the need for acetabuloplasty has been demonstrated the extent of the hip capsule is identified, particularly posteriorly, so that the bony section can be made parallel to the acetabular margin. An osteotomy is performed approximately 0.5–1 cm above the capsular attachment. The osteotomy is made under radiological control, directing the line towards the triradiate cartilage. When the osteotome is just short of the triradiate cartilage the acetabular roof is displaced downwards and laterally, restoring the normal contour of the acetabulum. The position is checked radiographically. Once a satisfactory displacement has been obtained, two triangular bone grafts from the iliac crest are inserted into the defect. They do not usually require fixation and are stable once inserted.

Test of stability

The same tests of stability as were previously applied during the process of open reduction are now repeated to check that the femoral head is stable within the new acetabulum and that realignment procedures such as a femoral osteotomy are not required (see p. 884).

Capsular repair and closure

These are the same as for open reduction.

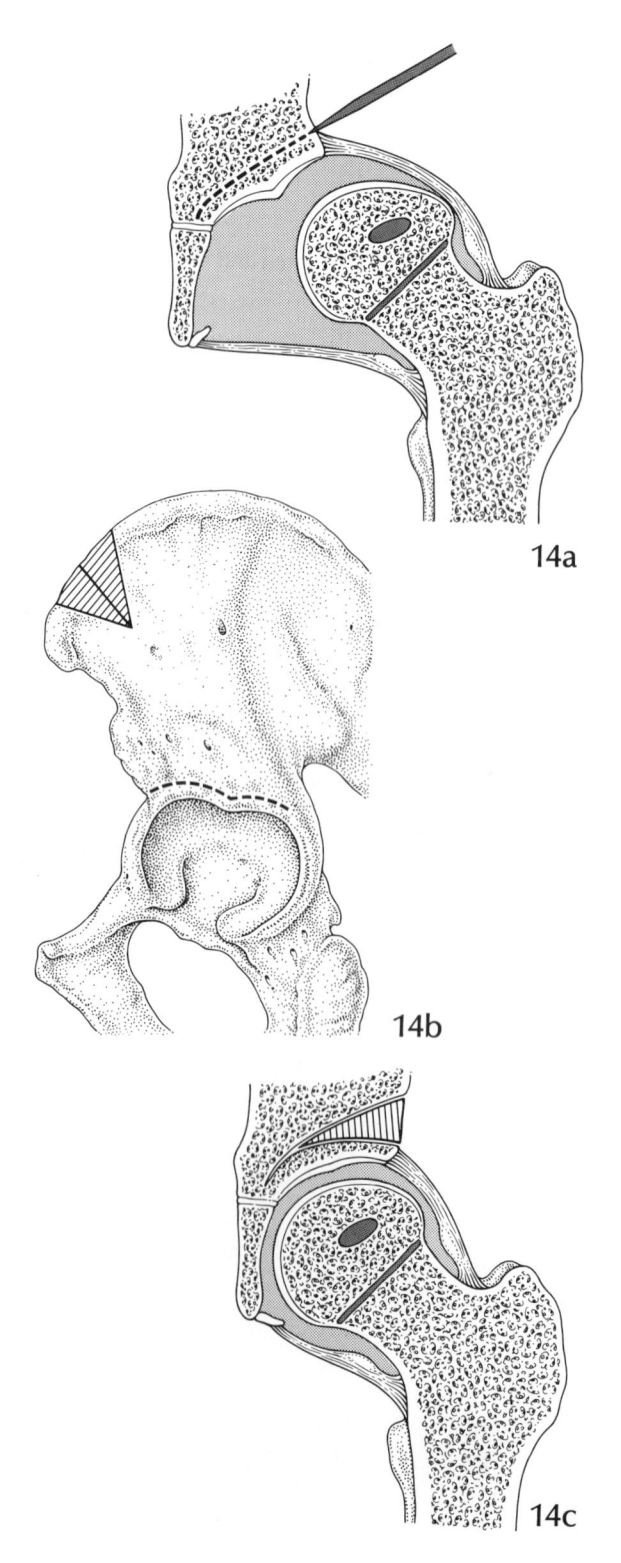

PELVIC OSTEOTOMY

Indications

The operations to be described here are the Chiari and lateral shelf acetabuloplasty, which have similar indications. (The technique of innominate osteotomy is described separately on pp. 893–899.) These two operations are used where there is evidence of disproportion between the femoral head and acetabulum with uncovering of the anterolateral segment of the femoral head. This may be observed in the following clinical situations.

1. Primary acetabular dysplasia with fixed subluxation over the age of 7 years.
2. Following primary treatment of congenital dislocation, either by conservative or operative methods, in which a concentric congruous reduction has not been maintained and a fixed subluxation with anterolateral uncovering of the femoral head has occurred.
3. In cases of Perthes' disease presenting over the age of 9 years, with disease in the early stages. Femoral osteotomy is often associated with residual shortening; lateral shelf acetabuloplasty will reduce the forces through the hip joint by enlarging the acetabular surface and prevent further subluxation from occurring. Where there is marked uncovering late in the disease process, Chiari osteotomy may be required as part of a reconstructive procedure.
4. In conditions producing avascular necrosis of the femoral head where flattening and overgrowth of the anterolateral segment has produced uncovering. Clinically, this uncovering can be felt as 'the lump sign'. Here the Chiari procedure, possibly associated with realignment femoral osteotomy, may be indicated for persisting symptoms.

The lateral shelf acetabuloplasty is a simpler procedure but cannot be expected to produce the same degree of lateral cover as the Chiari. In addition, where there has been a lateral displacement of the femoral head away from the midline, the advantage of the Chiari operation with its medial displacement is to bring the femoral head back into a more normal load-bearing position. The ideal indication for the lateral shelf, therefore, is an unstable lateral acetabular segment with moderate uncovering of the femoral head, or as an augmentation to the lateral segment of the femoral head at the time of the Chiari procedure. Where possible the Chiari operation should be reserved for the adolescent or older patient in view of the possible damage to the lateral acetabular epiphysis.

CHIARI OPERATION

Position of the patient

The patient should be lying flat either on a Hawley table or on a radio-translucent table so that an image intensifier may be used.

Approach

This is similar to the approach for congenital dislocation of the hip but in the older patient, where the iliac apophysis is fused, the muscles need to be detached from the iliac crest. Gluteus medius and minimus are detached posteriorly from the wing of the ilium all the way back to the sacroiliac notch so that the level of the osteotomy posteriorly may be easily identified.

880   Pelvis and hip

Dissection of the rectus femoris

15a & b

The rectus femoris is identified and the lateral margin dissected proximally in order to demonstrate the straight and reflected heads. The reflected head is dissected from the underlying capsule and detached medially from the point where it is attaching to the straight head.

Determination of the osteotomy level

The anterolateral uncovering of the femoral head (the lump sign) is noted, as it is this portion of the femoral head which must be covered by acetabular displacement. A 2 cm osteotome is inserted in the bone at the superior margin of the capsule to determine the level of the osteotomy. This is checked radiologically and the osteotome repositioned if necessary so that it is exactly at the superior and lateral point of the acetabulum. A careful dome-shaped osteotomy is performed. It is sometimes necessary to use a Gigli saw to complete its posterior part.

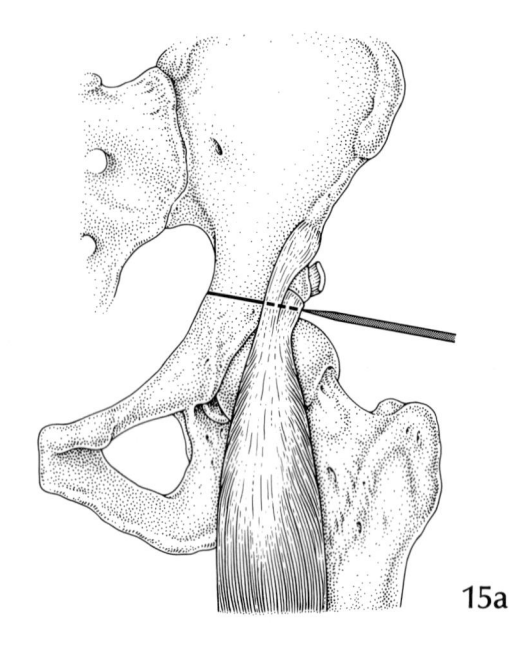

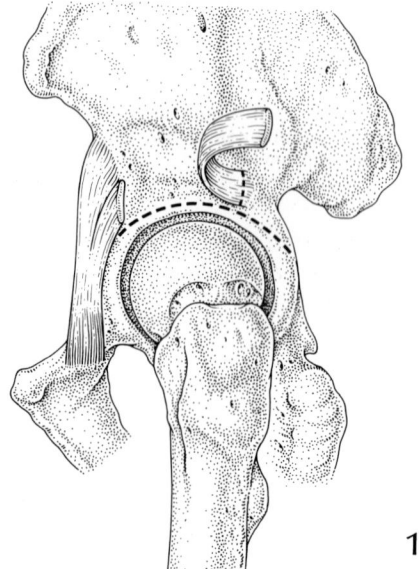

Displacement

16

It is the objective of the operation to produce cover of the anterolateral portion of the femoral head. The acetabular displacement is therefore medial and posterior. This is made easier by abducting the leg. The displacement is checked visually, by palpation, and image intensifier. If necessary the cover may be increased by the addition of a cancellous bone graft placed laterally.

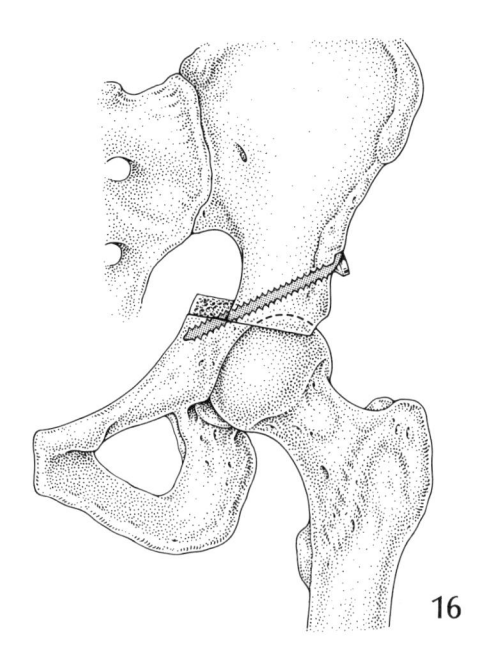

Fixation

A drill is inserted from above the osteotomy through the wing of the ilium into the cut surface of the lower fragment and checked radiologically. A cortical screw of suitable length is inserted.

The wound is closed in layers using strong sutures to reattach the tensor fasciae latae, and gluteus medius. Suction drainage is always required.

Postoperative management

The patient is nursed in bed for 2 weeks while the wound is healing on 'slings and springs'. Slings under the thigh and calf are suspended from springs and hold the hip at approximately 40° of flexion. Active extension and flexion exercises commence on the day after operation. Once the wound is healed the patient is mobilized on crutches, bearing no weight for 10 weeks.

LATERAL SHELF ACETABULOPLASTY

Position of patient

The same position is used as for the Chiari procedure.

Approach

This is similar to the Chiari procedure but the posterior mobilization of gluteus medius and minimus is not quite so extensive as it is not necessary to reach the sacroiliac notch.

Dissection of the rectus femoris

This is similar to the Chiari procedure except that the rectus femoris is detached from the straight head and reflected posteriorly, separating it from its capsular attachment to the extent that is necessary to enable the bone graft to be applied to the capsule. It is carefully preserved as it will have to be reattached.

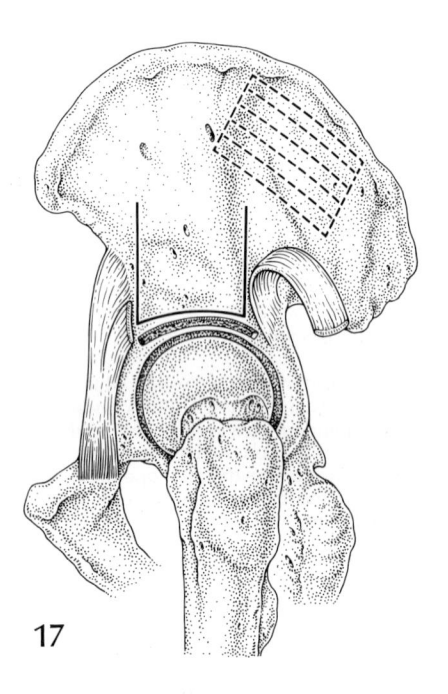

Identification of the lateral margin of the acetabulum

17

The capsule attachment to the lateral margin of the acetabulum is carefully identified, if necessary with the use of an image intensifier. Drill holes are made in the ilium directly above the acetabulum and directed parallel to the line of the capsule. An osteotome is then used to cut a slot on the superior margin of the acetabulum without deforming this margin; into this slot bone graft will subsequently be inserted. An osteotomy is now performed in a 'U'-shaped fashion on the outer table of the iliac bone directly above the hip joint and the flap created is hinged laterally on its proximal point. Care must be taken not to fracture this attachment. (N.B. If this fragment fractures and becomes unstable it is removed, the operation continued, and then the fragment is reattached with a single screw to hold the subsequent bone graft in position.) Bone graft is now obtained in corticocancellous slivers from the lateral table of the ilium and as much cancellous bone as possible obtained for use as a bone graft.

17

Bone graft

18a & b

Strips of corticocancellous bone are now inserted into the slot that has been cut in the ilium, are contoured to the capsule to which they are applied, and brought laterally to produce the cover required. They are trimmed at this point. The position of these grafts and the extent of the cover produced is checked by image intensifier. The remaining portions of bone are applied into the gap between the everted section of the lateral table of the ilium and the bone graft that has already been applied; this bone will be held in position by the rectus femoris.

18a

18b

Reattachment of rectus femoris

The rectus femoris is reattached to the straight head. As it is reattached the slightly unstable bone graft placed laterally over the femoral head will be stabilized into position and this stability can be further increased by accurately reapplying the anterior margin of gluteus minimus and suturing it, partly to the straight head of the rectus femoris and partly to the anterior inferior iliac spine.

Closure

The wound is closed in layers using strong sutures to reattach the tensor fasciae latae, and gluteus medius. Suction drainage is usually applied.

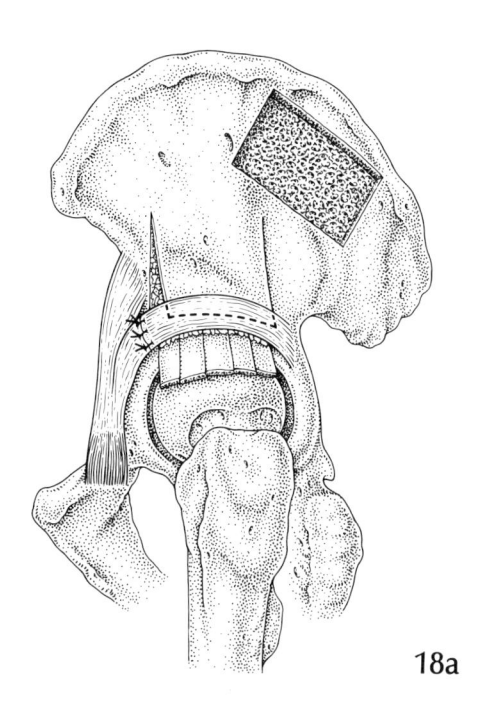

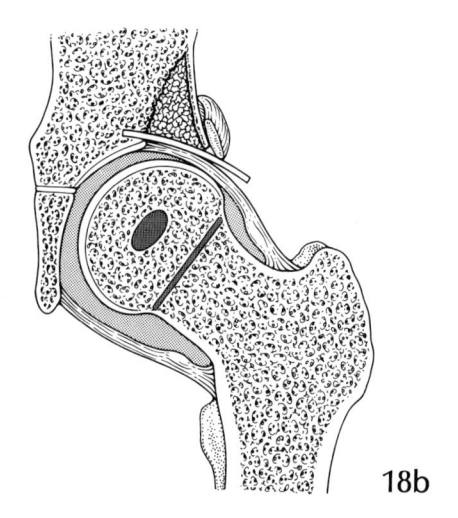

Postoperative management

A one-and-a-half hip spica is applied postoperatively and retained for a total period of 6 weeks to allow revascularization and incorporation of the bone graft. Then the plaster is removed and active mobilization started, initially with the use of crutches for a period of 6 weeks to allow consolidation of the graft. Once this has been confirmed radiographically, active free mobilization is encouraged.

FEMORAL OSTEOTOMY

Upper femoral osteotomy has been performed over many years for the correction of residual deformities of the proximal femur and also in an attempt to stabilize the hip after operative procedures on the joint. Previously it had been thought that the operation itself would reduce a hip but it is now recognized that it is largely a realignment procedure for a position that has already been achieved by open reduction of the joint or other procedures.

Indications

Femoral osteotomy is indicated for a number of different conditions and circumstances. These indications may be considered under a number of headings.

1. A correction of pre-existing deformity: coxa vara, coxa valga, or persistent anteversion of the femoral neck.
2. At the time of open reduction for a congenital dislocation of the hip where soft tissue tightness prevents easy reduction of the femoral head (see p. 875).
3. Realignment to stabilize a known position of the hip (a) after open reduction of congenital dislocation; (b) after containment of the femoral head in abduction in Perthes' disease or late in the disease process where hinge abduction is present to reverse the process of hinging; (c) after correction of acetabular dysplasia where adequate realignment cannot be obtained as the result of innominate osteotomy.

Technical considerations

After union of the osteotomy there will be considerable remodelling of the upper femur in response to the new position. As the result of this there is a tendency of varus position of the femoral neck to remodel into valgus, particularly when the operation has been performed under the age of 4 years. In view of this overcorrection into valgus, additional varus should be always added to a position of realignment in the young child. By contrast, in the child over 8 years the potential for remodelling is reduced and a normal neck–shaft angle of approximately 130° should be created at the time of operation.

In positioning the femoral shaft under the upper fragment it must be remembered that varus osteotomy displaces the greater trochanter laterally and the distal shaft must, therefore, be placed medially to restore Shenton's line of the neck; and when a valgus osteotomy is being performed, the shaft must be placed laterally.

Types of fixation

Where the femoral osteotomy is being performed as part of an operative procedure for which a hip spica will be required postoperatively, it is convenient to use a four-hole plate positioned anteriorly to stabilize the osteotomy and use an opening wedge technique. When, however, extension or flexion are required in addition to varus and rotation or if no plaster spica is to be used, a more secure method of fixation is required and a nail-plate, commonly 'Coventry' type, will allow early mobilization.

Operations

For all the operations to be described in this section a standard approach to the upper femur is used.

Position

The patient lies flat on his back so that the leg can be placed in the position from which realignment is to be made; no sandbag is used.

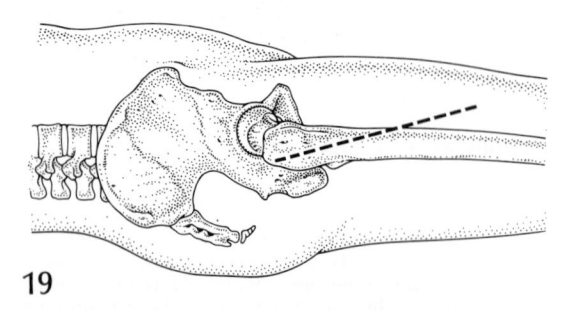

Incision

19

The incision is made obliquely forward from the posterior margin of the greater trochanter. It allows the fascia lata to be incised posteriorly to the tensor and avoids the bleeding associated with incision into this muscle.

Division of muscle

20

The fascia lata is split in the line of its fibres and separated by a self-retaining retractor. The tissue of the trochanteric bursa is incised in the mid-lateral point and reflected forwards to reveal the attachment of gluteus medius and the vastus lateralis. The lowest fibres of gluteus medius are incised to identify the attachment of vastus lateralis.

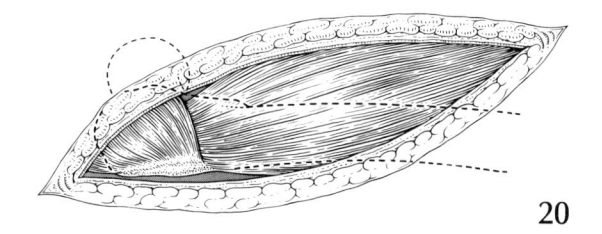

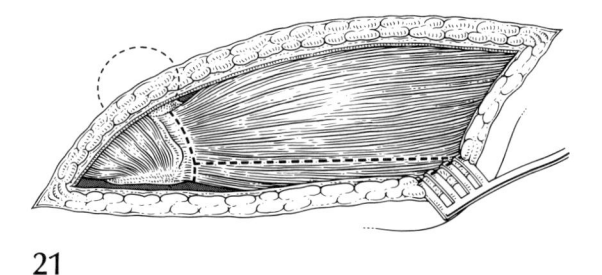

21

The vastus lateralis is incised parallel to its attachment on the inter-trochanteric line and a few millimetres distal to it. A longitudinal incision is made in the line of its fibres as posteriorly as possible. Both incisions divide the periosteum so that a clean edge is produced.

22

The femur is now exposed subperiosteally, elevating the vastus lateralis medially. Four Trethowan spikes are inserted, the most proximal of which should be placed at the junction of the femoral neck and shaft so that the medial border of the femoral neck may be identified. The anteversion of the femoral neck is now noted.

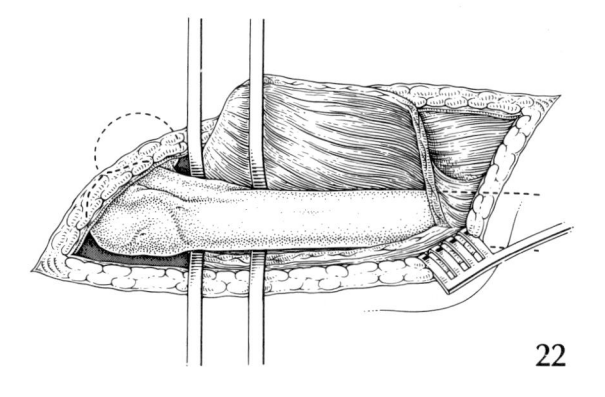

OSTEOTOMY USING A FOUR-HOLE PLATE

23

The leg is positioned so that the femoral head is in the desired position in relation to the hip joint and a small guide wire is inserted through the flat lateral cortex of the upper femur below the trochanteric growth-plate. The guide wire runs parallel to the inferior margin of the neck; and with the leg in the desired position for realignment, the guide wire is parallel to the floor. (At the end of the realignment osteotomy the guide wire in the upper fragment will still be in this position, but the distal femur and leg will be parallel to the opposite one and the patella will be pointing upwards.)

24

A drill hole of suitable size to accept the screw used to secure the osteotomy is now drilled in the anterior shaft just above the proposed line of osteotomy. This will be the second hole of the four-hole plate and is drilled at right angles to the floor and tapped if necessary.

The bone is now divided transversely to the axis of the shaft just below the screw hole previously made, and the periosteum is elevated from the medial and posterior surfaces of the distal fragment to allow rotatory alignment.

An osteotome is now inserted between the cut surfaces to act as a skid between the upper and lower fragments, and the leg now brought to the neutral position with the patella pointing upwards. The distal shaft is displaced slightly medially on the upper shaft to allow for the lateral displacement of the trochanter. When valgus osteotomy is performed, lateral displacement of the distal shaft is necessary.

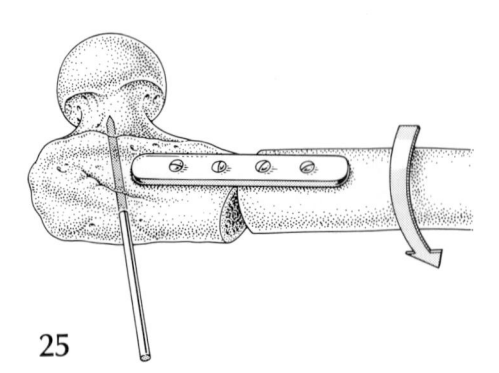

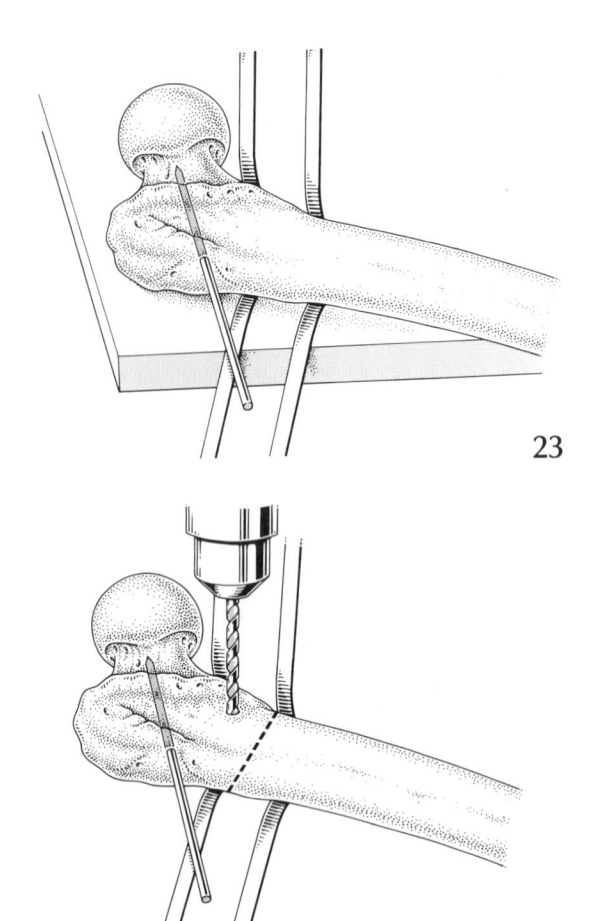

25

Once the desired position of the bones have been achieved, a four-hole plate is inserted by securing the second screw on the plate to the hole that has been drilled on the proximal fragment. The two holes on the distal fragment are now made with the drill at right angles to the floor and with the knee in the neutral position. Suitable screws are inserted.

The rotational element of the osteotomy is now fixed but the valgus/varus osteotomy may be altered by levelling the Steinmann pin and checking that the knee is in the neutral position. The top screw hole is now drilled and the screw inserted. The Steinmann pin is removed.

Closure

The vastus lateralis is reattached with a purse-string suture at the point of incision into the muscle. The fascia lata and subcutaneous tissues are closed in layers and a subcuticular polypropylene suture inserted into the skin.

Operations for congenital dislocation of the hip 887

COVENTRY SCREW AND PLATE FIXATION

26

A Kirschner wire is inserted through the same point as the Steinmann pin and passed up the femoral neck. Its length is measured.

The cortex is reemed and a screw of appropriate length inserted and tightened into position. The Kirschner wire is removed.

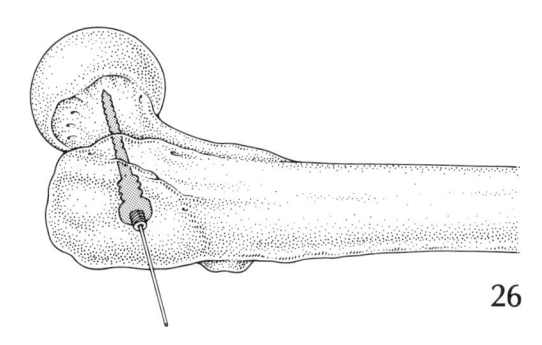

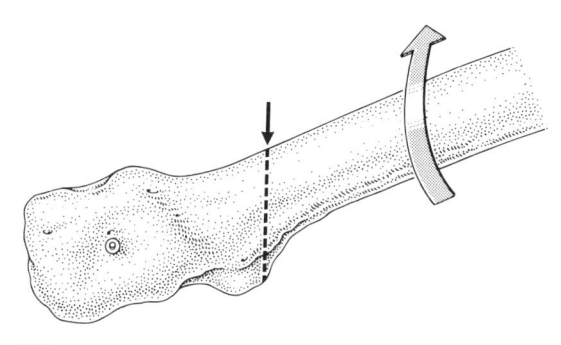

26

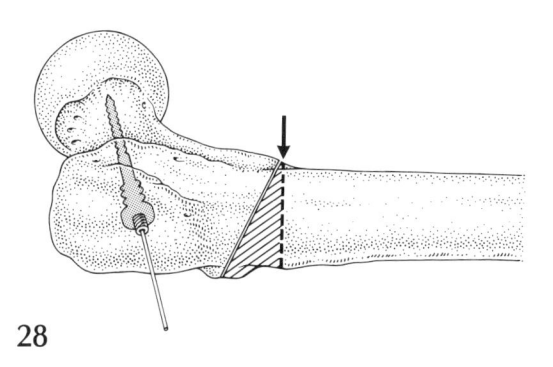

Osteotomy

27 & 28

In any femoral osteotomy whose aim is to realign the leg to a known position of the femoral head, an osteotomy of the femur is made with the leg held in the position from which realignment is required. Then the saw cut is made at right angles to the patient and vertical to the floor. This osteotomy is made at the level of the lesser trochanter and should not be complete. The leg is now turned to the neutral position and a second osteotomy performed at right angles to the distal shaft; this will result in a wedge of precisely the correct amount. Both osteotomies are now completed and the wedge of bone removed. Due to the plain surface of the distal fragment, any rotational correction is easily performed by bringing the patella to the neutral midline position.

27

28

29a & b

Once the necessary position has been obtained the Coventry plate is bent to fit and secured to the upper fragment by a nut and to the lower fragment with screws.
The wound is closed in layers.

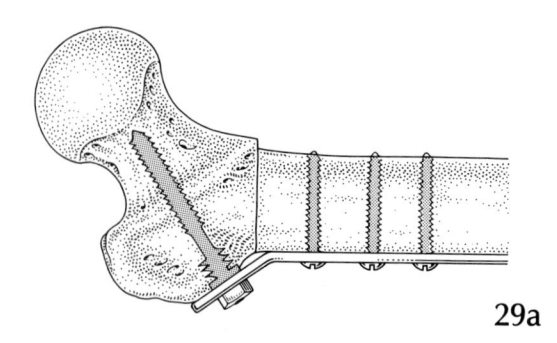

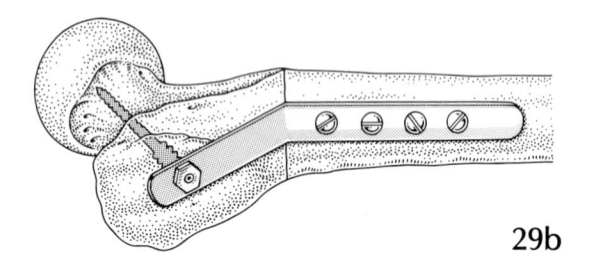

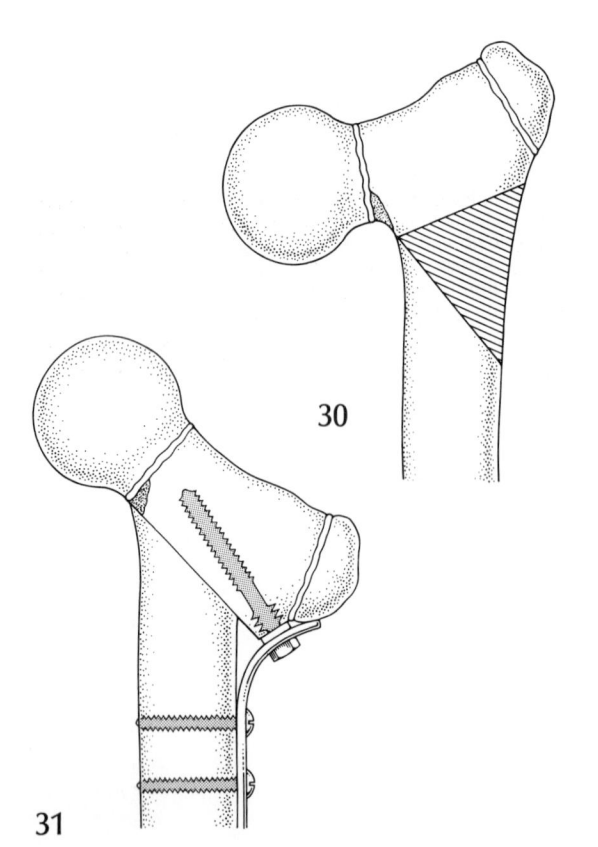

29a

29b

FEMORAL OSTEOTOMY FOR COXA VARA

30 & 31

For this condition the displacement described by Pauwels is used. The wedge to be removed is usually between 60° and 90°. The proximal level of osteotomy must reach the base of this femoral neck. The distal osteotomy is oblique to the shaft, in the line of the femoral neck. This produces a long line of osteotomy distally and allows the medial spike to be displaced under the medial fragment of the metaphysis. Fixation is usually by a Coventry screw-plate fixation.

The use of this operation in other conditions will be found in the chapter on 'High femoral osteotomy in childhood' (see pp. 900–908).

THE COLONNA OPERATION

This operation, which was initially described by Hey Groves[1] and subsequently reported in detail by Colonna[2] and Trevor[3], is a capsular arthroplasty and should always, therefore, be looked upon as a salvage procedure.

Indications

The indications for this operation have always been few and limited to the management of the older child with the high dislocation, particularly following previous surgery. With the advent of the new techniques of open reduction with femoral shortening the indications for the capsular arthroplasty are few; primary dislocation in the older child may now be treated by open reduction whereas previously it was treated by a Colonna operation. It is now possible to obtain a concentric reduction without undue pressure and the consequent risk of avascular necrosis.

There are at present two good indications for the Colonna operation.

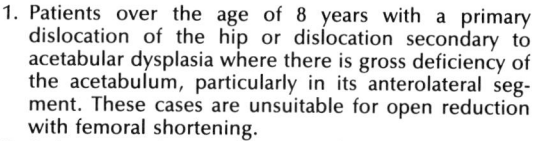

1. Patients over the age of 8 years with a primary dislocation of the hip or dislocation secondary to acetabular dysplasia where there is gross deficiency of the acetabulum, particularly in its anterolateral segment. These cases are unsuitable for open reduction with femoral shortening.
2. Patients over the age of 7 years with residual dislocation following surgery, where both acetabulum and femoral head are abnormal and a concentric reduction is therefore impossible to obtain.

It should be, however, stressed that this operation is not for the surgeon performing occasional surgery on the child's hip joint.

Anaesthesia and position

The operation is performed under general anaesthesia with an intravenous infusion running, as blood loss may be great during this procedure. The patient is positioned in the full lateral position with the dislocated hip upwards.

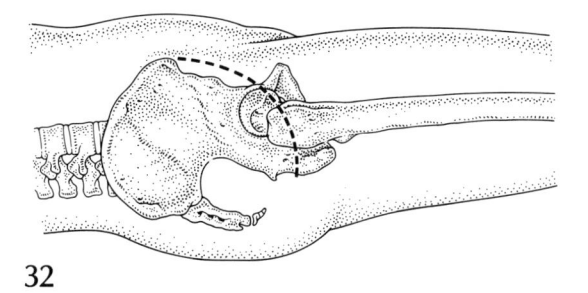

The incision

32

The operation is most easily performed through a curved transverse incision. This starts at the anterior superior iliac spine and passes obliquely down to cross the femur approximately 3–4 cm below the tip of the greater trochanter and then passes upwards and backwards in the line of the fibres of gluteus maximus. The superficial fascia and the fascia lata are divided transversely at the level of the incision. The gluteus maximus is split in the line of its fibres.

Dissection of muscle and capsule

33

The interval between the gluteus medius and the tensor fasciae latae is identified and dissected. At the femoral attachment the anterior fibres covering the attachment of the vastus lateralis are released and posteriorly the piriformis is identified. The greater trochanter is detached using an osteotome, dividing through the epiphysis not the growth-plate. Gluteus medius with its bony attachment is then mobilized and retracted proximally.

The gluteus minimus is now identified and dissected from the capsule so that the latter is now visible anteriorly, superiorly and posteriorly. The object of this part of the dissection is to obtain sufficient capsule to cover the entire femoral head completely. The deficiency is usually on the superior medial aspect of the femoral head; and here, as the capsule is mobilized from the edge of the acetabulum, sharp scissors are used to detach the capsule with the underlying articular cartilage. The remainder of the capsule is then freed from its acetabular attachments, the most difficult aspect of this problem being the posterior inferior aspect of the mobilization.

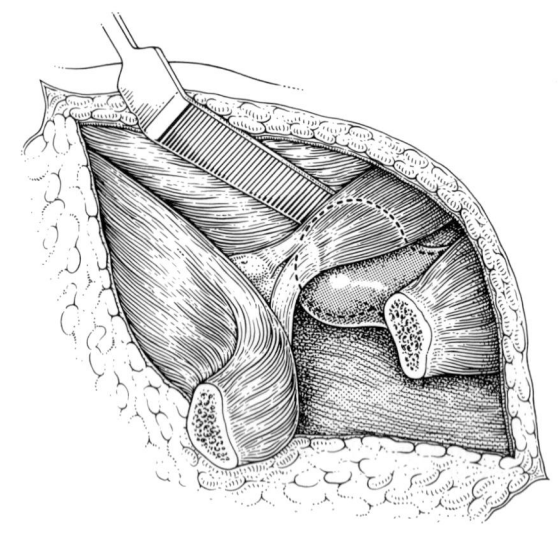

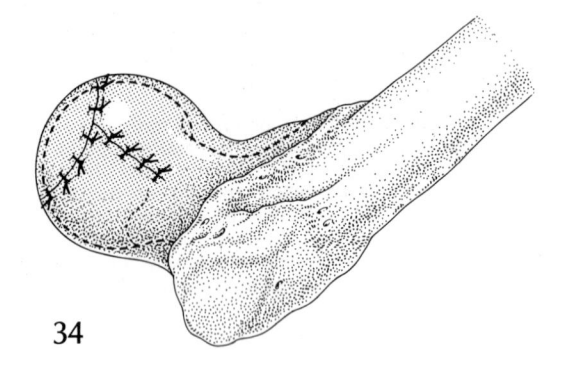

34

The cut surfaces of the capsule are now sutured over the femoral head so that it is covered completely.

Operations for congenital dislocation of the hip 891

Reaming of the acetabulum

35a & b

To obtain a good view of the acetabulum the leg is flexed to 90°, adducted and laterally rotated. By the use of curved gouges and small reamers the acetabulum is enlarged. As this enlargement commences the level of the acetabulum may be judged by noting the presence of the triradiate cartilage which should lie in the centre of the floor of the new acetabulum.

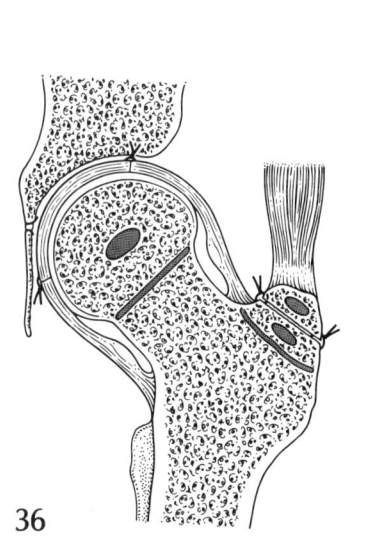

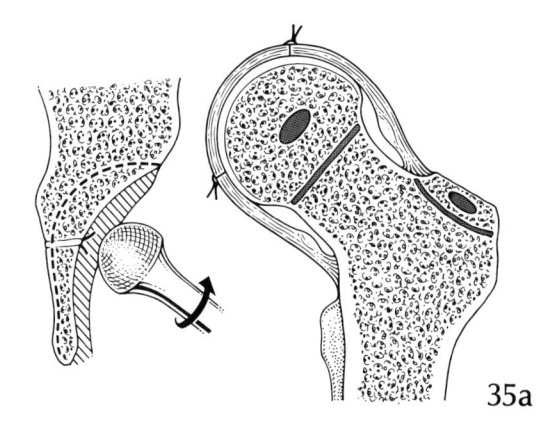

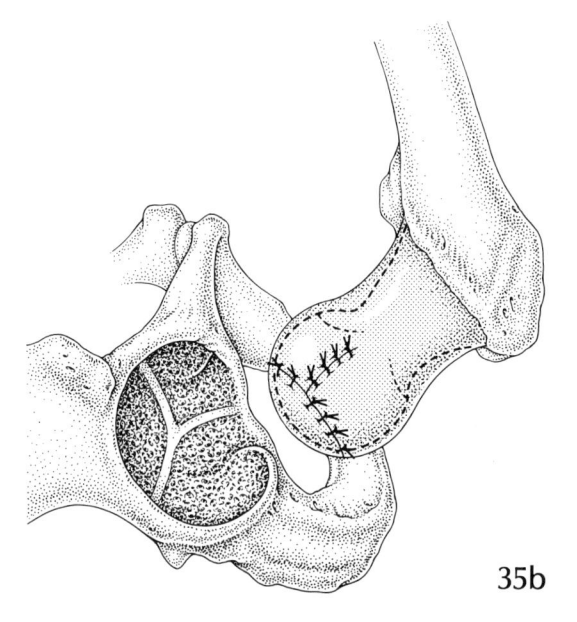

36

When an adequate size of the new acetabulum has been obtained the femoral head, covered by its capsule, is reduced into it and the position of maximum stability assessed. In the majority of cases stability of the femoral head in the neutral position is present but on occasions abduction and medial rotation are required to compensate for persisting anteversion and valgus in the femoral neck. If this is present, a subsequent realignment femoral osteotomy is indicated. The ideal timing for this is 2 weeks later. The capsular repair is then reinspected to be sure that the stitches remain intact and that the femoral head covered by its capsule is placed in the acetabulum.

Reattachment of greater trochanter

Holding the femoral head reduced in the position of maximum stability the greater trochanter is reattached with sutures to the upper shaft in its anatomical position.

Closure

The fascia lata is closed with particular attention to good sutures in the midline. The subcutaneous tissues and skin are closed in the usual way. A one-and-a-half hip spica is applied.

Postoperative management

Routine postoperative management is undertaken. In many of these children blood loss has been excessive and a careful check must be made to be sure that they do not become anaemic. Where a femoral osteotomy is indicated this is performed at 2 weeks after the Colonna operation.

The plaster is removed at 4 weeks and mobilization is started, initially on traction and subsequently with the use of a hydrotherapy pool. When the patient has obtained greater than 60° of flexion and 15° of abduction he may be mobilized on crutches without bearing weight. It is important for good long-term function[4] that the child should remain without weight-bearing for a period of 6 months. In many cases a raise will be required for the opposite shoe. Provided the radiographs are satisfactory at 6 months and show no evidence of avascular necrosis, progressive weight-bearing may be encouraged. Abductor exercises may be required at this stage.

References

1. Hey Groves EW. Reconstructive surgery of the hip. *Br J Surg* 1927; 14: 486–517.

2. Colonna PC. Capsular arthroplasty for congenital dislocation of the hip: indications and technique: some long-term results. *J Bone Joint Surg [Am]* 1965; 47-A: 437–49.

3. Trevor D. The place of the Hey Groves–Colonna operation in the treatment of congenital dislocation of the hip. *Ann R Coll Surg Engl* 1968; 43: 241–58.

4. Pozo JL, Cannon SR, Catterall A. The Colonna–Hey Groves arthroplasty in the late treatment of congenital dislocation of the hip: a long-term review. *J Bone Joint Surg [Br]* 1987; 69-B: 220–8.

Acknowledgement

Illustrations 2 and 3 are drawn after G. Lyth, and 5–9 and 11 after A. Barrett.

Illustrations by Philip Wilson

Innominate osteotomy

A. Catterall MChir, FRCS
Consultant Orthopaedic Surgeon, Charing Cross Hospital, London, and Royal National Orthopaedic Hospital, Stanmore, UK

Introduction

Indications

1. *During open reduction for congenital dislocation of the hip* Open reduction is indicated in the management of congenital dislocation of the hip when either the femoral head cannot be brought opposite the acetabulum by traction or when a concentric congruous reduction cannot be obtained by conservative means. At the time of open reduction a unique opportunity exists to assess the stability of the hip joint to axial load. Innominate osteotomy is indicated where a position of hip flexion is required to maintain the stability of the hip joint (*see* test of stability in the chapter on 'Congenital dislocation of the hip', p. 876).

2. *In acetabular dysplasia with subluxation, when acetabular realignment is indicated* Innominate osteotomy is indicated as a realignment procedure where arthrography has established a reducible subluxation, with flexion required for stability of the hip joint.

3. *In selected cases of Perthes' disease.*

Contraindications

Before an innominate osteotomy is performed the following requirements or prerequisites must be established.

1. A concentric position must be present between the femoral head and acetabulum.
2. There must be a free range of movement in the hip.
3. There should be no fixed deformity in the hip joint.

The operation is therefore contraindicated in the absence of concentricity or in the presence of fixed deformity or restricted movement.

Special requirements

The following equipment will be needed.

A Gigli saw
Two long periosteal elevators
Two deep retractors
O'Shaughnessy forceps
One pair of bone cutters
Two pairs of large towel clips

Operation

When the procedure is being performed as part of an open reduction, access to the hip joint will have already been obtained prior to the innominate osteotomy. Where the operation is performed without other procedures the following procedure is appropriate.

Position of patient

1

The operation is performed under general anaesthesia. The patient is placed with the operation side uppermost in the half-lateral position. A sandbag is placed under the buttock on the operation side.

Incision

The incision is made half-way between the greater trochanter and iliac crest, parallel to the iliac crest and curved downwards at its medial end. It is deepened through the superficial fascia, and the bleeding is controlled. The proximal flap is now retracted over the iliac crest and the remaining fat and fascia incised in the line of the iliac crest. The medial end of the distal flap is freed from the fascia lata.

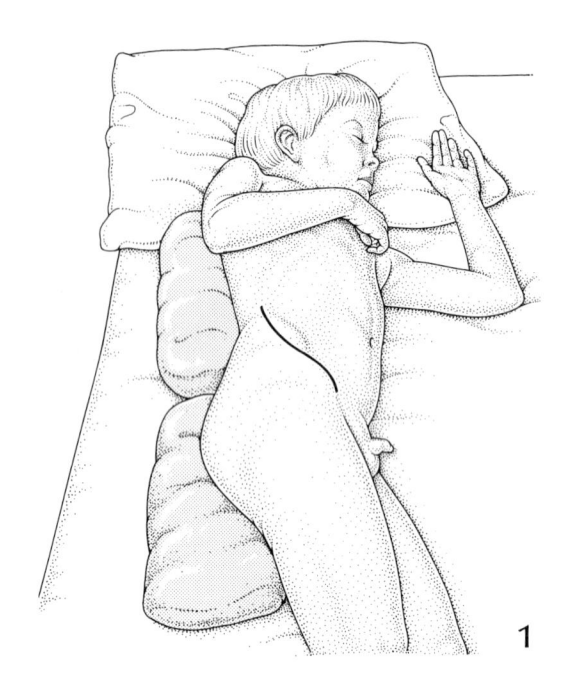

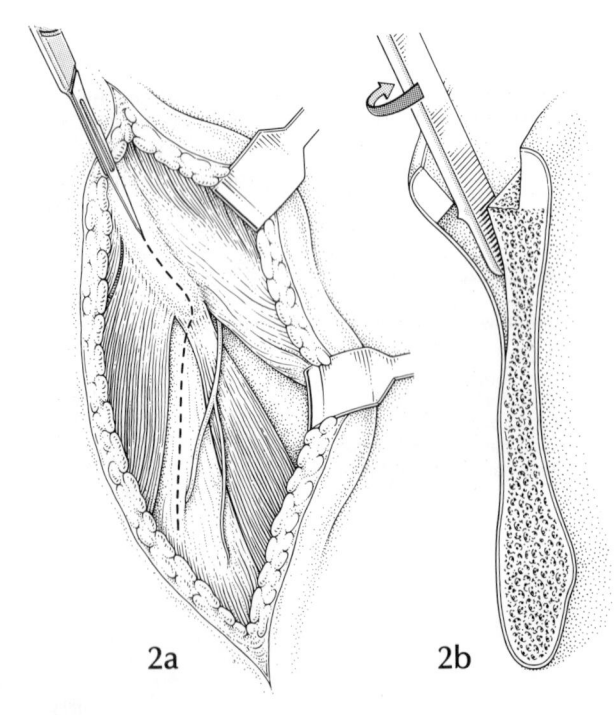

The fascia lata and iliac crest

2a & b

The interval between the sartorius and tensor fasciae latae is identified by a dense white area starting from the anterior superior iliac spine. This is incised and care must be taken to identify and preserve the lateral cutaneous nerve of the thigh. This is retracted medially. The interval is deepened and extended up to the anterior superior spine and the bleeding in the area controlled. The iliac apophysis is now split in the line of the crest and detached from it. The bulbous end of the apophysis passes down deeply towards the anterior inferior iliac spine. The apophysis will not detach from the bone until this has been completely divided. Some prefer to separate the whole apophysis to avoid the possibility of growth disturbance. In the adult, the muscles are detached from the iliac crest. The wing of the ilium is now exposed subperiosteally as far back as the sciatic notch.

Innominate osteotomy 895

Release of the capsule

3

Gluteus minimus is elevated from the capsule so that the attachments of the capsule, particularly posteriorly, can be identified. This allows the level of the osteotomy to be identified.

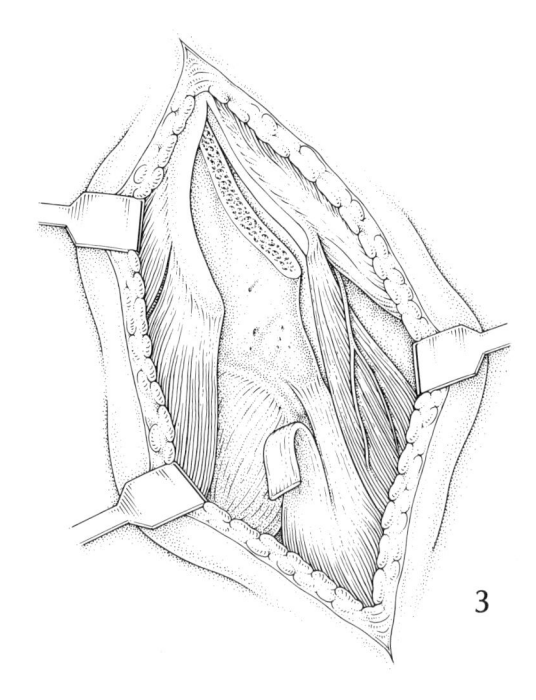

Release of the tendon of the psoas

4

The elevated periosteum from the medial side of the ilium is now incised to allow mobilization of the psoas muscle. Once the muscle has been mobilized a finger is passed under its deep surface and the tendon of the psoas identified by extending and medially rotating the hip. The hip is now flexed and a retractor placed under the deep surface. The tendon which lies in the substance of the muscle is now divided leaving the remainder of the muscle intact. Care must be taken not to damage the femoral nerve which is in a direct anterior and medial position to the psoas. When the hip is now brought into full extension no tightness can be felt in the deep surface of the muscle.

The stability of the joint to axial loading is now assessed. As the hip is flexed and abducted the prominence or lump of the anterolateral aspect of the femoral head can be felt to reduce into the acetabulum confirming that a reducible subluxation is present.

Dissection of the sciatic notch and passage of Gigli saw

5a, b & c

The sciatic notch is approached subperiosteally from the medial and lateral aspects. On the lateral side it may be visualized. A clean dissection is obtained by advancing the long periosteal dissector and then rotating it through 90°. The point of the O'Shaughnessy forceps is now passed from medial to lateral through the sciatic notch and then opened to receive the end of a Gigli saw. Care must be taken to ensure that there is no soft tissue between the forceps and the bone as the Gigli saw is passed through the sciatic notch.

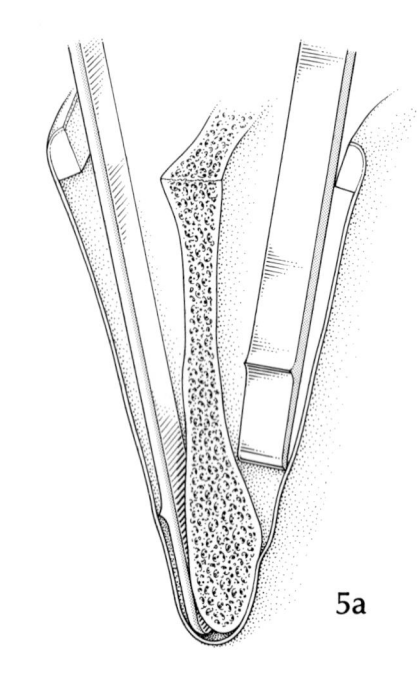

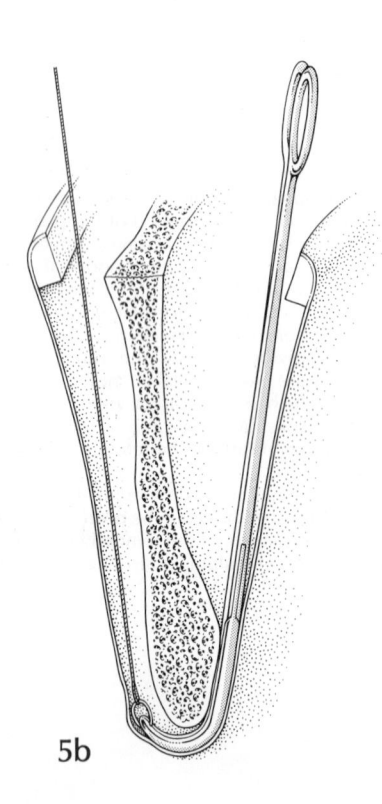

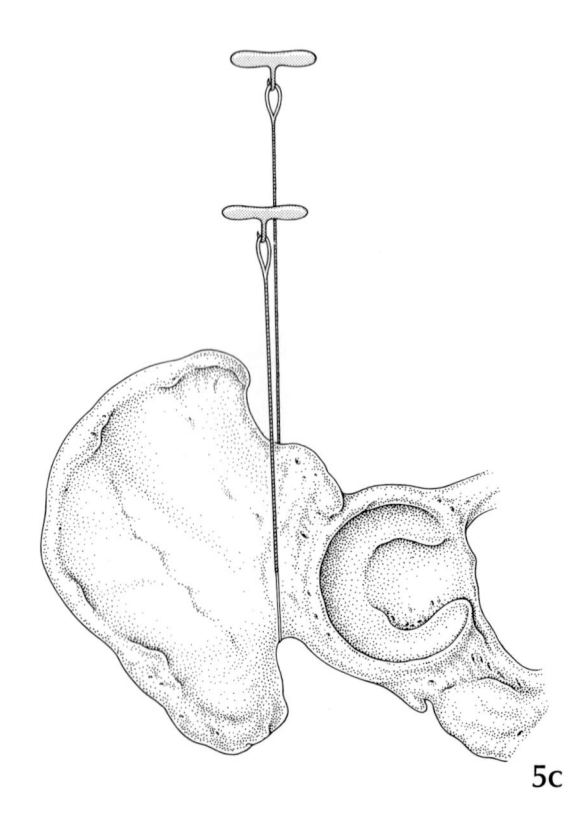

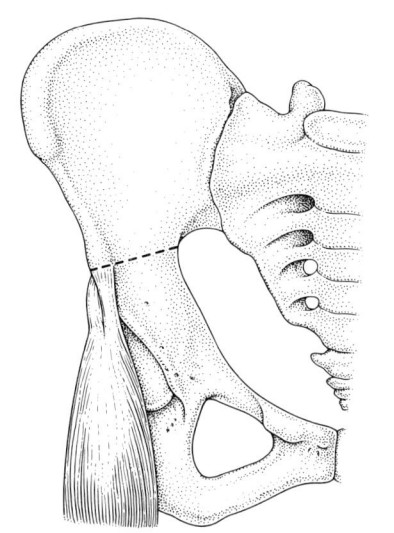

Osteotomy

6a & b

The pelvis is now divided in a line from the sciatic notch to the anterior inferior iliac spine.

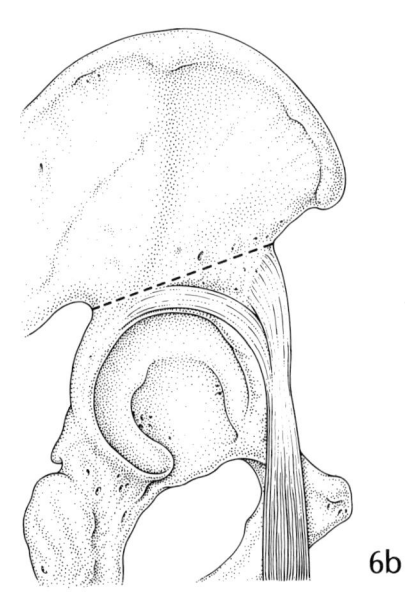

6a

6b

Displacement

7a, b & c

The object of the realignment is to produce an anterolateral buttress to prevent further subluxation or uncovering of the femoral head. This is achieved by rotating the acetabular fragment forward and laterally with the centre of the rotation at the posterior margin of the sciatic notch (arrowed in the illustration) and the symphysis pubis. The graft to fill the defect produced by the displacement is obtained from the iliac crest. This is best cut by large bone cutters before displacing the fragment.

Towel clips are secured into both fragments, the upper one to hold the wing of the ilium still while the lower acetabular fragment is moved. The lower fragment is now rotated forward and laterally; this process is facilitated by flexing, abducting and laterally rotating the leg. This is achieved by placing the foot of the operated leg on the opposite knee and then extending and abducting the hip by pressing down on the ipsilateral knee. As the displacement occurs care must be taken not to allow the acetabular fragment to slip backwards. The two pelvic fragments must be in contact at the sciatic notch. The position is stabilized by one or two Kirschner wires, or thin Steinmann pins.

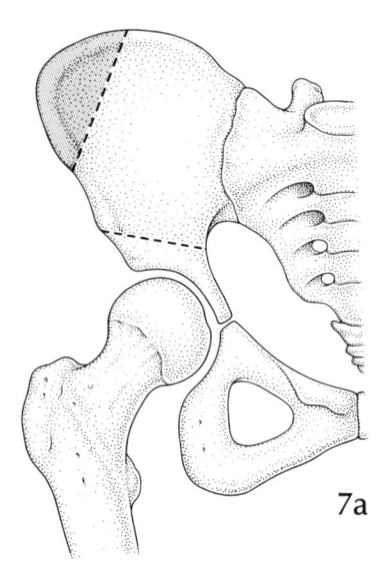

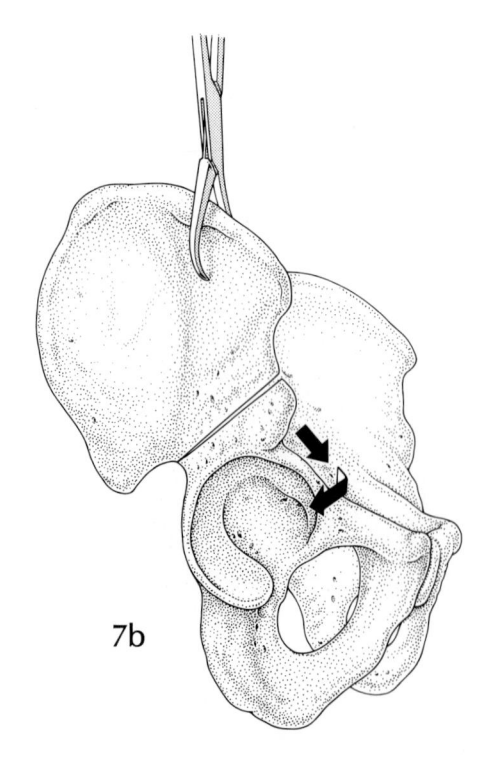

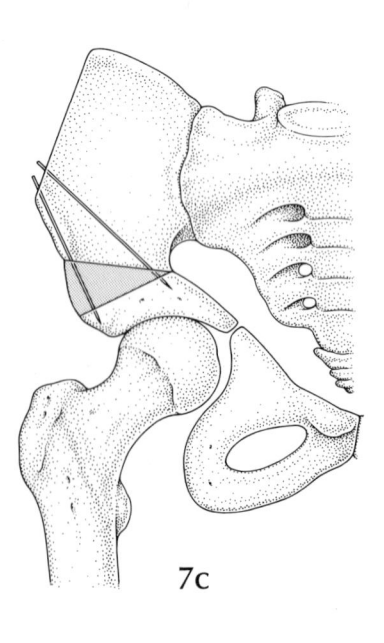

Closure

8a & b

When the osteotomy has been performed as part of an open reduction the capsule is repaired as described in the chapter on 'Congenital dislocation of the hip' (pp. 870–892). The iliac apophysis is approximated by strong interrupted sutures. The hip is flexed to reduce the tension as the layers are approximated. As the fascia over the thigh is repaired care must be taken not to include the lateral cutaneous nerve of the thigh in the sutures. The subcutaneous tissues are sutured and the skin closed, either with interrupted sutures or a continuous subcuticular wire stitch.

Postoperative management

In the younger child it is convenient to immobilize the child in a plaster hip spica as this results in less pain and an early discharge from hospital. At 6 weeks the child is readmitted for mobilization, usually for 3–5 days. In the older child, if adequate fixation has been obtained by the Kirschner wires or Steinmann pins, the patient may be nursed on 'slings and springs' until the wound is healed. Mobilization is then permitted, initially on crutches without weight-bearing for 6 weeks. After this time partial weight-bearing is permitted for 3–4 weeks. Provided that radiographs at this stage show union of the osteotomy and incorporation of the graft, full mobilization is then permitted.

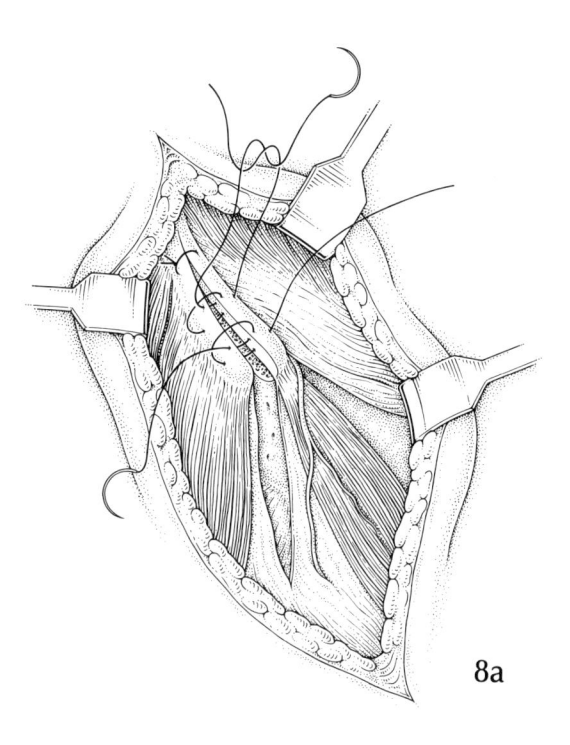

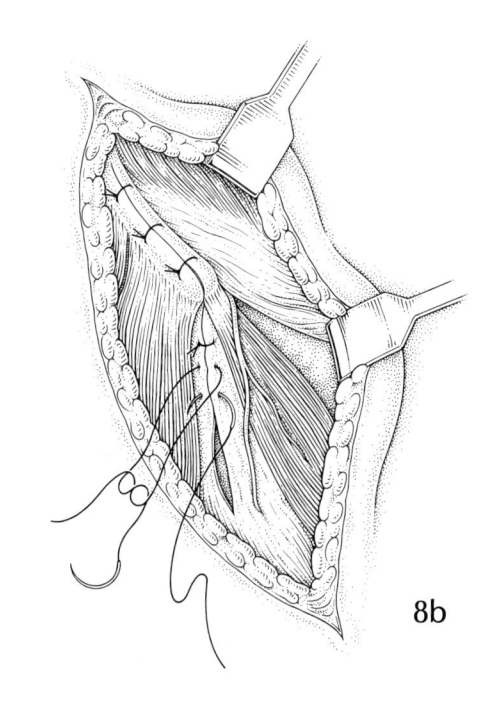

Illustrations by Paul Richardson after J. M. P. Booth

High femoral osteotomy in childhood

E. W. Somerville FRCS (Ed), FRCS
Emeritus Consultant Orthopaedic Surgeon, Nuffield Orthopaedic Centre, Oxford, UK

Introduction

During the past 20 years the importance of the shape of the upper end of the femur and the femoral head in relation to the development of the hip joint has become increasingly apparent. The object of the operation is to correct any faulty mechanics which may be present so that the hip joint may be allowed to develop normally. For this reason the operation is carried out in children, sometimes very young children, because it is only when growth is rapid that it can provide the maximum benefit.

Indications

Persistent fetal alignment of the hip (persistence of an excessive degree of anteversion of the neck of the femur)

In this condition, because of the excessive anteversion, there will be 90° of medial rotation but minimal or no lateral rotation when the hip is in extension. This may lead to secondary deformities of lateral tibial torsion and valgus foot, which are ugly and may cause clumsiness. It is not yet certain whether or not this condition predisposes to osteoarthritis. The object of the operation is to restore a normal arc of rotation, i.e. 45° medial rotation and 45° lateral, preferably before the secondary deformities have developed. The operation is therefore a simple rotation osteotomy.

Congenital dislocation of the hip

In this condition anteversion plays some part in the actual initial displacement and following the dislocation it increases still further. A not uncommon cause for gradual redisplacement is a recurrence of anteversion and the development of a valgus deformity. Even if there is no valgus deformity, creation of some varus improves the stability of the joint.

Details of the specific use for this condition will be found in the chapter on 'Congenital dislocation of the hip' (pp. 870–892).

Perthes' disease

In this condition there is no anteversion and no coxa valga but a small rotation and varus osteotomy will provide better cover of the femoral head, allowing early mobilization and weight-bearing instead of a prolonged period of splintage.

Congenital coxa vara

In this condition there is a congenital abnormality of the upper end of the femur which leads to a progressive varus deformity due to growth. This condition will not correct spontaneously and will need surgical correction in all cases.

Operations

ROTATION OSTEOTOMY

This operation is performed for persistent fetal alignment of the hip, congenital dislocation of the hip and Perthes' disease.

1

The child is placed on the operating table in the supine position without a sandbag under the hip. The limb is held in medial rotation by an assistant and a straight incision is made on the outer side of the thigh with its upper limit just below the prominence of the great trochanter. It is about 8 cm long and is slightly oblique forwards from above downwards so that when the rotation has been carried out the incision will become vertical. The degree of obliquity will be determined by the amount of rotation obtained at the osteotomy.

The iliotibial band is split in line with its fibres, exposing the fibres of the vastus lateralis. The fascia overlying the posterior part of the muscle belly is divided in length over the posterior fibres close to the linea aspera. The muscle fibres are separated by blunt dissection. This does less damage to the small blood vessels, reducing the amount of bleeding and thereby producing less ischaemia as compared with sharp division. The periosteum is exposed and is divided in length with a knife; small bone levers are introduced anteriorly and posteriorly to the bone inside the periosteum. There may be some difficulty with the posterior lever because of the linea aspera, which may need separating from the bone with a knife.

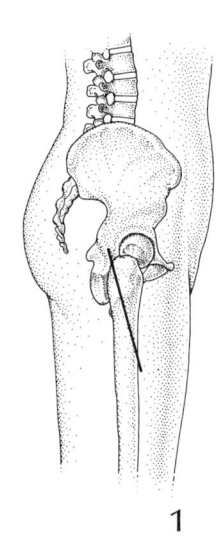

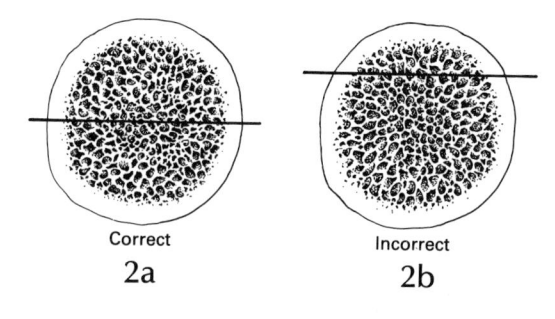

2a & b

A Steinmann pin is introduced into the lateral aspect of the upper femur just below the greater trochanter. It must traverse the diameter of the bone and penetrate through the opposite cortex.

3

To prevent sudden penetration of the pin it is wise to place over it a simple guard made from a metal tube of the appropriate length. A small Venable plate is slipped onto the pin through its upper hole and the plate laid along the bone. A second pin is introduced anterior to the plate and in line with the uppermost of the lower two holes and at the angle required for rotation. (In persistent fetal alignment 45°, in congenital dislocation of the hip 70° and in Perthes' disease 30°). Again it is of great importance that the pin traverse the diameter. The angle is checked by an assistant standing at the foot of the table in line with the femur with a goniometer set at the appropriate angle.

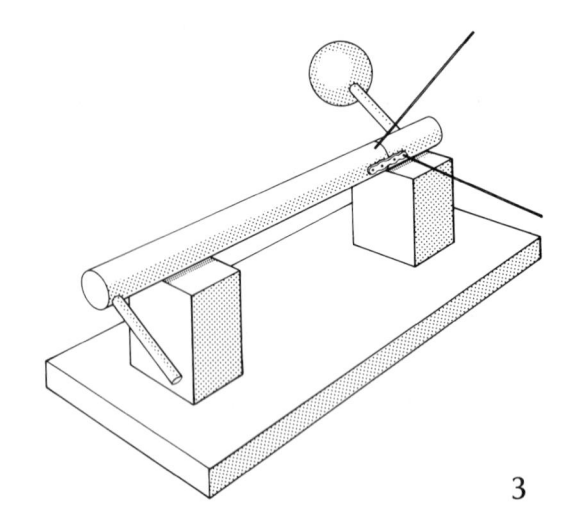

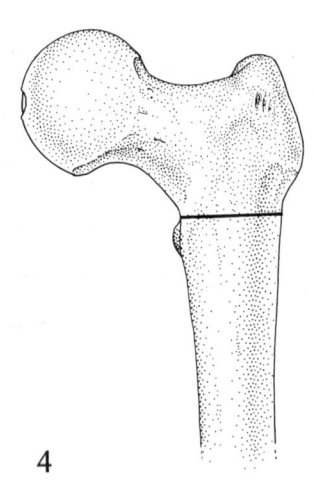

4

The plate is removed. A broad bone lever replaces the small one posteriorly and is rotated through 90° to ensure complete separation of the soft tissues so that they will not interfere with rotation. The small lever anteriorly is also turned on edge and the bone is divided with a saw. The division of the bone must be at right angles.

5

The distal fragment is then rotated until the pins are parallel. If there is difficulty in doing this it will be found that the pin has penetrated too far into the soft tissues on the medial side; if the lower pin is withdrawn a little the rotation can be performed easily. The plate is slipped back onto the pins.

The lowest hole is drilled first and screwed, which will ensure that the plate is properly placed. The lower hole in the upper part is similarly treated. The lower pin is removed and if the pin was of the right size it will not be necessary to drill the hole before the screw is inserted. Lastly the upper pin is removed and that hole screwed. The wound is closed in layers with care to put the minimum of stitches in the muscle and not to tie them tight to avoid ischaemia.

The operation can easily be performed bilaterally when necessary, but in a child under the age of 2 years it is better to operate on the two legs at an interval of 1 or 2 weeks.

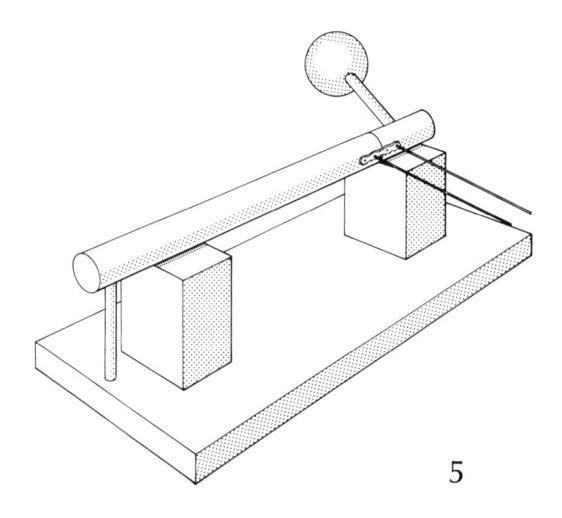

Postoperative management

A long hip spica is applied with the leg abducted 45°. In the small child the other leg should always be included down to the knee to prevent it adducting and being damaged.

The length of immobilization will depend on the age of the child. Under 6 or 7 years it will take 6 weeks, up to 12 years 8 weeks and after that 10 weeks to 3 months. As soon as the plaster is removed mobilization can be started, at first in the therapy pool then on dry land. Progress can be as rapid as the child can tolerate. After these operations the child will limp and it is always wise to warn the parents of this in advance so that they will not be disappointed. In a small child the limp will last only a few weeks but in a teenage child it may last many months and sometimes even as long as a year.

Prevention of complications

This is an operation which has no important complications provided it has been performed properly, but the following points are essential. The pins must pass through the diameter of the bone. The bone must be divided at a right angle. The lower screw must be inserted first to ensure the position of the plate, and if the bone is porotic, as is sometimes the case in the very young child, the screws should be introduced at different angles and not parallel to each other. While the operation can be performed at any age it is wise not to do it under 9 months of age since the bone is too small.

904   Pelvis and hip

ROTATION OSTEOTOMY COMBINED WITH VARUS

This operation may be required in the treatment of congenital dislocation of the hip and in Perthes' disease with the signs of a 'head at risk'.

In the younger child

The exposure and preliminary part of the operation are as described for rotation osteotomy, but special care must be taken to ensure that the top pin is introduced accurately into the lateral side of the femur and as near to the epiphyseal plate as is consistent with safety. In the upper part of the wound the white cartilaginous epiphysis of the greater trochanter will be visible and the pin is introduced immediately below this. The plate is slipped onto this pin and the second pin is introduced as previously described. The bone is divided as high as possible, allowing room for the introduction of the second screw. The end of the lower fragment is drawn out of the wound by adducting the leg and using the pin as a lever.

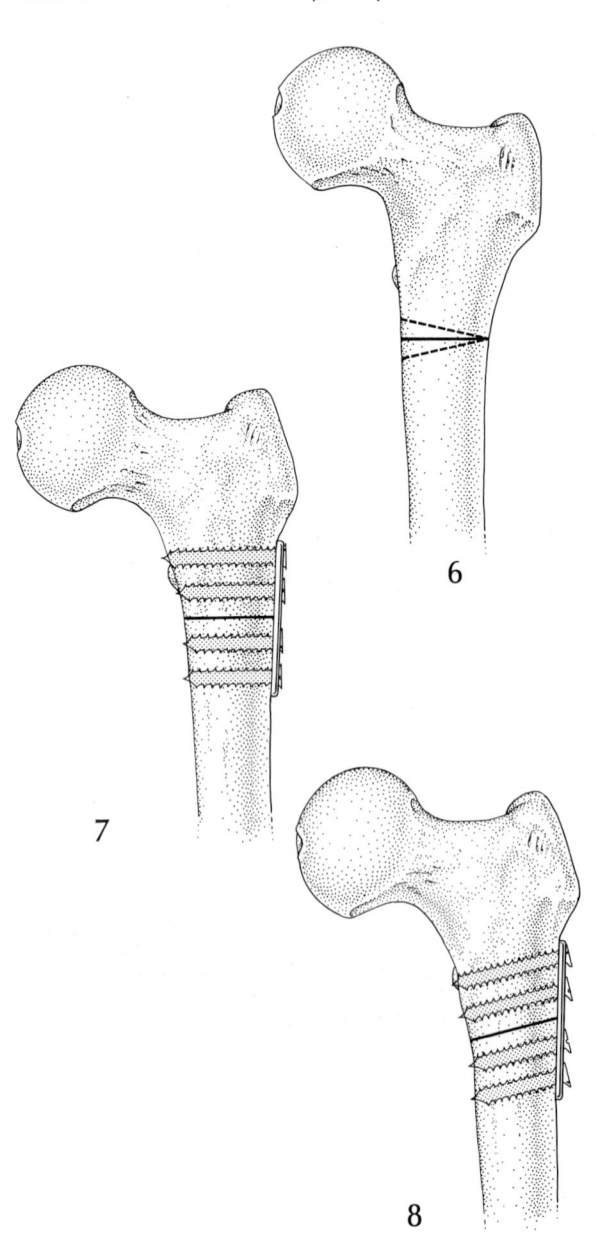

6

Using gouge-ended nibblers, a suitable amount of cortex is removed from the side of the bone where the point of the pin emerges, which when the lower fragment has been rotated will become the medial side. It is usual to remove sufficient bone to allow a varus angulation of 10° or 20°. The displacement is reduced, the pins held parallel to each other in the horizontal plane and the plate slipped on to the pins as previously described for rotation osteotomy.

7 & 8

There is often a flare of the greater trochanter sufficiently great so that when the necessary angulation has been achieved the outer side of the femur will be straight and it will be unnecessary to bend the plate.

If this can be done it gives a much better result cosmetically but if it is not possible the plate must be bent to the appropriate angle to fit accurately.

Although the production of varus by the removal of a wedge adds an extra manoeuvre, it makes the application of the plate and the introduction of the screws simpler than in a straight rotation osteotomy. This is because the fragments are more stable and there is little or no risk of losing or increasing the amount of rotation. Fixation and closure are the same as already described.

In the older child

This operation is a modification of the previous procedure which is employed in the relapsing congenitally dislocated hip.

Leg length must be taken more seriously into account. The production of varus will cause some shortening and a medial wedge will increase the shortening even further. In most cases this is of no great importance because the leg will be too long initially and it is desirable in these cases for the leg to be a little too short rather than a little too long. However, there are some cases where it is desirable to reduce the shortening to a minimum.

The preliminaries of the operation are as already described but in the older child the bone is often too hard for the wedge to be removed with nibblers and a saw must be used.

The pins are introduced as already described, preferably by hand, because they will get a much better grip on the bone than if they are introduced with a drill and this may be helpful in subsequent manipulations. If varus without rotation is required the pins are placed parallel and in the same plane; otherwise the manoeuvres are exactly the same as described below.

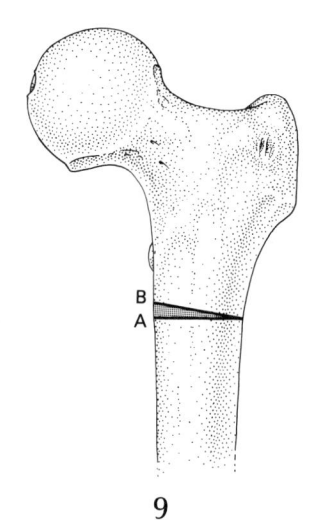

Removal of a medial bone wedge with rotation

9

The site of the osteotomy is selected as high as possible and a cut is made with the saw transversely half-way through the bone at A. This will be the lower cut. The upper cut is made at the required angle and is carried right through the bone at B. The angle of the wedge will be the angle of varus to be obtained. The lower cut is completed and the wedge is removed. If the lower cut is completed first it will be very difficult to control the upper fragment while completing the upper cut. The medial gap produced by removal of the wedge can then be closed, using the pins as levers, and the lower fragment can be rotated on the upper without further altering the angulation because the lower cut was made transversely. The plate, which in the larger child will need to be somewhat bigger, is applied in the manner described.

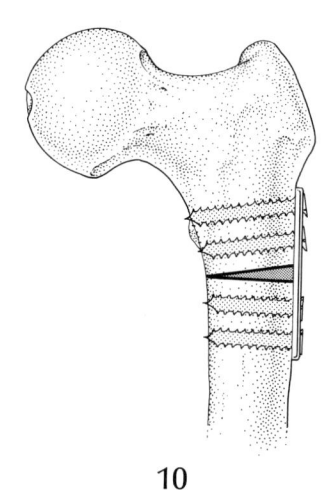

Reversed wedge osteotomy

10

If it is desirable to reduce the amount of shortening which will occur, a bone wedge as already described is removed in one piece from the medial side, is reversed and placed in the lateral side of the osteotomy, thus obtaining twice the angulation with half the wedge.

Opening wedge osteotomy

11

The degree of shortening can be reduced still further by not removing any wedge but opening the osteotomy on the outer side. A simple transverse cut is made as high as possible and the necessary degree of rotation obtained. The pins are separated to the required angle and the plate, bent as required, is applied to the pins and screwed in position.

In this operation and the previous one described, when angulation has been achieved the distance between the pins will have been increased and this increase must be allowed for when the screws are being introduced.

Up to the age of 12 years it is unnecessary to place any bone in the gap produced as it will fill in spontaneously. After this age it is probably wise to introduce a wedge of bone taken from the iliac crest.

Level of osteotomy

12

It is desirable, when producing varus, to make the osteotomy as high as possible. In many patients this can be done as described but in some it is difficult. In these cases the anterior surface of the upper end of the femur, including the base of the neck, is cleared. The angulation and rotation are obtained as described using the pins, but instead of the plate being threaded on to the pins it is placed anteriorly as high as possible with the upper screw passing through the base of the neck anteroposteriorly. Not infrequently the osteotomy can be carried out as much as 2 cm higher.

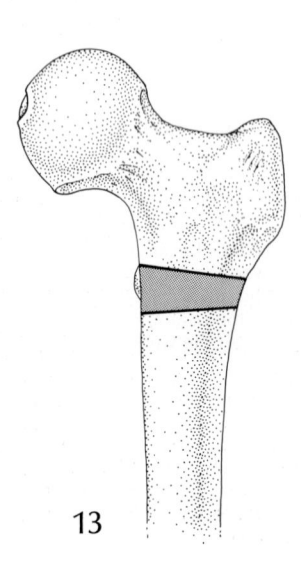

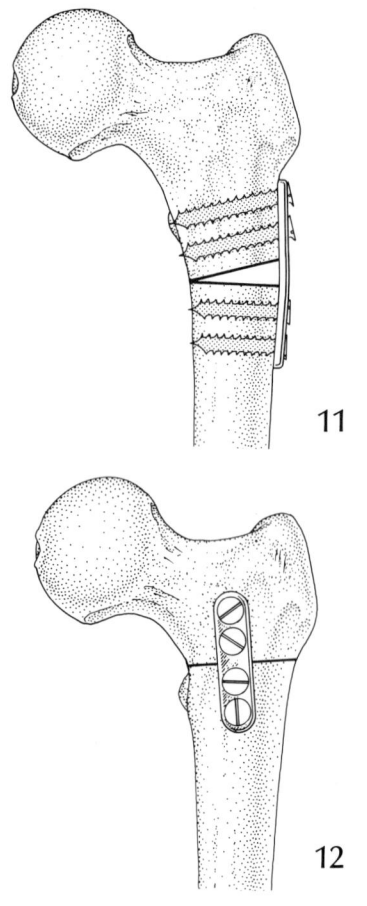

Shortening osteotomy

13

Occasionally the leg will have overgrown to a degree which makes it necessary to shorten it deliberately by more than will result from the varus and the wedge together. In such a case further shortening can be obtained by removing a trapezoid, with the base medial. The length of the opposite limb determines the degree of shortening to be obtained.

Other forms of internal fixation

Other forms of internal fixation have been described such as the Coventry plate and screw and the miniature nail–plate of Blundell-Jones. These have the advantage of making it possible to do the osteotomy a little higher but they are bulkier and, in the auther's opinion, the insertion of the appliance up the neck of the femur creates the risk of damage to the growth-plate if not placed with great accuracy.

Correction of congenital coxa vara

Congenital coxa vara is a growth defect of the upper end of the femur. In the most severe types complete absence of the upper end of the femur is simulated for a time after birth. In the less severe types growth of the capital side of the metaphysis is severely interfered with while the greater trochanter continues to grow normally. This results in an increasing varus deformity, the severity of which depends on the severity of the growth disturbance. Since this is a growth disturbance spontaneous correction will not occur and corrective osteotomy, which may have to be repeated, will be required. For this reason the initial osteotomy should not be performed too early.

ROBERT JONES VALGUS OSTEOTOMY

The child is placed on the operating table with a small sandbag under the hip to be operated on. An incision is made from above the tip of the greater trochanter along the line of the femur for about 10 cm. The anterior and lateral aspects of the greater trochanter and the upper end of the femur are exposed subperiosteally.

14

With a hand saw the bone is divided from just below the prominence of the greater trochanter downwards and medially to just above the lesser trochanter, strictly in the anteroposterior plane.

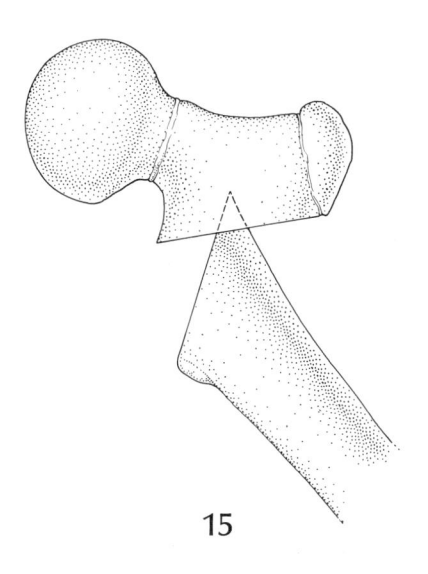

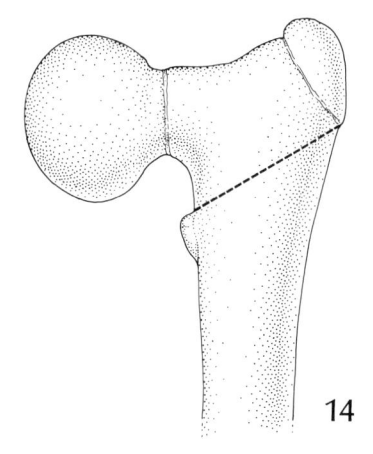

15

Posteriorly the periosteum is divided so that the lower fragment may be pulled downwards and angled so that the sharp spike can be driven into the medullary cavity in the proximal fragment below the midpoint of the neck.

This will permit the upper fragment to tilt downwards, allowing the wide abduction which is an essential part of the operation. Obtaining the necessary degree of abduction may be very difficult. In this case the introduction of a Steinmann pin into the upper fragment to stabilize it may help, but it may be necessary to tenotomize the adductors. This must be done with great care because if it is overdone all stability may be lost and it will be very difficult to maintain the required position. Rather than risk this it is better to shorten the bone by removing just enough of the spike to allow abduction with a tight fit. In this operation the use of internal fixation is difficult and unsatisfactory and is better avoided.

Postoperative management

A plaster spica is applied enclosing both legs in wide abduction even if only one side is being treated. It is difficult to achieve too much abduction. Union is usually sound in 2–3 months in the older child and sooner in the younger.

When union has occurred mobilization in bed and in a therapy pool can be started at once but, because of the wide abduction, may at first be slow; weight-bearing cannot be begun until adduction is almost complete.

Since this is a growth deformity some recurrence is inevitable (the younger the child at the time of operation the greater the recurrence). The parents must be warned in advance of the risk that the operation may need repeating when the child is older. By performing two operations rather than waiting until the deformity is very great before operating for the first time, the final deformity will be less.

908 Pelvis and hip

WEDGE OSTEOTOMY

16

An alternative operation is carried out through the same incision, exposing the anterolateral aspect of the upper end of the femur. With a mechanically operated reciprocating saw, an incomplete oblique cut is made from the prominence on the lateral aspect of the greater trochanter downwards towards the calcar but not extending through the calcar. A step is then cut. A wedge is removed as indicated by the shaded area.

The cuts are all completed, the periosteum is divided posteriorly and the wedge is closed with wide abduction.

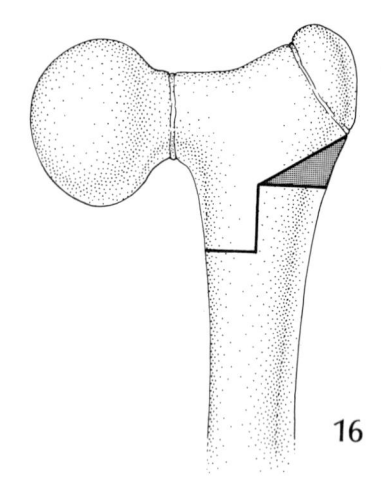

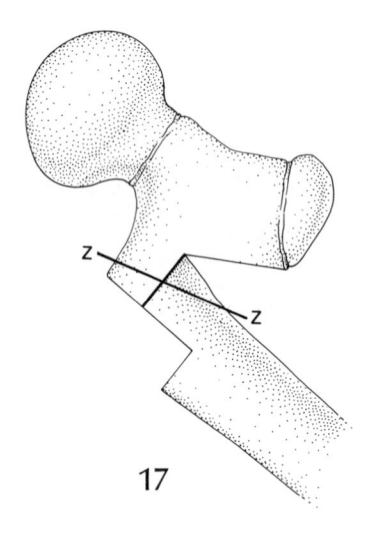

17

This operation usually retains a good degree of stability so that internal fixation should not be necessary, but it is not difficult to place a screw across the osteotomy if it is considered advisable (Z–Z).

In this operation the osteotomy is more difficult to cut and there is no increase in length, but in spite of this it is the simpler procedure and less prone to complications such as displacement.

Postoperative management

A plaster spica is applied enclosing both legs in wide abduction (90° between the two). Union usually occurs in 2–3 months. A check anteroposterior radiograph is taken to verify the position of the osteotomy. After 2 months the plaster is bivalved and a check radiograph out of plaster is taken.

If union is commencing, mobilization under physiotherapy supervision in hospital with daily pool therapy will rapidly restore the patient to normal activity. Weight-bearing begins when adduction is normal.

Illustrations by Peter Cox

Slipped upper femoral epiphysis

M. J. Griffith MChOrth, FRCS, FRCS(Ed)
Consultant Orthopaedic Surgeon, West Wales General Hospital, Carmarthen, UK

Introduction

The treatment of slipped upper femoral epiphysis is a controversial topic. Many questions remain unanswered. Surgical treatment will, at best, be misguided unless the surgeon has a clear three-dimensional concept of the deformity. An understanding of the surgical anatomy is an essential prerequisite to surgical intervention.

Surgical anatomy

1, 2, 3 & 4

The epiphysis slips backwards and downwards following the curved surface of the adolescent growth-plate. The slipped epiphysis lies directly behind the neck of the femur so that the appearance on routine anteroposterior radiographs is influenced by the effect of parallax. Radiographs taken with the leg in lateral rotation will show the epiphysis lying medial to the neck (varus). With the leg in medial rotation the epiphysis appears to lie lateral to the neck (valgus)[1].

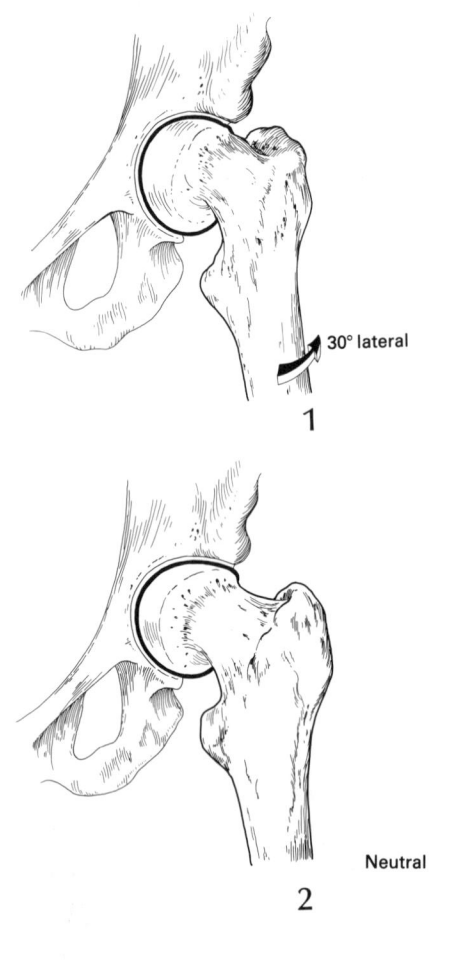

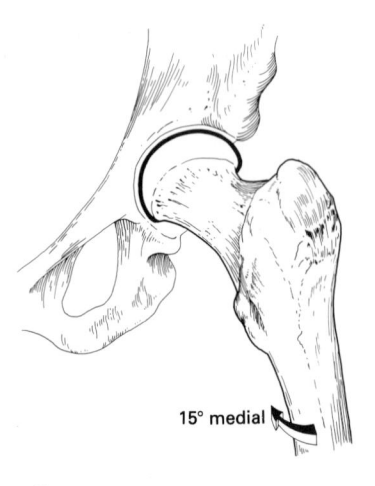

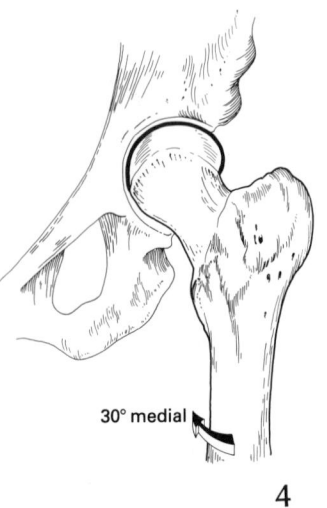

5 & 6

As the epiphysis slips backwards it strips the periosteum on the posterior aspect of the neck. New bone is laid down beneath the stripped periosteum, forming a bony beak at the back of the metaphysis. The exposed anterior aspect of the neck almost always resorbs. The only significant residual blood supply to the epiphysis is through the retinacular vessels that run in the periosteum on the back of the neck; any surgical intervention must preserve these vessels.

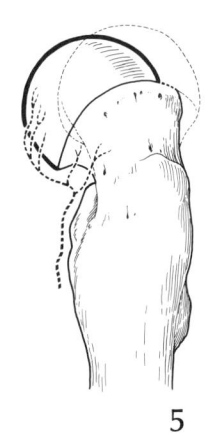

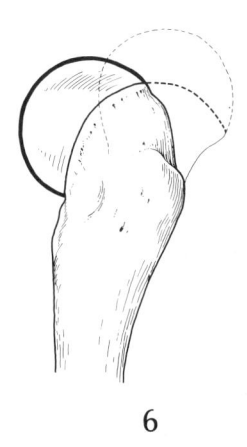

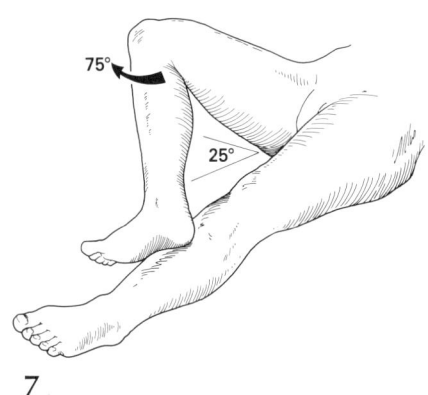

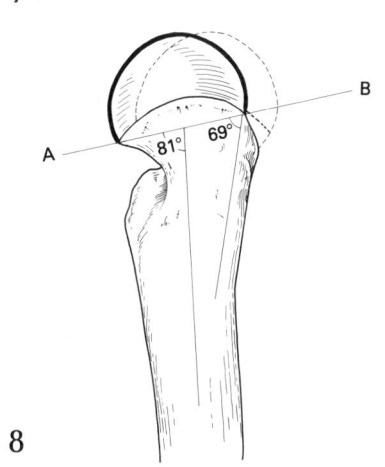

7 & 8

The severity of the slip is determined on frog lateral views of the hip. The patient lies supine and the X-ray tube is centred on the hip joint. The femur is laterally rotated 75° (90° minus anteversion angle) and elevated at an angle of 25° from the table (plane of inclination of the epiphysis on anteroposterior film), the knee is flexed to 90° and the lateral edge of the foot rested on the contralateral leg. The angle between the base of the epiphysis (A-B) and both the neck and the shaft of the femur are measured. In the normal hip the mean of these two angles is 90°. Subtracting the measured mean angle from 90° gives an accurate measure of the degree of slip[2]. Thus in Illustration 8 the degree of slip is $90° - \dfrac{81° + 69°}{2} = 15°$.

CHOICE OF TREATMENT

A number of factors determine the choice of treatment.

Severity of slipping

The functional result in patients with slight slipping does not deteriorate with the passage of time whereas those with severe slipping will show progressive impairment of function due to osteoarthritis[3]. Patients with up to 30° (about one-third diameter) slip do not require correction of the deformity and are regarded as acceptable (*see Illustration 8*). Patients with over 50° (about half diameter) slip have permanent restriction of movement and tend to develop premature osteoarthritis. They require correction of the deformity which is regarded as unacceptable. Between these two extremes there is a grey area where the treatment will depend on the existing functional disability and the individual surgeon's experience. The premature onset of osteoarthritis is a lesser evil than iatrogenic avascular necrosis or chondrolysis. The author is reluctant to correct deformities of less than 50° slip[4].

State of the growth-plate

The need for internal fixation and the choice of osteotomy depends on whether the growth-plate remains open or closed. An open growth-plate carries the risk of further slipping.

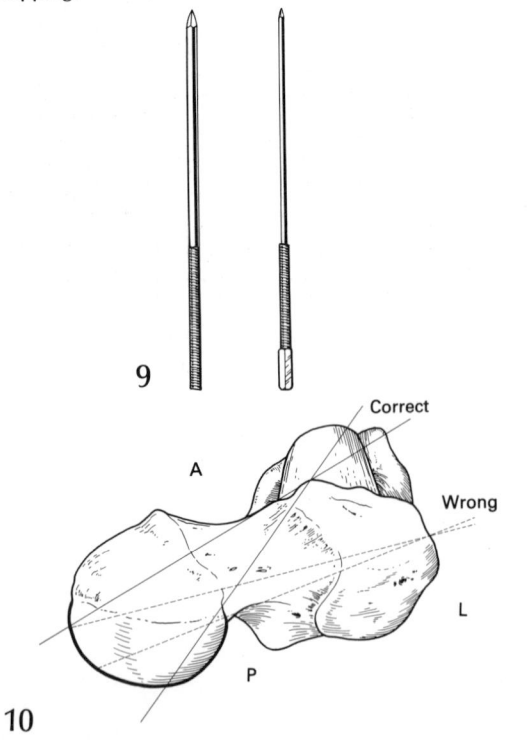

Presence of an acute component to the slip

This increases the vulnerability of the blood supply to the epiphysis.

Special considerations

Treatment may have to be modified if the patient has avascular necrosis, chondrolysis, osteoarthritic changes, renal failure or gross hormonal imbalance.

Specific treatment will be considered under four broad categories depending on whether the severity of the slip is acceptable or unacceptable and whether the growth-plate is open or closed.

Acceptable deformity with growth-plate open

Irrespective of whether the slip is gradual or acute these patients should be treated by urgent internal fixation to prevent further slipping. Bone graft epiphysiodesis[5] is equally effective and should be considered when rapid closure of the growth-plate is required. The reader should consult the original paper and that of Melby *et al*[6].

TECHNIQUE OF PINNING *IN SITU*

9 & 10

The procedure is performed on a radiotranslucent operating table. The patient lies in the prone position and the affected leg draped to allow its free movement. An image intensifier is placed so as to give an anteroposterior picture of the hip.

Through a lateral approach the femur is exposed immediately below the greater trochanter. A fine threaded pin in which the thread stands proud of the wire, such as a Moore's (left) or Crawford Adams pin (right), is recommended as it is easier to remove at a later date. The pin is introduced through the anterolateral cortex just below the trochanteric ridge and drilled towards the epiphysis. Once the pin just crosses the growth-plate on the anteroposterior radiograph, the leg is placed in the frog lateral position and a true lateral radiograph of the neck and epiphysis obtained. Provided the pin lies in a suitable direction it can then be advanced to lie just below the articular cartilage.

Two further pins are then introduced in the same manner so that the tips of the pins engage different segments of the epiphysis. The hip should then be screened with the image intensifier to ensure as far as possible that pin penetration of the joint has not occurred.

Common errors of technique

1. The use of a fracture table. It is impossible to obtain true lateral radiographs with the shoot-through technique which is done on a fracture table. This makes pin placement even more difficult and increases the risk of pin penetration of the joint. There are also theoretical risks to blood supply of the epiphysis in the use of a fracture table.
2. Failure to appreciate that the epiphysis slips behind the neck. The technique is quite different to that used for a femoral neck fracture. The pin should be introduced from the anterolateral cortex (see Illustration 10); and if the slipping is severe, from the anterior aspect of the femur.
3. Multiple entry holes. These should be avoided as far as possible because they may so weaken the femur as to result in a subsequent fracture.
4. Pin placement in the distal one-third of the epiphysis may endanger the retinacular vessels in moderate or severe slipping.

Postoperative management

When the slipping is gradual the patient may be allowed up, with partial weight-bearing, in 2–3 days and resume full weight-bearing in 10–14 days. When the slipping is acute, the patient should rest in bed for 10 days and then avoid weight-bearing for 4–6 weeks. Patients should remain under surveillance and avoid contact sports or strenuous activities until the growth-plate is closed.

Acceptable deformity with growth-plate closed

No treatment is required and the patient is reassured.

Unacceptable deformity with growth-plate open

It is generally agreed that the more severe degrees of slip require correction of the deformity. Closed reduction, either by manipulation under anaesthesia or traction, carries an unacceptable risk to the blood supply of the epiphysis and should not be undertaken[1]. Some improvement in the range of hip movement is achieved by removal of the exposed anterior surface of the metaphysis (osteoplasty). In the author's experience this part of the neck almost always absorbs spontaneously, rendering the procedure unnecessary. In the rare cases where this does not occur, as judged on a true lateral radiograph, an osteoplasty as described by Heyman, Herndon and Strong[7] may be indicated in patients with moderate slipping (30°–50°).

Anatomical reduction is most accurately achieved by open replacement of the femoral epiphysis[8]. The initial results included a significant incidence of avascular necrosis but more recent results[9] have shown a very low incidence of complications.

The procedure demands meticulous attention to detail and should only be undertaken if the surgeon has a clear understanding of the deformity to be corrected and is confident that he can protect the residual blood supply to the epiphysis. The procedure should not be attempted if the growth-plate is closed or nearly closed as the retinacular vessels then become inseparable from the femoral neck and part of the blood supply to the head is across the old growth-plate[10]. In the author's opinion this is the procedure of choice provided these criteria are met.

Many surgeons are fearful of open replacement and prefer a corrective subcervical osteotomy for severe gradual slipping. The biplane trochanteric osteotomy[11,12] is a well-established procedure for severe gradual slipping. It is free of risk to the capital blood supply and gives good early clinical results. Nevertheless, it is a difficult operation with a tendency to overcorrect the varus and undercorrect the posterior tilt. The procedure may be complicated by chondrolysis or significant shortening, and there are doubts about the long-term results[13].

The severe acute or acute-on-chronic slip is fraught with dangers. Closed reduction either by gentle manipulation or traction is associated with an unacceptable incidence of avascular necrosis. If the surgeon considers open replacement too hazardous then the epiphysis should be carefully pinned *in situ* and a definitive subcervical osteotomy either by the biplane or geometric technique deferred until the growth-plate is closed.

914 Pelvis and hip

OPEN REPLACEMENT OF FEMORAL EPIPHYSIS[8]

11

The patient lies on his side with the affected leg uppermost. The hip is exposed through a lateral incision made over the proximal femoral shaft and then curving into the buttock.

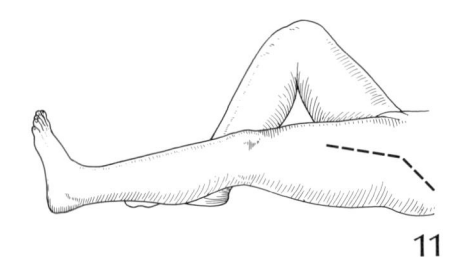

12

The greater trochanter is divided from below up through its growth-plate and with the attached abductors retracted proximally.

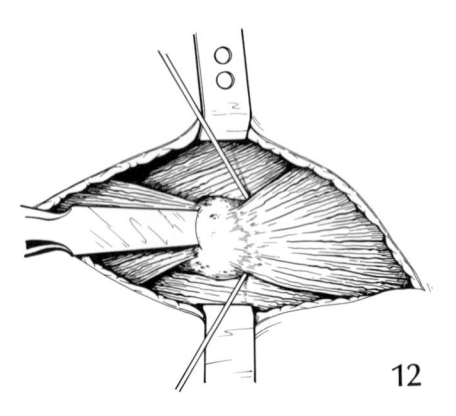

13

A T-shaped incision is made in the capsule down its lateral aspect and round the acetabular rim. The blood supply to the femoral head runs on to the femoral neck through the base of the posterior flap into the neck.

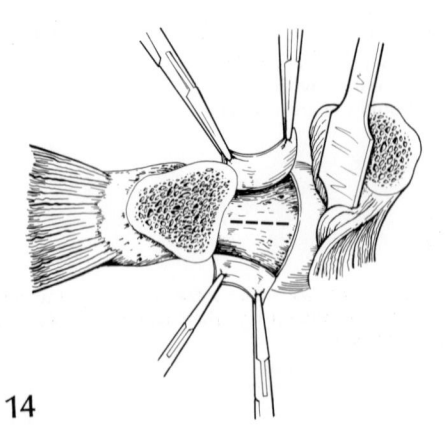

14

The periosteum of the neck is incised along its lateral margin between the pale avascular anterior part and the red vascular posterior surface, and round the anterior edge of the neck–head junction.

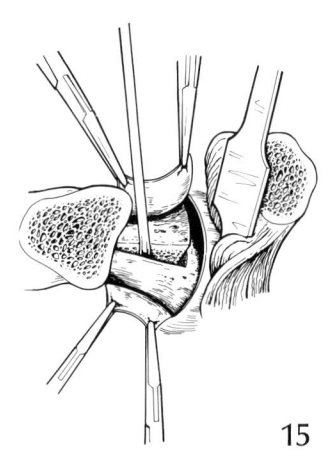

Slipped upper femoral epiphysis 915

15 & 16

The posterior periosteum carrying the capital blood supply is carefully stripped from the back of the neck, preserving its attachment to the rim of the head proximally and the capsule distally. Using a wide gouge as a shoehorn through the remains of the growth-plate, the head is gently prized backwards off the neck, exposing the posterior beak of new bone.

The first osteotomy cut is made in the long axis of the neck to remove this beak.

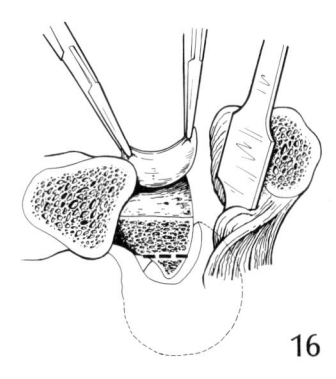

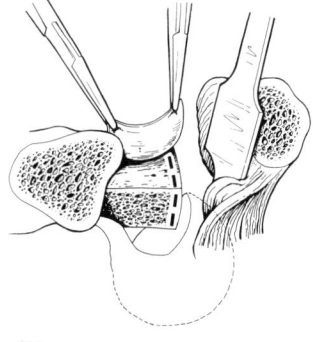

17

The second osteotomy cut curves across the metaphysis to remove the remains of the growth-plate and shorten the neck by 3–4 mm.

The inside of the epiphysis is gently curetted to remove the rest of the growth-plate.

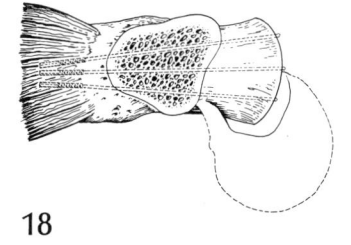

18

Three Crawford Adams pins are drilled up the neck to present at the metaphysis. The head is reduced and the pins driven home.

19 & 20a & b

The head should sit squarely on the neck in the lateral view, and with about 20° of valgus to the neck on the anteroposterior view.

The trochanter is reattached with a screw.

Postoperative management

Light skin traction is applied to the leg for 1 month and immediate hip flexion encouraged. After 1 month the patient is allowed up without bearing weight until radiographs show bony union of the epiphysis, usually about 3 months after operation.

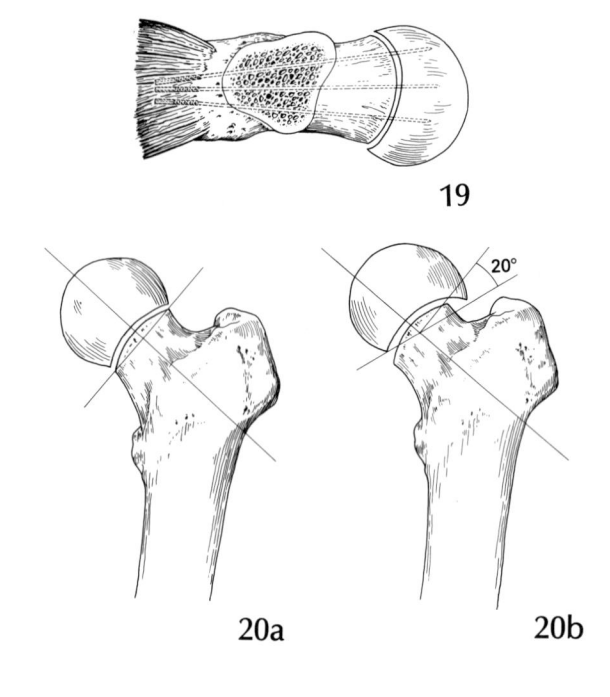

BIPLANE TROCHANTERIC OSTEOTOMY[11,12]

Preoperative measurement of desired correction

Clinical measurement of loss of abduction, flexion and medial rotation gives a very crude estimate of the degree of correction required. The different components of the deformity are best determined radiologically.

Varus

21

Southwick recommends an anteroposterior film of the pelvis taken with both legs in a neutral position. The axis of the epiphysis (a–a) and a line at right angles to this down the neck of the femur (A–B) are drawn. The long axis of the shaft is drawn (B–C) and the angle A–B–C measured. The difference between the normal and abnormal sides represents the amount of correction needed on the anterior aspect of the femur.

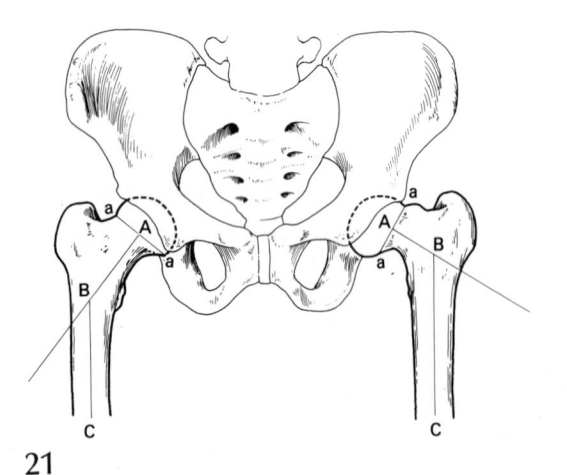

Posterior angulation

22

Comparable frog lateral radiographs are taken of both hips. If positioning is difficult the pelvis may be tilted to give an accurate lateral film of the proximal end of each femur. Southwick draws the axis of the head (x–x) and the vertical to it (X–Y) and measures the angle between X–Y and the long axis of the shaft (X–Z). The difference between the normal and abnormal sides represents the amount of correction needed on the lateral aspect of the femur.

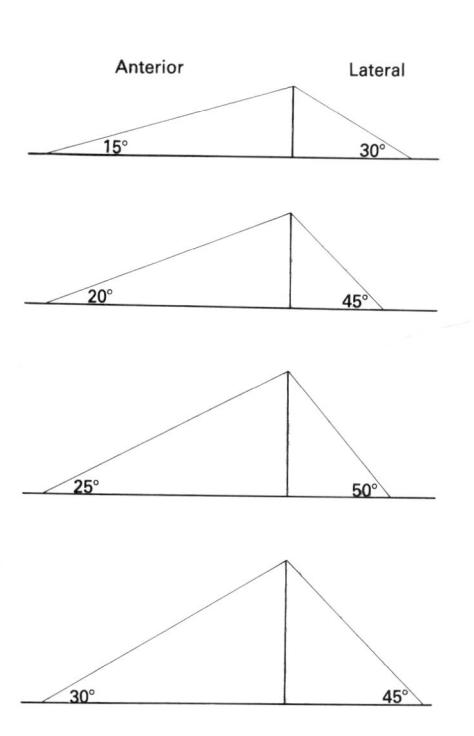

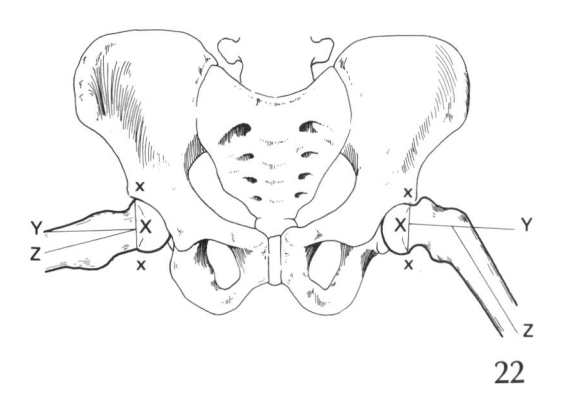

Lateral rotation

Correction of the varus and posterior tilt restores normal rotation. If the posterior tilt exceeds 60° Southwick prefers to undercorrect the deformity lest excessive shortening occurs, and to compensate for this by medial rotation of the shaft of the femur according to the range of movement achieved at the time of operation.

23

A piece of metal foil is cut as a template, the anterior part corresponding to the measured angle of valgus required and the lateral part to the flexion required. The hypotenuse of the lateral triangle should be 2 cm long to ensure good bony contact when the wedge is closed.

Surgical technique

The patient lies supine with the leg draped free. The anterolateral aspect of the upper femoral shaft is exposed through a lateral incision in line with the posterior edge of the greater trochanter, the lesser trochanter identified round the front of the shaft, and the psoas tendon detached.

At the junction of the relatively flat anterior surface and the rounded lateral surface of the upper femur, an orientation mark is made with an osteotome, and at the level of the lesser trochanter a second mark made at right angles to the first, representing the vertical and horizontal lines on the template. The template is bent and applied and the edges of the intended osteotomy marked.

24

A threaded Steinmann pin is drilled from the base of the greater trochanter distally and medially towards the lesser trochanter in line with the anterior edge of the intended osteotomy. Keeping to the guide lines, the wedge of bone is removed. The wedge should not be larger than necessary for good bony apposition. The greater the wedge the more shortening is produced.

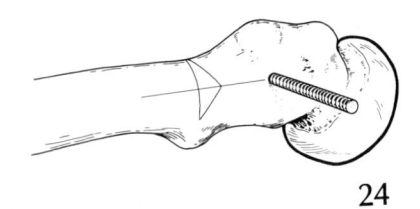

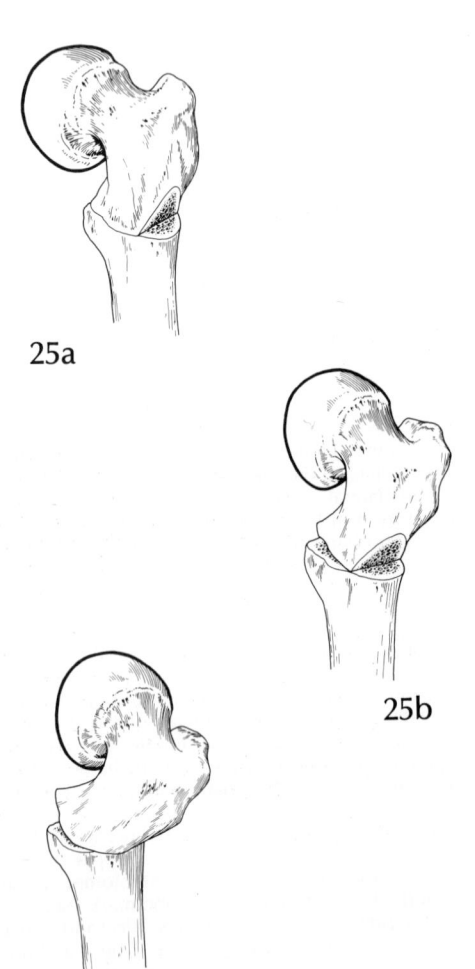

24

25a

25b

25c

25 a, b & c

The transverse part of the osteotomy is continued through the shaft of the femur.

The proximal fragment is controlled by a pin and the osteotomy closed anterolaterally by flexion and abduction of the limb. This opens a gap posteromedially.

The position is stabilized either by two pins in each fragment brought out through the wound and fixed to an external bar, or a plate and screws with or without compression. The range of hip movement is checked and should show at least 90° of flexion in neutral rotation and 30° of abduction. The skeletal fixation is supplemented by a plaster of Paris hip spica.

The spica is removed after about 8 weeks. Union of the osteotomy occurs in 8–12 weeks, by which time the affected growth-plate has become closed. Weight-bearing is then allowed.

Unacceptable deformity with growth-plate closed

Operations on the femoral neck are contraindicated and correction of the deformity has to be undertaken in the intertrochanteric region. Southwick's biplane trochanteric osteotomy is the established operation of choice. The author has used an alternative geometric flexion osteotomy on 14 patients. In one patient there was failure of fixation due to placement of two screws in the trochanteric growth-plate, and this required further surgery; another patient developed chondrolysis. The remaining patients regained an almost full range of pain-free movement, although one has radiological evidence but no symptoms of early osteoarthritis 13 years later. The operation has only been used after closure of the growth-plate for fear of subsequent slipping.

GEOMETRIC FLEXION OSTEOTOMY[1]

Theoretical considerations

The metaphyseal surface of the proximal femoral growth-plate may be represented by one-quarter of a cylinder. The epiphysis slips round the curved surface of this cylinder. The centre of rotation lies in the middle of the intertrochanteric region, as seen on the lateral radiograph, and in a plane parallel to the slope of the original growth-plate as seen on the anteroposterior view (this can be best measured on the normal hip).

The aim of the operation is to remove a wedge of bone with its apex at the geometric axis of rotation of the epiphysis and thus rotate the epiphysis back to its normal relationship to the acetabulum and femur.

Surgical technique

26a & b

The anterior surface of the proximal end of the femur is exposed. A wedge of bone is removed from the intertrochanteric region, the apex of the wedge lying along the axis of rotation of the epiphysis. The proximal surface of the wedge is cut first. The line of division is in the intertrochanteric region and usually inclines medially and distally at 70° to the long axis of the shaft of the femur. The oscillating saw should be held at right angles to the anterior surface of the femur and should pass only half-way through the shaft at this stage.

The distal surface of the wedge is then cut so that the wedge is equal to the angle of rotation of the epiphysis. The apex of the wedge should be half-way through the shaft of the femur and should lie in the anteversion plane – that is, it should be a little more posterior on the lateral than on the medial side of the shaft. The cortex on the medial side of the shaft is then divided completely, leaving the posterolateral cortex intact. This facilitates application of the osteotomy plate. The osteotomy plates are made to provide angles of correction of 45°, 50°, 60° and 70°.

27

If the osteotomy is made distal to the axis of rotation of the epiphysis, either inadvertently or because the patient has an excessively long valgoid femoral neck, a secondary deformity of the femur will occur.

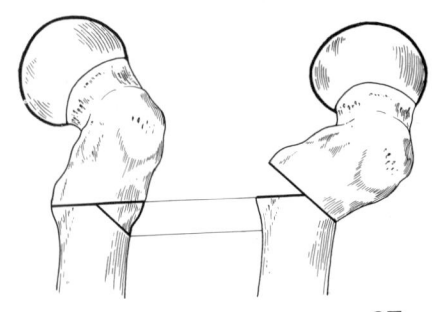

28

The appropriate plate is screwed to the proximal fragment so that the long axis of the plate lies at right angles to the osteotomy surface. The posterolateral cortex is then divided. Once the femur is completely divided, the proximal fragments tend to move into abduction. The shaft of the femur is abducted a similar amount and flexed to align it to the osteotomy plate, to which it is fixed with three screws. Care should be taken to avoid rotation of the shaft of the femur.

Postoperative management

After operation the hip is held in a flexed position by light Hamilton Russell traction and early gentle movement of the hip is encouraged. At 6–8 weeks the patient is allowed to walk with crutches, but weight-bearing is prohibited until the osteotomy is united.

References

1. Griffith MJ. Slipping of the capital femoral epiphysis. *Ann R Coll Surg Engl* 1976; 58: 34–42.
2. Billing L, Severin E. Slipping epiphysis of the hip: a roentgenological and clinical study based on a new roentgen technique. *Acta Radiol* 1959; Suppl 174.
3. Oram V. Epiphysiolysis of the head of the femur: follow-up examination with special reference to end results and social prognosis. *Acta Orthop Scand* 1953; 23: 100.
4. Boyer DW, Mickelson MR, Ponseti IV. Slipped capital femoral epiphysis: long-term follow-up study of one hundred and twenty-one patients. *J Bone Joint Surg [Am]* 1981; 63-A: 85–95.
5. Heyman CH, Herndon CH. Epiphysiodesis for early slipping of the upper femoral epiphysis. *J Bone Joint Surg [Am]* 1954; 36-A: 539–55.
6. Melby A, Hoyt WA Jr, Weiner DS. Treatment of chronic slipped capital femoral epiphysis by bone-graft epiphyseodesis. *J Bone Joint Surgery [Am]* 1980; 62-A: 119–125.
7. Heyman CH, Herndon CH, Strong JM. Slipping femoral epiphysis with severe displacement – a conservative operative treatment. *J Bone Joint Surg [Am]* 1957; 39-A: 293.
8. Dunn DM, Angel JC. Replacement of the femoral head by open operation in severe adolescent slipping of the upper femoral epiphysis. *J Bone Joint Surg [Br]* 1978; 60-B: 394–403.
9. Colton CL. Slipped upper femoral epiphysis. In: Catterall A, ed. *Recent advances in orthopaedics* No. 5. Edinburgh: Churchill Livingstone, 1987: 61–77.
10. Crock HV. A revision of the anatomy of the arteries supplying the upper end of the human femur. *J Anat* 1965; 99: 77–88.
11. Southwick WO. Osteotomy through the lesser trochanter for slipped capital femoral epiphysis. *J Bone Joint Surg [Am]* 1967; 49-A: 807–35.
12. Southwick WO. Compression fixation after biplane intertrochanteric osteotomy for slipped upper femoral epiphysis. *J Bone Joint Surg [Am]* 1973; 55-A: 1218–24.
13. Ireland J, Newman PH. Triplane osteotomy for severely slipped upper femoral epiphysis. *J Bone Joint Surg [Br]* 1978; 60-B: 390–3.

Illustrations by Gillian Oliver

Correction of flexion contracture of the hip

B. Helal MChOrth, FRCS
Honorary Consultant Orthopaedic Surgeon, The Royal London Hospital and The Royal National Orthopaedic Hospital, London, and Enfield Group of Hospitals, UK

S. C. Chen FRCS
Consultant Orthopaedic Surgeon, Enfield Group of Hospitals, UK

Introduction

In cerebral palsy the hip joint may become flexed due to contractures of the iliotibial tract, rectus femoris muscle, iliopsoas and gluteal muscles. Usually the flexion contracture is associated with either an adduction deformity due to contractures of the adductor muscles or with a medial rotation deformity due to overactivity of the medial rotator muscles of the hip. It is important to establish clearly the type of deformity present in the hip, for the typical spastic scissor gait of a child suffering from cerebral palsy can be due to a simple flexion contracture, or to a contracture producing both flexion and medial rotation, or flexion and adduction of the hip. Severe cases can secondarily affect the lumbar spine producing, in longstanding cases, a fixed scoliosis due to pelvic tilt. Mild cases can be treated by regular stretching and exercises in the physiotherapy department.

Operations

RELEASE OF A TIGHT ILIOTIBIAL TRACT
(Yount procedure[1])

The tensor fasciae latae muscle flexes and abducts the hip while at the same time it flexes the knee and laterally rotates the tibia. When this muscle becomes contracted, deformities will occur in the direction of its actions.

Incision

1

The skin is incised along the lateral aspect of the knee, extending from the joint line to just above the femoral condyle.

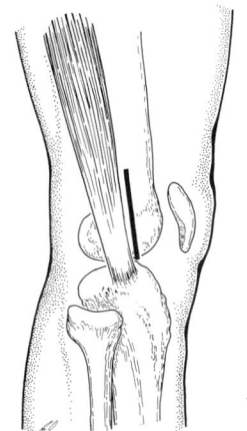

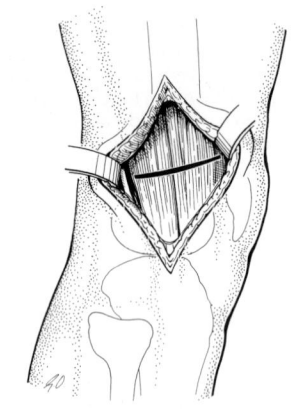

Procedure

2

The iliotibial tract and fascia lata are exposed and both these structures divided transversely backwards to the lateral head of the biceps femoris and forwards to just above the upper pole of the patella. Care should be taken not to damage the quadriceps tendon and muscles and the lateral popliteal nerve.

Postoperative management

A plaster cast is applied from the foot to the upper thigh with the knee in full extension. The patient can walk with the plaster cast on for 2 weeks. Then the plaster is removed and physiotherapy to mobilize the knee can commence. A removable backslab is applied for 3 more weeks during the day for walking, and this is used as a night splint for 6 months before discarding it completely.

ILIOPSOAS TENOTOMY

An iliopsoas tenotomy is necessary when the hip is flexed more than 15° but less than 45°, and passive stretching cannot correct the deformity. An adductor tenotomy may have to be done at the same time, for an associated adductor deformity.

Incision

3

The attachment of the iliopsoas to the lesser trochanter of the femur is found through a medial approach. A vertical incision is made on the medial aspect of the thigh, 2 cm distal to the pubic tubercle.

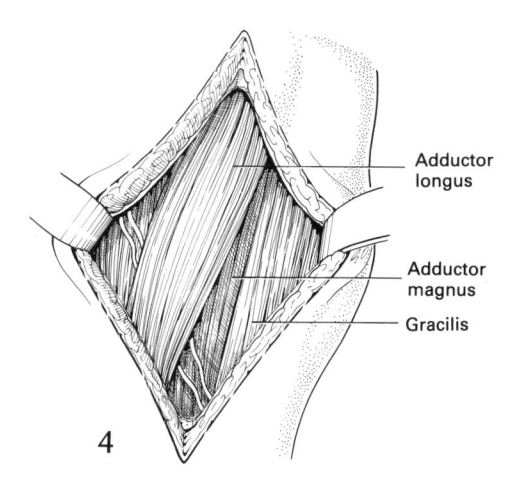

Procedure

4

The adductor longus and gracilis muscles are identified. The tissue plane between the adductor longus and brevis anteriorly and the gracilis and adductor magnus posteriorly is identified and the muscles separated, taking care to protect the branches of the obturator nerve and blood vessels in this area.

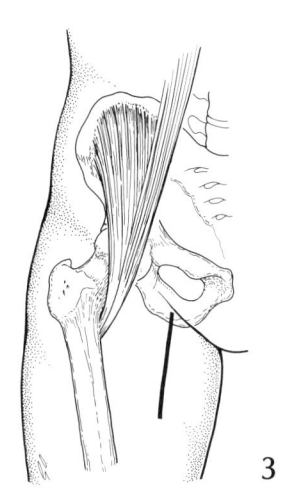

5

The lesser trochanter is identified, and the iliopsoas is detached. The tendons of the adductor longus, brevis and magnus can be cut at the same time if necessary.

Postoperative management

Hip abduction and extension exercises are commenced early. Full weight-bearing is permitted after a few days. The patient is encouraged to sleep prone at night.

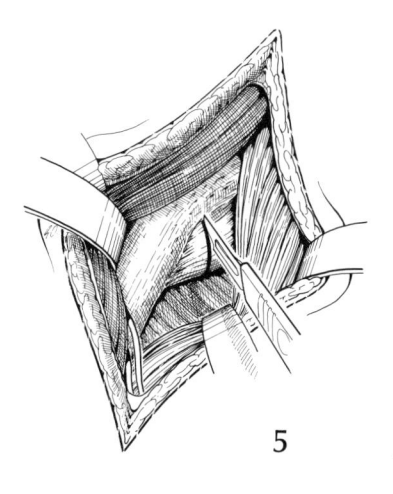

SOUTTER OPERATION FOR HIP FLEXION CONTRACTURE[2]

In severe flexion contracture of the hip there is extensive involvement of the sartorius, rectus femoris, tensor fasciae latae and glutei. These have to be released if full correction is to be achieved. An iliopsoas tenotomy is almost always necessary.

Incision

6

The incision runs from the anterior part of the iliac crest to the anterior superior iliac spine and downwards for about 12 cm towards the lateral side of the patella.

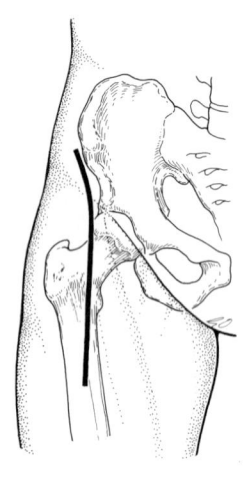

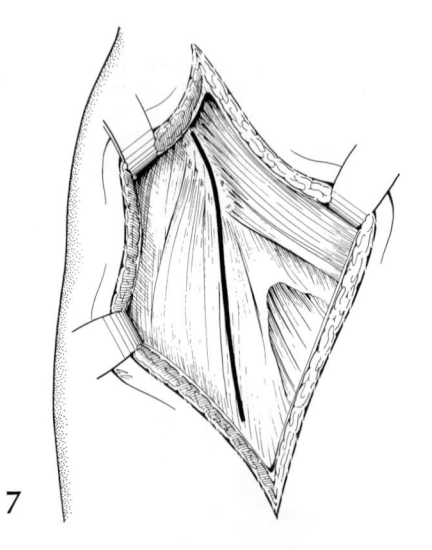

7

The skin and subcutaneous tissue are reflected distally and backwards to expose the crest of the ilium and deep fascia. The deep fascia is incised from the anterior superior iliac spine downwards and backwards to the greater trochanter.

Release

8

The sartorius, tensor fasciae latae and glutei are released from their attachments to the ilium, with a combination of sharp and blunt dissection deep to the deep fascia on the lateral side of the ilium. The hip is extended and the released structures allowed to retract. The subcutaneous tissue and skin only are sutured.

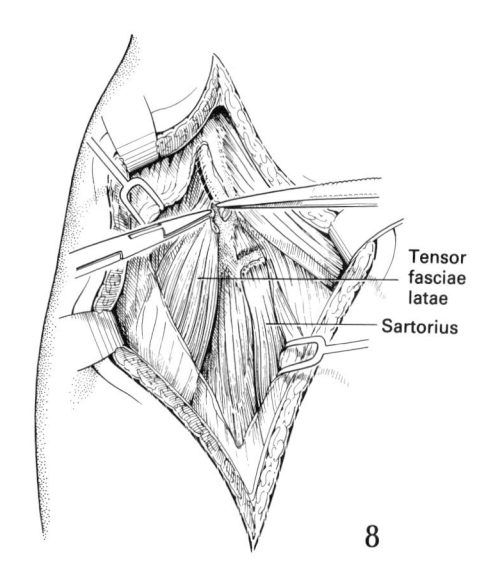

Postoperative management

Skin traction is applied to the affected leg for 3 weeks. Hip abduction and extension exercises are commenced and full weight-bearing is permitted after this period. The patient should be encouraged to sleep prone at night.

References

1. Yount CC. The role of the tensor fasciae femoris in certain deformities of the lower extremities. *J Bone Joint Surg* 1926; 8: 171–93.

2. Soutter R. A new operation for hip contractures in poliomyelitis. *Boston Med Surg J* 1914; 170: 380–1.

Illustrations by Peter Cox after F. Price

Adductor release (with or without partial anterior obturator neurectomy)

W. J. W. Sharrard MD, ChM, FRCS
Emeritus Consultant Orthopaedic Surgeon, Royal Hallamshire and Children's Hospital, Sheffield;
Professor of Orthopaedic Surgery, University of Sheffield, UK

Preoperative

Indications and assessment

Before adductor release the range of abduction must be assessed with the hips and knees extended to ensure that any contracture of the gracilis, which is frequently affected, is recognized. Abduction of the hip is limited to 40° or less owing to strong and probably spastic adductor muscle in the presence of weaker hip abductors in cerebral palsy, myelomeningocele, poliomyelitis or other paralytic conditions and is the main indication for the operation. If abductor power is greater than MRC Grade 3 (antigravity) and there is minimal radiological subluxation of the hip, adductor release only is needed, often only of adductor longus and gracilis. If abductor power is less than Grade 3 and/or there is more than one-third subluxation of the femoral head, adductor release should be combined with neurectomy of the anterior branch of the obturator nerve. Adductor longus, gracilis, adductor brevis and, in severe contracture, adductor magnus, may need to be released until a full range, or as full a range of abduction as possible, is achieved. If the hip has been completely dislocated before operation, it may reduce. The operation may be combined with iliopsoas tendon lengthening or recession by the medial approach (see the chapter on pp. 936–939).

The operation can be performed at any age in a child or an adult and is often needed bilaterally.

A radiograph of the hips should be taken before operation.

Anaesthesia and position of patient

General anaesthesia is normally needed. In children thought to be unfit for general anaesthesia because of severe respiratory dysfunction, local anaesthesia can be used. The degree of limitation of abduction is confirmed under anaesthesia. The patient is placed supine with a small sandbag under the buttocks. After skin preparation the limbs are enclosed in stockinette to just above the level of the knee. A vertical narrow drape is used to cover the genitalia and other towels are applied to leave the upper medial aspects of the thigh exposed. The operative area may be covered by transparent adhesive. The lower limbs should be free to allow the hips to be manipulated in all directions.

A diathermy plate should be placed to give adequate skin contact, usually under the back or upper part of the buttock.

Operation[1]

Incision

1

A 3–4 cm incision, depending on the size of the patient, is made parallel to the groin crease and 2.5–3 cm below it, centred over the adductor longus tendon. The subcutaneous tissue is divided down to, but not through, the deep fascia and is mobilized proximally for about 2 cm and distally for 1 cm to expose the fascia over the proximal end of the adductor muscle.

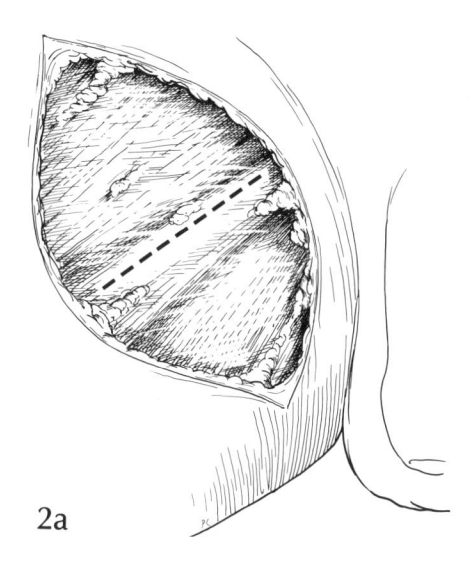

Exposure

2a, b & 3

A vertical incision is made along the line of the adductor longus, which is usually identifiable by the prominence of its tendon. The fascia is undermined medially and laterally to expose the gracilis medial to and the pectineus and adductor brevis lateral to the adductor longus. The muscles and tendons can be identified by their shape. The adductor longus arises by a thick oval tendon attached to the pubis and rapidly expanding into a broad fleshy belly. The gracilis arises by a thin flattened aponeurosis, vertically disposed and taking origin from the medial margins of the lower half of the body of the pubis and the ischium. The flat muscle lies immediately below the surface of the skin with a thin covering layer of fascia, and can easily be obscured beneath a medially placed retractor. The pectineus arises by a muscular origin anteriorly. It does not normally require division and is separated and retracted forward to expose the adductor brevis beneath it.

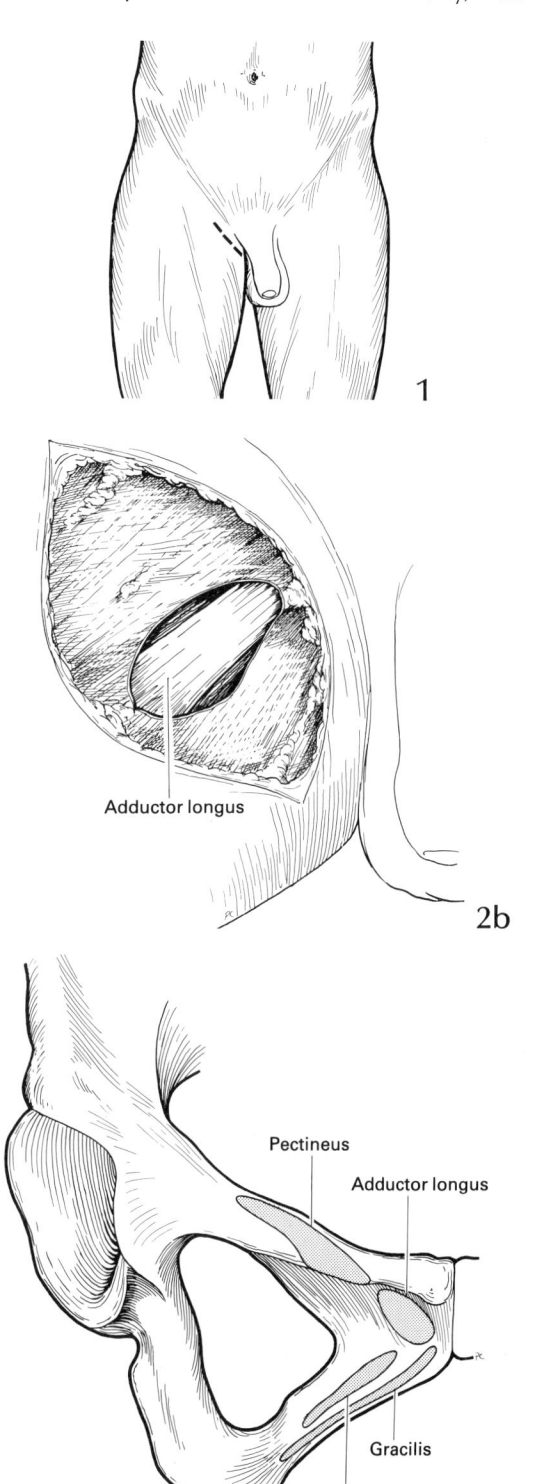

928 Pelvis and hip

Musculotendinous division

4a, b & c

The uppermost part of the adductor longus is defined by passing a MacDonald blunt dissector behind its tendon and uppermost muscular fibres. It is divided transversely 1 cm from its origin by cutting through the tendon onto the blunt dissector. The distal muscle should retract distally when it has been completely divided; only occasionally a small vessel may require coagulation by diathermy.

The aponeurosis of the gracilis is defined by blunt dissection on its medial and lateral sides. The aponeurosis is wide, extending well posteriorly. It is divided by a slightly oblique cut parallel and 1 cm distal to its origin. At its most posterior attachment, a small vessel is always encountered which needs to be coagulated by diathermy. The distal muscle should retract distally. Complete division of the adductor longus and gracilis is confirmed by abduction of the hip with the knee extended. The range of abduction should now be considerably improved. If the abduction range is more than 65°–70°, no further adductor release is required. If it is still limited, the adductor brevis and possibly the adductor magnus muscle, exposed beneath the divided adductor longus and gracilis, are palpated.

Some lengthening of the adductor brevis can be made without incision by teasing its fibres with a blunt dissector whilst slowly stretching them by abducting the hip further. The adductor magnus rarely requires division except in very severe adduction deformity. If the hip was dislocated or severely subluxated before operation, a radiograph may be taken to check whether reduction has been achieved.

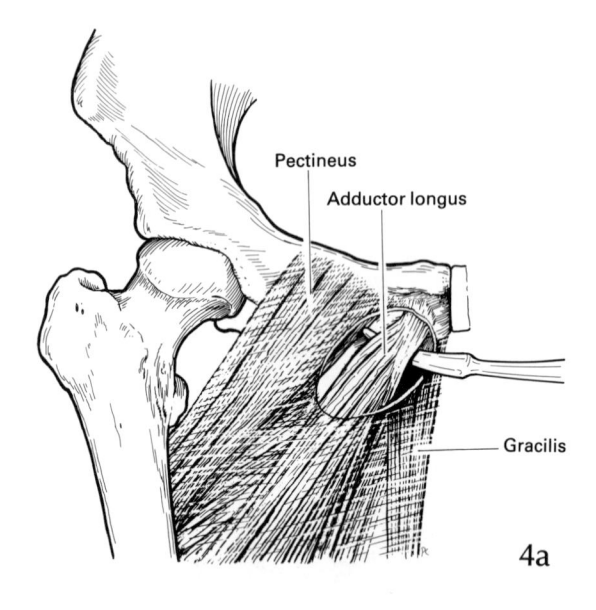

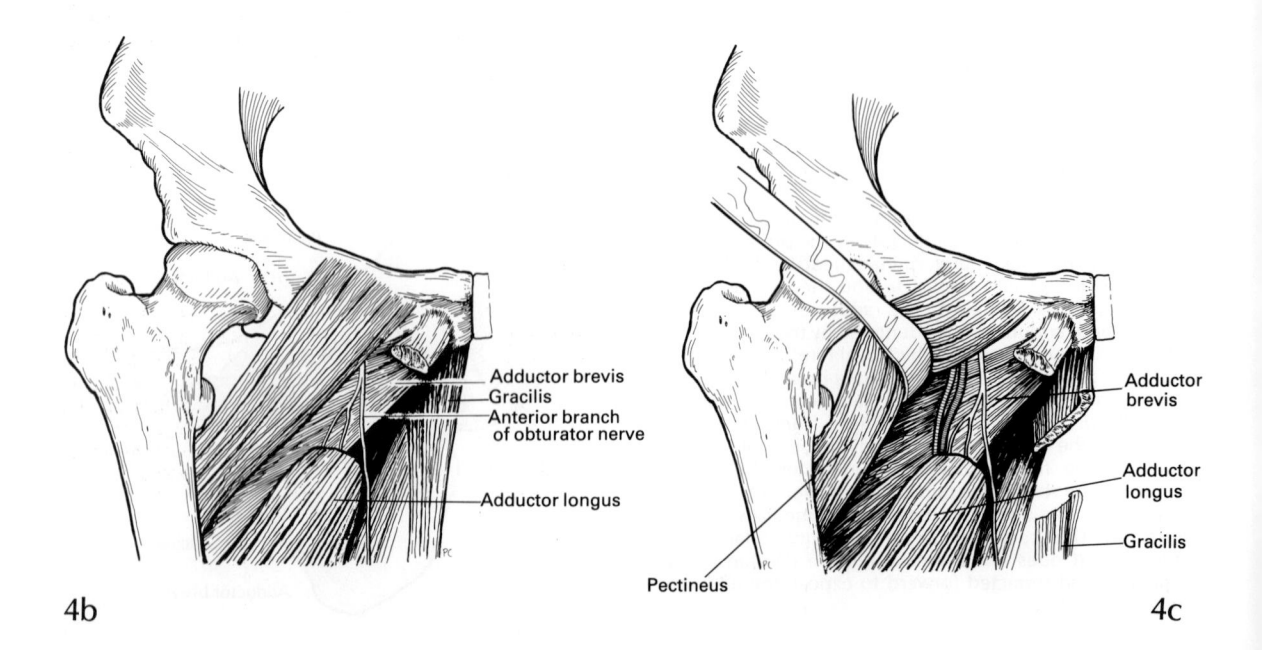

Additional procedure – posterior adductor transfer

If adduction deformity is associated with hip flexion deformity, owing to weakness of hip extension and abduction, adductor release and iliopsoas lengthening or recession may be combined with posterior transfer of the adductors. The approach is similar, except that the skin incision is extended posteriorly by an additional 2 cm. The origins of the adductor longus and gracilis and, if desired, adductor brevis are detached close to the pubic ramus[2]. The upper 5 cm of the muscles are mobilized, retaining their nerve supply. The tendons of origin are moved posteriorly and attached to the ischial tuberosity or to the common tendon of origin of the hamstrings with strong unabsorbable sutures using a Mayo's cutting needle. Care must be taken to ensure that adductor tightness is not reproduced in the attempt to attach the tendons of origin to the bone; if there is a tendency for this to occur, it is better to attach the tendons to the common tendon of origin of the hamstrings.

Partial neurectomy of the obturator nerve

5

The anterior branch of the obturator nerve passes obliquely across the surface of the adductor brevis accompanied by branches of the obturator artery and vein. It may present as a single nerve dividing into two branches or as two separate branches. If necessary, it can be identified by gently pinching it with non-toothed dissecting forceps and noting twitching of the adductor muscles. If there are two nerve branches, the posterior branch of the obturator nerve should be identified on the posterior aspect of the adductor brevis to confirm that one of the anterior branches is not a posterior branch taking an anomalous course on the anterior surface of the muscle.

The nerve is separated from its accompanying vessels and retracted by blunt hooks. Artery forceps are applied proximally and distally and the nerve divided with removal of 1–1.5 cm of nerve. If the artery or vein are accidentally divided, brisk bleeding may occur, but the vessel can be coagulated by diathermy without important after-effects.

The posterior branch of the obturator nerve should not be divided, but it may be crushed in cases of severe adductor spasticity.

Wound closure

6

After diathermy of any outstanding smaller vessels, the wound is closed in three layers. The deep fascia is closed by vertical interrupted sutures and serves to limit haematoma formation. The subcutaneous fat is closed transversely by a continuous or interrupted suture and the skin is closed by interrupted sutures or a continuous subcuticular suture. A suction drain is not normally needed in children but is advisable in adolescents or adults for 48 hours.

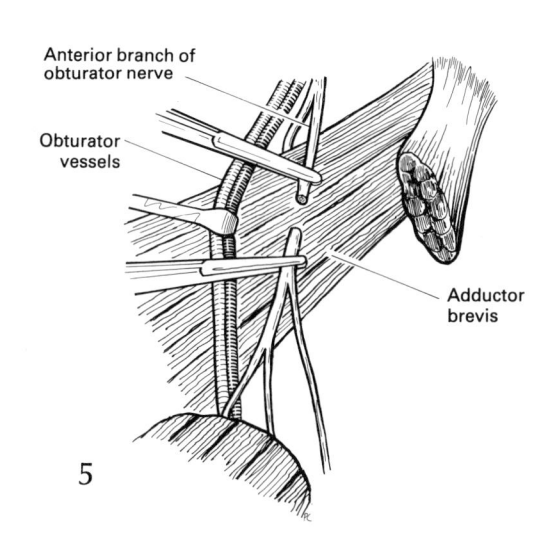

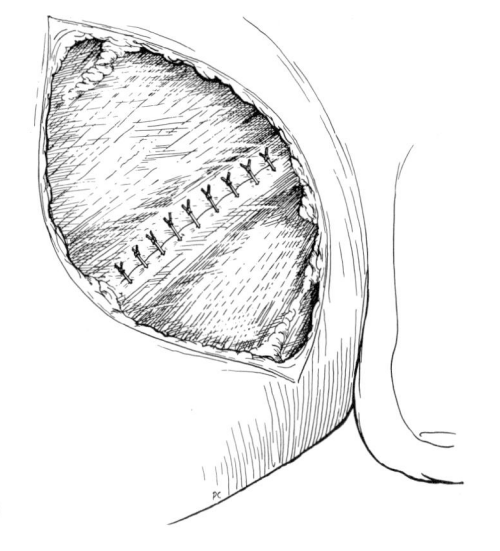

Immobilization

7

If the hip joint was not dislocated or markedly subluxated before operation and spasticity is not severe, no plaster immobilization is necessary in a child below the age of 10 years. The limbs can be maintained in abduction by a pillow between the thighs.

If the hip joint has been unstable, the lower limbs are immobilized in a groin-to-ankle or groin-to-toe plaster cast with the knees extended and both hips abducted as far as possible. The plaster casts are connected by two metal, wood or plaster bars.

Spasm can be limited by oral diazepam or baclofen for 2–3 days or longer if necessary.

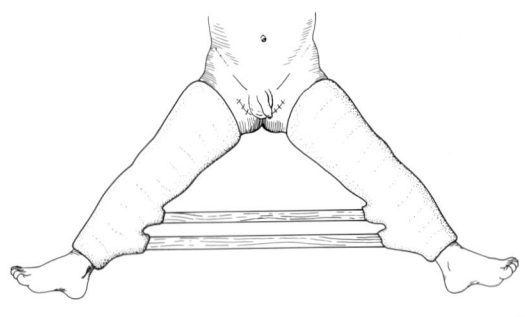

Postoperative management

The patient, if a child, can usually return home after 2 or 3 days. Sutures, if not absorbable, are removed after 10–12 days. If plaster casts have been needed, they are retained for 2–3 weeks in children below the age of 5 years, 3–4 weeks in children between the ages of 5 and 10 years and 4–5 weeks in patients over this age. Physiotherapy is given to encourage active and passive movements, including hip flexion, in joints not immobilized by plaster. After removal of plaster casts physiotherapy to encourage passive and active abduction should be instituted immediately.

References

1. Banks HH, Green WT. Adductor myotomy and obturator neurectomy for the correction of adduction contractures of the hip in cerebral palsy. *J Bone Joint Surg [Am]* 1960; 42-A, 111–26.

2. Root L, Spero CR. Hip adductor transfer compared with adduction tenotomy in cerebral palsy. *J Bone Joint Surg [Am]* 1981; 63-A, 767–72.

Illustrations by Peter Cox after F. Price

Hip flexor release: iliofemoral approach

W. J. W. Sharrard MD, ChM, FRCS.
Emeritus Consultant Orthopaedic Surgeon, Royal Hallamshire Hospital and Children's Hospital, Sheffield;
Professor of Orthopaedic Surgery, University of Sheffield, UK

Preoperative

Indications and assessment

The main indication for hip flexor release is flexion deformity of the hip of between 20° and 80°, arising from the activity of strong hip flexors in the presence of weak hip extensors in cerebral palsy, myelomeningocele, poliomyelitis and other paralytic conditions in which the deformity is due to musculotendinous contracture rather than bony deformity.

Before operation an assessment should be made of the part contributed to the flexion deformity by the iliopsoas, tensor fasciae latae, sartorius and rectus femoris. An increase of flexion on medial rotation of the hip suggests tightness of the iliopsoas or sartorius or both. An increase of hip flexion when the knee is flexed indicates tightness of the rectus femoris. An increase of hip flexion when the hip is adducted suggests tightness of the tensor fasciae latae. In most cases, the iliopsoas is likely to be the predominantly short tendon.

When there is more than 45° of fixed flexion, the hip tends to fall into abduction and lateral rotation. When the hip is adducted, the true degree of flexion deformity becomes apparent. Inability to adduct to neutral even when the hip is allowed to flex indicates that there is an abduction or a combined flexion and abduction deformity, often owing to contracture in the tensor fasciae latae.

Anaesthesia and position of patient

General anaesthesia is needed. An intravenous infusion should be begun. One or two units of blood may be needed during the operation. The patient is placed supine with a small sandbag under the buttock of the affected side. The skin is prepared. The limb is enclosed in stockinette to above the knee. Drapes are placed to expose the upper third of the thigh, the anterior superior iliac spine and the anterior half of the iliac crest. The operative area is covered either by stockinette or a transparent adhesive drape. When there is a marked flexion deformity, the limb may need to be held in semi-flexion until some correction has been obtained. Stockinette is applied to the opposite limb so that it can be flexed fully to perform a Thomas' test during the operation.

A diathermy plate is placed to give adequate skin contact, usually under the back or upper part of the buttock.

Operation

Incision

1

The incision is made along the outer side of the anterior third of the iliac crest, immediately lateral to the anterior superior iliac spine and obliquely along the line of the sartorius in the upper third of the thigh. The subcutaneous tissue is divided in the same line down too deep fascia. A vein running transversely just distal to the anterior superior iliac spine may need to be coagulated. The incision must not be made too deeply just distal to the anterior superior iliac spine to avoid dividing the lateral cutaneous nerve of the thigh as it emerges from beneath the inguinal ligament.

To avoid postoperative breakdown of the skin over a prominence, the incision should not cross directly over the anterior superior iliac spine.

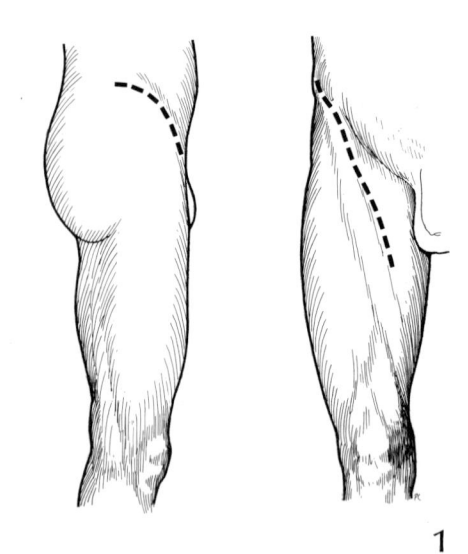

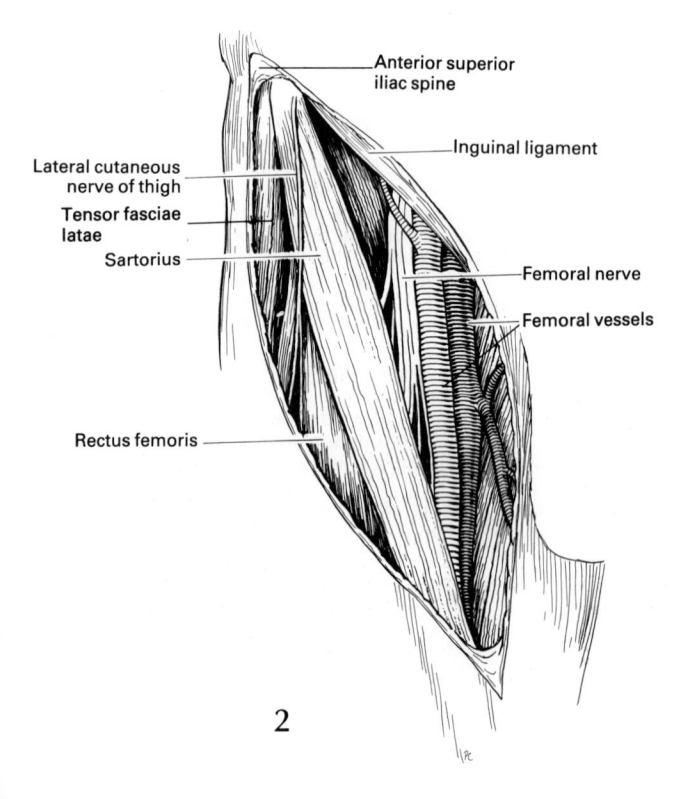

Exposure

2

The deep fascia is incised from the anterior superior iliac spine distally along the proximal half of the sartorius, which can often be seen through the fascia. The lateral cutaneous nerve of the thigh lies immediately beneath the fascia just distal and medial to the anterior superior iliac spine, running obliquely distally and laterally, and should be preserved. In the incision of the thigh, small cutaneous branches of the femoral nerve may be encountered and their division should, if possible, be avoided. The aponeurosis on the inner and outer side of the tensor fasciae latae is defined up to its origin from the iliac crest from which it is detached in its anterior two-thirds, and sometimes completely, if it is found to be contributing significantly to the flexion deformity.

Division of sartorius

3

The origin of the sartorius from the anterior iliac spine and an adjoining 1 cm of the inguinal ligament medial to it is defined over a distance of 2 cm. The sartorius tendon is divided obliquely to allow for the possibility of suture with elongation at the end of the operation. A number of vessels require coagulation with diathermy. The conjoint tendon of rectus femoris at the junction of its straight and reflected heads is found beneath the sartorius. If it is tight, the tendon is defined by blunt dissection and also divided obliquely. If, with the knee extended, the rectus femoris is not tight, it should be left untouched, but, as release of hip flexors continues, especially after release of the iliopsoas tendon, its tension should be reviewed and division made if necessary.

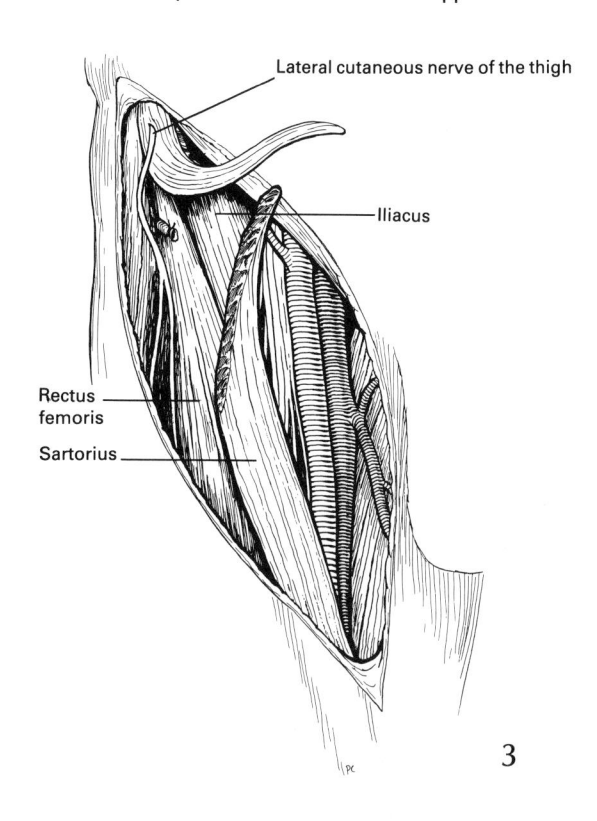

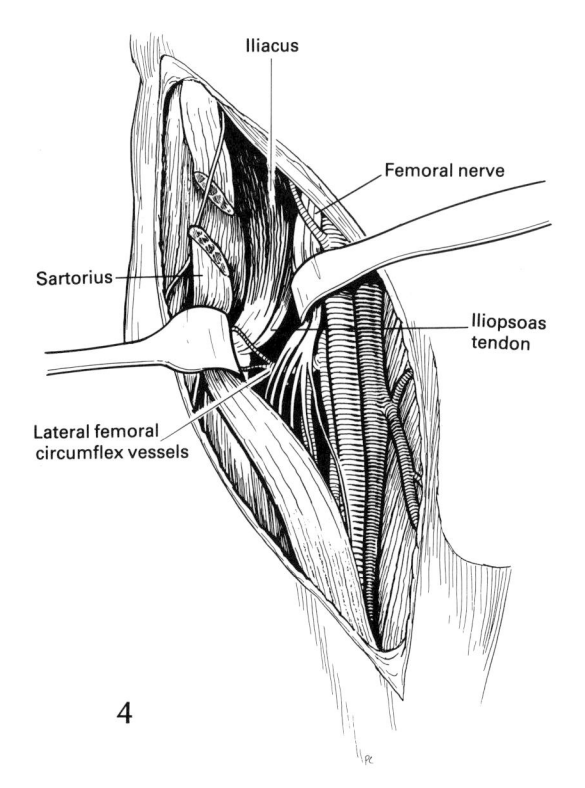

Anterolateral approach to the iliopsoas tendon

4

A thin layer of fascia immediately medial to the origin of the sartorius, attached to and just distal to the inguinal ligament, is incised and opened up with a haemostat to expose the femoral nerve as it emerges from beneath the inguinal ligament lying on the medial part of the iliacus muscle. The same fascial plane is extended distally to expose the branches of the femoral nerve. The hip is allowed to flex a little so that the nerve and its branches may be freed and retracted forwards and medially. In the distal third of the incision, the lateral femoral circumflex vessels cross the wound from the medial to the lateral side and must be divided and ligatured to allow further retraction of the femoral nerve and vessels to expose the iliopsoas tendon.

934 Pelvis and hip

Division of iliopsoas tendon

5

The lesser trochanter should be palpated deeply on the medial side of the femur with the hip laterally rotated to facilitate this.

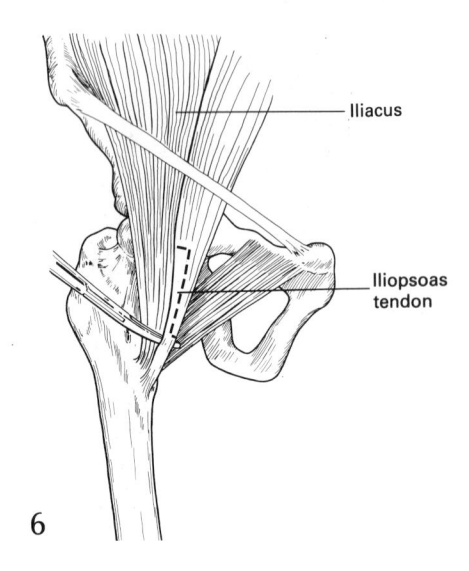

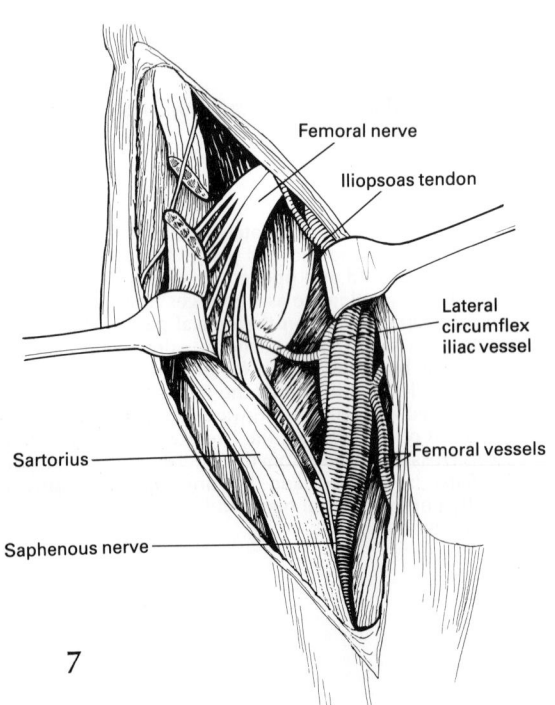

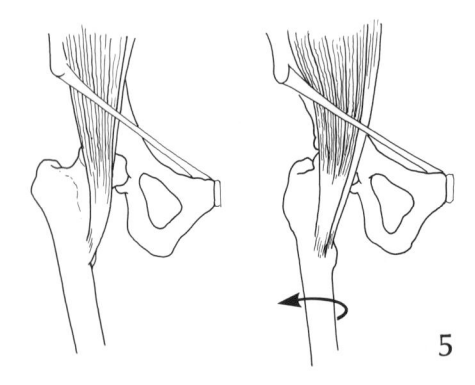

Iliacus

Iliopsoas tendon

6

If the lesser trochanter is not too posteriorly situated and lateral rotation and flexion of the hip allows it to be brought into view with the aid of deep retractors, elongation of the iliopsoas tendon or recession of it can be done as described on pp. 936–939.

If the lesser trochanter lies posteriorly, as it often does in paralytic conditions of the hip, adequate exposure by this approach is difficult or impossible. In that event, it is better to expose the iliopsoas tendon between the femoral nerve and the femoral vessels.

Alternative approach to the iliopsoas tendon

The femoral nerve and its proximal branches are exposed as in the preceding section. The most medial branch, the saphenous nerve, is traced distally by blunt dissection until it crosses the femoral artery. The femoral vessels are then exposed by opening the femoral sheath from this level proximally up to the level of the inguinal ligament.

7

The proximal part of the femoral nerve is retracted gently to the lateral side and the femoral vessels are retracted medially. The superficial circumflex iliac vessels arising from the lateral side of the femoral vessels are identified, divided between haemostats and either ligated or coagulated with diathermy. About 1 cm more distally, the profunda artery, and slightly more distally still, the profunda vein are exposed; the lateral femoral circumflex vessels passing laterally are identified with extreme gentleness and divided between haemostats and double ligated. The femoral and profunda vessels can then be easily retracted medially to expose the iliopsoas tendon deeply, passing down to the lesser trochanter. The tendon is defined, freed and lengthened or recessed as described on pages 936–939.

Femoral nerve

Iliopsoas tendon

Lateral circumflex iliac vessel

Sartorius

Femoral vessels

Saphenous nerve

Additional release

After division of the tensor fasciae latae, sartorius, rectus femoris and iliopsoas, an assessment is made of the degree of correction of the flexion deformity by flexing the opposite hip fully. If further correction is prevented by tightness of the femoral vessels and nerve, no further release of soft tissue is indicated and any additional correction can only be achieved by division and shortening of the femur. If the vessels and nerve are not unduly tight, the remaining flexion deformity may be due to tightness of the iliofemoral ligament which can be divided to provide a further, but limited amount of correction. Excessive division of the anterior capsule of the hip should be avoided lest it should result in anterior dislocation of the hip.

8

Wound closure

The tensor fascia latae is left unsutured. The sartorius is sutured with lengthening, either by attaching its obliquely cut ends to each other by two or three sutures or by suturing the distal end of the tendon to any available deep fascia. The rectus femoris tendon is similarly treated. It may be possible to close a layer of deep fascia, but, more usually in marked flexion deformity, it is only possible to suture the deep layer of superficial fascia and to close the skin with interrupted sutures or a continuous subcuticular suture. In children over the age of 6 years, one or two suction drains are inserted.

Immobilization

The hip is immobilized in maximum extension, neutral abduction and neutral rotation in a hip spica plaster cast extending to the toes on the operated side and to the knee on the opposite side.

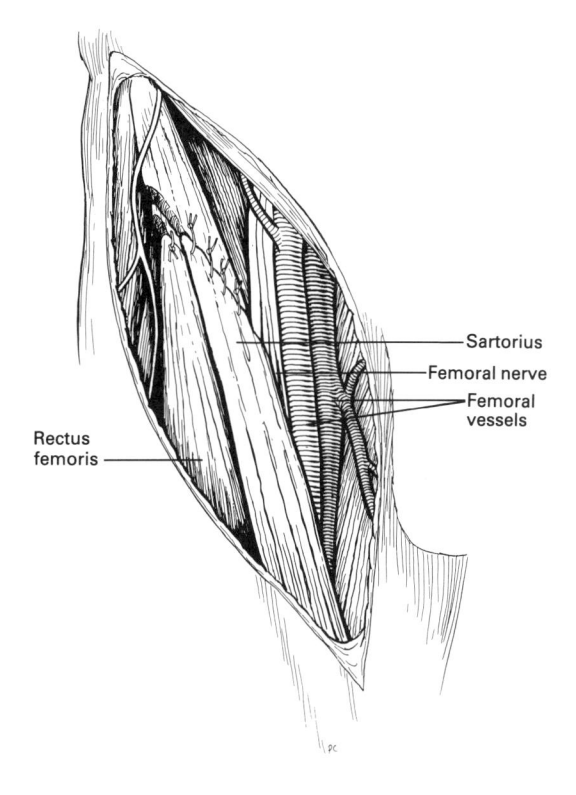

Postoperative management

Intravenous dextrose saline infusion is continued for 24 hours, or, if necessary, additional blood is given if there was substantial loss during the operation. The circulation to the toes is kept under observation as is the upper thigh for any evidence of haematoma. Paralytic ileus is a rare but possible complication. Plaster immobilization is continued for 3½ to 4 weeks; it is not normally necessary to remove the sutures, even if they are non-absorbable, until the plaster cast is removed. Mobilization and physiotherapy treatment is started immediately after removal of the plaster spica.

Illustrations by Peter Cox after F. Price

Iliopsoas tendon lengthening or recession: medial (Ludloff) approach

W. J. W. Sharrard MD, ChM, FRCS
Emeritus Consultant Orthopaedic Surgeon, Royal Hallamshire Hospital and Children's Hospital, Sheffield; Professor of Orthopaedic Surgery, University of Sheffield, UK

Preoperative

Indications and assessment

The main indication for operation on the iliopsoas tendon is flexion deformity of the hip of 20°–40° owing to strong and possibly spastic iliopsoas and hip flexor muscles in the presence of weaker hip extensors in cerebral palsy, myelomeningocele, poliomyelitis or other paralytic conditions. Flexion and adduction deformity are often combined together so that adductor and flexor release are both needed, possibly combined with posterior transfer of the adductors to the ischium. If so, this approach is the recommended one. Assessment is made as described in the chapter on 'Hip flexor release: the iliofemoral approach' (pp. 931–935) and should confirm that there is no excessive tightness of the tensor fasciae latae or sartorius.

Anaesthesia and position of patient

General anaesthesia is needed. The degree of fixed flexion and adduction should be confirmed under anaesthesia. The patient is placed supine with a small sandbag under the affected hip. The approach to the iliopsoas tendon is made easier if the hip is flexed and laterally rotated during the operation. Skin preparation and the application of drapes is as for adductor release (see chapter on 'Adductor release' pp. 926–930).

Operation

Incision

1

The incision is the same as for adductor release with a distal extension of the medial end of the incision to allow sufficient distal mobilization of the lower flap.

Exposure

The deep fascia is incised and the muscles exposed as for adductor release (see p. 927). If adductor release is required, this is done first. If only iliopsoas lengthening or recession is needed, it can be performed through this approach if the adductors are relaxed and the knee semiflexed to allow their retraction.

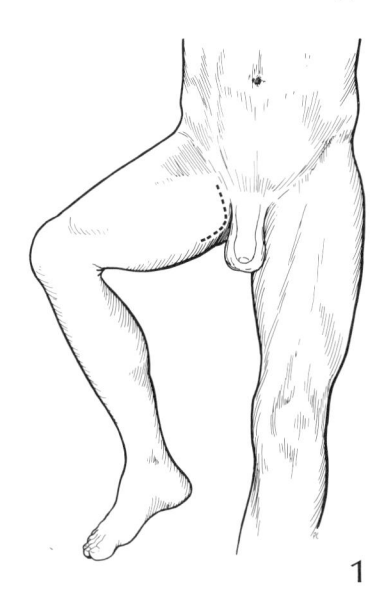

Approach to the iliopsoas tendon

2

The approach, originally attributed to Ludloff[1], was described for iliopsoas release by Keats and Morgese[2]. The plane between the adductor longus and pectineus anteriorly and the gracilis and adductor brevis posteriorly is opened up by blunt dissection. The iliopsoas tendon and the lesser trochanter are obscured by a layer of fat. The lesser trochanter is palpated beneath this fat layer on the posteromedial aspect of the femur and its position confirmed by rotation of the thigh.

3

Deep retractors are placed to expose the lesser trochanter, which is covered by a layer of fascia and fat which needs to be lightly incised: one or two small vessels need to be coagulated. The direction of the iliopsoas tendon as it passes from the pelvis to the lesser trochanter needs to be appreciated: the tendon runs almost vertically from above downwards and backwards. Once the plane of the tendon has been defined, it can be cleared proximally to visualize 5–7 cm of its length. Branches of the medial femoral circumflex vessels cross the tendon about 1 cm above the lesser trochanter and may need to be divided and coagulated by diathermy.

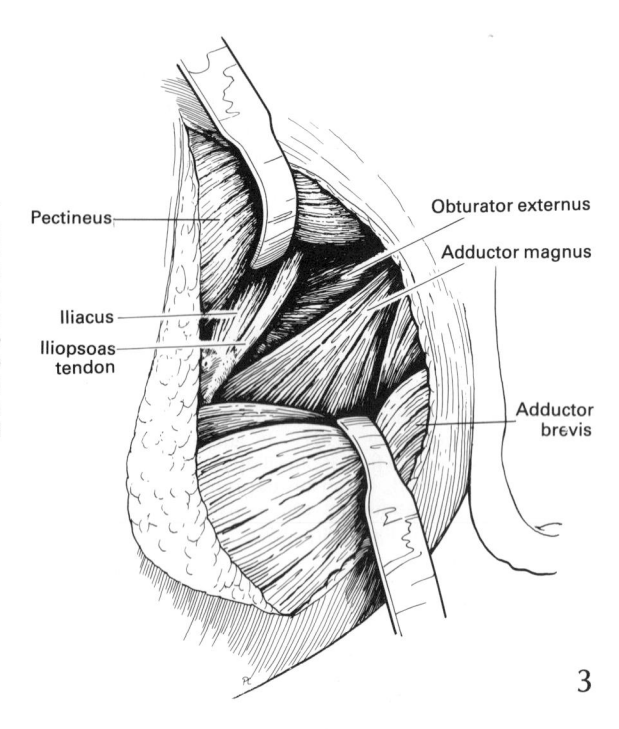

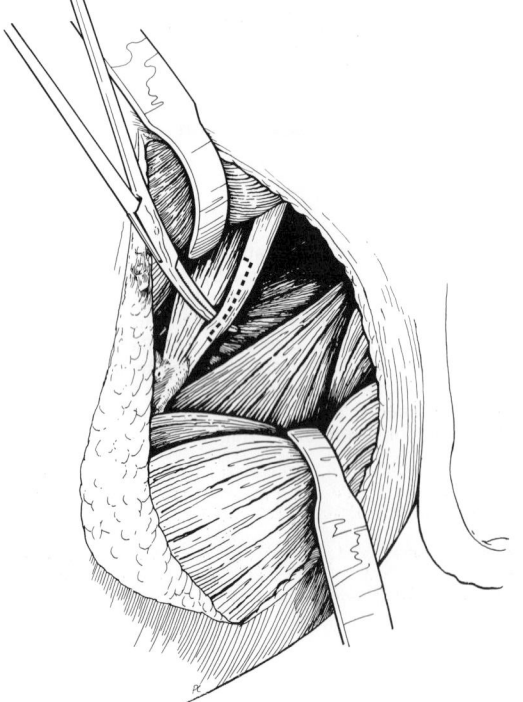

Procedure

4

The tendinous part of the iliopsoas tendon needs to be defined from the muscular fibres of the iliacus which lie lateral to the tendon and are inserted into it and to the femur just above the lesser trochanter. The iliopsoas tendon is often present as two bands: a more superficial one attached to the lesser trochanter and a deeper one which passes more posteriorly to be attached to the shaft of the femur. A pair of long-handled curved artery forceps is insinuated between the tendon and the femoral shaft just above the lesser trochanter to lift it up and to allow the precise definition of its deep surface.

5

If sufficient tendon is available, it can be divided by a Z-incision over a distance of 4–5 cm. If there are two well-defined bands they can be used as the two portions of tendon for lengthening, dividing the anterior band from the lesser trochanter and the deep band as far proximally as possible. Before the two portions of the tendon are divided, the ends should be secured by Kocher's forceps. The proximal portion is likely to retract into the depths of the wound proximally. Confirmation of correction of the flexion deformity is made by flexing the opposite hip fully (Thomas' test). The ends of the tendon are approximated and sutured to each other by two or three stout non-absorbable sutures using a small curved needle.

If the iliopsoas tendon is too short or exposure of a sufficient length is not possible, the iliacus fibres are not separated from the tendon. The iliopsoas tendon is divided just above the lesser trochanter and allowed to stretch. If the iliacus fibres prove to be too tight, they can be sectioned as well but it is usually better to leave the iliacus to prevent too much proximal displacement of the iliopsoas tendon. Alternatively, the proximal end of the tendon can be sutured more proximally to the anterior aspect of the hip capsule near the base of the femoral neck as an iliopsoas recession[3].

Because the dissection takes place between muscle planes, blood loss is minimal and blood transfusion is not normally required.

Wound closure

The wound is closed in the same way as for adductor release (see p. 929). If the preoperative flexion deformity was 30° or less and the hip is not significantly unstable, no plaster fixation is required. A crêpe hip spica bandage is applied. If there is more severe deformity or hip instability a plaster hip spica may be needed (see chapter on 'Hip flexor release: iliofemoral approach', pp. 931–935).

Postoperative management

Rest in bed either prone or supine is needed for 3 weeks, with pillows between the thighs if plaster is not used. If there is considerable spasm in spastic patients, diazepam is a useful drug for its control after operation. Gentle passive hip movements and active hip extension exercises can be started on the second or third day. The skin sutures are removed after 10–12 days. Active mobilization and return to preoperative activities can start after the third week.

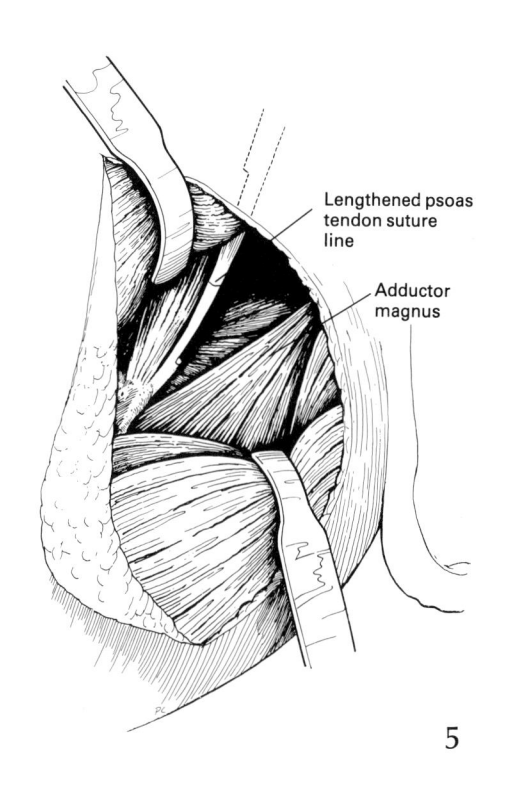

References

1. Ludloff K. Zur blutigen Einrenkung der angeborenen Hüftluxation. *Z Orthop Chir* 1908; 22: 272–6.

2. Keats S, Morgese AN. A simple anteromedial approach to the lesser trochanter of the femur for the release of the iliopsoas tendon. *J Bone Joint Surg [Am]* 1967; 49-A: 632–6.

3. Bleck EE. Postural and gait abnormalities caused by hip-flexion deformity in spastic cerebral palsy: treatment by iliopsoas recession. *J Bone Joint Surg [Am]* 1971; 53-A: 1468–88.

Illustrations by Peter Cox after F. Price

Proximal hamstring release

W. J. W. Sharrard MD, ChM, FRCS
Emeritus Consultant Orthopaedic Surgeon, Royal Hallamshire Hospital and Children's Hospital, Sheffield;
Professor of Orthopaedic Surgery, University of Sheffield, UK

Preoperative

Indications and assessment

The indication for this operation is limited to shortness of the hamstring muscle in the absence of significant flexion deformity of the knee in cerebral palsy or other paralytic conditions. The effect is to cause limitation of hip flexion, so that the patient's length of stride is much reduced and he has to walk with flexed knees or with rotation of the pelvis or both. He cannot sit with the knees extended. The degree of shortness is assessed either by determining the range of straight-leg raising, that is flexion of the hip with the knee extended, or the limitation of extension of the knee when the hip is flexed to a right angle. Straight-leg raising of less than 35° or limitation of extension of the knee by 35° or more when the hip is flexed is an indication for operation. If there is more than 20° of limitation of knee extension when the hip is extended, distal hamstring release is preferable (see pp. 981–984). Proximal hamstring release is also contraindicated when there is marked lumbar lordosis, which may be increased by proximal hamstring release.

Anaesthesia and position of patient

General anaesthesia is needed. The shortness of the hamstring is confirmed under anaesthesia. The patient is placed prone with the pelvis elevated on sandbags and the hip flexed 30°–40° by breaking the operating table. A diathermy pad is applied. The skin is prepared. The lower limbs up to the level of the mid-thigh are covered by sterile stockinette and drapes are placed to expose the distal part of the buttock and the upper half of the posterior aspect of the thigh. The operative area may be covered by a transparent adhesive drape.

Operation

Incision

1

A transverse incision is made in the natal fold 2.5 cm distal to the ischial tuberosity over medial two-thirds of the posterior aspect of the thigh. The incision is deepened through subcutaneous fat, which is often thick, down to the deep fascia from which it is mobilized proximally and distally for 6 or 7 cm in each direction.

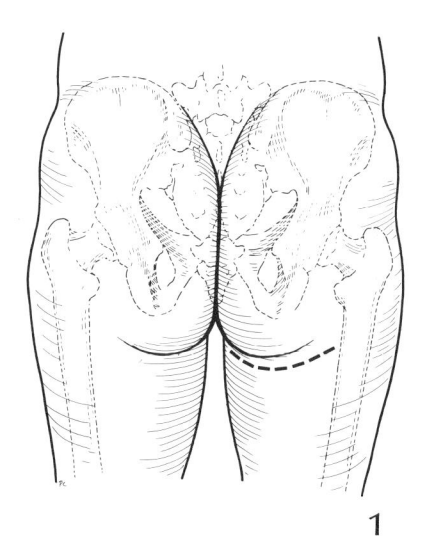

Exposure of the hamstring tendons

2

The lower border of the gluteus maximus is defined, separated from the deep fascia and mobilized upwards and laterally. Care must be taken to avoid damage to the sciatic nerve which lies deep to the gluteus maximus. The ischial tuberosity is palpated and the site of the hamstring tendons arising from it and running distally is established. A vertical incision is made through the deep fascia overlying the tendons which are cleared over a distance of 6 or 7 cm and their origin from the ischial tuberosity is defined. The long head of biceps arises in common with the semitendinosus from the inferomedial facet of the ischial tuberosity, and the semimembranosus arises from the superolateral facet expanding into an aponeurosis closely associated with the other two tendons. The sciatic nerve should be identified and a tape passed beneath it with which to retract it laterally. Occasionally the nerve may present in its two main branches at this level.

Musculotendinous division

3

The more superficial tendon arising from the ischial tuberosity is the common tendon of the long head of biceps and semitendinosus. It is divided by a long incision as oblique as possible, the proximal end of the distal fragment being held by Kocher's forceps to prevent its excessive distal retraction. The tendon and upper aponeurosis of the semimembranosus is similarly exposed and divided. If the adductor magnus tendon is tight, it, too, can be divided at its attachment to the ischial tuberosity and allowed to retract. The tips of the elongated hamstring tendons are sutured by thick non-absorbable sutures. The tendons should not be allowed to retract or there is a danger of excessive lengthening and the production of pelvic lordosis. Bleeding is not usually significant and any small vessels can be coagulated by diathermy.

Wound closure

The deep fascia is closed vertically by interrupted or continuous non-absorbable sutures and the subcutaneous tissue is closed by absorbable interrupted sutures in a transverse line. The skin is closed by interrupted sutures or continuous subcuticular sutures. A simple adhesive dressing is applied.

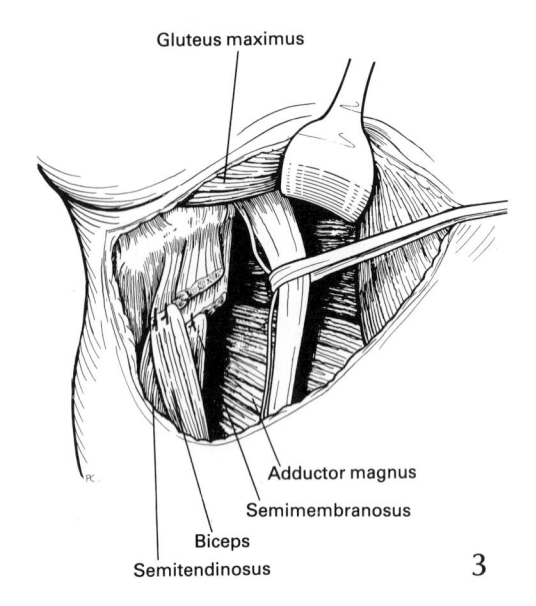

Postoperative management

For the first 24 hours, the patient is nursed supine. After this the patient is encouraged to sit in bed with the hips progressively flexed by 20° more per day whilst the knees are kept straight by means of a draw sheet. He is allowed to lie in a straight supine posture at night. In younger children, in whom it may be difficult to keep the knees extended, or in patients with considerable spasm, a plaster backslab or a plastic splint may be needed to keep the knees extended, and diazepam may help to limit muscle spasm.

The sutures are removed on the tenth to twelfth day. By the end of the second week, straight-leg raising should reach 90° and walking can be resumed, using, if necessary, a simple brace to maintain knee extension for 2 or 3 weeks.

Further reading

Reimers J. Contracture of the hamstrings in cerebral palsy: a study of the three methods of operative correction. *J Bone Joint Surg [Br]* 1974; 56-B: 102–9.

Seymour N, Sharrard WJW. Bilateral proximal hamstring release of the hamstrings in cerebral palsy. *J Bone Joint Surg [Br]* 1968; 50-B: 274–7.

Illustrations by Robert Lane and Gillian Lee

Total hip replacement arthroplasty

Kevin Hardinge MChOrth, FRCS
Hunterian Professor, Royal College of Surgeons of England; Honorary Lecturer, Victoria University of Manchester; Consultant Orthopaedic Surgeon, Centre for Hip Surgery, Wrightington Hospital, Wigan, UK

Introduction

Cemented total hip replacement is firmly established as a highly successful procedure giving total relief of pain and good movement in painful osteoarthritis from a variety of causes for periods up to 15 years. Infection rate is low and the chief problem is component loosening. Longer-lasting prostheses wear more, producing particles which cause inflammation and bone resorption leading to loosening. New, low-wear materials will be required in future. The early promise of uncemented prostheses, which should be easy to revise in the absence of cement, has been marred by slow recovery from operation and persistent thigh pain.

Indications

Total hip replacement aims to eradicate pain and stiffness in the operated hip and restore a physiological gait. To obtain this goal there must be optimum conditions for joint visualization, cementation, implant orientation and correction of leg length inequality.

The total hip arthroplasty, using a stemmed femoral component and an ultra-high molecular weight polyethylene (UHMWPE) acetabular cup, has the longest record of proven benefit in the treatment of degenerative arthrosis of the hip. The components are bonded to the bone by methylmethacrylate cement and this bond depends upon an intimate interdigitation of the cement with cancellous bone, producing sound mechanical interlocking – the bond responding well to compression but poorly to tension and shear.

A femoral component with a head of small diameter is an essential feature of the Charnley low-friction arthroplasty as the low frictional torque reduces shear at the cement–bone interface of both the acetabular component and the femoral stem. The small-diameter component needs precise orientation to minimize postoperative dislocation.

944 Pelvis and hip

Primary osteoarthrosis

1a & b

The total hip arthroplasty was originally indicated for 'idiopathic' osteoarthrosis in old patients because of the limited lifespan of the procedure: these patients may have loss of joint space, sclerosis of bone and marginal osteophytes, leading to pain and stiffness. However, the success of the operation in this group of patients has led to the application of the technique to a greater variety of pathological abnormalities.

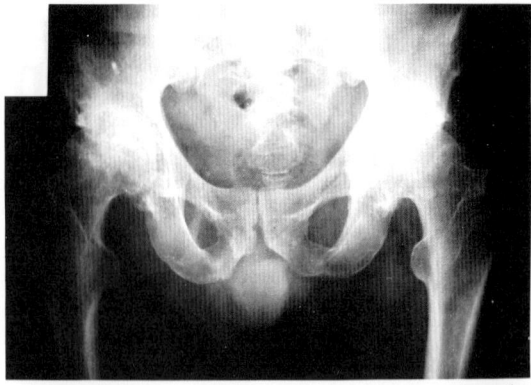

1a

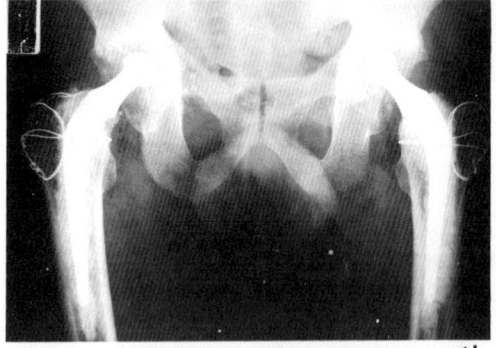

1b

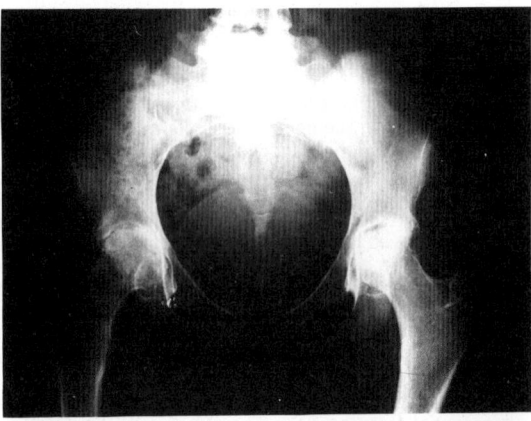

2a

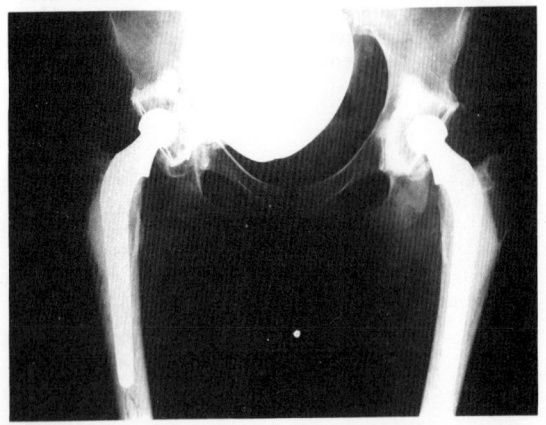

Rheumatoid arthritis

2a & b

The earliest alternative application was for rheumatoid arthritis where the hip degeneration can be severe. Many of these patients are young but the alternative to operation can be a wheelchair existence. The lady depicted in the illustration was 27 years old, having suffered with rheumatoid arthritis since the age of 11 years. The arthroplasties have been performed using the direct lateral approach. It is noteworthy that the pre-operative film shows that Shenton's line is almost intact, thus leg length discrepancy is not marked. The post-operative film shows complete restoration of Shenton's line; good walking ability was restored.

2b

Ankylosing spondylitis

3a & b

Ankylosing spondylitis affects young adults presenting usually with pain and stiffness in the spine. Spontaneous fusion of the hip was frequently seen formerly and was possibly due to prolonged immobilization. The preoperative illustration shows fusion of the sacroiliac joints, which is diagnostic of ankylosing spondylitis; the hips have also fused, in addition to the symphysis pubis. Note how Shenton's line is intact, indicating that the hips have fused in the anatomical position[1]. The mobilization of this fusion and conversion to total hip arthroplasty can be a difficult technical procedure, but it is certainly made easier by the wide exposure gained from trochanteric osteotomy. The postoperative radiograph shows the appearance after bilateral total hip arthroplasty where trochanteric osteotomy has been employed to facilitate the exposure and femoral neck section.

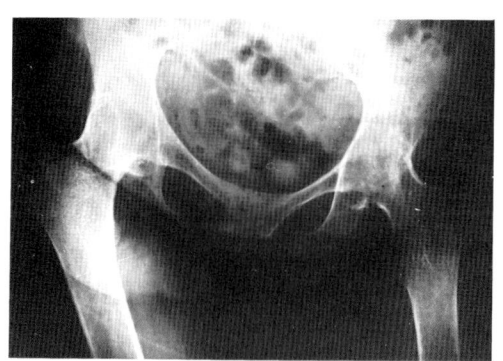

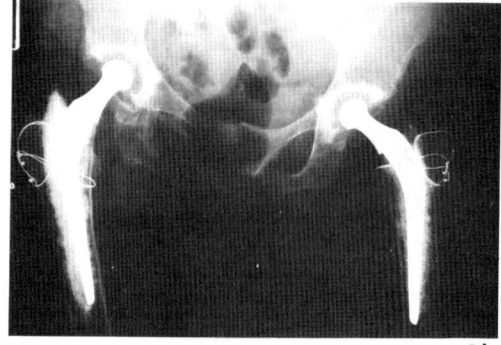

946 Pelvis and hip

Protrusio acetabuli

4, 5a & b

Stress fracture of the medial wall of the acetabulum with subsequent healing can occur idiopathically or in rheumatoid arthritis, Paget's disease, ankylosing spondylitis or osteoarthritis. It is typified radiologically by the medial wall of the acetabulum being shown to have protruded past the ilio-ischial line (Y–Y). The medial acetabular wall may become fragmented and total hip replacement may be technically difficult because of the lack of constraint on the fixation of the prosthetic cup. Grafting the medial wall with slices taken from the femoral head constitutes a useful method of containing the cement.

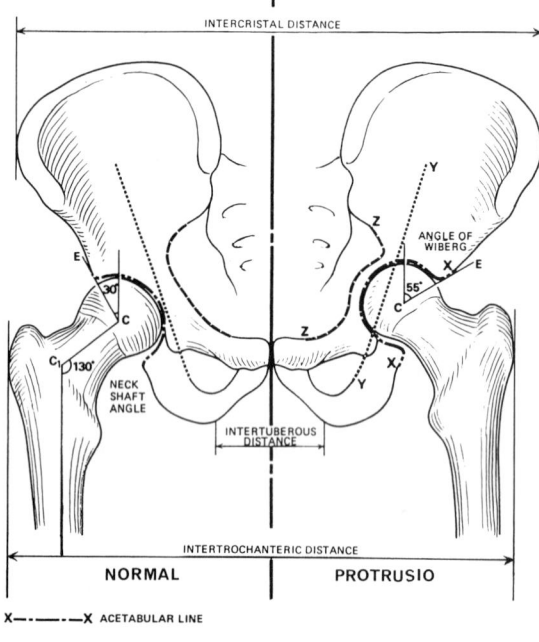

4

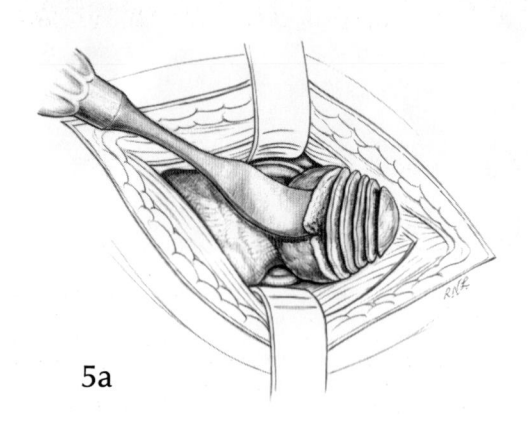

5a

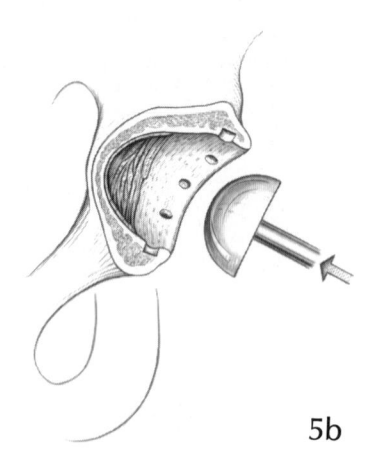

5b

6a & b

This method was used in a 67-year-old man who had suffered gradually increasing pain and stiffness in the hips for 10 years, having enjoyed an exceptional level of physical activity until the age of 50 years[2]: he had medial migration of the acetabular walls, with thick sclerotic bases to the acetabula. As a result of the bone graft allowing the cup to be lateralized to the face of the pelvis, Shenton's line was restored, and the patient has become much more mobile.

The bone graft has become incorporated with the fragmented medial acetabular wall and remodelled so the the pelvic brim (ilio-pectineal line) is restored to normal.

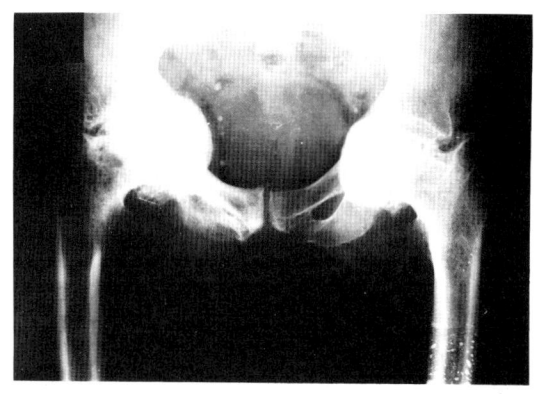

6a

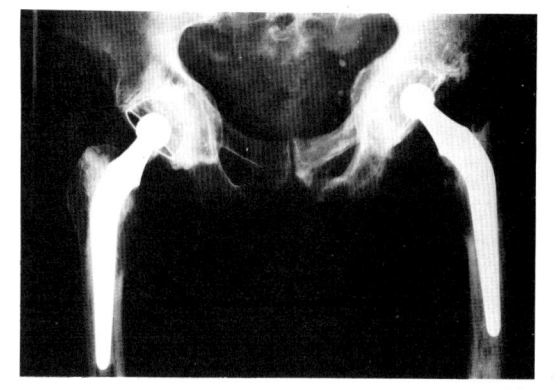

6b

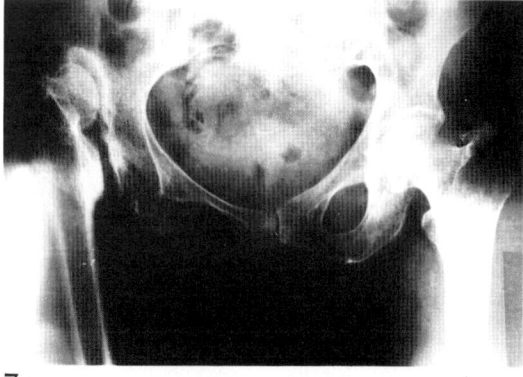

Congenital dislocation of the hip

7a & b

Congenital dislocation of the hip occurs when there is variable disproportion between the head of the femur and the acetabulum. In many cases the head has never been in the true acetabulum, and indeed moulds a false acetabulum on the side of the ilium. Secondary degenerative arthrosis can supervene in the third and fourth decade and impose a severe restriction on walking as a result of pain and stiffness. The acetabulum in these cases is abnormally small and a bone graft, taken from the head of the femur and bolted to the side of the ilium, can provide an improved bone cover for the prosthetic acetabular cup. Clearly, in these cases a wide exposure is mandatory and can be obtained using a trochanteric osteotomy.

7a

7b

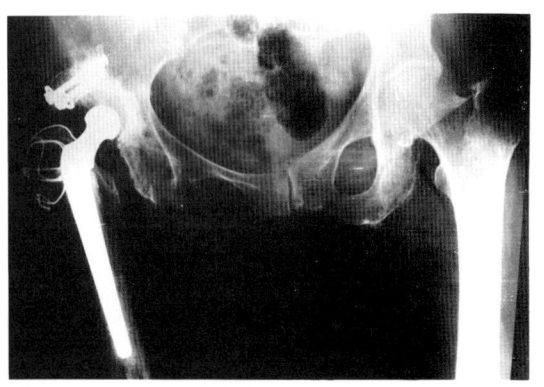

948 Pelvis and hip

Degenerative hip conditions due to old sepsis

8a & b

Septic arthritis and tuberculous hip disease lead to a variable damage of the articular surfaces. This joint damage can lead, after full healing of the primary infection, to a secondary degenerative arthrosis or to a spontaneous fusion in the healing process. In this case, after a tuberculous infection of both hips in childhood, there has been spontaneous fusion of the right hip in marked abduction with ossification of the sacrospinous ligament, and a severe degenerative arthrosis of the left hip in marked adduction. The right hip was not painful because it was fused. The left hip was very painful and was the primary reason for the patient's referral. There was flexion contracture of both hips and lumbar lordosis. It is important to note that the symptoms in the left hip are due to the position of marked adduction producing a subluxation that is *secondary* to the deformity of the right hip. It could be incorrect to offer a total hip arthroplasty for the left hip alone as it would still function in marked adduction and would be in danger of dislocating.

It was necessary to correct the primary deformity; in this case, converting the right hip to a total arthroplasty with correction of the abduction deformity, so that the subsequent arthroplasty of the left hip could function in a more neutral position. The pelvic tilt and lordosis were thus reduced and mobility increased.

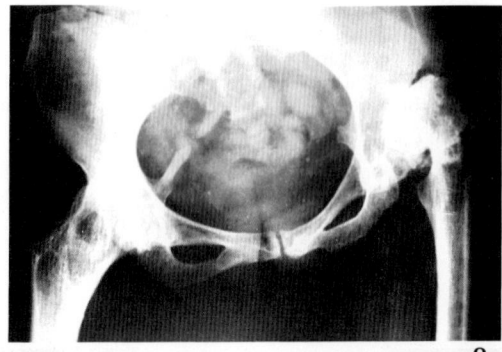

Criteria for arthroplasty after infection

Clearly it is important to avoid reactivation of a pre-existing septic or tuberculous infection as the total hip arthroplasty would fail. It is vital to ensure that the previous infection is cured and this can be achieved with a high level of certainty using clinical, radiological and haematological criteria[3].

Clinically, the patient must have a clear-cut history of the infective condition and have recovered from it. This course of events may have entailed from 1 to several years in hospital or under treatment, but been followed by complete subsidence of the infection and the restoration of walking with useful function. The history must also reveal that the period of recovery and improvement in function has lasted several years. If the patient's symptoms are due to the supervention of secondary arthritis there will also typically be a gradual decline in overall function over a period of years. The onset of pain and stiffness will have been in the remote past and both will have gradually increased in severity. Physical examination shows stiffness of the joint without local signs of inflammation and an absence of spasm.

The radiographs show sound bony ankylosis in these cases with spontaneous fusion of the joint or, if the joint is mobile, loss of joint space, sclerosis of joint surfaces and marginal osteophytosis. The haematological tests should show a normal erythrocyte sedimentation rate and white cell count. It is important to repeat the radiographs and blood tests after a 6-month period when it should be possible to establish that the patient's symptoms are due to secondary degenerative arthrosis, and that total hip arthroplasty is a safe procedure.

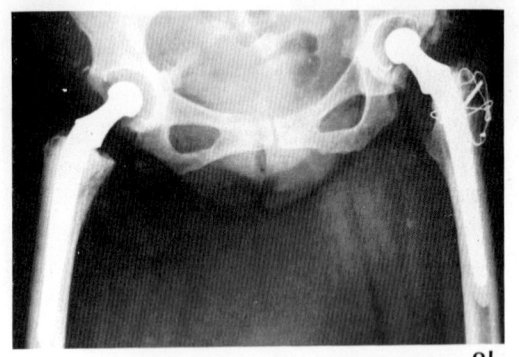

8a

8b

9a & b

Where septic arthritis before skeletal maturity has led to severe bone destruction and limb shortening, it is not always possible to restore the leg length fully, because of tension in the pelvifemoral intermuscular septa. In a similar way, active movement will not be full and a limp will persist as a result of the overall limb-length discrepancy. It must be emphasized to the patient that total hip arthroplasty in the presence of severe bone destruction cannot fully restore movement and limb length, and must be considered 'a limited goal' procedure. There can, however, occasionally be quite gratifying results after septic arthritis of the hip in infancy has caused loss of the head of the femur. The illustration shows a hip that had always been mobile, and it was possible to restore leg length by total hip arthroplasty.

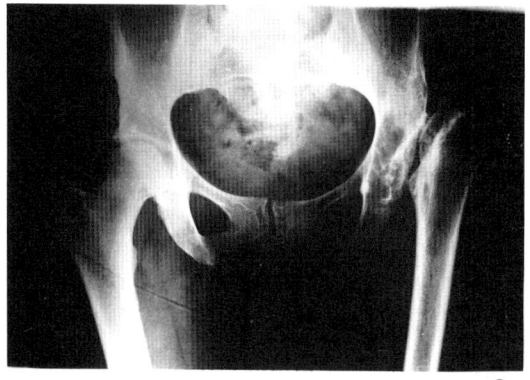

9a

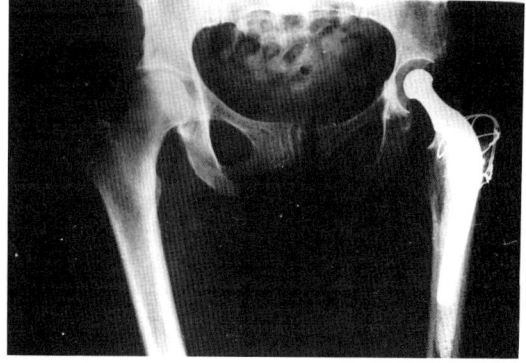

9b

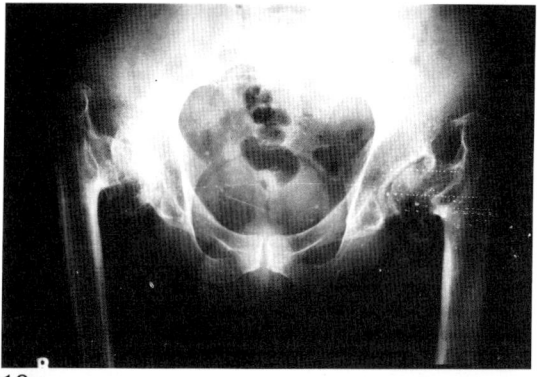

Congenital hip dysplasia other than dislocation

10a & b

Infantile coxa vara can present as an idiopathic condition or may be present in association with craniocleidodysostosis. Both these conditions, and also multiple epiphyseal dysplasia, can lead to a severe secondary degenerative arthrosis in the fourth and fifth decade: the patient illustrated could not abduct the hip, so that ankle separation was limited to 12 cm. Considerable improvement in function can be bestowed by total hip arthroplasty, but it is necessary to improve exposure by performing trochanteric osteotomy in these cases of distorted anatomy.

The secondary degenerative arthrosis that follows Perthes' disease and slipped upper femoral epiphysis does not require variation in surgical technique, and will not be considered separately.

10a

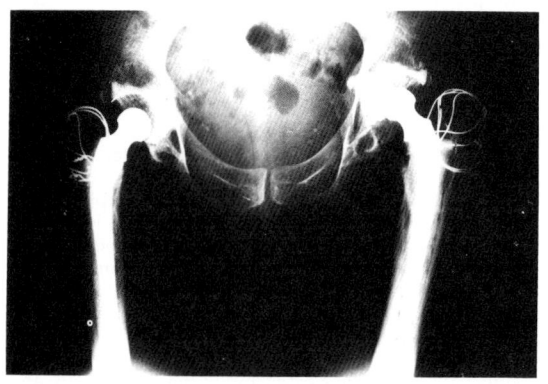

10b

950   Pelvis and hip

Failed previous surgery

11a & b

The success and dependability of the total hip arthroplasty in primary and secondary arthrosis has led to wide application in cases where surgery has failed.

In the decade before successful total hip arthroplasty, a variety of surgical methods were employed to treat osteoarthrosis. The illustration shows the result of attempted fusion of the hip in osteoarthrosis by the use of a transarticular pin (which broke) and an ischiofemoral graft (which also fractured). Movement of the joint still occurred, and caused severe local pain. Impressive relief of pain resulted from conversion of the unsound fusion to a total hip arthroplasty, when, to improve exposure, a trochanteric osteotomy was performed[4,5].

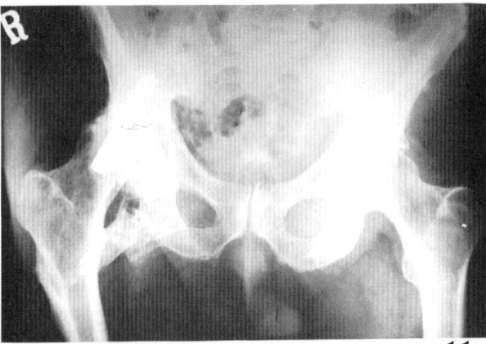

11a

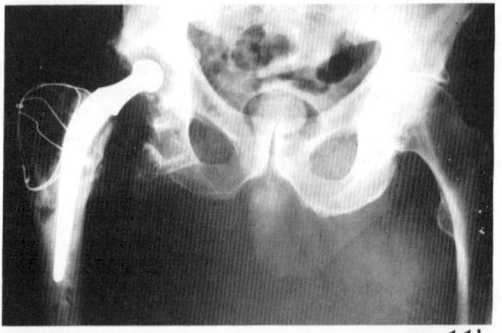

11b

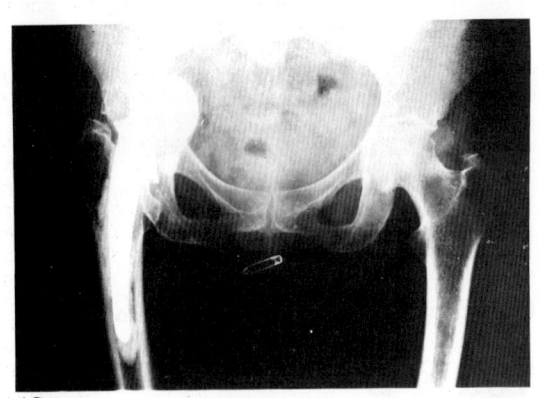

12a & b

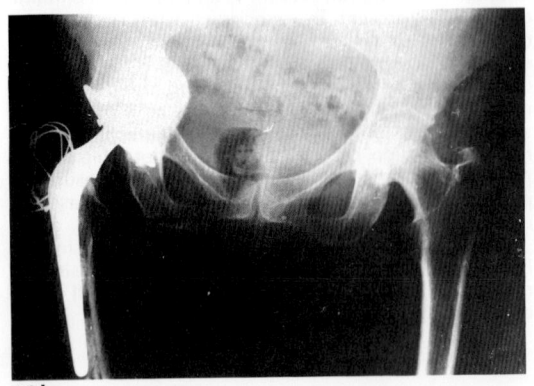

Femoral head replacement after fracture of the neck of the femur has been the method of choice where wide separation of the capital fragment has occurred and reduction is poor. On occasion the femoral replacement can loosen, migrate upwards, erode the acetabulum and penetrate the pelvis. In one patient there was a large defect of the base of the acetabulum and the femoral head was not available to use for grafting. When the total hip arthroplasty was performed, a metallic reinforcement ring was used to support the prosthetic acetabular cup, and when placed into the acetabulum prevented migration of the cement used for fixation. Before the total hip arthroplasty, this patient had had severe leg length discrepancy due to migration of the prosthetic head which had occurred within 12–18 months of operation. After this relatively short history and previous normal leg length, it was possible to restore equality.

The original indication for total hip arthroplasty was severe degenerative osteoarthrosis of the hip in the elderly. Yet a large group of patients in their seventh decade had pain in the hip, stiffness and a limp due to shortening of the limb as a result of destruction of the joint surfaces. Initially, the procedure was confined to the elderly because it was felt that the lifespan of the implant was limited to at most 10 years, but the success of the early results led to a cautious extension of the time period, and use in the younger patient.

12a

12b

Surgical approaches

General principles

Surgical exposure of the hip joint must take account of muscle innervation and blood supply and must avoid, if possible, detachment of muscle insertions, since detachment prolongs recovery time and increases morbidity. Thus, the advantage of any approach that minimizes muscle detachment must be contrasted with the disadvantage that may arise from limited exposure which may necessitate heavy soft tissue retraction. Poor visibility of the joint cavity may similarly lead to poor orientation of the implants so that movement may be compromised or instability and dislocation occur.

Orientation of the implant to the bony pelvis is certainly facilitated if the patient is placed in the supine position. In this way the anterior superior iliac spine and the greater trochanter can be palpated through the surgical drapes and thus implant orientation can be facilitated by alignment to the horizontal plane, and leg length equalization promoted by direct comparison to the contralateral limb. The supine position is used in the original technique of McKee, Müller and Charnley while the lateral decubitus position is employed for the posterior approaches to the hip joint.

An appreciation of the development of the various surgical approaches to the hip joint in an historical sense serves to emphasize their original indication and can illustrate potential shortcomings. For example, Moore's southern exposure[6] was originally described for insertion of the self-locking femoral head prosthesis, and while it is adequate for this purpose it does not give a sufficient view of the acetabulum for total hip arthroplasty. In addition, the acetabulum is anteverted or anteriorly disposed to a varying extent, and necessitating as it does the lateral decubitus position, the posterior approach of Moore does not facilitate accurate orientation of the implant.

The anterolateral approach of Watson-Jones[7] was originally described for open reduction of fractures of the neck of the femur; although it gives good exposure of the neck of the femur, exposure of the acetabulum depends upon heavy retraction of the soft tissue and can be associated with damage to the femoral vein, artery and nerve, particularly in obese patients or those with well-developed musculature. Similarly access to the femur is possible only with the femur held in strong lateral rotation, adduction and flexion, so that orientation of the femoral component may be difficult.

The lateral approach with trochanteric osteotomy, the patient lying in the supine position, has always been associated with Charnley[8]. Trochanteric osteotomy has been the traditional approach used in hip surgery in Manchester, having been brought from Boston, Massachusetts, by Platt where he had worked with Brackett and also visited Whitman in New York. It has the advantage of a wide exposure of the hip for correction of deformity, implant orientation, and leg length equalization.

Trochanteric osteosynthesis remains a difficult problem, particularly with scarred tissue and osteoporotic bone. In Charnley's hand the level of complication was accepted, but trochanteric osteotomy has not been widely practised, except by a few devotees[9].

The direct lateral approach[10] developed from that described by McFarland and Osborne[11], offers the advantages of the supine position, without trochanteric osteotomy, and adequate exposure of the acetabulum and femur for implant orientation and leg length equalization, but is suitable only for the patient without severe deformity or marked leg length inequality (the 'anatomical' hip). These patients account for 85 per cent of primary arthritic hips. It has distinct advantages in this respect over the anterolateral and posterior approaches.

Anterior approaches to the hip were described by Smith-Petersen[12] and others. They were used exclusively for the original cup arthroplasty and by Wagner[13] for his double-cup arthroplasty. The approach has not gained popularity with other surgeons because of the need for extensive detachment of tendinous insertions and retraction of muscle, with potential damage to vital structures such as femoral artery and nerve, and because of traction exerted on the lateral cutaneous nerve of the thigh, causing numbness or meralgia paraesthetica. Whereas the Smith-Petersen approach can be recommended for operation on the innominate bones (Chiari and Salter osteotomy), it is not recommended for total hip arthroplasty as better exposures exist.

POSTERIOR APPROACH

Anatomical considerations

13

The muscles covering the posterior aspect of the hip joint form two layers. The outer layer, the 'pelvic deltoid of Henry'[14], is the gluteus maximus, the largest muscle in the body; the fascia lata covers the gluteus medius and the tensor fasciae latae forms a continuous muscle sheath. This outer layer can be incised at different points, each of which changes the surgical approach.

The Moore or southern exposure splits the gluteus maximus at the junction of the anterior and intermediate thirds, and because of poor access to the acetabulum is not advised for total hip arthroplasty.

The Gibson approach[15] is in the inter-nervous plane between gluteus maximus (inferior gluteal nerve) and gluteus medius (superior gluteal nerve). Whereas the Gibson approach detaches gluteus medius and minimus from the greater trochanter, the further refinement of Marcy and Fletcher[16] leaves the gluteus medius and minimus insertions intact and effects dislocation by strong flexion and medial rotation.

The deep layer of muscle consists of the short lateral rotators of the hip, the piriformis, the superior gamellus, the obturator internus, the inferior gamellus and the quadratus femoris. The sciatic nerve runs down through the operative field between the layers closely applied to the posterior capsule of the hip joint.

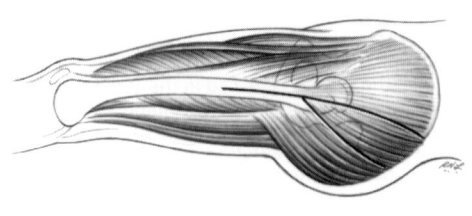

13

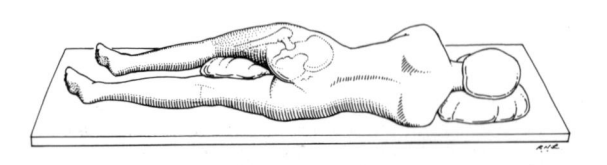

Position of patient

14

The patient is placed in the true mid-lateral position with the affected limb uppermost. The limb is draped free to allow for movement and manipulation during the procedure.

14

Incision

15

The greater trochanter forms the landmark for the incision and the posterior edge can be palpated through the drapes.

The incision is 12–15 cm long, curved and centres on the greater trochanter. Its starts 6–8 cm above and posterior to the greater trochanter, in line with the posterior superior iliac spine, and passes towards the trochanter in the same direction as the fibres of the gluteus maximus. The incision curves over the posterior aspect of the greater trochanter and continues down along the shaft of the femur for 6–8 cm.

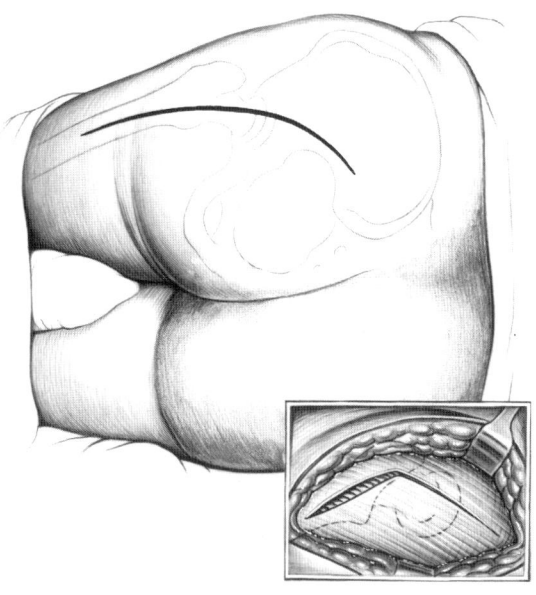

Superficial dissection

16

The fascia lata on the lateral aspect of the femur is incised and this fascial incision is developed proximally and enters the plane between gluteus maximus and gluteus medius. The fibres of the gluteus maximus are coarser than gluteus medius and the plane is developed between them to split the fascia and open it up. In this way the blades of the retractors are placed on the gluteus maximus and gluteus medius to avoid traction on the sciatic nerve which will not be exposed in this procedure, although it can be palpated in the fat lying in the posterior aspect of the deeper space.

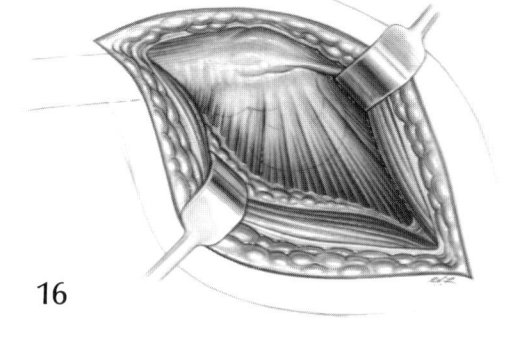

Deep dissection

17

The space between the gluteus medius and gluteus maximus is floored by the short lateral rotators which cover the posterior aspect of the hip joint. The thigh is medially rotated to stretch the short lateral rotators and to distance the deep incision from the sciatic nerve.

Stay sutures are inserted into the piriformis and obturator internus tendons before their insertion to leave a skirt of tendon inserted into the femur for later suture. The tendons are divided to expose the neck of the femur and laid over the sciatic nerve to protect it. Part of quadratus femoris may need to be divided, at which point troublesome bleeding from the lateral circumflex femoral artery can be encountered.

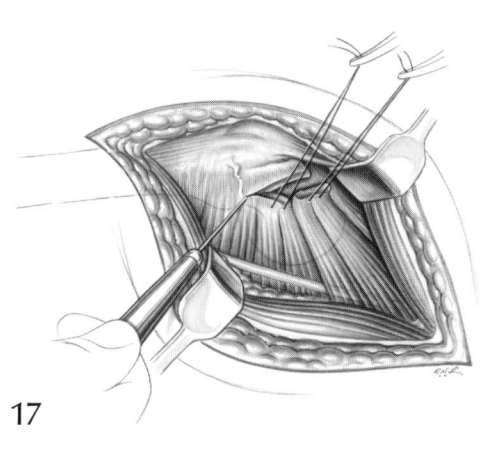

18

The capsule of the hip joint is now exposed and is longitudinally incised; if the hip is stiff part of the posterior capsule is excised to permit dislocation by medial rotation of the femur. With excision of the capsule and placement of the Hohmann's retractors, the acetabulum is exposed.

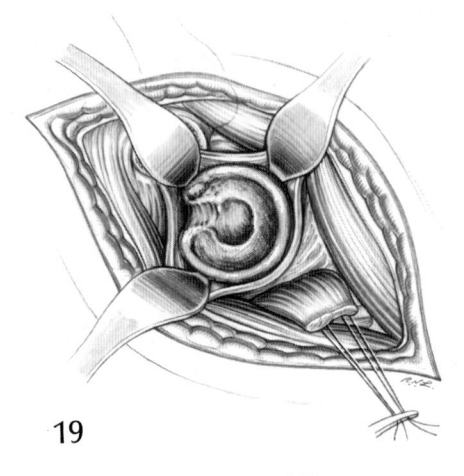

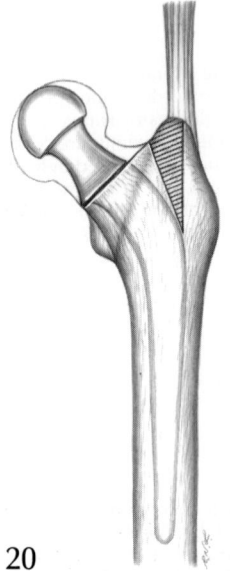

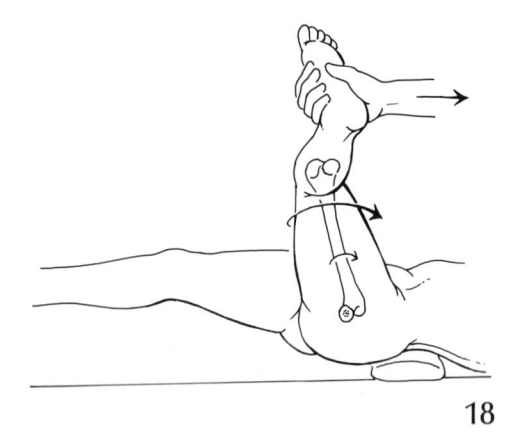

19 & 20

The femoral head is excised by Gigli saw or oscillating saw and the femur is prepared for insertion of the prosthesis by removal of bone at the trochanteric fossa.

21

Clearly alignment of the acetabular component depends upon the patient being firmly secured in the true lateral decubitus position, whilst the femoral prosthesis is inserted with the femur held in full medial rotation.

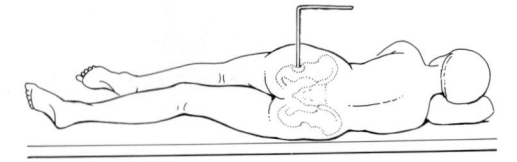

THE ANTEROLATERAL APPROACH

Anatomical considerations

The fascia lata covers all the thigh and hamstring muscles; it covers the sartorius and then splits into a deep and superficial layer to enclose the tensor fasciae latae and the gluteus maximus. The gluteus medius is covered by the fascia lata on its superficial surface only and is not enveloped by it.

The anterolateral approach develops the intermuscular plane between the tensor fasciae latae and the gluteus medius. The origins of the two muscles are almost continuous but they diverge towards their insertions.

The tensor fasciae latae arises superficially from the anterior portion of the outer lip of the iliac crest and inserts into the iliotibial band; whereas the gluteus medius, arising from the outer surface of the ilium between the anterior and posterior gluteal lines, inserts deeply into the anterior and lateral aspects of the greater trochanter. They share a common nerve supply from the superior gluteal nerve.

To exploit this intermuscular plane, the overlying fascia is incised below the posterior margin of the tensor fasciae latae, so that, because the fascia lata envelops the tensor muscle, retracting the fascia takes the muscle up with it. The nerve supply lies in the interval and can be damaged inadvertently as the capsule is exposed.

Position of patient

The patient is placed in the supine position, although some proponents place a small pillow beneath the buttocks on the operative side[17] or slightly tilt the table to raise the buttocks[18].

Incision

22

The incision begins 2 cm distal and 2 cm posterior to the anterior superior iliac spine, curves distally and laterally to the apex of the greater trochanter, and extends down over the greater trochanter to end 6 cm distal to the vastus lateralis ridge.

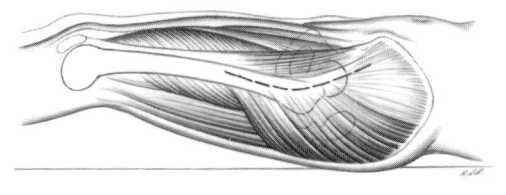

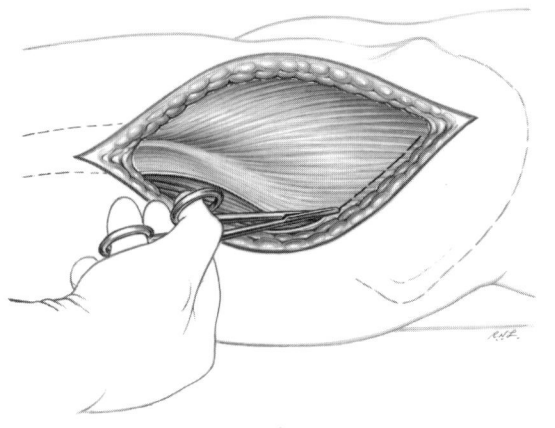

Superficial dissection

23

The deep fascia is incised over the femur distally to the greater trochanter, and the incision continued proximally keeping to the palpable posterior lower border of the tensor fasciae latae. As the cut edge of the fascia lata, with its contained tensor fasciae latae, is brought forwards, the anterior border of the gluteus medius is exposed. The plane between the two muscles is now developed by blunt dissection using the fingers. There are blood vessels in this plane that need to be coagulated.

24

A retractor placed on the anterior border of the gluteus medius muscle border retracts the muscle posteriorly to expose the fat lying on the hip capsule.

The femur should now be fully rotated laterally to stretch the capsule. The upper border of the vastus lateralis is thus exposed at the anterior surface of the femoral neck and reflected for 1 cm, extending down to the vastus lateralis ridge laterally.

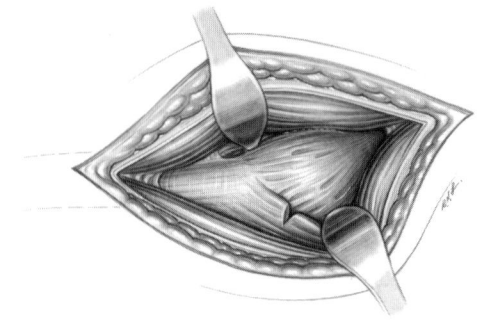

Deep dissection

25

The capsule is visible at this stage and further exposure is only possible with full lateral rotation of the femur and release of the neck of the femur to allow the neck to fall backwards. This is necessary to facilitate exposure of the acetabulum and femoral reaming.

A stay suture is placed into the anterior border of gluteus medius tendon, leaving a skirt of tendon attached to the trochanter for later reattachment. The exact amount of gluteus medius that needs to be detached in this way will vary with the stiffness of the hip and anatomical distortion, but this clearly represents a limitation of the surgical exposure.

A complete capsulectomy is then performed, including the fibres of the reflected head of rectus femoris and vastus lateralis apex inferiorly. Anterior dislocation can now be facilitated by removal of the osteophytes with nibblers followed by traction, lateral rotation and adduction; the neck is sectioned at the desired level with a Gigli saw.

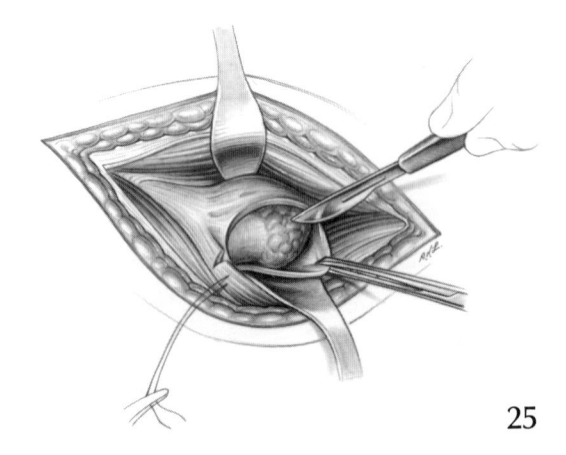

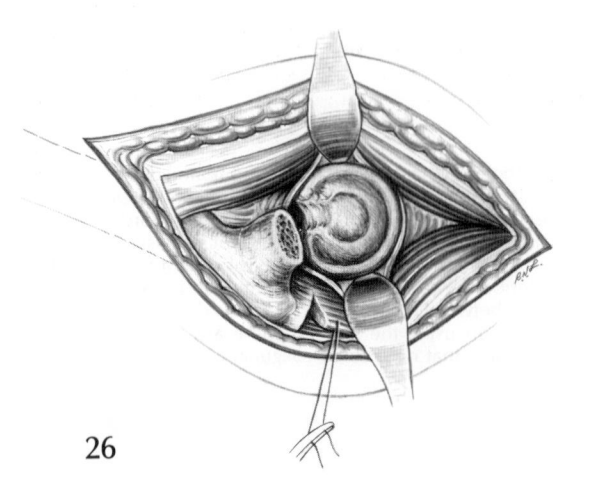

26

The exposure of the acetabulum is then completed by Hohmann retractors placed anteriorly, posteriorly and inferiorly, whilst access to the femur is promoted by full lateral rotation after partial detachment of the gluteus medius insertion.

THE DIRECT LATERAL APPROACH

Anatomical considerations

The direct lateral approach, with or without trochanteric osteotomy, and with the patient lying in the supine position, offers the optimum conditions for joint visualization, adequate cementation, implant orientation and correction of leg length discrepancy.

If there has been a previous arthroplasty, previous surgery such as an intertrochanteric osteotomy, arthrodesis or if there is severe anatomical deformity such as occurs in osteoarthrosis secondary to congenital hip dysplasia or coxa vara, then trochanteric osteotomy gives the preferred wide exposure to the hip joint and ilium to deal with the distorted anatomy. Trochanteric osteosynthesis remains a difficult procedure and problems can occur postoperatively with trochanteric detachment, wire breakage and trochanteric bursitis. If the degenerative arthrosis has occurred in a hip that has an 'anatomical' appearance, then trochanteric osteotomy is not necessary.

A strong physiological gait should be possible in this group of patients if an attempt is made to restore Shenton's line, thus ensuring that all of the pelvifemoral muscles are able to act in a normal fashion. There has been a tendency in the past to concentrate on abductor power only; it must be realized, however, that strong hip function is dependent upon all of the muscle groups that act around the hip joint. If the centre of the axis of rotation of the total hip replacement (the locus) is sited at the centre of the head of the femur, and thus Shenton's line is restored, then excellent function can be expected to return as a result of rehabilitation.

Optimum joint visualization with the patient in the supine position ensures the following.

1. Accurate implant orientation – which permits a maximum range of movement without instability leading to dislocation
2. Adequate cementation – with pressurization in an attempt to ensure a long-term bond that will reduce implant loosening
3. Leg length equalization – the use of bony landmarks enables direct comparison to aid accurate correction of leg length which, combined with correct lateralization, helps to produce a physiological gait.

The gluteus medius tendon blends into the greater trochanter by a crescentic insertion. Taking a pair of blunt forceps it is possible to demonstrate the mobile tendon of the gluteus medius insertion as it merges with the periosteum of the greater trochanter.

Position of patient

The patient is placed in the supine position, with the greater trochanter lying at the edge of the table, thus freeing the buttock muscles from the table. In this way if there are 10 cm or so of subcutaneous fat this is made to hang over the edge of the table so that the actual bony edge of the trochanter is lying at the table edge.

Incision

27

A curved longitudinal incision is made which has the greater trochanter at the midpoint. From the midpoint it proceeds distally along the lateral midline of the shaft of the femur. Proximally it curves posteriorly and ends at a vertical line dropped through the anterior superior iliac spine. If the patient is heavily muscled, it may be necessary to extend this incision slightly more proximally in the posterior direction. The incision will usually be 24 cm in length.

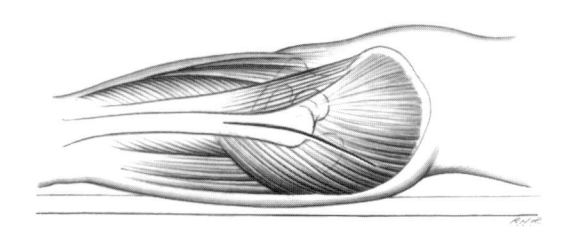

Superficial dissection

28

The gluteal fascia and iliotibial band are exposed in line with the skin incision. It is useful to go straight down to the greater trochanter and palpate the bony landmark before exposing the deep fascia.

The incision of the deep fascia begins over the middle of the trochanter and passes distally, the tissue layer being recognized by bulging of the vastus lateralis, with the fascia here being incised, once again, in the lateral midline of the femur. The deep fascial incision is completed by passing proximally and posteriorly in the direction of the fibres of the gluteus maximus, thus splitting them[19].

The trochanter is then exposed and any soft tissue adhesions on the front of the gluteus medius or the gluteus maximus are freed by blunt dissection.

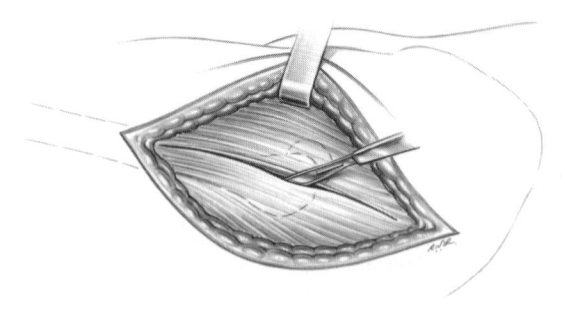

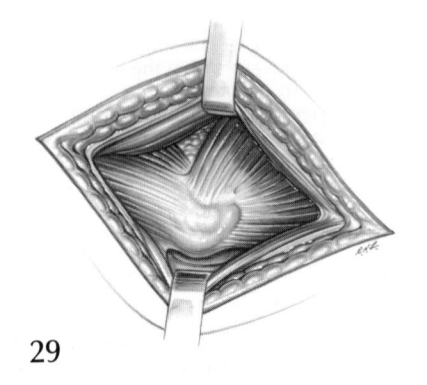

29

There may be a bursa over the trochanter and this must be incised and partially excised to expose the gluteus medius insertion into the greater trochanter. The initial-incision retractor is now inserted, the anterior blade beneath the deep fascia anteriorly at the level of the anterior border of the gluteus medius, and the posterior blade at the level of the gluteus maximus insertion into the posterior aspect of the femur. Tension on the bow of the initial-incision retractor enables the deep fascia to be distracted and the greater trochanter exposed.

Deep dissection

30

In the average subject the incision of the gluteus medius tendon is approximately 1 cm from the musculotendinous junction anteriorly. The incision extends distally to leave the anterior border of the gluteus medius where it borders the vastus lateralis intact, and it divides the vastus lateralis at the junction of the anterior quarter and intermediate half (thus preserving its innervation) for a distance of approximately 6 cm. Posteriorly, the incision of the gluteus medius tendon is extended to the apex of the trochanter and then passes horizontally in a proximal direction so that it splits the fibres of gluteus medius for a distance of 3 cm from the apex of the trochanter. This avoids the innervation of the muscle, that is, the superior gluteal nerve, which is some distance away.

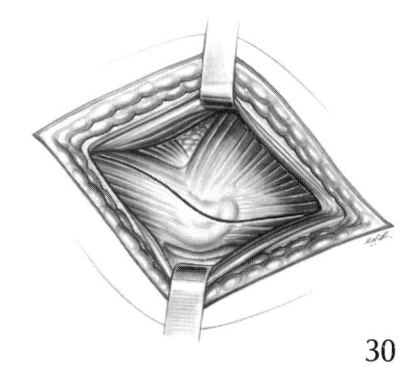

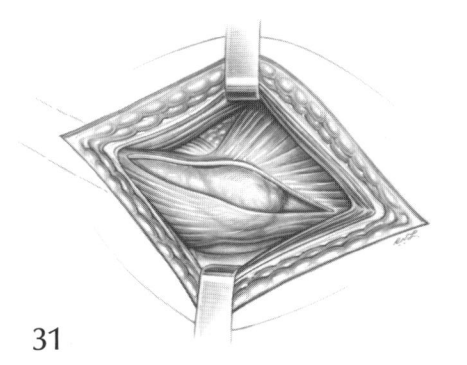

31

Using a cutting diathermy the tendinous insertions of the gluteus medius and minimus are then lifted from the greater trochanter; mild adduction of the thigh causes the neck of the femur to come into view as the gluteus medius muscle opens up anteriorly, while the thick tendinous posterior portion is undisturbed. Using the cutting diathermy the neck of the femur is exposed and the ligament of Bigelow is separated from the prominent ridge on the front of the neck of the femur. Further adduction allows the capsule of the hip joint to come into view. The capsule is incised circumferentially until the posterior aspect of the head of the femur is reached (in the left hip at the 4 o'clock position and in the right hip at the 8 o'clock position), where a radial incision is made into the capsule of the joint down to the edge of the acetabulum.

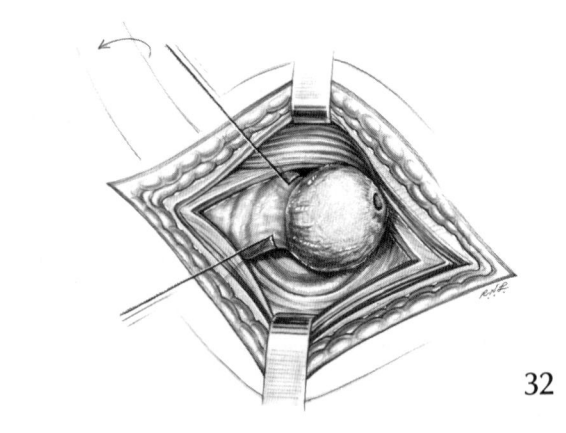

32 & 33

Further adduction of the thigh then brings the head of the femur into view, and gentle further adduction combined with some lateral rotation usually allows dislocation to occur. It will occasionally be necessary to put a curved cholecystectomy-type forceps underneath the neck of the femur to produce gentle traction on the neck to aid dislocation. Dislocation occurs when full adduction of the thigh takes place so that the femur is hanging over the contralateral extended leg. With the tibia in the vertical position neutral section of the neck of the femur is accomplished using the Gigli saw. This takes advantage of the anatomical observation that the trochanter is a posterior structure and the undisturbed part of the gluteus medius is isolated from the femoral neck section.

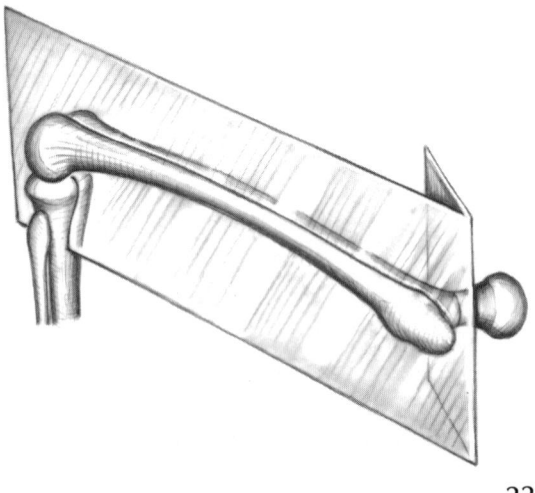

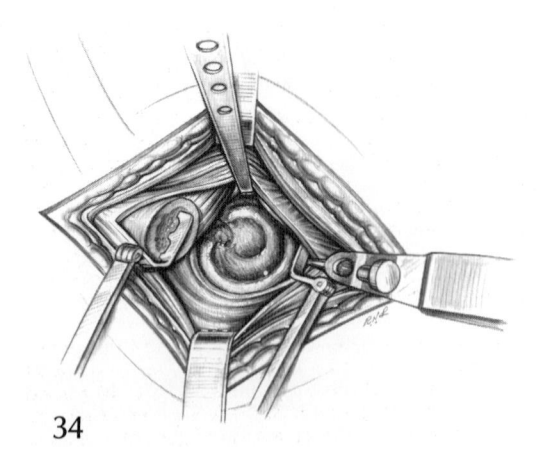

34

The capsule on the superior aspect of the acetabulum is then retracted using a pin retractor (superior capsular retractor) which is hammered firmly home into the innominate bone (in the left hip at the 3 o'clock position, in the right hip at the 9 o'clock position). The blades of the horizontal retractor engage distally with the stump of the cut end of the neck of the femur and proximally with the pin of the superior capsular retractor. Distraction of the horizontal retractor exposes the acetabulum. The anterior capsular retractor is then placed underneath the anterior capsule at the 12 o'clock position in both hips and, by means of the chain, attached to the upper or anterior blade of the initial-incision retractor.

35

The remains of the ligamentum teres is dissected and excised using cutting diathermy. A Hohmann's retractor may be placed into the obturator foramen if prominent synovium obscures the lower lip of the acetabulum. Correlation of the radiographs and the anatomical findings at operation will give an indication of the thickness of the medial wall of the pelvis. A large curette can be used to remove bone from the fovea or insertion of ligamentum teres so that the glistening medial wall of the pelvis is exposed. Preparation of the acetabulum, removing the fibrocartilage and sclerotic bone, is carried out using the deepening and expanding reamers as in the original Charnley technique, or 'potato-grater' reamers. The Charnley technique necessitates a pilot hole to be drilled into the fovea whereas a 'potato-grater' reamer does not. The acetabulum is prepared, removing all fibrous tissue and sclerotic bone, so that raw, bleeding corticocancellous bone is obtained. A series of 5 mm holes is drilled through the cortico-cancellous bone to a depth of 8 mm to augment the keying of the cement into the acetabulum. Lavage is used to remove all fat, blood and debris.

The orientation of the pelvis is then ascertained using the bony landmarks of the anterior superior iliac spines for orientation in the coronal plane, and also the degree of rotation. The acetabular gauge is then placed in the acetabulum to ascertain the cup size required. Familiarization takes place for the correct orientation of the cup and to ensure that full bony cover occurs. The trimming of the cement injection flange is performed at this stage. Mixing of the cement is then permissible and this is pressurized into the acetabulum using either a dome-shaped pressurizer or the inflatable pressurizer of Ling. The cup is then inserted and pressed until full bony cover takes place in its favoured orientation. Excess cement is removed. The cup holder remains on the cup until the cement is set fully, firm pressure being applied continuously.

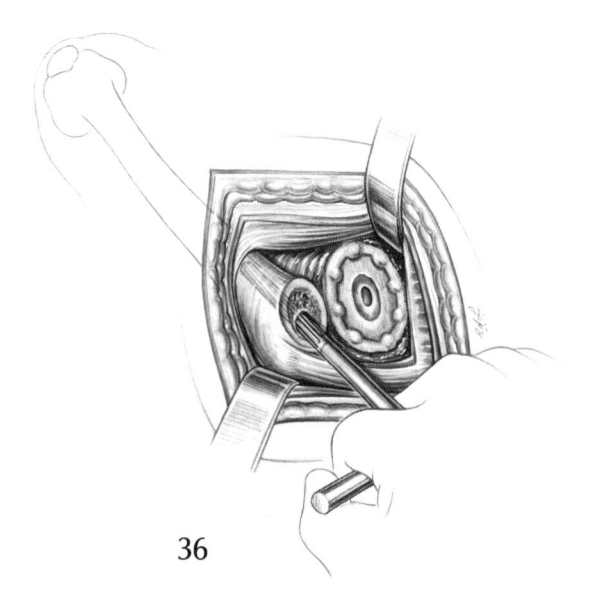

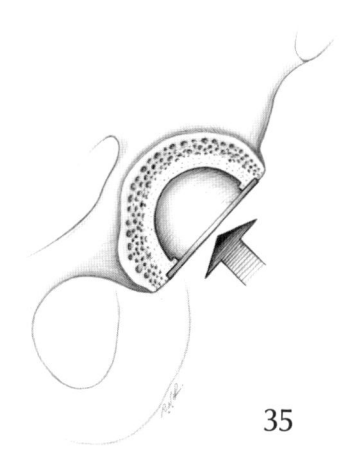

Preparation of the femur and insertion of the prosthesis

36

The bone on the lateral aspect of the neck of the femur, from the cut end of the femoral neck into the trochanteric fossa, is removed using Trotter's forceps to obtain neutral entry into the shaft of the femur (that is, no valgus or varus). Rotatory taper reamers are passed down the shaft of the femur until they bite into the corticocancellous bone. A blunt curette is used to remove the loose swarf and weak cancellous bony trabeculae. A trial prosthesis is inserted that will fit easily into the shaft of the femur. It is mandatory to have this trial prosthesis lying with the neck in the neutral plane with no anteversion or retroversion. A trial reduction takes place and the range of movement of the trial prosthesis is decided. It is important to ensure that the prosthesis is stable in adduction. This can only be performed with the patient in the supine position. Flexion, rotation and abduction are also assessed. At this stage the equalization of leg length can be determined to a high degree of accuracy using the bony landmarks of the anterior superior iliac spines, the patellae and the medial malleoli, comparison being made with the normal side. Having determined that the range of movement and leg lengths are satisfactory, the trial prosthesis is removed and the femoral cement restrictor is inserted to a distance of 13.5 cm from the calcar to prevent excessive migration of the femoral cement.

The first stage of the soft tissue repair of the anterior aspect of the hip joint now takes place. A braided Mersilene suture (Ethicon, Edinburgh, UK) is passed anteriorly through the neck of the femur to reattach the ligament of Bigelow and the tendon of gluteus minimus.

37

The ligament of Bigelow is attached to a horizontal ridge on the front of the neck of the femur at its midpoint. The gluteus minimus is attached to the outer aspect of this ridge. When these sutures have been passed through the neck of the femur the cement is mixed and is then pressurized into the shaft of the femur. The cement can either be inserted using a cement piston gun, preferably, or less favourably by finger packing, a femoral vent being necessary with the latter technique. The stem of the prosthesis is then inserted into the pressurized cement in the neutral axis *vis-à-vis* valgus/varus, with the neck of the prosthesis being maintained in the neutral plane *vis-à-vis* anteversion/retroversion. The hip joint socket and surrounding soft tissues are then irrigated with isotonic saline or chlorhexidine solution to clear debris, and when the cement is set the hip is reduced.

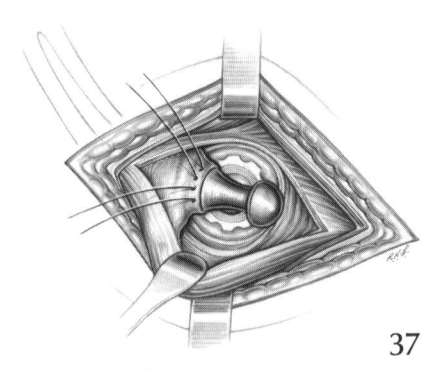

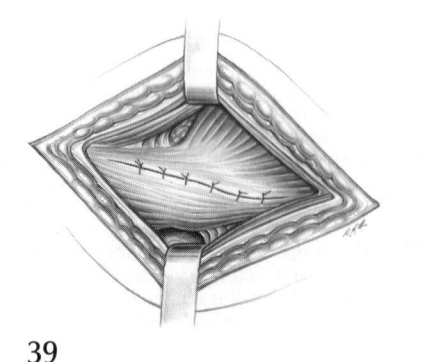

Closure

38 & 39

The ligament of Bigelow and gluteus minimus are reattached to their insertions. Closure of the gluteus medius is performed with a series of interrupted non-absorbable sutures. This is a tendinous closure and allows early mobilization. The deep fascia is similarly closed with non-absorbable interrupted sutures. Two drains are inserted beneath the deep fascia and one subcutaneously. These are removed at 48 hours.

Postoperative management

The patient begins active movement of the legs in flexion and extension as soon as consciousness returns. Adduction of the hip is avoided for 4 weeks postoperatively.

Standing is allowed at 48 hours when the drains have been removed, and usually the intravenous infusion is terminated. Standing and walking are accomplished using two elbow crutches. These elbow crutches are usually retained for 6 weeks after operation, some two of which are spent in hospital. Patients are allowed to go home when they can get out of bed, arise from a chair and climb stairs using two elbow crutches, which varies from 10 to 14 days postoperatively depending on age, general fitness and recovery from surgery.

Total hip replacement arthroplasty 963

TROCHANTERIC OSTEOTOMY

The patient position, skin incision and superficial dissection is the same as for the lateral approach.

Deep dissection

40 & 41

The trochanter is elevated using a Gigli saw passed through the trochanteric fossa to leave the gluteus medius and minimus insertions undisturbed; it is secured in position with a superior capsular retractor. Dislocation is achieved by adduction and slight lateral rotation, as previously described (see *Illustration 32*), and the insertion of the implants follows the same pattern.

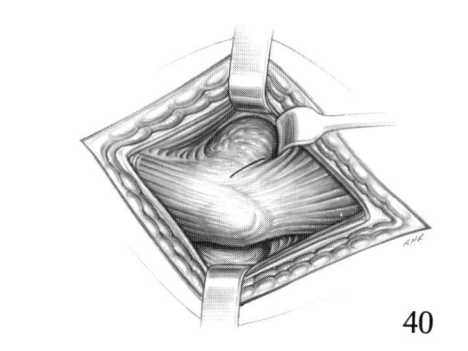

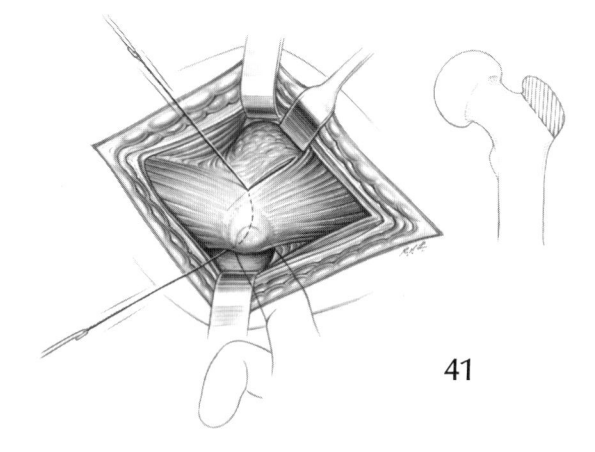

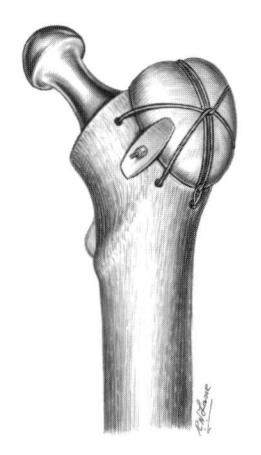

40

41

42

Trochanteric osteosynthesis is achieved by securing the trochanter back onto the trochanteric bed by wires and staples. It is important to locate the trochanter accurately and to hold it securely during the healing phase. During this time, approximately 6 weeks, the patient needs to have protected weight-bearing using elbow crutches.

42

Acknowledgement

Illustrations 4, 5a and 5b are reproduced from the Journal of Bone and Joint Surgery, 1987; 69-B: 229–33, by kind permission of the Editor.

References

1. Hardinge K. Reconstructive surgery of the hip in ankylosing spondylitis. In: Kelly WN, Harris ED, Ruddy S, Sledge CB, eds. *Textbook of rheumatology*. Philadelphia: Saunders, 1981: 1973–9.
2. Hirst P, Esser M, Murphy JCM. Hardinge K. Bone grafting for protrusio acetabuli during total hip replacement: a review of the Wrightington method in 61 hips. *J Bone Joint Surg [Br]* 1987; 69-B: 229–33.
3. Hardinge K, Cleary J, Charnley J. Low friction arthroplasty for healed septic and tuberculous arthritis. *J Bone Joint Surg [Br]* 1979; 61-B: 144–7.
4. Hardinge K, Williams D, Etienne A, McKenzie D, Charnley J. Conversion of fused hips to low friction arthroplasty. *J Bone Joint Surg [Br]* 1977; 59-B: 385–92.
5. Hardinge K, Murphy JCM, Frenyo S. Conversion of hip fusion to Charnley low friction arthroplasty. *Clin Orthop* 1986; 211: 173–9.
6. Moore AT. The Moore self-locking vitallium prosthesis in fresh femoral neck fractures: a new low posterior approach (the southern exposure). *Am Acad Orthop Surg Instr Course Lect*. 1959; 16: 309.
7. Watson-Jones R. Fractures of the neck of the femur. *Br J Surg* 1936; 23: 787–808.
8. Charnley, J. *Low friction arthroplasty of the hip: theory and practice*. Berlin: Springer-Verlag, 1979.
9. Eftekhar N. Charnley "low friction torque" arthroplasty: a study of long-term results. *Clin Orthop* 1971; 81: 93–104.
10. Hardinge K. The direct lateral approach to the hip. *J Bone Joint Surg [Br]* 1982; 64-B: 17–9.
11. McFarland Osborne G. Approach to the hip. *J Bone Joint Surg [Br]* 1954; 36-B: 364–7.
12. Smith-Petersen MN. Approach to and exposure of the hip joint for mold arthroplasty. *J Bone Joint Surg [Am]* 1949; 31-A: 40–6.
13. Wagner H. Surface replacement arthroplasty of the hip. *Clin Orthop* 1978; 134: 102–30.
14. Henry AK. *Extensile exposure*. 2nd ed. Edinburgh: Churchill Livingstone, 1973.
15. Gibson A. Posterior exposure of the hip joint. *J Bone Joint Surg [Br]* 1950; 32-B: 183–6.
16. Marcy GH, Fletcher RS. Modification of the postero-lateral approach to the hip for the insertion of femoral head prosthesis. *J Bone Joint Surg [Am]* 1954; 36: 142–3.
17. McKee, GK, Watson-Farrar J. Replacement of arthritic hips by the McKee–Farrar prosthesis. *J Bone Joint Surg [Br]* 1966; 48-B: 245–59.
18. Müller ME. Total hip prostheses. *Clin Orthop* 1970; 72: 46–68.
19. Brady LP. Lateral oblique incision for the Charnley low friction arthroplasty. *Clin Orthop* 1976; 118: 7–9.

Illustrations by Philip Wilson after F. Price

Girdlestone's pseudarthrosis of the hip

E. W. Somerville FRCS (Ed), FRCS
Emeritus Consultant Orthopaedic Surgeon, Nuffield Orthopaedic Centre, Oxford, UK

Introduction

During the past 30 years the treatment of arthritis of the hip has become more precise. High femoral osteotomy with internal fixation is an operation of value in the younger patient when degenerative changes are not advanced. When gross changes have developed in rheumatoid arthritis or osteoarthritis, total hip replacement is the procedure of choice. In such circumstances it is easy to forget the value of other well-tried procedures, such as arthrodesis and pseudarthrosis.

Girdlestone developed the use of the pseudarthrosis operation in the treatment of osteoarthritis from its previous use in tuberculosis of the hip joint. In this condition a complete joint clearance combined with excision of the head and neck of the femur was found to lead to healing of the disease and still allow a mobile and painless joint. A similar operation in osteoarthritis was found to provide a mobile and painless joint although this joint was subsequently unstable. Nevertheless, it allowed walking with a stick and sitting in comfort which, in the elderly patient for whom the operation was advocated, provided an excellent result.

Indications

There are certain indications for this operation.

It is particularly useful as a salvage operation following failure of an arthroplasty. The scarring which will have resulted from the previous operation greatly improves the stability of the joint, and in these patients a very satisfactory result is often obtained.

In ankylosing spondylitis the problem of restoring mobility to the hip joint is great. In such a case Girdlestone's pseudarthrosis gives comparatively good results, and after the operation a range of movement sufficient to allow sitting in comfort and for the legs to be separated adequately for nursing purposes is usually obtained. There is also a sufficient range of movement to allow walking, but it is probable that the patient will need to use either two sticks or crutches. Nevertheless, in such cases the patient is usually well satisfied with the result.

Contraindications

Generally speaking the operation is contraindicated in young patients where other procedures will probably be of greater value, but occasionally, as the result of very severe trauma, the results of pseudarthrosis in these patients have been good.

Pseudarthrosis performed bilaterally, except in the case of ankylosing spondylitis, as already mentioned, produces a degree of bilateral instability which is extremely disabling, so that the operation is contraindicated when arthritis is bilateral, unless it is combined with some other procedure to provide stability in the other hip.

Limitations

Pseudarthrosis is an operation which, although successful when carried out in the right patient, has strict limitations. It is an operation which relieves pain and preserves mobility, but at the same time produces an unstable hip. The degree of instability will usually condemn patients to using one stick, sometimes two, for the rest of their lives, although they usually manage to walk indoors without support. The pain which has been relieved by the operation is often rapidly forgotten, but the instability continues to be a source of great annoyance. Before this operation is carried out it is of the greatest importance that the nature of these limitations should be made perfectly clear to the patient and, because patients so easily forget, it is wise to explain this to the relatives as well.

Results

In 1950, Taylor[1] reported the results obtained in 93 patients. In 83 the results were considered to be satisfactory, in seven they were poor and three patients died as a result of the operation.

966 Pelvis and hip

Operation

Approach

1

The operation may be carried out through any of the standard approaches to the hip joint. Girdlestone used the anterior Smith-Petersen approach, but the Gibson lateral approach is often preferable to this, particularly if a severe flexion contracture is present.

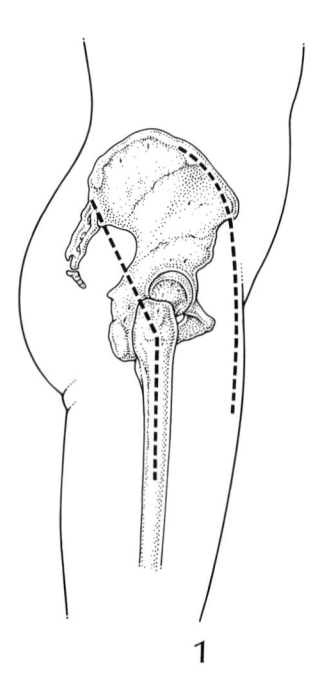

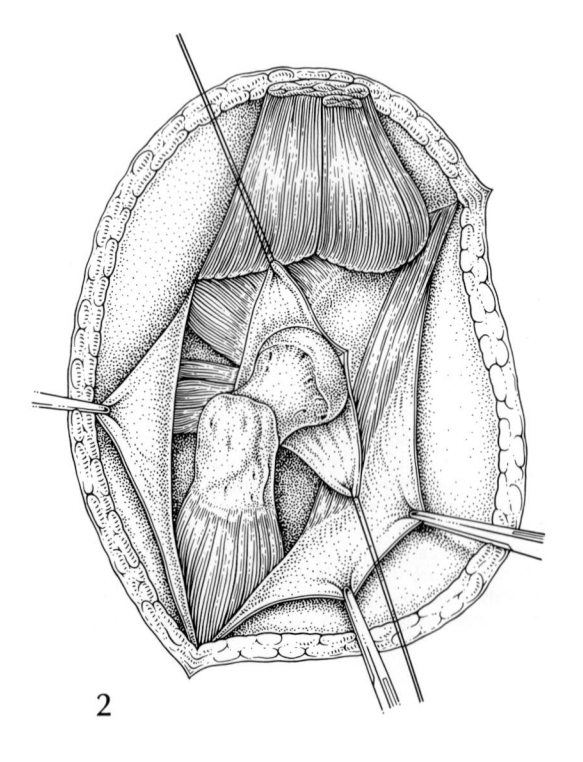

Exposure of joint capsule

2

Whatever approach is used the capsule of the joint is exposed and the anterior and superior portions are widely excised, allowing the hip to be dislocated arteriorly.

Division of neck of femur

3 & 4

The neck of the femur is divided along the intertrochanteric line, care being taken to see that none is left protruding. This division may be carried out either with a Gigli saw or an osteotome, provided that care is taken to avoid splintering. The lip of the acetabulum is examined, and if it is found to be prominent, it must be excised flush with the side of the pelvis so that no protruding spur is left which might make contact with the upper end of the femur, since this invariably causes pain and stiffness. It is not necessary to interpose soft tissue between the pelvis and the upper end of the femur deliberately.

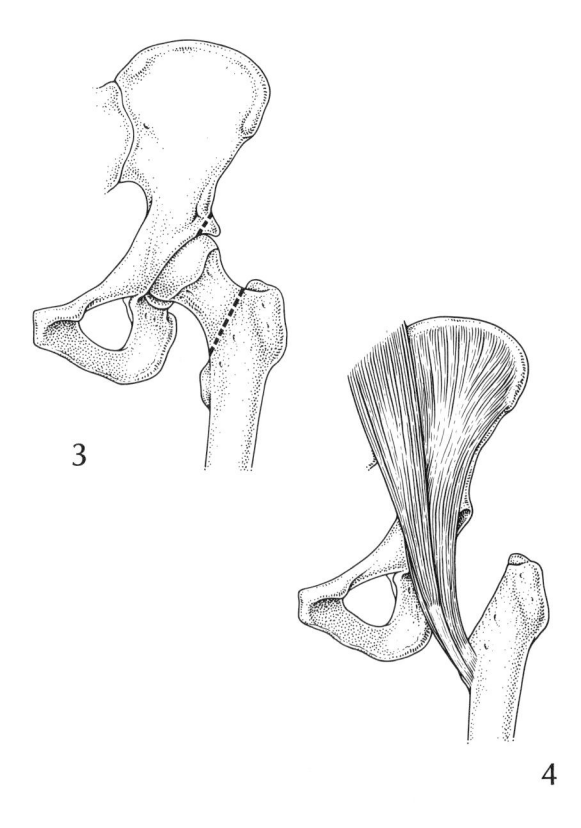

Useful modifications

5 & 6

There are two modifications to this operation which can be often usefully employed at this stage. There is a tendency for the leg to lie in lateral rotation because the fulcrum of the head of the femur has been removed, and the psoas muscle acts as a powerful lateral rotator. To reduce this tendency to lateral rotation the lesser trochanter can be removed with the psoas attached to it, and this can be displaced upwards and reattached to the raw surface at the base of the neck of the femur; or what is simpler still, the lesser trochanter can simply be excised and the iliopsoas will reattach itself in a more suitable position. After this the leg will lie more easily in neutral rotation.

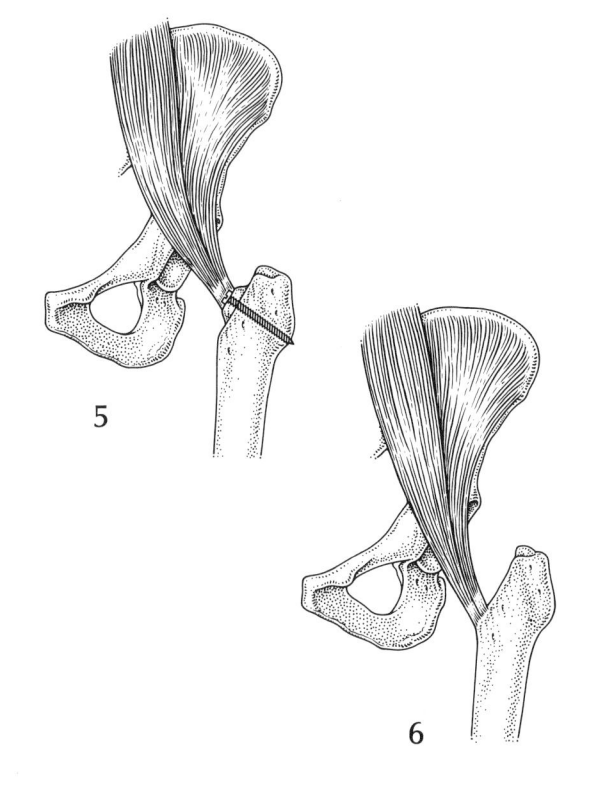

968 Pelvis and hip

Traction

7

Postoperatively, the leg is suspended in traction which is usually obtained by adhesive strapping to the skin with a 19 kg weight, although fixed traction can often be used provided it is carefully attended. If an anterior incision has been used, the leg is most satisfactorily suspended on a Thomas' splint with the knee flexion piece, but if the lateral incision has been employed it is better to use simple modified Russell traction and thereby avoid pressure from the ring of the splint on the wound. If there is a tendency for the leg to lie in lateral rotation this must be controlled, or the deformity will become fixed and make walking more difficult later. Usually a medial rotation bandage will be adequate, although of course this has the disadvantage of producing some circulatory constriction, which should be avoided in view of the risk of thrombophlebitis after such hip operations; traction by means of a Steinmann pin, which can also control rotation, may be better.

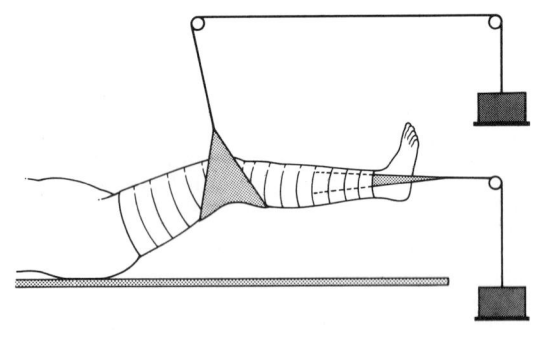

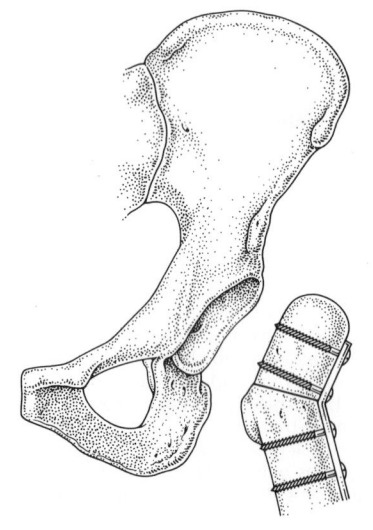

Batchelor's modification

8

The operation has been modified by Batchelor[2]. In this operation, after excision of the head and neck of the femur, an osteotomy is carried out at the level of the lesser trochanter, and the fragments are joined together with a plate in valgus position. This is said to improve stability when walking.

Postoperative management

Balanced traction, as descibed, is maintained for 3 weeks, after which time it is replaced by a simple form of traction with the leg lying on the bed over a pillow. From the beginning, quadriceps, foot and calf exercises will have been regularly carried out. Now with simple traction, hip and gluteal exercises are started. At 6 weeks from the time of the operation, the fixed traction is removed and removable extensions are applied, so that the patient can start getting up and can have hydrotherapy and sling exercises in the gymnasium and start walking between the bars. Classically a bucket-top caliper with knee flexion hinge is used when walking is started, a plaster of Paris cast being taken for this at the time the stitches are removed, so that the caliper will be ready by the time the patient is able to get up. Such a caliper is helpful to many patients, but to some a caliper is quite intolerable however well it may have been fitted, and in these patients there is no point in insisting on the caliper being used — they will get on very much better without it. A certain degree of shortening always occurs after this operation, usually amounting to 25–38 mm, which is compensated for by a 19 mm raise on the heel of the shoe, tapering to 6 mm at the toe. About 1 week after getting up, the patient will be allowed to start standing and walking between bars, and as soon as it is possible he should start with elbow crutches, which he will have to use for approximately 3 months. By this time the patient should be able to graduate to the use of two sticks. At 6 months the patient is encouraged to walk with the knee hinge unlocked and gradually during the next 2 or 3 months progressively to give up the caliper altogether and practise walking with one stick only in the opposite hand.

References

1. Taylor RG. Pseudoarthrosis of the hip joint. *J Bone Joint Surg [Br]* 1950; 32-B: 161–5.

2. Batchelor JS. Pseudoarthrosis for ankylosis and arthritis of the hip. *J Bone Joint Surg [Br]* 1949; 31-B: 135.

Illustrations by Philip Wilson

Arthrodesis of the hip

J. Crawford Adams MD, MS, FRCS
Consulting Orthopaedic Surgeon, St Mary's Hospital, London, UK

Introduction

Arthrodesis of the hip is carried out much less often now than it was two or three decades ago. The main reason for this is the successful development of total replacement arthroplasty, which has revolutionized the treatment of osteoarthritis and rheumatoid arthritis of the hip, for which arthrodesis was formerly often advocated. A secondary reason is the dramatic decrease in the incidence of tuberculous arthritis in the western world – a benefit of the general improvement of living standards and the large-scale elimination of tuberculosis by antibacterial drugs. Arthrodesis is nevertheless still a useful method of treatment in certain special situations.

Indications

The present indications for arthrodesis of the hip may be summarized as follows.

1. For certain cases of destructive arthritis of the hip in which conditions are unsuitable or difficult for replacement arthroplasty – particularly in cases of tuberculous arthritis or pyogenic arthritis with much destruction of bone.
2. For certain cases of major disintegration of the hip from trauma – as for instance in central dislocation of the hip, especially in a young person.
3. For certain cases of slipped upper femoral epiphysis complicated by avascular necrosis of the femoral head and consequent disorganisation of the joint.
4. For certain cases of untreated or relapsed congenital dislocation of the hip in which the femoral head is displaced high up on the ilium – especially when an ill-developed lateral wall of the pelvis offers poor support for the socket of a replacement hip.
5. Very occasionally, for a hip that lacks muscle control from selective paralysis, in order to provide stability.

None of the above conditions is an absolute indication for arthrodesis, and much will always depend upon other factors – especially upon the age of the patient, upon the requirements of his or her occupation and leisure activities, and upon the patient's religious or cultural habits.

So far as age is concerned, arthrodesis of the hip is much more acceptable to a young adult patient than to the elderly. In general, it is more suitable for an active patient than for one with a sedentary occupation. Arthrodesis is always much more readily acceptable to a patient whose hip is already partly stiff – as for instance in a case of fibrous ankylosis – than to one who has retained a good range of movement.

The advantages of arthrodesis are that it abolishes pain completely; that the result is permanent; and that it provides good stability for the limb. Disadvantages – accentuated if the position of the fused hip is imperfect – are that it throws a strain upon the corresponding knee and upon the lumbar region of the spine. Sitting has to be modified, and squatting is precluded. Sexual function is not seriously prejudiced, provided that the other hip is fully mobile.

Contraindications

Arthrodesis of the hip should be avoided if the opposite hip shows significant impairment of mobility; or if the knee on the same side is disordered. It should usually be avoided in those whose national or religious habits demand the adoption of a squatting position.

A cautious attitude should be adopted towards hip arthrodesis in children. While the epiphyseal plate at the upper end of the femur is still open there is a strong tendency for progressive adduction to occur after hip fusion, to the extent that corrective osteotomy may be required. When practicable, therefore, arthrodesis should be deferred until growth is complete.

Position for arthrodesis

It is fundamentally important that the hip be fused in the optimal position: fusion in an incorrect position may badly mar the patient's functional ability for the remainder of his or her life. The optimal position for hip fusion is: 15°–20° of flexion; no adduction or abduction; and no medial or lateral rotation. If the limb on the affected side is short, it is a mistake to try to gain length by fusing the hip in abduction. An abducted position severely prejudices the integrity of the opposite hip and of the lumbar spine.

Technique

Of the many techniques of hip arthrodesis that have been described, there are two that have stood the test of time rather more successfully than the others. These are: (1) intra-articular arthrodesis with nail fixation and iliofemoral graft[1,2]; and (2) ischiofemoral arthrodesis by nail and graft[3]. These two methods will be described.

INTRA-ARTICULAR ARTHRODESIS WITH ILIOFEMORAL GRAFT

In this technique the hip joint is opened, the remains of articular cartilage are removed to expose vascular subchondral bone, the parts are reassembled in the required position, the hip is locked by a long nail transfixing the joint, and a bridge of bone is constructed by grafts between the wing of the ilium and the greater trochanter of the femur.

Preoperative

It is important to establish that the arterial circulation in the limb is adequate. Extensive atheroma in the proximal limb arteries presents a hazard. In elderly men, any prostatic obstruction should be dealt with before the hip operation is undertaken: otherwise acute obstruction may be precipitated.

Anaesthetic

General anaesthesia is usually to be preferred, but the operation may be done under spinal or epidural anaesthesia.

Position of patient

The patient is placed supine upon the raised platform of the orthopaedic table, the footpieces being in position to accept the feet at the appropriate stage of the operation: that is, while the hip is fixed with a transfixion nail.

The whole length of the affected limb should be draped in a sterile occlusive tube (e.g. stockinette) to facilitate handling of the limb during the operation.

Operation

Incision

1

The anterior (Smith-Petersen) approach to the hip is used. The skin incision follows the anterior half of the iliac crest to the anterior superior spine, whence it extends vertically downwards into the thigh for about 12.5 cm.

Deep dissection

2

The deep fascia is incised in the line of the incision, revealing in the proximal part of the thigh the line of separation between the sartorius medially and the tensor fasciae latae laterally. These muscles are separated and retracted apart. The sartorius may be divided. More proximally, the tensor fasciae latae muscle is stripped from the outer aspect of the wing of the ilium, and a large gauze pack is inserted to hold it away. Deep to this layer, the gap between the iliopsoas muscle medially and the rectus femoris laterally is developed, with care to avoid damage to laterally directed branches of the femoral nerve. A leash of vessels crossing laterally to the rectus muscle needs to be divided. The rectus muscle is detached and retracted downwards and medially to expose the capsule of the hip joint, the front of which is excised.

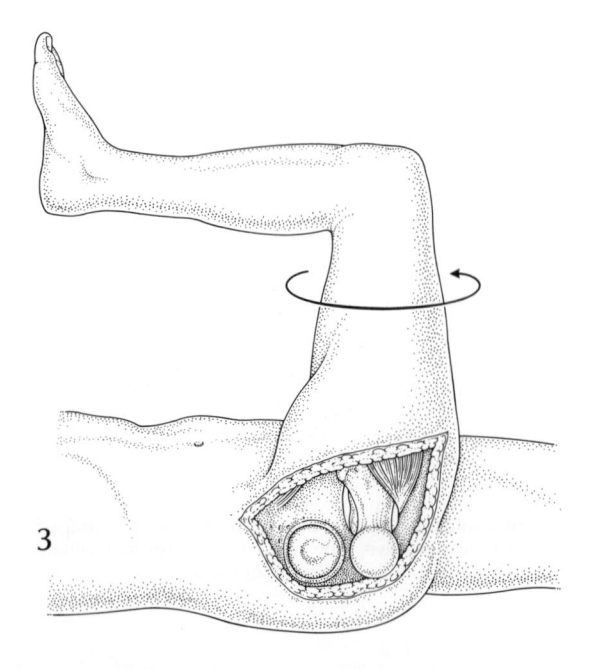

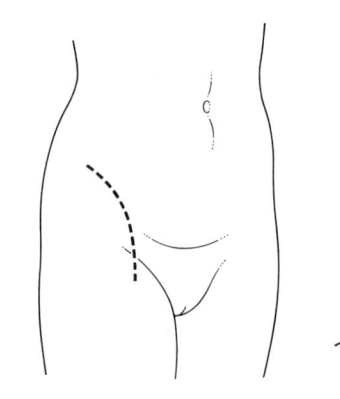

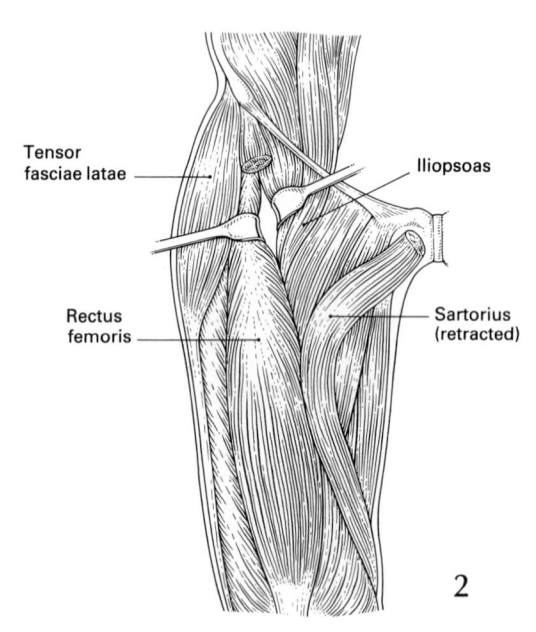

Dislocation of hip

3

The hip is dislocated by first flexing the thigh and then rotating the limb laterally. If dislocation is impeded by large osteophytes these may be chiselled away, and dislocation may be further aided by a stout skid or gouge inserted between the femoral head and the acetabulum to serve as a lever, or by a large hook around the femoral neck. Strong rotational force must not be used for fear of breaking the shaft of the femur.

Rawing of articular surface

4

The limb is laid on its outer side in order to direct the femoral head towards the operator. With chisels and gouges, or, if preferred, by a powered burr, all the articular cartilage is removed from the femoral head and from the acetabulum. The subchondral bone is lightly imbricated to leave a rough, oozing surface.

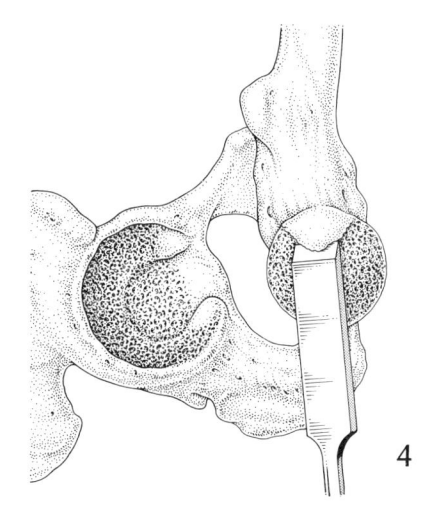

Introduction of guide wire

5

A guide wire is introduced into the lateral aspect of the femoral shaft 2–3 cm distal to the commencing flare of the greater trochanter, and is so directed within the femoral neck that its point emerges through the femoral head at its superior (weight-bearing) surface. The point is left almost flush with the surface of the bone at this stage.

Reduction of dislocation and adjustment of position of hip

6

The dislocation is reduced by guiding the femoral head towards the acetabulum and then rotating the limb medially and extending it. The feet are then strapped to the footpieces of the orthopaedic table, and by adjustment of the push-pull attachments both hips are brought to the neutral position so far as abduction/adduction is concerned. (If the limbs are of equal length the feet will now be level.) The footpieces may now be raised as far as is necessary to ensure that the hip rests in a position of flexion of 15°–20°.

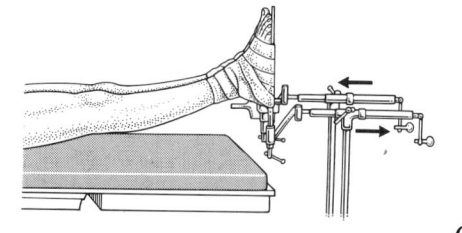

Locking of hip by transfixion nail

7

The length of the trifin nail required is calculated by determining the length of guide wire contained within the femur (by measuring the length protruding) and adding 3 cm for penetration of the acetabular roof. The guide wire is advanced across the joint to emerge, ideally, from the brim of the pelvis at the iliopectineal line, where its tip may be felt by a finger directed along the inner aspect of the ilium. The chosen three-flanged hip nail is driven in over the guide wire, with care to ensure that the wire is not inadvertently driven on with the nail. An impactor is used to correct any 'rebound' of the femoral head that might have left a space between the femoral head and the acetabulum. Alternatively, two AO cancellous screws may be used to secure the femur and acetabulum under compression.

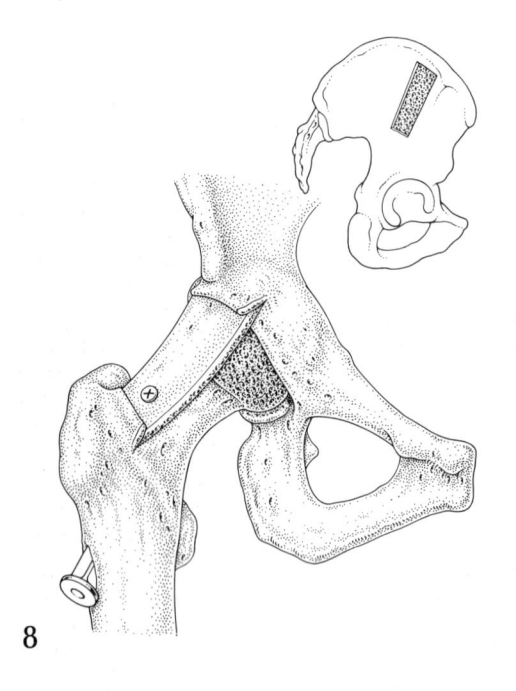

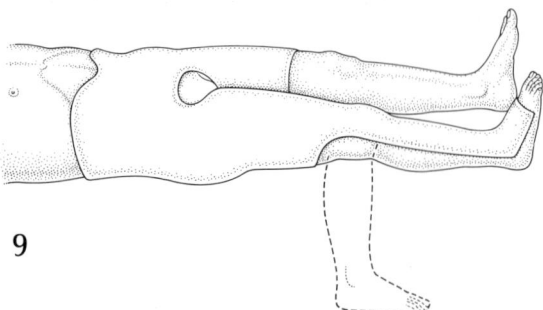

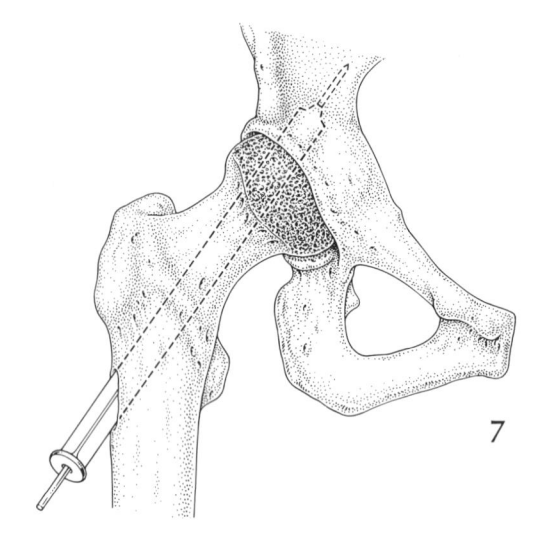

Iliofemoral grafting

8

A graft cut from the outer aspect of the ilium just below the crest is trimmed appropriately and inserted in a precise fit between the ilium and the greater trochanter of the femur, being engaged in slots cut in the ilium just above the hip joint, and in the medial aspect of the greater trochanter. Additional sliver or chip grafts are laid about the main graft to fill up any crevices. The graft may be secured by a screw transfixing it to the base of the femoral neck.

Closure and plaster

9

The wound is closed in layers, with provision for suction drainage. A double plaster hip spica is applied: this extends to include the foot of the limb operated upon, and to just above the knee on the opposite side. The plaster may be bivalved posteriorly below the lower thigh, to permit knee flexion exercises.

Postoperative management

After a week the patient may be got out of bed and encouraged to walk with crutches, minimal weight being taken on the affected side. A closer-fitting plaster may be applied after 2 or 3 weeks, when the sutures are removed. The spica should remain for 12 weeks when a radiograph out of the spica will show if fusion has occurred. If this is not certain, a short hip spica extending to above the knee may be used with full weight-bearing until fusion is solid.

Arthrodesis of the hip 975

ISCHIOFEMORAL ARTHRODESIS

In this technique the hip is first transfixed by a long three-flanged nail. Without exposure of the hip joint itself, the interval between the femur and the ischium is then bridged by a rigid tibial graft inserted through a drill hole in the femur and driven on to enter a hole drilled in the ischium.

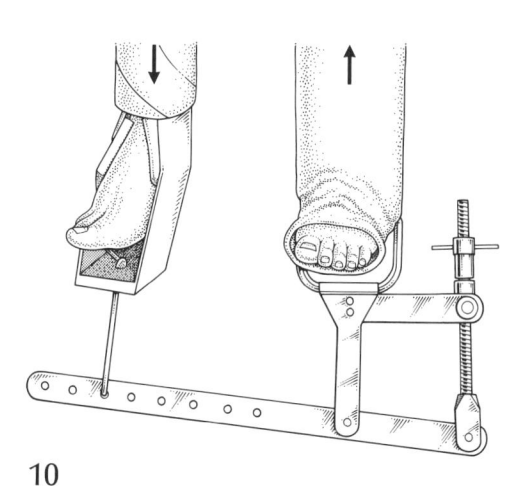

Special contraindications

Since in this operation the hip joint itself is not opened, the technique is inappropriate if the hip shows a fixed deformity that cannot be overcome in the way now to be described.

Preoperative

Correction of fixed deformity

10

Moderate adduction or abduction deformity, and a flexion deformity not exceeding 30°, may usually be corrected by the push-pull method described by Roger Anderson[4] in 1932 and known as 'well-leg traction' because traction is exerted against, or sometimes upon, the well leg.

In the correction of fixed adduction deformity – the usual pattern – a full-length plaster of Paris splint is applied to the well leg, with the knee almost fully extended. The plaster includes the foot, and the Roger Anderson well-leg traction apparatus is incorporated in it. Through the lever arm of the apparatus sustained traction is then applied to the disordered limb, usually through the medium of skin strapping, though a lower tibial Steinmann pin may be used if desired. The correcting force acts on the hip by a parallelogram of forces. If the fixed deformity is severe and of long duration, correction may be aided by tenotomy of the taut adductor tendons.

If abduction deformity is to be corrected the system is reversed, the plaster splint and the apparatus being applied to the disordered leg and traction to the well leg. Again, tenotomy of contracted tendons or muscles may be carried out if necessary.

If correction of fixed deformity is to be achieved by this method it will usually be gained within a week. If the deformity resists correction beyond this time, either the hip must be opened to correct the deformity before ischiofemoral arthrodesis is undertaken, or this method of arthrodesis must be abandoned in favour of intra-articular arthrodesis.

10

976 Pelvis and hip

Operation

Position of patient

11

Because of the fundamental requirement that the hip be fused in precisely the optimal position, the first stage of the operation should be carried out with the patient supine upon the orthopaedic table and the feet strapped to the push-pull footpieces. By appropriate adjustment of the footpieces, the correct position of the hip can be assured before the joint is transfixed with a long nail. For the second stage of the operation the patient must be turned to the prone position. (It is impracticable to adjust the position of the hip with the patient prone.)

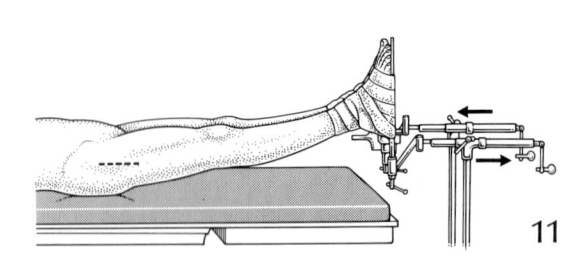

FIRST-STAGE OPERATION: TRANSFIXION OF HIP BY THREE-FLANGED NAIL

Incision

12

In this first stage a lateral incision is made immediately below the prominence of the greater trochanter to expose the lateral aspect of the upper part of the shaft of the femur. A second incision is made over the anterior part of the crest of the ilium, through which the iliacus muscle is stripped away from the inner aspect of the pelvis by a blunt periosteal elevator. The purpose of this incision is to allow a finger to reach the brim of the pelvis to palpate an emerging guide wire, inserted in the manner now to be described.

Insertion of guide wire

13

Through the lateral incision a small hole is made with a gouge or drill in the cortex of the femur 2.5 cm below the outward flare of the greater trochanter, and slightly behind the mid-lateral line of the bone. This allows the insertion of a long (30 cm) guide wire, which is directed obliquely upwards, medially and slightly forwards towards a doubly-gloved finger inserted deeply in the iliac wound. The wire is best introduced in the chuck of a powered drill. Edged forwards by degrees, its point should be felt as it emerges through the bone of the pelvic brim. If necessary the position of the guide wire may be checked radiographically, but this is not essential if the tip of the wire is palpated as described.

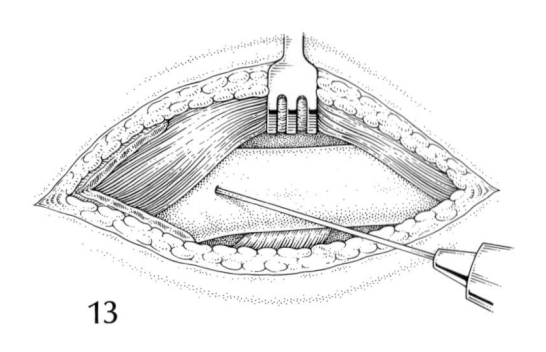

Arthrodesis of the hip 977

Driving of nail

14

By measurement of the length of guide wire still protruding from the femur the length that is within the bone is calculated, and hence the length of nail required to transfix the hip joint and to enter strong iliac bone is determined. The chosen three-flanged nail, held in a Smith-Petersen punch, is then driven in over the guide wire, with special care to ensure that the guide wire is not inadvertently driven forward with the nail. To prevent this, the wire should be rotated after every few hammer blows, and the length of wire protruding remeasured.

The incision over the crest of the ilium is now closed. The lateral incision is closed temporarily with towel clips.

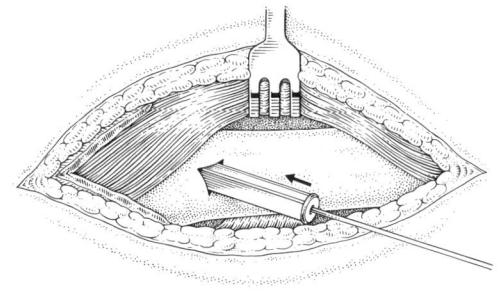

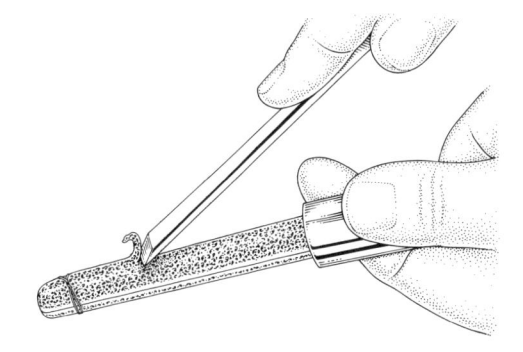

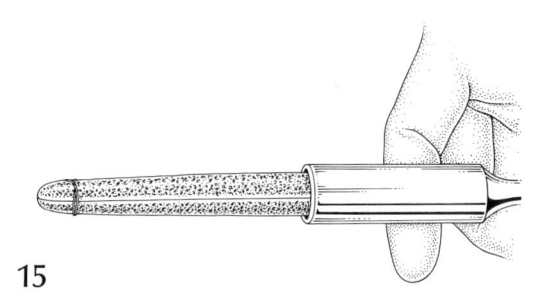

Cutting and preparation of bone graft

15

The bone graft is cut from the subcutaneous surface of the tibia. Twin parallel or tandem grafts exactly 12.5 mm wide and 10 cm long are required. The anterior and posteromedial corners of the tibia must be preserved to minimize the risk of fracture. After extraction, the two grafts are wired together cortex to cortex, and one end is finely tapered to a blunt point over a length of 1.5 cm. Finally the composite graft is rounded with a chisel or with a powered burr so that it forms a cylindrical peg exactly 12.5 mm in diameter.

978   Pelvis and hip

SECOND-STAGE OPERATION: INSERTION OF BONE GRAFT

For the second stage of the operation the patient is turned and placed prone upon the operation table, with care not to apply any undue force to the hip, the position of which has been locked with the nail. Fresh drapes are placed in position.

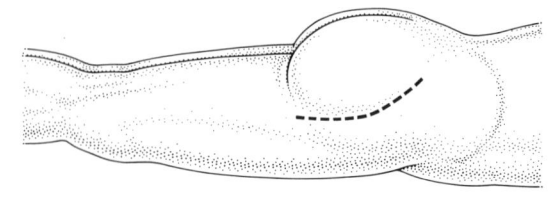

Incision

16

The existing lateral incision is prolonged upwards and medially across the buttock, towards the posterior superior spine of the ilium.

The deep exposure

17

The gluteus maximus is split in the direction of its fibres and its femoral insertion is detached. The two sides are retracted apart to expose, more deeply, the short posterior muscles of the hip – namely the obturator internus and gemelli above, and the quadratus femoris below. The sciatic nerve is identified lying on these muscles before disappearing proximally beneath the piriformis muscle. The nerve must be carefully protected. The interval between the inferior gemellus above and the quadratus femoris below is opened up. In the gap thus created the tuberosity of the ischium is first palpated and then exposed by blunt dissection.

Drilling of channel for bone graft

18

The drill enters the lateral aspect of the femur 2 cm below the head of the transfixion nail (already inserted) and in a plane slightly anterior to the mid-lateral axis. The pilot hole, 9.5 mm (3/8 inch) in diameter, is directed towards the tuberosity of the ischium under direct vision: it passes almost horizontally, with a slight posterior inclination. When the drill has penetrated the femur it is carefully advanced to strike the outer aspect of the ischium (usually 5 cm distant from the femur), which is then penetrated by the drill. (If desired, a guide wire may first be introduced into the ischium and the hole then made by a cannulated drill passed over the guide wire.) When the pilot hole has been made it is enlarged to 11 mm (7/16 inch). The femoral hole is further enlarged to 12.5 mm (1/2 inch) in diameter but the ischial hole is left undersize to ensure a jam-fit of the graft.

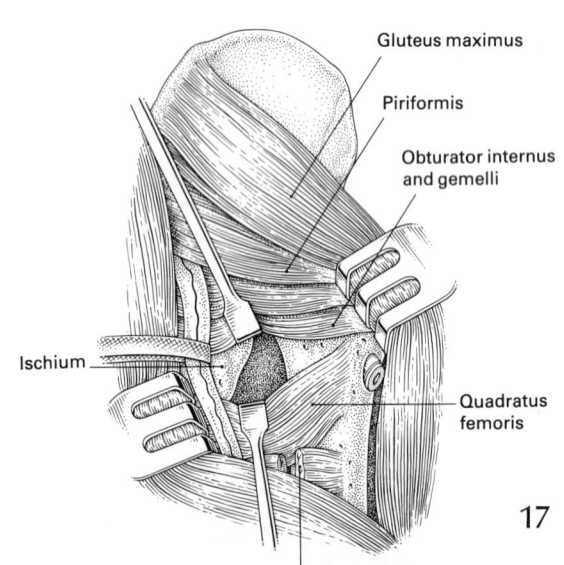

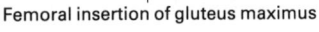

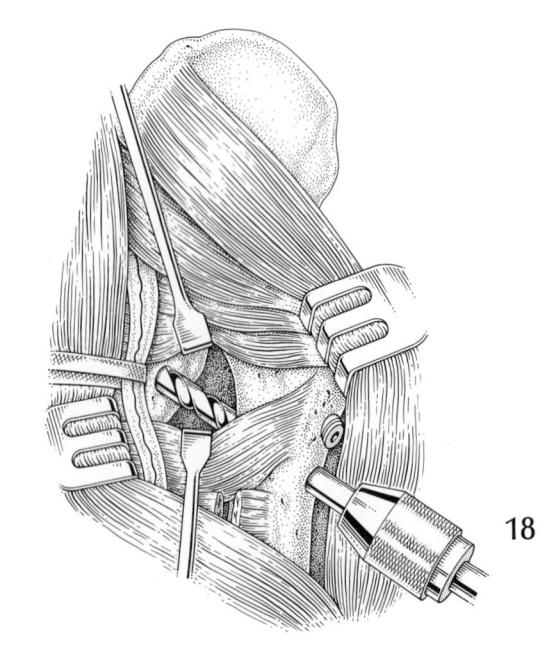

Insertion of graft

19

The prepared graft, with the point carefully tapered, is held in the hollow end of a Smith-Petersen punch and driven through the hole in the femur and on into the ischial tunnel. It should preferably penetrate right through the ischium, which has a depth of about 2.5 cm. The graft is impacted so that its outer end is flush with the lateral cortex of the femur. The wound is closed in layers.

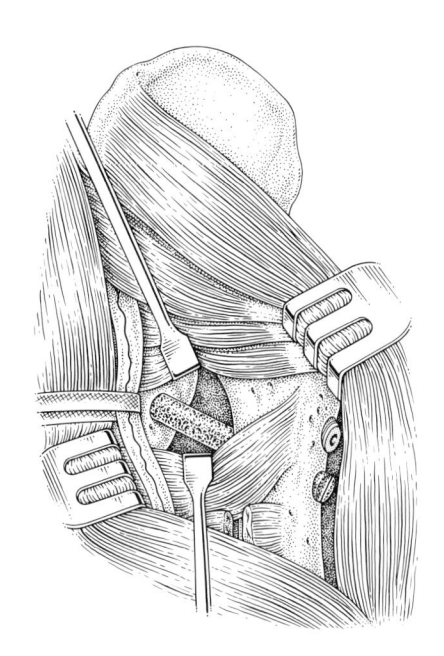

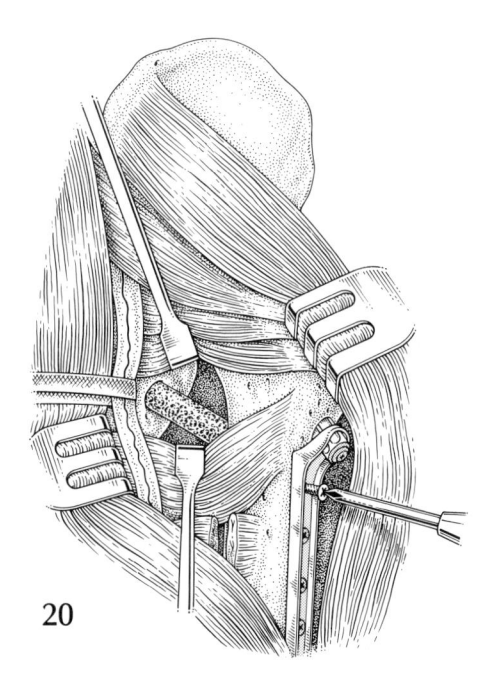

Alternative fixation

20

Some surgeons recommend the use of a two-piece nail–plate in preference to a plain three-flanged nail, in order to forestall the risk of fracture of the femoral shaft through the drill hole. If this is the case the plate component of the nail–plate is screwed in place after the graft has been driven home.

Postoperative management

21

The patient is turned back to the supine position on the orthopaedic table; the feet are strapped to the adjustable footpieces of the table, or the feet may be held by an assistant while the pelvis rests upon a portable support. A close-fitting plaster spica is applied, extending high up on the thoracic cage and including the thigh on the affected side to just above the knee. (Since the graft as well as the nail provides stability this minimal spica is adequate.) Walking with crutches is encouraged after 3 or 4 days, with some weight being taken upon the affected limb. Knee movements are practised with the patient prone. The plaster spica is changed as necessary to maintain a snug fit: it is retained for a total of 8 weeks.

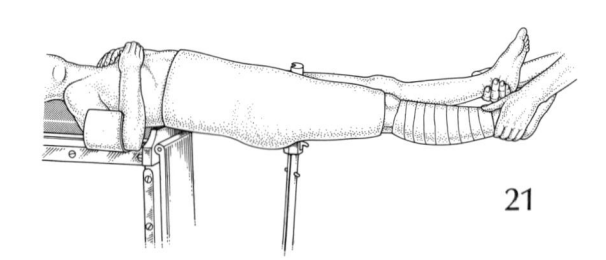

Special complications

The most frequent complication has been fracture of the graft near the point where it enters the ischium. This has occurred usually about 2 months after the operation. It may be in the nature of a stress fracture. If the nail remains firm, and the hip immobile, the fracture will often heal spontaneously, often with the formation of abundant callus. Exceptionally, if the nail loosens and the fracture fails to heal, regrafting and fresh nailing may be required. The incidence of primary incorporation of the graft has been about 90 per cent. It is followed many months later by obliteration of the acetabulofemoral joint space. Fracture of the femur through the drill hole has been a rare complication. In the author's experience it has occurred only in frail women.

References

1. Watson-Jones R, Robinson WC. Arthrodesis of the osteoarthritic hip joint. *J Bone Joint Surg [Br]* 1956; 38-B: 353–77.

2. Wiles P. The surgery of the osteoarthritic hip. *Br J Surg* 1958; 45: 488–97.

3. Adams JC. *Ischio-femoral arthrodesis*. Edinburgh: Livingstone, 1966.

4. Anderson R. New method for treating fractures utilising the well leg for counter-traction. *Surg Gynecol Obstet* 1932; 54: 207–19.

Distal hamstring release

W. J. W. Sharrard MD, ChM, FRCS
Emeritus Consultant Orthopaedic Surgeon, Royal Hallamshire Hospital and Children's Hospital, Sheffield;
Professor of Orthopaedic Surgery, University of Sheffield, UK

Preoperative

Indications and assessment

A flexion deformity of the knee of 20°–50° due to moderate imbalance of muscle activity at the knee in paralytic conditions such as cerebral palsy, poliomyelitis and spina bifida is the main indication for distal hamstring release, though it may be used in other non-paralytic lesions associated with knee flexion contracture.

Distal hamstring release is ideally performed when there are strong knee flexor muscles associated with an active but weak quadriceps muscle with a power of MRC Grade 3 or 4. The assessment of the degree of knee flexion contracture is best made with the patient prone. Sometimes, one or more of the hamstring tendons or gracilis tendon may be more severely affected, but it is more usual to find that all the hamstring tendons require release.

Before performing a hamstring release, a check should be made on the presence of any contractures at the hip or foot. Knee flexion may arise as a secondary consequence of hip flexion deformity, which puts the hamstring muscles under tension and which should be corrected first.

Anaesthesia and position of patient

General anaesthesia is needed. The limb is normally exsanguinated by an Esmarch bandage, and a pneumatic tourniquet cuff is applied as proximally as possible and inflated with the knee extended. The operation is performed with the patient prone. A diathermy plate is applied.

The skin is prepared. A sterile stockinette is applied to the level of the upper calf. Drapes are applied to leave the knee and lower third of the thigh exposed. The operation area can be covered by a transparent adhesive drape, though is does not mould well to the contours of a knee with a flexion deformity and it may be easier to leave the skin undraped, or to cover it with stockinette stuck to the skin with adhesive solution and to incise the stockinette.

982 Thigh and knee

Operation

Incisions

1

The operation is done through two vertical incisions, posteromedial and posterolateral. The posteromedial incision is made along the line of the semitendinosus tendon, which is usually the most prominent medial hamstring tendon, extending for a distance of 12–15 cm in the lower third of the thigh and across the back of the knee to end by curving slightly forwards. The posterolateral incision is made for a similar distance over the biceps tendon, extending distally to the level of the head of the fibula.

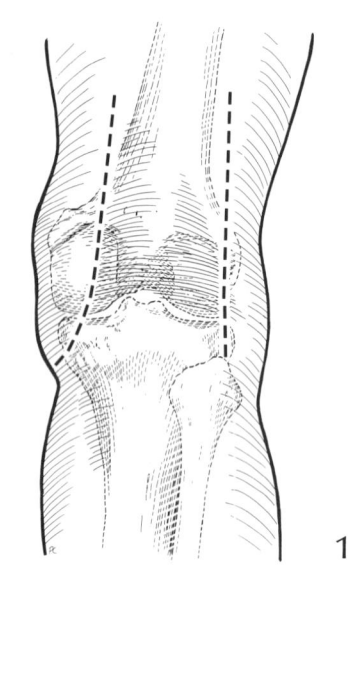

Exposure of the medial tendons

2

The incision is deepened through the subcutaneous tissue; a few subcutaneous veins need to be identified and coagulated. The tendons to be exposed are the semitendinosus, gracilis and semimembranosus. The semitendinosus and gracilis tendons are enclosed in sheaths of paratenon, often associated with a considerable amount of fat which may make the tendons difficult to find, isolate and uncover. Both tendons are fairly superficial and can become hidden under a retractor.

The semitendinosus is usually the most prominent tendon and is exposed by a vertical incision along its sheath for as much of its extent as the incision allows. Additional length can be exposed by allowing the knee to flex and retracting the distal end of the incision. It is differentiated from the gracilis tendon in that it is more substantial, oval and does not have muscle fibres along most of its length.

The gracilis tendon lies medial to the semitendinosus. It is finer and muscle fibres extend on one side of the tendon along the upper half of its extent.

The semimembranosus muscle and tendon lies deep to the semitendinosus. It is in the form of a flat aponeurosis on the superficial surface of a substantial bulk of muscle fibres which extend well distally. It narrows to about half its width from above downwards.

The tibial (medial popliteal) nerve, which lies between and deep to the semimembranosus and biceps muscles proximally and becomes more superficial distally, should be identified by careful blunt dissection to avoid injury to it.

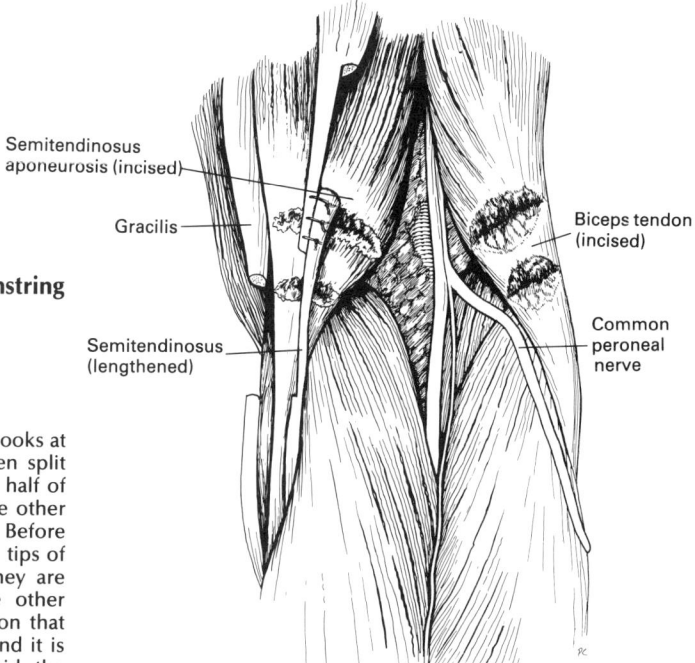

Musculotendinous release of the medial hamstring tendons

3a, b & c

The semitendinosus tendon is lifted up by single hooks at each end to put it under some tension. It is then split longitudinally by incising it along its length. One half of the tendon is divided transversely distally and the other half of the tendon proximally to form a Z-incision. Before the tendon is divided, a stay suture is put into the tips of each tendon slip to avoid losing them when they are released. They are not resutured until all the other tendons have been released. The length of tendon that will need to be divided is sometimes deceptive and it is wise to lengthen as much as possible to avoid the embarrassment of being unable to approximate the tendon ends when the deformity has been corrected.

The gracilis tendon can either be split longitudinally in the same way as the semitendinosus or simply divided and allowed to retract without suturing it.

The aponeurosis of the semimembranosus is lengthened by several transverse incisions into it, without cutting the muscle fibres beneath. The muscle and tendon will stretch easily when the knee is extended. There is no need to suture it.

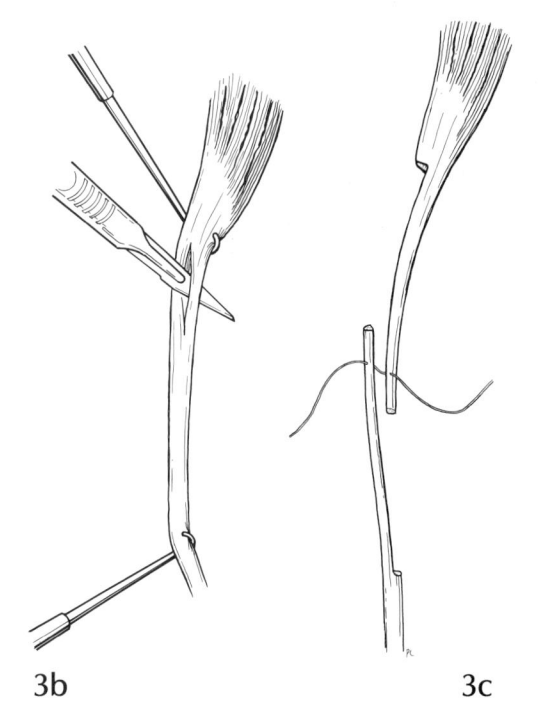

Exposure and release of the biceps femoris

The biceps tendon is exposed through the posterolateral incision over a length of 7–10 cm by a vertical incision through the thin fascia overlying it. It is formed of a substantial bulk of muscle fibres extending well distally on the surface of which a thick but flattened tendon arises, which is exposed down to the point at which it divides to enclose the lateral ligament of the knee. Immediately medial and posterior to the biceps tendon, the common peroneal nerve should be identified by careful blunt dissection. Distally it approaches close to the tendon and must be seen and retracted out of harm's way before the biceps tendon is incised. The biceps tendon can be lengthened by multiple transverse incisions into it in its proximal part leaving the muscle fibres to stretch in the same way as the semimembranosus, or the tendon can be separated from its attached muscle fibres and lengthened by a Z-incision, dependent on the amount of lengthening that is required.

Correction of knee flexion deformity and tendon suture

The knee is now extended as far as possible, watch being kept on the tension on the tibial and common peroneal nerves. There may be need to divide the deep fascia of the posterior aspect of the thigh lying beneath the subcutaneous tissue if it has not already been released sufficiently. If there is still incomplete extension of the knee, a small amount of further correction may be obtained by posterior capsulotomy of the knee. The posterior capsule is exposed by dissecting carefully beneath the tibial nerve and the popliteal vessels, with care being taken not to damage the medial or lateral geniculate vessels. The capsule is divided transversely at the joint line. It is doubtful whether this manoeuvre, by itself, is justified, since, if the capsule and ligaments of the knee are short, only division of the medial, lateral, and possibly the cruciate ligaments is likely to provide significant further improvement in knee extension.

The slips of the divided semitendinosus tendon are approximated under moderate physiological tension and sutured side-to-side to each other with 3 or 4 non-absorbable sutures. The gracilis and biceps tendons are similarly sutured only if they have been lengthened by Z-incisions. If not, no other tendon sutures are required.

Wound closure

The subcutaneous layer of each incision is closed with interrupted non-absorbable sutures after putting in suction drains to the deep layers. The skin is sutured with non-absorbable intermittent sutures or absorbable subcuticular sutures. Dressings are applied and mutual pressure applied to the posterior aspect of the thigh and popliteal fossa whilst the tourniquet is released and removed. The toes need to be observed for the adequacy of circulation in them before the plaster is applied. If the circulation is not adequate the knee should be allowed to flex until the blood supply is restored. The corrected position is held by a plaster cast applied from the top of the thigh, as near to the groin as possible, down to the toes, over an adequate layer of plaster wool, particularly over the front of the knee and the back of the heel which are likely to be subject to pressure. The suction drain tubes are brought out of the top of the plaster cast and are not sutured to the skin, so that they may be removed after 48 or 72 hours by directly pulling on them without the need to remove the plaster.

Postoperative management

The circulation in the toes is kept under observation. If the toes become swollen and the circulation in them diminishes, the plaster should be split immediately and the knee allowed to flex if necessary to restore circulatory flow. The plaster cast is changed on the tenth day and any non-absorbable sutures removed. This is best performed under sedation or general anaesthesia in young children. If some flexion deformity remains, further correction may be possible. The plaster cast is retained for 4–5 weeks, after which active mobilization and physiotherapy is begun to encourage the return of active knee extension and the maximum range of knee movement.

Illustrations by Philip Wilson after P. Henry

Transfer of the hamstrings to the quadriceps in the adult

J. A. Fixsen MChir, FRCS
Consultant Orthopaedic Surgeon, The Hospital for Sick Children, Great Ormond Street, London, and St Bartholomew's Hospital, London, UK

Introduction

Indications

Transfer of the hamstring muscles to the quadriceps can be used to reinforce a weak or paralysed quadriceps muscle. However, several criteria must be fulfilled if the operation is to be a success.

1. Both biceps femoris and semitendinosus muscles must be of power 4 or more on the Medical Research Council scale.
2. The biceps femoris muscle should not be transferred on its own as this can lead to lateral instability and dislocation of the patella[1].
3. Transfer of the biceps femoris and semitendinosus should not be performed unless one other knee flexor is active and the gastrocnemius is also functioning to flex the knee and prevent genu recurvatum.
4. The patient should have active hip flexors and extensors. If the hip flexors are weak the patient will have difficulty in clearing the floor with the foot. This is a serious contraindication to the operation.
5. Any flexion deformity at the hip or the knee must be corrected before performing the transfer. Valgus or varus at the knee and equinus at the foot should also be corrected.

Operation

The operation is performed under general anaesthesia with the patient supine. A tourniquet placed high as possible on the thigh is used to provide a bloodless field.

Incisions

1

The first incision is made over the anteromedial aspect of the knee centred on the patella and long enough to expose the patella, quadriceps tendon and patellar tendon when retracted laterally.

2

The second incision is made longitudinally over the lateral side of the lower third of the thigh extending distally to the head of the fibula. The deep fascia is divided.

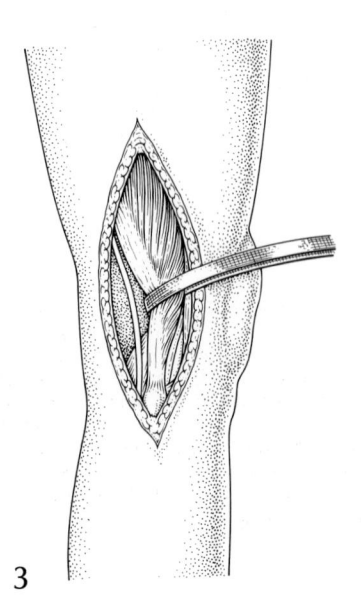

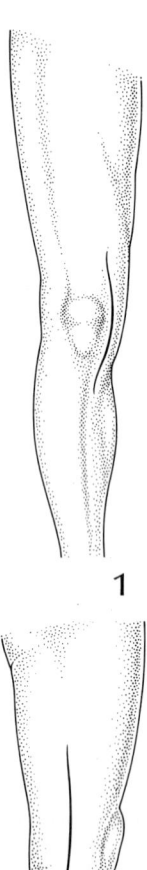

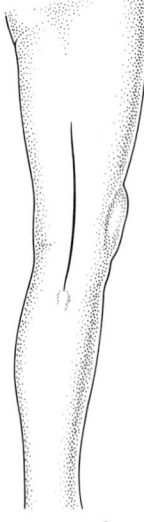

3

The biceps femoris tendon is dissected out, taking particular care not to damage the lateral popliteal nerve which lies immediately behind the tendon and winds round the neck of the fibula.

4

The biceps tendon is divided distally at its insertion on the lateral aspect of the head of the fibula, taking care not to damage the lateral ligament of the knee joint which it surrounds. A slip of the tendon inserts onto the lateral tibial condyle and must also be divided.

The tendon and muscle belly are mobilized proximally, detaching the short head from the femur as far proximally as the entry of its nerve and blood supply on the medial side will permit. A wide subcutaneous tunnel is made as obliquely as possible from the first to the second incision so the pull of the tendon after transfer is as straight as possible.

5

A third incision is now made on the medial side of the lower third of the thigh extending as far distally as the medial tibial condyle. The semitendinosus tendon, which is round with no muscle belly, is found lying behind the sartorius and gracilis muscles. It is divided at its insertion on the tibia and mobilized proximally to the mid-thigh. Blunt finger dissection is very useful for this. A second oblique subcutaneous tunnel is made from the first to the third incision so that the semitendinosus tendon can be transferred to the patella. Both tendons are passed through their respective tunnels. It is most important to make sure that they can move quite freely in the tunnels and their line is as straight as possible.

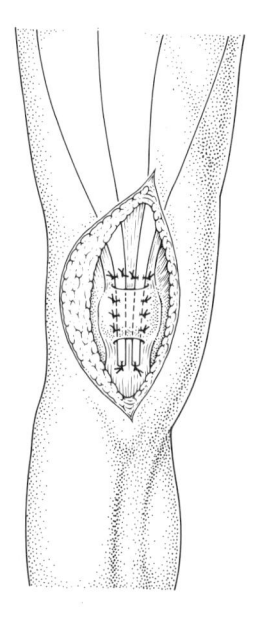

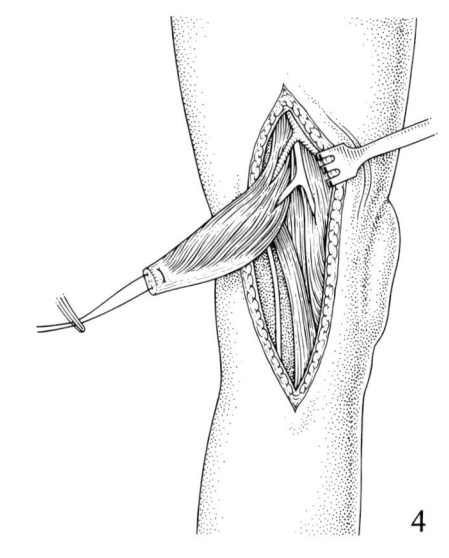

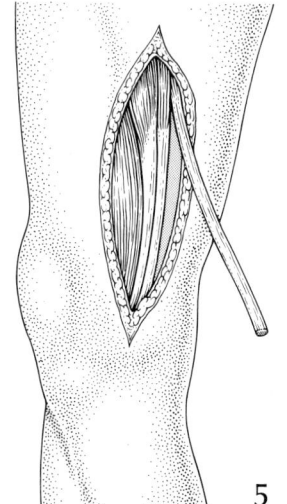

6

A subperiosteal tunnel is made on the anterior surface of the patella and the two tendons passed through it. Alternatively, the periosteum may be raised as two longitudinal flaps and the tendons placed beneath them. With the knee in extension the tendons are then firmly sutured with non-absorbable sutures to the patella and its periosteum, to the quadriceps tendon proximally and the patellar tendon distally. The tourniquet is removed and haemostasis obtained. The wound is closed in layers, usually without drainage.

Postoperative management

A long-leg plaster is applied for 3 weeks with the knee in extension but not hyperextended. Care must be taken during this period not to stretch the transferred muscles by flexing the hip.

At 3 weeks the plaster is removed and physiotherapy started to mobilize the knee and re-educate the transferred muscles. Protective splintage is retained until adequate muscle control of the knee has been achieved. Some surgeons prefer to retain a protective orthosis and night splintage for up to 6–12 months postoperatively.

Complications

Provided the initial criteria described have been adhered to, good control of the knee without an orthosis should be obtained. Lateral instability of the patella should not occur if both tendons are transferred. Serious genu recurvatum should not develop if the gastrocnemius and semimembranosus are working adequately.

Reference

1. Schwartzmann JR, Crego CH Jr. Hamstring-tendon transplantation for the relief of quadriceps femoris paralysis in residual poliomyelitis: follow-up study of 134 cases. *J Bone Joint Surg [Am]* 1948; 30-A: 541–9.

Illustration by Peter Cox after F. Price

Proximal gastrocnemius release

W. J. W. Sharrard MD, ChM, FRCS.
Emeritus Consultant Orthopaedic Surgeon, Royal Hallamshire Hospital and Children's Hospital, Sheffield;
Professor of Orthopaedic Surgery, University of Sheffield, UK

Preoperative

Indications and assessment

This operation may be used for equinus deformity due to gastrocnemius tightness, for which the indications are the same as in distal gastrocnemius release (see p. 1169). It may also form part of an operation for the release of knee flexion deformity, in association with distal hamstring release (see pp. 981–984). It is particularly indicated in combined equinus and knee flexion deformity in neglected cases of cerebral palsy or for equinus deformity when there is weakness of ankle dorsiflexion to less than MRC Grade 3, indicating the need for gastrocnemius release combined with partial gastrocnemius neurectomy.

Anaesthesia and position of patient

This is the same as for distal gastrocnemius release (see p. 1169). A pneumatic tourniquet is applied to the upper thigh.

Thigh and knee

Operation

Incision

1

A transverse incision is made in the popliteal fossa parallel with the skin creases from a point 1 cm lateral to the biceps tendon to 1 cm medial to the semitendinosus tendon. If the operation is combined with lengthening of the hamstring tendons, the gastrocnemii may be exposed through the incisions used for that operation. The incision is deepened through the deep fascia and a small flap retracted proximally.

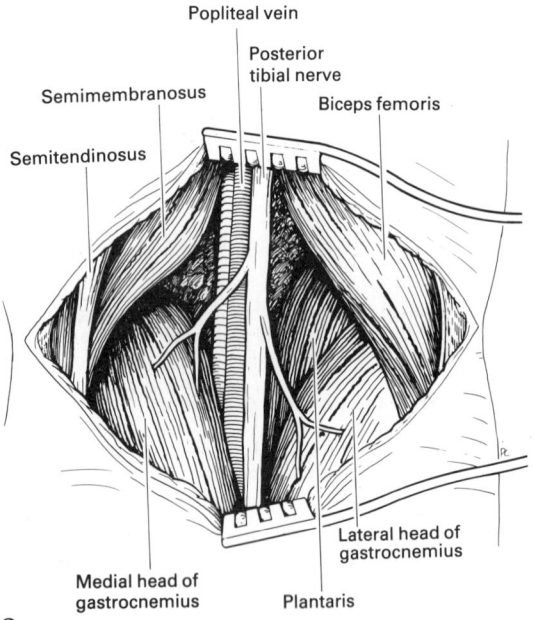

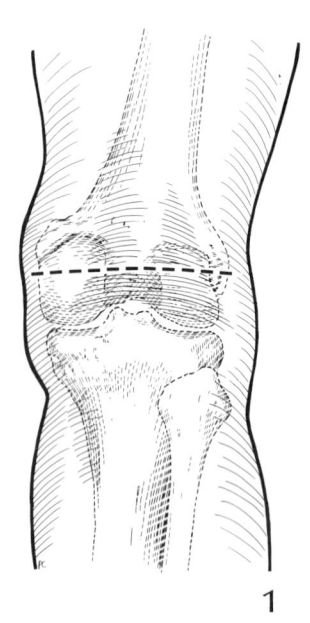

Exposure of gastrocnemius origins

2

The posterior tibial nerve is identified by blunt dissection in the fat of the popliteal fossa and its motor branches to the heads of the gastrocnemii traced to the point where they enter the muscle. One or two of the branches to each head are divided with removal of a small amount of nerve to effect a partial denervation.

By blunt dissection, the medial and lateral heads of the gastrocnemius are exposed with care to avoid injury to the popliteal vein which lies immediately deep to the posterior tibial nerve. On the lateral side of the incision, the common peroneal nerve should be exposed and retracted.

Musculotendinous division

3

The origins of the medial and lateral heads of the gastrocnemius from the lower end of the femur are defined. The medial head arises from the femoral shaft above the medial femoral condyle, whilst the lateral head arises from the lateral side of the lateral femoral condyle more distally. A curved clamp is passed beneath each origin which is divided transversely near its attachment to the bone and mobilized distally. The plantaris origin arising immediately proximal to the lateral head is also divided. The medial and lateral genicular vessels pass medially and laterally, respectively, proximal to the gastrocnemius heads and care is needed to avoid damage to them or to the posterior tibial nerve.

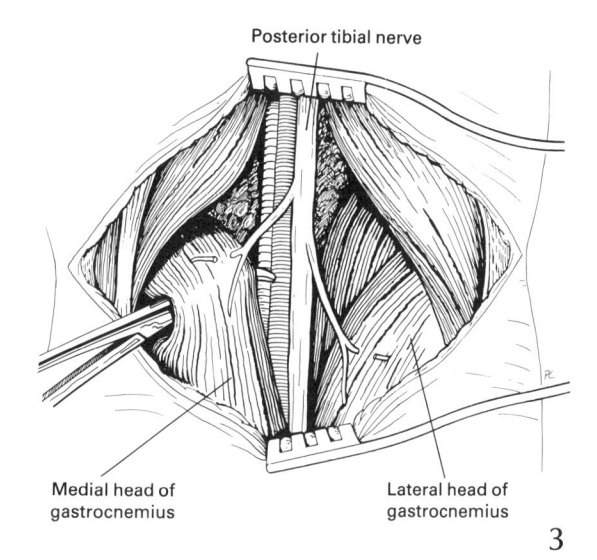

4

The two gastrocnemius heads are freed so that they move freely distally when the ankle is dorsiflexed with the knee extended and the equinus deformity corrected.

Wound closure

It is advisable to release the tourniquet at this point to identify and coagulate by diathermy or ligate any bleeding vessels. The wound is closed by interrupted or continuous non-absorbable sutures to the deep fascia and interrupted absorbable sutures to the subcutaneous fat. The skin is closed by a subcuticular suture or interrupted non-absorbable sutures and a plaster cast is applied from the groin to the toes with the knee fully extended and the ankle dorsiflexed as fully as possible.

Postoperative management

The postoperative management is the same as for distal gastrocnemius release (see p. 1171).

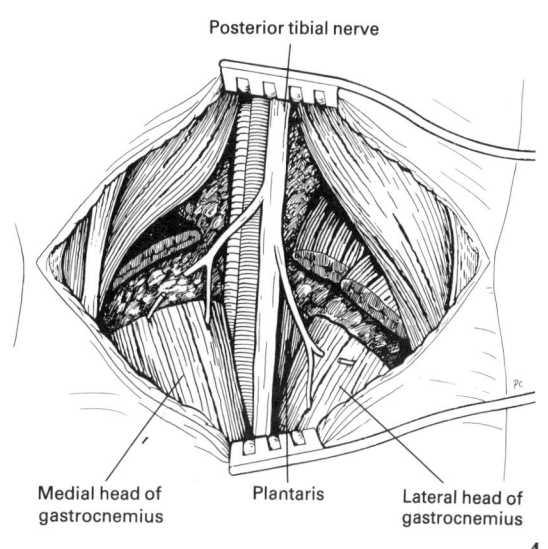

Further reading

Silfverskiold N. Reduction of the uncrossed two-joint muscle of the leg to one-joint muscle in spastic conditions. *Acta Chir Scand* 1924; 56: 315–30.

Illustrations by Philip Wilson after P. Henry

Supracondylar osteotomy of the femur

J. A. Fixsen MChir, FRCS
Consultant Orthopaedic Surgeon, The Hospital for Sick Children, Great Ormond Street, London, and St Bartholomew's Hospital, London, UK

Introduction

Osteotomy of the lower end of the femur in the supracondylar region can be used to correct valgus or varus, flexion or extension deformities mainly in children but also in adults. Rotational deformities can be corrected at this level but the author prefers to correct pure rotational deformity in the subtrochanteric region. In children, fixation by staples is sufficient but in adults a plate and screws can be used. When the femur is very small or delicate the two-stage osteotomy–osteoclasis described by Moore[1] can be used. This method avoids the problems of inadequate fixation in a small or soft bone and the danger of losing control of a small bony fragment close to the joint. At the first stage the required wedge of bone is removed leaving the cortex at the apex intact. The bone wedge is cut into chips and replaced in the gap left by the wedge. Two to three weeks later closed osteoclasis is performed, bending or cracking the intact cortex to close the gap and correct the deformity while retaining stability without internal fixation.

Varus and valgus deformities can be corrected at any age. It is tempting to correct severe soft tissue flexion deformity at the knee in conditions such as arthrogryposis, spina bifida and lumbar agenesis by supracondylar osteotomy. Unfortunately this produces a forward angulation of the epiphyseal plate which with growth results in a very ugly and functionally awkward deformity of the femur. Osteotomy should be avoided until near maturity in these patients.

In the adult, extension supracondylar osteotomy may be indicated rarely for old poliomyelitis. The main indication in the adult is for valgus deformities resulting from osteoarthritis or trauma. Although rigid fixation and early movement can be achieved by use of an angled blade–plate and screws placed on the lateral aspect of the femur, as described for supracondylar fractures (see pp. 242–251), fixation with one or two staples and a high cylinder plaster of Paris cast for 6 weeks postoperatively will give good results and the exposure is much less extensive.

Preoperatively the deformity must be carefully assessed and measured clinically and radiologically in the weight-bearing position. This is vital to achieve the right amount of correction.

Operation

The correction of a valgus deformity by medially based wedge will be described.

To correct other types of deformity the position of the base of the wedge is altered accordingly. To correct a varus deformity by removal of a laterally based wedge a lateral approach is used.

1

The patient lies supine under general anaesthesia. A high thigh tourniquet may be used. A medial longitudinal incision, approximately one quarter the total length of the thigh, is made, extending proximally from the apex of the medial femoral condyle.

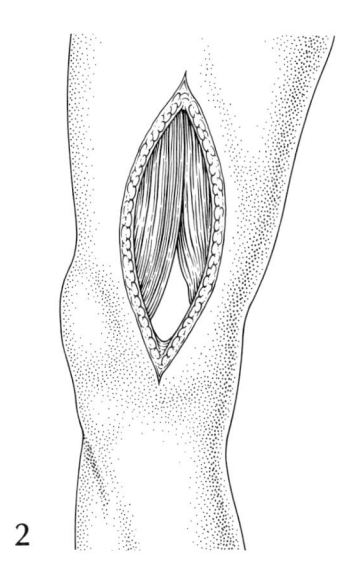

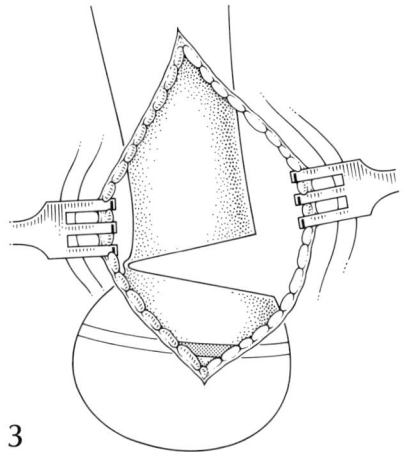

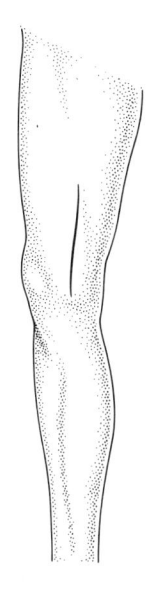

2

The deep fascia is divided and the vastus medialis exposed. To avoid damaging the muscle it is lifted forwards developing the plane between it and the adductor magnus. The femur is exposed and a longitudinal incision made in the periosteum on the medial side. The periosteum is raised and the supracondylar region is exposed widely by retracting the periosteum with bone levers. The epiphyseal plate can be clearly seen and care taken not to damage it either when removing the wedge of bone or inserting the fixation device.

3

A medially based wedge of bone is then removed proximal to the epiphyseal line making sure there is sufficient room to insert the fixation device, staple or plate, without damaging the epiphyseal plate. The wedge can be removed with a power saw or an osteotome and multiple drill holes. It is most important to leave the periosteum and the apex of the wedge intact to retain control of the bony fragments when the wedge is closed. The exact size of the wedge required must be measured from a weight-bearing radiograph and accurately marked out on the bone to ensure that the right amount of bone is removed. To avoid undesirable rotational deformity the bone can be marked above and below the wedge so that the surgeon can check rotational alignment at the end of the operation.

4

In children two or three staples are inserted to hold the wedge closed. It is advisable to start the points of the staples in small drill holes. This avoids displacing the osteotomy when the staples are hammered in. It also ensures that they are inserted evenly as the cortical bone of the proximal fragment is usually harder than that of the distal.

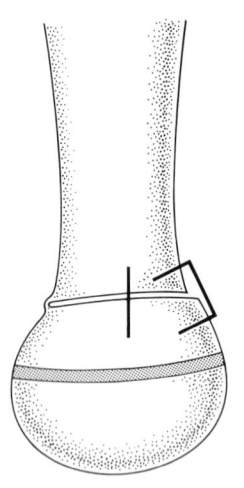

4

Postoperative management

The wound is closed in layers. Suction drainage is not usually necessary. A long leg plaster is applied with the knee in a few degrees of flexion. The foot may or may not be included in the plaster depending on the surgeon's preference. It is normally not necessary to immobilize the hip in a single spica unless the femur is very short. The plaster is retained until union occurs, usually 6 weeks in children and 8–10 weeks in adults. Weight-bearing in the plaster is allowed as soon as the surgeon feels it is safe, usually after 1 week.

Complications

The commonest error is failure to obtain the right amount of correction. Care in the clinical and radiological measurement of the correction required when the limb is weight-bearing should avoid this. Some surgeons use a sterile template to measure the angle for the wedge. In young children and patients with soft porotic bone adequate fixation can be difficult and the two-stage osteotomy–osteoclasis method is very useful.

Damage to the epiphyseal plate while it is still open must be avoided.

Reference

1. Moore JR. Osteotomy-osteoclasis: method for correcting long-bone deformities. *J Bone Joint Surg* 1947; 29: 119–29.

Illustrations by Gillian Oliver after B. Hyams

Rupture of the quadriceps mechanism

B. Helal MChOrth, FRCS
Honorary Consultant Orthopaedic Surgeon, The Royal London Hospital and The Royal National Orthopaedic Hospital, London, and Enfield Group of Hospitals, UK

S. C. Chen FRCS
Consultant Orthopaedic Surgeon, Enfield Group of Hospitals, UK

Introduction

The quadriceps mechanism can be disrupted at one of three levels depending on the age of the patient.

1. Rupture of the ligamentum patellae in children and young adults.
2. Fracture of the patella in young adults.
3. Rupture of the quadriceps tendon in the middle and older age groups.

RECENT RUPTURE

RUPTURE OF LIGAMENTUM PATELLAE

This occurs usually at the attachment of the ligamentum patellae to the inferior border of the patella as a result of a severe flexion injury against resistance. A haemarthrosis is present but the gap in the tendon may only be palpable after administration of a general anaesthetic. The treatment is always surgical.

Incision

1

A slightly curved anterior midline vertical incision is made over the knee from above the patella to below the tibial tuberosity.

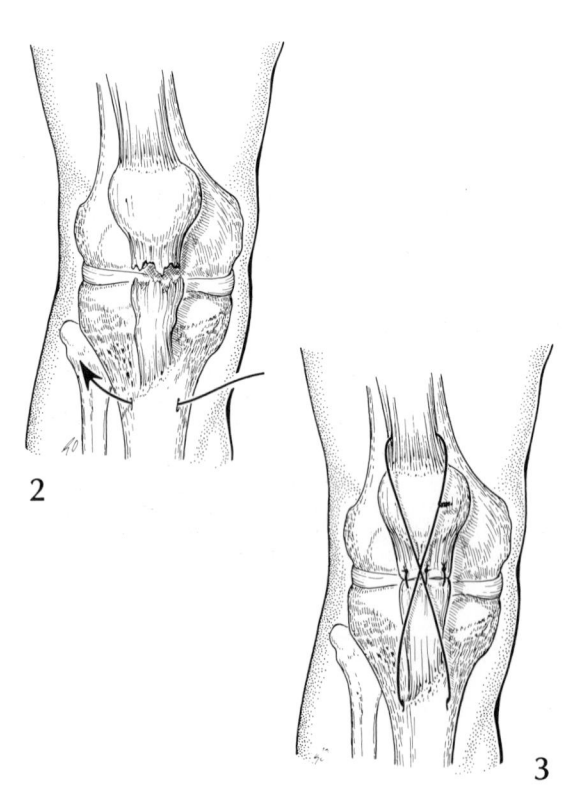

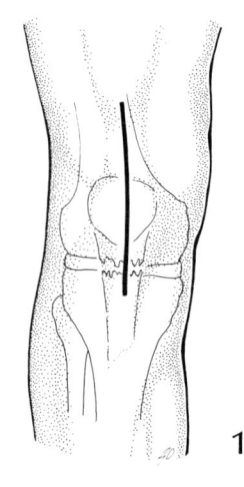

Procedure

2 & 3

A horizontal drill hole is made in the tibia at the level of the tibial tuberosity. A steel wire, 1.2 mm diameter, is threaded through the drill hole and passed across into the quadriceps tendon just above the patella, forming a figure-of-eight stitch. This stitch is tightened so that the ruptured ligamentum patellae is brought together. The tendon is stitched back using thick synthetic slowly absorbable sutures (polydioxanone-PDS). The subcutaneous tissue and skin are then closed.

Postoperative management

A well-padded crêpe bandage is applied over the knee and static quadriceps exercises including straight-leg raising exercises are commenced immediately. At 1 week, gentle knee flexion exercises can begin. The patient should walk on crutches at the end of 2 weeks but weight-bearing on the affected leg should not begin until 3 weeks have elapsed. Once the quadriceps muscles can lift the leg against gravity and some resistance, and the knee will flex to 90°, the crutches can be discarded for a walking-stick, which in its turn is discarded with the return of power and mobility.

RUPTURE OF QUADRICEPS TENDON

Incision

4

A midline vertical incision is made over the knee.

The surgeon must identify and ascertain the extent of the rupture of the quadriceps tendon. The rupture is usually across the musculotendinous junction of the quadriceps and the edges are ragged.

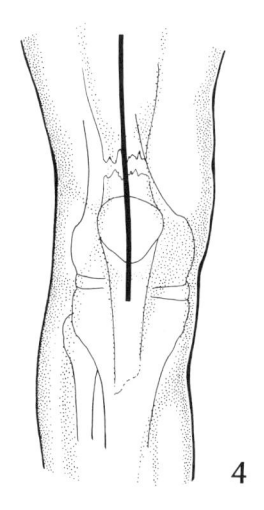

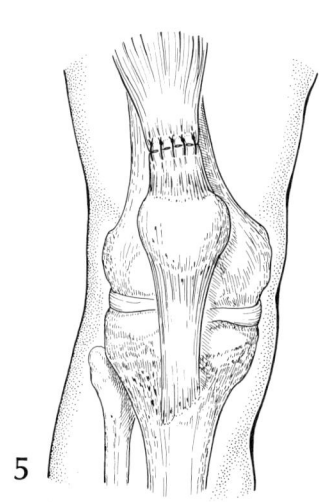

Repair

5

The ruptured muscle is stitched with interrupted thick synthetic, slowly absorbable sutures (polydioxanone-PDS). The wound is closed in layers.

Postoperative management

A plaster cylinder is applied from the ankle to the upper thigh and static quadriceps exercises are started the following day. At the end of 1 week straight-leg raising exercises are started and at the end of 2 weeks partial weight-bearing with the leg in plaster is allowed, using crutches. At the end of 4 weeks the plaster cylinder is removed and knee flexion exercises commenced. Unprotected weight-bearing is allowed when the knee can flex to 90° and the quadriceps muscles are strong.

OLD RUPTURE

OLD RUPTURE OF LIGAMENTUM PATELLAE
(modified Kelikian, Riashi and Gleason technique[1])

In old rupture, the quadriceps muscle becomes contracted. This has to be overcome and the patella brought down to its normal position before the ligamentum patellae can be replaced. The operation is carried out in two stages.

Stage 1

6 & 7

A vertical midline incision is made over the knee. The incision is deepened and the knee joint entered. The patella and the quadriceps muscle are freed so that any adhesions are broken down, enabling the patella to move freely.

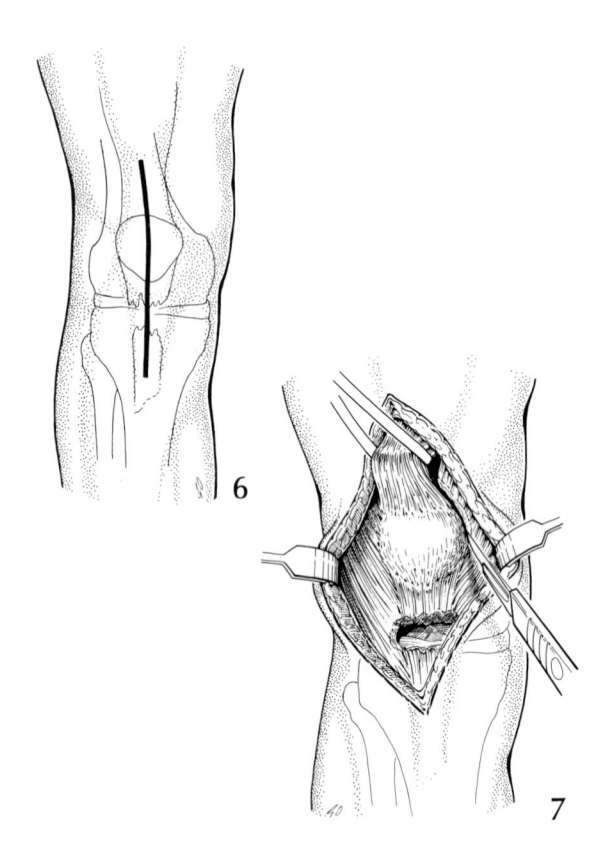

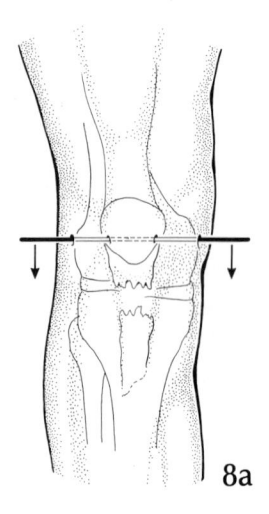

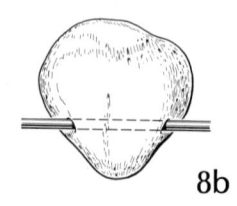

8a & b

A skeletal pin (Steinmann or Denham pin) is passed transversely across the lower third of the patella. It is important to position the pin accurately as the pin track is later enlarged in Stage 2 to accommodate the semitendinosus tendon.

The skin incision is closed and traction applied to the skeletal pin in order to stretch the quadriceps muscle. Traction is continued until the patella is brought down to its normal level, the position being checked by radiography. This usually takes up to 2 weeks. In the meantime, the patient is encouraged to perform static quadriceps exercises.

Stage 2

9a, b & 10

The skeletal pin is removed.

A longitudinal incision is made on the posteromedial aspect of the thigh. The semitendinosus tendon is identified and cut at the musculotendinous junction. Another small incision is made at the insertion of the semitendinosus tendon and the severed tendon withdrawn through this incision.

A third incision, a vertical midline incision, is made along the line of the initial incision in Stage 1.

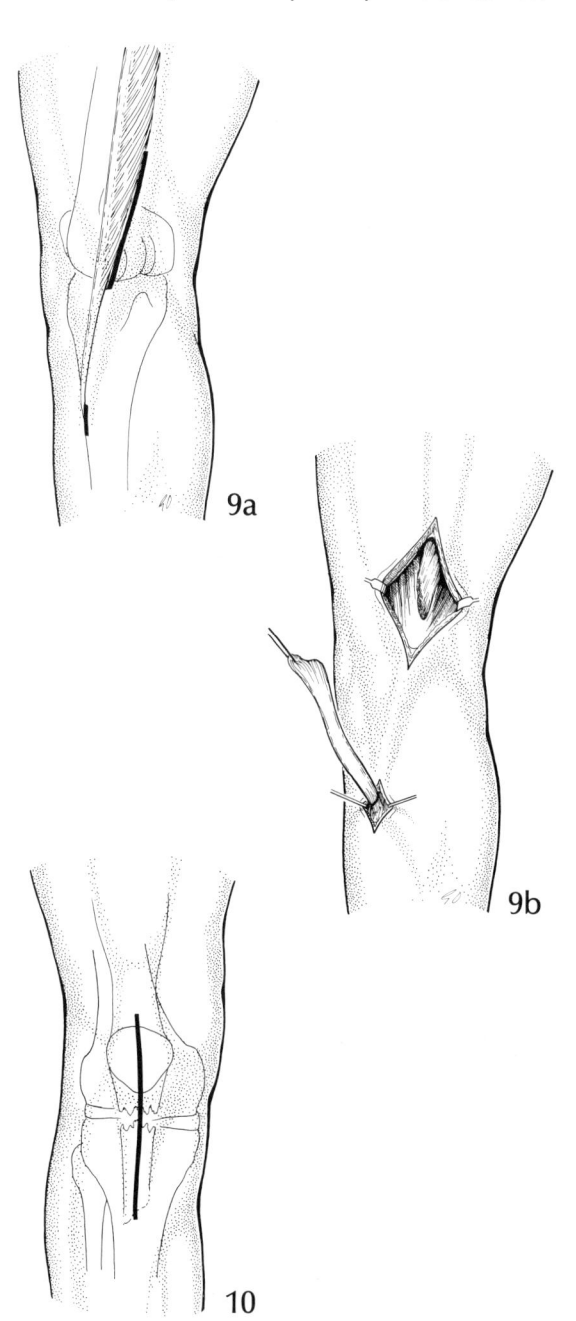

11

A transverse hole is drilled across the tibia at the level of the tibial tuberosity. This hole must be of adequate size to accommodate the semitendinosus tendon. The pin track in the patella is enlarged in a similar manner.

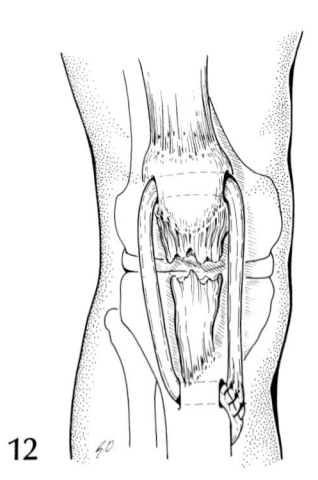

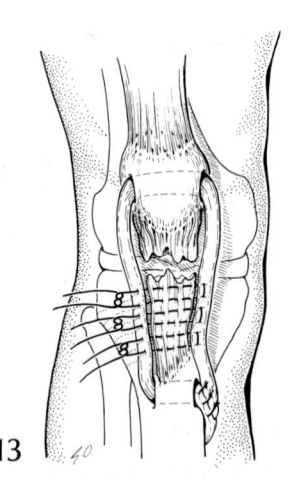

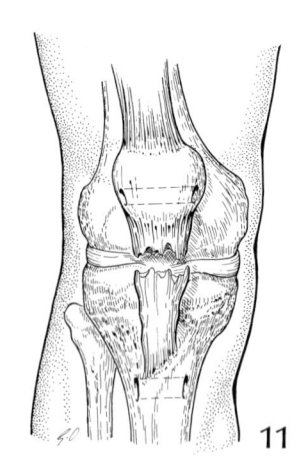

12 & 13

The semitendinosus tendon is passed subcutaneously from its insertion into the front of the tibia. It is threaded through the holes in the tibia and patella. The tendon is tightened and stitched back to itself as shown. The crumpled ligamentum patellae is pulled up and stitched to the two parts of the semitendinosus tendon with thick synthetic, slowly absorbable, sutures (polydioxanone-PDS).

Postoperative management

A plaster cast is applied from the toes to the upper thigh with the knee in extension. At the end of 6 weeks, the plaster cast is removed and passive and active knee exercises started.

OLD RUPTURE OF QUADRICEPS TENDON

Here again, the quadriceps muscle may be contracted.

Incision

14

A curved incision is made along the front of the knee extending from the lower thigh to the lower pole of the patella and the ruptured quadriceps tendons exposed.

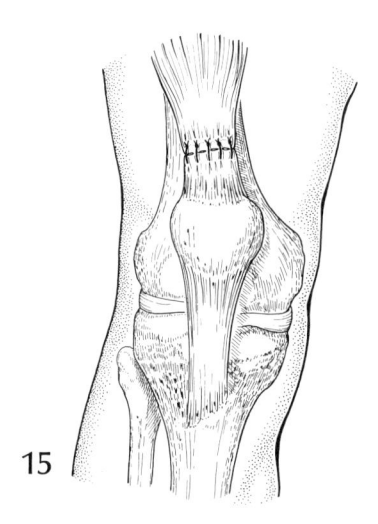

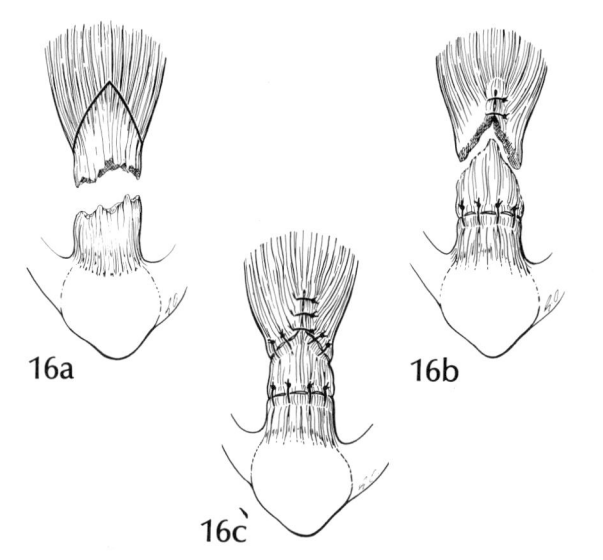

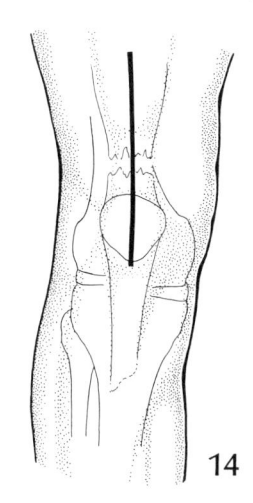

Repair

15

If the ruptured ends can be approximated with the knee fully extended, the ends are sutured together with interrupted thick chromic catgut sutures.

Lengthening and repair

16a, b & c

If, however, the ruptured ends cannot be approximated, the quadriceps tendon can be lengthened by an inverted V-Y-plasty. An inverted V-inc'sion is made completely through the proximal segment of the quadriceps tendon 1 cm proximal to the ruptured end.

The ruptured ends are sutured with interrupted thick chromic catgut sutures.

The inverted V-incision is closed converting it into an inverted Y.

Postoperative management

A plaster cast is applied from the toes to the upper thigh with the knee in extension. At the end of 6 weeks, the plaster cast is removed and passive and active knee exercises started.

CONTRACTURE IN INFANCY

Repeated injections into the quadriceps, e.g., of antibiotics in the neonatal period, can lead to the muscle becoming fibrosed and contracted. This results in an inability to flex the knee. The fibrosis may occur in the deep fascia and in the quadriceps muscle.

Incision

17

The fibrosed part of the quadriceps should be sought. A longitudinal incision is made over the anterior part of the lower thigh to include the fibrosed area of the quadriceps.

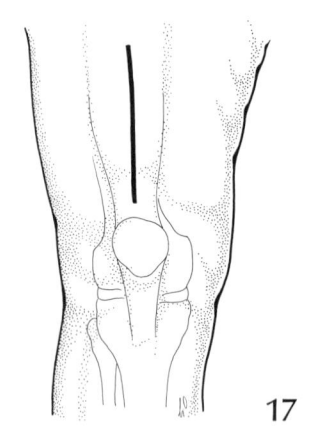

Release

18 & 19

The deep fascia is incised transversely across the front and sides of the thigh. Knee flexion should be assessed. If it is still restricted, the fibrosed parts of the quadriceps muscle are excised. This is rarely necessary. Usually the vastus intermedius is involved, but the rectus femoris and vastus lateralis may also be involved. The wound is then closed.

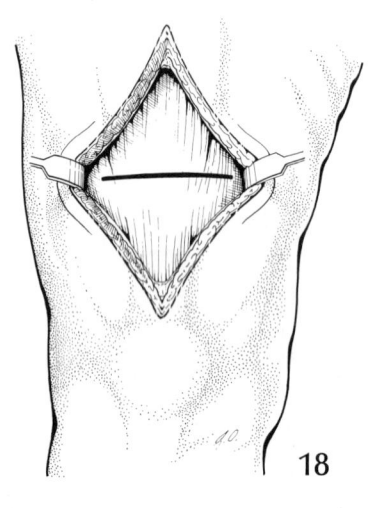

Postoperative management

A plaster cast is applied from the toes to the upper thigh with the knee flexed to 90°. The plaster cast is removed at the end of 3 weeks and passive and active exercises started.

Reference

1. Kelikian H, Riashi E, Gleason J. Restoration of quadriceps function in neglected tear of the patellar tendon. *Surg Gynecol Obstet* 1957; 104: 200–4.

Further reading

Thompson TC. Quadricepsplasty to improve knee function. *J Bone Joint Surg* 1944; 26: 366–79.

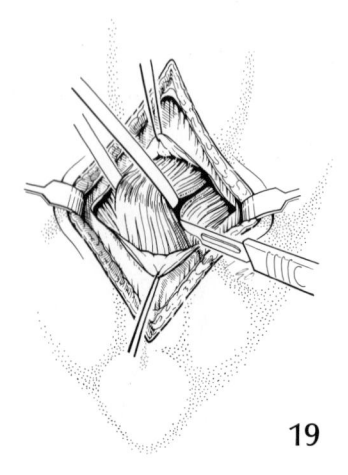

Illustrations by Philip Wilson after P. Henry

Quadricepsplasty in the adult

J. A. Fixsen MChir, FRCS
Consultant Orthopaedic Surgeon, The Hospital for Sick Children, Great Ormond Street, London, and St Bartholomew's Hospital, London, UK

Introduction

Indications

This operation can be used to correct limitation of flexion of the knee due to soft tissue scarring in the anterior aspect of the thigh involving the quadriceps muscle and its expansion. The commonest cause of such scarring and fibrosis are fractures of the femoral shaft, extensive soft tissue wounds of the thigh and immobilization following trauma. At operation limitation of flexion is usually found to be due to one or more of the following factors, all of which block the distal movement of the patella[1].

1. Fibrosis of the intermedius.
2. Adhesion of the patella to the femoral condyles.
3. Fibrosis and shortening of the lateral expansions of the vasti with adherence to the femoral condyles.
4. Actual shortening of the rectus femoris muscle, but this is rare.

Thompson, when describing the operation in 1944, commented that success depends on[2]:

1. whether the rectus femoris has escaped injury;
2. how well the rectus femoris can be isolated from the scarred parts of the quadriceps mechanism; and
3. how well the muscle can be developed by active use postoperatively.

Patients should have had a thorough course of active conservative treatment, including manipulation under anaesthesia to mobilize the knee, before considering this operation. The procedure is rarely indicated if the patient can flex his knee to 70° or more, and in the majority of patients considered for operation flexion is less than 30°.

1004 Thigh and knee

Operation

The operation is usually performed under general anaesthesia. The patient lies in the supine position. A tourniquet can be used to facilitate the dissection in the early part of the operation if it is possible to place it high enough on the thigh to avoid the operation site. It must be removed before completing the operation to allow careful haemostasis and remove any tethering effect it may have on the quadriceps mechanism. Careful haemostasis using diathermy is essential throughout the operation.

1

A straight or slightly curving S-shaped anterior longitudinal incision is made through the skin, subcutaneous tissue and superficial fascia from the distal pole of the patella to the mid-thigh. The precise position and length of the incision are determined by the site of the scarring.

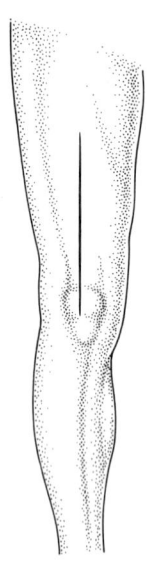

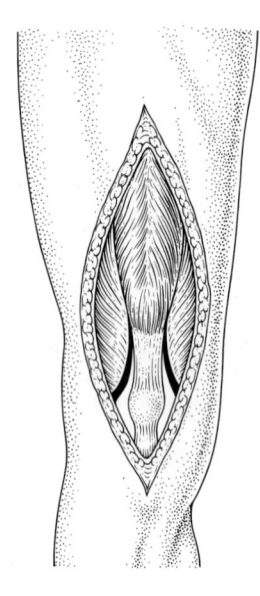

2

The rectus is then separated out by dividing the deep fascia on each side of the muscle to separate it from the vastus medialis and lateralis. The incisions are continued distally into the medial and lateral expansion of the capsule of the knee as far as is necessary to overcome any contracture. If the tendon of the rectus femoris has been obliterated by scarring it is necessary to fashion a new one by making a longitudinal strip out of scar tissue to replace it.

3

The scarred vastus intermedius which commonly binds down the rectus femoris and patella to the femur is excised completely, preserving the integrity of the rectus femoris and, if possible, a fibrous or periosteal covering over the anterior aspect of the femur. Following each step in the release of the quadriceps mechanism, the knee can be flexed to gauge how much flexion has been achieved. After removal of the scarred vastus intermedius the knee should be flexed to at least 110° to break down any intra-articular adhesion. If the rectus femoris is the sole remaining tight structure preventing flexion it can be lengthened but this will result in some permanent loss of active extension. If the patella itself is severely damaged on its articular surface, Nicoll[1] advises that it should be removed, but Hesketh[3] warns that this will weaken the quadriceps tendon and adversely affect postoperative mobilization.

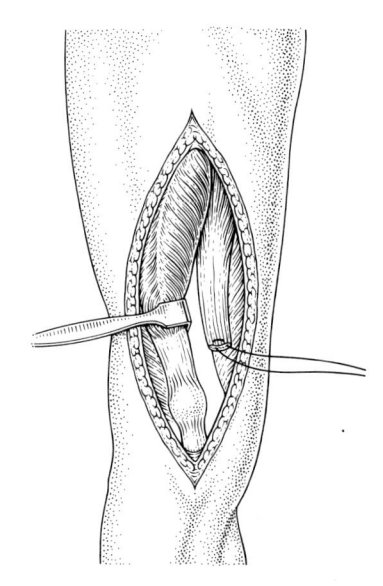

4

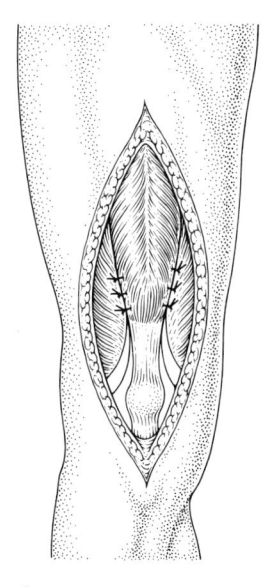

If the vastus medialis and lateralis are severely scarred, subcutaneous tissue and fat should be interposed between them and the rectus femoris. If they are reasonably normal, they may be sutured back to the sides of the rectus as far as the distal third of the thigh. The incisions in the capsule of the knee and lateral expansions are left open. If a tourniquet has been used this should be removed and careful haemostasis obtained. The wound is then closed with suction drainage.

Postoperative management

There is a variety of regimens for treatment of the limb postoperatively. Thompson immobilizes the leg in a Thomas' splint with a Pearson kneepiece. Balanced traction is applied and continued for 3 weeks. Active and passive stretchings are started as soon as possible after surgery. This is a slow and painful process and considerable determination on behalf of the patient and the physiotherapist are necessary to mobilize the knee at this stage. The author prefer Nicoll's method of immobilizing the knee in plaster in flexion of about 20°–30° less than that obtained at operation for the first 48–72 hours. The plaster and drain are then removed and the knee exercised during the day. At night it is immobilized in extension provided the range of flexion is being maintained during the day. Once the wound is healed, a gentle manipulation under anaesthesia may be necessary if flexion is being lost. The constant passive motion (CPM) machine can also be very useful in the postoperative management.

Complications

All authors writing on the subject of quadricepsplasty stress that the postoperative mobilization of the knee is usually slow and painful and requires determination and fortitude on the part of the patient. Hesketh[3] recommends that the operation should not be offered to patients over 55 years, unless they are unusually determined. The variety of postoperative regimens for mobilizing the knee also points to the difficulty of regaining the range of movement obtained at the time of operation by this extensive soft tissue procedure. Pool therapy is often helpful in regaining movement. An initial extension lag is almost invariable but usually disappears gradually over a period of up to a year, except in those patients where the rectus femoris has been lengthened, when some permanent loss of active extension is the rule.

References

1. Nicoll EA. Quadricepsplasty. J Bone Joint Surg [Br] 1963; 45-B: 483–90.

2. Thompson TC. Quadricepsplasty to improve knee function. J Bone Joint Surg 1944; 26: 366–79.

3. Hesketh KT. Experiences with the Thompson quadricepsplasty. J Bone Joint Surg [Br] 1963; 45-B: 491–5.

Illustrations by Gillian Oliver

Diagnostic arthroscopy of the knee

George Bentley ChM, FRCS
Professor of Orthopaedic Surgery, The Institute of Orthopaedics, University of London; Honorary Consultant Orthopaedic Surgeon, Royal National Orthopaedic Hospital, Stanmore and the Middlesex Hospital, London, UK

Anthony J. B. Fogg FRCS
Consultant Orthopaedic Surgeon, Princess Margaret Hospital, Swindon, UK

Introduction

Endoscopic examination of the knee joint was first performed by Professor K. Tagaki in 1918, primarily for the assessment of tuberculosis. Eugen Bircher[1] of Switzerland reported the first European series in 1921 and the procedure was popularized by Watanabe in the 1950s[2,3] and by Jackson in the 1970s[4,5] and 1980s[6].

Arthroscopy is now routinely used in the diagnosis of knee joint injuries and disorders and as a prelude to endoscopic procedures, providing the surgeon with a method of accurate intra-articular assessment without the attendant risks of open arthrotomy.

1008 Thigh and knee

Anatomy

1, 2 & 3

With practice, a more extensive view of the interior of the joint can be achieved than is possible by arthrotomy. The structures visible through the routine anterolateral approach are as follows:

1. Articular surfaces of patella, patellar groove, femoral condyles and tibial condyles.
2. Anterior two-thirds of the medial meniscus and its posterior horn.
3. Entire lateral meniscus.
4. Anterior cruciate ligament.
5. Retropatellar fat pad and synovial folds.
6. Popliteus tendon.
7. Suprapatellar pouch.
8. Medial patellar plica.
9. Lateral and most of the medial femoral recess.

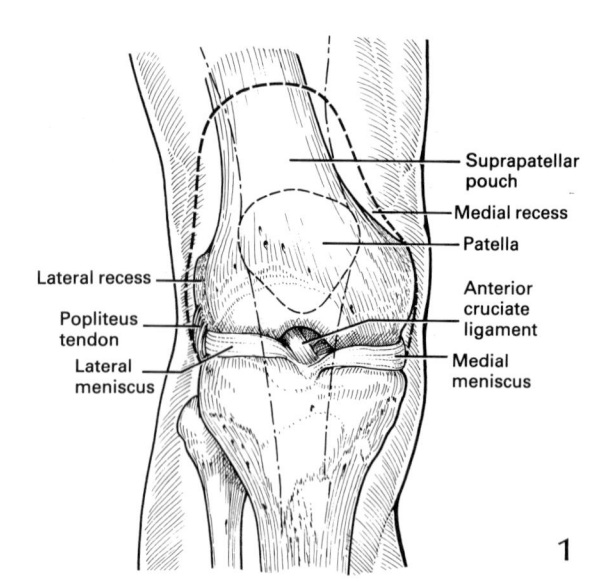

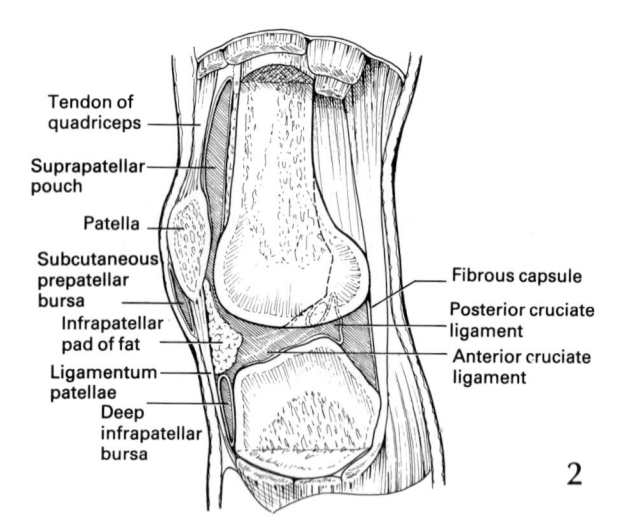

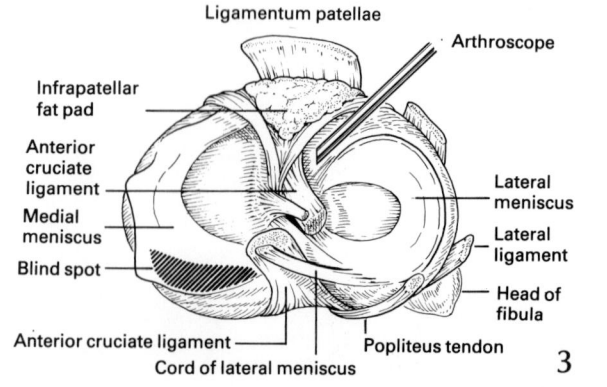

Preoperative

Indications

Arthroscopy should always be used in conjunction with a thorough history and clinical examination of the patient and is not an adequate substitute for either. Plain radiographs of the knee are an essential prerequisite: anteroposterior, weight-bearing and lateral views of the knee with views of both patellae at 30° of flexion are ideal. The procedure is used for the following purposes:

1. Confirmation of suspected meniscal lesions prior to arthroscopic or open surgery.
2. Assessment of anterior cruciate ligament integrity.
3. Diagnosis of acute injuries associated with haemarthrosis.
4. Investigation of anterior knee pain.
5. Evaluation of chondromalacia patellae and estimation of patellar 'tracking'.
6. Localization of loose bodies.
7. Assessment of osteochondritis dissecans.
8. Diagnosis and assessment of osteoarthritis.
9. Diagnosis of inflammatory joint disease and synovial biopsy.
10. Assessment of articular cartilage and synovium before and after treatment (e.g. tibial osteotomy, synovectomy, osteochondral grafting).
11. Examination of knee joint prostheses.

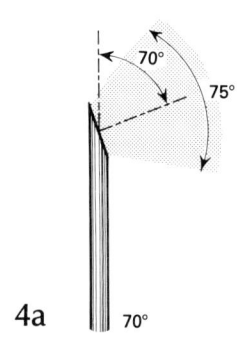

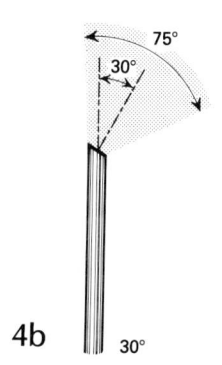

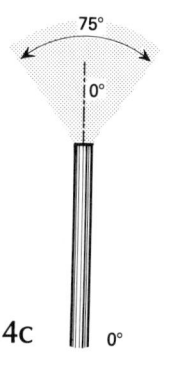

Equipment

4a

The rod lens system designed by Professor Hopkins of Reading University can provide the modern surgeon with a 4 mm, wide-angle (75°) viewing lens giving sharp bright images.

4b

The preferred instrument for general use is the 30° fore-oblique arthroscope.

4c

0° telescopes are available for the novice and give a straight-ahead view which allows for easier orientation. Visualization of certain areas is, however, impossible with the 0° telescope.

A 70° telescope provides greater access to the posteromedial and posterolateral joint compartments and is a useful addition to the experienced arthroscopist.

Modern arthroscope design has incorporated the bridge of the old cystoscope-based instrument into a stainless steel sheath down which sharp and blunt trocars are passed prior to insertion of the telescope. The risk of breakage of the telescope has consequently been reduced. Narrow diameter (2.7 mm) telescopes are available for paediatric use. A fibre-optic cold light source with a 150 watt lamp provides adequate illumination for routine examination. More powerful 250 watt sources are essential for television and video documentation.

Still slide photographs are obtainable using camera and flash attachments.

All diagnostic arthroscopy sets are equipped with at least one blunt hook with which to manipulate the menisci and cruciate ligaments and assess the articular cartilage for fissuring and softening.

Sterilization

The arthroscope is sterilized according to the manufacturers' instructions. The telescope may be subjected to flash autoclaving with great care, or gas sterilization using carboxide (88 per cent) and ethylene oxide (12 per cent) can be used (4 hour cycle at 71°C) in a gas autoclave. All parts of the instrument can be sterilized by immersion in an activated glutaraldehyde solution for 20 minutes provided that they are thoroughly washed in sterile water before use, and this is the commonly used method.

Anaesthesia

General anaesthesia

This is the preferred method in the majority of cases, and has advantages for both the surgeon and the patient. It allows for the comfortable use of a tourniquet, avoids the need for multiple injections of local anaesthetic, and presents the surgeon with a totally relaxed patient. Under a general anaesthetic, the joint is readily unlocked or manipulated for the purpose of improving the surgeon's view and arthrotomy can be performed if necessary.

Local anaesthesia

This method should be employed only by the experienced surgeon with confidence in his technique. It precludes the use of a tourniquet and, where multiple incisions are contemplated, is best conducted with the smaller diameter telescope. Each entry site is infiltrated with 0.5 per cent bupivacaine containing 1/100 000 adrenaline. A similar concentration of anaesthetic can be added to the irrigation fluid and the joint left for 5 minutes before proceeding. Femoral nerve block will facilitate this procedure and reduce postoperative pain.

Examination under anaesthesia

In an anaesthetized, fully relaxed patient, no diagnostic arthroscopy is complete without a thorough clinical examination of the knee. The examination should preferably be carried out prior to application of tourniquet and drapes and should include an assessment of the range of movement, collateral ligament stability, Lachman's test, pivot shift or 'jerk' test, anterior and posterior drawer signs, and patellar stability.

Tourniquet

A high thigh pneumatic tourniquet is applied to the leg prior to draping. Unless it is essential to assess the vascularity of the synovium arthroscopically, the leg is exsanguinated by elevation and/or application of a 'roll-on exsanguinator' and the tourniquet inflated to approximately twice systolic blood pressure.

It is considered useful to flex the knee as much as possible before inflation. This minimizes 'tightness' in the quadriceps muscles and allows greater freedom of movement of instruments within the joint.

Preparation and position

The leg should be shaved preoperatively and the skin prepared as for an arthrotomy. Although gaining in popularity as a day case procedure, the operation should be carried out in a fully equipped operating theatre under routine aseptic conditions. Because of the inevitable contact of the surgeon's mask, eyelash or hood with the eyepiece of the arthroscope, and the unavoidable spillage of irrigating fluid, it is impossible to keep the procedure completely sterile. Careful handling of the instruments by the eyepiece or handles and avoidance of contact with the barrel will help to minimize the introduction of potentially infective agents into the joint. The use of a video camera also reduces the risk, but the operator must be aware of potential contamination of the instruments, especially if the procedure proves difficult.

With the patient supine on the operating table, the limb is cleaned with an appropriate antiseptic solution such as 0.5 per cent chlorhexidine in 70 per cent alcohol and draped in such a manner that the hip and knee can both be flexed towards 90° and the perineum can remain completely isolated. Single-handed operators can use table-mounted thigh rests to assist control of the limb if necessary.

5

To avoid entanglement of the operatives with essential lengths of cable and tubing used during the procedure, it is wise to spend a short time in planning the positioning of personnel and equipment before embarking on diagnostic arthroscopy. Special attention should be paid to the positioning of the light source to avoid undue tension on the cable, and also to the provision of irrigation control which should be sterile and within easy reach of the surgeon.

The investigation is most comfortably performed sitting on a mobile stool with the table elevated to an appropriate height and the leg supported by the foot in the operator's lap. Where video photography is available, the operator stands or sits facing the television screen.

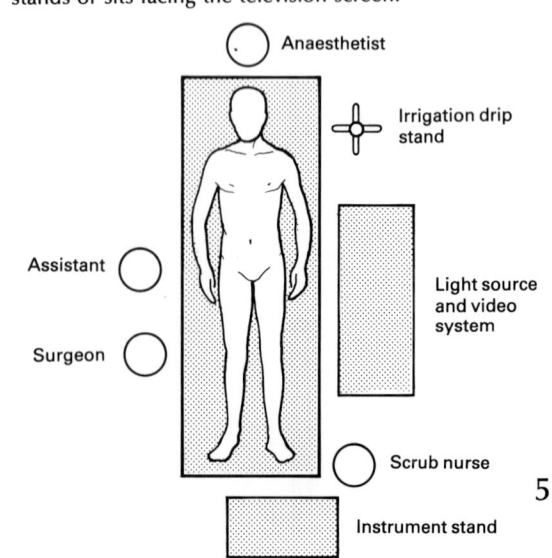

Operation

Aspiration and irrigation

Prior to insertion of the arthroscope, any effusion or haemarthrosis in the joint is aspirated using a large bore irrigation or hypodermic needle and syringe, introduced via a lateral suprapatellar approach. Wide-bore, disposable trocars and cannulae are commercially available and serve equally well as fluid entry or exhaust portals.

Approach and assembly

6a & b

The anterolateral approach is the most useful for routine initial arthroscopic examination of the knee. With the knee flexed to 90°, it is easy to locate the small depression in the joint line to the lateral side of the patellar tendon with a fingertip. With a size 10 blade, a 5 mm transverse stab incision, 5 mm above the lateral tibial condyle (to avoid the lateral meniscus) and 5 mm lateral to the patellar tendon, is made in the skin and extended down through the joint capsule. The arthroscope sheath with the sharp trocar is then introduced and directed medially, upwards and backwards towards the intercondylar notch, using gentle pressure and a rotational force. Once the capsule is penetrated, the tip lies just above the anterior horn of the lateral meniscus. The blunt trocar is now substituted for the sharp trocar.

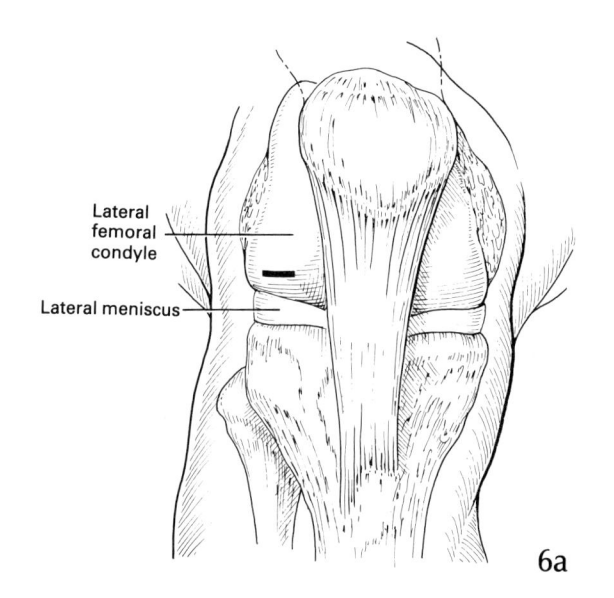

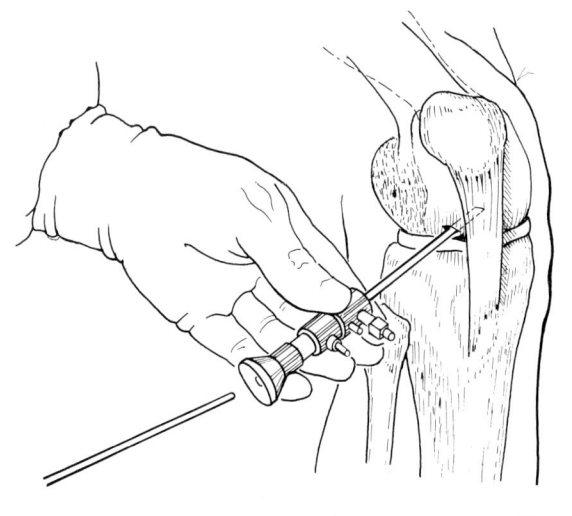

6c

The knee is extended and, with a sudden controlled push, the tip is introduced beneath the patella into the suprapatellar pouch. The trocar is removed and replaced by the telescope, which is locked into the sheath. The light cable, VDU and video systems are attached and the distension and irrigation system assembled. Distension of the joint is achieved by a sterile 'giving-set' connected from a 1 litre bag of normal saline (suspended 1 metre above the knee) to the inlet tap on the arthroscope sheath. A drainage tube is connected to the outlet tap of the arthroscope and led to a bowl beneath the table. For diagnostic procedures it is often not necessary to use continuous irrigation but the joint can be irrigated at intervals by alternate use of inlet and outlet taps. The joint may be filled prior to insertion of the arthroscope by a wide-bore needle if preferred. Continuous irrigation may be performed by this method also. Examination of the joint commences. With practice it is easier to view the TV monitor directly than to use the eye-to-telescope method.

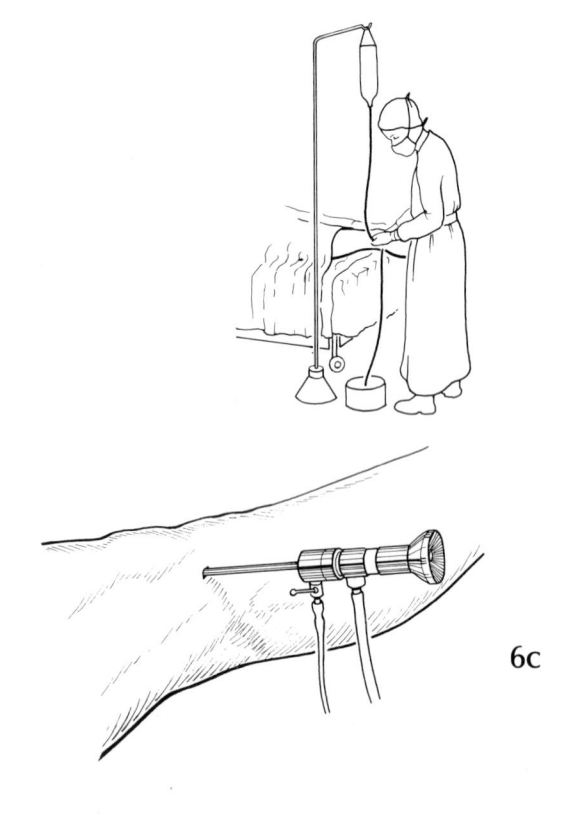

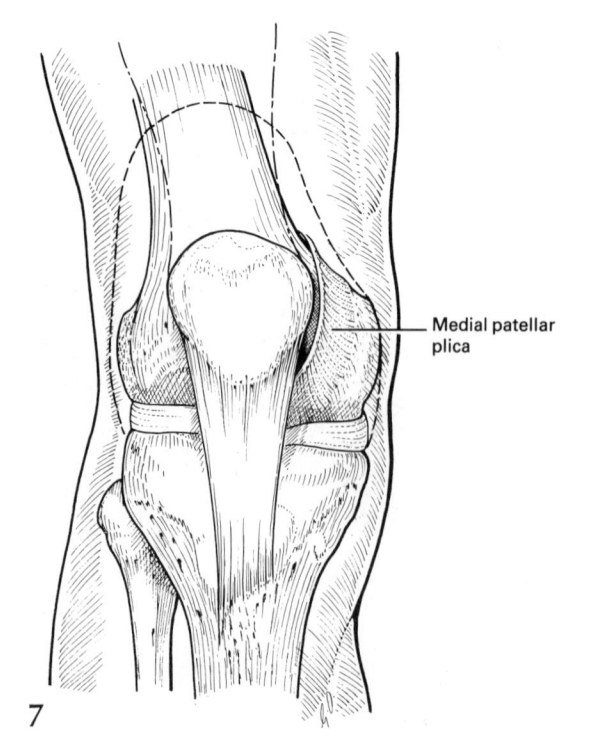

7

With the knee extended the arthroscope is pushed gently towards the apex of the pouch and gradually withdrawn, inspecting the synovium en route (*Plate 11**). At the superior medial pole of the patella and running upwards and backwards to the femur is the medial suprapatellar plica which very occasionally divides the pouch into two distinct cavities and may obscure the presence of loose bodies. This structure is not to be confused with the more common medial patellar plica (medial synovial shelf or Aoki's band) (*see Illustration 7*), which runs in the coronal plane from the medial side of the joint to insert distally below the inferior pole of the patella into the infrapatellar fat pad (*Plate 12*). This latter structure, although infamous, rarely causes symptoms. When pathological, it is visible as a thickened, fibrous crescentic band which can be seen to impinge between the patella and femur as the knee is flexed and may cause a groove in the medial femoral condyle. These structures can be further assessed by probing them with an irrigation needle or arthroscopy hook. Biopsy of the synovium, especially in the absence of a tourniquet, is deferred until completion of the examination to avoid bleeding and interference with the visual field.

*Colour plates 11–30 are on pages 1033–1036.

Patellofemoral joint

By withdrawing the instrument and rotating it to direct the line of vision upwards, the undersurface of the patella can be inspected. The lateral half of the patella can be examined easily by carefully running the arthroscope along its length and, by pushing the patella laterally and tilting it towards the examiner, the median ridge, the medial articular cartilage and the most medial (odd) facet can be visualized.

Aoki's band is best seen by directing the arthroscope medially and upwards at this juncture. Further assessment of the patellar articular cartilage can be gained by probing with a blunt hook introduced through an anteromedial stab incision, special note being taken of any areas of softening, 'blistering' or fissuring on the medial or odd facets suggestive of chondromalacia patellae.

The relationship of the median patellar ridge to the intercondylar groove of the femur is now inspected during an arc of flexion of 0–60°. In normal subjects, the ridge strikes just lateral to the floor of the groove and gradually comes to lie centrally by approximately 60° flexion (*Plate 13*).

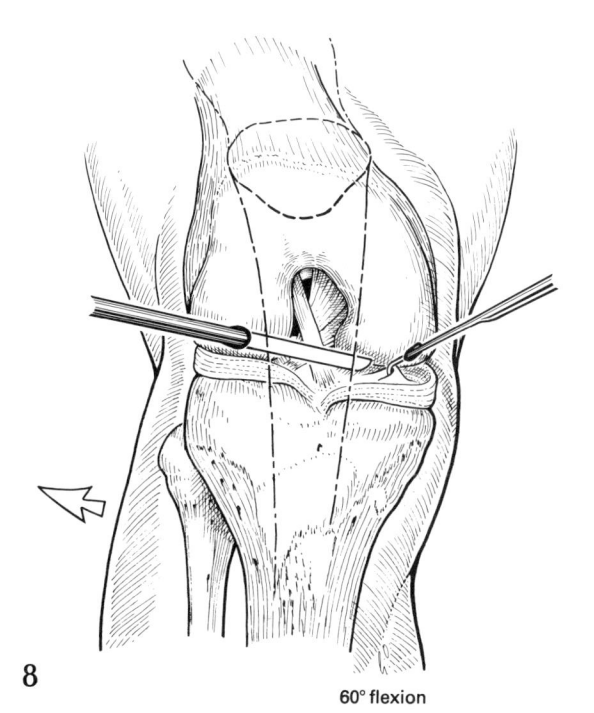

Infrapatellar fat pad

The infrapatellar fat pad is occasionally traumatized (Hoffa's syndrome) or caught between the patella and femoral condyles during violent extension (hurdler's knee). The normal pad can be seen easily as a fatty globular structure immediately below the patella with a covering of synovium containing a fine plexus of blood vessels (*Plate 14*). The alar fold can also be seen. Occasionally, if introduced too medially, the arthroscope penetrates the suspensory ligament of the patella, impeding visualization. This is remedied by reinsertion of the instrument in a more posterior direction.

Medial compartment

8

By turning the arthroscope downwards after examination of the patellofemoral joint, the rolled edge of the medial femoral condyle can be identified and followed downwards to gain entry to the medial compartment. The knee is now placed in 60° of flexion and a valgus/lateral rotation strain applied. The meniscosynovial attachment is readily identifiable and, as the telescope is very slightly withdrawn, the sharp free edge of the medial meniscus and the anterior horn are seen (*Plate 15*). Further inspection of the femoral and tibial condyles is also possible and particular note should be made of irregularities in the articular cartilage of the femoral condyle where it abuts on the anterior horn in full extension. 'Abrasions' of the cartilage are frequently associated with meniscal tears. The anterior two-thirds of the medial meniscus are easily inspected but the posterior third is not so readily visualized, although its free edge may be seen beneath the femoral condyle if a considerable valgus strain is applied to the knee in 30° flexion. At the junction of the two parts, a 'flounce' or 'kink' is regularly noted (*Plate 16*). This is a normal finding, unless excessive, in which case a detachment of the posteromedial portion may be present. The inspection is assisted by introducing a blunt probe through the anteromedial portal and lifting the free edge to explore for inferior cleavage tears (*Plate 17*). The hook can also be used to try to displace the meniscus into the joint, as may occur with a peripheral detachment (*Plate 18*). By placing the hook into the meniscosynovial junction and rotating the knee laterally, large flap tears previously hidden beneath the femoral condyle may emerge. Further information about the posterior horn is gained by accessing the posteromedial compartment.

8

60° flexion

Intercondylar notch and anterior cruciate ligament

9 & 10

By gently withdrawing the tip of the arthroscope from the anteromedial compartment, the anterior cruciate ligament will present itself as a silver striated bundle, covered with synovium. Blood vessels are arranged longitudinally along the length of the ligament which travels posteriorly and laterally, tapering towards its attachment on the medial surface of the lateral femoral condyle (Plate 19). The ligament is occasionally bifurcate but is still distinguishable from a partial tear by the presence of an intact synovial membrane. The integrity of the ligament can be assessed under direct vision while the assistant performs the anterior drawer test. The ligament may also be probed with the hook.

To gain access to the posteromedial compartment, the knee is flexed 10° and, under direct vision, the telescope is passed over the anterior cruciate ligament and between it and the posterolateral edge of the medial femoral condyle (see Illustration 10). This manoeuvre is occasionally hampered by the presence of excessive synovial folds or osteophytes but, in the majority of cases, gives the surgeon a rewarding view of the posterior horn of the medial meniscus and an area behind the medial tibial condyle where a loose body may be concealed. The back of the meniscus can be examined in greater detail by substituting the 70° lens at this stage. The instrument is now withdrawn and, if rotated medially and slightly upwards, may identify a raised area on the lateral aspect of the medial femoral condyle corresponding to the attachment of the posterior cruciate ligament. This structure is otherwise not seen through the anterolateral approach unless there is a complete rupture of the anterior cruciate ligament. In a proportion of such cases where diagnosis has been delayed, the anterior cruciate ligament may be identified running posteriorly and medially to become adherent to the posterior cruciate ligament.

The arthroscope is rotated downwards so that the anterior cruciate ligament again enters the field. The ligamentum mucosum (infrapatellar synovial fold) sometimes impedes passage of the instrument across the notch and may be confused with the ligament itself. By keeping the anterior cruciate in constant view, orientation is not lost and the telescope can gradually be withdrawn and moved laterally into the lateral compartment of the joint.

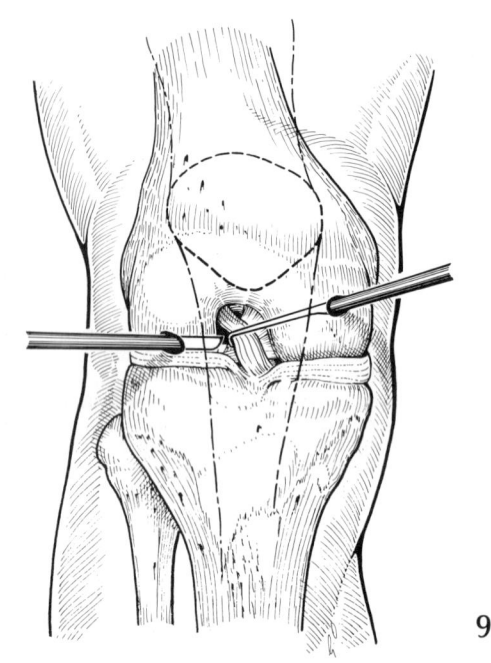

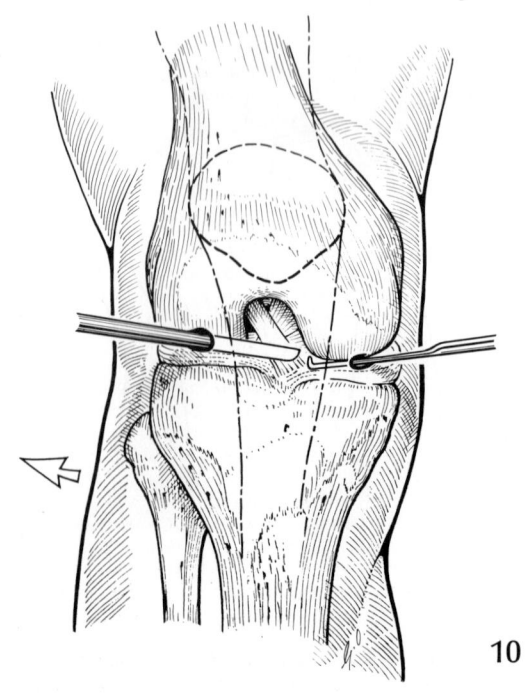

9

10° flexion

10

10° flexion

Lateral compartment

11

With the knee flexed to 30° and the foot placed across the table onto the opposite leg, a varus strain can be applied to the knee joint, thereby opening up the lateral compartment for inspection. An alternative method is to place the foot over the edge of the operating table with the knee in 30° flexion and apply a varus strain with the surgeon's thigh against the patient's foot, using the table edge as a fulcrum.

The first structure visible is the free edge of the posterior horn of the lateral meniscus lying under the lateral femoral condyle (*Plate 20*). This is easily visualized on its inferior surface by passing the arthroscope directly beneath it into a small recess where loose bodies may lodge. It may also be inspected by elevating the meniscal margin with a hook introduced through the anteromedial portal.

By advancing the instrument under direct vision between the anterior cruciate ligament and the medial edge of the lateral femoral condyle, the posterolateral compartment is entered. The superior and posterior surfaces of the posterior horn of the lateral meniscus and the back of the lateral femoral condyle are now easily seen. Use of the 70° telescope will again provide a more detailed inspection. The instrument is now withdrawn back into the joint and the sharp edge of the lateral meniscus followed laterally and anteriorly. During this manoeuvre the popliteus tendon is usually seen running obliquely downwards and medially behind the posterior third of the meniscus towards its insertion on the posteromedial aspect of the tibia (*Plate 21*).

Occasionally it is difficult to see the attachment of the anterior horn of the lateral meniscus and, if serious doubt exists, then an entry from the anteromedial portal should be made.

Lateral gutter

If difficulty is encountered in traversing the intercondylar notch, then a bucket-handle tear of either meniscus should be suspected. In this instance, the lateral compartment is best reached by returning the telescope to the suprapatellar pouch with the knee in extension and passing the tip down into the lateral gutter, adjacent to the lateral surface of the lateral femoral condyle. While here, the gutter can be inspected for loose bodies (*see Plate 22*) and, by guiding the instrument backwards through the synovial folds, a different perspective of the popliteus tendon may be obtained. In cases of suspected lateral patellar instability, one should assess the degree of 'overhang' between the lateral margin of the patella and the lateral femoral condyle by turning the tip of the instrument upwards and observing the relationship during flexion. The lateral joint compartment can then be entered by withdrawing the tip of the arthroscope and directing it medially.

After inspection of the lateral compartment, including visualization of the articular surfaces, the procedure is at an end.

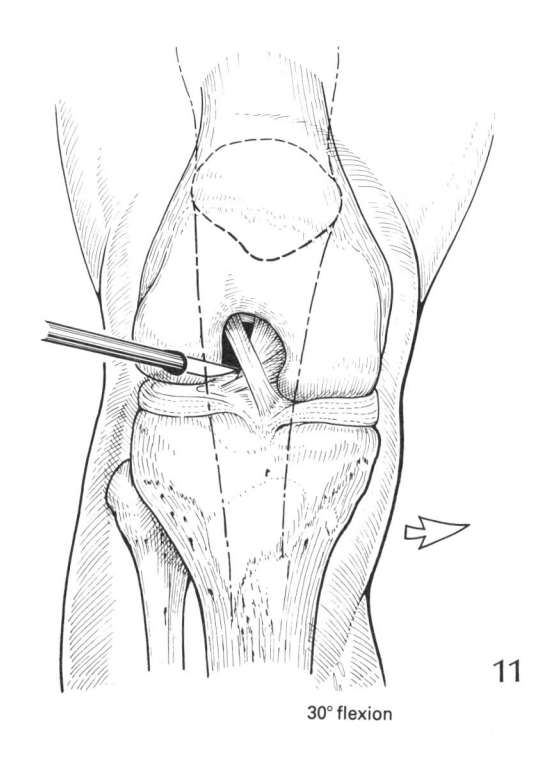

11
30° flexion

Wound closure

Fluid is expressed from the joint at the end of the procedure down the empty sheath which is then withdrawn completely. The skin is closed using sterile skin 'closure strips' or fine microfilament nylon sutures through skin and subcutaneous tissues and the wound dressed with non-adhesive material. The knee is supported with a compression bandage of wool and crêpe extending from the tibial tuberosity to the lower thigh.

If the surgeon wishes to proceed to arthrotomy at the end of the arthroscopy, the leg should be prepared anew and draped in the usual manner and the surgeon and assistant should change gloves and gowns.

Postoperative management

Straight-leg raising should commence immediately postoperatively and flexion and weight-bearing should begin within 24 hours, following reduction of the compression dressing. The patient may be discharged when recovered from the anaesthetic. Sutures, if used, are removed 10 days postoperatively, at which time full activity may be able to recommence, depending on the findings.

Alternative approaches

Anteromedial approach

12

As a visual portal, this approach (labelled 2 in illustration) is not recommended unless there is considerable suspicion of an anterior horn lesion of the lateral meniscus. If the arthroscope is to be introduced through this approach, then a stab incision approximately 1 cm above the tibial plateau and 1.5 cm medial to the edge of the patellar tendon will allow an acceptable view of the anterior horn of the lateral meniscus, the posterior attachment of the medial meniscus and the intercondylar notch. The anteromedial approach is, however, the routine portal of entry for arthroscopic surgical instruments including the blunt hook or probe. To facilitate the choice of site of entry, a hypodermic needle can first be inserted under direct vision until the ideal position is obtained and a stab incision then made at this point.

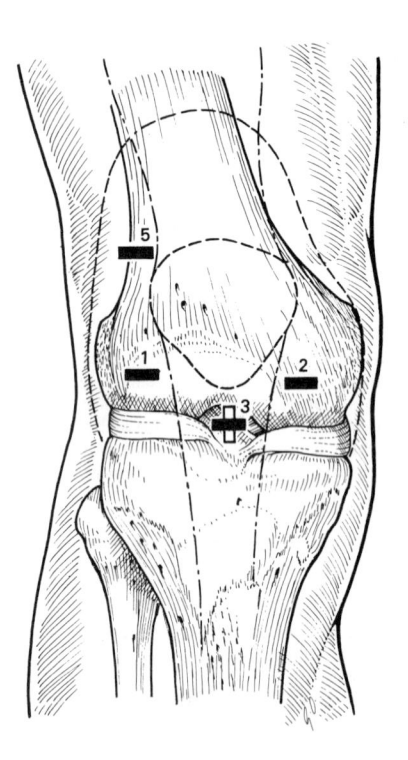

Central approach

This route (3), popularized by Gillquist[7], allows more detailed inspection of the posterior compartments of the knee. A transverse skin crease stab incision is made in the midline, 1 cm below the inferior pole of the patella through skin and subcutaneous fat. The patellar tendon is then incised along the length of its fibres and the trocar and sheath directed upwards and backwards through it.

The suprapatellar pouch can be examined with the knee in extension and the rest of the joint inspected with the knee flexed and appropriate strains applied. The posteromedial compartment is accessed by guiding the instrument between the anterior cruciate ligament and the medial femoral condyle. With a 70° lens, the posterior cruciate ligament can be seen if the tip is rotated laterally and downwards. Tension can be introduced into the ligament by applying medial tibial rotation. The authors of this approach claim to reduce significantly the numbers of unseen tears of the posterior horn of the medial meniscus, this being the most common diagnostic error when using the standard anterolateral approach.

Posteromedial approach

13

This approach (4), described by Dashefsky[8], allows optimal examination of the 'blind area' of the medial meniscus. Entry is gained under direct vision by inserting the telescope through a stab wound in the posteromedial angle of the joint, with the knee in 90° of flexion. Initial passage of a hypodermic needle into a fluid-filled joint will reassure the surgeon that the extracapsular structures remain undamaged. The posterior aspect of the meniscus, posterior cruciate ligament and the inferior recess are best visualized with the knee flexed to 90°.

Lateral suprapatellar[9] (approach 5), *posterolateral* and *medial suprapatellar* approaches are all described but have no place in routine diagnostic arthroscopy.

Note. It is very unwise for the novice to embark on any but the routine anterolateral approach until total familiarity with intra-articular landmarks and common abnormalities has been achieved. Proficiency at 'visual triangulation' is also essential before proceeding to any arthroscopic surgical procedure, and this is most rapidly achieved by regular use of the blunt hook introduced via the anteromedial portal.

Biopsy

This can be achieved under direct vision using either a specially adapted 2.7 mm telescope with attached biopsy forceps or by directing, under vision, a second instrument through the anteromedial or lateral suprapatellar portals.

Photography

Normal and pathological features can be documented on both still photographs and video tape. The former method requires a modified single lens reflex camera and a flash attachment, operated by a non-sterile member of the team. Three shots at different exposures are recommended. Video tape recording not only allows the surgeon a greater freedom of movement, but is extremely valuable as a teaching aid and provides a more dynamic record of intra-articular pathology. Sterilizable video cameras have now achieved a high level of sophistication and compactness.

Pathological findings

Tears of the meniscus (semilunar cartilage)

The edge of the meniscus is a sharp, clearly defined border although the edge, especially of the lateral meniscus, may be slightly fibrillated over the age of 25 years. Degenerated menisci are more fibrillated and have a rough edge with fibrils floating into the joint. These may conceal a horizontal tear and should be carefully examined with a blunt hook (*Plate 23*). Bucket-handle tears can be confusing, especially if one end is free or the handle is displaced into the centre of the joint. Peripheral detachment can be recognized if care is taken to ensure that the arthroscopic view extends out to the junction of the synovium and the meniscus and the junction is probed with the blunt hook. The stability of the meniscus can then be checked. The doubtful area of the posterior one-third of the meniscus can be viewed partially from the intercondylar notch, but generally speaking a small cleft, fibrillation or irregularity of the meniscus can be seen when there is a posterior tear. A normal-looking meniscus which is stable on probing usually is normal and not a cause of symptoms.

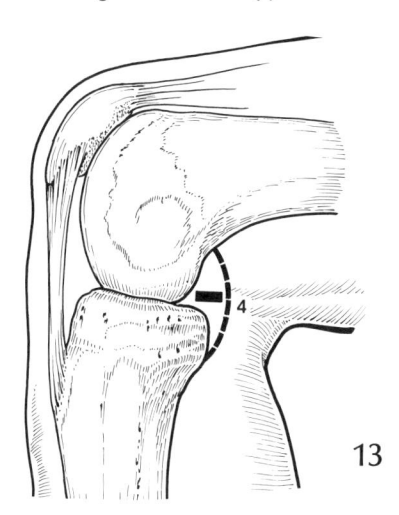

A discoid lateral meniscus (*Plate 24*) may be difficult to recognize but can be defined by exerting pressure on the lateral joint line, thus moving the meniscus edge further towards the centre of the joint.

Synovial membrane

This is visible throughout most of the joint and covers the intra-articular structures such as the infrapatellar fat pad and cruciate ligaments. Normally a thin vascularized film, it is hypertrophied when the joint is inflamed from any cause (*Plate 25*) and can be biopsied under vision by a forceps passed through the anteromedial portal.

Articular cartilage

Chondromalacia patellae is easily recognized at all stages and careful probing of the cartilage surface will indicate softening (*Plates 26, 27* and *28*). In osteoarthritis pitting of the femoral condyle (*Plate 29*) is an early change, whilst in the later stages erosion of the tibial articular surface is seen with multiple tears of the meniscus (*Plate 30*).

Osteochondritis dissecans

Sometimes it is difficult to see any change in the articular cartilage arthroscopically, even with a clearly defined bony defect on the radiographs. Probing the affected area will indicate any soft or unstable cartilage.

References

1. Bircher E. Die Arthroendoskopie. *Zentralbl Chir* 1921; 48: 1460.

2. Watanabe M, Takeda S. The number 21 arthroscope. *J Jap Orthop Assoc* 1960; 34: 1041.

3. Watanabe M, Takeda S, Ikeuchi H. *Atlas of arthroscopy*. 2nd ed. Tokyo, Igaku: Shoin Ltd, 1969.

4. Jackson RW, Abe I. The role of arthroscopy in the management of disorders of the knee; analysis of 200 consecutive examinations. *J Bone Joint Surg [Br]* 1972; 54-B: 310–22.

5. Jackson RW, Dandy DJ. *Arthroscopy of the knee*. New York: Grune and Stratton, 1976.

6. Jackson RW. The scope of arthroscopy. *Clin Orthop* 1986; 208: 69–71.

7. Gillquist J, Hagberg G, Oretop N. Arthroscopic examination of the posteromedial compartment of the knee joint. *Int Orthop* 1979; 3: 13–8.

8. Dashefsky JH. Arthroscopic visualization of the 'blind area' in the posteromedial compartment of the knee. *Orthop Rev* 1976; 5: 51.

9. Dandy DJ. *Arthroscopic surgery of the knee*. Edinburgh: Churchill Livingstone, 1981.

Illustrations by Peter Cox

Arthroscopic surgical procedures

Ian Stother MA, FRCS(Ed), FRCS(Glas)
Consultant Orthopaedic Surgeon, Glasgow Royal Infirmary and The Glasgow Nuffield Hospital, Glasgow, UK

Introduction

The range of surgery performed on the knee joint is very large. Arthroscopic surgery is by definition intra-articular surgery. In theory it should be possible to carry out any intra-articular procedure through the arthroscope; indeed, the range of arthroscopic surgical procedures is continually increasing, and includes not only procedures such as meniscectomy but also such diverse procedures as the insertion of prosthetic ligaments and abrasion arthroplasty for degenerative arthritis.

Arthroscopic surgery offers a number of advantages. Firstly, the surgical incisions and subsequent scars are small. Secondly, the postoperative recovery is usually rapid when compared with the equivalent open operation. Thirdly, arthroscopy allows access to all areas of the joint without extensive scarring.

1020 Thigh and knee

Triangulation

1 & 2

The basic technique used in arthroscopic surgery is triangulation. The arthroscope is inserted through one incision or portal. The operating instrument is usually inserted through a separate incision and manipulated into the field of view of the arthroscope. Most surgeons use a 25° or 30° telescope for arthroscopic surgery. Sometimes two instruments are used simultaneously (see chapter on 'Arthroscopic meniscectomy', pp. 1043–1055). Before the actual operating instruments are inserted it is recommended that a hypodermic needle or probe be inserted along the proposed route to check that access to the site of operation is possible.

Distension of the joint

It is essential that all the surgical manoeuvres are carried out under direct vision (either via the telescope itself or via a television monitor attached to the arthroscope). To achieve this the knee joint must be distended with either gas or liquid (see chapter on 'Diagnostic arthroscopy of the knee', pp. 1007–1018).

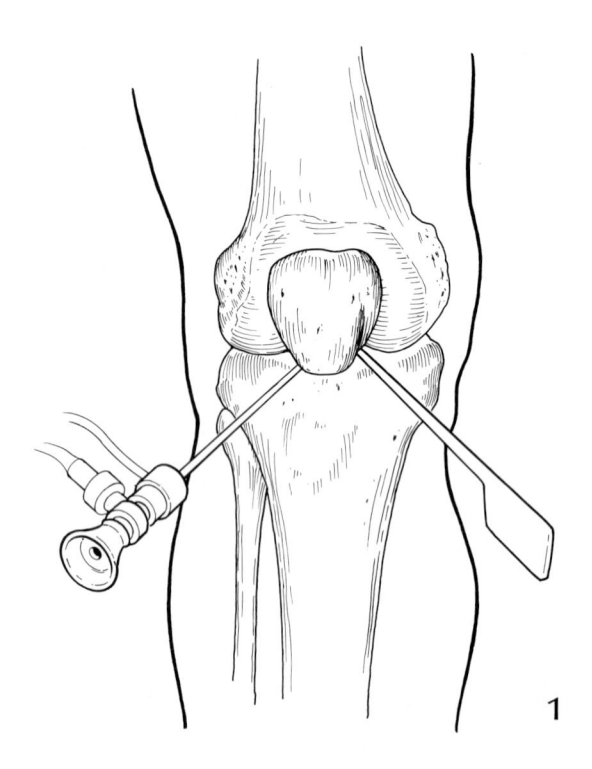

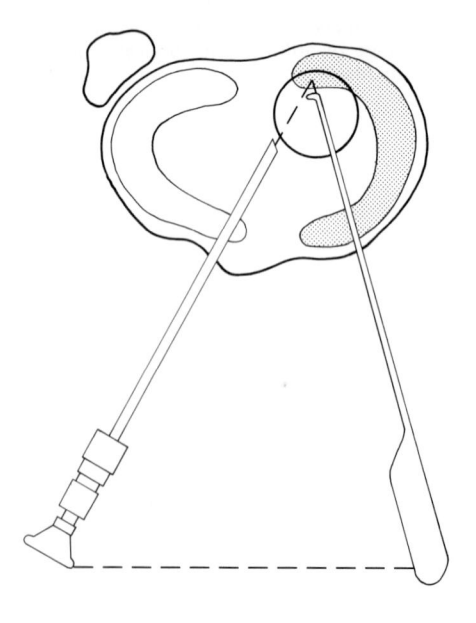

Arthroscopic surgical instruments

The equipment needed for diagnostic arthroscopy is required (*see* chapter on 'Diagnostic arthroscopy of the knee', pp. 1007–1018). In addition many special instruments are also available. There are two major types of instrument; hand instruments and power instruments.

In general both groups of instruments serve the same functions. Power instruments are potentially more dangerous than hand instruments and should probably only be used by experienced arthroscopic surgeons.

It is useful to have instruments of different diameters. Small (2.7 mm) diameter instruments are useful to reach the posterior parts of the medial meniscus. Curved instruments also make access easier on occasion. All the instruments serve a number of basic functions:

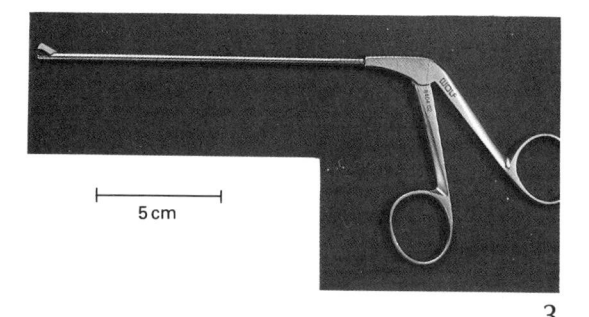

Cutting instruments

3, 4 & 5

Small scissors (*Illustrations 3* and *4*). Small knife (preferably with retractable blade) (*Illustration 5*). 'Draw knives' which cut towards the operator as the knife is withdrawn are useful for short bucket-handle tears.

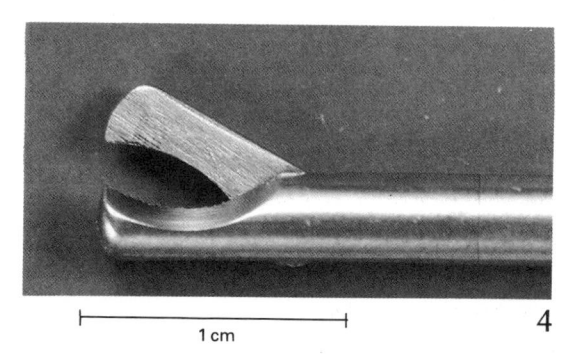

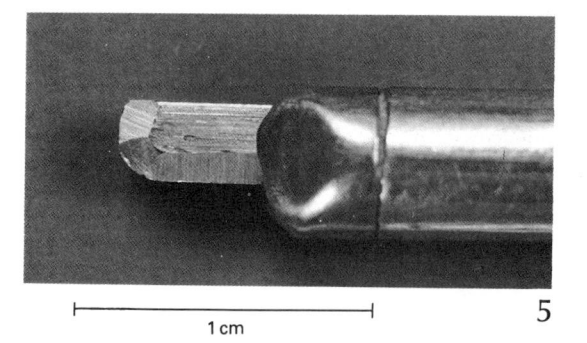

1022 Thigh and knee

Grasping instruments

6 & 7

Various grasping forceps are available. It is helpful if they have teeth in the jaws and ratchet handles.

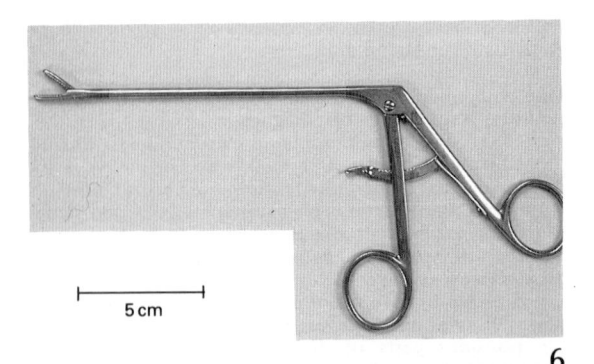

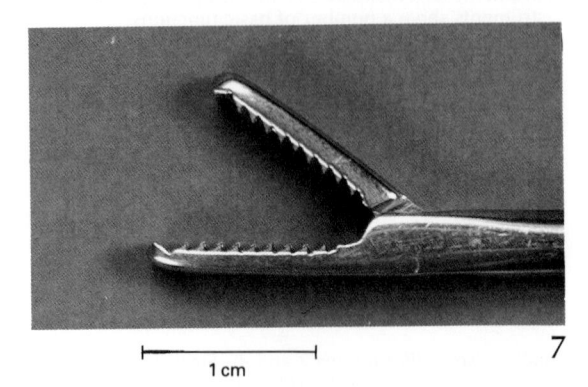

Nibbling instruments

8 & 9

Pituitary rongeurs of small size and with different head angles are useful for degenerate meniscus and articular cartilage flaps.

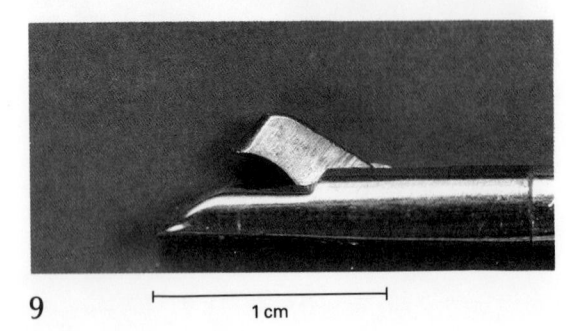

9

Punch forceps in several sizes are useful for trimming and cutting. Side-cutting punch forceps may be easier to manipulate into the desired position near the back of the joint, and at the front of the joint.

During arthroscopic surgery it may be necessary to insert the telescope and instruments through several different portals, and to exchange the position of the telescope and instruments.

Operative procedures

Surgery of the synovium

SYNOVIAL BIOPSY

Indications

A diagnostic procedure for chronic effusion or synovitis of the knee joint.

Serology for the various causes of chronic synovitis should be performed preoperatively. These include tests for rheumatoid arthritis, *Salmonella* and *Shigella* antibody titres, and on occasion the antituberculin titre and tests for syphilis.

Preparation of the patient

The operation may be performed under local or general anaesthesia. The patient is placed supine on the operating table. A mid-thigh tourniquet placed well clear of the suprapatellar pouch reduces bleeding and aids viewing in the presence of synovitis. Some surgeons prefer not to inflate the tourniquet as this allows a better appreciation of the synovial colour and vascularity.

The skin is cleaned and drapes applied to give a sterile operating field.

Insertion of irrigation cannula

This is inserted laterally above the patella. Usually there will be an effusion and a sample of this should be sent for culture.

As much effusion as possible should be drained. The joint should then be distended with normal saline. A sample should then be drained and if it is turbid the joint should be drained and re-filled until clear fluid emerges.

Insertion of the arthroscope

The arthroscope is inserted in the anterolateral portal. A stab skin incision is made with the knee flexed and then the arthroscope inserted and the knee extended so the scope enters the suprapatellar pouch. The view here may be very limited in the presence of florid synovitis.

Assessment of the synovitis

Continuous irrigation with clear saline entering via the arthroscope is usually required. All compartments of the joint should be inspected. An area of florid synovitis should be chosen for biopsy. Any invasion of the joint surfaces and their state should be carefully documented.

Insertion of the biopsy forceps

10

It is usually convenient to biopsy synovium in the suprapatellar pouch. Pituitary rongeurs make suitable biopsy forceps. It is easiest to insert the forceps through a stab incision made directly through skin and joint capsule some distance from the proposed biopsy site. This makes it easier to manipulate the forceps into the field of view by triangulation.

The telescope passes from an anterolateral portal across the patellofemoral joint in the extended knee. The rongeurs are inserted in a midpatellar medial position. *Plate 31** shows the biopsy being taken; two or three bites of abnormal synovium should be sent for histology.

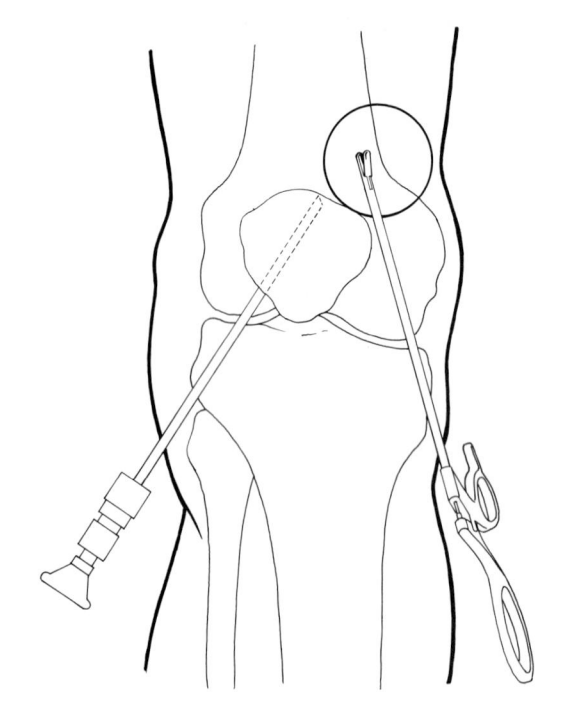

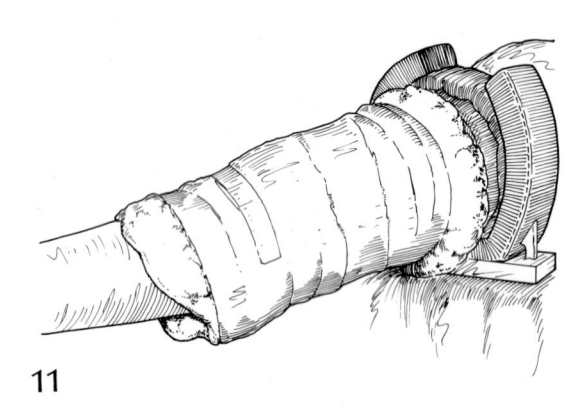

Closure of wounds

11

The fluid is drained from the knee joint. The skin incisions are closed with single sutures. A padded crêpe compression bandage is applied.

Postoperative management

The patient starts quadriceps exercises on recovery from the anaesthetic and mobilizes weight-bearing as comfort allows as soon as straight-leg raising can be performed with minimal lag. Knee flexion can be started at the same time. The speed of recovery depends upon the extent of the synovitis. If the recovery is very slow this may be because of a haemarthrosis. If this is suspected the dressings should be removed and the haemarthrosis aspirated after 48 hours. The sutures can be removed after 7 days.

*Colour plates 31–43 are on pages 1037–1039.

DIVISION OF A SYNOVIAL FOLD OR SHELF

Indications

Pathological synovial folds usually catch against the femoral condyle, often at the junction of the patellar and tibial surfaces where the articular cartilage heaps up. The folds can usually be detected clinically as a fibrous band which suddenly snaps over the femoral condyle during flexion or extension.

There may be a history of direct trauma to this area of the knee. The folds may be asymptomatic, but removal is indicated if the abnormal movement of the fold causes pain or a feeling of instability.

Preparation of the patient

The approximate position of the fold should be marked on the skin preoperatively. The patient is placed supine on the operating table. General or spinal anaesthesia should be used. A mid-thigh tourniquet should be in position and inflated to control bleeding. The skin is cleaned and drapes are applied to give a sterile operating field. The knee is distended with normal saline inserted via the suprapatellar pouch.

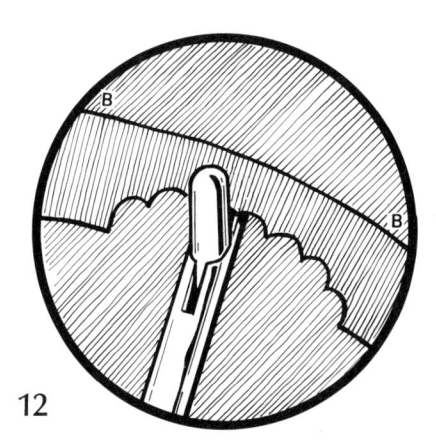

Insertion of the arthroscope

The arthroscope should be inserted on the side opposite the fold visualized, anteromedially for lateral folds and anterolaterally for medial folds.

Definition of the fold

The fold must be palpated, both through the skin and also with a probe inserted into the joint. Abnormal folds are firm or hard and do not stretch out of the way of a probe (see *Plate 32*). The probe may be inserted anteriorly or from the suprapatellar pouch. The presence of an erosion of the femoral condyle should be sought (see *Plate 33*).

Division of the fold

12

A length of 1 cm or more of the abnormal fold is removed. The base of the fold (marked B–B) must be excised so that no tight band remains.

The excision is often most easily achieved using punch forceps – either end-cutting or side-cutting. A power meniscotome with a rotating side-cutting blade and suction is also very suitable. Scissors may also be used to divide the fold, but once the initial cut has been made the tension in the fold is relaxed and subsequent excision is more difficult.

The joint is irrigated and drained. The instruments are removed. The joint is palpated through the skin to check that the fold no longer catches. If it still catches, then a further length of fold must be removed. A check should be made that a length of the base of the fold has been excised. If these measures fail to stop the fold catching, a lateral release may be helpful if the fold is on the lateral side.

Closure of wounds

As for Synovial biopsy (p. 1024).

Postoperative management

As for Synovial biopsy (p. 1024).

Thigh and knee

EXCISION OF SYNOVIAL TAGS

Indications

Pedunculated synovial tags, often of abnormal synovium, e.g. localized villonodular synovitis, may interpose between the joint surfaces and cause episodes of locking or giving way. They may mimic a loose body or a tag of torn meniscus.

Preparation of the patient

The patient is placed supine on the operating table. General or spinal anaesthesia is required. A mid-thigh tourniquet may be useful to control bleeding. The skin is cleaned and the leg draped to provide a sterile operating field. The joint is distended with isotonic saline.

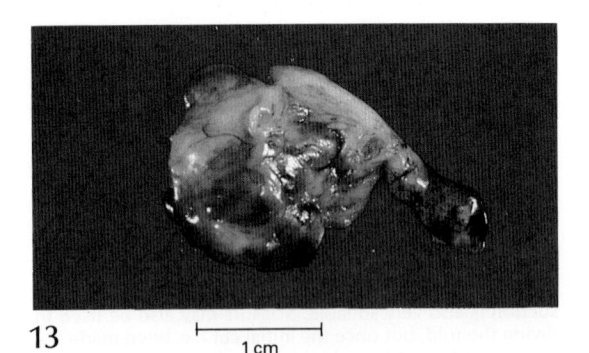

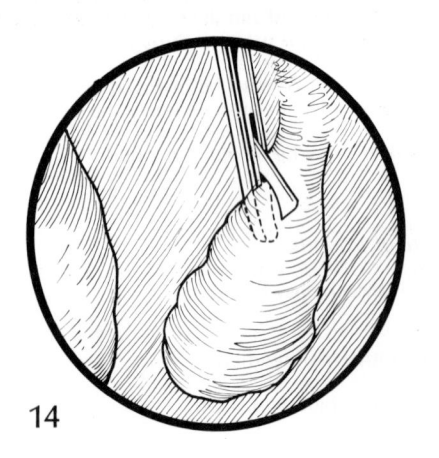

Insertion of the telescope

The arthroscope is inserted anterolaterally. Synovial tags are commonly associated with the fat pads and interfere with the front of the joint (see *Plates 34a, 34b*). If they cannot easily be defined from an anterolateral insertion of the telescope then it should be reinserted in the mid-patellar lateral position. Tags may also jam between the patella and its groove (see *Plate 35a, 35b*).

Definition of the synovial tag

The size of the tag and the position of its base should be defined with a probe (see *Plate 36*). If the telescope is in the anterolateral portal the probe may be inserted through a high anteromedial portal. If the telescope is in the midpatellar lateral portal the probe can be inserted anteromedially or anterolaterally.

13

Tags which cause symptoms are probably at least 1 cm in diameter, and if they have been catching between the articular surfaces they are often oedematous and bruised.

Removal of the synovial tag

Pedunculated tags can often be removed by putting scissors in place of the probe and subtotally dividing the base. The scissors are then removed and a pair of grasping forceps or rongeurs are inserted to grasp the tag across its base.

14

The telescope views from anterolaterally and scissors have been inserted from a high anteromedial portal for a medial tag. Large tags may be removed piecemeal with rongeurs. Care must be taken to remove the whole of any abnormal tag (see *Illustration 13*). A check must be made for the presence of two or more tags. The excised tissue should be sent for histology.

Closure of wounds

As for Synovial biopsy (p. 1024).

Postoperative management

As for Synovial biopsy (p. 1024).

SYNOVECTOMY

Indications

As for open synovectomy (see chapter on 'Synovectomy of the knee', pp. 1109–1112).

The range of movement and stability of the joint as well as the state of the joint surfaces shown on the radiograph and the presence of synovial thickening and an effusion should be noted. Marked instability or stiffness are contraindications.

Equipment

Some form of power instrumentation with a rotary cutting head and suction is required. Large volumes of irrigation fluid are also needed.

Preparation of the patient

As for Excision of synovial tags (pp. 1026).

The operation

A tourniquet should be applied. A telescope is inserted in the anterolateral portal. A power shaver may be inserted supermedially to shave the suprapatellar pouch. All hypertrophic synovium should be excised, although some areas will inevitably be inaccessible. Some tissue may be more easily removed with pituitary rongeurs. The medial gutter should be accessible with the superomedial insertion of the shaver. The lateral gutter may require a superolateral insertion. The area around the anterior cruciate ligament may be accessible via an anteromedial portal. All shaving must be done under direct vision. The operation is a long one.

Closure of wound

As for Synovial biopsy (p. 1024).

Postoperative management

A compression bandage is applied for 48 hours, and then the leg is gradually mobilized. A continuous passive motion machine may be useful in the postoperative period.

Surgery of the articular cartilage

SURGERY OF OSTEOCHONDRITIS DISSECANS

Diagnosis of the condition is primarily radiological. Diagnostic arthroscopy is useful to determine whether or not the articular cartilage is breached and to see if there is an unstable area of joint surface.

In young patients with open epiphyses the initial treatment is conservative. In older patients and in young patients who do not respond to conservative measures diagnostic arthroscopy is indicated. Further treatment depends upon the findings:

1. Where the osteochondritic areas have separated and formed loose bodies they should be removed unless they are very large, when an attempt may be made to fix them back in place (see chapter on 'Loose bodies in the knee', pp. 1073–1078).
2. Where the osteochondritic area is unstable and the articular cartilage is breached the abnormal area should be fixed rigidly after freshening the base (see Fixation of osteochondritic fragments, below).
3. Where the osteochondritic area is covered by intact articular cartilage, treatment may consist of immobilization alone, or immobilization after drilling – the latter especially if the base of the abnormal area is very sclerotic on the radiograph (see Removal of fixation devices used to treat osteochondritis dissecans, p. 1028).

Fixation of osteochondritic fragments

Indications

See previous section. It should be noted that even after arthroscopic surgery a period of immobilization is required. The main advantage of the arthroscopic technique is therefore reduced scarring.

Preparation of the patient

As for Excision of synovial tags (p. 1026).

Insertion of the telescope

A 25° or 30° telescope should be inserted anterolaterally.

Definition of the abnormal area

The area to be inspected can be identified from radiographs. If the articular surface is not breached then the abnormal area is often slightly dulled and shows some loss of normal contour (see *Plate 37*).

The suspect area should then be probed via the anteromedial portal. Instability can often be demonstrated by abnormal movement of an area of the articular surface. If there is a breach in the articular surface a probe can be inserted into this and the breach extended to allow the osteochondritic fragment to be elevated on a hinge of articular cartilage (see *Plate 38*). It is important not to detach the fragment completely.

Fixation of the fragment

15

Using a small curette, the base of the deficit is freshened via the same portal as the probe.

The fragment is replaced in its bed. It may be fixed there with Smillie pins or small screws. Two or preferably three should be inserted. The position for inserting the pin holder or screwdriver should be piloted with a hypodermic needle. The skin and capsular incision should allow the instruments easy access so that the pin or screw is not displaced. The Smillie pin holder is a good instrument to use as the pins can be withdrawn almost completely into the instrument until the latter is positioned. With flexion and extension of the knee it is often possible to insert all the pins or screws through the same skin incision. After insertion of the pins or screws the head of the fixation device should be slightly below the articular surface. The stability of the fixed fragment should be checked with a probe.

Closure of wound

As for Synovial biopsy (p. 1024).

Postoperative management

The knee should be immobilized in a plaster cylinder for 6 weeks during which time the patient remains non-weight-bearing. After removal of the plaster the knee is mobilized gradually but the patient should remain non-weight-bearing for a further 6 weeks. The fixation device should be removed after 3 months.

Removal of fixation devices used to treat osteochondritis dissecans

Indications

Fixation devices should be removed when healing has occurred. It is the author's practice to remove pins or screws about 3 months after insertion and before full weight-bearing is allowed.

Radiographs should be taken immediately prior to operation to check the position of the pins or screws.

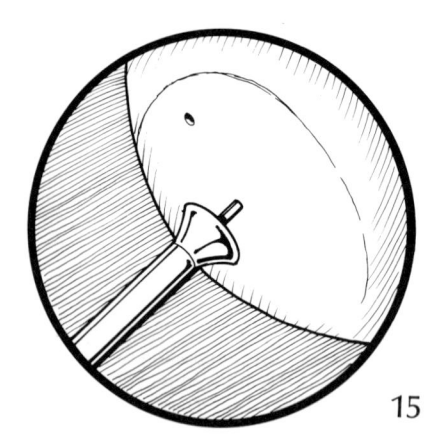

15

Preparation of patient

See Excision of synovial tags (p. 1026).

Location of the pins or screws

The arthroscope should be inserted anterolaterally if the area of osteochondritis is in the usual place on the medial femoral condyle. The knee should be flexed and extended to bring the pins or screws into view. They may have become covered with articular cartilage.

A large diameter hypodermic needle should be inserted anteromedially to gain access to the pins. If they are covered with articular cartilage they may be visible as dark areas beneath the joint surface.

The overlying cartilage may need to be moved away with the edge of the needle to expose the pins. The needle may also be used to tease articular cartilage out of the grooves in the pins or the slots in the screws (see *Plate 39*).

Removal of the pins or screws

The needle should be removed. Smillie pins can usually be removed using pituitary rongeurs. Small bone nibblers are sometimes useful. Screws should be removed with an appropriate screwdriver with screw-retaining clip.

The stability of the osteochondritic area should be checked after removal of the fixation. If it is loose it also should be removed. If the fragment is stable the state of its articular cartilage should be noted.

The joint should be irrigated.

Closure of wound

As for Synovial biopsy (p. 1024).

Postoperative management

The patient mobilizes fully weight-bearing as soon as he has adequate muscle control. A radiograph of the knee should be taken to check the union of the osteochondritic fragment after a further 6 weeks.

Drilling of osteochondritis dissecans

Indications

See Surgery of osteochondritis dissecans (p. 1027).

Preoperative preparation

See Excision of synovial tags (p. 1026).

Insertion of telescope

A standard anterolateral insertion of a 30° telescope should be suitable for osteochondritis in the common sites.

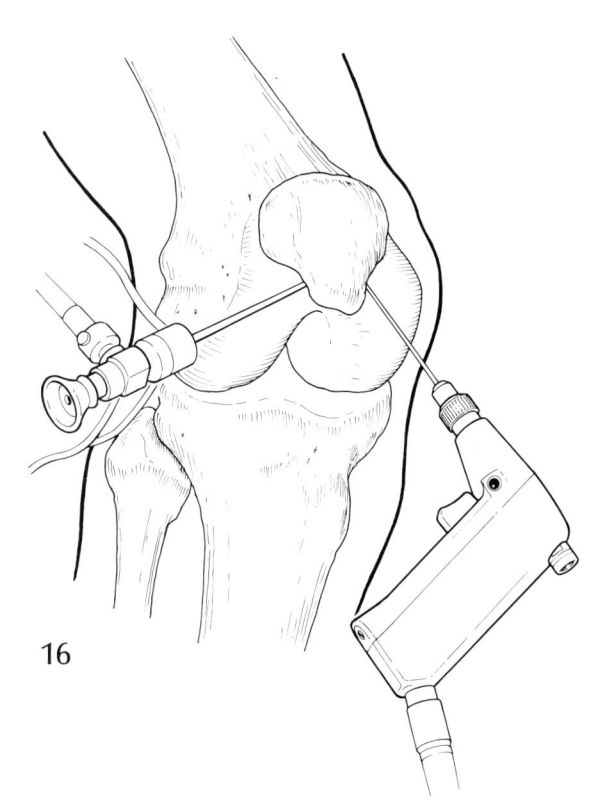

Definition of the abnormal area

The suspect area can be approximately located from radiographs. If the articular surface is not breached (which it must not be for this procedure) the abnormal area is slightly dulled. There is a slight loss of normal contour. The affected area often lies slightly below the normal surrounding area.

On probing (via an anteromedial portal), the articular surface is slightly soft and there may be a jog of movement between the normal and abnormal areas if the abnormal area is pressed with the probe.

16

Drilling of the abnormal area

Usually access via an anteromedial portal is suitable. Access may be piloted using a hypodermic needle. The actual drilling is most easily performed using a short Kirschner wire or toe pin with a shaped end, inserted into a small power drill. Only a puncture wound needs to be made in the skin. The drilling must be done under direct vision and no undue pressure applied.

The pin can usually be felt to penetrate the sclerotic base of the lesion. Multiple drill holes are made 3–4 mm apart. It may be necessary to insert the drill through more than one puncture.

Closure of wound

As for Synovial biopsy (p. 1024).

Postoperative management

The knee should be immobilized in a plaster cylinder for 6 weeks and the patient should remain non-weight-bearing during this time.

After 6 weeks the plaster is removed and the knee mobilized. The state of the articular surface should be checked radiographically after 6 weeks and 3 months.

16

SURGERY OF CHONDROMALACIA PATELLAE

Shaving of chondromalacia patellae

Indication

Shaving is indicated when chondromalacia patellae involves less than one-third of the articular surface. It should be noted that the results of this operation are not consistently good. Surgery is only indicated if conservative measures have failed and the patient has moderate or severe symptoms.

At diagnostic arthroscopy the patellar groove should not be involved. The aetiology of the chondromalacia should be determined whenever possible. If there is a patellar tracking problem this should be identified and corrected to prevent recurrence.

Preparation of patient

See Excision of synovial tags (p. 1026).

Insertion of telescope

Anterolateral insertion of the telescope is usually satisfactory. A 70° telescope may be useful to assess extent of the condition. Probing of the articular surface to assess softening is important. The probe may be inserted via the suprapatellar pouch or anteromedially. Where there are areas of fibrillation the probe can be inserted down to the subchondral bone.

Assessment of the abnormal area

The severity and extent of the condition must be assessed.

Removal of the fibrillated articular cartilage

This may be carried out using pituitary rongeurs. Instruments which are straight and instruments angled upwards at the tip are useful. They should be inserted in place of the probe. Fibrillated cartilage should be removed as completely as possible leaving a sharp edge to the deficit. Alternatively a power shaver may be used. The joint should be extensively irrigated to remove the articular cartilage debris.

Closure of wound

Wounds should be closed with single sutures and a compression bandage applied. The sutures are removed at 7–10 days.

Postoperative management

Static quadriceps exercises should commence at once. Crutches should be used for 3–4 weeks. The flexed knee should not be loaded for this period. (In theory this should allow fibrous tissue to fill the defect in the patella.)

Removal of loose and foreign bodies

Removal of loose and (rarely) foreign bodies from the knee joint utilizes one of the main advantages of arthroscopic surgery. Through one or two portals the whole of the knee joint is accessible. This is important for the removal of loose and foreign bodies which by definition may move within the joint.

Foreign bodies are much less common than loose bodies. Small pieces of needle may puncture the skin and break off in the joint. If they cannot be located they should be sought in the articular cartilage (especially in children) and in the sheath of the popliteus tendon (see Plate 40). Rust staining may be a useful guide to the location.

There are three stages to the removal of a loose or foreign body. It must be (a) located, (b) trapped and (c) removed. A search must then be made to seek for additional loose bodies and also their origin.

Indications

Loose bodies almost always cause locking and giving way – not pain, which is usually from the origin of the loose body and may not be helped by its removal.

Many, but not all, loose bodies are radio-opaque. Preoperative radiographs are important to determine the number, size and position of any loose bodies. Serial radiographs will show whether or not radio-opaque bodies are truly loose, i.e. they are seen in different positions on different occasions. If a body is in a fixed position it may well be stuck to the synovium and may not be causing any symptoms.

Preparation of the patient

As for Excision of synovial tags (p. 1026).

Insertion of the telescope

A routine anterolateral insertion of a 30° telescope is used first. It is best to have a 70° telescope available.

Locating the loose body

Loose bodies may be found in many sites. If a loose body is not easily seen the following sites should be inspected:

17

1. Lateral gutter.
2. Medial gutter (via an anteromedial insertion).
3. Intercondylar notch.
4. Posterior compartments (via a 70° telescope inserted anteromedially or anterolaterally). *Illustration 17* and *Plate 41* show a 70° telescope across the notch and a needle being used to triangulate the loose body in the posterolateral compartment.
5. Under the lateral meniscus and around the popliteus sheath.
6. Any folds within the suprapatellar pouch.

Trapping the loose body

Once the loose body has been seen it is important to try not to lose it again. The surgeon should therefore stop irrigation via the telescope.

Loose bodies in the medial and lateral gutters and in the suprapatellar pouch can usually be impaled with a needle inserted transcutaneously (*see Plate 42*). If the loose body is too hard to impale, then one or more needles may be inserted behind the loose body to prevent its escape.

Removal of the loose body

Some form of grasping instrument needs to be used. The author routinely uses pituitary rongeurs, but other instruments such as artery forceps and Kochers forceps may also be used.

The grasping instrument should be inserted some distance from the loose body, so that it is not disturbed by the insertion of the graspers. Access to the suprapatellar pouch, medial recess and lateral recess is easily achieved. If the proposed portal of entry is dubious it can be piloted with a hypodermic needle inserted first.

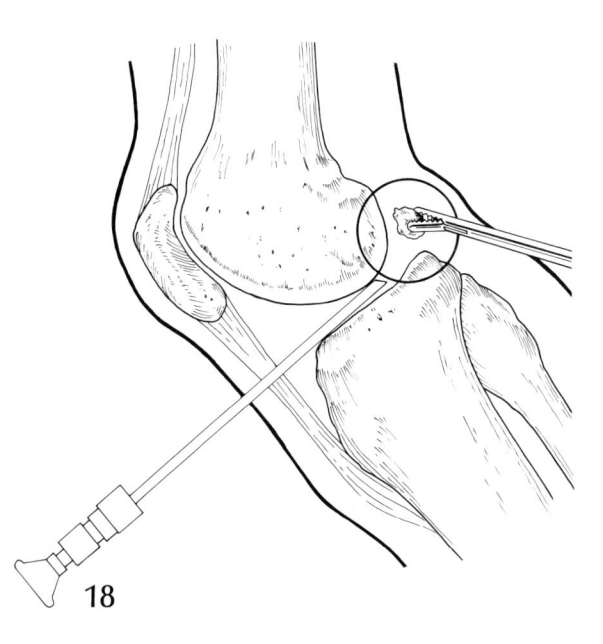

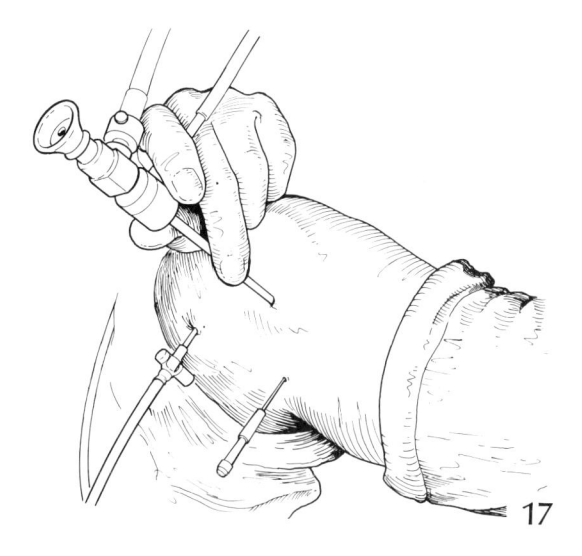

Access to loose bodies in the posterior compartment

Loose bodies in the posterior compartments can usually be located using a 70° telescope inserted across the intercondylar notch.

18

The loose body can often then be removed with rongeurs inserted posteromedially or posterolaterally (*see also Plate 43*). (*see* chapter on 'Diagnostic arthroscopy of the knee', pp. 1007–1018). These portals should be piloted with a hypodermic needle viewed into the joint. It is important to angle the needle and then the grasping forceps forwards, towards the patella and away from the popliteal fossa.

If access across the intercondylar notch is difficult, e.g. in an arthritic knee, it may be necessary to insert the telescope posteromedially or posterolaterally. In this case the grasping instrument can be inserted through an extension of the same incision. Angled rongeurs are useful in this situation.

Checks

After removing the loose body always check for (a) further loose bodies and (b) the origin of the loose bodies.

Closure of wound

As for Synovial biopsy (p. 1024).

Postoperative management

Quadriceps exercises are started on recovery from the anaesthetic and the patient is mobilized when he has muscle control.

Lateral release

Indications

These are not well defined, but as an isolated procedure lateral release may be indicated in recurrent subluxation of the patella, excessive lateral pressure syndrome and perhaps chondromalacia patellae. *See also* the section on Division of a synovial fold or shelf (p. 1025).

Preoperative preparation

As for Excision of synovial tags (p. 1026).

Insertion of telescope

The arthroscope may be inserted anterolaterally or (perhaps better) anteromedially.

The release

19

The lateral release must extend from the joint line up to the vastus lateralis muscle. The release should be a little away from the patella. A skin incision about 2 cm long is made at about the level of the middle of the patella and is deepened through the subcutaneous fat. The capsular release is started with a scalpel. Branches of the lateral geniculate vessels are tied. The capsular release is extended up and down with scissors or a Smillie knife. The inner edge of the blade is inserted deep to the capsule. The synovium may be left intact.

The incision is extended up to the muscle and then down to the joint line. As the incision is extended the irrigation fluid escapes and it is usually necessary to complete the incision by feel rather than under direct vision.

Before closure the joint should be flexed and extended. In flexion the cut capsular edges should separate. Any tethers should be divided.

Closure of wound

Skin closure only is performed, using monofilament polyamide sutures. A compression bandage is applied.

Postoperative management

A haemarthrosis is said to be relatively common after this procedure, so bandaging should be retained for 5 days. A large haemarthrosis should be aspirated. Knee flexion should commence as soon as comfort allows or at any rate after 1 week.

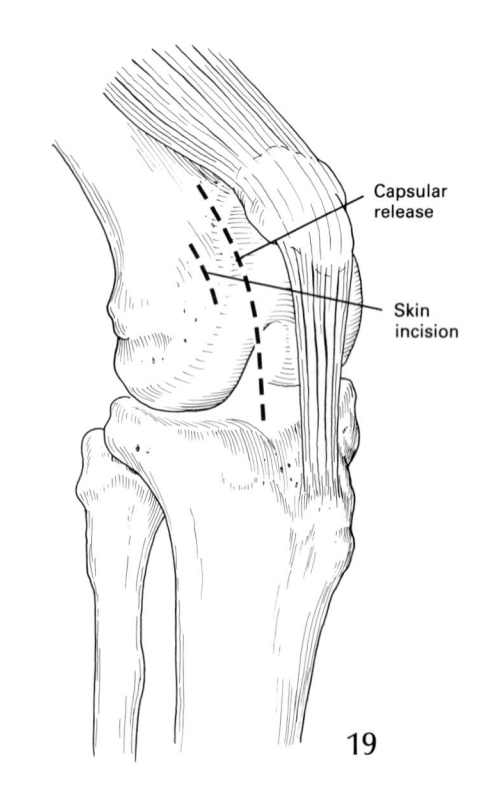

19

Further reading

Dandy DJ. *Arthroscopic surgery of the knee.* Edinburgh: Churchill Livingstone, 1981.

Jackson RW. Current concepts review – arthroscopic surgery. *J Bone Joint Surg [Am]* 1983; 65-A: 416–9.

Sherman OH, Fox JM, Snyder SJ, Del Pizzo W, Friedman MJ, Ferkel RD, Lawley MJ. Arthroscopy – 'no problem surgery' – an analysis of complications in 2640 cases. *J Bone Joint Surg [Am]* 1986; 68-A: 256–65.

Stother IG, Illingworth G, Ayoub M. Arthroscopic removal of loose bodies from the knee. *J R Coll Surg Edinb* 1984; 29(4): 246–8.

Vaughan-Lane T, Dandy DJ. The synovial shelf syndrome. *J Bone Joint Surg [Br]* 1982; 64-B: 475–6.

Diagnostic arthroscopy of the knee

Plate 11. Synovial membrane of suprapatellar pouch, characterized by small ridges produced by the underlying capsular fibres and by the fine arterioles running just beneath the surface.

Plate 12. Arthroscopic view of the patellofemoral joint with the patella uppermost. A medial synovial shelf or plica can be seen which lies between the edges of the two articular surfaces and usually slips medially out of the articulation as flexion proceeds.

Plate 13. View of the patellofemoral joint showing the patella lying in the femoral groove, slightly laterally placed, with the knee flexed to 30°.

Plate 14. Normal infrapatellar fat pad covered with thin synovial membrane containing fine blood vessels on the fatty base.

Plate 15. Free edge of the medial meniscus with slight fibrillation of the femoral condyle. The normal kinking of the junction of the anterior two-thirds and the posterior one-third is seen.

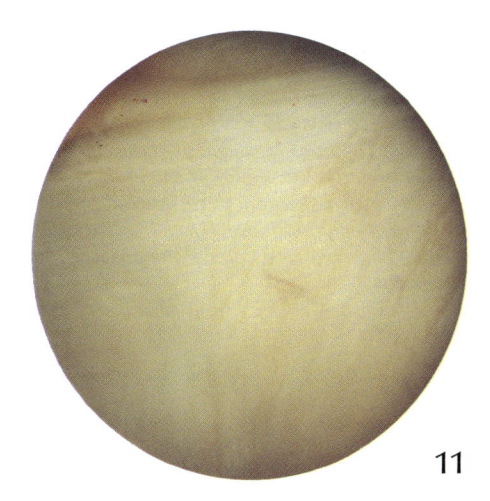

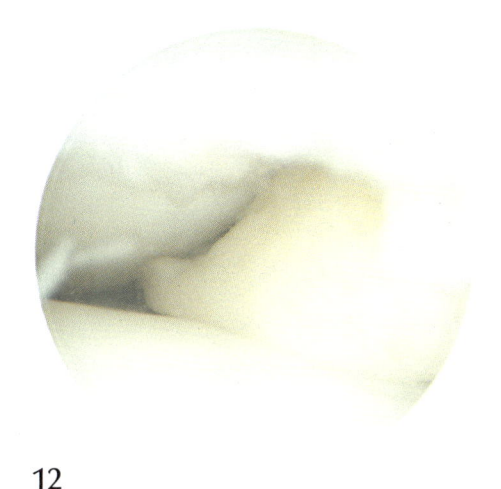

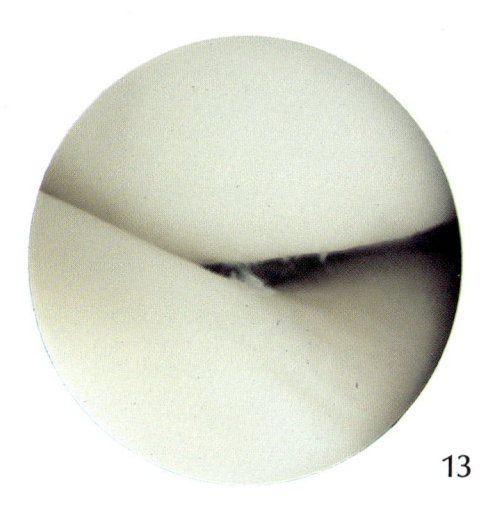

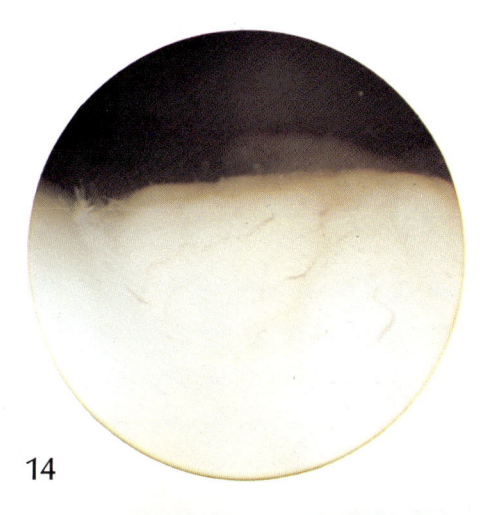

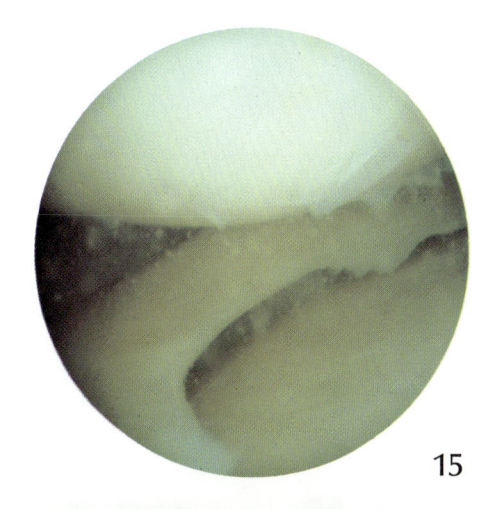

1034 Diagnostic arthroscopy of the knee

Plate 16. Normal kinking of the inner edge of the medial meniscus.

Plate 17. A hook placed beneath the free edge of the medial meniscus to exclude a concealed posterior horn tear.

Plate 18. The hook is placed over the top of the meniscus and pulled towards the centre of the joint to assess its stability.

Plate 19. Normal anterior cruciate ligament with fine arteries in the synovial membrane which covers the surface.

Plate 20. Normal free edge of the posterior horn of the lateral meniscus.

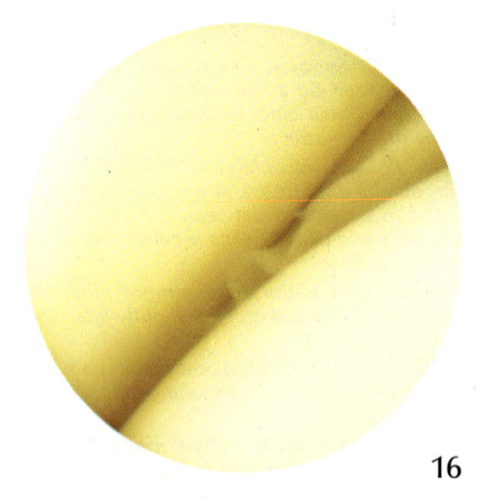

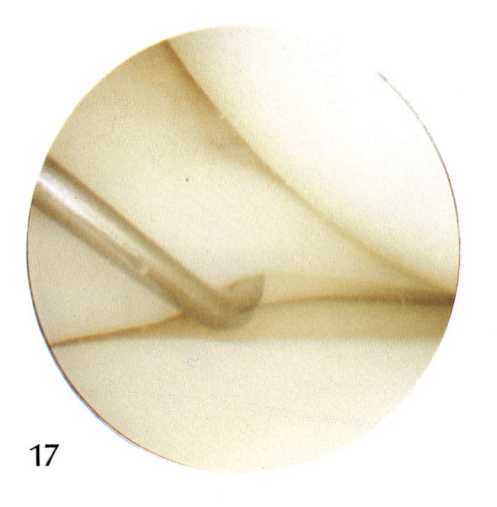

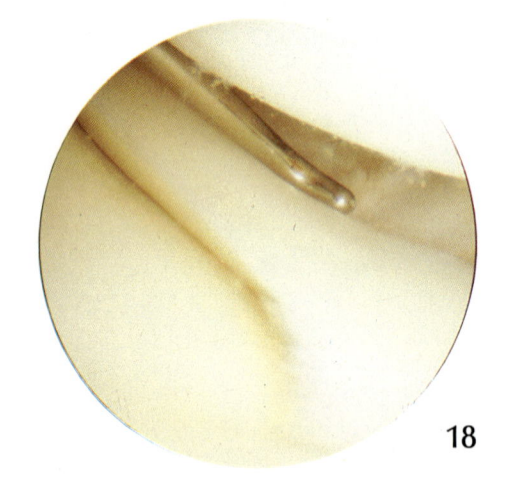

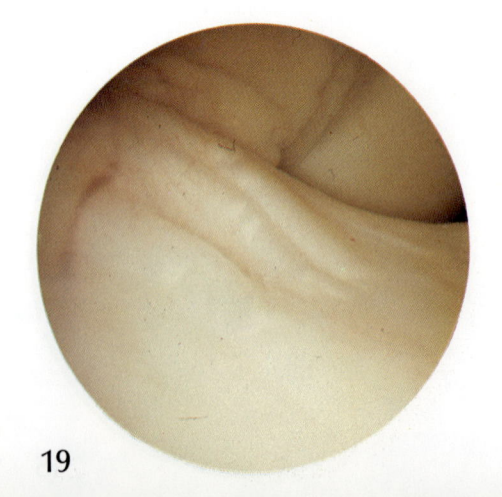

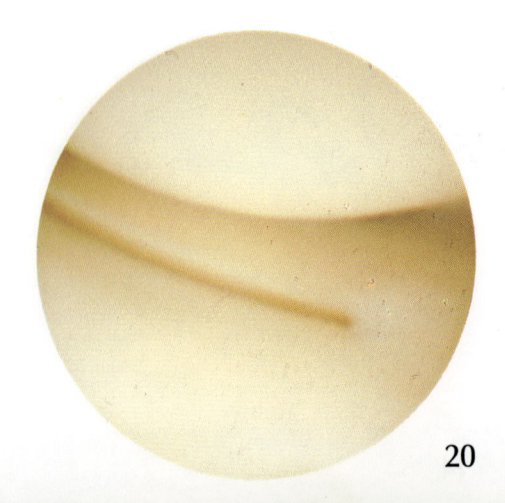

Diagnostic arthroscopy of the knee 1035

Plate 21. The posterolateral compartment of the knee with the hook placed over the posterior edge of the lateral meniscus, in the gap between it and the popliteus tendon which can be seen running obliquely downwards and medially.

Plate 22. Osteocartilaginous loose body in the lateral parafemoral gutter.

Plate 23. Horizontal tear of the medial meniscus.

Plate 24. Discoid lateral meniscus showing the edge near the intercondylar area.

Plate 25. Typical hypervascular synovial villus in rheumatoid arthritis.

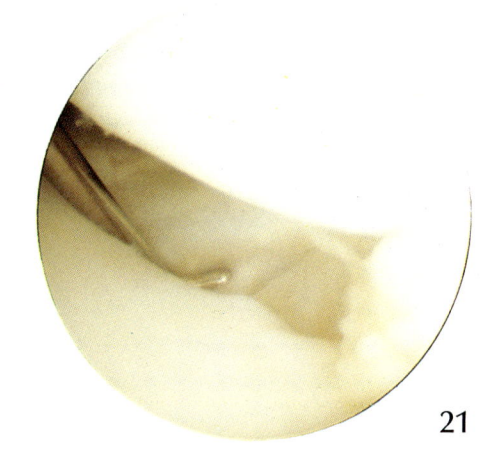

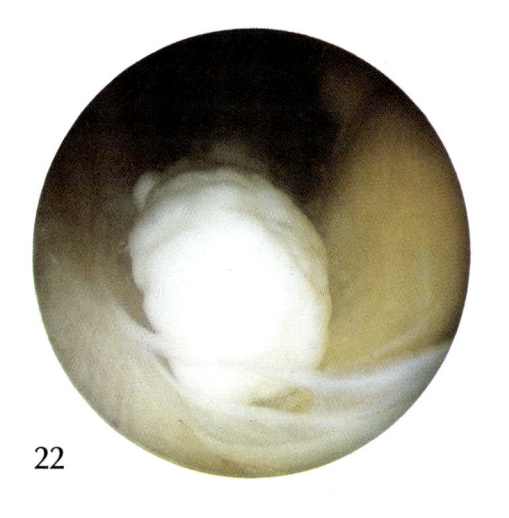

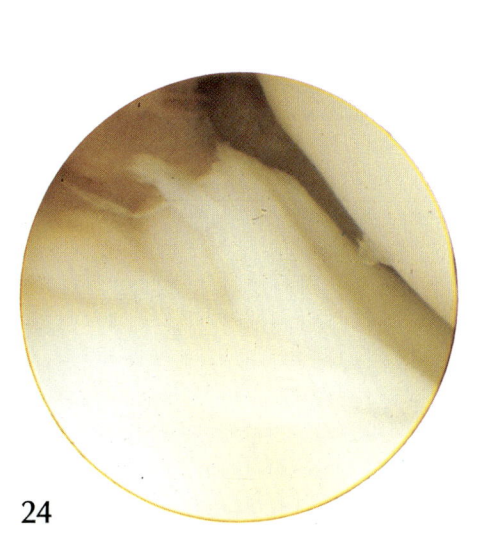

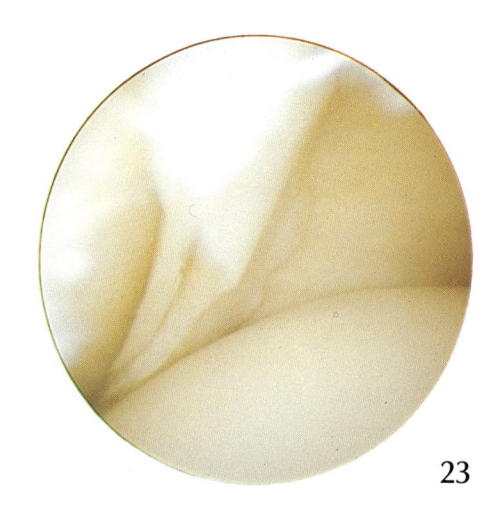

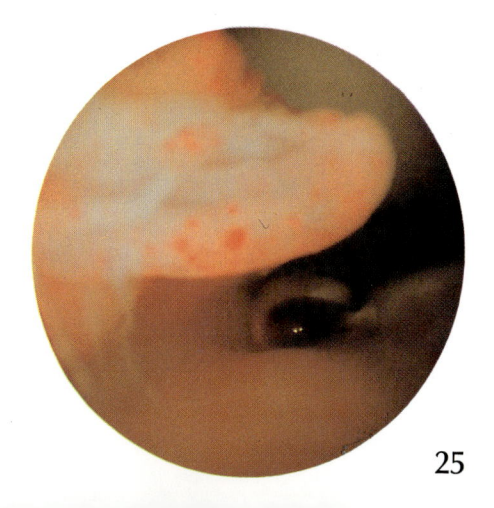

1036 Diagnostic arthroscopy of the knee

Plate 26. Grade I chondromalacia patellae.
Plate 27. Grade II chondromalacia patellae.
Plate 28. Grade III chondromalacia patellae.
Plate 29. Osteoarthritic, pitted femoral condyle.
Plate 30. Advanced osteoarthritis with erosion of the medial femoral and tibial articular surfaces and multiple tears of the medial semilunar cartilage.

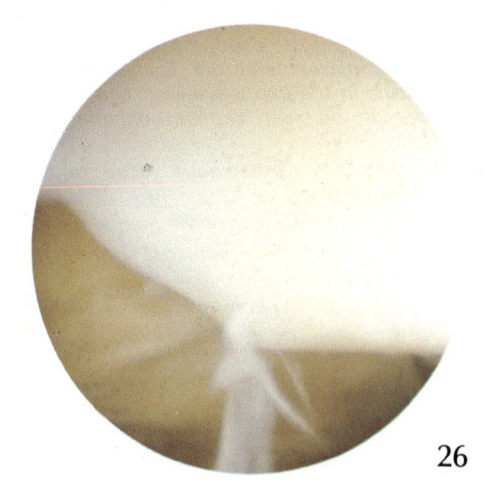

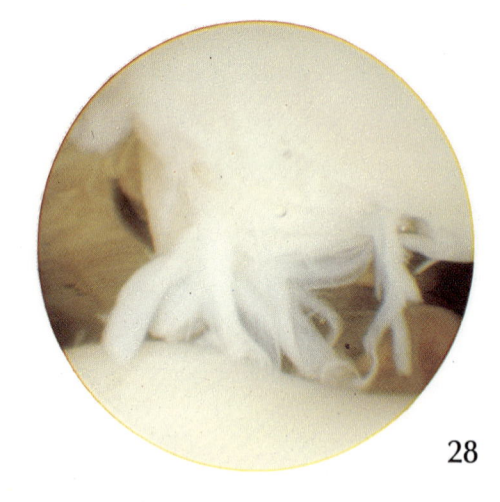

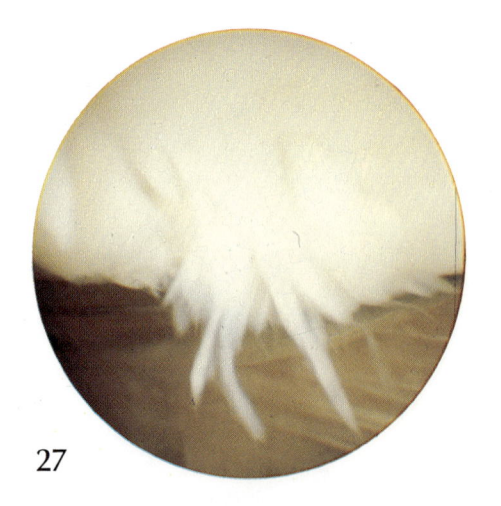

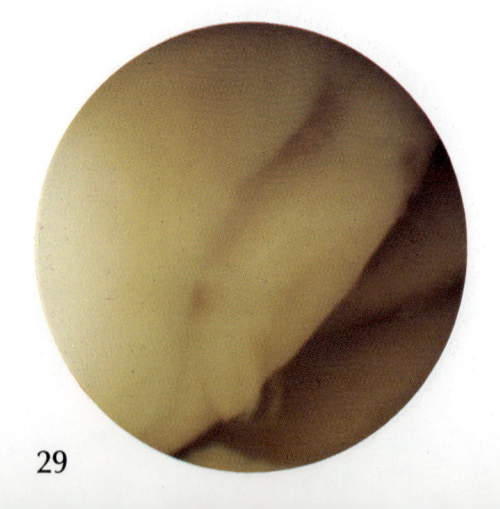

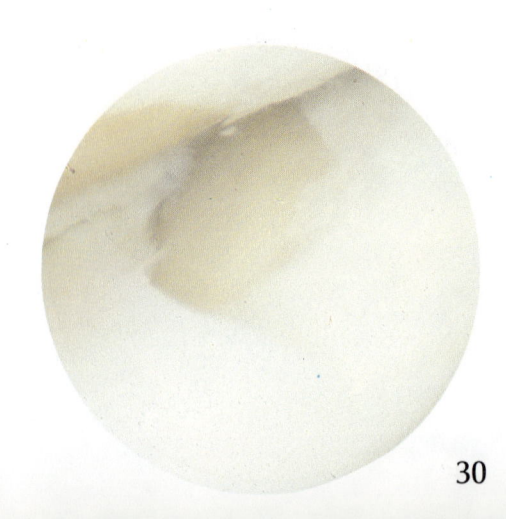

Arthroscopic surgical procedures

Plate 31. Synovial biopsy.
Plate 32. Palpation of abnormal synovial fold using a probe.
Plate 33. Erosion of the femoral condyle.
Plates 34a, b. Synovial tag and associated fat pad.

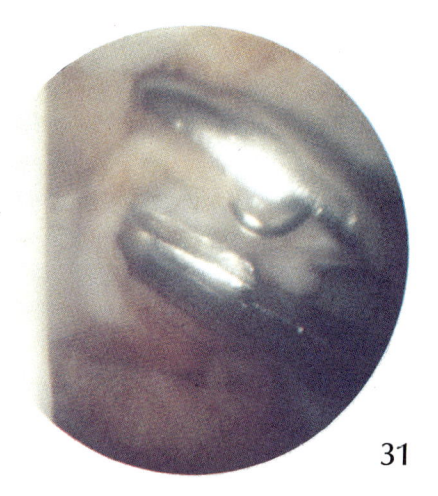

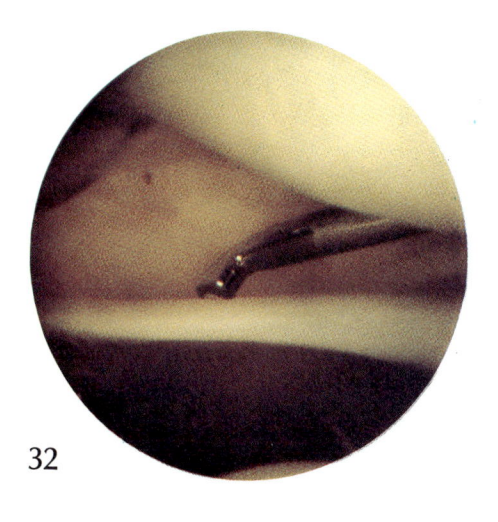

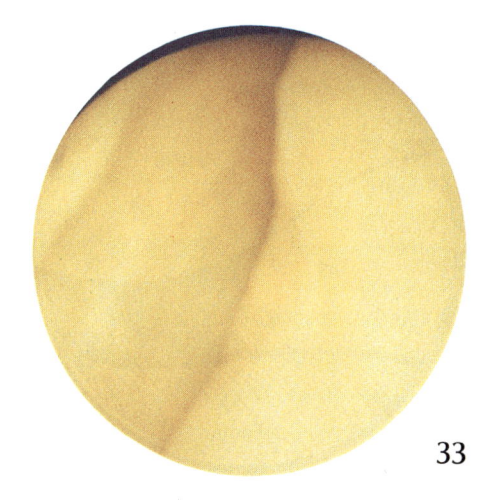

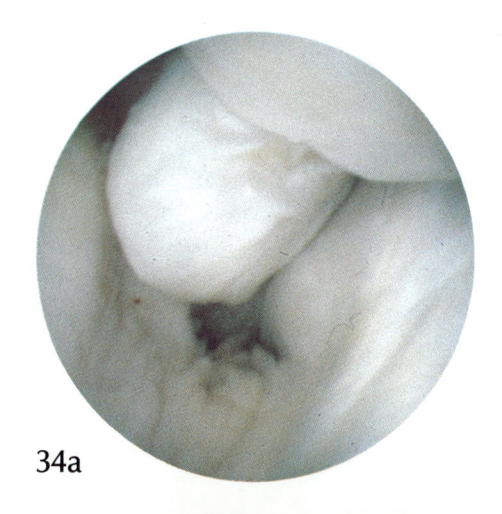

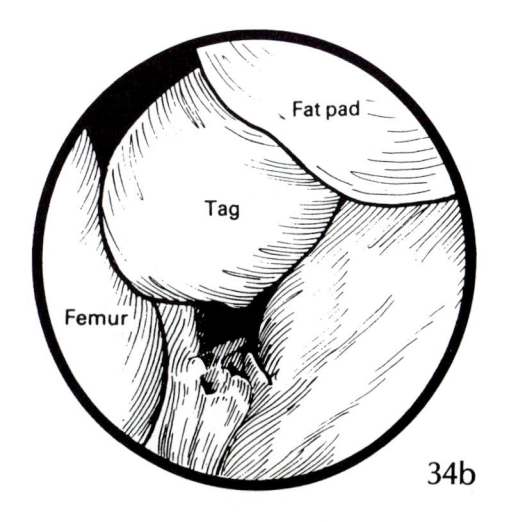

1038 Arthroscopic surgical procedures

Plates 35a, b. Synovial tag jammed between the patella and its groove.
Plate 36. Defining the synovial tag by means of a probe.
Plate 37. Appearance of the abnormal articular cartilage in osteochondritis dissecans.
Plate 38. Probing a breach in the articular cartilage to elevate, and therefore define, the osteochondritic fragment.

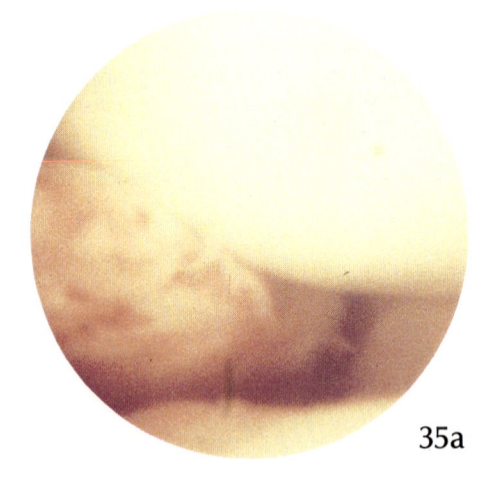

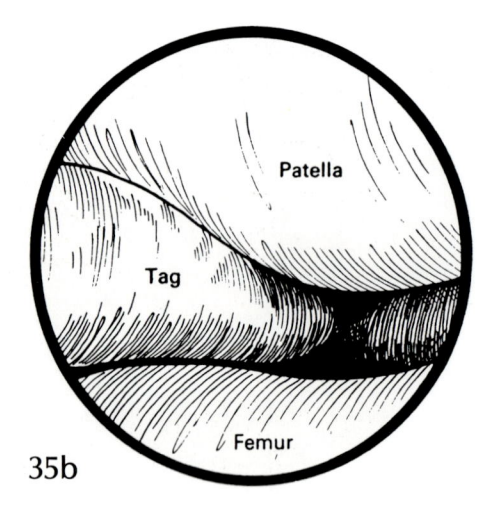

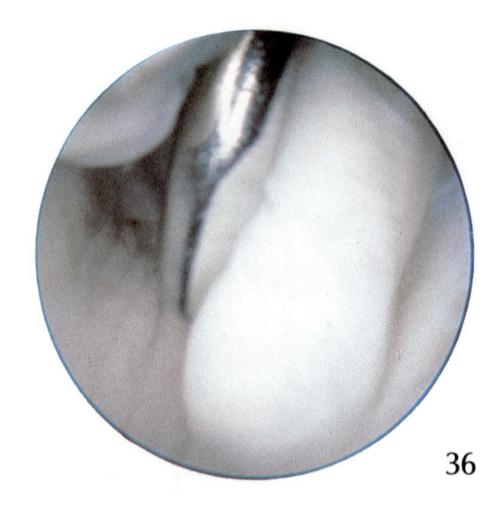

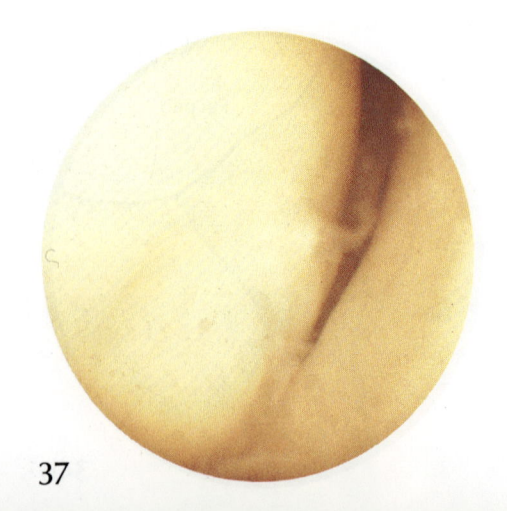

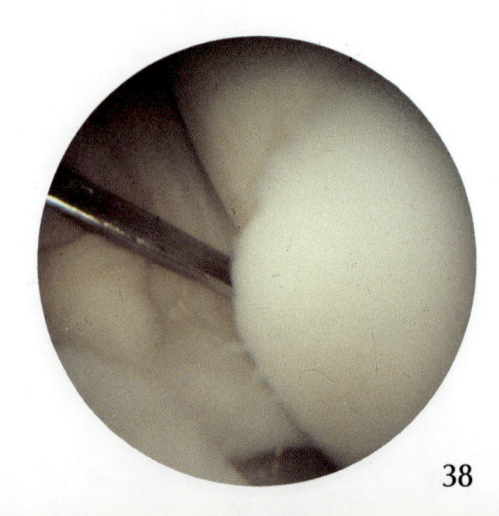

Plate 39. Screw head exposed after the removal of articular cartilage.
Plate 40. Metallic foreign bodies in the sheath of the popliteus tendon.
Plate 41. Triangulation of a loose body in the posterolateral compartment using a needle.
Plate 42. A loose body impaled with a needle inserted transcutaneously.
Plate 43. Removal of the loose body using rongeurs.

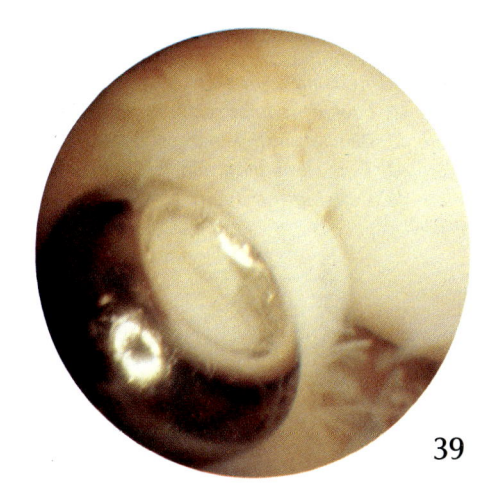

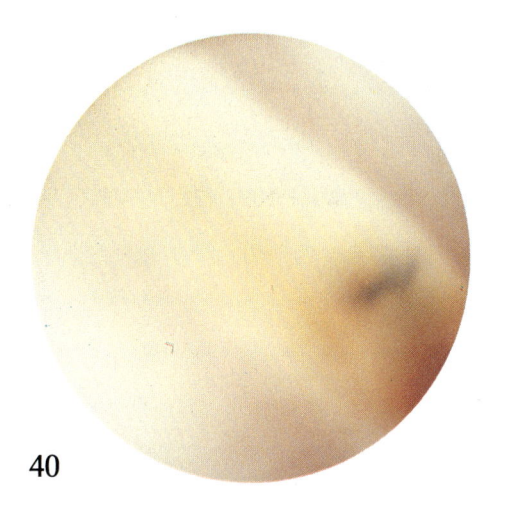

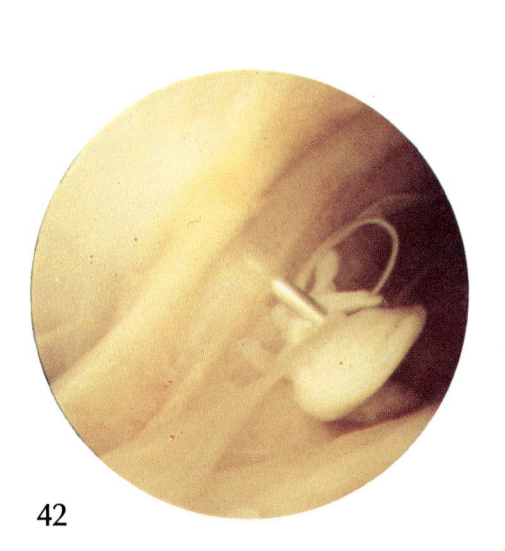

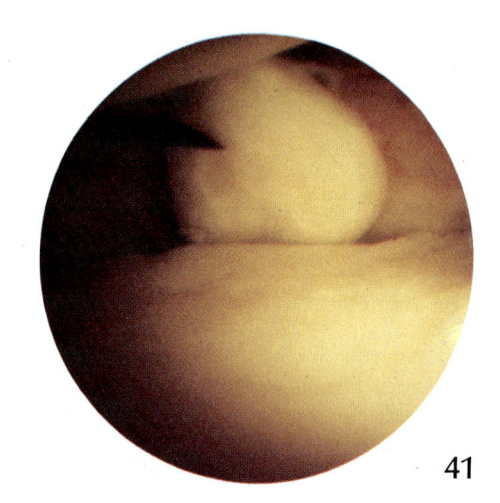

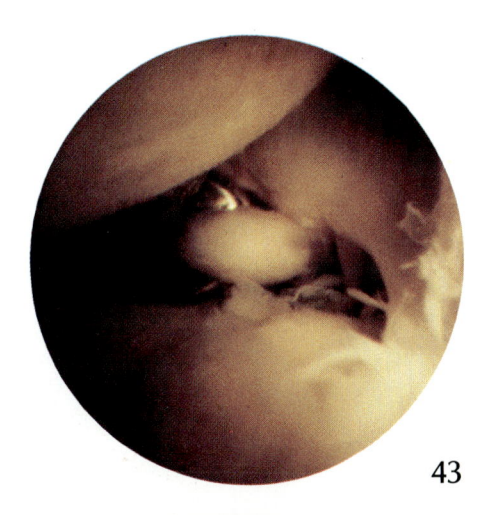

Arthroscopic meniscectomy

Plate 44. Defining the junction of a full bucket-handle tear and the rim using a probe.
Plate 45. Lower blade of scissors placed under the tear.
Plate 46. Division of the meniscus–tear junction.
Plate 47. Tags remaining after excision of the tear.
Plate 48. Defining the points of attachment of a tag using a probe.

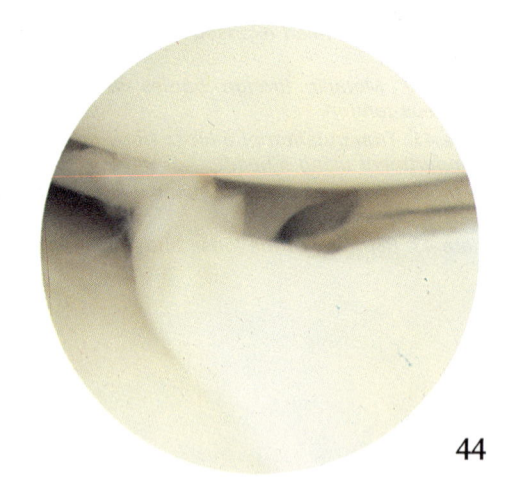

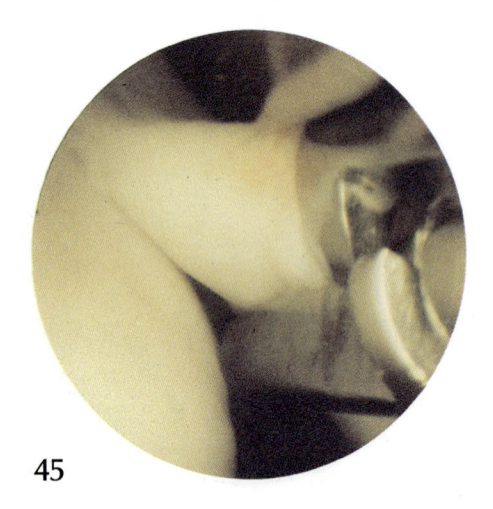

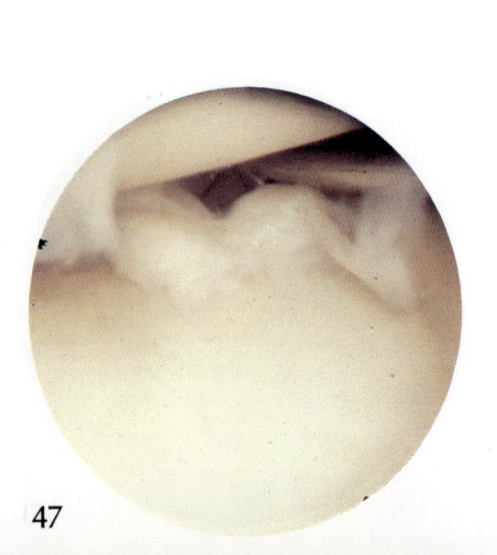

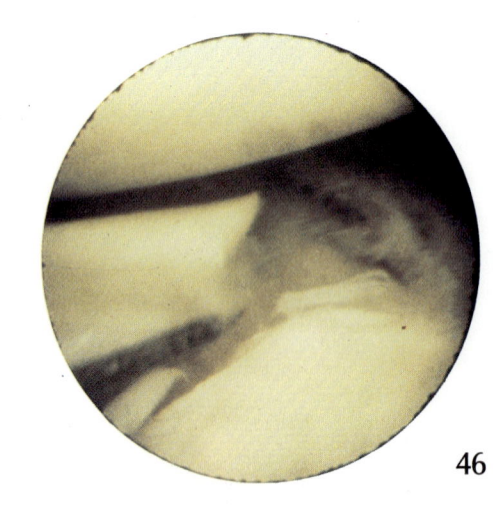

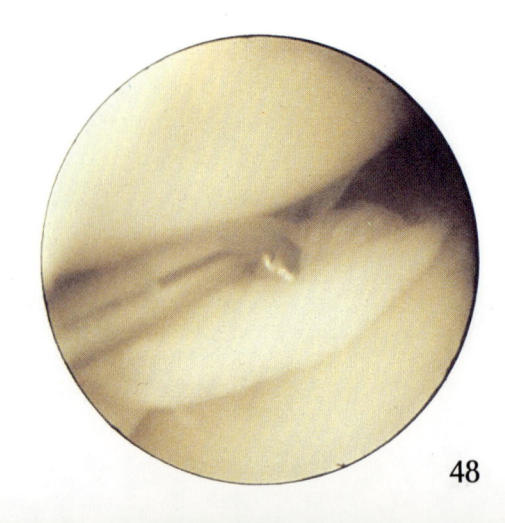

Arthroscopic meniscectomy 1041

Plate 49. Avulsion of a tag using rongeurs.
Plate 50. Appearance after avulsion of a tag.
Plate 51. Using punch forceps to trim the remains of an excised tear.
Plate 52. Using a hook to define a posterior third bucket-handle tear.
Plate 53. Dividing a tear with scissors passed across the intercondylar notch.

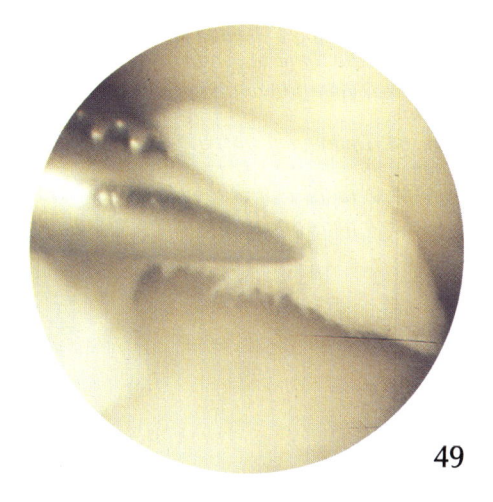

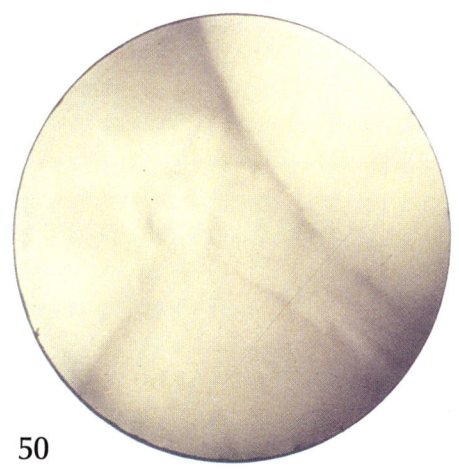

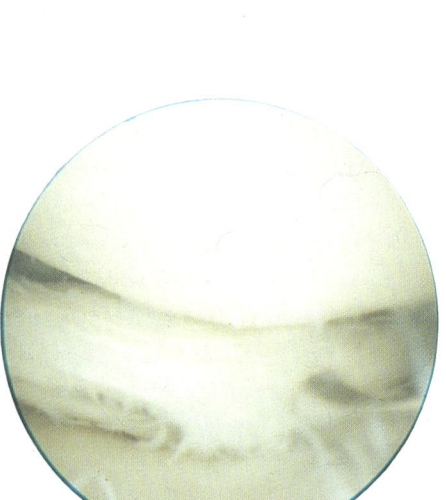

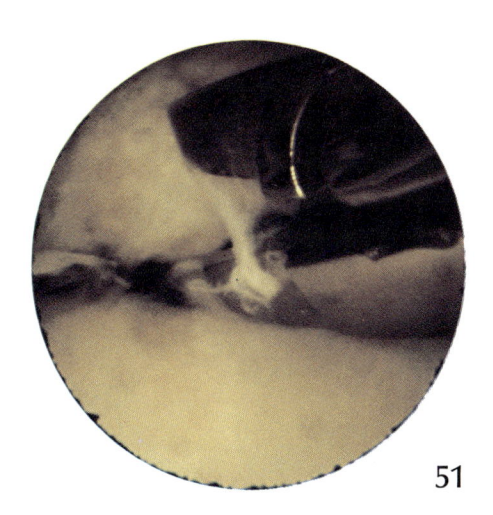

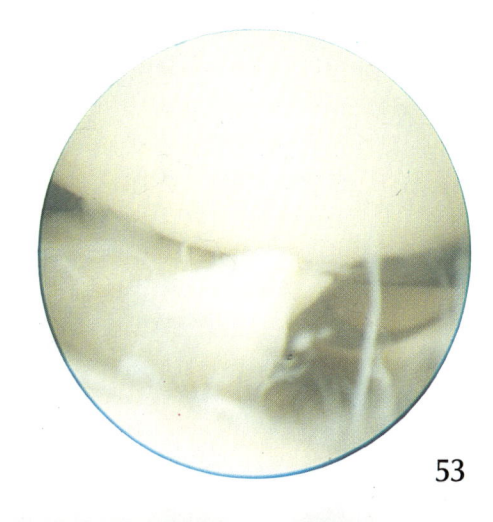

Plate 54. Hingeing a divided tear forwards with a hook to lie in front of the femoral condyle.
Plate 55. Dividing the anterior attachment of the tear using scissors.
Plate 56. Defining a posterior horn cleavage tear using a probe.
Plate 57. A radial tear of the lateral meniscus.
Plate 58. A parrot-beak tear of the lateral meniscus.

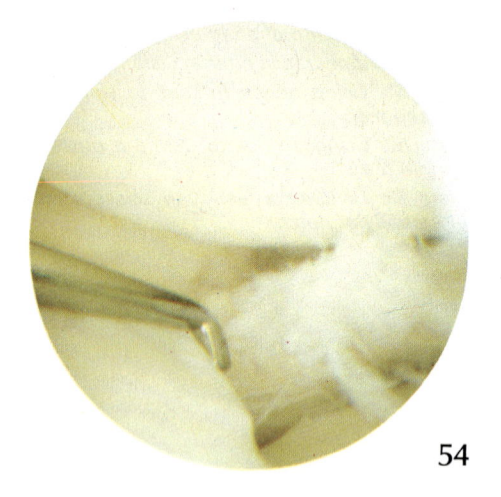

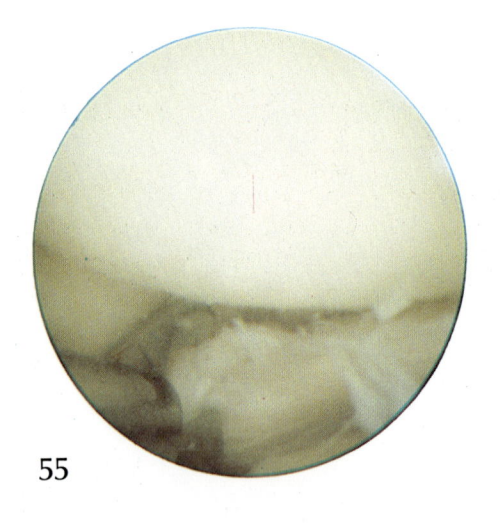

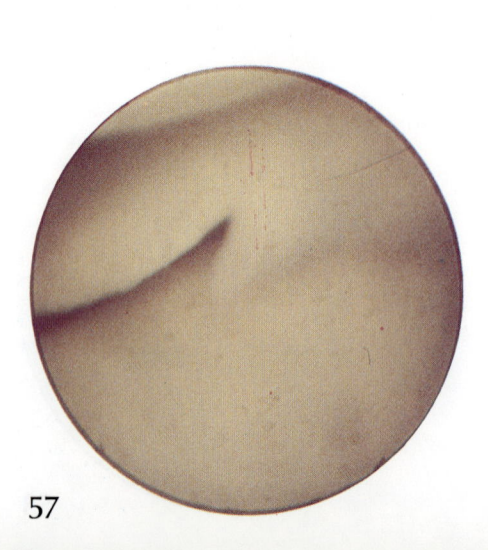

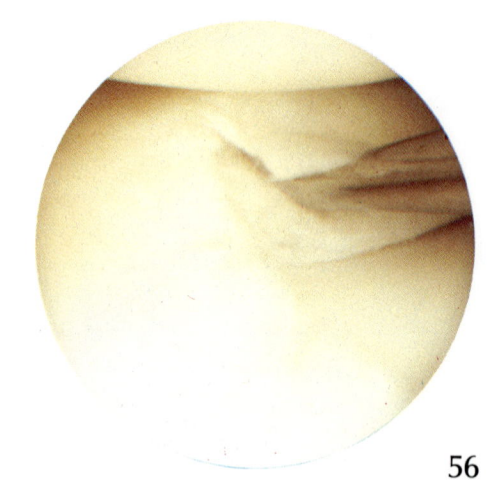

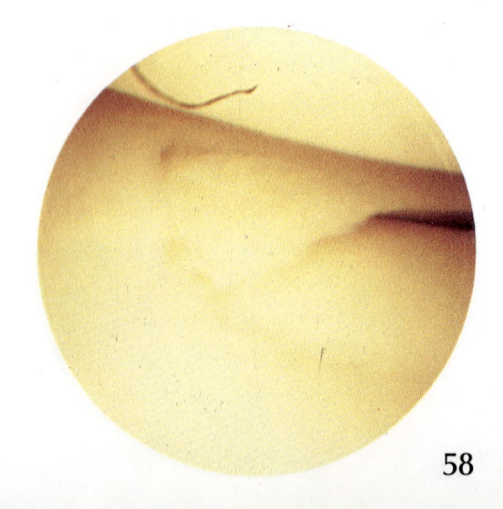

Illustrations by Peter Cox

Arthroscopic meniscectomy

Ian Stother MA, FRCS(Ed), FRCS(Glas)
Consultant Orthopaedic Surgeon, Glasgow Royal Infirmary, Glasgow, UK

Introduction

Meniscus pathology is a common cause of knee morbidity. Initial diagnostic arthroscopy allows precise assessment of the site and extent of meniscus damage. It therefore allows logical treatment of meniscus tears. The main treatment options to be considered are:

1. No procedure.
2. Meniscal suture (see chapter on 'Arthroscopic meniscal repair', pp. 1056–1061).
3. Partial meniscectomy.
4. Total meniscectomy (see chapter on 'Open meniscectomy of the knee', p 1062–1072).

Arthroscopic partial meniscectomy is considered in this chapter. The long-term results of partial meniscectomy are better than those of total meniscectomy[1] and closed partial meniscectomy allows a more rapid early recovery[2].

Basic technique

Arthroscopic meniscectomy has three essential stages:

1. Definition of the abnormal area
2. Excision of the abnormal area
3. Trimming of the remaining rim.

These stages are carried out by the 'double puncture' or 'triple puncture' technique.

1

In the double puncture technique the arthroscope is inserted through one skin puncture or portal, usually the anterolateral, and one or more instruments are inserted through a second portal, often the anteromedial.

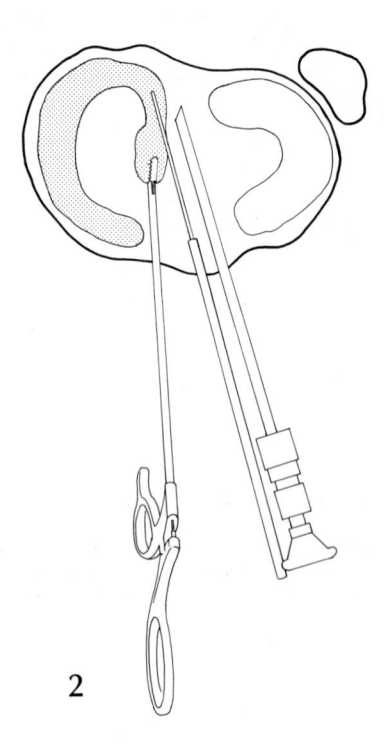

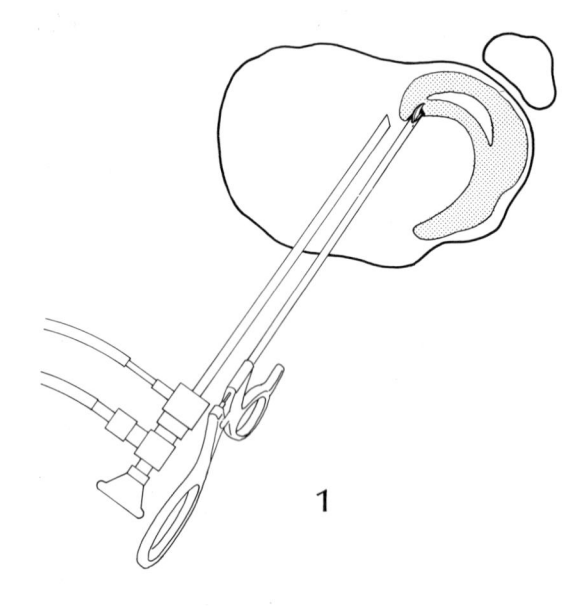

2

In the triple puncture technique, three portals are used, one for the telescope and two for instruments – most commonly one grasping and one cutting instrument.

Hand instruments

The equipment needed for diagnostic arthroscopy is required (see chapter on 'Diagnostic arthroscopy of the knee', pp. 1007–1018).

In addition special hand instruments are required for performing three basic functions – cutting, grasping and nibbling. Curved instruments are useful for access to the horns of the menisci.

Power instruments

Various power instruments are available. Most have a rotating cutting blade or burr and an attached suction mechanism for removing debris. On the whole these instruments are an alternative to hand instruments. With the possible exceptions of synovectomy and patellar shaving, power instruments do not increase the range of surgery.

Special diathermy cutting instruments are also available.

EXCISION OF A FULL BUCKET-HANDLE TEAR OF THE MENISCUS

Medial bucket-handle tears

Indications

The procedure is indicated for locked knee or recurrent giving way.

Preparation of the patient

A general or spinal anaesthetic is administered. The patient lies supine on the operating table and the knee ligaments are examined under anaesthesia. A mid-thigh tourniquet is applied (optional). The skin is cleaned and drapes are applied to give a sterile operating field.

Insertion of the telescope

3

The knee is distended with irrigation fluid inserted via the suprapatellar pouch. A 30° telescope is inserted via an anterolateral portal. Irrigation is continued via the telescope.

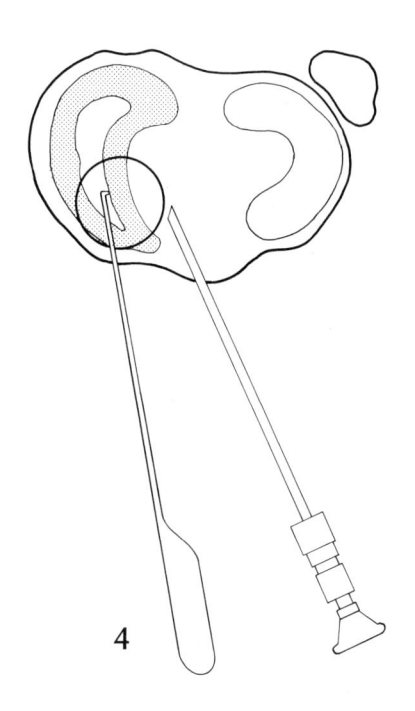

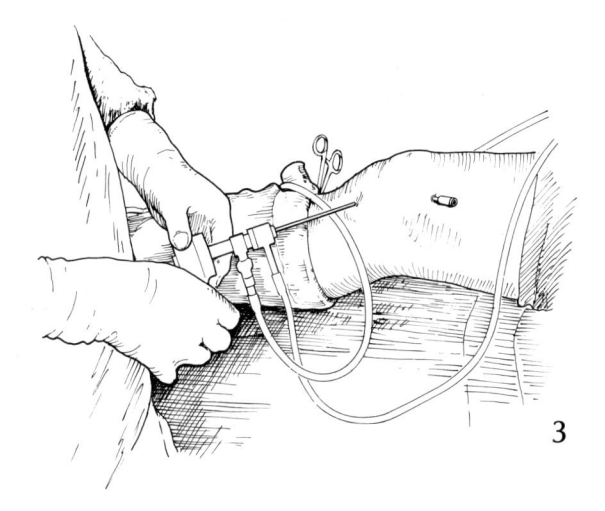

Defining the tear

4

The bucket-handle tear will be either displaced or undisplaced. The junctions of the tear and the rim are defined with a probe inserted via an anteromedial portal. *Plate 44** shows the hook between the bucket-handle tear and the rim, and *Illustration 4* is a plan view of this.

**Colour plates 44–48 are on pages 1040–1042.*

5

If the tear is displaced it may be reduced with the probe whilst a valgus force is applied. To do this the leg may be dropped over the side of the table onto the operator's knee.

Excising the tear

Ideally each end of the bucket-handle tear should be divided as close as possible to the rim so that one large fragment is removed, leaving no tags to trim. If at all possible the tear should be reduced with the probe.

If the tear can be reduced, its posterior attachment should be divided first. The telescope remains in the anterolateral portal. A probe is manipulated across the intercondylar notch from the anteromedial portal to the posterior horn of the meniscus. The probe is then replaced with a small pair of hook scissors and the posterior attachment of the tear is divided. The completeness of the division is then checked with the probe.

The anterior attachment of the tear is then approached. Initially the telescope should remain in the anterolateral portal and the probe should be manipulated through the anteromedial portal. If access to the anterior attachment of the tear is difficult, the insertions of the telescope and probe should be reversed.

Occasionally a third portal further anteromedially may be required. The site for such a portal can be piloted with a hypodermic needle. Such an approach may enable the meniscus to be divided from the angle between the rim and the tear.

Once access to the anterior attachment of the tear has been achieved with the probe then the probe should be replaced with a pair of scissors or a small knife and the attachment subtotally divided. The cutting instrument is then removed and a pair of grasping forceps gently inserted and the torn fragment of meniscus seized. With a twisting action the tear is completely detached from the rim and removed.

6

If the tear cannot be reduced or if the fat pad is becoming oedematous and tending to obscure the anterior attachment of the tear then the anterior attachment should be divided first.

The probe is manipulated through an anteromedial portal into the position where it is desired to divide the meniscus. The probe is then replaced with scissors or a knife. *Plate 45* and *Illustration 6* show a pair of scissors with the lower blade under the tear. The meniscus-tear junction is divided (*Plate 46*). The completeness of division is checked with the probe.

The cut anterior end of the bucket handle is seized with grasping forceps inserted in the anteromedial portal. The tear is then gently displaced into the intercondylar notch.

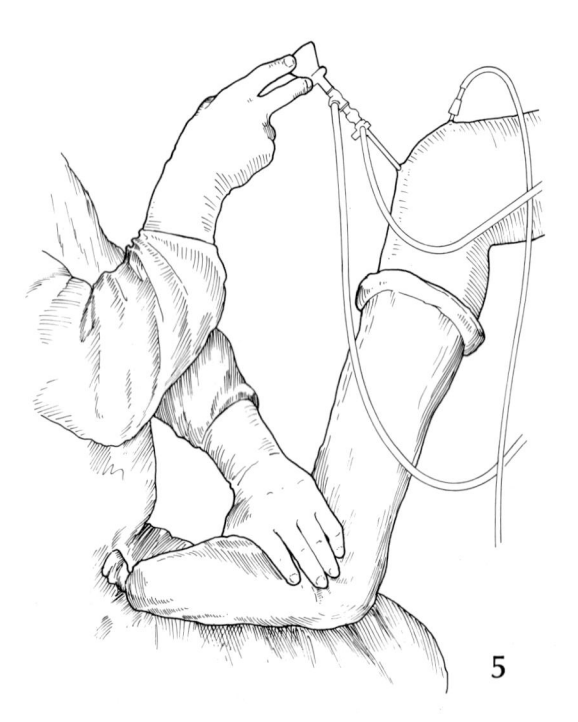

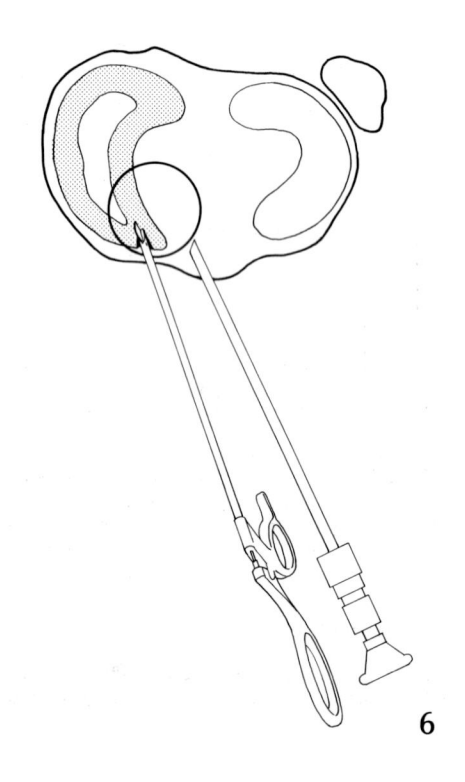

7

The telescope is moved across the intercondylar notch to view the posterior end of the tear. Scissors or a retractable bladed knife are inserted via a third portal, usually placed medial to the graspers.

The cutting instrument is manoeuvred posteriorly to divide the posterior end of the tear under direct vision. The bucket-handle tear can be kept under tension with the graspers. Care must be taken not to damage the anterior cruciate ligament. The torn fragment is then withdrawn from the joint in the graspers.

Checking the remaining rim

8

The size of the excised fragment is a good guide as to the likelihood of any remaining tags to be trimmed. Ideally the excised bucket-handle tear should measure about 2 cm in length. Any tags such as those seen in *Plate 47* may be excised as described below.

Closure of the wound

The joint should be irrigated. Skin wounds are closed with single sutures or sterile wound closure strips.

Postoperative management

A wool and crêpe bandage is applied. When the patient can achieve straight-leg raising he is mobilized with a walking stick and discharged home, usually within 24 hours.

Sutures are removed at 1 week. Most sedentary workers can return to work at or before this time. If the quadriceps are poor at this time a course of physiotherapy should be given. Final review is usually 6 weeks after operation, when the patient's knee should be clinically normal.

Lateral bucket-handle tears

The procedure for excision of a bucket-handle tear from the lateral meniscus is similar, except that the knee should be opened into varus.

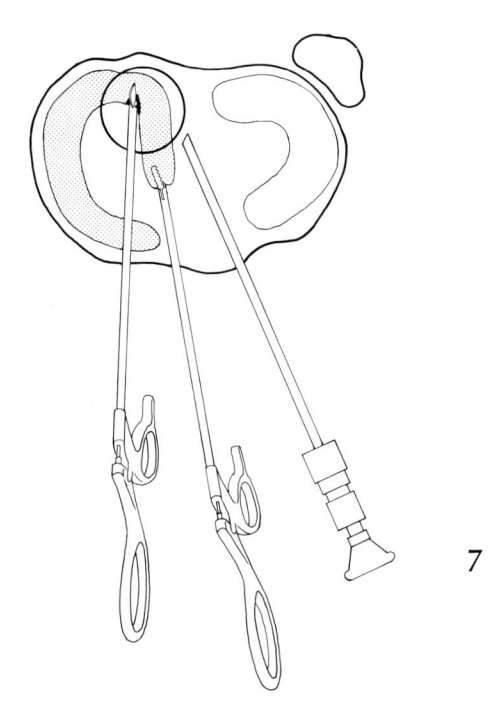

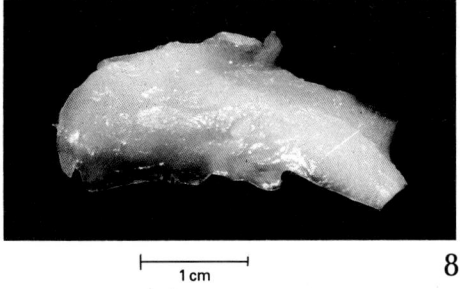

Thigh and knee

EXCISION OF TAG TEARS

Indications

The tags must be large enough to cause mechanical symptoms of pain and tenderness medially. Minor fraying of the meniscus edge is not an indication for surgery.

Preparation of the patient

As for Excision of a full bucket-handle tear, p. 1045.

Insertion of the telescope

A routine anterolateral insertion is used.

Defining the tear

9

The free and attached ends of the tag must be defined using an anteromedially inserted probe, as shown in *Illustration 9* and *Plate 48*. Sometimes tags are the ends of a transected bucket-handle tear. If a tag is seen antero medially it is important to check for a second tag at the posterior horn.

Occasionally a tag of meniscus from the lower surface of the meniscus will fold underneath the meniscus and cause a palpable joint line swelling mimicking a cystic meniscus. Such tags can be retrieved by careful probing under the meniscus.

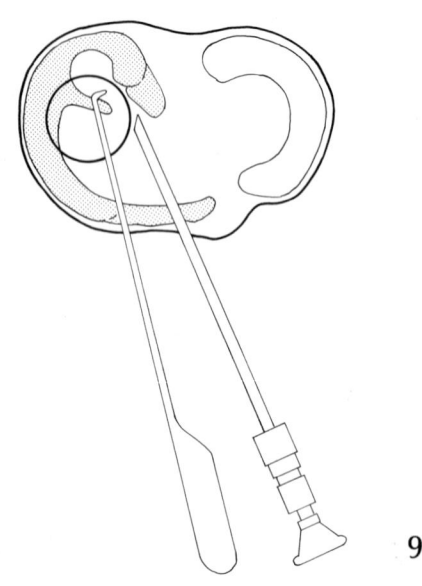

Excising the tear

If the tag has a broad base this should be divided subtotally with scissors, which can usually be inserted in place of the probe. Once the width of the base of the tag has been reduced the tag can be avulsed or excised using rongeurs or grasping forceps inserted in place of the probe, as shown in *Plates 49* and *50*.

Tags at the posterior horn can be pulled forwards with a probe and excised using angled rongeurs or grasping forceps, inserted either anteromedially across the intercondylar notch or occasionally posteromedially with the telescope across the notch.

Checking the remaining rim

The surgeon should always check for a second tag. Any sharp angles should be trimmed using punch forceps (*Plate 51*).

Closure of the wound

As for Excision of a full bucket-handle tear, p. 1047.

Postoperative management

As for Excision of a full bucket-handle tear, p. 1047.

EXCISION OF POSTERIOR THIRD BUCKET-HANDLE TEARS

Indications

10

Tears such as those shown in *Illustration 10* are often associated with ligament injuries and cause intermittent giving way when they sublux in front of the femoral condyle. In young patients with recent short tears, consideration should be given to suturing the tear (*see* chapter on 'Arthroscopic meniscal repair', pp. 1056–1061).

The longer the tear, the longer the duration of symptoms and the older the patient, the greater the indication for excision. These tears are among the most difficult to gain access to, especially on the medial side.

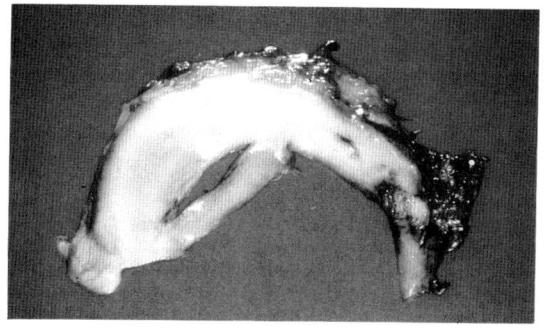

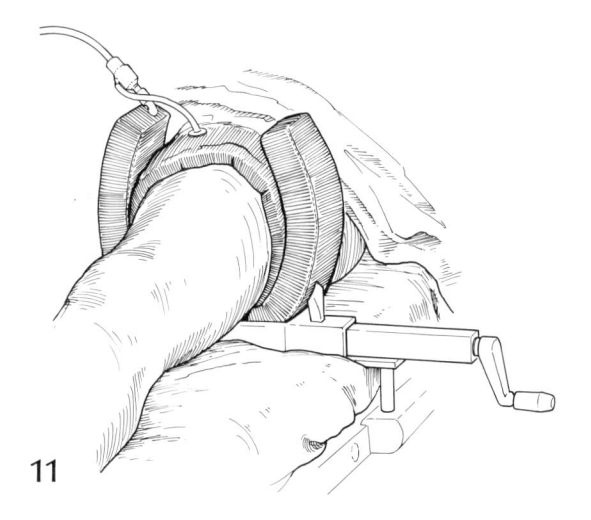

Preparation of the patient

11

As for Excision of a full bucket-handle tear, p. 1045. It is always useful to have a leg holder to immobilize the thigh in order to gain access to the posterior third of the meniscus.

Insertion of the telescope

As for Excision of a full bucket-handle tear, p. 1045.

Defining the tear

12

Using a hook, the tear can often be subluxated forward in front of the femoral condyle (*Plate 52*) but usually slips back immediately. It is important to try and define the ends of the tear and to check the ease of access to each end.

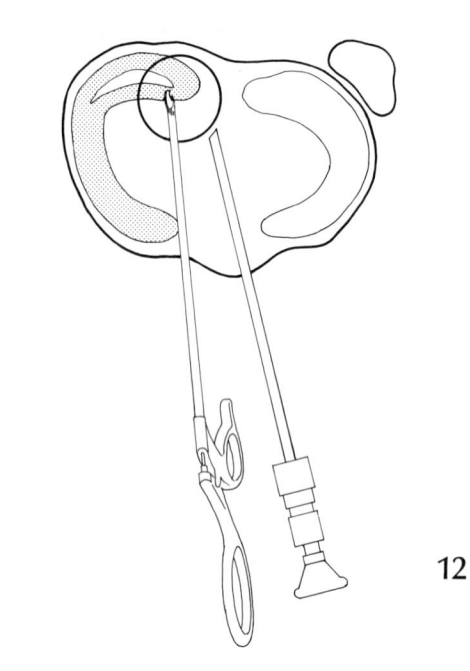

Excising the tear

It is often easiest to divide the posterior end first, provided the knee is not arthritic and there is access to the posterior horn across the intercondylar notch. If a small pair of scissors can be passed across the notch, the tear can be divided right to its edge (*Plate 53*). Once divided, the tear can be hinged forwards with a hook to lie in front of the femoral condyle (*Plate 54*). Grasping forceps can then be inserted anteromedially to put traction on the cut end of the tear.

13

Using a third incision medial to the graspers, small scissors or a sheathed knife can be used to cut the anterior attachment of the tear while gentle traction is applied with graspers (*Plate 55*).

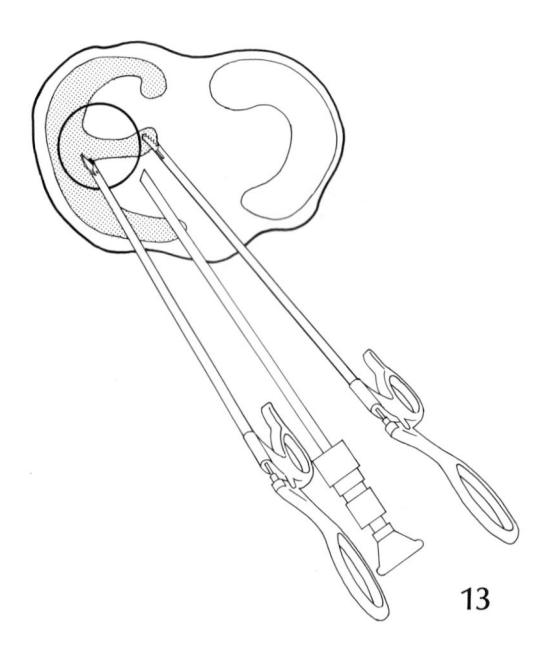

Checking the remaining rim

The rim should be checked with a hook. Small posterior horn tags can be ignored. The anterior edge of the excision should be as smooth as possible and should be trimmed with punch forceps, or perhaps with powered instruments. On the lateral side care should be taken to leave a popliteus bridge.

Closure of the wound

As for Excision of a full bucket-handle tear, p. 1047.

Postoperative management

As for Excision of a full bucket-handle tear, p. 1047.

Arthroscopic meniscectomy

EXCISION OF POSTERIOR HORN CLEAVAGE TEARS

Indications

So-called cleavage or degenerative tears of the posterior horn of the medial meniscus have been associated with both pain and mechanical symptoms. Mechanical symptoms are usually due to tag tears which can be excised as outlined previously. Where the meniscus is degenerate but there are no major tags, there may be a place for removing the abnormal tissue for relief of pain.

Preparation of the patient

As for Excision of a full bucket-handle tear, p. 1045.

Defining the tear

14

Visualization of the tear requires the knee to be opened into valgus. The abnormal area should be defined with the probe as shown in *Illustration 14* and *Plate 56*. Occasionally a posteromedial insertion of the arthroscope may be useful.

Excising the tear

15

The degenerate meniscus is soft and fragmented. It therefore needs to be removed piecemeal. Access to the posterior third from the anteromedial portal can be limited and it can be difficult to open instruments such as punch forceps and rongeurs. Side-cutting punches and powered rotating instruments may make the operation easier. Care must be taken not to damage the articular surface.

Bites of abnormal meniscus should be removed until a stable peripheral rim remains. The ends of the area should be contoured back to the normal meniscus edge. The loose bites of meniscus should be flushed out down the arthroscopic sheath or removed with a suction probe.

Checking the remaining rim

A small rim of meniscus should be left *in situ*, even if it is somewhat degenerative. There should, however, be no remaining tags.

Closure of the wound

As for Excision of a full bucket-handle tear, p. 1047.

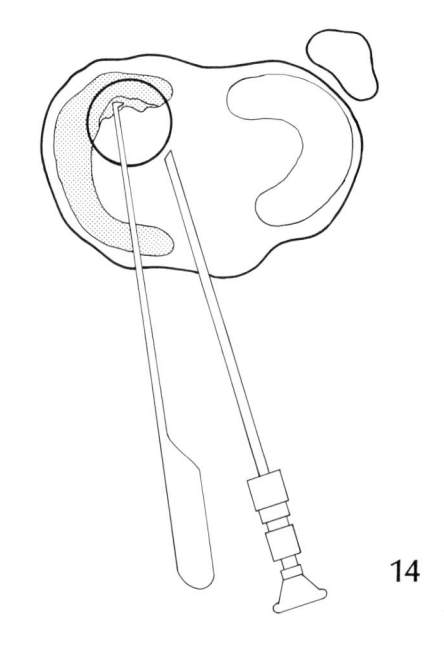

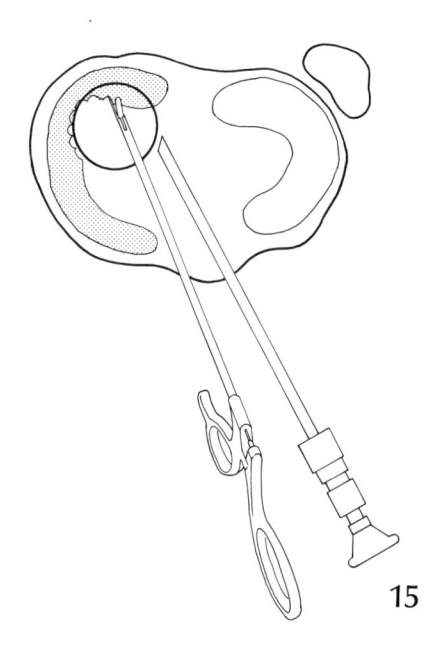

Postoperative management

As for Excision of a full bucket-handle tear, p. 1047.

RADIAL TEARS OF THE LATERAL MENISCUS

Indications

These tears, as shown in *Plate 57* indicate instability of the posterior third of the lateral meniscus. The tears themselves should be 'saucerized' and the posterior third of the lateral meniscus should either be stabilized with a suture or excised. Stabilization is preferable, as excision usually requires removal of the popliteus bridge which is functionally undesirable.

Preparation of the patient

As for Excision of a full bucket-handle tear, p. 1045.

Defining the tear

16

The edges of the tear should be defined using a hook, placing the hook into the popliteus groove. Usually the posterior third of the meniscus can be subluxated forwards in front of the femoral condyle.

Excising the tear

The margins of the tear should be 'saucerized'. Lateral cutting punches are useful for this. Next either the posterior third should be sutured to the capsule (see chapter on 'Arthroscopic meniscal repair', pp. 1056–1061) or alternatively the posterior third should be removed using large punch forceps.

Checking the remaining rim

The surgeon should ensure that no large tags can cause symptoms by interposition.

Closure of the wound

As for Excision of a full bucket-handle tear, p. 1047.

Postoperative management

As for Excision of a full bucket-handle tear, p. 1047.

16

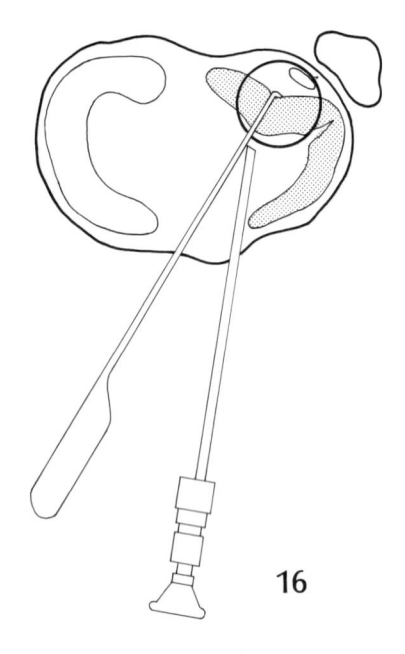

SURGERY OF TORN CYSTIC LATERAL MENISCUS

In such cases there is both intra-articular and extra-articular pathology. The tear can be excised arthroscopically, but the area of cystic change extends outside the periphery of the meniscus and often involves a considerable length of the meniscus itself. To excise the abnormal tissue therefore often involves both breaching the continuity of the meniscus edge and removing a large part of the meniscus itself. Where extensive cystic changes are found at diagnostic arthroscopy, and where the tear itself is complex and involves a considerable length of the meniscus, an open complete lateral meniscectomy is often the easiest operation to perform. Alternatively, resection with a powered meniscotome may be performed.

Care must be taken not to mistake a flap tear of the inferior surface of the lateral meniscus, which has come to be extruded peripherally, for a small meniscus cyst.

If a partial arthroscopic meniscectomy is performed for a cystic lateral meniscus the procedure is as described in the next section. In the author's experience, recurrence of symptoms after partial meniscectomy for cystic degeneration is quite common.

EXCISION OF PARROT-BEAK TEARS OF THE LATERAL MENISCUS

Indications

17

Tears such as those shown in *Plate 58* and *Illustration 17* may cause lateral pain and also recurrent instability, in which case the abnormal area of lateral meniscus should be removed.

Parrot-beak tears are complex tears of the posterior half of the lateral meniscus. They extend obliquely through the substance of the meniscus. They are sometimes associated with cystic changes in the affected area. The tears can be excised arthroscopically but care needs to be taken to remove the whole of the abnormal area.

Preparation of the patient

As for Excision of a full bucket-handle tear, p. 1045.

Insertion of the telescope

The 30° telescope should be inserted anterolaterally through a portal as close to the patellar tendon as possible. The probe should be inserted anteromedially. Where the lateral femoral condyle is very convex, care should be taken not to insert the probe too low. It is often helpful to reverse the positions of telescope and probe.

Defining the tear

The upper surface of the tear usually does not indicate the extent of the meniscal involvement. The tear itself and the inferior surface of the meniscus should be probed to assess the posterior extent of the tear.

Excising the tear

Care must be taken to excise the whole of the abnormal area of meniscus. Usually the posterior and inferior part of the tear has a very broad base, so the tear cannot be treated like a tag tear. Instead the posterior component of the tear needs to be excised piecemeal with punch forceps or power instruments (see *Illustration 15*). It may also be necessary to trim the anterior or superior part of the tear with punch forceps. The base of the tear needs to be carefully probed. Some of these tears extend to the capsular margins of the meniscus. In this case, or if cystic changes in the meniscus are encountered as bites of meniscus are being removed, consideration can be given to performing a subtotal meniscectomy, removing the posterior half of the meniscus (behind the tear) piecemeal with punch forceps. The remaining rim of the anterior part of the meniscus is often gently sloping towards its capsular attachment and requires little trimming.

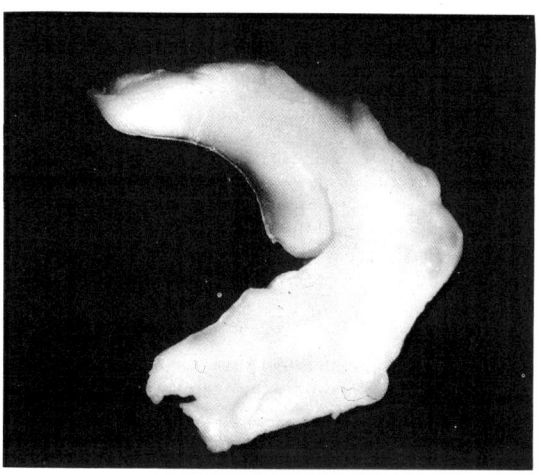

After removing the meniscus piecemeal, the portions of the meniscus should be flushed out of the joint, either down the telescope sheath or through a sucker.

Checking the remaining rim

If possible, a rim of the posterior part of the meniscus should be left *in situ* to preserve meniscal function. If such a rim is left, a hook should be placed over it into the popliteal groove and traction applied. If the rim can be subluxated forwards in front of the femoral condyle the rim should be removed or sutured, otherwise it may interpose between the joint surfaces and cause instability.

Closure of the wound

As for Excision of a full bucket-handle tear, p. 1047.

Postoperative management

As for Excision of a full bucket-handle tear, p. 1047.

1054 Thigh and knee

SURGERY OF THE DISCOID LATERAL MENISCUS

Indications

The only definite indication for surgery is the presence of mechanical symptoms together with the finding of a torn discoid meniscus.

Such tears commonly involve the central area of the meniscus. If the discoid meniscus is a complete one, the tear may involve only the upper surface or the lower surface, one surface of the meniscus remaining intact.

Preparation of the patient

As for Excision of a full bucket-handle tear, p. 1045. If the patient is a child, the normal arthroscope and instruments are quite suitable.

Insertion of the telescope

As for Excision of a full bucket-handle tear, p. 1045.

Defining the tear

It is very important to determine exactly the size of the meniscus and the location of any tears. In complete discoid menisci the inferior surface of the meniscus must be viewed. The telescope may be easier to manoeuvre under a discoid meniscus from the anteromedial portal.

Two main types of tear occur:

18, 19 & 20

1. There is separation of the thickened medial margin of the meniscus (a 'perforated' discoid meniscus).
2. There is a 'flap' tear of one surface of an imperforate meniscus. *Illustrations 19* and *20* show the intact upper and torn lower surface of such a meniscus.

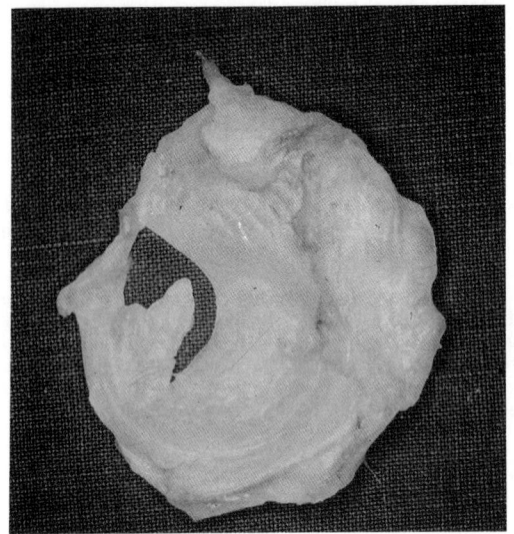

Excision of the medial part of a perforated discoid meniscus

The operation is similar to excising a displaced bucket-handle tear, except that the 'bucket handle' is bulky and its attachments more extensive than usual.

The space occupied by the inner edge of the meniscus is large and access to it is tight. The anterior end of the inner edge of the meniscus should be divided first. Because of the difficult access the cutting instrument may be best introduced from the anteromedial portal.

The procedure is essentially that described for Excision of a full bucket-handle tear, p. 1046.

Closure of the wound

As for Excision of a full bucket-handle tear, p. 1047.

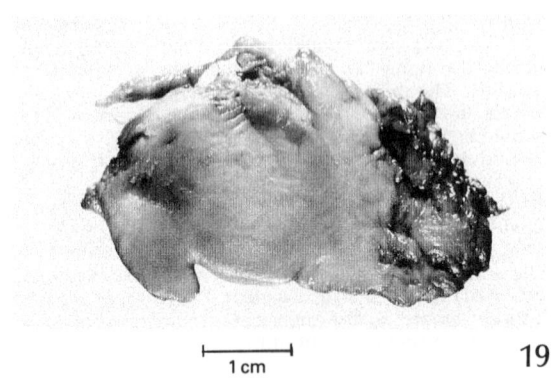

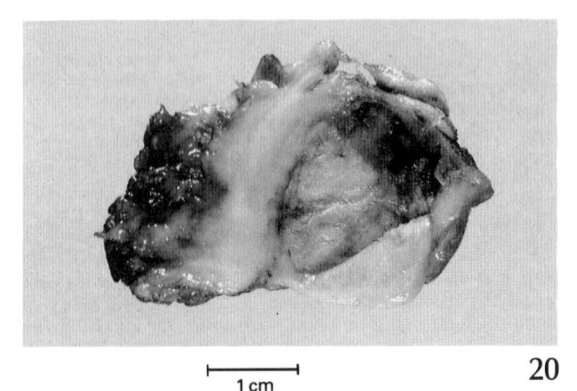

Postoperative management

As for Excision of a full bucket-handle tear, p. 1047.

Excision of a superior surface flap tear

Such a tear usually has a broad base. The base can be divided with scissors or a knife inserted on the same side of the patellar tendon as the tear. The tear can then be grasped and removed.

The remainder of the discoid meniscus may be left *in situ*. Alternatively it may be trimmed creating a bucket-handle type of tear, which is then excised to leave a relatively normal rim.

If such a procedure is undertaken and becomes difficult it should be abandoned and an open total meniscectomy carried out rather than damage the joint surfaces. The large volume of tissue which needs to be removed may be dealt with more quickly by power instruments, provided the anatomy is carefully defined first.

Excision of an inferior surface flap tear

If there is a flap tear of the inferior surface then the options are:

1. Arthroscopic partial meniscectomy, fashioning a 'normal' meniscus by excising the central area (as for Excision of a superior surface flap tear, above).
2. Open total meniscectomy.

References

1. Tapper EM, Hoover NW. Late results after meniscectomy. *J Bone Joint Surg [Am]* 1959; 51-A: 517–26.

2. Dandy DJ. Early results of closed partial meniscectomy. *Br Med J* 1978; i: 1099–100.

Illustrations by Peter Cox

Arthroscopic meniscal repair

Robert W. Jackson MD, MS (Tor), FRCS(C)
Chief of Staff/Surgery, Orthopaedic and Arthritic Hospital, Toronto; Professor of Surgery, University of Toronto, Canada

Sanford S. Kunkel MD
Orthopaedic Surgeon, Methodist Hospital, Indiana, USA

Introduction

Since Thomas Annandale published his description of the surgical repair of a torn semilunar meniscus one century ago, the pendulum of opinion has swung back and forth in regard to the ideal method of treatment of a meniscal disruption. In the early part of this century the trend was towards removal of the entire meniscus, based on the theory that this would allow nature to produce a fibrous replica of the original. In spite of the trend towards total meniscectomy, some voices of moderation pointed out that partial removal of the mobile or damaged portion of the meniscus was probably the better method of treatment[1,2]. Eventually, the thought evolved that total removal of the meniscus might actually be the precipitating cause of the degenerative changes that were seen so frequently after total meniscectomy[2-4], a theory that was soon supported by numerous clinical studies[5-7]. Further support came from biomechanical studies which demonstrated the importance of the meniscus in several ways, including load distribution, lubrication and stability[8-10]. The trend then quickly moved towards partial meniscectomy, usually under arthroscopic control, as the 'gold standard' of treatment[7,11,12].

It was then logical, that if retention of the peripheral portion of the meniscus produced better results than total meniscectomy, preservation of the entire meniscus, through successful repair of the torn structure, might result in a virtually normal knee. This concept was supported by the good clinical evidence obtained in follow-up after primary suturing of both torn collateral ligaments and torn menisci[13,14]. Several studies of a clinical nature and some of an experimental nature endorsed the fact that a torn meniscus could indeed heal itself given the right conditions[15,16].

The first arthroscopic repair of a torn meniscus was carried out by Ikeuchi in 1969[17]. Since that time there has been considerable interest in this minimally-invasive arthroscopic technique for two important reasons. First, the morbidity with an arthroscopic procedure is generally less than with an open procedure. Secondly, the selection, preparation, and stabilization of many meniscal tears is easier. Arthroscopy not only allows the surgeon to see further back in the joint, but also to see better (due to the fibre-light illumination and the magnification) than with open techniques[18]. Moreover, tears that are situated towards the centre of the knee are accessible to arthroscopy, whereas only those that are at the periphery of the meniscus can be repaired by open procedures. Coincident with the clinical interest in closed meniscal repair, came scientific evidence in dogs and humans to support the concept[19,20]. Now, with favourable medium term results, meniscal repair is becoming a standard method of treatment for suitable cases.

Indications

The ideal indication for meniscal repair would appear to be a vertical tear in the vascular outer third of the meniscus, longer than 1.5 cm in length and inherently unstable, in a young athletically-orientated individual, with no other pathology in his knee. A further strong indication for repair would be the meniscal lesion that exists in association with ligamentous instability, such as that following torn anterior cruciate or medial collateral ligament. Various studies have shown that lesions suitable for repair are present in only 20 to 30 per cent of all knees with torn menisci, with 70 per cent of those lesions existing in the medial compartment and 30 per cent in the lateral compartment.

Contraindications

1

Contraindications to repair are somewhat relative. A surgeon might not wish to repair a knee in an older individual (35 years plus) if the tear was relatively short (less the 1.5 cm) and stable, or where there was associated ligamentous instability and no attempt was going to be made (for whatever reasons) to stabilize the joint. Further contraindications include the various types of meniscal tears other than vertical – such as horizontal cleavage tears, radial tears, flap tears, or degenerative tears of the posterior horn. Also, most surgeons would agree that a tear in the inner two-thirds of the meniscus (Zone B), in the avascular or white zone, would best be treated by partial meniscectomy, as the chance of successful healing is greatly reduced in this area. By contrast, a tear in the vascular zone (Zone A) can be successfully treated by suture.

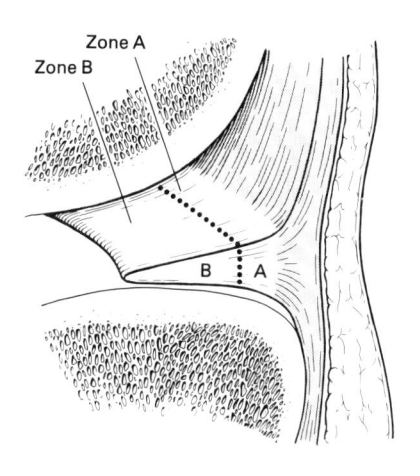

Special investigations

The role of arthrography remains to be established. Some surgeons feel that an arthrogram can give useful information regarding the integrity of the inner portion of the meniscus and demonstrate better than arthroscopy the position of the tear in terms of its relative vascularity. Most competent arthroscopists, however, feel that this information can easily be obtained at arthroscopy and that the arthrogram is no longer of any significant value in assessing the lesion preoperatively. Arthrography might be of some value in the postoperative evaluation of healing; however, the overall usefulness of this technique is doubtful.

Magnetic resonance imaging promises to clarify the location and extent of tears preoperatively.

Experimental studies using fluorescent dyes injected intravenously, and viewed with ultraviolet light under arthroscopic control, are being carried out in an effort to visualize the vascularity of the meniscus, and thus select the most suitable cases for repair. Such studies have not as yet been successful.

Technique

The important stages involved in successful arthroscopic meniscal repair can be described as follows.
1. Selection of the case for treatment.
2. Preparation of the tissues to obtain the maximum biological healing response.
3. Fixation or stabilization of the meniscal fragments to allow healing to occur. Stabilization techniques involve either inside-out techniques or outside-in techniques relating to the placement of sutures.

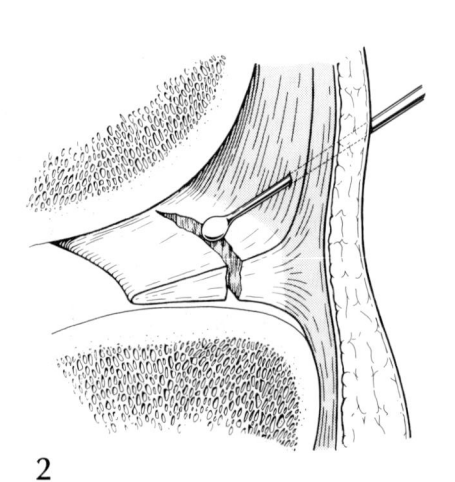

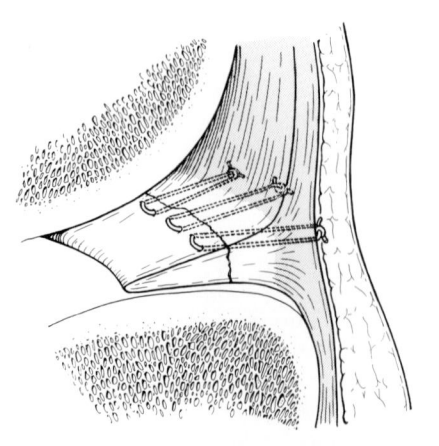

Selection

Selection of appropriate cases is by arthroscopy. The lesion should be in the vascular periphery of the meniscus, of more than 1.5 cm in length, unstable and vertical.

Preparation

2

The peripheral rim should be debrided of scar tissue and the synovial area should be abraded or otherwise stimulated, to promote a maximum vascular response during the healing phase. This may be carried out using rotating burrs, rasps, or punch forceps, either from the anterior approach under direct vision or through additional posterior portals. The vascular peripheral side of the defect obviously deserves the most attention in order to promote vascularity to the area. Some recent evidence suggests that vascular access channels can be made from the peripheral vascular area to lesions that are more central in the meniscus. However, clinical experience in this area is still meagre and these techniques are not commonly practised, for fear of weakening the inner meniscal tissue by creating stress-risers. Recent evidence also suggests that an autogenous fibrin clot placed in the healing area can enhance the repair process. Again however, long-term studies to prove or disprove the effectiveness of clot placement are not available.

Stabilization

3

Whether the technique is from inside out, or outside in, most surgeons feel that sutures should be placed approximately 2 to 3 mm apart, either on the inferior or superior border of the meniscus, and in such a way that stability and firm apposition of the internal fragment to the peripheral rim is obtained at the conclusion of the procedure. Some controversy exists as to whether the suture material should be placed horizontally or vertically to the plane of the meniscus. Those advocating vertical placement suggest that the circular orientation of the peripheral fibres of the meniscus can best withstand the tension of a suture if it is placed vertically. Most sutures placed by arthroscopy are horizontal, because it is easier to do. The suture material that is most commonly used is an absorbable material, either polyglactin 910 or PDS (polydioxanone) of either 0 gauge or 2/0 gauge strength.

'Inside-out' technique

4

In this technique the sutures are placed from anterior portals through cannulae. The suture material is usually attached to a long, thin, and relatively malleable needle which can be passed through the inner fragment, across the defect, through the peripheral rim, and out through capsule and other soft tissues surrounding the knee. This can be done through a single-channel cannula or double-channel cannula, forming a loop of tissue on the inner fragment which is then pulled tight and tied outside the capsule, thus holding the meniscal fragment against the peripheral rim. Sufficient sutures are placed to obtain good stability, usually 2 to 3 mm apart.

One of the major problems associated with passing sutures from inside out is the risk of damage to extra-articular structures such as the sartorial branch of the saphenous nerve on the medial side, the peroneal nerve on the lateral side, and the popliteal vessels posteriorly. Most arthroscopists now prefer to dissect down to the capsule in the posterior regions of the joint so that these vital structures will not be compromised by inadvertent passage of the suture through the structures or by tying the suture around them.

Once appropriate sutures have been placed, they should be tied extracapsularly, and therefore buried subcutaneously. Early attempts at bringing sutures out through the skin, and tying them over a bolster, was complicated by infection in several instances.

A retractor is commonly inserted through a posterior incision which dissects down to the capsular layer. The tip of the malleable needle strikes the retractor and is deflected outwards to an area where there is no danger. A common tablespoon is of good shape to provide such deflection and act as a retractor posteriorly.

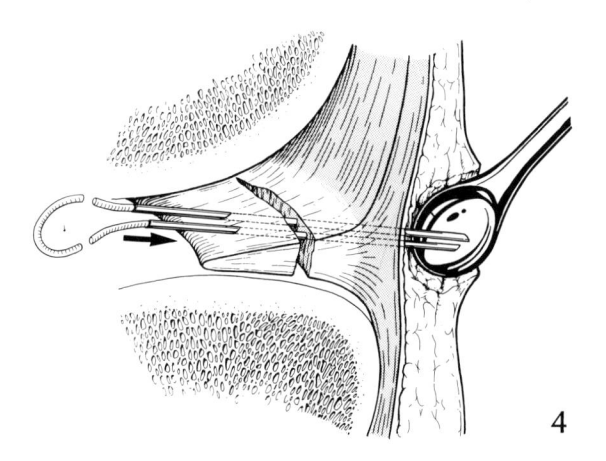

1060 Thigh and knee

'Outside-in' technique

5a, b, c & d

In this technique needles are passed from the exterior through the peripheral rim and then through the mobile inner fragment. This is usually carried out with a number 18 spinal needle through which suture material can be threaded. The advantage of this technique is that with the knee appropriately flexed and a knowledge of surface anatomy, one can choose the appropriate sites for penetration of the skin and thus avoid the neurovascular structures that are at risk with blind placement from the inside-out technique.

Once the spinal needles have been placed under arthroscopic control, two stabilization techniques are possible. One method involves suture material passed through the needle and threaded through a second needle and withdrawn so that it becomes a loop inside the joint. The second method involves passing a suture into the joint where it is retrieved, and pulled out through an anterior portal. Then a knot is tied in the end of the suture material, and it is then pulled back into the joint so that the knot abuts against the mobile fragment and pulls it firmly against the peripheral rim. Again, with the outside-in technique, dissection is carried out so that the sutures are tied over the capsule and not left exterior on the skin surface.

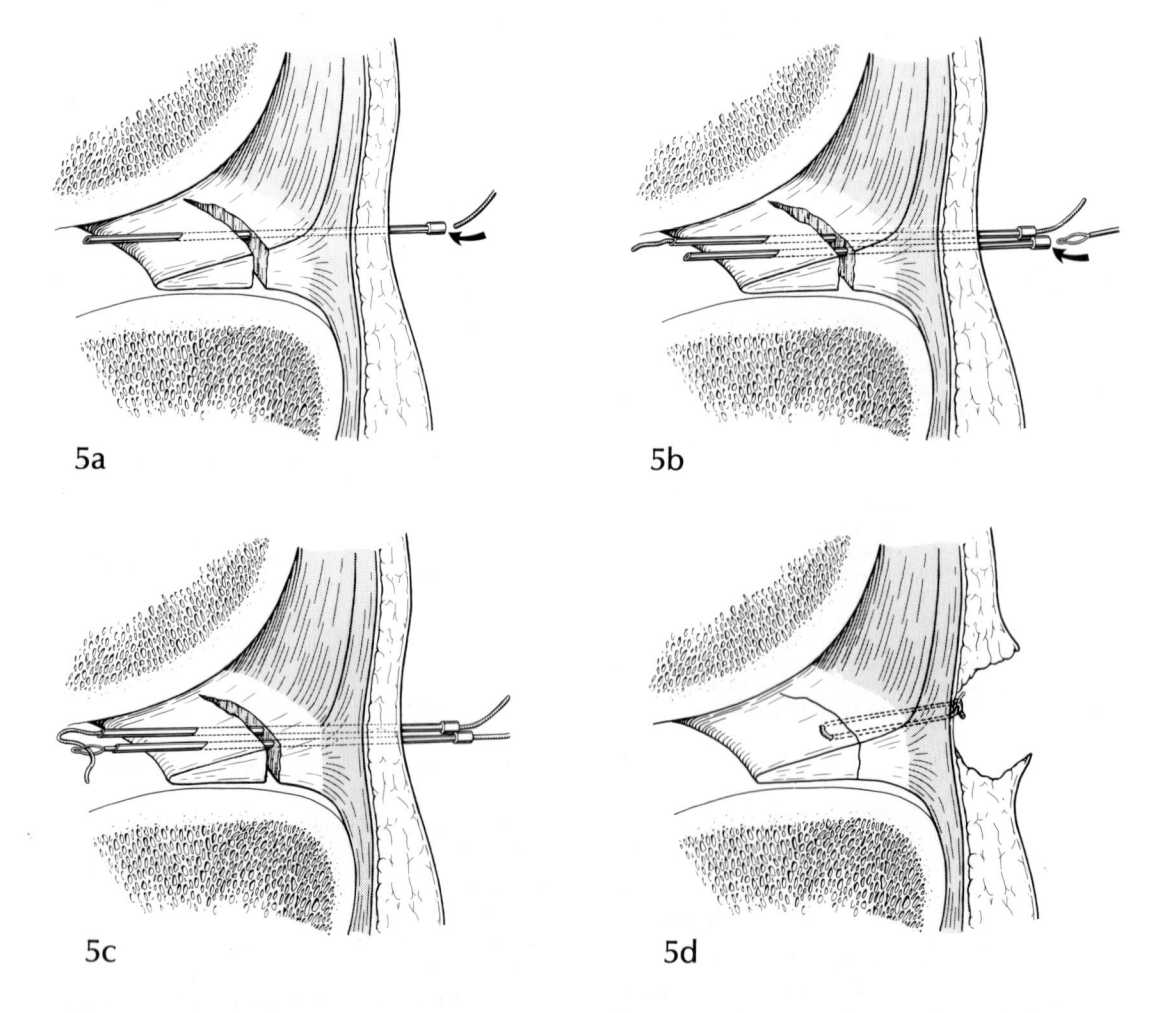

5a

5b

5c

5d

Postoperative management

Most authors recommend immobilization of the knee at 30° to 40° to avoid weight-bearing strains during the initial healing phase. Immobilization is maintained from 4 to 6 weeks. Other authors have advocated tying the sutures with the knee in full extension and immobilizing the limb in this position with immediate full weight-bearing. They argue that in this position there is little stress on the periphery of the meniscus, and if there is no pivoting or weight-bearing in flexion, the repaired area is not stressed and the patient is able to maintain function during the immobilization phase. It now appears that primary healing does occur within 4 to 6 weeks; however, consolidation of the repair probably does not occur for many months. Consequently, it is recommended that the individual be restricted from running and impact-loading for at least 4 months, and from squatting, pivoting, or other sporting activities for at least 6 months after the repair has been done.

Complications

Major complications include damage to neurovascular structures, sepsis and postoperative stiffness. On the medial side, the sartorial branch of the saphenous nerve has been damaged, through the formation of scar tissue, through the actual perforation by needles, or by tying a suture over the nerve structure. On the lateral side, similar problems have been encountered with the peroneal nerve. The disastrous effect on the lateral side is one of peroneal nerve palsy which has a far greater significance than mere sensory loss.

The most serious complications to date have been damage to the popliteal artery and vein, either through perforation by the passage of sutures or through sutures encircling the vessels and obstructing the circulation to the lower leg. Cases of amputation have been reported following this complication.

Knee infections can occur at any time but deep joint infection or pyarthrosis has been reported largely in association with sutures that were tied externally over bolsters, for a long enough period of time which allowed the ingress of bacteria to the joint. A septic knee should be treated in the usual fashion with arthroscopic lavage, appropriate distension-irrigation of the joint, and antibiotics.

Flexion contractures have been reported, presumably due to an inadvertent suture imbrication of the posterior capsule which prevents the knee from coming into full extension. For this reason, some authors advocate tying sutures with the knee in full extension. The use of absorbable sutures might minimize this complication, as any loss of extension might be regained once the suture material has been absorbed.

References

1. Cargill AO'R, Jackson JP. Bucket handle tear of the medial meniscus: a case for conservative surgery. *J Bone Joint Surg [Am]* 1976; 58-A: 248–51.

2. Dandy DJ, Jackson RW. Meniscectomy and chondromalacia of the femoral condyle. *J Bone Joint Surg [Am]* 1975; 57-A: 1116–9.

3. Fairbank TJ. Knee joint changes after meniscectomy. *J Bone Joint Surg [Br]* 1948; 30-B: 664–70.

4. Tapper EM, Hoover NW. Late results after meniscectomy. *J Bone Joint Surg [Am]* 1969; 51-A: 517–26.

5. Dandy DJ, Jackson RW. The diagnosis of problems after meniscectomy. *J Bone Joint Surg [Br]* 1975; 57-B; 349–52.

6. Gillquist J, Oretorp N. Arthroscopic partial meniscectomy: technique and long term results. *Clin Orthop* 1982; 167: 29–33.

7. McGinty JB, Geuss LF, Marvin RA. Partial or total meniscectomy: a comparative analysis. *J Bone Joint Surg [Am]* 1977; 59-A: 763–6.

8. Frankel VH, Burstein AH, Brooks DB. Biomechanics of internal derangement of the knee: pathomechanics as determined by analysis of the instant centers of motion. *J Bone Joint Surg [Am]* 1971; 53-A: 945–62.

9. Kurosawa H, Fukubayashi T, Nakajima H. Load-bearing mode of the knee joint: physical behaviour of the knee joint with or without menisci. *Clin Orthop* 1980; 149: 283–90.

10. Seedhom BB, Dowson D, Wright V. Functions of the menisci: a preliminary study. *J Bone Joint Surg [Br]* 1974; 56-B: 381–2.

11. Dandy DJ. Early results of closed partial meniscectomy. *Br Med J* 1978; 1: 1099–1100.

12. Jackson RW, Rouse, DW. The results of partial arthroscopic meniscectomy in patients over 40 years of age. *J Bone Joint Surg [Br]* 1982; 64-B: 481–5.

13. Hughston JC, Barrett GR. Acute anteromedial rotatory instability: long term results of surgical repair. *J Bone Joint Surg [Am]* 1983; 65-A: 145–53.

14. Price CT, Allen WC. Ligament repair in the knee with preservation of the meniscus. *J Bone Joint Surg [Am]* 1978; 60-A: 61–5.

15. DeHaven KE. Peripheral meniscus repair: an alternative to meniscectomy. *J Bone Joint Surg [Br]* 1981; 63-B: 463.

16. King D. The healing of semilunar cartilages. *J Bone Joint Surg* 1936; 18: 333–42.

17. Ikeuchi H. Meniscus surgery using the Watanabe arthroscope. *Orthop Clin North Am* 1979; 10: 629–42.

18. Johnson LL. *Arthroscopic surgery, principles and practice*, 3rd ed. St Louis: Mosby, 1986.

19. DeHaven KE. Meniscus repair in the athlete. *Clin Orthop* 1985; 198: 31–5.

20. Rosenberg TD, Scott SM, Coward DB, Dunbar WH, Ewing JW, Johnson CL, Paulos LE. Arthroscopic meniscal repair evaluated with repeat arthroscopy. *Arthroscopy* 1986; 2(1): 14–20.

Illustrations by Peter Cox after P. Archer

Open meniscectomy of the knee

Adrian N. Henry MCh, FRCS, FRCSI
Formerly Senior Consultant Orthopaedic Surgeon, Guy's Hospital, London, UK

Introduction

Indication

Lesions of the menisci are but one cause of symptoms of mechanical derangement of the knee joint. It is essential that an accurate preoperative diagnosis be made concerning the state of the menisci since adequate visualization of the menisci at arthrotomy is not possible and removal of a normal meniscus is undesirable. Confirmation of the clinical diagnosis should be obtained by arthroscopy or magnetic resonance imaging. The descriptions of the operations which follow relate to total meniscectomy. Current practice places much more emphasis on conservative operations on the menisci, such as removal of torn fragments or repair of peripheral detachments, under arthroscopic control.

Preoperative preparation

It is unnecessary and undesirable to shave the part prior to operation. An exsanguinating tourniquet is used, the skin prepared and the part towelled off as for other operations on the knee joint.

Operations

MEDIAL MENISCECTOMY

Incision

1

With the end of the table lowered and the knee flexed 90° with a pad beneath it, a slightly oblique, vertical, medial, parapatellar incision of approximately 5 cm in length is made one thumb's-breadth medial to the border of the patella and patellar tendon and just crossing the upper margin of the tibial plateau distally.

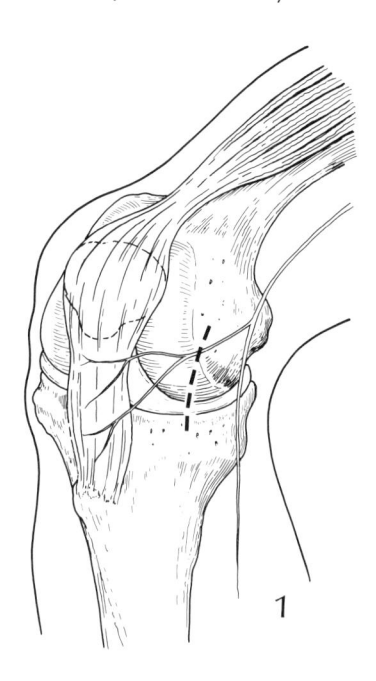

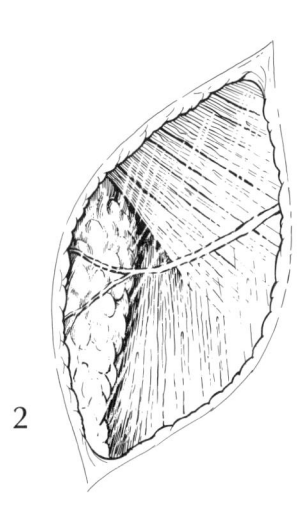

Exposure

2

The infrapatellar branch of the saphenous nerve is sought in the subcutaneous fat immediately superficial to the fibrous capsule. This nerve crosses the operative field at an inconstant level and if identified should be resected wide of the incision by sharp division.

3

Next, the two layers of the fibrous capsule are divided in the same direction and length as the skin incision. The synovial membrane is also opened in a similar manner at the upper end of the incision to avoid damage to the meniscus. A medium-sized Langenbeck retractor is placed in the lateral edge of the incision, retracting the infrapatellar fat pad laterally.

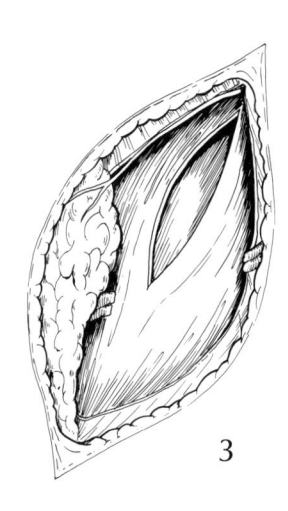

4

A Stamm or similar retractor is inserted into the medial aspect of the incision, retracting the fibrous and synovial capsules medially. This retraction exposes the anterior horn of the medial meniscus together with the distal insertion of the anterior cruciate ligament and part of the articular cartilage of the medial femoral condyle on its lateral aspect.

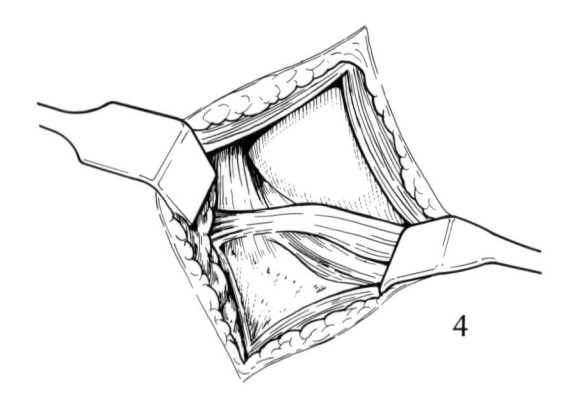

Mobilization of anterior horn of the medial meniscus

5

A blunt hook is inserted under the free margin of the anterior horn to emerge through the coronary ligament on the inferior aspect of the meniscus.

6

Using the plane of the hook as a guide, a scapel with rounded tip incises the coronary ligament at the tip of the hook and is directed in a horizontal plane laterally and then vertically to detach the anterior horn of the meniscus. Care must be taken to avoid damage to the anterior cruciate ligament.

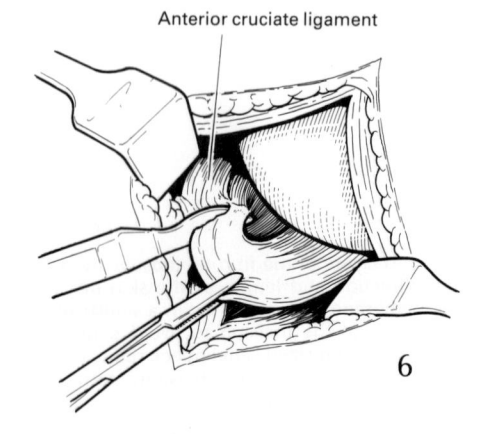

Excision of medial meniscus

7

The detached anterior horn is now gripped by Kocher's forceps and, with the scalpel, the meniscus is divided along its periphery just inside its attachment to the synovial membrane.

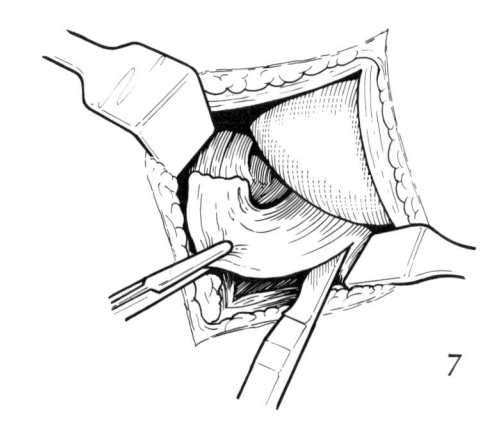

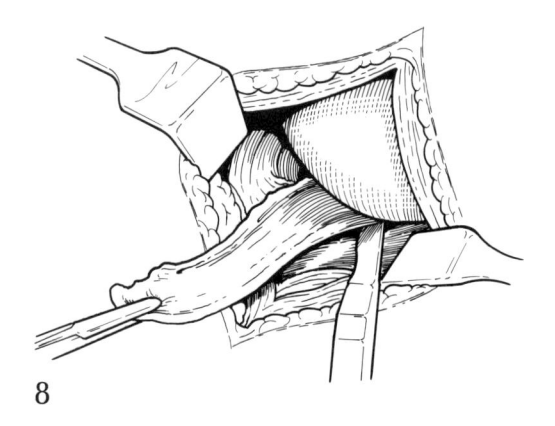

8

This division continues along the periphery of the meniscus at the same time as the Kocher's forceps are exerting a laterally directed pull on the meniscus. Mobilization of the periphery of the meniscus is continued posteromedially until the structure displaces into the centre of the joint.

9

Finally, the attachment of the posterior horn is divided and the meniscus removed.

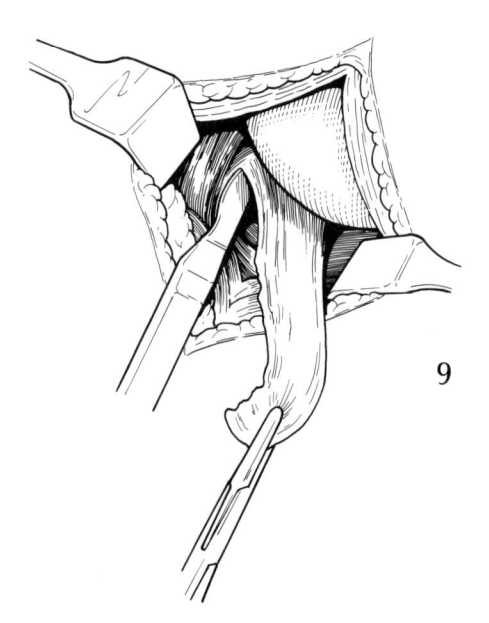

Closure

10

The synovial membrane is closed by a continuous haemostatic plain catgut or polyglactin 910 suture.

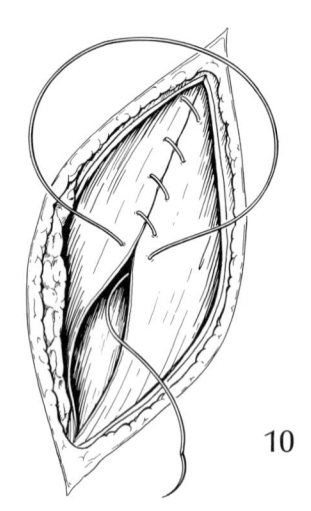

11

The two layers of the fibrous capsule are closed together with interrupted chromic catgut polyglactin sutures. Skin may be closed by interrupted sutures or a continuous subcuticular stitch of nylon or polypropylene.

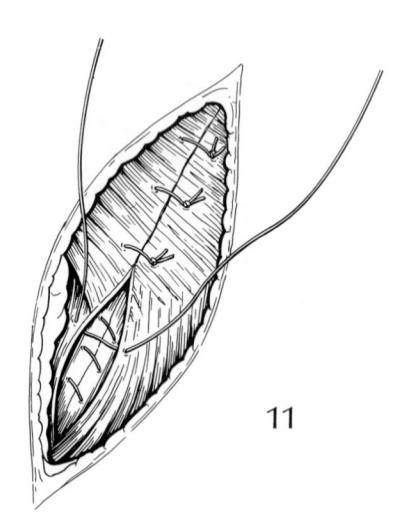

Postoperative management

A two-layer wool and crêpe bandage is applied from ankle to groin before removal of the tourniquet. On regaining consciousness the patient is immediately instructed to start quadriceps exercises and these are continued with bedrest until 48 hours postoperatively, when the patient may begin partial weight-bearing on crutches. The compression bandage is maintained for 10–14 days when the sutures are removed and flexion exercises may then be commenced in addition to continuing the quadriceps drill. At this stage crutches may be discarded and the patient may gradually resume normal activity, which should be possible at approximately 4–6 weeks after operation depending on his occupation.

LATERAL MENISCECTOMY

Incision

12

Without lowering the end of the table, the knee is flexed 120°. A horizontal incision is made in the skin from the lateral edge of the patellar tendon to the fibular collateral ligament and approximately 0.5 cm above the level of the lateral tibial plateau.

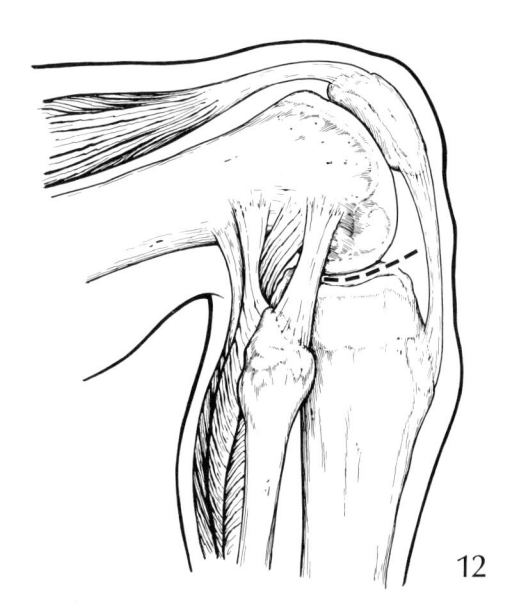

Exposure

13

After retraction of the skin edges the fibres of the iliotibial tract are divided in the direction in which they run, which is approximately similar to that of the skin incision. The tract is divided throughout the same length as the skin incision.

14

The edges of the iliotibial tract are retracted by a self-retaining retractor. This exposes the extrasynovial lateral infrapatellar fat pad in the anterior half of the wound and the synovial membrane in the posterior half. An incision is made in the latter and carried forward through the fat pad almost to the patellar tendon.

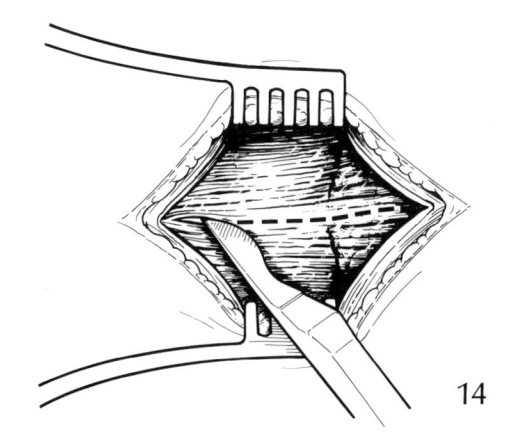

15

A medium-sized Langenbeck retractor is then inserted into the anterior end of the wound, retracting the fat pad. This exposes the anterior aspect of the lateral meniscus.

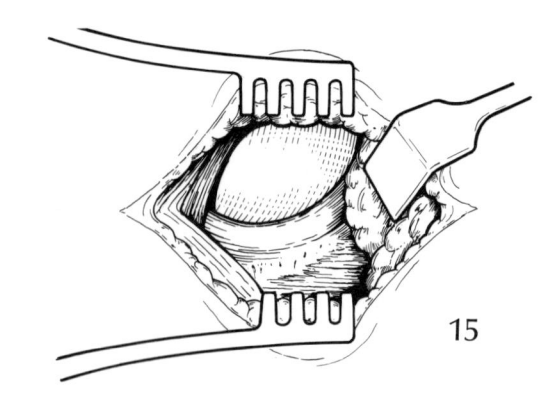

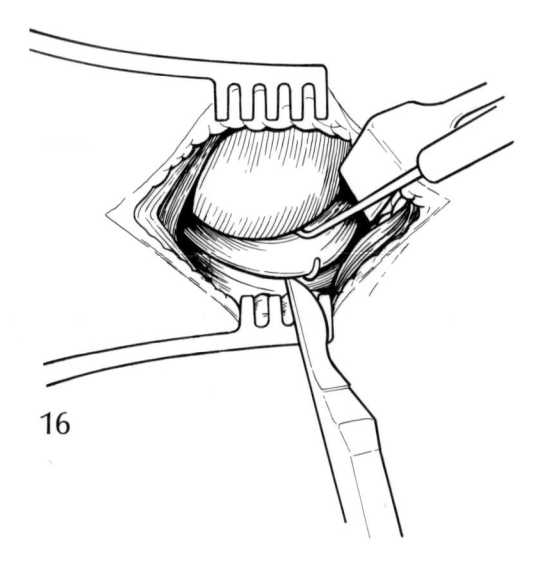

Mobilization of the meniscus

16

A blunt hook is inserted under the anterior horn of the lateral meniscus, as in medial meniscectomy, and the anterior horn mobilized in a similar manner.

17

After the anterior horn has been gripped by Kocher's forceps, the meniscus is detached from the synovial membrane by a scalpel and a small Langenbeck retractor is inserted into the posterior end of the wound to retract the popliteal tendon and the leash of lateral inferior geniculate vessels running just anterior to it.

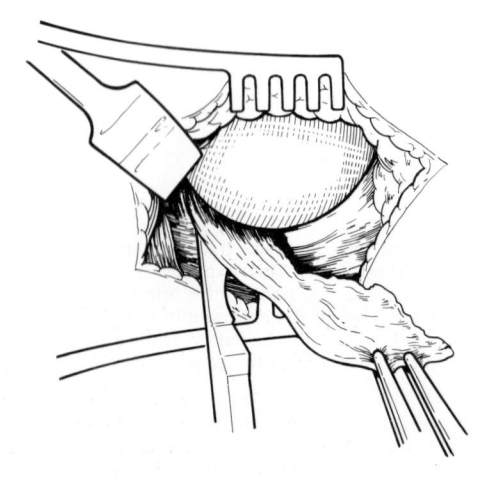

18

The peripheral attachment of the meniscus is deficient surrounding the popliteal tendon and is continued posteriorly by a loose tenuous attachment to the posterior horn. The peripheral attachment is divided posteriorly beyond the popliteal tendon, at the same time exerting an anterior strain by the Kocher's forceps on the meniscus. The extreme attachment of the posterior horn from the tibia is divided with removal of the whole meniscus.

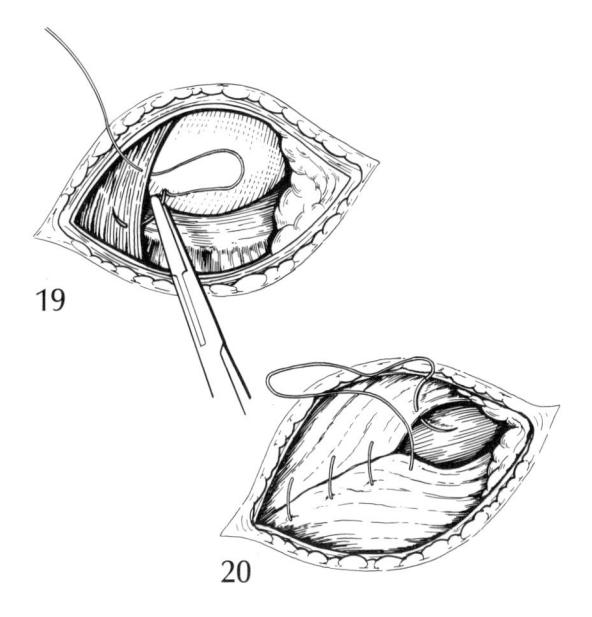

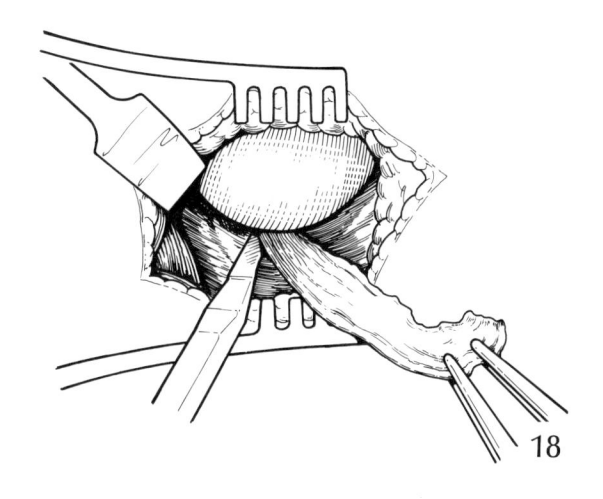

Closure

19 & 20

The synovial membrane is closed with a continuous haemostatic plain catgut or polyglactin suture, particular attention being paid to inclusion of the lateral inferior geniculate vessels in the initial stitch.

21

The iliotibial tract is closed with interrupted chromic catgut or polyglactin and the skin is closed according to the surgeon's choice.

Postoperative management

The postoperative programme for lateral meniscectomy is similar to that for the medial side. However, the incidence of postoperative haemarthrosis is greater following lateral meniscectomy owing to haemorrhage from the lateral inferior geniculate vessels. This complication must be watched for and dealt with at an early date by aspiration or evacuation of the haematoma or haemarthrosis, otherwise the patient's postoperative recovery is delayed.

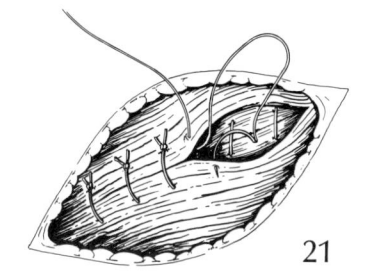

1070 Thigh and knee

EXCISION OF RETAINED POSTERIOR HORN OF MEDIAL MENISCUS

Occasionally the posterior horn of the meniscus may become detached during the procedure of medial meniscectomy. If the retained fragment is large and mobile it should be removed through a separate posteromedial incision. The patient should be placed supine on the table with a sandbag under the opposite buttock and the knee flexed 90° to expose the posteromedial corner of the knee joint.

Incision

22

An oblique incision is made in the skin approximately 2.5 cm in length on the posteromedial aspect of the knee joint.

Exposure

After retraction of the skin edges the important posteromedial component of the medial capsule is exposed and an incision made through this structure in the direction of its fibres. Deep to the fibrous capsule the synovial membrane is exposed and divided in a similar manner. Small Langenbeck retractors are inserted to expose the posterior horn of the medial meniscus and this is removed by peripheral division as during medial meniscectomy.

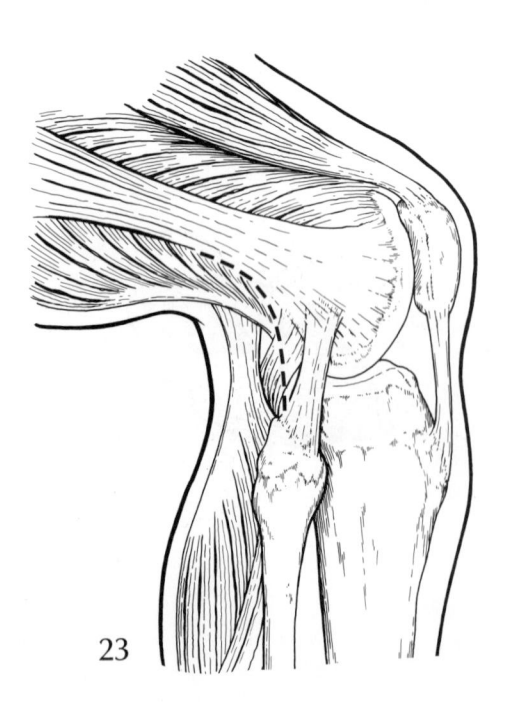

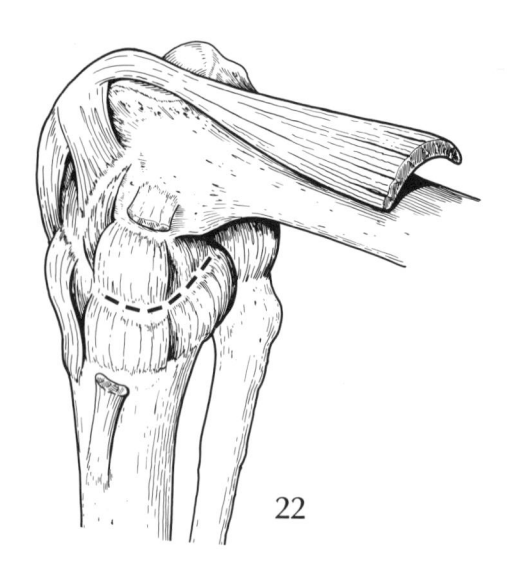

Closure

Closure is carried out in a similar manner to that for the anterior incision during medial meniscectomy, particular care being taken to repair the posteromedial capsular ligament.

EXCISION OF POSTERIOR HORN OF LATERAL MENISCUS

Position of patient

The patient is positioned on his side with the affected knee uppermost and flexed 70°.

Incision

23

The skin is incised along the posterior border of the iliotibial tract for approximately 5 cm distal to the styloid process of the fibula.

Exposure

24

The posterior margin of the iliotibial tract is freed from the fascia overlying the biceps muscle.

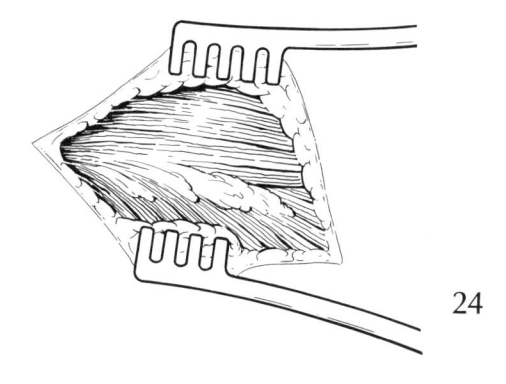

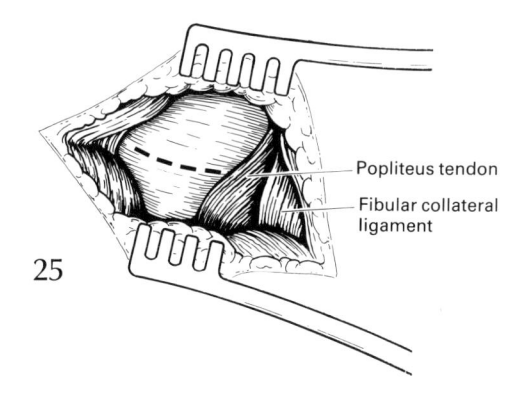

25

The iliotibial tract is retracted superiorly and the biceps muscle inferiorly. After separation of these structures the fibular collateral ligament is seen running vertically in the distal part of the incision, and just deep to the ligament the popliteal tendon runs obliquely upwards and forwards.

26

Both these structures are retracted to reveal the underlying synovial membrane which is divided horizontally just above the posterior horn of the lateral meniscus.

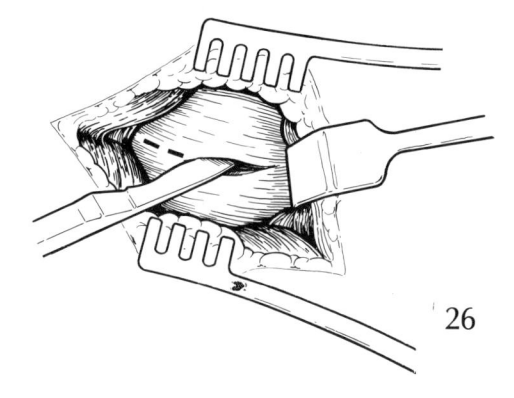

1072 Thigh and knee

27

Langenbeck retractors are inserted to show the posterior horn of the meniscus. This is then detached peripherally and at its insertion to the tibial intercondylar area.

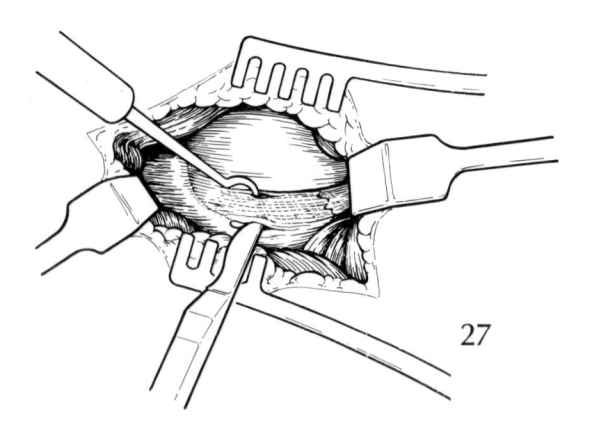

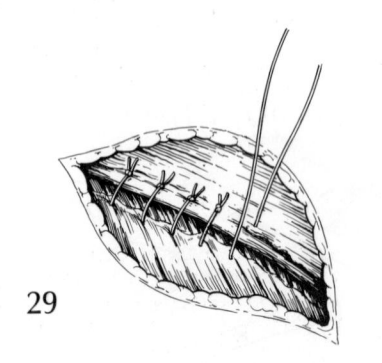

Closure

28 & 29

Closure is effected in layers in similar fashion to closure of other meniscectomy incisions.

Illustrations by Peter Cox after B. Hyams

Loose bodies in the knee

Paul Aichroth MS, FRCS
Consultant Orthopaedic Surgeon, Westminster Hospital and Westminster Children's Hospital, London; Queen Mary's Hospital, Roehampton, UK

Introduction

Loose bodies form in the knee joint in a variety of different conditions. The majority are due to the following conditions.

Osteochondritis dissecans

A fragment of articular cartilage and subchondral bone separates from a joint surface. This condition may be considered an ununited osteochondral fracture of the femoral condyle. Rarely is the patellar surface involved.

Acute osteochondral fractures

A fragment is avulsed from the femoral condyle in a severe knee injury. Also, fragments separate by shearing stresses from the lateral margin of the femoral groove of the femur and the patella in twisting injuries.

Osteoarthritis

Rarely, an osteophyte separates from the articular margin and becomes free in the joint. The cartilage component may increase in size as the articular cartilage proliferates.

Synovial osteochondromatosis

Metaplasia of the synovial membrane results in the formation of a multitude of small chondromatous bodies. The cartilaginous material then ossifies and the bodies become radio-opaque. These may float free in the synovial cavity. The posterior synovial pouch is frequently involved.

Avascular necrosis of bone

Loose fragments of necrotic bone together with hyaline cartilage separate in steroid arthropathies, caisson disease and other conditions where massive necrosis of the femoral condylar bone occurs. Loose fragments shed from a necrotic femoral condyle are an increasing problem in the post-renal transplantation arthropathies.

Symptoms and signs of a loose body

The loose body may sometimes be palpated in the parapatellar or suprapatellar region. The knee joint becomes internally deranged only when the fragment becomes jammed between the joint surfaces. It produces the following.

1. Pain
2. Locking of the joint during movement
3. Synovial effusion.

Indications for removal

Loose bodies may be present in the knee joint singly or in large numbers. They may remain asymptomatic but if the above symptoms of an internal derangement occur they should be removed. A patient may present with pain and disability in an osteoarthritic knee and on X-ray examination loose bodies are found. Episodes of locking will necessitate an arthrotomy or arthroscopy to remove the loose fragments; but, in the absence of locking, the joint may be treated by conservative means.

Arthroscopic removal of loose bodies

The removal of loose bodies may be undertaken arthroscopically as described in the chapter on 'Arthroscopic surgical procedures' (see pp. 1019–1032). It may be very simple to remove the loose body in the anterior compartment after appropriate visualization, localization and then extraction using the pituitary rongeur or spiked grasping forceps. However, the loose body may move to a difficult position or to the posterior recesses. It will then become much more difficult and before embarking on such an arthroscopic procedure the operator must be conversant with all arthroscopic approaches to the knee.

Arthrotomy may be indicated if there are multiple or very large loose bodies.

OPEN REMOVAL

Preoperative

The position of the loose body should be determined by palpation. The fragment in the suprapatellar pouch is best approached with the knee extended. Fragments seen radiologically to be lying on the tibial plateau are usually not palpable, and these, together with loose bodies posteromedially and posterolaterally, are best approached with the knee flexed over the end of the table. An Esmarch bandage is applied to exsanguinate the limb and a pneumatic cuff is inflated around the upper thigh. The knee should be palpated again and the joint position arranged as indicated above. A radiograph must be taken in the anteroposterior and lateral planes – with the knee in the position in which it will be opened – if the fragment cannot be felt with certainty.

These careful preoperative precautions must be undertaken to avoid the situation where the joint is opened with one incision and the fragment has moved to another area, where a second incision is required.

Operations

LOOSE BODY REMOVAL FROM THE SUPRAPATELLAR POUCH AND ANTERIOR CAVITY

The skin of the knee, the thigh and the leg is prepared and towelled in such a way that the knee may be flexed. An incise drape may be used. If the loose body can be palpated it should be transfixed with a sterile needle through the skin.

Incision

A vertical parapatellar incision is recommended. Ideally, this should be over the loose body if it can be palpated or in the appropriate position if the site of the fragment has been identified radiologically. When the fragment is due to osteochondritis dissecans, or osteochondral fracture, the parapatellar incision may be extended inferiorly to allow inspection of the condylar crater from which the loose body came. After skin incision, the parapatellar aponeurosis is opened in the same line. The synovium is then exposed and should be incised in the same line, with the incision entering the joint cavity. The loose fragment sometimes pops through, with a rush of synovial fluid, but more commonly it is obscured from view by a synovial fold.

Technique

1 & 2

As soon as the fragment is sighted a large curette should be positioned behind it so that there is little chance of the body being squeezed by the approaching broad forceps and moved to another part of the joint. If this technique fails, and the loose body moves, then it may be retrieved by palpating the area through the skin and pushing it back into view. Flexing and extending the joint may be helpful but, if this fails, syringing the joint cavity with a large quantity of normal saline may be successful.

The above manoeuvres are usually successful, but if they are not a second glove may be donned, and the joint cavity explored with the finger. A further radiograph may be helpful, or the arthroscope inserted through the wound may reveal the site of the loose fragment.

Closure

The synovium is closed with a fine chromic catgut or polyglactin 910 (Vicryl, Ethicon, Edinburgh, UK) continuous suture. Interrupted 1/0 or 2/0 chromic catgut or Vicryl sutures will approximate the patellar expansion and the subcutaneous tissues. The skin is closed with intradermal nylon or Prolene (Ethicon, Edinburgh, UK) reinforced by surgical tapes.

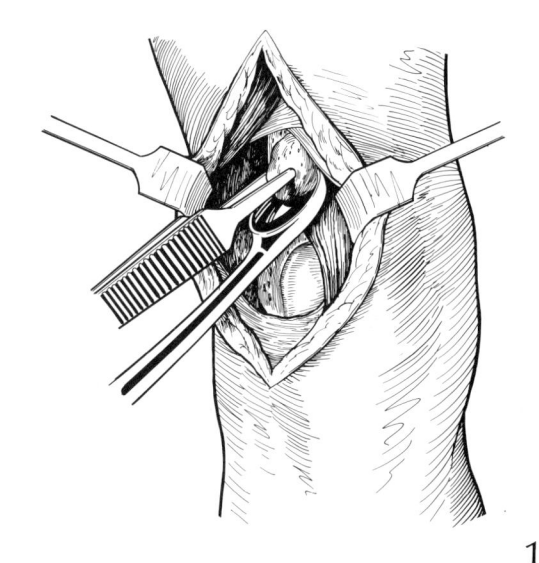

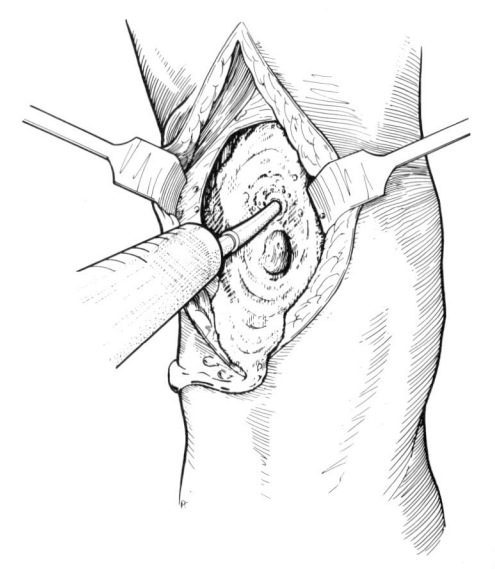

Dressing

3

The limb is wrapped in cotton wool from the thigh to above the ankle and compression bandages applied. Side slabs of plaster of Paris within the layers of bandage will give extra support and strength. The patient can walk, weight-bearing, after 48 hours and begin knee flexion after 5 days. Sutures should be removed after 14 days if the wound is satisfactory.

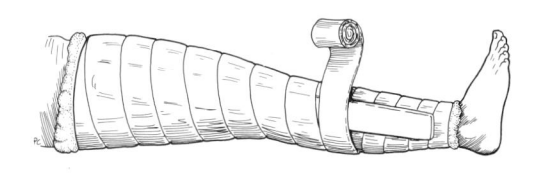

REMOVAL FROM THE POSTERIOR COMPARTMENT

The posterior cruciate ligament and its synovial reflection separates the posterior aspect of the knee into two compartments. It is therefore essential to identify the particular compartment containing the posterior loose body.

Posteromedial approach

4

The knee is flexed and a vertical incision is made, centred on the joint line posteromedially. The oblique fibres of the posteromedial capsule behind the medial collateral ligament are exposed. This layer is incised vertically, and after entering the synovium the posterior horn of the medial meniscus and the posterior compartment is exposed.

Posterolateral approach

5

The knee is flexed and a posterolateral curved incision is made anterior to the fibular head and the biceps femoris tendon. The lateral popliteal nerve is behind these two structures. The popliteus tendon is seen between the biceps tendon and the lateral collateral ligament. This is retracted posteriorly, the capsule and synovium are incised and the posterior compartment opened.

TREATMENT OF OSTEOCHONDRITIS DISSECANS

6

Osteochondritis dissecans may be considered a subchondral or osteochondral surface fracture. Some lesions will heal and others will remain ununited in a crater and will later separate as a loose body. Eighty-five per cent affect the medial femoral condyle and 70 per cent are situated in the classic site on the intercondylar region of the medial femoral condyle. Fifty per cent of patients with such a lesion give a history of substantial trauma, and as a group they are excellent athletes.

Arthroscopic procedures

The fragment may be removed and the crater curetted using arthroscopic techniques. Alternatively, the fragment may be drilled under direct arthroscopic inspection using powered instruments.

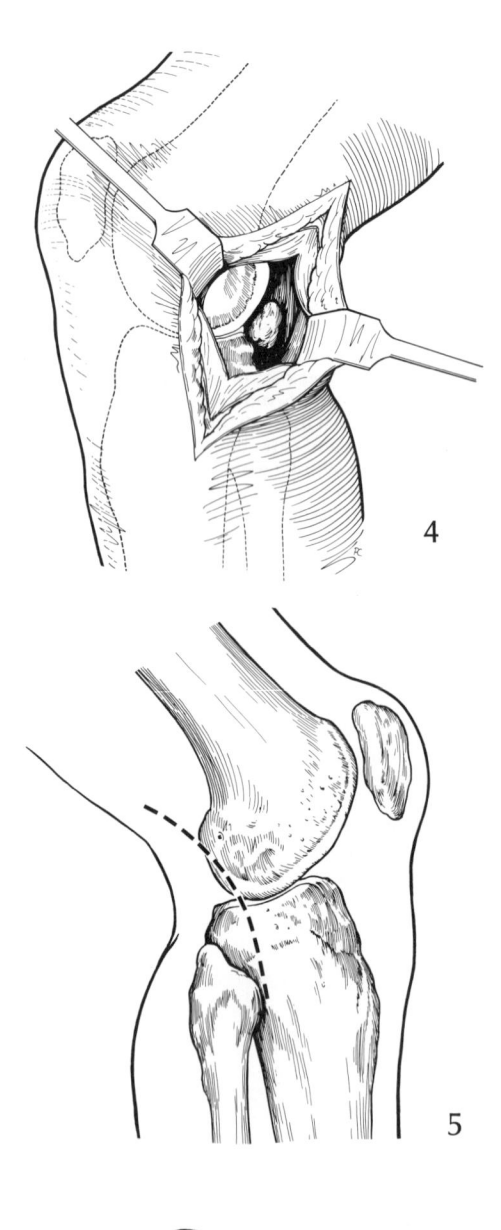

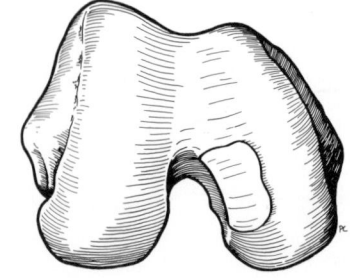

Osteochondritis dissecans with the fragment *in situ*

7 & 8

If the fragment remains in its crater, and the symptoms are slight, then it should be left alone. Arthroscopy is useful to confirm the fixity of the fragment and to exclude any other internal derangement. Regular clinical and radiological follow-up will be required to confirm the healing or separation of the fragment. If the knee locks or regularly gives way, it is likely that the fragment is hinging or moving in its crater. Arthrotomy is then required with approaches similar to those used in meniscectomy. If the fragment is loose in its crater, it should be excised and the crater curetted. All fibrous tissue should be removed and drilling performed to expose bleeding bone. This allows the proliferation of fibrocartilaginous material in the crater and produces a remarkably smooth surface.

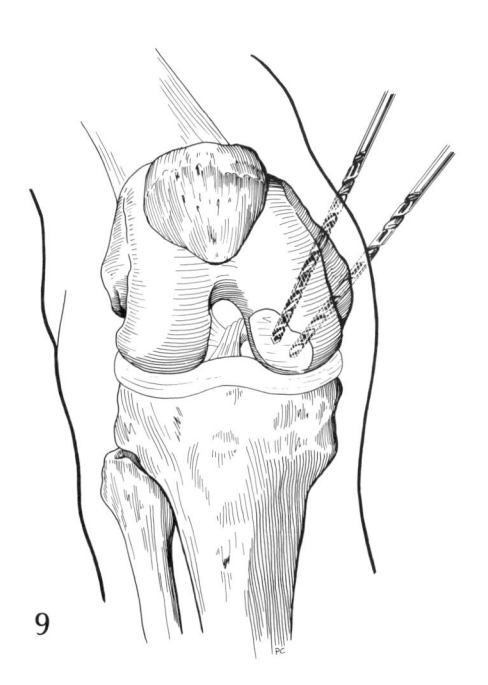

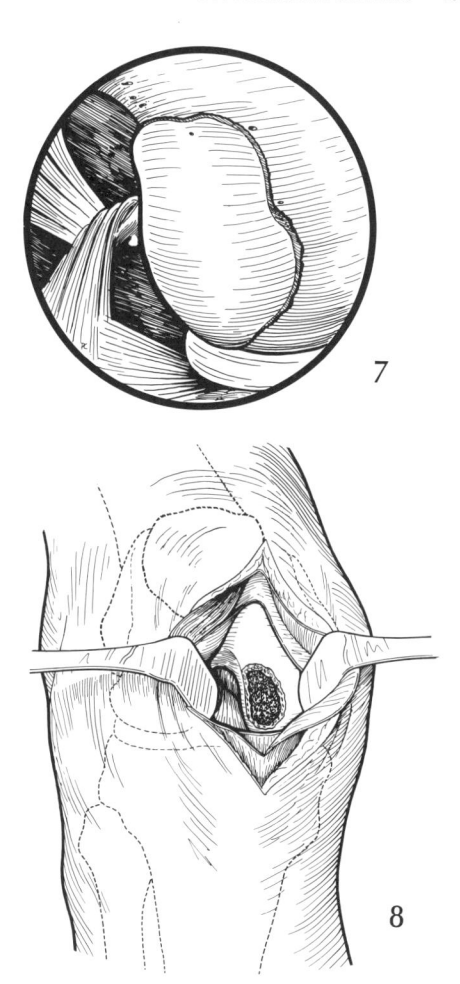

9

If at arthrotomy the fragment is found very tightly *in situ* or the fragment is not visible from the intact cartilaginous surface (the fracture being entirely subchondral), then the bony fragment may be drilled from the condylar side. The twist-drills traverse the pseudarthrosis but do not pierce the condylar surface cartilage and so stimulate healing and revascularization from the subchondral bone. Alternatively, the fragment may be drilled at arthroscopy with a fine bone wire on a power drill.

Osteochondritis dissecans with a loose body

The loose body should be removed as described above and the crater from which it came should be inspected and curetted. There is no definite indication for replacement of the loose fragment using internal fixation for it is only rarely possible to produce enough stability of the fragment with a good fit of the articular surfaces and bony apposition to allow union to occur.

1078 Thigh and knee

TREATMENT OF THE ACUTE OSTEOCHONDRAL FRACTURE

Osteochondral fractures are sustained in severe injuries to the knee joint. Avulsion or shearing off of a fragment is associated with a rapid large haemarthrosis, and oblique, tunnel and sky-line radiographs may be required for its detection. Small fragments should be removed at arthrotomy but larger fragments (2 × 2 cm or more) may be repositioned accurately and internally fixed.

Technique

10

The crater is approached as above (p. 1074) and is debrided. The fragment is similarly prepared and is repositioned with the correct orientation. Two or more Smillie pins are inserted to transfix the fragment with their heads punched just beneath the cartilage surface. The wound is closed and dressed as above (p. 1075). Alternatively, small Herbert screws with reverse threads are ideal and produce good fixation with compression.

Postoperative management

A compression bandage of wool and crêpe is applied from ankle to groin and the leg is elevated for 24 hours. Quadriceps exercises begin as soon as pain allows and weight-bearing in the bandages with crutches at 48 hours.

The knee is mobilized when the wound is healed at 2 weeks after operation. Minimal weight-bearing on crutches is recommended until the fragment unites. A further arthrotomy may then be required after 1 year to remove the pins or screws.

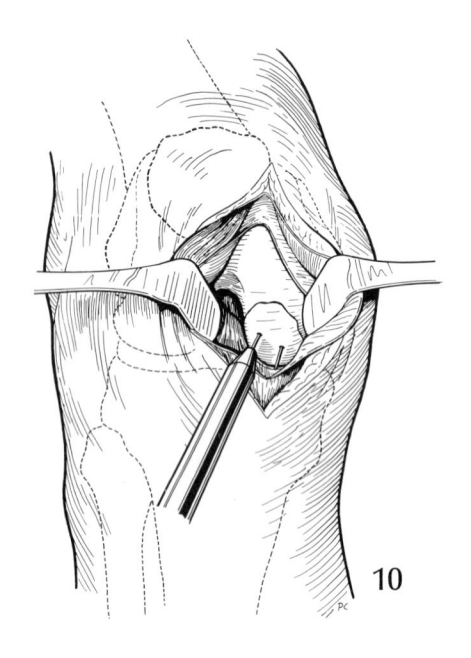

SYNOVIAL OSTEOCHONDROMATOSIS

This is a poorly understood condition in which the whole synovial lining is involved. Symptoms are frequently severe and on opening the joint vast numbers of loose bodies gush out. A synovectomy will be required (see pp. 1109–1112) and a posterior synovial mass may require excision through the popliteal fossa via a formal posterior approach.

Illustrations by Peter Cox

Repair and reconstruction of knee ligament injury

Paul Aichroth MS, FRCS
Consultant Orthopaedic Surgeon, Westminster Hospital and Westminster Children's Hospital, London; Queen Mary's Hospital, Roehampton, UK

Introduction

Injury to a knee ligament may be partial or complete. A sprain or partial tear of the medial collateral ligament may occur in isolation and is very painful. The stability of the ligament, however, remains intact and treatment is that of pain relief and then full rehabilitation. Temporary splintage may be required in the most painful stage.

The complete tear of a knee ligament is rarely in isolation. O'Donoghue described his 'unhappy triad' of medial collateral ligament tear, anterior cruciate avulsion and an injury to the medial meniscus.

The assessment of a knee ligament injury must include a full history and a detailed clinical examination. The type of injury sustained often indicates the structures damaged. For example, a dashboard injury to the knee is frequently associated with a tell-tale anterior bruise and abrasion on the tibial tubercle, and a posterior cruciate ligament tear is detected when undertaking posterior drawer and Lachman tests.

Clinical examination of the knee must be undertaken carefully to assess the medial and lateral collateral stability by means of a valgus and varus strain in a few degrees of flexion. Cruciate ligaments are assessed by anterior and posterior drawer signs with the knee at right angles, and, more importantly, by the Lachman test, in which the tibia is brought forwards and backwards on the femur in 20° flexion. Rotary instability of the knee joint must also be assessed, and anterolateral rotary instability with a 'pivot shift' and a jerk is present in an anterior cruciate ligament tear with associated capsular laxity.

Posterior cruciate ligament laxity is best assessed with the knee at right angles when a posterior sag of the tibia on the femur is noted. The posterior drawer sign is positive at this angle, and a posterior drawer or posterior Lachman manoeuvre may also be positive with the knee at 20° flexion. Rotary instability may also be detected with a posterior cruciate ligament injury if the posteromedial and posterolateral structures are damaged in association. There may be a reverse pivot shift or, alternatively, a hyperextension lateral rotation sign if the great toe is lifted high. Immediately following a knee injury, swelling, tenderness and general irritability may prevent movement and adequate examination. The sight of a strong athlete walking into the examination room with a complete rupture of the medial and cruciate ligaments must not fool the surgeon. In these circumstances it is vital to assess the knee ligament structures and their integrity by examination under anaesthesia. At the same time an arthroscopy is undertaken to elucidate any problem of internal derangement fully. There is an associated haemarthrosis in most patients with an acute injury of this type, and at arthroscopy patient and copious irrigation is required to obtain a good view of all internal structures. A hook is always necessary to assess the stability of the menisci and anterior cruciate ligament. The meniscal damage may be treated arthroscopically at this stage.

The presence of clinical physical signs together with the results of examination under anaesthesia and arthroscopy will allow a plan of surgical action to be made. Early and accurate diagnosis is necessary so that appropriate treatment may avoid the need for reconstruction later.

Operations

MEDIAL COLLATERAL LIGAMENT REPAIR

Examination under anaesthesia is undertaken to assess knee ligamentous damage fully. Arthroscopy is also performed to elucidate any internal derangement. A plan of repair and reconstruction is then made and any meniscal damage may be treated arthroscopically.

After exsanguination, a high thigh tourniquet is applied. The knee is flexed over the end of the table or is maintained in this position with a knee rest.

Incision

1a & b

A long, curved, medial parapatellar incision is made. The middle portion of the incision is situated in the appropriate place for formal medial arthrotomy. The superior part of the incision is curved posteriorly to allow access to the more posterior portions of the joint and its posteromedial capsule.

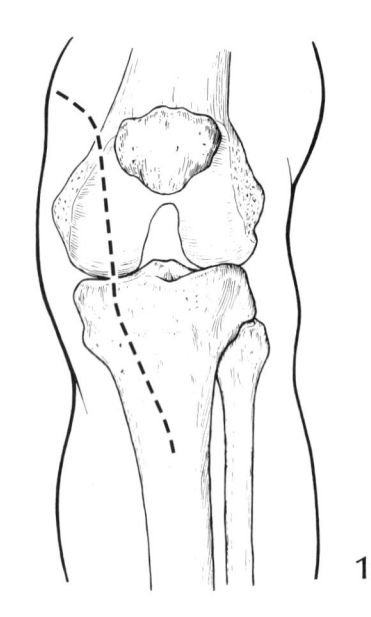

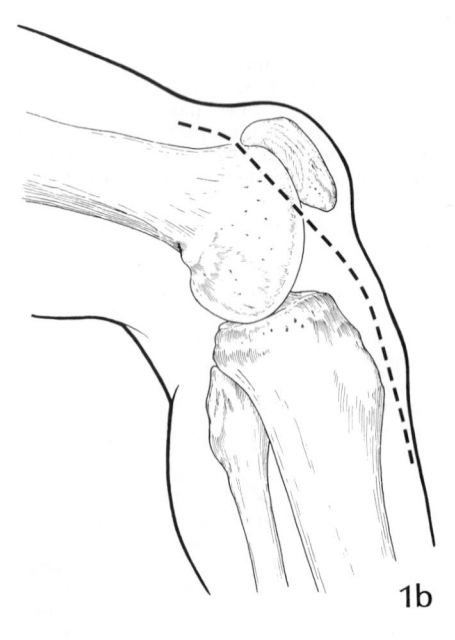

Exploration

2

The whole of the medial capsule and medial collateral ligament is exposed. A swab is used to wipe away the superficial areolar tissue which is frequently infiltrated by blood or oedema. It is important to explore as far as the posterior aspect of the capsule as this structure is frequently ruptured behind the medial collateral ligament. It may be obvious that the superficial part of the medial collateral ligament is ruptured from the femur above or the tibia below.

The superficial collateral ligament is then incised in the line of its fibres to expose the deep layer of the medial collateral ligament beneath. The deep ligament may be ruptured at the midpoint of its attachment to the medial meniscus or it may be shredded and stretched at this site.

The medial meniscus may be torn peripherally and an assessment must be made to determine whether it is to be repaired or removed. If removal is indicated, a formal anteromedial arthrotomy is made through the capsule and a routine meniscectomy undertaken unless prior arthroscopic treatment has been performed. If the anterior cruciate is to be repaired or reconstructed, this must be planned before the medial collateral ligament and medial capsule repair sutures are finally tightened.

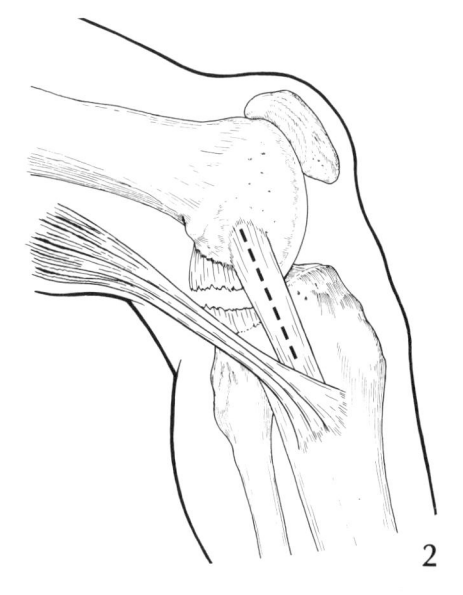

Technique of repair

3a & b

The exact reposition site for the superior attachment of the medial collateral ligament must be identified. However, it is ideal to repair the posterior capsule and also the posterior oblique fibres of the medial collateral ligament initially. Sutures of 1/0 Dexon (Davis and Geck, Gosport, UK) or Vicryl (Ethicon, Edinburgh, UK) are recommended. The sutures should be placed obliquely to bring the superior fibres in this repair more anterior.

Superior or inferior reattachment of the medial collateral ligament must be accurately undertaken with sutures which pass through the bone. The bone is drilled with an awl or fine drill entering the bone surface at 45°. A stout trocar/small-radius needle is used to pass the sutures through interconnecting holes in the bone to reattach the collateral ligament tightly. If, however, a main portion of the medial collateral ligament has been avulsed from the bone, it may be reattached using a barbed staple of the Richards type.

Tears of the midpoint of the deep medial collateral ligament may require attachment to the medial meniscus, and the peripheral edge can be used to receive the suture material. Shreds in this position are again brought into a more anterior position with appropriate placement of the sutures. It should be noted that the tibia is rotated medially whilst the sutures are tightened and the layers are advanced anteriorly.

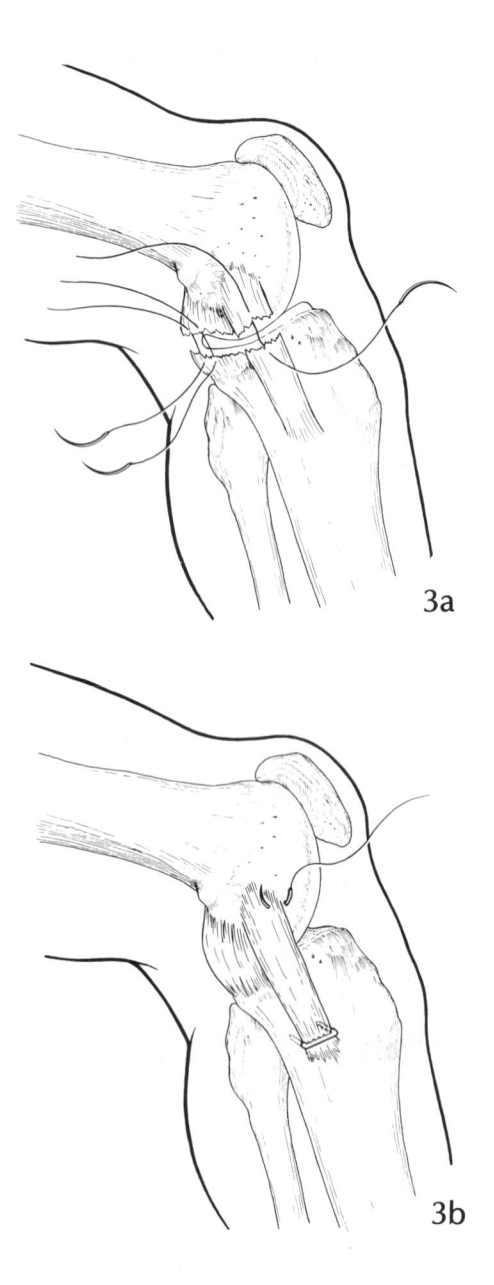

3a

3b

Postoperative management

The wound is closed with suction drainage and the limb is placed in a cast in some 30°–40° flexion with the tibia rotated medially. At 5–6 weeks the cast is removed and physiotherapy is continued, followed by progressive rehabilitation. However, if the repair is thought to be strong and tight, the surgeon may decide that gentle early restricted movement is possible followed by a brace. In this situation, a constant passive motion machine may be used with the movement setting between 30° and 80° of flexion. When the wound is quiescent and movement may be maintained, a brace is applied with a setting at approximately 20°–80° of flexion. This must be maintained for 6 weeks after operation and during this period the patient does not bear weight and remains on crutches.

POSTERIOR CRUCIATE LIGAMENT REPAIR

This is a large structure which may be torn in isolation or in combination with any other knee ligament. The posterior capsule is frequently injured and the combination may constitute a posteromedial or posterolateral instability. The tibia is posteriorly displaced on the femur, the ligament is either pulled off the bone or, frequently, a bone fragment is avulsed from its inferior tibial attachment.

After exsanguination of the limb, a high thigh tourniquet is applied and the patient is positioned prone.

Incision

4

An S-shaped incision is made across the popliteal fossa with the inferior limb on the medial side. The deep fascia is divided in the same line and the posterior cutaneous nerve of the calf is preserved.

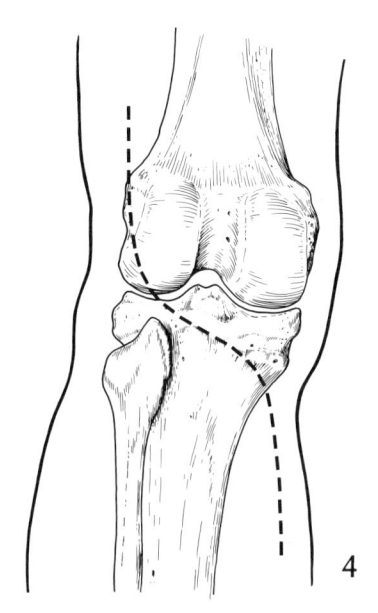

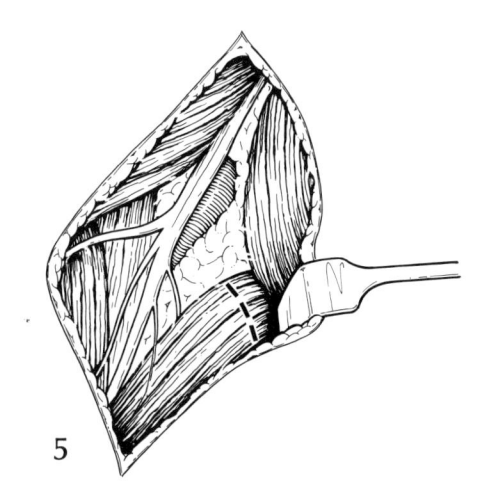

Dissection

5

The medial head of gastrocnemius is isolated and dissected superiorly to its attachment on the back of the femoral condyle. It is divided transversely near its attachment to the bone. The medial edge of the muscle is then dissected free and the whole structure retracted to the lateral side.

Repair

6

The medial superior genicular vessel may be over the site of the capsule incision and require division after ligation. The middle genicular vessel must be similarly ligated. A vertical incision is made through the capsule and posterior oblique ligament near the midline, and the posterior cruciate and its bone fragment detachment can be seen. The bone fragment may then be screwed back into the bed from which it has been avulsed using a cancellous screw. If the ligament has been torn above the bone it may be sutured back and multifilament Dacron (du Pont de Nemours and Company, UK) sutures may be used, passing through bony tunnels. However, midsubstance posterior cruciate tears are best reconstructed using a tendon transfer of semitendinosus and gracilis as discussed below.

Postoperative management

The capsular incision is repaired and the medial head of the gastrocnemius resutured. The wound is closed with drainage and the knee is placed in a cast in a few degrees of flexion for 5–6 weeks. Vigorous rehabilitation emphasizing active movement follows. Sporting activity is forbidden for 6 months.

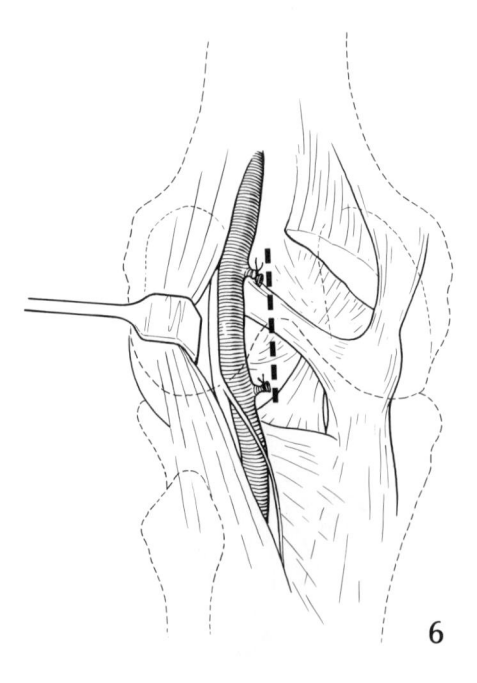

ANTERIOR CRUCIATE LIGAMENT REPAIR

Rupture of the anterior cruciate ligament may occur in isolation or with medial collateral ligament and medial meniscus injuries. If an anterior cruciate ligament injury occurs in isolation, full counselling of the patient is necessary to determine his or her future physical and sporting aims. Many patients may wish to avoid a major repair or reconstruction at this stage and simply concentrate on muscle rehabilitation.

With midsubstance tears the ligament is frequently so torn and shredded that repair is not possible, and reconstruction using a tendon transfer of semitendinosus and gracilis is necessary.

If the cruciate is avulsed with a bone fragment, a good repair may be effected by fixation of this bone portion with a screw or other fixation device. From time to time the cruciate is avulsed from either the superior or inferior attachments with a small fragment of bone removed. If the bone avulsion fragment is small, then a screw cannot be used and the fragment, together with the ligament, is reattached with sutures.

When the anterior cruciate is ruptured from its upper attachment it is best repaired by an 'over the top technique' taking the sutures through the intercondylar region and over the top of the lateral femoral condyle. The most appropriate repair suture consists of a heavy 2/8 circle, round-bodied, taper-cut needle swaged to a loop of multifilament polyester.

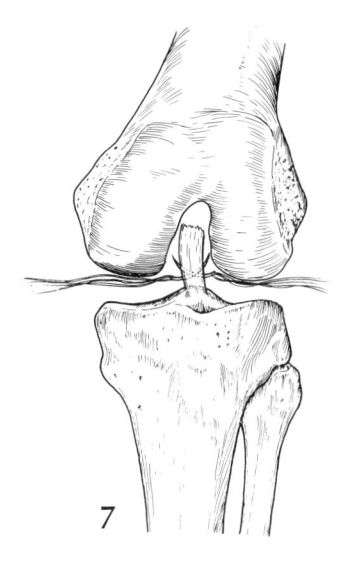

Technique of repair

7

A routine medial arthrotomy incision is made, and two sutures and needles are positioned in the upper attachment of the anterior cruciate as shown.

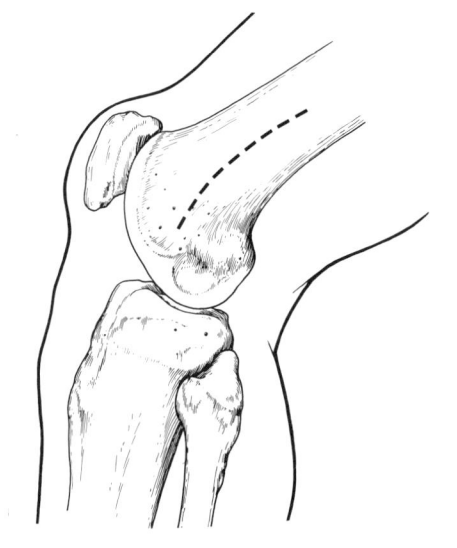

8

An incision is made over the lateral femoral condyle and the supracondylar region. The iliotibial tract is incised in the same line, and, using a self-retaining retractor, the posterior aspect of the femoral condyle is palpated and the lateral gastrocnemius muscle identified. The lateral gastrocnemius is then separated from the posterior capsule.

9

A director is then passed through the posterior capsule and through the intercondylar region. A tape may be taken along the same path by attaching it to the notch in the director. The four ends of the Dacron sutures are attached to this tape and brought through the posterior capsule and over the top of the condyle.

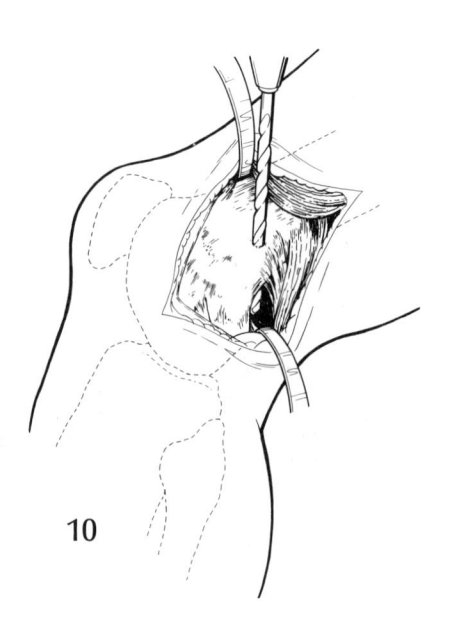

10

An oblique hole is then drilled in the supracondylar bone just above the attachment of the lateral gastrocnemius. Sutures are tied tightly through this bone tunnel with the knee in flexion and lateral rotation.

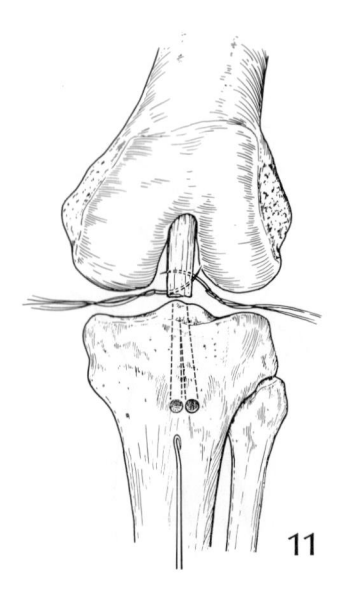

11

The inferior attachment of the anterior cruciate ligament may also be repaired using the same two sutures. The Dacron fibres are then brought through two bone tunnels drilled in the tibia. A hook is used to pull the Dacron suture through these holes and they are then tied tightly on the surface of the medial upper tibia.

Postoperative management

A cast is applied for 5–6 weeks in 40° flexion with the tibia in lateral rotation.

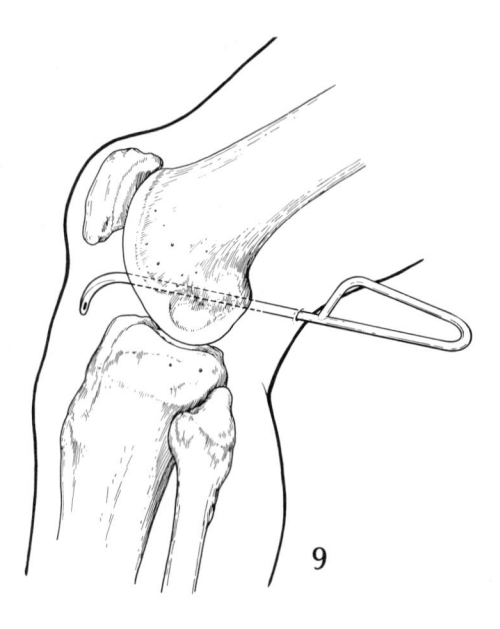

ANTERIOR CRUCIATE REPAIR/RECONSTRUCTION USING TENDON TRANSFER FOR ACUTE INJURY

The large majority of anterior cruciate injuries occur in the midsubstance or at the upper end without bone avulsion. The diagnosis will be made by examination under anaesthesia and confirmed arthroscopically. Sometimes the arthroscope will show a bruised but essentially intact synovium over the anterior cruciate ligament. When the ligament is apparently partially torn or is very lax, dissection with a hook reveals the extent of the cruciate ligament damage. The anterior cruciate ligament is in two portions, anteromedial and posterolateral. One or other, or both, portions may be ruptured. If one portion is intact it may still be considered necessary to reconstruct the ligament using tendon transfers, as the laxity may be substantial.

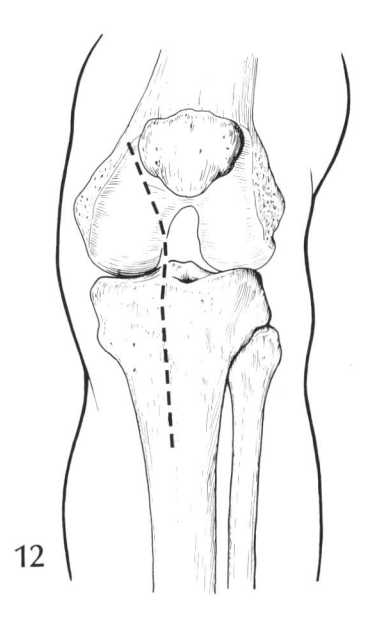

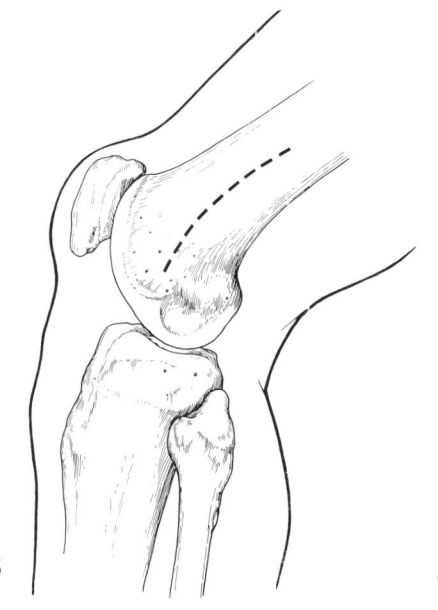

Incision

12 & 13

A medial parapatellar incision with inferior extension to allow access to the pes anserinus is made. A routine medial parapatellar arthrotomy is also undertaken through the upper end of this incision. A lateral incision is made to allow access to the lateral supracondylar region.

Dissection of pes anserinus

14, 15 & 16

The semitendinosus and gracilis tendons are identified by careful dissection of the whole pes structure. They are traced back into the posteromedial thigh and the maximal length is achieved by means of a special rotary tenotome or by open dissection superiorly. A small incision is made in the posteromedial thigh. The tendons are dissected free and isolated; they are then separated from surrounding muscle and cut off as high as possible.

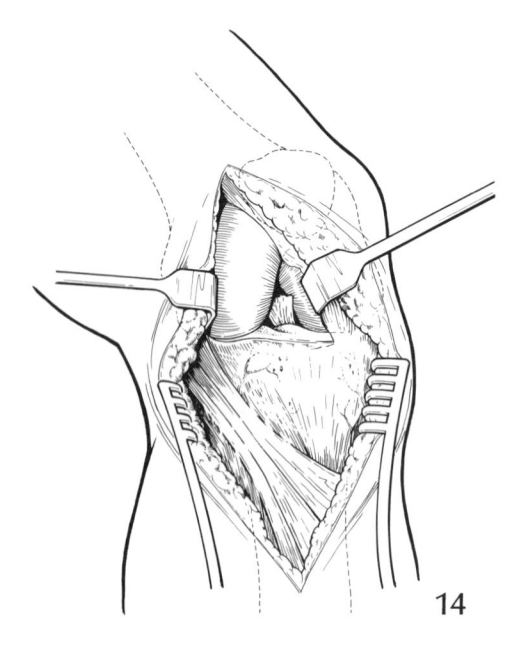

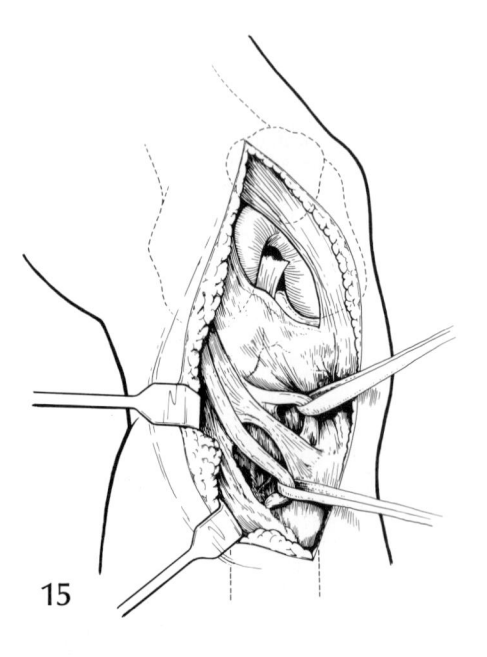

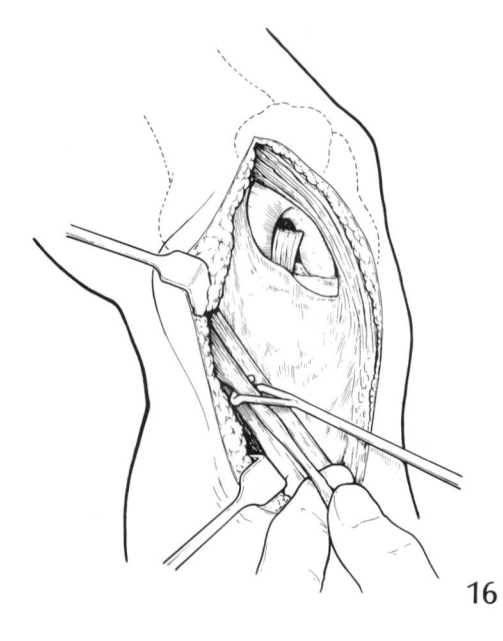

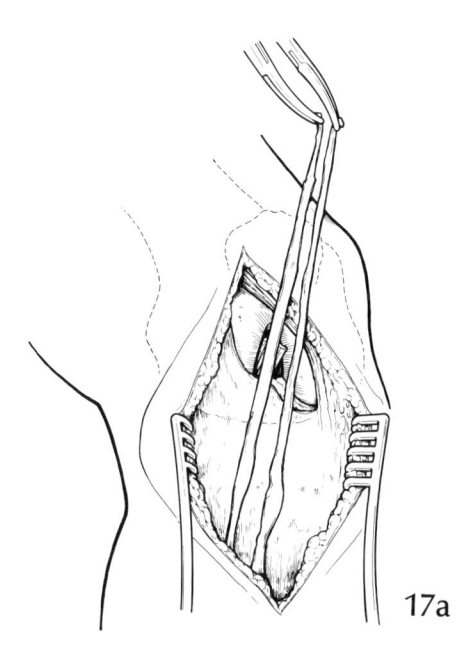

17a & b

The gracilis and semitendinosus tendons are sutured together. A Bunnell-type suture is then inserted superiorly.

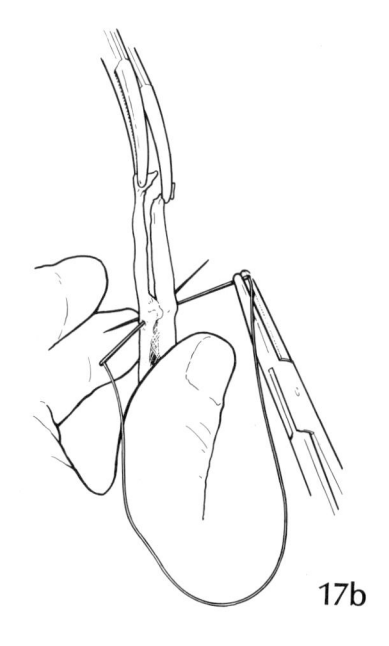

18

A jig is used to drill a tibial tunnel. The drill enters the tibia just above the insertion of the two tendons and emerges from the tibial plateau at the normal inferior attachment of the anterior cruciate ligament – just at, and slightly posterior to, the bifid anterior tibial spine. This point is often better felt than observed.

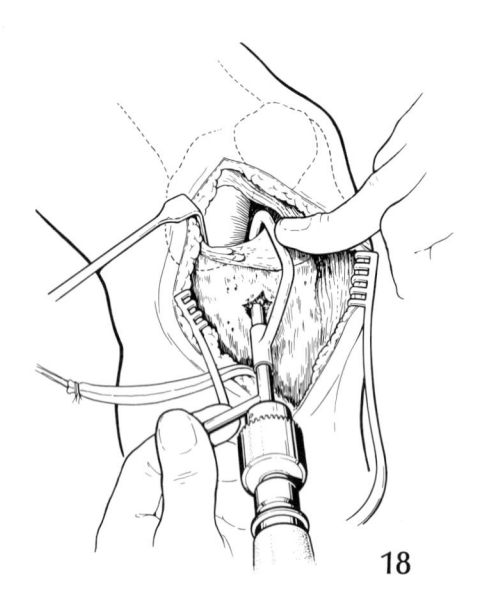

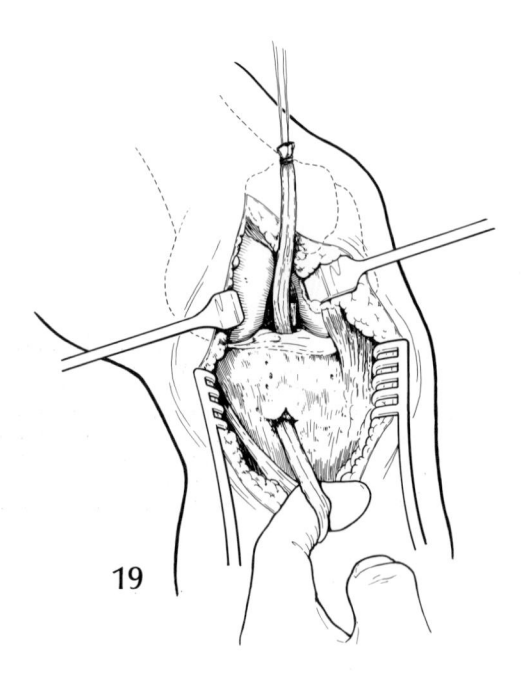

19

The conjoined tendons are then brought through the tibial tunnel. This is best effected by passing a malleable hook down the tibial tunnel and thereby bringing through the leading Bunnell suture. The conjoined tendons then follow.

Lateral dissection

20

The incision follows the line of the supracondylar and condylar regions of the lateral femur. The iliotibial tract is split along the same line.

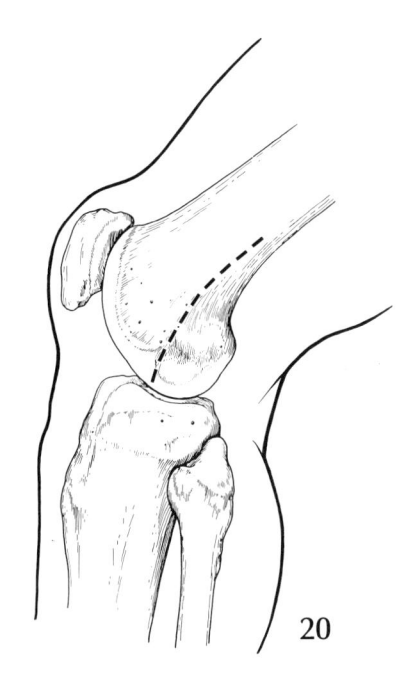

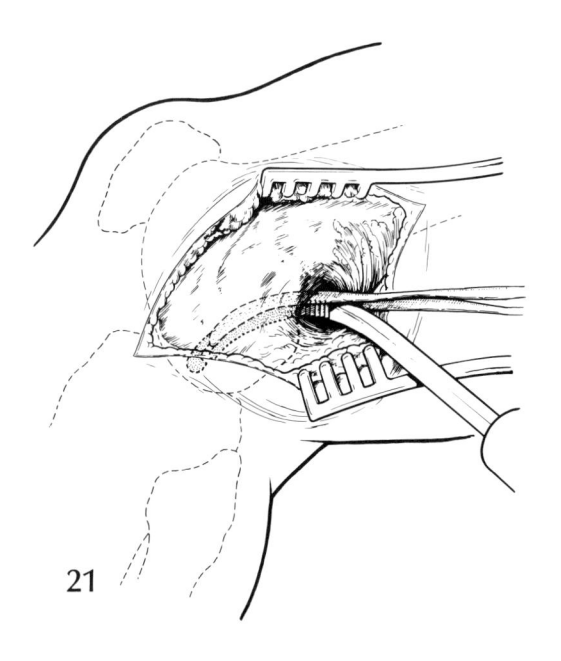

21

Dissection then proceeds beneath the lateral gastrocnemius, separating it from the lateral capsule. A curved director is passed through the intercondylar region and over the top of the lateral femoral condyle. A tape may be taken through the same path and the Bunnell suture attached. Alternatively, a long curved artery forceps may be similarly positioned and the conjoined tendon is brought through and over the top of the lateral femoral condyle.

1092 Thigh and knee

22, 23a, b & c

The conjoined tendons are then strongly attached to the exposed supracondylar bone using two barbed staples. The whole procedure may be undertaken with arthroscopic assistance, and then smaller incisions are used.

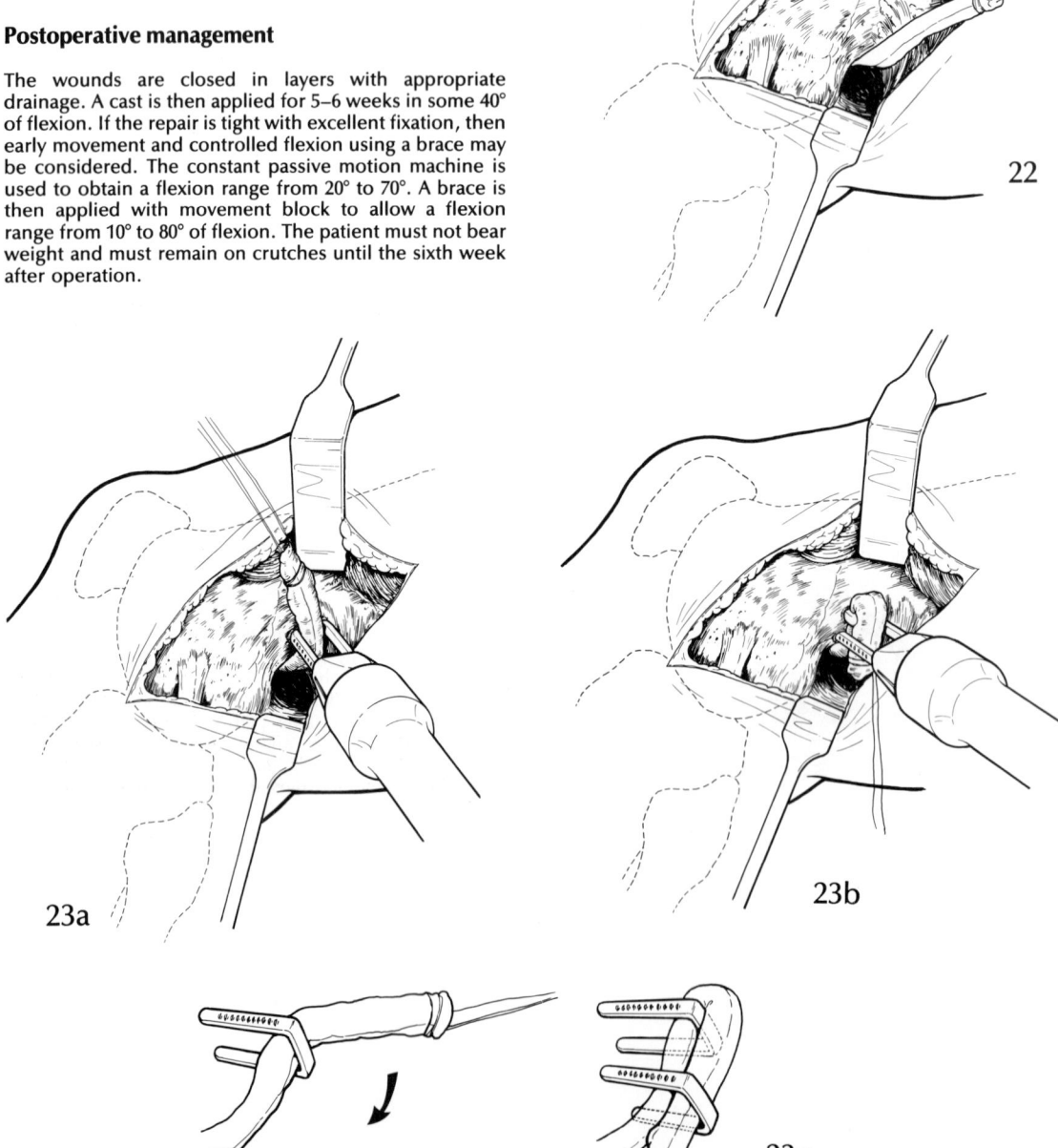

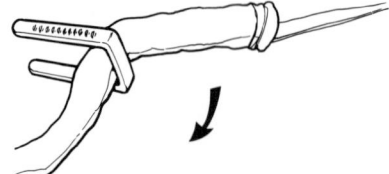

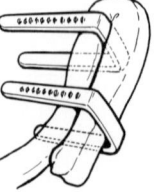

Postoperative management

The wounds are closed in layers with appropriate drainage. A cast is then applied for 5–6 weeks in some 40° of flexion. If the repair is tight with excellent fixation, then early movement and controlled flexion using a brace may be considered. The constant passive motion machine is used to obtain a flexion range from 20° to 70°. A brace is then applied with movement block to allow a flexion range from 10° to 80° of flexion. The patient must not bear weight and must remain on crutches until the sixth week after operation.

POSTERIOR CRUCIATE REPAIR/RECONSTRUCTION USING TENDON TRANSFER FOR ACUTE INJURY

Incision

24

Surgical exposure will depend upon the extent of the posterior reconstruction. The lateral structures may require repair or reconstruction and this should be undertaken before the posterior cruciate procedure. A long medial incision is required for posterior cruciate ligament reconstruction.

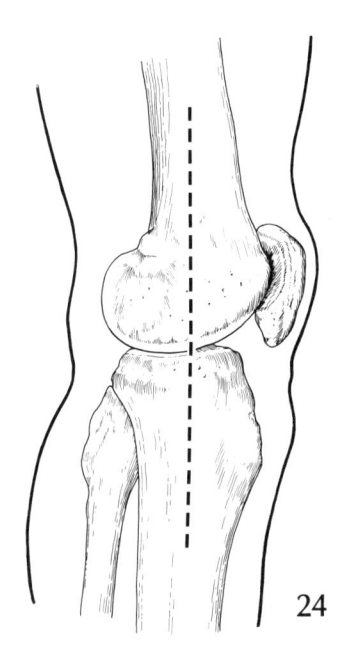

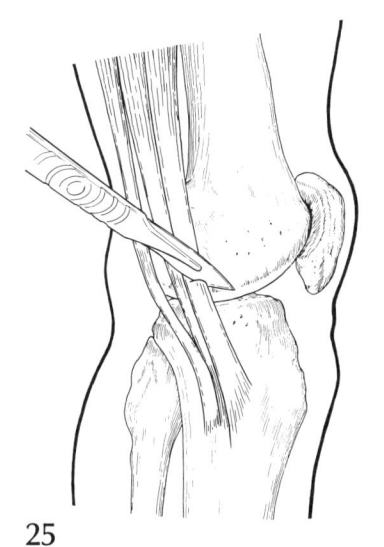

Posterior dissection

25

The knee is flexed and the pes anserinus defined. The semimembranosus tendon is then divided near its insertion, allowing easier access to the popliteal fossa. The tendons of semitendinosus and gracilis are then isolated and traced upwards. They are separated from muscle over their longest length and cut off as high as possible. They are best sutured together as a combined tendon transfer.

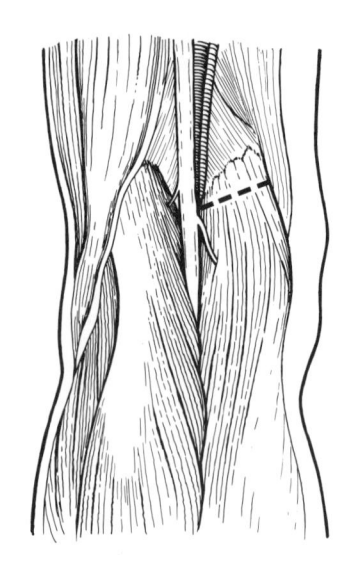

26 & 27

The origin of the medial gastrocnemius is then divided near its femoral attachment and the muscle belly is retracted laterally. The popliteal vessels are now easily visualized in the popliteal fat and areolar tissue. They are tethered to the site of the posterior tibial dissection by the middle genicular vessel and above by the superior medial genicular vessels. These two vascular leashes should be carefully identified, ligated and divided. Once these vessels are cut, the popliteal vascular bundle may be gently retracted laterally. The posterior capsule in the intercondylar region is palpated and divided vertically in the midline. Some of the upper border fibres of popliteus may obstruct the upper tibial bone at this site and they should be dissected laterally with a periosteal elevator.

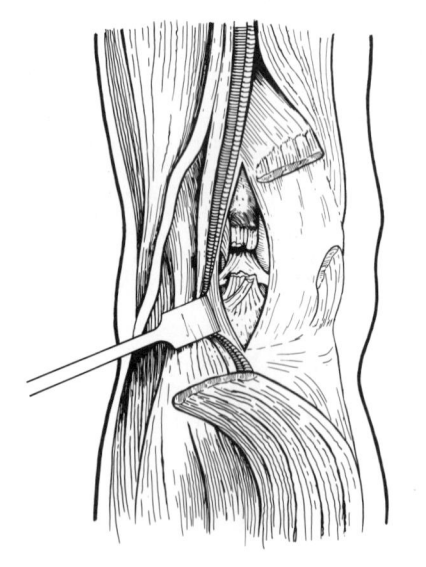

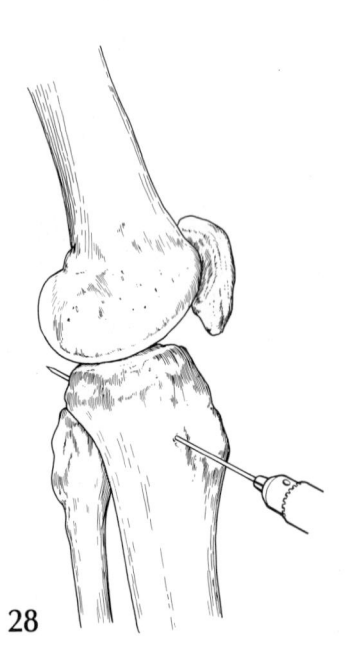

28

The tibial tunnel is drilled.

The drill enters the medial tibia above the pes anserinus insertion to exit at the upper posterior tibia in the midline at the normal insertion of the posterior cruciate ligament. A guide wire with cannulated drill is ideal in locating this site. The combined tendons are pulled through this tunnel on the end of a stout suture. This suture is then passed anteriorly and superiorly through the intercondylar region and into the knee joint cavity.

A medial parapatellar incision is then made and the suture is picked up as it emerges at the end of a director or a long curved artery forceps.

29 & 30

The femoral tunnel is drilled. This emerges at the apex of the intercondylar region at a point resembling 1.30 pm in the right knee and 11.30 am in the left knee. The combined tendons are then drawn through the knee to emerge at the apex of the intercondylar notch. They are taken through the femoral tunnel to emerge in the medial supracondylar region where the combined tendon is fixed to the bone with a double-barbed Richards staple technique after appropriate tensioning.

In chronic posterior cruciate laxity a prosthesis may be used and is routed in a similar fashion.

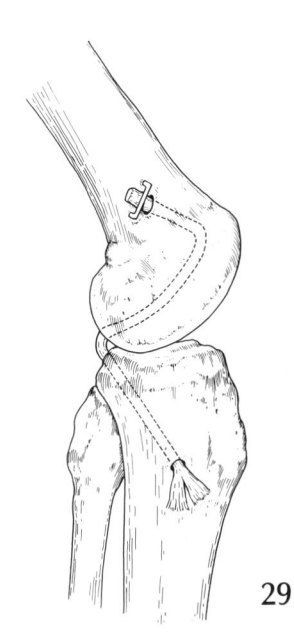

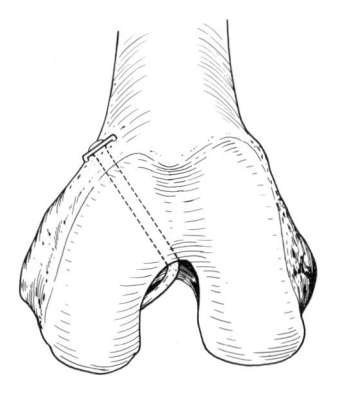

RECONSTRUCTION FOR CHRONIC ANTERIOR CRUCIATE DEFICIENCY (combined intra/extra-articular technique)

There have been many attempts at reconstruction of the chronic anterior cruciate-deficient knee. Tendons, iliotibial tract and prosthetic materials have all been used with various degrees of success. The extra-articular reconstruction of MacIntosh prevents anterorotary instability but stretches in time. It is, however, incorporated in this reconstruction and the long strip of iliotibial tract is tubulated and taken over the top of the lateral femoral condyle. (The 'over-the-top' route produces a more isometric positioning of the neoligament.) The tube then passes through the knee and into a tibial tunnel, accurately re-routing this structure. It has been found necessary, however, to augment this iliotibial tract with prosthetic material, and a Dacron prosthesis is thought to be best at the present time.

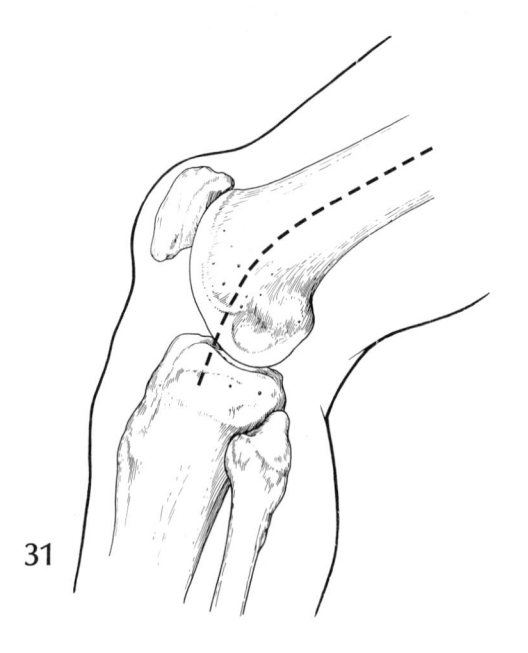

Incision

31

The lateral incision passes superiorly from a point 10 cm above the supracondylar region, laterally along the line of the shaft, through the midcondylar point, and finishes inferiorly at Gerdy's tubercle – the prominence on the upper, lateral tibial plateau where the iliotibial tract is inserted.

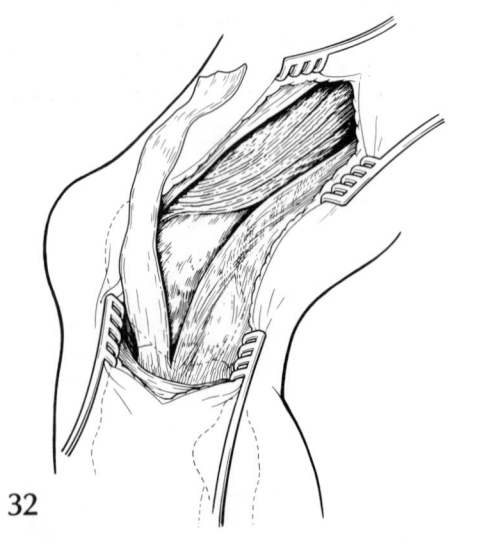

32

A strip of iliotibial tract is raised and detached, using appropriate skin retraction superiorly. The ribbon of iliotibial tract should be 2–2.5 cm broad and is left attached to Gerdy's tubercle inferiorly.

33

A MacIntosh extra-articular tenodesis procedure is now undertaken with the iliotibial tract passed beneath the lateral collateral ligament. The lateral collateral ligament must be isolated both anteriorly and posteriorly by extrasynovial dissection, and the iliotibial tract is placed beneath. With the knee in flexion and full lateral rotation, the iliotibial tract is kept very tight and four sutures are positioned to attach the iliotibial tract to this lateral collateral ligament. The sutures are positioned but are not tied at this stage.

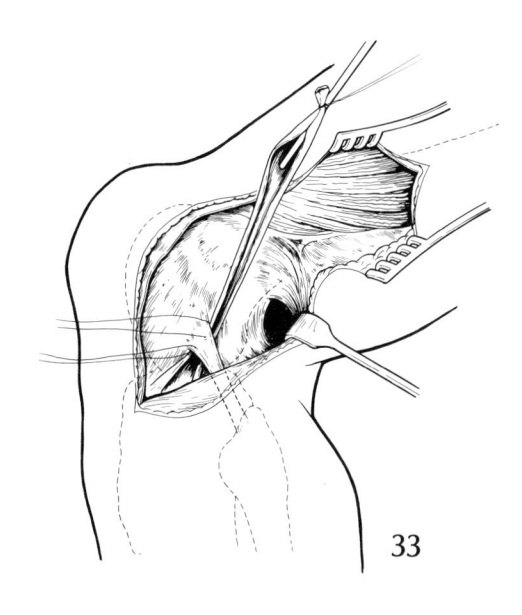

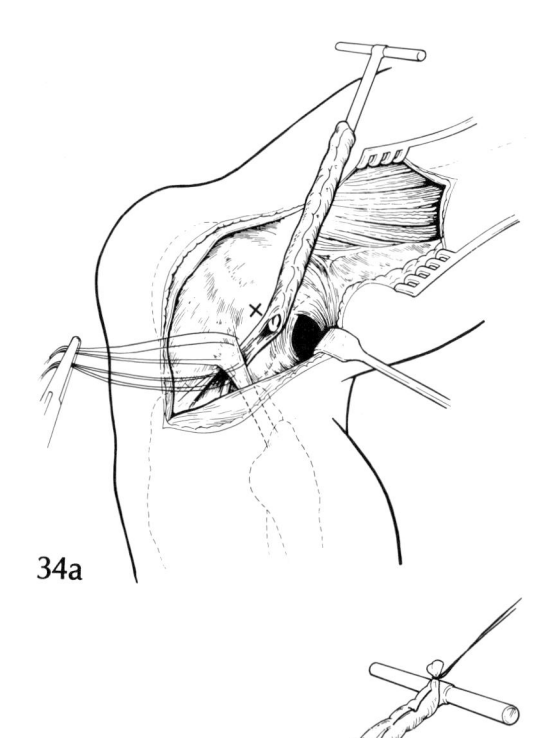

34a & b

The iliotibial tract is now tubulated from its end point to point 'X' (see also Illustration 33). This is best undertaken by bringing its two sides together over a T-shaped cannula. A fine but strong, absorbable suture is recommended and a running, interlocking stitch has been found preferable.

35

The leading loop of the prosthesis may be hooked and drawn through the iliotibial tract. Attached to this loop is a flexible probe which follows the loop into the tube of iliotibial tract from its distal to its proximal end. The end of the probe is now sutured to the free end of the iliotibial tract by an encircling stitch so that the tube and prosthesis may be pulled together over the top of the condyle by traction on the end loop.

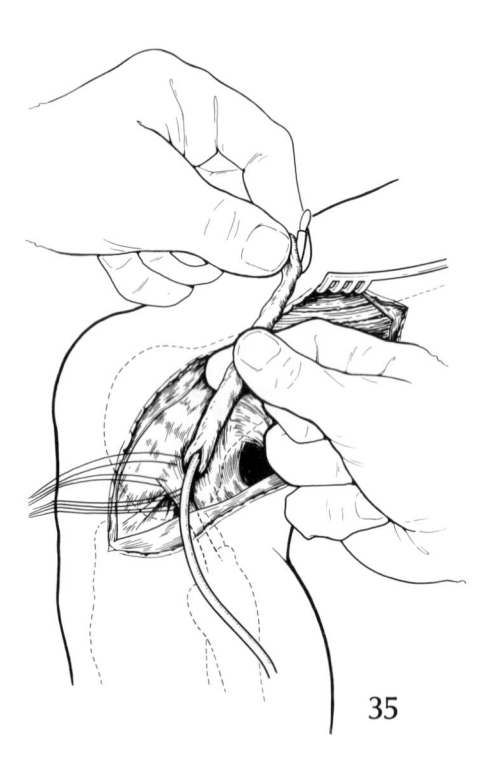

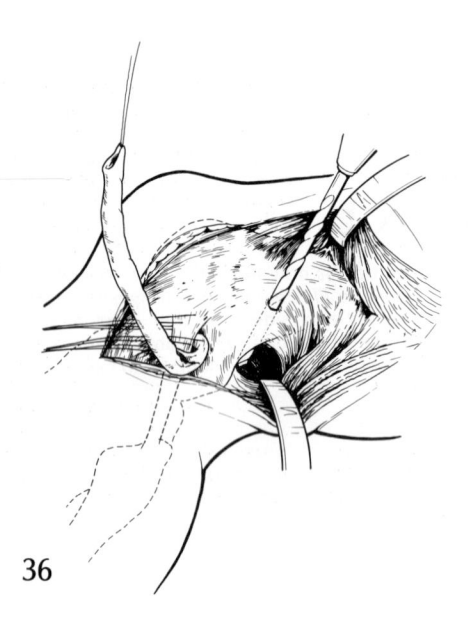

36

A drill hole is made in the supracondylar midpoint, emerging posteriorly just above the capsule at the origin of the lateral gastrocnemius muscle.

37

The ligament is now passed through this bony tunnel and a toggle is inserted in the loop.

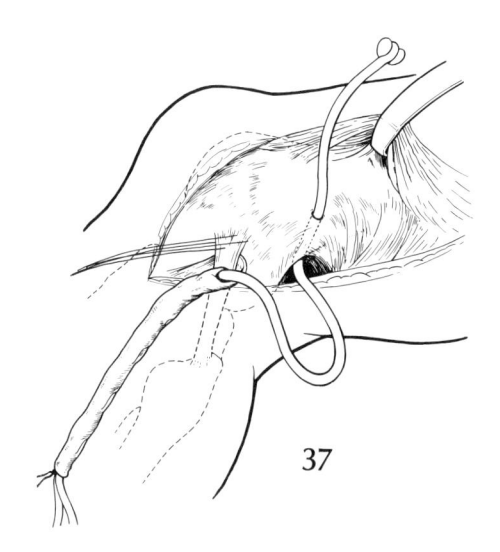

38

Attention must now be turned to the dissection of the posterior capsule extending into the intercondylar region. The fibres of the lateral gastrocnemius are identified, and dissection continues medially beneath this muscle, exposing the posterior capsule. Using sharp and blunt dissection, the intercondylar region is reached with instruments keeping close to the posterior capsule. A director is now passed through the intercondylar region and into the knee joint as indicated in *Illustration 39*. A routine medial parapatellar arthrotomy is made and extended inferiorly to the medial and inferior aspect of the tibial tubercle. The ruptured cruciate is noted in the intercondylar fossa.

The iliotibial tract tube, which is filled with prosthesis, is now ready to be passed behind the lateral femoral condyle, through the intercondylar region and into the knee joint cavity. The tube of iliotibial tract is tightened around the end of the prosthesis by a transfixion suture which encircles the tube and the prosthesis. The leading loop of the prosthesis is then attached to the director and passed into the knee joint cavity.

39

Using a tibial drill guide, a hole is made with the 6 mm drill through the anteromedial tibia. Superiorly it emerges in the normal tibial attachment for the anterior cruciate – between the two prominences of the anterior tibial spine. The upper end of the tibial hole on the tibial plateau surface should be opened and smoothed with a high speed burr and a fine curette. The prosthesis and iliotibial tract tube is now pulled through the intercondylar region and secondarily pulled through the tibial tunnel to the outside.

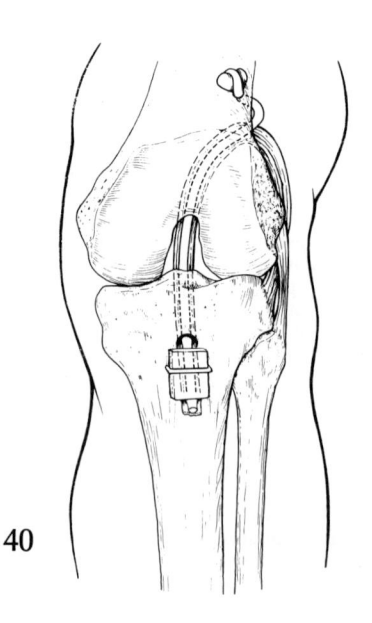

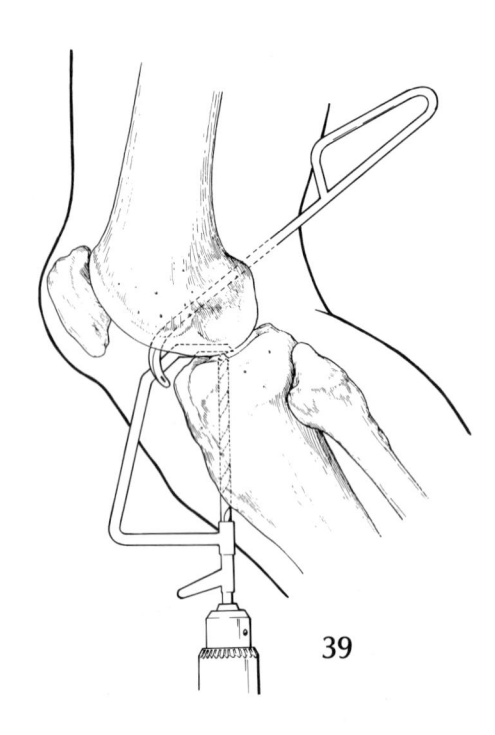

40

A bone block of cortical bone 1 × 2 cm in size is raised from the upper medial tibia, just below the exit hole of the tibial tunnel.

The toggle is positioned in the proximal loop of the prosthesis in the supracondylar position, and the prosthesis is pulled tight with the tibia rotated laterally on the femur and drawn posteriorly. The tubed prosthesis is put into the depression where the bone block was raised and the bone block is returned and stapled in position with the composite ligament under tension. The four stay sutures anchoring the iliotibial tract to the lateral collateral ligament are tightened and tied.

Postoperative management

The lateral wound is closed with drainage. The medial parapatellar wound is closed in the usual way.

The limb is then placed in the constant passive motion machine with a range of movement from 30° to 60°. At 1 week a brace is applied blocking movement from 30° to 70° of flexion. The brace is maintained until the sixth week after operation. After removal of the brace, increasing physiotherapy is given to mobilize and strengthen the knee joint to the maximum. The patient usually returns to some jogging, cycling and swimming at approximately 3 months. At 6 months some gentle recreational games may be considered, and at 1 year the patient may return to all field contact sports.

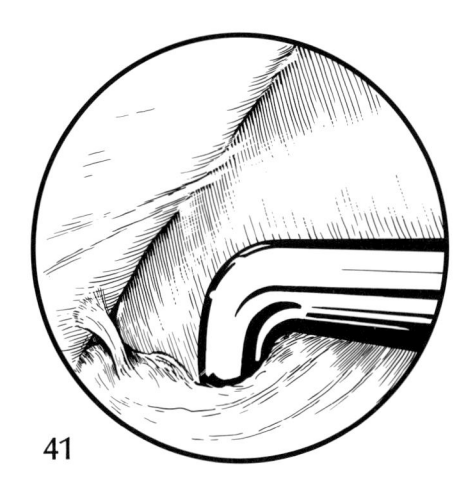

41

The 6-month arthroscopic appearance of the ligament is seen. The hook is prodding the midpoint of the ligament.

Illustrations by Peter Cox after B. Hyams

Recurrent dislocation of the patella

Paul Aichroth MS, FRCS
Consultant Orthopaedic Surgeon, Westminster Hospital and Westminster Children's Hospital, London; Queen Mary's Hospital, Roehampton, UK

Introduction

Dislocation of the patella occurs in both children and adults. Subluxation of this bone is more common in the teenager and frequently produces problems of diagnosis and management.

Patellar dislocations are most commonly lateral although medial and intra-articular positions have been recorded. The dislocation may be congenital or acquired, and the latter may be recurrent, or even persistent.

1

Anatomically there is a natural tendency towards lateral subluxation of the patella and to this may be added the following aetiological factors.

1. Abnormal weakness of the medial capsule following trauma.
2. An extreme valgus knee.
3. Flattening of the articular surface of the lateral femoral condyle and of the patella.
4. Lateral insertion of the patellar tendon, giving an increased Q angle.
5. Patella alta.
6. Anteversion of the femoral neck.
7. Contracture of vastus lateralis.
8. Familial joint laxity.

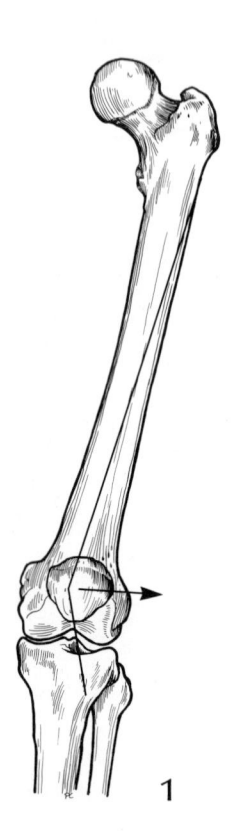

DISLOCATION IN CHILDREN

The dislocation may become recurrent and then habitual if the patella dislocates with every flexion and extension movement. Persistent dislocation is present when the patella is constantly displaced to lie lateral to the femoral condyle, and this may occur when there is gross vastus lateralis contracture – sometimes due to frequent neonatal antibiotic injections into the thigh.

Congenital dislocation is rare, but may be the cause of a flexion contracture of the knee in the newborn. An acquired dislocation may be totally painless, especially if it is persistent, but the child frequently falls, the joint 'gives way' and the knee cap may be described as being 'out of place'. Pain is less common in childhood.

Most children with recurrent dislocations in the first decade of life exhibit some generalized abnormalities such as familial joint laxity or local joint features, as described above.

Indications for operation

The above-mentioned symptoms associated with recurrent or persistent dislocation of the patella provide the indications for operative correction and repair. In doubtful cases, careful assessment of patellar instability under general anaesthesia must be performed. Recurrent dislocation of the patella may produce a loose body due to osteochondral fracture, chondromalacia patellae due to patellar malalignment and osteoarthritis in later life.

A soft tissue procedure is recommended in the child because any operation which disturbs the tibial tubercle will cause a genu recurvatum owing to disturbance of the anterior epiphyseal growth-plate.

Simple lateral patellar release is inadequate in the child and distal transplantation of the patellar tendon may produce severe chondromalacia patellae. A combined patellar release and medial repositioning of the patellar tendon is advocated.

Preoperative preparation

The physiotherapist should teach all the quadriceps-strengthening exercises. The presence of a loose body must be determined radiologically and if present should be removed arthroscopically.

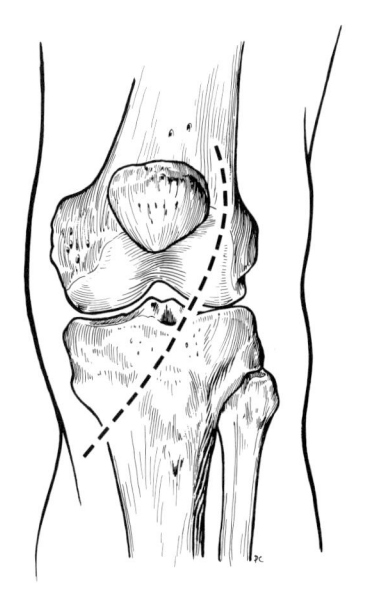

PATELLAR RELEASE AND REPOSITIONING (GOLDTHWAITE–ROUX OPERATION)

After exsanguination of the limb by means of an Esmarch bandage, a very high pneumatic tourniquet is inflated. The skin is prepared from the tourniquet cuff to the ankle. An incise drape may be applied.

Incision

2

A lateral parapatellar incision starts well above the patella and proceeds inferiorly and then medially, crossing the tibial tubercle. If the operation is being performed for persistent dislocation or vastus lateralis contracture, a very high thigh incision will be required to allow adequate release of the vastus lateralis muscle.

Lateral patellar release

3

The lateral capsule of the patellar expansion is incised in the same line, from the suprapatellar region to the tibial tubercle. When the knee is flexed and the lateral release is adequate, the two sides of this capsular incision will widely separate. The synovium may be left intact but in the persistent dislocation and in some recurrent dislocations this lateral synovium is so tight and thick that it must be similarly incised and released.

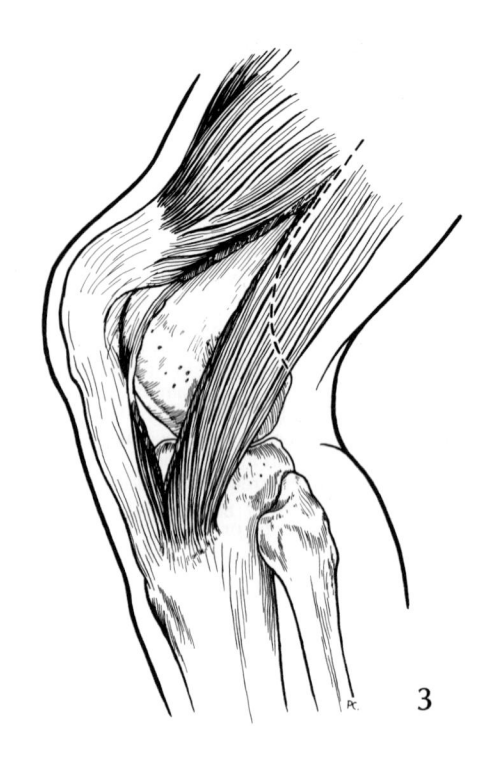

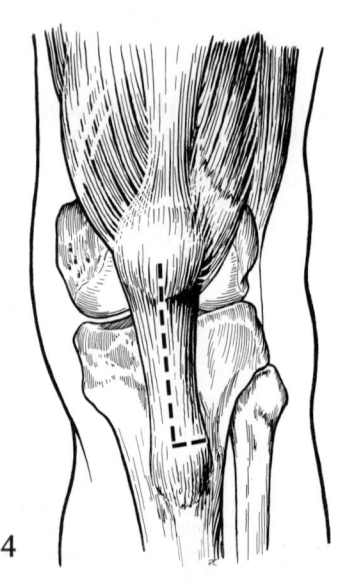

Longitudinal division of the patellar tendon

4

The patellar tendon is isolated throughout its length and divided longitudinally. The distal attachment of the lateral half is divided at the tibial tubercle.

Half-tendon transposition

5, 6 & 7

The lateral half of the patellar tendon is then transposed medially beneath the rest of the tendon, or sometimes superficial to it, thus pulling the patella over to the medial side.

The transposed half-tendon is then implanted beneath an osteoperiosteal flap. The flap is raised with an osteotome and the half-tendon is anchored with two or more thick polyglactin 910 sutures (Vicryl, Ethicon Ltd, Edinburgh, UK).

The tension is adjusted to prevent any lateral displacement of the patella on full flexion and the sutures are tied. In the adult a staple may also be added to anchor the patellar strand beneath the osteoperiosteal flap. However, this is not recommended in the child owing to the proximity of the upper medial growth-plate.

The medial patellar expansion is sutured with plication to the medial patellar tendon.

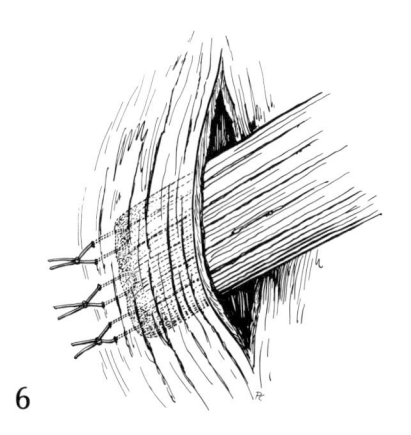

Closure

A vacuum drain is used and the wound is closed with an intradermal skin suture and adhesive tapes. A well-padded cylinder plaster is applied.

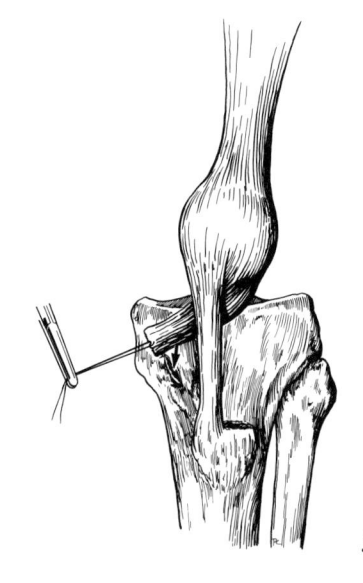

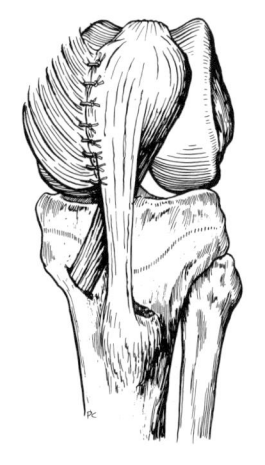

Postoperative management

The limb is elevated for 24 hours. Mobilization without weight-bearing may then commence and be followed after 2 weeks by weight-bearing with crutches or sticks.

The cylinder plaster cast is retained for 4 weeks with an optional change of plaster at 2 weeks to remove the sutures. The physiotherapist will be required to mobilize and strengthen the knee.

DISLOCATION IN TEENAGERS AND ADULTS

Symptoms and signs

The patient may present with a fully dislocated patella but more commonly there are episodes of 'giving way', with pain and subsequent knee effusion. Pain and tenderness over the medial capsule may be confused with a medial internal derangement of the knee. The most important signs are pain and apprehension of the patient when lateral movement of the patella is attempted: this apprehension causes the patient to tense his quadriceps, thus preventing the dislocation from occurring. With a very lax patella, substantial subluxation or dislocation may be demonstrated with only minor pain. In doubtful cases, assessment of patellar stability must be made under general anaesthesia.

Radiographic signs

8, 9 & 10

1. A tangential osteochondral fracture may be seen in the patellar sky-line view.
2. A loose body may be found or an area of osteochondritis dissecans may be present on the anterior aspect of the lateral femoral condyle.
3. Patella alta: the patella is high in most cases of dislocating or subluxing patellae. With the knee flexed at 30°, measurement A is greater than measurement B (Blackburne's method).
4. Hughston's view taken with the knee flexed at 45° shows the patella with a lateral tilt.
5. Patellar alignment in various positions of knee flexion is best assessed in the tangential view of the patella with the knee flexed at 30°, 60° and 90°. The lateral positioning of the patella is then easily seen and subluxation in flexion or extension may be assessed[1].

Treatment

The symptoms described above may occur so regularly that gross inconvenience is produced and correction is indicated. It is now known that degenerative changes are not as great as previously expected in recurrent dislocation of the patella; therefore, an occasional patellar dislocation does not constitute a definite indication for operation and a 'wait and see' policy may be adopted.

Multiple soft tissue operations have been suggested but the release/repositioning operation described above is recommended. A simple lateral patellar release (see *Illustration 3*) may be undertaken in patients with simple subluxation of the patella.

Bony procedures such as the Hauser operation have been used for many years. It is now known that the incidence of retropatellar osteoarthritis is increased markedly following this tibial tubercle transposition – especially if there is distal reimplantation of the tubercle, thus tightening the patellar tendon. In addition, there is an unacceptably high incidence of anterior compartment syndromes associated with this procedure, and it should be avoided.

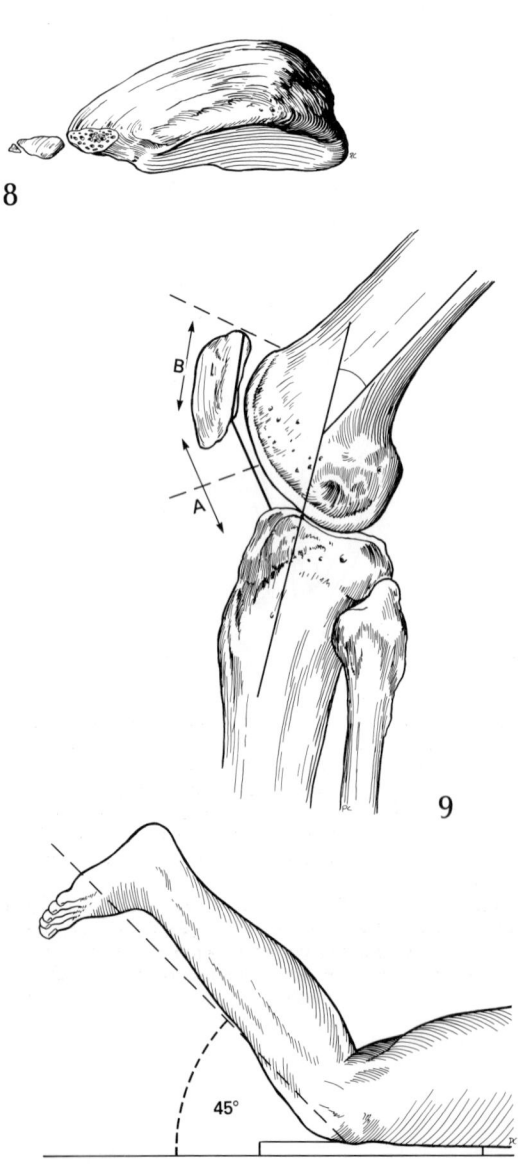

PATELLOFEMORAL OSTEOARTHRITIS

PATELLAR DECOMPRESSION AND REALIGNMENT (MAQUET OPERATION)

Retropatellar osteoarthritis associated with lateral subluxation of the patella may be relieved by the Maquet operation. This has the effect of correction of the malalignment together with decompression of the patellofemoral joint by forward and medial positioning of the tibial tubercle.

11

The skin incision is long and extends from the level of the lower patella, down the anteromedial aspect of the leg, passing 1 cm posterior to the tibial crest. Holes are drilled through the tibia which is then split with an osteotome along the lines connecting the drill holes. Care must be taken not to fracture across the distal end of this split tibia. A full-thickness bone graft is taken from the iliac crest or from the adjacent tibia.

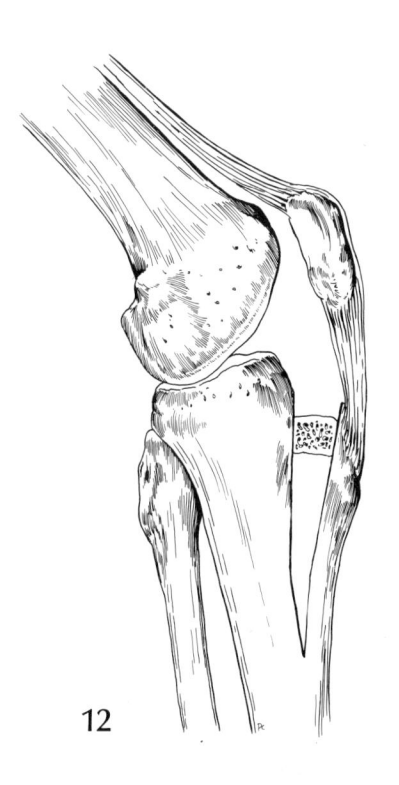

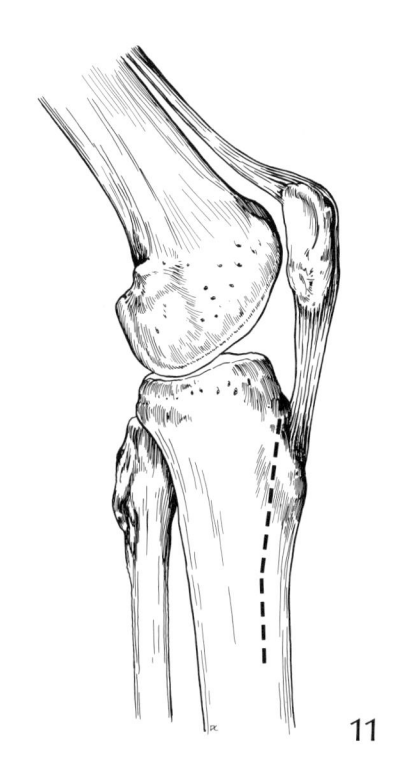

12

The anterior tibial fragment remains attached distally and the iliac crest graft is inserted behind this fragment, pushing it forwards and medially by a variable amount depending on the pathology. Care must be taken to avoid skin tension by mobilizing the edges if necessary. If tension is too great the thickness of the bone graft will be reduced. The wound is closed with adequate vacuum drains.

The leg is supported in a compression bandage for 1 week, and the patient begins walking after 48 hours. Knee flexion may be started within 7 days because fixation is firm but full weight-bearing is restricted for 1 month.

1108 Thigh and knee

THE TRILLAT OPERATION

The distal insertion of the patellar tendon may be moved medially with a sliver of tibial tubercle bone and distal periosteum in the mature patient. This operation is not recommended in the child with an open tibial tubercle growth-plate.

13

A midline longitudinal skin incision is made and deepened to expose the extensor apparatus. Incisions are made along the medial and lateral borders of the patellar tendon, distally on each side of the tibial tubercle extending into the periosteum inferior to the tubercle. An osteotome then raises a sliver of tibial tubercle some 5–7 mm and the bone inferiorly is raised as an osteo-periosteal flap.

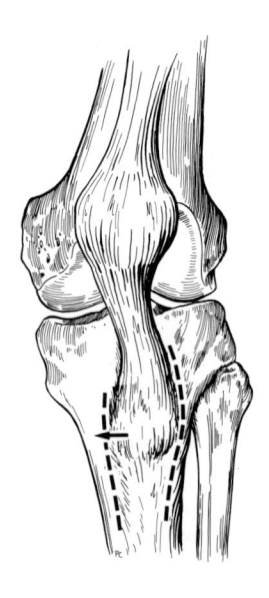

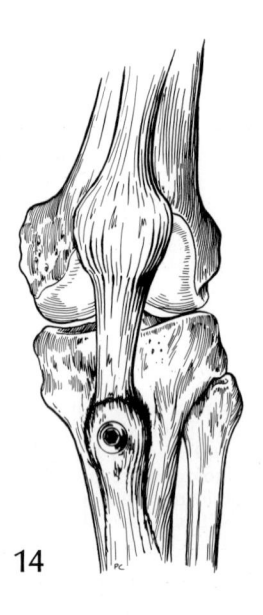

14

The patellar tendon and tubercle are then moved medially and a screw may be used to fix the position of the tibial tubercle in its definitive more medial position.

Postoperative management

The leg is enclosed in a plaster of Paris cylinder and elevated for 24 hours. Weight-bearing with crutches then begins with gentle quadriceps exercises daily. After 6 weeks mobilization under physiotherapy supervision is begun. Full activities are restricted for 3 months.

References

1. Dowd GSE, Bentley G. Radiographic assessment in patellar instability and chondromalacia patellae. *J Bone Joint Surg [Br]* 1986; 68-B: 297–300.

Illustrations by Gillian Oliver after G. Lyth

Synovectomy of the knee

W. Waugh MChir, FRCS
Emeritus Professor of Orthopaedic and Accident Surgery, University of Nottingham;
Honorary Consultant Orthopaedic Surgeon, Harlow Wood Orthopaedic Hospital, Nr Mansfield, Nottinghamshire, UK

Introduction

Indications

Synovectomy is indicated when there is a persistent chronic, or intermittent, synovitis (with effusion and thickening) which is producing pain and disability.

The pathological conditions in which this situation arises are as follows.

Rheumatoid arthritis

Synovectomy will relieve pain but there is no clear evidence that it will prevent further destruction of the knee joint. Operation should only be considered when medical treatment of at least 3 months' duration has failed to relieve pain and swelling. The best results will be achieved at a stage of the disease when the radiographs are normal (or show only peripheral erosions). Once there is extensive loss of articular cartilage and bony collapse, arthroplasty, using one of the modern designs of knee replacement, will be more likely to produce a painless, stable and mobile joint. Synovectomy may, however, be preferable in younger patients even in the more advanced stages of the disease.

Pigmented villonodular synovitis

Excision of localized nodules is satisfactory, but in the diffuse type of the disease recurrence is common and an extensive synovectomy is only justified when the symptoms are causing serious disability.

Tuberculosis

Operation may be considered when antituberculous treatment fails to produce resolution of the synovitis.

Preoperative considerations

There are four controversial points which should be discussed before the operation is described.

Amount of synovial tissue to be removed

It is technically impossible to carry out a total synovectomy, but through an anterior incision the synovium in the suprapatellar pouch, in the lateral recesses and in the intercondylar notch can be removed. Fortunately in rheumatoid arthritis this operation seems to produce regression of the remaining tissue, possibly as a response to injury.

One or two incisions?

It has been suggested that two short incisions (anteromedial and anterolateral) allow adequate exposure with less damage so that knee movement recovers more quickly. A long midline incision gives equally good access, and provided it is carefully closed, movements can be started after a few days; it also can be used for a subsequent knee replacement operation, which may eventually be necessary.

Should the menisci be removed?

Erosions frequently occur on the margins of the tibial condyles; if these are to be cleared, the menisci have to be removed. It is, however, important to remember that meniscectomy removes an essential part of the load-bearing mechanism of the knee and is likely to be followed by progressive degenerative changes. This has to be weighed against the theoretical advantages of a more thorough synovectomy. Generally it is better to retain the menisci.

Mobilization or immobilization?

Although the operation inflicts considerable damage to the knee joint, movement can be started after 3 or 4 days provided skin healing is satisfactory and there is no haematoma. Immobilization for 3 weeks seems to carry no special advantages; recovery of movement is delayed and manipulation is nearly always necessary.

Operation

A pneumatic cuff tourniquet is applied to the upper thigh after exsanguination.

Towelling

After skin preparation with chlorhexidine in spirit a plastic drape is applied. The foot can be completely isolated by wrapping it up in a large sheet of plastic drape. The leg is lifted so that the table below it can be covered with a towel. The rest of the body is excluded by towels applied from below and above and clipped around the thigh. The knee should then be flexed and extended to make sure that the towels are secure.

Incision

1 & 2

A midline incision is used and it should extend from at least 10 cm above the upper pole of the patella to 5 cm below the tibial tuberosity. The joint is entered on the medial side by division of the capsule opposite the patella (and about 1 cm from its medial border) in the line of the skin incision. The approach is extended proximally by separating vastus medialis from the rectus femoris with scissors. Distally the soft tissues and periosteum over the upper part of the tibia are divided and stripped laterally and medially by sharp dissection. It is important to preserve the soft-tissue flaps in this part of the incision to allow closure at the end of the operation.

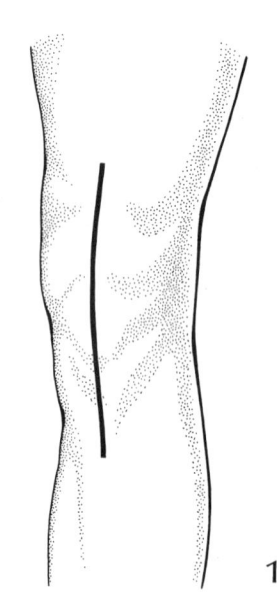

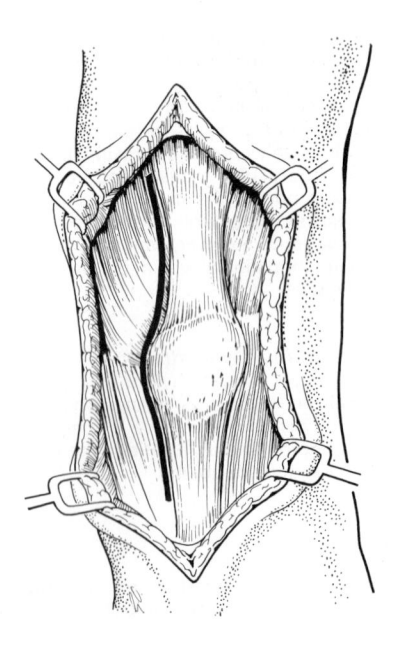

Dislocation of patella

3

Separation of vastus medialis from the rectus femoris is continued proximally and any adhesions in the joint divided until the patella can be turned so that its articular surface faces directly forward. It may be necessary to detach (by sharp dissection) the medial quarter of the patellar ligament before this can be done. The knee is then flexed to beyond a right angle and when this is done the patella can be turned over so that its articular surface faces outwards; the whole of the articular surface of the femur can now be seen. The joint is inspected with particular reference to the state of the synovial membrane and the articular cartilage.

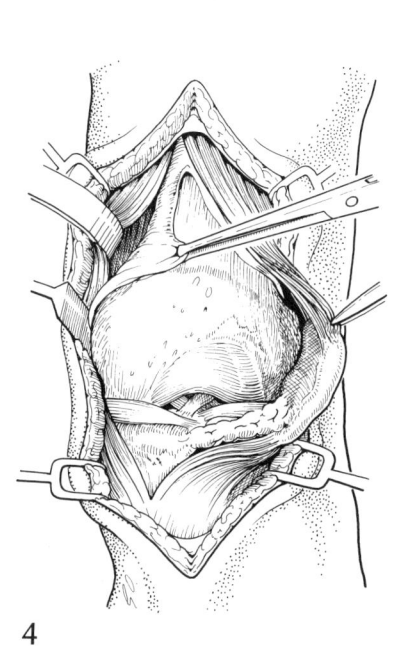

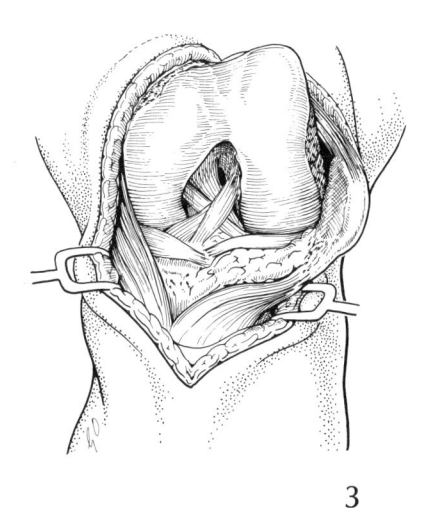

Excision of affected synovial membrane

4

The knee is straightened and the plane of dissection between the synovium and capsule found. This is begun most easily in the suprapatellar pouch; tissue forceps are applied to the capsule and synovium and the dissection carried out with Mayo scissors. The suprapatellar pouch is excised – the dissection starting from medial to lateral and then extending back across the femoral reflection. As much synovial membrane is removed from the paracondylar gutters as possible. The affected tissue is often removed piecemeal.

Special attention should now be paid to the articular margins around the patella and femoral condyles. The synovium must be carefully removed from these areas (particularly if there is any articular invasion) and all pannus should be stripped off the underlying cartilage. Erosions should be curetted and bone nibblers may be used to remove fragments of tissue. The intercondylar notch is often an area of active synovitis and affected tissue should be stripped off the cruciate ligaments in the hope of avoiding their subsequent destruction by the disease.

The joint should now be thoroughly examined and any remaining tags of tissue removed.

The tourniquet is removed and the wound packed with large swabs. After waiting for the reactive hyperaemia to subside, bleeding vessels (usually in the capsule) are sealed by diathermy.

Closure

One or occasionally two suction drains are inserted. The capsule should be closed with interrupted black silk stitches and the skin with interrupted nylon.

Dressings

5

If a standard pressure bandage is applied the knee will tend to flex over the mass of wool behind the knee. It is better to use a very thick (5 cm) strip of wool down the front of the leg and encircle this with a few turns of plaster wool. A crêpe bandage is applied from toes to groin followed by a plaster back splint (not including the foot).

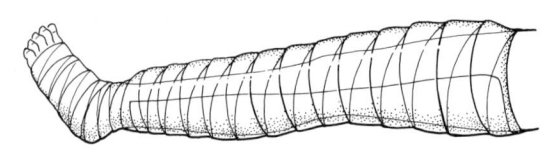

Postoperative management

This will vary with the amount of swelling in the knee and the response of the patient. Quadriceps and foot exercises are started immediately after operation. The splint and drains can be removed after 2 days and knee flexion exercises started after 4 or 5 days. The wound is then left exposed. Walking with crutches is allowed after 1 week. Manipulation should only rarely be necessary: it is best carried out (with due care) between the second and third weeks after operation.

Complications

Infection

The risks are decreased by careful operative technique, haemostasis and suction drainage.

Wound breakdown and skin necrosis

This is avoided by not undermining the skin more than necessary and careful suturing.

Haemarthrosis

The wound should be inspected at 48 hours after operation and any collection of blood aspirated.

Stiffness and extensor lag

These should be avoided by early movement and quadriceps exercises and, if necessary, manipulation. Primary wound healing is essential to achieve this.

Illustrations by Peter Cox

Tibial osteotomy for arthritis of the knee

J. P. Jackson FRCS
Emeritus Orthopaedic Surgeon, University Hospital, Nottingham, and Harlow Wood Orthopaedic Hospital, Mansfield, UK

Introduction

Indications

Tibial osteotomy is indicated for the relief of pain in osteoarthritis of the medial compartment of the knee in younger patients. The object of the operation is to realign the limb so that weight-bearing is transferred to the more normal part of the joint. Whilst the operation has been employed with some success in both valgus and varus knees, for the best and most consistent results to be obtained certain factors should be considered.

Contraindications

1. The degree of deformity There is a limit to the deformity that can be successfully corrected if a wedge is to be removed proximal to the tibial tuberosity. Correction of a tibiofemoral angle of more than 5° may weaken the proximal fragment so that fracture into the joint occurs.

2. Excessive collapse of the joint surface Bony collapse of more than 0.5 cm implies that the joint is too disorganized to benefit from the operation.

3. Limited movement The knee should flex to more than 90° and there should not be a flexion contracture of more than 10° before operation.

4. Valgus deformity Whilst many patients with a knock-knee deformity have benefited from this procedure, division through the tibia leaves a very oblique joint-line and a better result may be obtained by osteotomy of the femur. In general, patients with a valgus deformity present late when there is already considerable joint damage and a good result already compromised.

Assessment

The operation is best carried out by removal of a wedge of bone above the tibial tuberosity. This method has the advantage of being very stable and leading to early union. A curved osteotomy through the tibial tubercle may be required if for any reason, such as the presence of cysts, there is need for considerable correction.

The wedge size

1

This is calculated from the standing film. Full-length films which show both hip and ankle joints give a more accurate assessment. The object of the operation is to move the line of weight-bearing of the limb away from the affected side so that it passes across the more normal tibiofemoral compartment. In effect, this means moving the centre of the ankle joint so that it comes to lie beneath the opposite compartment from its preoperative position. The wedge removed should be sufficient in size to produce slight overcorrection of the deformity. The operation is carried out with the use of a tourniquet.

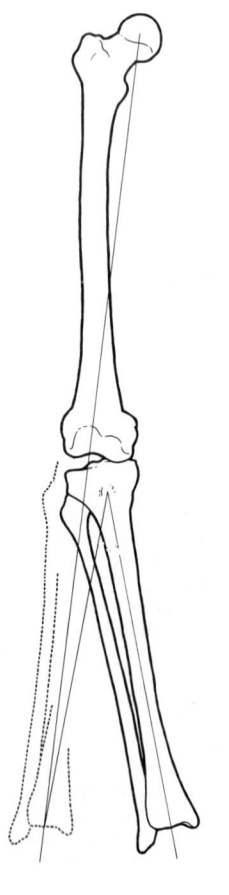

Operation

Division of the fibula

2

The limb is draped so that it is free and can be picked up and manipulated by the surgeon. The fibula can either be osteotomized in the shaft or the head can be excised. If the head is to be removed, then this is usually done as part of a lateral approach to the tibia. Section of the shaft of the fibula is easier and allows the tibia to be approached from the front, through a separate incision. The wedge can then be cut more easily and measured more accurately.

To approach the fibula the interval between the peronei and the calf muscles is defined. If the bulge of the peronei is felt, the intermuscular septum is just behind; this can be followed down to the bone without significant bleeding.

A vertical incision is employed and this should be centred on a point about 15 cm below the proximal tip of the fibula, or lower. The object of osteotomy at this site is to avoid precipitating a compartment syndrome, which has been found to be more common when bone division is above this level. The osteotomy should be oblique so that bone ends slide on each other and remain in contact, facilitating union.

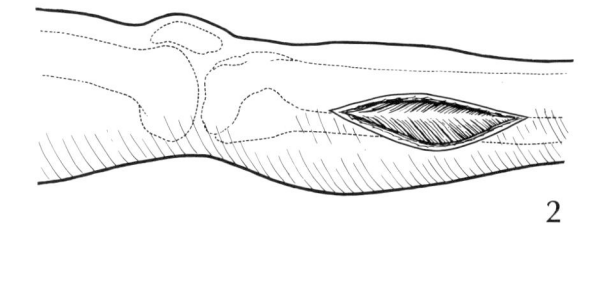

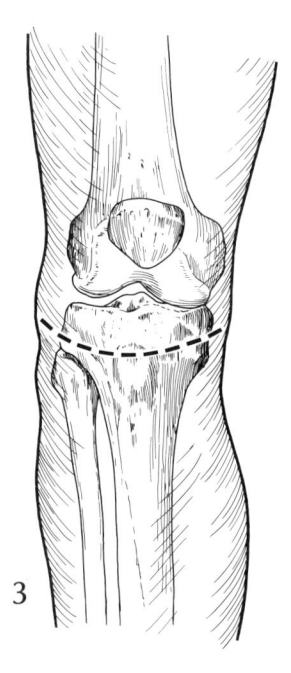

Incision

3

The tibia is best approached from the front by a transverse incision centred on the upper part of the tibial tubercle. If for any reason it is necessary to enter the knee joint (i.e. to remove loose bodies) a medial parapatellar incision is used.

Incision of capsule and periosteum

4

The incision is deepened through superficial tissues and the tibial tubercle and anterior capsule are displayed.

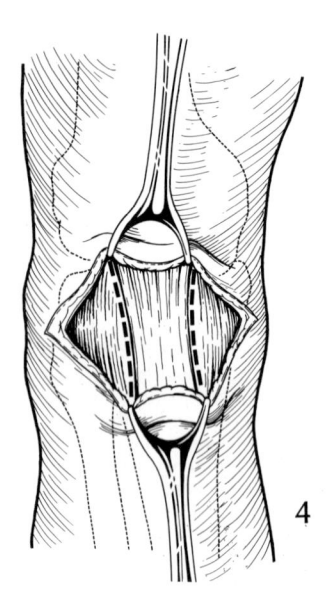

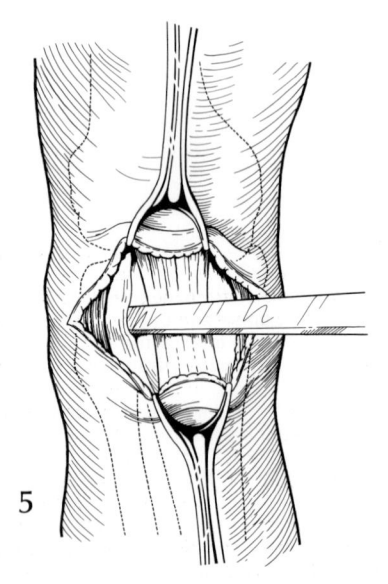

5

The tendon is isolated by two longitudinal incisions. The periosteum is then reflected medially round to the posteromedial border of the tibia and then to the posterolateral border. Care must be taken as the area just below the tibiofibular joint is entered, since the anterior tibial artery is very vulnerable. In addition, the recurrent branch of this vessel runs upwards to the patella and may also be injured. Bleeding from these arteries may cause increased compartmental pressure. A spike should not be placed behind the lateral border of the tibia as it may well cause damage to the vessels.

Insertion of Steinmann pins

6

Before the bone is cut, two Steinmann pins should be placed in position. The upper one must pass through the proximal fragment parallel to the proposed saw cut, but at a sufficient distance above it, so that there is no danger of cutting out, when compression is applied. The lower pin is positioned parallel to the proposed lower saw cut. The angle between the two pins will be that of the wedge which is to be removed. In fat patients particularly or if the surgeon is in any doubt, the two pins should be passed under X-ray control. It is essential that they are accurately placed, so that when the bone wedge is removed the pins will lie parallel, and compression can be evenly applied.

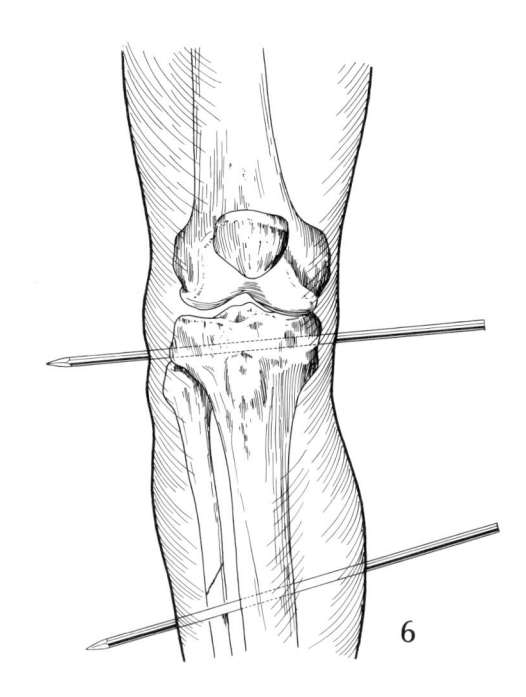

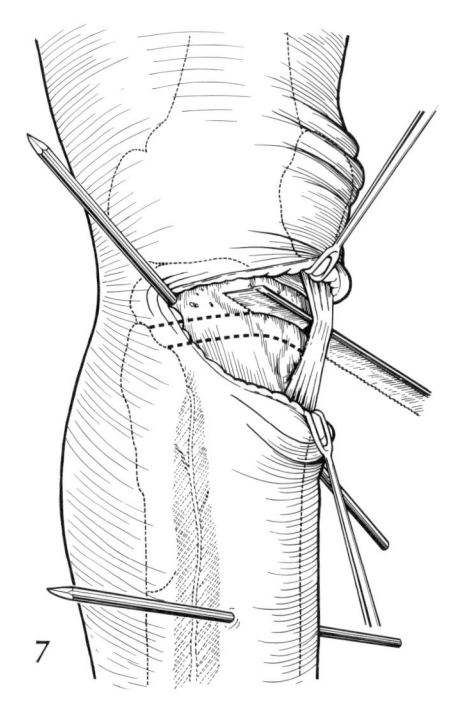

Division of the tibia

7

The tibial tendon is held forwards with the aid of a hook. The initial saw cuts are made with a keyhole saw, and will mark the exact dimensions of the wedge. In order to make the lower cut, it may be necessary to detach the tibial tendon insertion partially. Complete detachment is unwise, as this can jeopardize the success of the operation. The cuts are deepened as far as possible onto and through the posterior cortex. The structures behind the tibia can be protected by a Watson Cheyne dissector passed from the lateral side. Care must be taken to remove the cortex cleanly, as otherwise the bone ends may be held apart by small spicules of bone. Bone nibblers can be very helpful in smoothing off the posterior cortex. Once all bone has been satisfactorily removed, the wedge can be closed, and compression applied to the two Steinmann pins. When the bone is adequately compressed, the alignment of the tibia can be checked to see that correction has been obtained.

Insertion of staples

8 & 9

The final step is to insert two staples. On the medial side, the surface is sloping and an angled staple will fit best. The lateral surface usually has a step so that a stepped Coventry staple will fit more comfortably. Pre-drilling of the point of entry of the staple into the cortical bone of the distal fragment with a 3.5 mm drill will facilitate entry and prevent tilting of the staple. When the staples are judged to be correctly placed, the compression is released and the Steinmann pins withdrawn. Trial flexion and extension of the knee is now carried out to confirm that the osteotomy is firmly fixed. A third staple may sometimes be thought necessary. Finally, the wound is closed in layers. Suction drainage is advisable.

Postoperative management

A well-padded plaster cylinder is applied which should include the foot. Allowing the foot to fall into plantar flexion results in a significant rise of pressure in the anterior tibial compartment. The limb is elevated for 24 hours, or longer if the swelling is excessive. The patient is allowed up after the suction drainage is discontinued and swelling controlled. After 1 week the plaster is removed and changed for a lightweight cast-brace. This is applied with the limb in the corrected position. Once the patient is comfortable in the brace, full weight-bearing should be encouraged with knee flexion. With this regimen, satisfactory union is obtained at the end of 6 weeks. The brace is removed and the patient encouraged to walk normally.

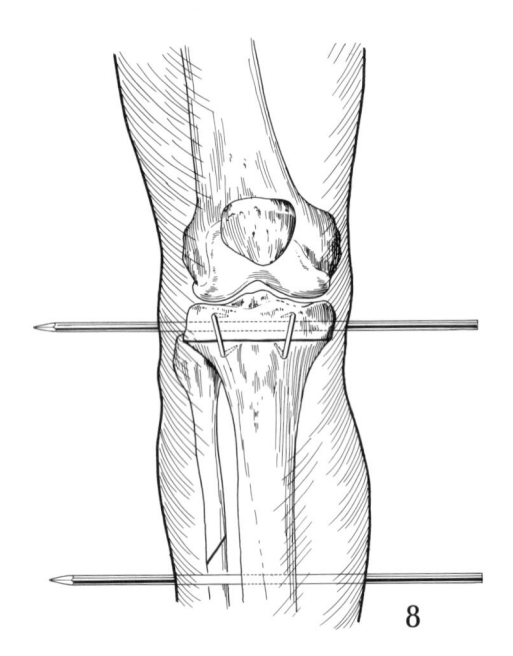

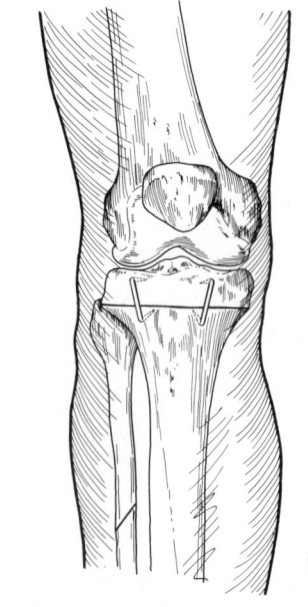

Illustrations by William Thackeray

Arthroplasty of the knee

Russell E. Windsor MD
Assistant Professor, Orthopaedic Surgery, Cornell University Medical College, New York; and Assistant Attending Orthopaedic Surgeon, The Hospital for Special Surgery and The New York Hospital, New York, USA

John N. Insall MD
Professor of Orthopaedic Surgery, Cornell University Medical College, New York; and Director, The Knee Service, The Hospital for Special Surgery, New York, USA

Introduction

Indications

Total knee arthroplasty is recommended for patients with severe *unremitting knee pain* due to: rheumatoid panarthritis (regardless of age), gonarthrosis, post-traumatic osteoarthritis, failure of high tibial osteotomy and arthritis associated with gout, psoriasis, or pigmented villonodular synovitis. A less common indication is *severe patellofemoral osteoarthritis* in an elderly patient. Usually, patchy articular degeneration is found at arthrotomy and the results of arthroplasty in this type of degenerative arthritis are better than any other method.

Total joint arthroplasty for a painful neuropathic joint is controversial, but it is feasible, provided that a surface replacement can be used, the joint is thoroughly debrided with a complete synovectomy and correct alignment and stability is achieved. Metal-backed components with long intramedullary stems are recommended for this situation.

Contraindications

A sound *painless arthrodesis* is an absolute contraindication to total knee arthroplasty. Long-term *painful ankylosis* in a young patient due to trauma or previous infection is also not recommended for arthroplasty. The chances of regaining movement and eradicating pain are unpredictable, and the high likelihood of postoperative complications in these patients make arthroplasty a poor choice. Arthrodesis in this situation is the preferred procedure. Gross quadriceps weakness, and genu recurvatum associated with muscle weakness and paralysis will severely compromise the function of the knee. Total knee arthroplasty in these knees, even if a constrained prosthesis is used, will fail early because of the excessive stresses placed upon the implants. The operation should also not be done in an actively *infected knee*. However, later arthroplasty is feasible after the infection is eradicated by thorough debridement and antibiotic therapy.

Preoperative

Planning

Before total knee arthroplasty is performed, the surgeon must appropriately plan the operation. This entails proper patient selection and choice of prosthetic design. If severe deformity is present, a custom-made implant may be needed, or consent for autologous bone grafting obtained.

Surgical preparation

A broad-spectrum antibiotic, such as cephalosporin, is administered preoperatively. General endotracheal or epidural anaesthesia may be used. The patient is placed in the supine position. A thigh tourniquet is applied and the knee is washed with antiseptic solution and draped thinly so as not to interfere with positioning of surgical instruments. The anterior superior iliac spine should be easily palpated through the drapes to allow assessment of alignment during surgery.

If a bilateral arthroplasty is required, the procedures should be done sequentially. After completion of the first arthroplasty, the dressings are applied and the second knee is prepared and draped. The instruments are re-sterilized. This method, in our opinion, is much safer than using the instruments simultaneously for both knees, as we feel the chances for infection are less.

Operation

Incision

1

The limb is exsanguinated with an Esmarch bandage and the tourniquet is inflated to a pressure of 350–400 mmHg. A midline longitudinal incision should be used[1]. Although medial and lateral parapatellar incisions are acceptable, a midline incision generally offers a clear exposure and requires less dissection of the medial and lateral skin flaps. However, if other surgical scars are present, the incision should be modified so that the risk of skin necrosis is minimized.

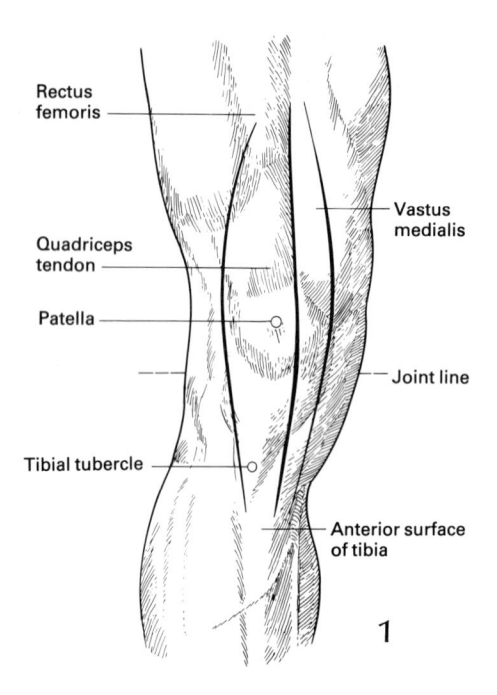

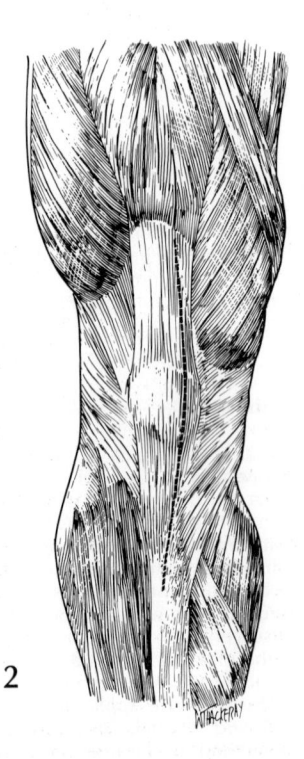

Capsular incision

2

A medial arthrotomy is performed in a straight line through the medial patellar retinaculum. The incision crosses the medial border of the patella, with care taken not to cut the patellar tendon. The distal aspect of the incision should lie 1 cm medial to the tibial tubercle to preserve a cuff of tissue so that inadvertent avulsion of the tibial tubercle will be prevented. Partial resection of the fat pad may be necessary to obtain sufficient exposure of the proximal tibia.

The proximal tibia is exposed by subperiosteal dissection of the pes anserinus and semimembranosus tendons. The latter tendon is not necessarily dissected off its insertion in cases of severe valgus deformity. A periosteal elevator or scalpel may be used. The patella is everted and the knee is flexed.

Correction of deformity and soft-tissue release

Usually, adaptive changes occur in the ligaments of the knee in cases of longstanding arthritis. Loss of cartilage and bone is symmetrical in rheumatoid arthritis, whereas it is frequently asymmetrical in osteoarthritis.

3a, b & 4

In a varus deformity, the medial collateral ligament is contracted and the lateral collateral ligament is stretched. In order to obtain normal mechanical alignment, the shortened collateral ligament must be released. The distal insertion of the medial collateral ligament and pes anserinus insertion are released by subperiosteal dissection along with the semimembranosus insertion. Medial osteophytes are removed and care is taken not to disrupt the ligament proximally. The release is done progressively as the situation requires, starting with osteophyte removal initially and proceeding to distal ligament release. It is sometimes necessary to release the deep fascia investing the soleus and popliteus muscles.

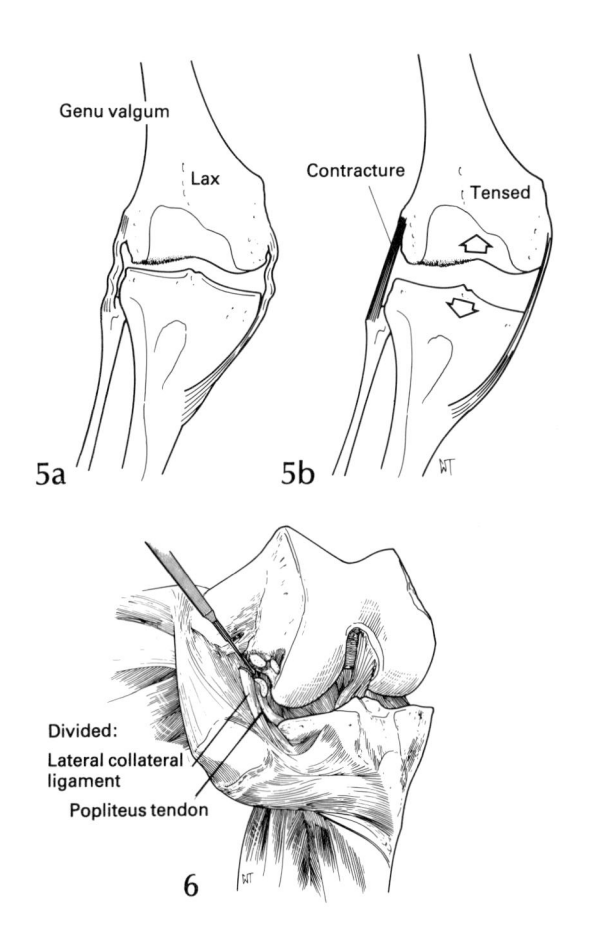

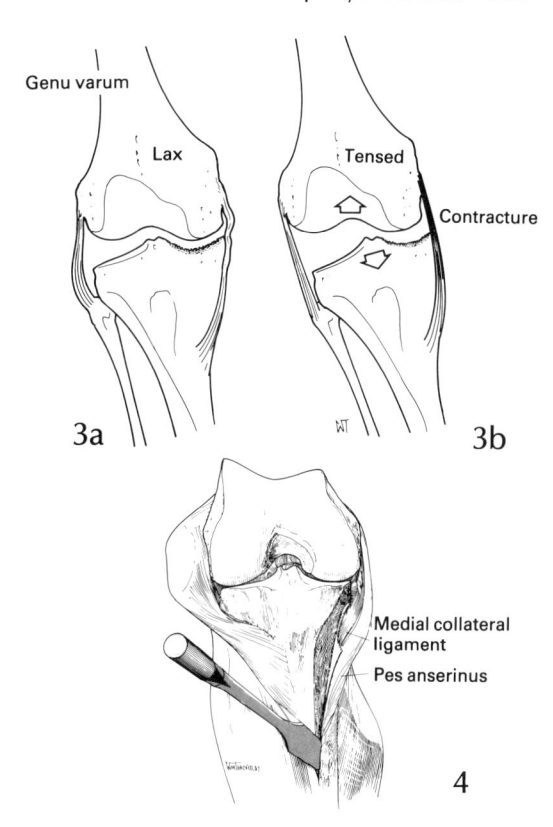

5a, b & 6

A fixed valgus deformity presents a shortened lateral collateral ligament and an attenuated medial collateral ligament. The lateral collateral ligament and popliteus tendon may be released proximally off the femur when the knee cannot easily be corrected to normal valgus alignment. In severe cases, the lateral head insertion of the gastrocnemius muscle is released subperiosteally and the iliotibial band is incised in a horizontal direction across its fibres. Stability will be achieved by obtaining a tight fit with the spacer in flexion to maintain tension on the medial collateral ligament.

Flexion contracture frequently accompanies fixed varus or valgus deformities and must also be addressed. This may be considerable in severe cases of rheumatoid arthritis. Resection of the posterior femoral condyles will correct mild contractures. However, posterior osteophytes should be removed initially and, in the severest cases, the femoral origins of the medial and lateral heads of the gastrocnemius muscles must be released. In cases of valgus deformity and flexion contracture, the surgeon and patient should be aware of the potential for a peroneal nerve palsy. If it occurs, it is best treated by removing the dressing and flexing the knee[2]. It is now rarely seen in cases which use continuous passive motion as the knee begins flexion immediately.

Implant design Given adequate soft-tissue release, most knees will not require a constrained prosthesis. We seldom use constrained devices except where the collateral ligaments have been totally destroyed by trauma or in a severe flexion contracture which requires bone resection above the femoral origins of the collateral ligaments. In the latter case, soft-tissue release may be inadequate, and a subsequently large femoral bone resection may compromise the collateral ligament insertions. Regardless of the implant design used, certain general principles should be followed to assure a successful surgical outcome[3]. Certain steps are the same whether a severe or mild deformity is present.

7a, b & 8a, b

The operation requires a transverse proximal tibial resection, followed by a resection of the posterior and anterior aspects of the femoral condyles to obtain a rectangular space in flexion. The rectangular space (flexion gap) may be obtained by collateral ligament release, or by lateral rotation of the cutting block on the femur. Further ligament release may be still necessary depending on the deformity of the knee.

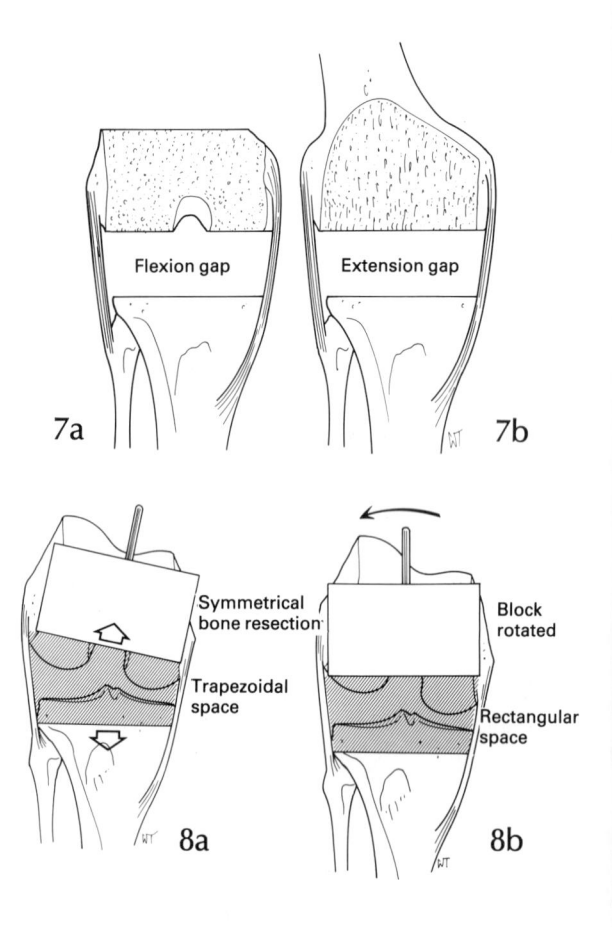

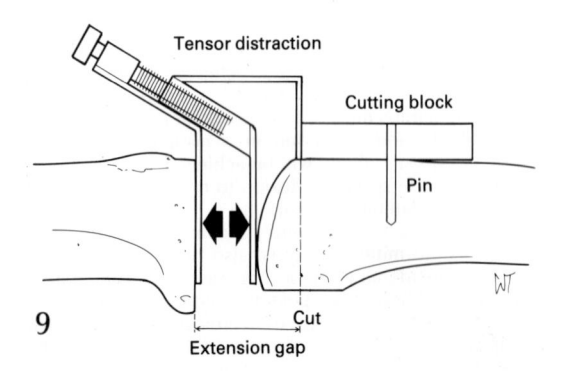

9

When the ligaments have been balanced, an extension gap is created by a tensor and distal femoral cutting block. The extension gap should equal the flexion gap; the distal femoral resection should be made in 7°–10° valgus while collateral ligament tension is kept relatively equal. Final chamfering and sculpting of the femur and tibia are performed according to the dimensions of the prosthetic design that is used.

Flexion gap

10, 11 & 12

The proximal tibia is transected perpendicular to the longitudinal axis of the shaft with the assistance of a cutting block and alignment bar which is affixed to bone. The lower end of the bar is placed on the lower tibia in line with the malleoli; the upper end of the bar is placed with the lateral edge in line with the centre of the tibial tubercle. The tibial surface is cut flat with an oscillating saw; no more than 5 mm of the proximal tibia should be resected in order to preserve strong trabecular bone stock. The femoral cutting block is placed and resection of the anterior and posterior aspects of the femoral condyles is performed. A rectangular space in flexion is obtained.

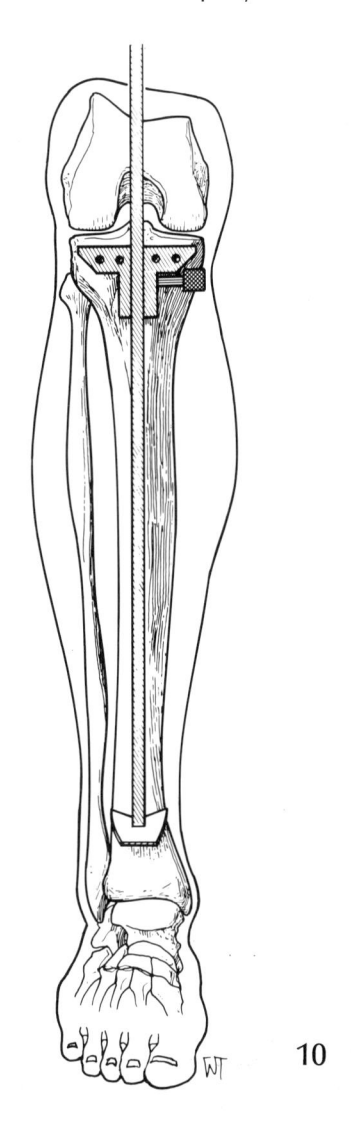

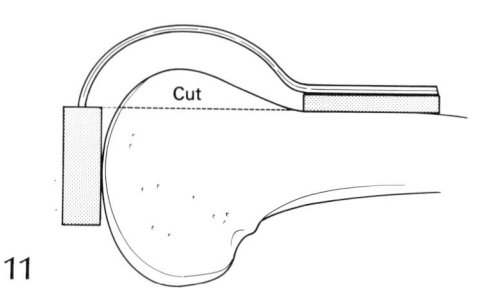

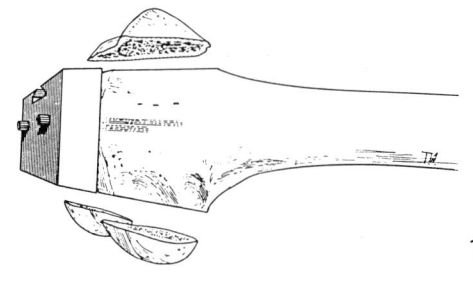

13 & 14a, b

A spacer block is placed in the rectangular gap with a suitable thickness to tense the collateral ligaments in flexion. The tibial resection is concurrently assessed by an alignment rod that is placed through the spacer. This rod should fall midway between the medial and lateral malleoli of the ankle joint if a transverse tibial resection is present. The surgeon must protect the collateral ligaments with retractors during these steps so that inadvertent transection of the collateral ligaments by the reciprocating saw is prevented.

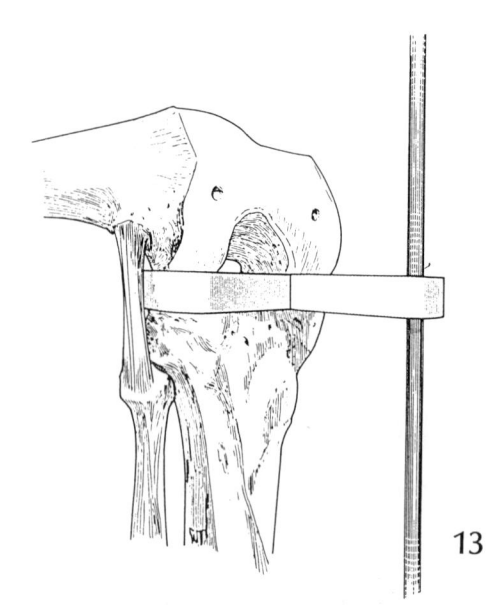

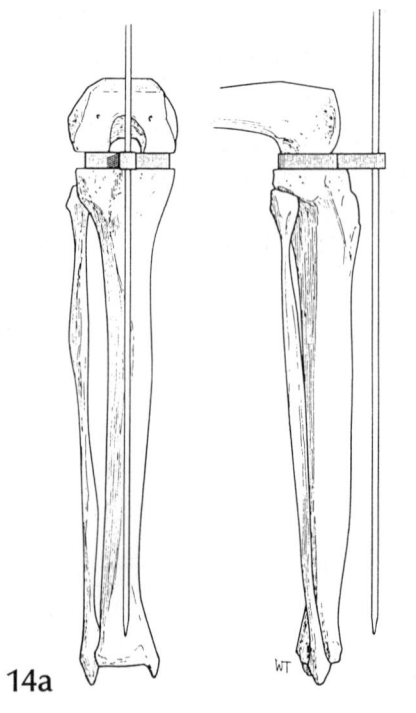

Extension gap

15a & b

After the surgeon has appropriately sized the flexion gap with a spacer, an extension gap must be created equal in dimension to the flexion gap. The collateral ligaments should be balanced. A tensor device (*see Illustration 9*) is used to tense the collateral ligaments[4]. An alignment rod which can be affixed to the device, should fall two to three fingers'-breadth medial to the anterior superior iliac spine in order to obtain 7°–10° of valgus. If the iliac crest is not easily palpable, a preoperative radiograph of the hip should be done so that an external marker can be applied over the centre of the femoral head. In this instance, the alignment rod should fall directly over this marker to assure correct alignment. The tensor must not be used to release the collateral ligaments any further. If the alignment rod falls medial to the femoral head, further lateral ligament release is required. If the rod is located lateral to the femoral head, the mechanical axis is in varus or neutral and more medial collateral ligament release should be performed.

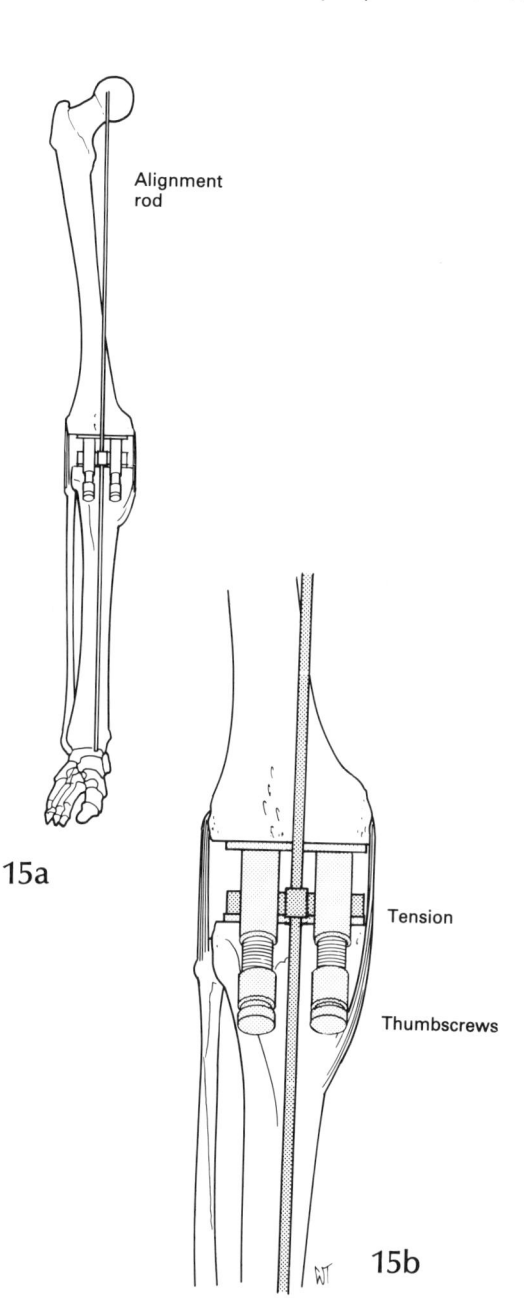

16, 17 & 18

When the correct alignment is obtained with appropriate ligament balance, a distal femoral cutting block is attached to the tensor and affixed by pins to the femur (see *Illustration 9*). The distal femur is transected with a reciprocating saw at an angle of 7°–10° of valgus. The same spacer block that was used to size the flexion gap is placed in the extension gap to check the fit, alignment and collateral ligament tension.

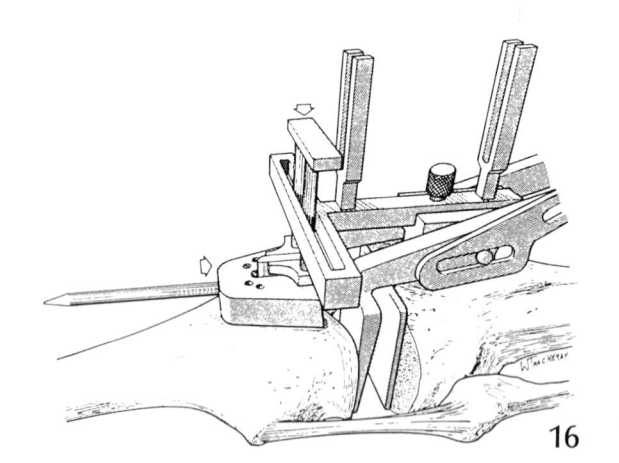

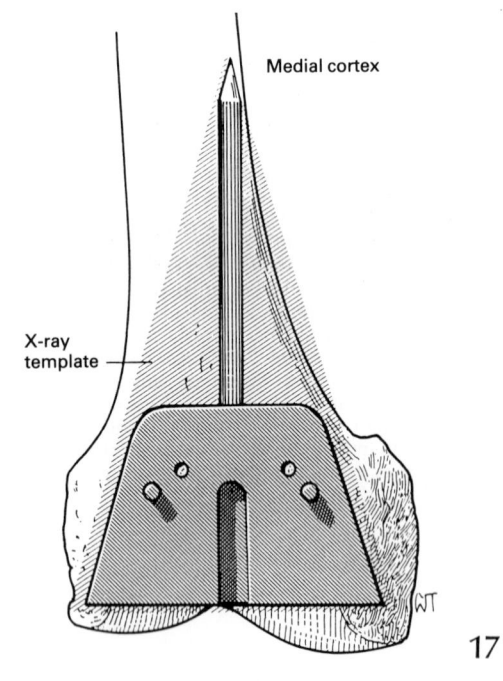

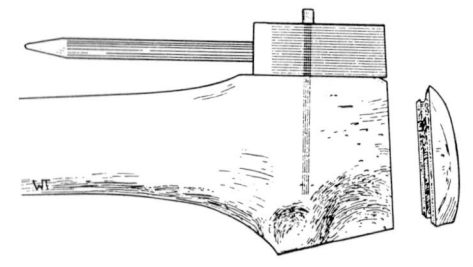

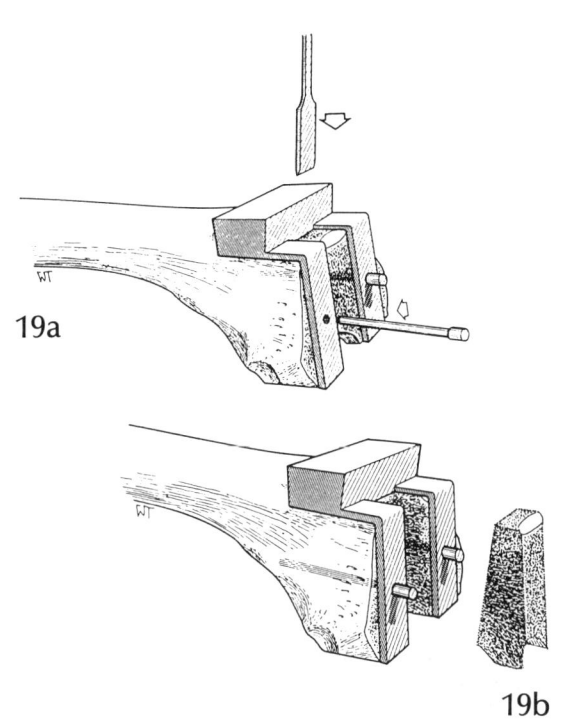

Final preparation of the femur, tibia and patella

19a, b, 20 & 21

The distal femur is prepared by placing a notch-cutting guide onto the distal femur, so that the intercondylar notch is resected to a depth equal to the dimension of the prosthesis. The anterior and posterior aspects of the distal femur are chamfered with the aid of a guide to complete the preparation of the femur.

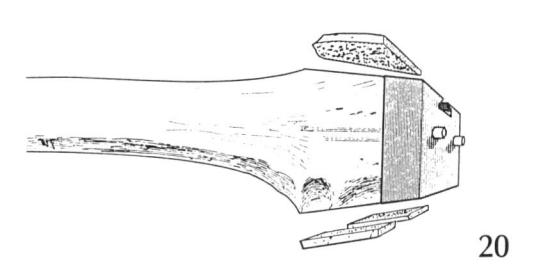

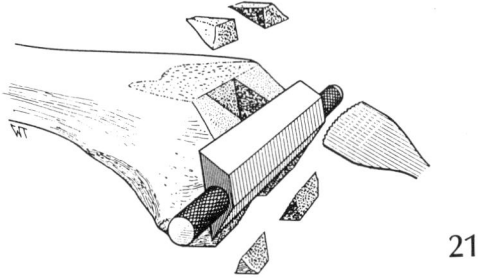

1128 Thigh and knee

22a, b, 23, 24 & 25

A central fixation hole is made in the proximal tibia so that the central peg of the tibial component is correctly aligned with the tibial tubercle. Tibial component malrotation must be avoided by aligning the handle of the jig with the tibial spine, as excessive medial rotation will pose the risk of postoperative patellar dislocation.

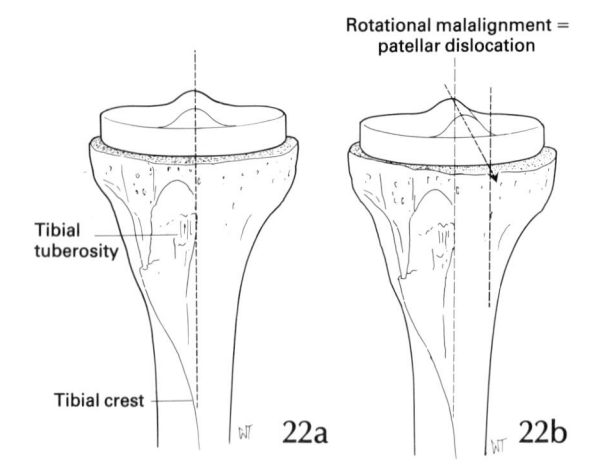

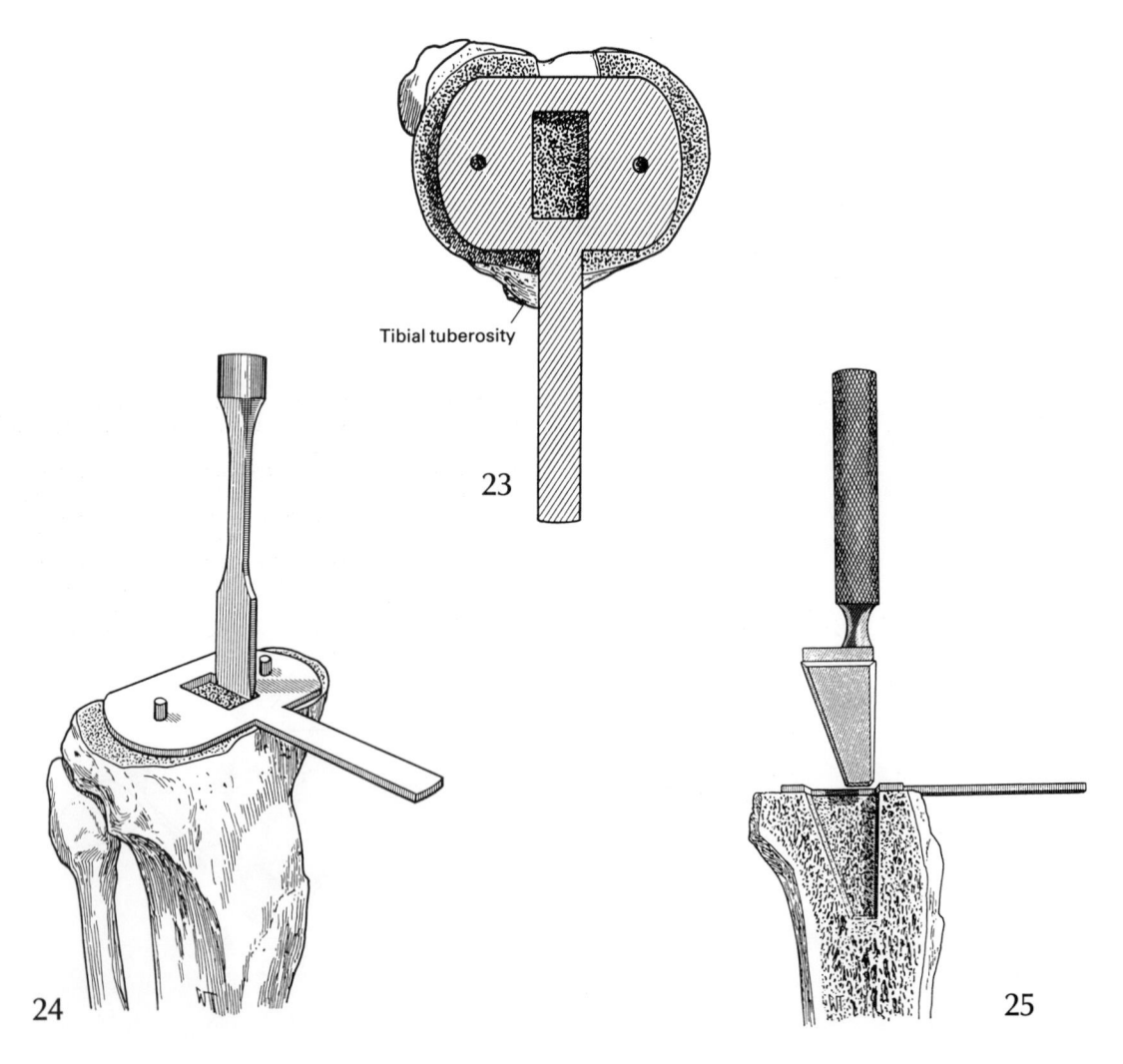

26

The patella is resurfaced in all cases where possible. The patella must be of sufficient size to accept a prosthesis, otherwise it is impractical to resurface it. The resection is done by eye, with the patella held everted. The resection is carried from the medial to lateral articular surfaces. A patellar thickness of 1–1.5 cm should remain to provide adequate fixation of the prosthesis. This may not be possible in rheumatoid knees because of loss of bone, and is then best avoided. A central fixation hole is made with a gouge.

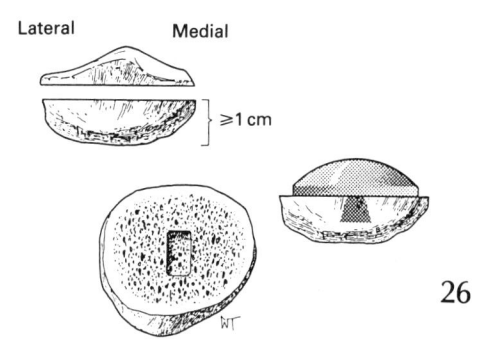

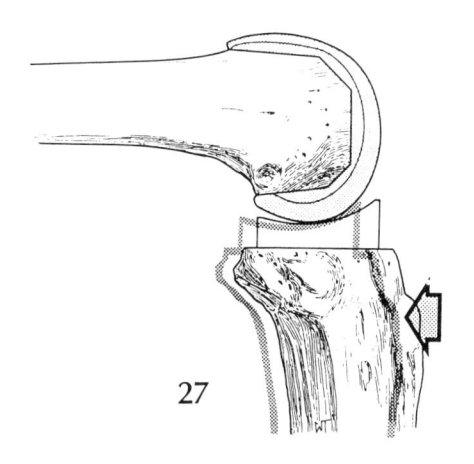

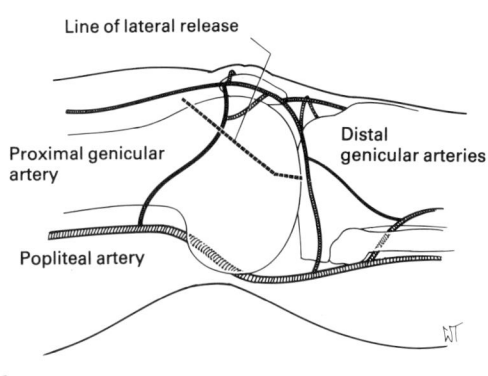

27 & 28

Trial prostheses are positioned onto each respective bony surface and the knee is reduced. Alignment and ligament balance are rechecked and the tibial component thickness should equal that of the spacer block that was used to size the flexion and extension gaps. Patellar tracking is evaluated and a lateral retinacular release is performed if there is a tendency for the patella to mistrack laterally.

The tourniquet is released, and haemostasis is maintained by means of cauterization. The limb is re-exsanguinated and the tourniquet re-inflated. The trabecular surfaces are cleansed by pulsatile saline lavage in order to remove blood and bone debris.

29, 30 & 31

The femoral and patellar components are affixed simultaneously to each respective dried surface with acrylic cement. Only sufficient cement is used to fill the gaps between the prosthetic components and the bone. Where there is loss of bone on the tibia this may be made up by bone grafts taken from the resected segments. (In this situation, weight-bearing is restricted by crutch-walking for 3 months after operation.) The tibial component is then inserted with a separate batch of cement. Excess acrylic is removed by scalpel or curette. The knee is reduced and brought into extension after the cement hardens and the wound is irrigated with an antibiotic saline solution and suction drains are placed in the knee. The wound is closed in layers with interrupted vertical mattress sutures. A bulky Robert Jones dressing is applied to the limb.

Postoperative management

Intravenous broad-spectrum antibiotics are continued postoperatively for 48 hours and suction drainage is used for 24 hours. Continuous passive motion, if available, is initiated in the recovery room, and a lighter postoperative dressing will then be required. If the situation dictates against early movement, a bulky Robert Jones dressing is used and kept in place for 2 days; active assisted flexion is begun on the second postoperative day. The patient stands and begins walking with assistance on the second or third postoperative day. The patient is discharged when he or she can climb stairs, walk with a stick and bend the knee to 90°. Active resisted quadriceps exercises are not recommended for 6 months to prevent inadvertent disruption of the extensor mechanism.

We consider that some form of postoperative prophylaxis against deep venous thrombosis should be given. We obtain a venogram on the fifth postoperative day. Warfarin prophylaxis is begun if there is a known risk of deep venous thrombosis. If thrombosis is present in the thigh or the patient is symptomatic, heparin therapy is started, followed by warfarin, and the patient remains on the latter medication for 2 to 3 months. Some surgeons, however, use salicylates postoperatively in a twice-daily dosage of 650 mg.

Complications

Complications may be divided into medical and mechanical. The medical complications include: deep venous thrombosis, pulmonary embolism, skin necrosis, and postoperative infection. Antibiotic prophylaxis, careful handling of soft tissues during surgery, and medical prophylaxis against clot formation will minimize these problems. Mechanical complications include: improper mechanical alignment (especially neutral or varus) owing to insufficient ligament release, malrotation of the tibial component with subsequent patellar dislocation, instability owing to inadvertent transection of the medial collateral ligament, component loosening, and peroneal nerve palsy. Careful attention to proper surgical technique will minimize these difficulties and assure proper function of the knee.

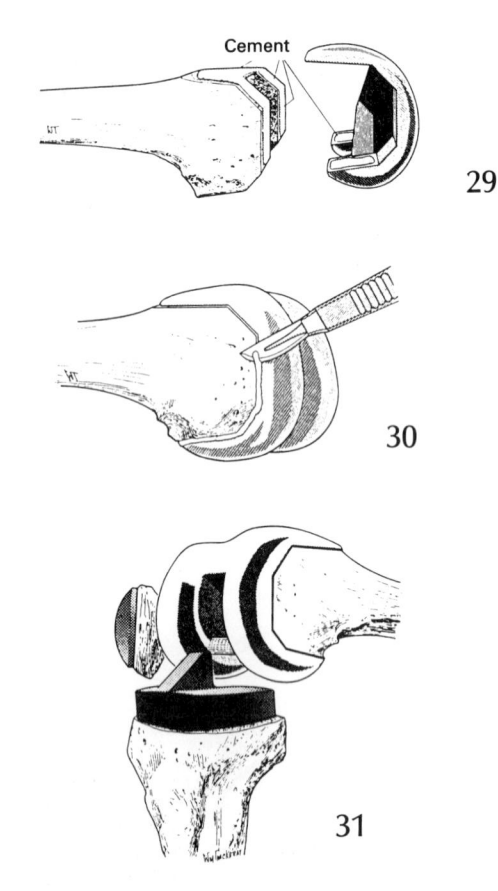

References

1. Insall J. A midline approach to the knee. *J Bone Joint Surg [Am]* 1971; 53-A: 1584–1586.

2. Rose HA, Hood RW, Otis JC, Ranawat CS, Insall JN. Peroneal-nerve palsy following total knee arthroplasty. *J Bone Joint Surg [Am]* 1982; 64-A: 347–51.

3. Insall JN, ed. *Surgery of the knee*. New York: Churchill Livingstone, 1984.

4. Freeman MAR, Insall JN, Besser W, Walker PS, Hallel T. Excision of the cruciate ligaments in total knee replacement. *Clin Orthop* 1977; 126: 209–12.

Acknowledgement

Illustrations 12–14, 16–21, 23–27 and 29–31 are reproduced with permission from Insall JN, Burstein AH, Freeman MAR. *Principles and Techniques of Knee Replacement*, published by the New York Society for the Relief of the Ruptured and Crippled.

Illustrations by Gillian Oliver after F. Price

Compression arthrodesis of the knee

The late Sir John Charnley CBE, FRS, FRCS, FACS
Formerly Emeritus Professor of Orthopaedic Surgery, University of Manchester, Honorary Orthopaedic Surgeon, Centre for Hip Surgery, Wrightington Hospital, Wigan; Consultant Orthopaedic Surgeon, King Edward VII Hospital, Midhurst, Sussex, UK

Introduction

Indications

The pathological conditions suitable for treatment by knee fusion are varied though the procedure is now rarely performed. They range from painless mechanical instability in paralytic and traumatic conditions, to painful and stiff knees in chronic arthritis and destructive processes such as tuberculosis and failed prosthetic replacement. Cancellous bone graft may be required to fill any gaps between the bone ends after failed prosthetic replacement.

Contraindications

The involvement of other joints in chronic arthritis, especially the opposite knee and one or both hips, makes it difficult for a patient to cope with a stiff knee. Ideally knee fusion should therefore be done only in patients whose other joints in the lower extremities are normal. There are many cases where a knee disability so dominates the clinical picture that there is no alternative but to fuse the knee in the presence of other abnormal joints, and in these cases the patient will be greatly benefited though still remaining disabled to some extent.

In very rare instances bilateral fusion of the knees can produce remarkable benefit if both hips are normal, and if the patient fully understands all that this operation entails. Usually a combination of an arthrodesis of one knee and an arthroplasty of the other produces a better result.

Preoperative

Anaesthesia

Any form of anaesthesia can be used for this operation except a local anaesthetic, since a tourniquet on the thigh is essential.

Position of patient

The patient lies supine on an ordinary operating table.

Tourniquet

This should be applied high in the thigh. It can be applied, unsterile, before skin preparation and draping.

Draping

The skin is prepared with Hibitane in spirit (ICI Pharmaceuticals, UK). Adhesive plastic drape is then applied.

1132 Thigh and knee

Operation

Incision

1

Generally, a transverse incision is the best. When in tuberculosis excision of the suprapatellar pouch is needed then a longitudinal incision is better. It is unnecessary to excise the suprapatellar synovia of non-tuberculous chronic arthritis.

The knee should be flexed to 90° with the heel on the table. The skin incision is made exactly at the level of the joint line in the plane of the head of the tibia. The incision should be carried medially and laterally about 1 cm posterior to the central axis of the limb.

Incision of capsule

The capsule of the joint should be incised in the same line as the skin without undercutting. The capsular incision should go down to the bone of the tibia all the way round just below the level of the menisci. The patellar tendon is divided at this level.

The front of the capsule should be reflected upwards as a flap containing the patella. This may require short relaxing incisions at the lateral and medial extremities of the capsule.

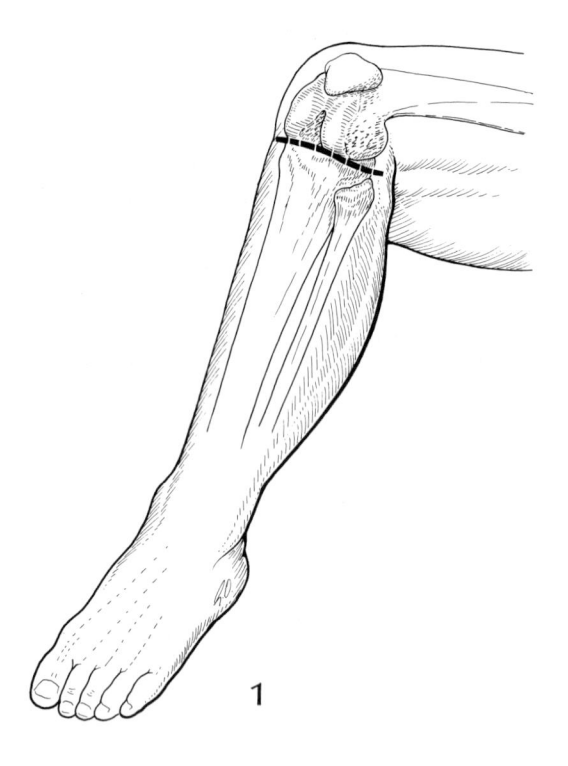

Subluxating the joint

2

Division of the capsule and the medial, lateral and cruciate ligaments is complete when the knee can be fully flexed with the heel touching the buttock. The head of the tibia is thereby slightly subluxated forwards. A bone lever passed behind the head of the tibia, using the lower end of the femur as a fulcrum, will help in this forward subluxation of the tibia and will also protect the popliteal structures when the saw is used on the upper end of the tibia. It should be emphasized that to present the upper end of the tibia easily to the saw: (a) the skin incision should not be at a higher level than the upper end of the tibia, and (b) full flexion of the knee should be secured.

Patella

A decision must be made on the fate of the patella. Ideally it is best excised since residual pain sometimes can arise in patellofemoral arthritis but the majority of cases do well with the patella left *in situ*.

Resecting upper end of tibia

3

With the knee in full flexion two retractors pull the medial and lateral parts of the skin incision downwards so that the head of the tibia projects clear of the wound. The bone lever guarding the popliteal fossa helps to push forward the tibia. With the tibia held vertically the saw is started at right angles to the long axis of the tibia and about 1 cm below the level of the articular surface of the tibia. An amputation saw with a deep blade of 7.5 cm is suitable.

Having started the cut, the tibia should be inspected in two planes with the saw resting in the cut, to make sure that the saw is completely at right angles to the long axis of the bone. No tilt or inclination of the saw should be given at this stage if some fixed flexion is desired in the final result.

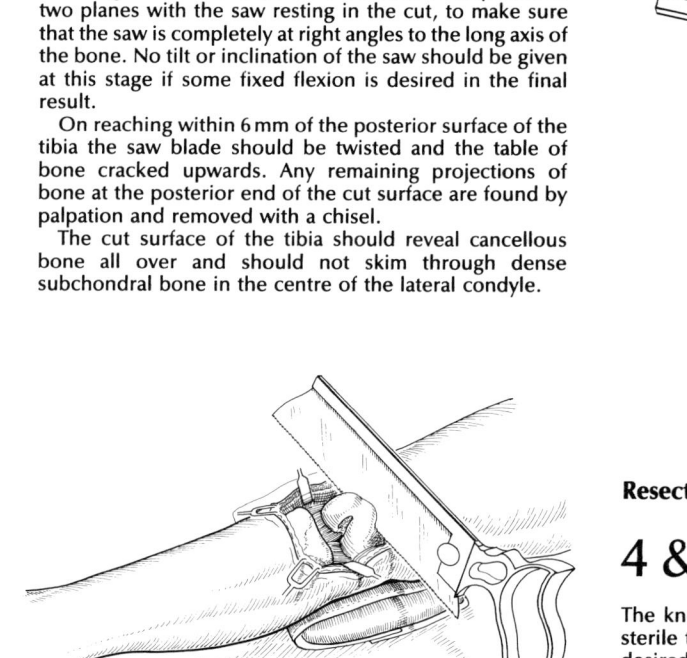

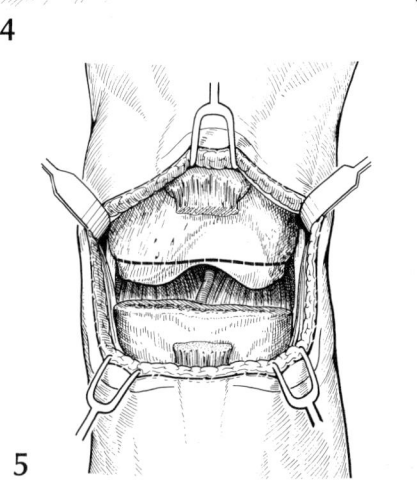

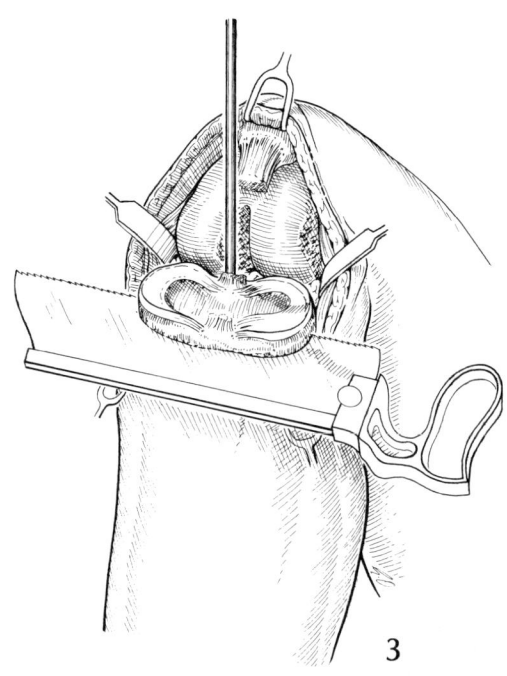

On reaching within 6 mm of the posterior surface of the tibia the saw blade should be twisted and the table of bone cracked upwards. Any remaining projections of bone at the posterior end of the cut surface are found by palpation and removed with a chisel.

The cut surface of the tibia should reveal cancellous bone all over and should not skim through dense subchondral bone in the centre of the lateral condyle.

Resecting lower end of femur

4 & 5

The knee is extended and a small sandbag wrapped in a sterile towel is put behind the popliteal fossa to give the desired amount of flexion with the heel resting on the table.

The author prefers to have not more than 5° of flexion at this stage. It is not possible to be more accurate than plus or minus 5° between the position on the table and the end result; with 5° of flexion on the table the end result can range from a completely straight knee to one flexed at 10°. If, on the other hand, 10° of flexion on the table is used the end result can be flexed as much as 15° or 20° and this, in the author's opinion, is a disadvantage in walking.

An assistant holds the foot, applying some traction to open the space between the bones, and makes sure that the tibia is in the desired alignment as seen in the anteroposterior plane. The surgeon applies the saw to the front surface of the femur at the level of the intercondylar notch. The plane of the saw blade must be strictly parallel to the cut surface of the tibia as seen in the open wound with the axis of the tibia in the chosen position.

Flexing of knee in sawing

6

When the saw has penetrated about 2.5 cm into the femoral condyles, the knee is flexed to facilitate the final sawing off of the lower end of the femur. The tibia can be displaced backwards under the femoral condyle to give support to the femoral condyles during this sawing.

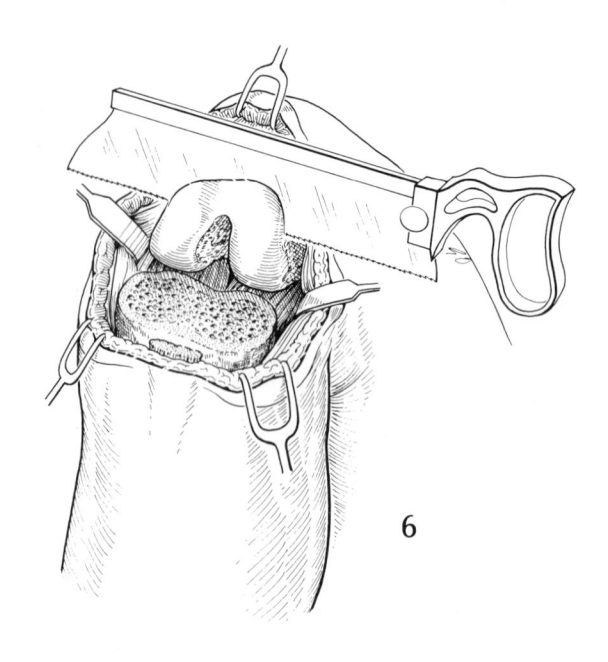

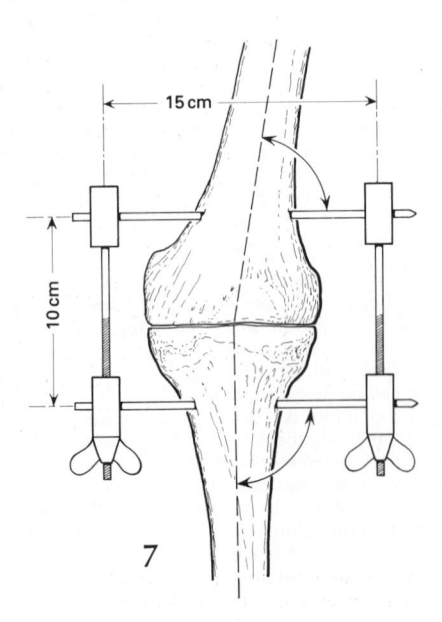

Inserting the tibial pin

7

The tibial pin should always be inserted first. The placing of the tibial pin is easy since this must be at right angles, in two planes, to the long axis of the tibia. The femoral pin has to be inserted at an angle to the long axis of the femur and this is difficult to assess if attempted first.

The tibial pin should pass across the tibia about 3.5 cm below the cut surface. The pin should be sited carefully half-way between the anterior crest and the posterior surface of the tibia.

Inserting the femoral pin

The Charnley compression clamps are now applied to the distal pin to act as a guide for the second pin in the femur. The blocks in the clamps should be separated the full distance of 10 cm. Care should be taken to place the pin in the femur half-way between the anterior and posterior cortices.

Tightening the clamps

An assistant holding the foot should put the posterior edges of the cut bone surface in contact by pushing in the axis of the tibia, while leaving the anterior edges gaping slightly so that the surgeon can be sure that no soft parts are trapped posteriorly between the bone surfaces.

As soon as the tightening of the clamps has reached the point where the cut surfaces are first drawn into full apposition, the process of applying mechanical compression can be started. With 4 mm Steinmann pins, and with the clamps separated laterally from each other by 15 cm the Charnley clamps will give 50 kg of compression force if both are tightened 12 half turns. This is because the screw threads are 6.2 mm (0.25 inch) Whitworth; any other type of thread would need a different calibration. If the bones are of normal density, and if the pins are well placed, the tightening of the clamps should give sufficient rigidity for the fixation to hold with nothing more than a compression bandage.

Checking rotation

If any error in rotation has been incurred, as indicated by the position of the foot, this is easily altered at this stage by the ability of the simple Charnley pattern of clamps to permit rotary adjustment. The compression is released, the rotatory error corrected and the clamps are retightened.

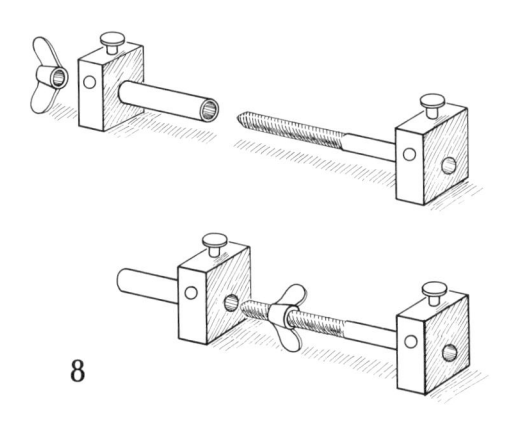

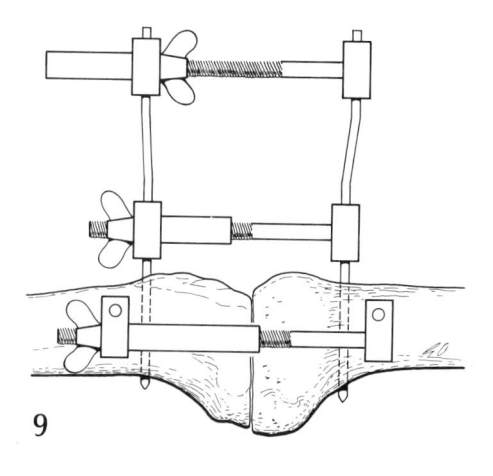

Additional fixation

8 & 9

If the rigidity of the fixation is not considered satisfactory, or if the bone is osteoporotic, additional fixation against movement in the plane of flexion–extension may be considered advisable and can be obtained either by (a) external support or (b) additional fixation. External support by means of a Thomas' splint is mechanically superior to a plaster cylinder. Additional internal fixation is most conveniently added by using two more 4 mm Steinmann pins and mounting a second pair of Charnley compression clamps to make a 'side-pin compression unit'. The two pins are driven into the tibia and femur from the front, making sure that the points merely penetrate the posterior cortices without projecting into the popliteal fossa. The first clamp is then slid along the pins to within about 1.2 cm of the skin and fixed by tightening the set-screws on the clamp. The second clamp is now re-assembled to act as a 'pusher' rather than a compressor, as indicated in the diagram. The 'pusher' clamp is applied to the free ends of the pins and adjusted to hold the free ends apart. Tightening the compression clamp near to the knee will then apply compression as well as lock any tendency of the knee to move in the flexion–extension plane.

Closing the wound

A few interrupted stitches of polyglactin 910 are inserted into the capsule and the patellar tendon.

The skin punctures round the pins should be inspected to avoid unequal tension. If unequal tension in the skin is present appropriate incisions should be made, and if necessary one or two fine skin sutures inserted.

Dressings

10

A pressure dressing is applied, completely burying the whole compression unit in 'fluffed up' wool, and then compressing everything with a crêpe bandage applied over all.

The tourniquet is then removed.

It is important never to strain the arthrodesis by lifting the limb by the foot during this bandaging. Lifting the foot can allow the knee to sag backwards and crush the cancellous bone. The limb should be lifted at the centre of gravity, by a hand under the upper part of the calf.

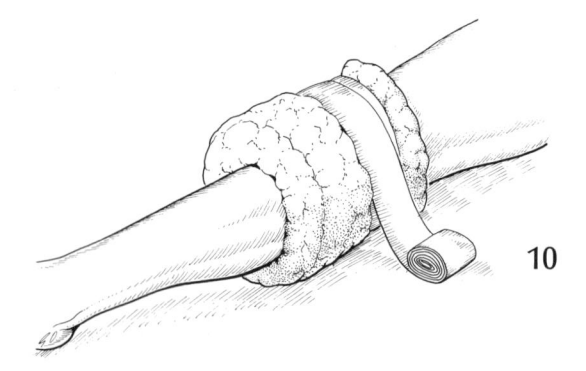

Postoperative management

The compression unit should be left in position for 1 month. It is usually unnecessary to retighten the clamps if the bone is soft, because retightening will merely cause the pins to cut through the bone with further loss of pressure. A check radiograph of the anteroposterior plane should be taken at 10–14 days and this should show the pins deflected by the same amount that they were at the end of the operation if the bone is of good quality. If the deflection has diminished at 10–14 days, in the presence of good bone, then the clamps should be retightened, which can be done without anaesthesia.

The patient is confined to bed for 4 weeks while the compression unit is in position.

At the end of 4 weeks the clamps should be removed from the nails and the knee tested for movement with the nails in position. The accuracy of detecting movement is increased by leaving the pins to act as pointers.

If fibrous movement should be present the clamps should be reapplied for another 2 weeks. In most cases the knee will be quite solid at 4 weeks.

A close-fitting plaster cast is applied for another 4 weeks after the pins have been extracted, and the patient is allowed to take full weight on the foot. This cast prevents excessive external leverage being exerted on the fusion site.

Patients are usually able to rehabilitate completely in the 4 weeks following removal of the plaster. The total time of disability is 3 months (4 weeks of compression, 4 weeks of walking in the plaster cylinder and 4 weeks of walking without plaster).

Complications

The author never found it necessary to use suction drainage after this operation. Occasionally the dressings may drip blood soon after the tourniquet has been removed. If this should happen it is not necessary to take the dressings down; the limb should be steeply elevated, an extra pressure bandage applied over the existing dressings, and the foot of the bed should be raised.

Sepsis in pin tracks was never any trouble in the author's experience. If the patient is confined to bed during the whole time the pins are *in situ*, and if the pins are not *in situ* for more than 6 weeks, superficial sepsis clears up in a few days.

Illustrations by Gillian Lee

Massive replacement for tumours of the lower limb

H. B. S. Kemp MS, FRCS
Consultant Orthopaedic Surgeon, The Middlesex Hospital, London, and The Royal National Orthopaedic Hospital, Stanmore, UK

John T. Scales OBE, FRCS, CIMechE
Emeritus Professor of Biomedical Engineering, The Royal National Orthopaedic Hospital, Stanmore, UK

Introduction

Benign tumours of the appendicular skeleton can generally be treated by curettage with or without adjuvant therapy such as cryosurgery, and by marginal excision. Nevertheless, extensive or recurrent benign tumours may require wide resection and conservative reconstructive surgery.

In the field of malignant tumour surgery, where amputation was originally accepted as the only method of treatment, considerable advances have been made in conservative management. Although initially this was limited to such tumours as chondrosarcoma, the introduction of cytotoxic therapy and, in particular, the regime advocated by Rosen et al.,[1] not only led to a marked improvement in the prognosis but also facilitated the surgery required to preserve the affected limb. In contemporary surgical management of malignant tumours of the lower limb there are four generally accepted methods of treatment.

1. Resection and autogenous bone grafting
2. Resection and allografting (using cadaveric bone)
3. Resection and rotational approximation of the femur and tibia
4. Resection and prosthetic replacement.

In the UK, as a sequel to the pioneering work of Burrows, Wilson and Scales[2], the method of choice and the management of such lesions is that of prosthetic replacement.

Indications

In the lower limb, massive replacement is indicated for tumours of the proximal femur, the distal femur and the proximal tibia. Benign tumours and osteoclastomas that are too extensive for local curettage or have been affected by a pathological fracture and malignant tumours such as osteosarcomas, parosteal osteosarcomas, periosteal osteosarcomas, chondrosarcomas, malignant fibrous histiocytomas and Ewing's sarcomas may all be suitable for such replacements.

Contraindications

Tumours that have widely infiltrated locally and, in particular, those that have invaded subcutaneous tissue and skin are rarely suitable for such treatment, though there are instances where a vascularized musculocutaneous pedicle may be rotated to cover a skin defect.

Occasionally, patients are shown to have extensive medullary involvement. Such patients are probably most suitably treated by disarticulation, though the occasional individual may be suitable for total replacement of the affected bone. However, such surgery is only applicable to tumours affecting the femur or humerus.

Preoperative

Assessment

Patients presenting with tumours suitable for conservative resection and prosthetic replacement, regardless of whether they require cytotoxic therapy, should have a full medical and dental assessment in order to exclude or treat any pre-existing infection. Routine radiographs of the lesion and the lungs should be obtained. In addition, computed tomographic (CT) scans of the lesion and the lungs, radionuclide skeletal scans and magnetic resonance imaging (MRI) scans of the affected limb should be performed. The reasons for such detailed radiological investigations are to determine the local extent of involvement of the affected bone, to exclude the extremely rare occurrence of a 'skip' lesion and to assess whether the tumour is contained within the periosteum. In addition, it is necessary to determine the presence of pulmonary and other secondaries and to exclude the rare manifestation of multiple skeletal metastases. If it is considered that the tumour is resectable, measurement films are then taken so that a custom-built prosthesis can be manufactured.

Biopsy

A biopsy should always be performed as the last procedure before a tumour is resected, in that, at least theoretically, such a procedure may convert an intracompartmental lesion into an extracompartmental lesion. However, a biopsy is essential to determine the precise histological nature of the lesion. In the majority of patients, adequate material can be obtained by needle biopsy, though very occasionally core biopsy is necessary. Positioning of the biopsy site is critical to enable the biopsy scar to be excised *en bloc* when definitive surgery is performed. All too frequently, biopsies performed by the referring hospital seriously prejudice the surgical management. Bone biopsy, if incorrectly performed, carries a considerable morbidity. Consequently it is preferable that the biopsy should be performed by an individual aware of the implications of surgical resection and prosthetic replacement (*see* chapter on 'Techniques of bone biopsy' pp. 91–99).

Prosthesis

Design and manufacture

Major prostheses are individually designed and custom-built for each patient. In order to manufacture these prostheses measurement films, CT and MRI scans are required. Routine radiographs produce a variable degree of magnification. Radiographs of the appendicular skeleton enlarge the image between 10 and 15 per cent. To correct for this error a radio-opaque linear scale is placed alongside the limb that is to be radiographed. Anteroposterior and lateral views of the affected bone including the articular surfaces and views of the unaffected contralateral bone are required for accurate measurement and design. The CT and MRI scans are necessary in order to determine the soft tissue and intramedullary extent of the tumour.

Stainless steel is a suitable material for prosthetic manufacture, though for technical reasons it is now rarely used. Cobalt–chromium–molybdenum alloys, titanium (T1–T5), and titanium alloy (TAl) are preferred, for only these alloys possess adequate fatigue and endurance properties required for the manufacture of the highly stressed, shaped and cross-sectionally contoured intramedullary stem employed in the fixation of the prosthesis to the bone. The optimal length of the intramedullary stem is 14 cm, and it is grouted into the prepared medullary cavity using injected polymethylmethacrylate bone cement. In preparing the cavity, reaming must be minimal and the resultant cavity should not exceed the diameter of the pin by more than 2 mm. Antibiotic cement should be used where there have been previous surgical procedures or if the patient is on cytotoxic drugs. Titanium alloys possess the additional advantage that, to date, no adverse tissue responses have been reported in implants.

The weight-bearing surfaces of orthopaedic components usually have a concavo-convex configuration. Ultra-high-density polyethylene (RCH 1000) is the most commonly used material for the concave component, while the convex component is made of metal or ceramic alumina.

All prostheses eventually become surrounded by a sheath of fibrous tissue. The various muscles detached in the process of dissection become adherent to this capsule. However, in certain situations, it is necessary to obtain a more accurate fixation of the tendons: for instance, in reconstituting the rotator cuff at the shoulder, the prosthesis is sheathed in a polyester locknit mesh which facilitates the reattachment of the muscles of the rotator cuff. At the hip, the abductors are attached to the prosthesis; and at the knee, the patellar tendon is reconstituted using artificial tendons of several layers of folded mesh. It is also possible to use such material to extend tendons and to repair muscle and fascial defects.

Extending or growing prosthesis

The rationale behind the use of an extending prosthesis is that the loss of growth of the relevant growth-plate can be compensated for by the periodic lengthening of the prosthesis. These prostheses have a specific complication: occasionally abundant soft tissue scarring in the adolescent may in some instances produce contractures and limit repeated extension. In addition, the size of the prosthesis used in a child may be inadequate to maintain the mature adult weight. Consequently a further prosthetic replacement sometimes becomes necessary prior to or with the completion of growth. However, such a prosthesis is of particular importance in the lower limb in order to maintain equal length of the two legs.

1

The prosthetic component that replaces the bone deficit is similar in design to that used in adult prostheses. The articulating portion of the prosthesis is connected to the shaft segment by a piston which contains an anti-rotation device so that only extension can take place. At present, two methods are employed to extend the piston. In one method, a distraction tool is used to draw the piston out of the shaft; then tungsten–carbon ball-bearings are introduced through a port at the side of the prosthesis, which is normally closed by a threaded plug. The disadvantage of tungsten–carbon ball-bearings is that maximum loading will occur over a minimal contact area. In consequence, even such a hard material is subjected to stress fracturing. The alternative method of maintaining extension is the use of C-ring sections which can be fitted round the piston between the jaws of the distraction tool.

On the opposite side of the joint, where, for instance, the growth-plate has been preserved in the proximal tibia, the tibial spines are removed, the plateau is reamed and the reamer is carried through the epiphysis, the growth-plate and into the metaphysis. The cavity is progressively enlarged to allow the insertion of a polyethylene sleeve. This lies distal to the growth-plate in intimate contact with the medullary bone. In this particular instance, the component which is inserted into this sleeve is similar to the tibial component of the constrained hinge joint, but it is mounted on a floating table with lugs which fit into grooves cut into the tibial plateau. Under the table there is a medullary rod which fits into the polyethylene sleeve. Subsequently, as growth occurs, this intramedullary rod is progressively extruded. Despite the creation of a defect in the growth-plate there is no clinical evidence of a synostosis occurring between the epiphysis and metaphysis, and unconstrained growth occurs.

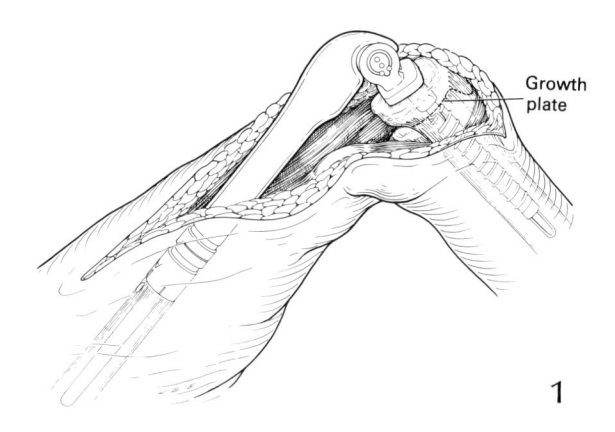

Preoperative management

Patients with malignant tumours are initially treated by the oncologist and admitted to a randomized therapeutic trial[3]. The patients usually receive three cycles of treatment prior to surgery. The rationale for this is that the tumour response to chemotherapy can then be assessed by the histopathologist and an alternative drug regime can be administered, when appropriate, to patients with resistant tumours.

The major risk of massive prosthetic replacement is infection. This applies particularly to the patient who is immunologically suppressed as a sequel to chemotherapy. For this reason patients are given antibiotics intravenously prior to surgery and this regime is continued until the wound has healed. The reason for giving antibiotics intravenously is to maintain a constant blood level. If the patient receiving chemotherapy has a tunnelled central line *in situ*, these lines may have been previously colonized by pathogens, so a separate intravenous line should be used for the antibiotics.

1140 Thigh and knee

Principles of tumour surgery

Enneking et al.[4] have propounded the guidelines for the resection of tumours based on a staging system.

1. Intracapsular excision: a debulking procedure performed within the pseudocapsule
2. Marginal excision: *en bloc* resection performed extracapsularly within the reactive zone (not applicable to bone tumours)
3. Wide excision: *en bloc* excision performed through normal tissue beyond the reactive zone but within the compartment of origin
4. Radical excision: an *en bloc* resection including the compartment of origin.

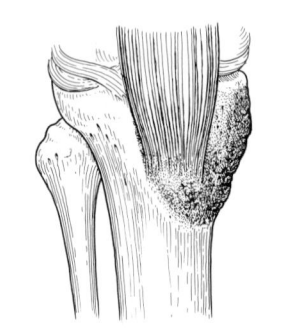

Marginal excision

2

Marginal excision of bone is not feasible. A benign tumour is removed by curettage and subsequent resection is made of the reactive bone that surrounds it.

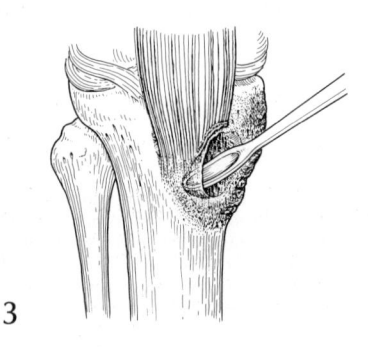

3

Curettage through a small window inevitably leaves a residual tumour behind.

4 & 5

The fenestration of a bone should be as extensive as the parameters of a lesion. The reactive margin of a lesion should then be removed with gouges.

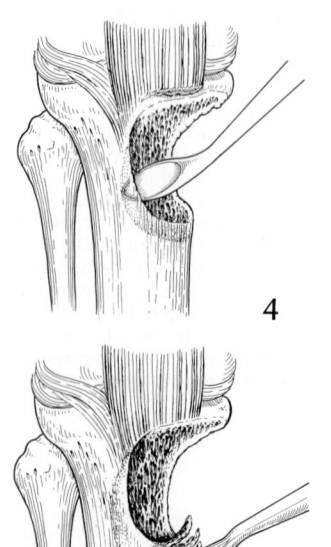

Wide excision

6

Occasionally, even relatively malignant tumours, such as periosteal osteosarcomas, may be resected by wide excision provided the patient is treated by adjuvant chemotherapy.

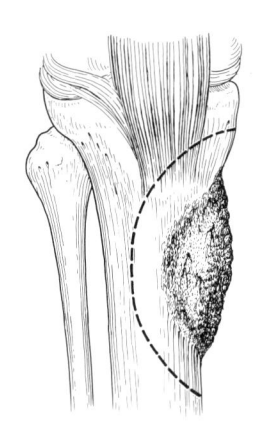

7

Large defects are partially or completely replaced by new bone formation.

Malignant bone tumours

Only Enneking's last two methods are applicable to malignant bone tumours, though at best the surgeon can only achieve a wide margin of resection. The approach to malignant bone tumours in the UK differs in two aspects to Enneking's principles. First, it is believed that in almost all sarcomas the periosteum constitutes a distinctive barrier to tumour spread. In consequence an intact periosteum modifies the staging of the tumour. This does not apply to Ewing's sarcoma which freely permeates the periosteum to involve the soft tissues. Second, in performing a wide resection, if Enneking's principles are followed, a margin of 2 cm of normal tissue is removed with the tumour. While this represents the ideal, it cannot necessarily be obtained in that bone anatomically has 'bare areas' as instanced by the distal femur in its relation to the popliteal fossa. Consequently, an attempt to achieve such a margin posteriorly would result in the resection of the neurovascular bundle, subcutaneous tissue and skin. Sarcomas rarely involve the neurovascular bundle by direct spread; fascial layers, periosteum, epineurium and the adventitia of major arteries are relatively resistant to invasion and, as a result, arterial resection and replacement is only rarely required[5].

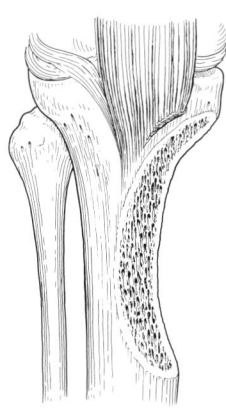

1142 Thigh and knee

Operation

Limb salvage surgery should be performed in an ultra-clean air theatre. The surgeon and his assistants should be hooded and fully gowned in impervious material.

REPLACEMENT OF PROXIMAL FEMUR

Position of patient

The patient is placed on the operating table with the affected side uppermost. The skin should be scrupulously prepared and the patient should be doubly draped with impervious towelling. The incision site is covered with an adhesive drape once the skin has been effectively dried.

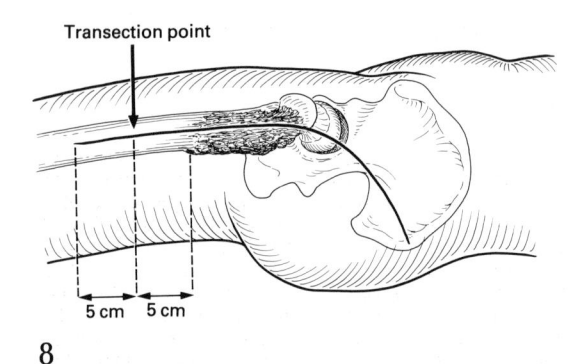

8

Incision

8

Although any of the standard approaches are acceptable, whenever possible we favour the posterior or lateral approach. The proposed point of transection is marked on the skin. The incision is made over the gluteus maximus in line with the muscle fibres, passing downward and forward to the anterior border of the greater trochanter. It is then carried downward in line with the femur to 5 cm beyond the point where it is intended to transect the affected bone.

9 & 10

Using a muscle-splitting technique, the incision through the gluteus maximus is deepened and the fascia lata is incised along the line of the femur anteriorly. The insertion of gluteus medius and minimus into the greater trochanter, when the latter is unaffected by tumour, can be detached in continuity with the fascia lata by removing a thin sliver of the trochanter with an osteotome. If the insertion has to be sacrificed the tendinous insertions of these muscles are transfixed with stay sutures. The underlying musculature is systematically excised so that some 2 cm of normal tissue surrounds the tumour.

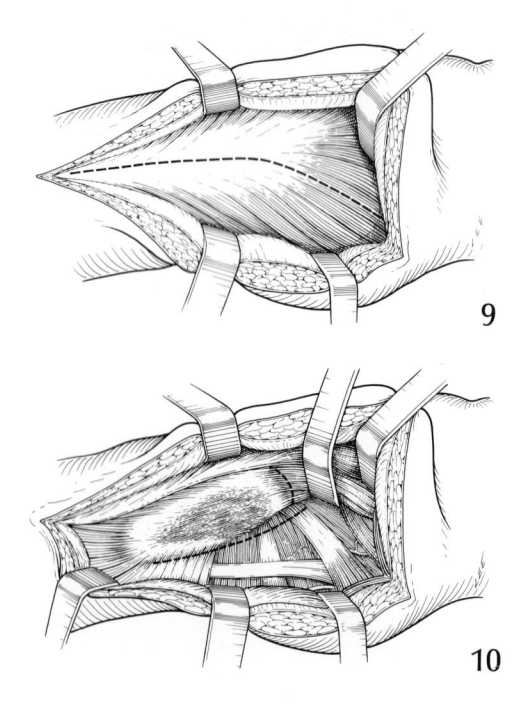

9

10

11

When the tumour has been completely freed, the femur is divided at the site of election. It is sometimes easier to divide the femur at an early stage and complete the dissection in a retrograde manner. The capsule of the hip joint is incised circumferentially. The femoral head is gently distracted and the ligamentum teres is divided. When the femur has been transected a sample of the distal medullary contents is taken so that an imprint can be examined to determine that full clearance of the affected bone has been obtained.

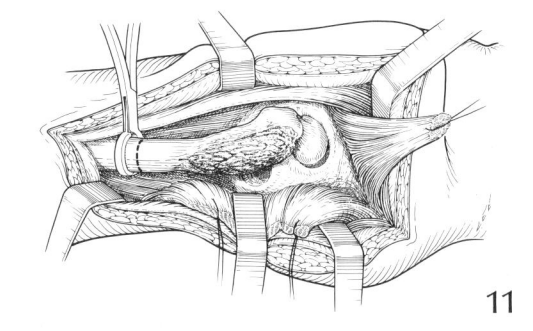

Insertion of prosthetic replacement

12

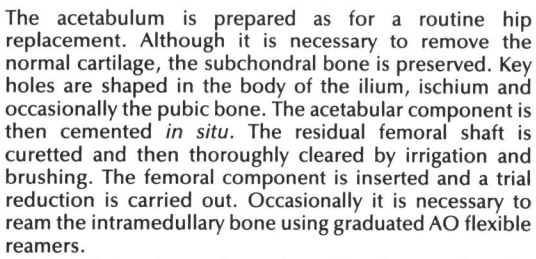

The acetabulum is prepared as for a routine hip replacement. Although it is necessary to remove the normal cartilage, the subchondral bone is preserved. Key holes are shaped in the body of the ilium, ischium and occasionally the pubic bone. The acetabular component is then cemented *in situ*. The residual femoral shaft is curetted and then thoroughly cleared by irrigation and brushing. The femoral component is inserted and a trial reduction is carried out. Occasionally it is necessary to ream the intramedullary bone using graduated AO flexible reamers.

When it has been shown by trial reduction that the desired length of femur has been resected, cement is injected into the femoral canal. Because of the length of the canal, in order to achieve adequate filling, it is necessary to use a cement gun with a long nozzle of the appropriate diameter. The nozzle that is normally used corresponds to the diameter of the medullary lumen so that cement insertion is under pressure. For this reason, the prosthesis needs to be inserted as soon as the cement is of appropriate consistency because such a long column of cement offers a mechanical resistance as the stem is introduced. As far as the orientation of the prosthesis is concerned, this is normally done by relating the prosthesis to the linea aspera. When the linea aspera is defective it is advantageous to put a small drill hole anteriorly in the residue of the femur for orientation. When the cement has polymerized, the prosthesis is articulated with the acetabular cup.

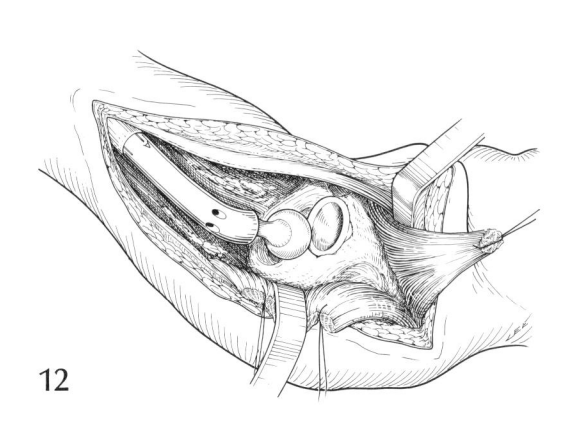

13 & 14

Originally the wound was closed in layers, the tendinous insertions of the gluteus medius and minimus being stitched in to the fascia lata with the hip in abduction, but this presented problems in terms of function. Now, a hole drilled through the neck of the femoral component allows a polyester tape to be stitched to the tendons of the muscles, providing more adequate fixation. The wound is closed in the normal manner after obtaining haemostasis. The wound should be drained using a superficial and deep drain.

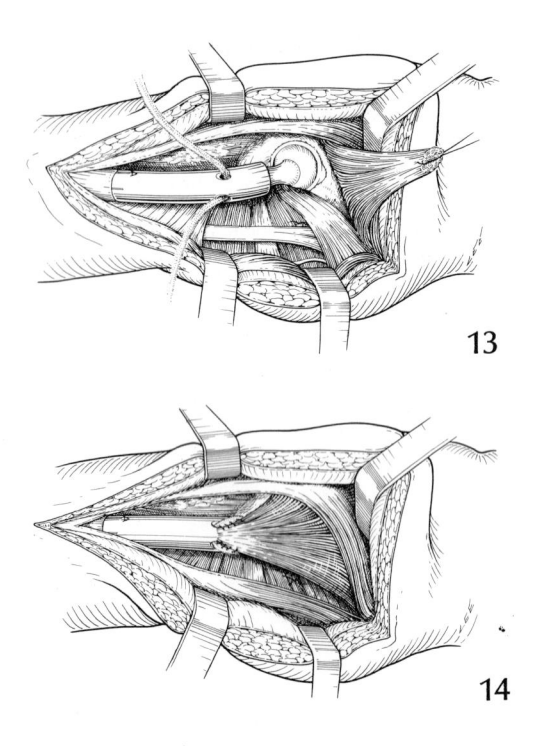

Postoperative management

The patient is nursed with the leg in abduction and supported on balanced slings. Physiotherapy is commenced on the second postoperative day and consists essentially of isometric contractions. Eventually, when adequate muscle tone has been achieved the patient is mobilized in an anti-rotation and anti-adduction splint for 12 weeks using crutches. At this stage all active movements are encouraged by intensive physiotherapy.

Function

Lateral rotation without the reattachment of the rotators is increased to some 60°. Because there is no control over the prosthesis at the point where the greater trochanter was, these patients will walk, in the majority of cases, with a positive Trendelenburg gait. However, with the reattachment of the abductors, most patients can walk with a negative gait or a slight lurch; many patients will be able to run with a negative Trendelenburg gait.

Massive replacement for tumours of the lower limb 1145

REPLACEMENT OF DISTAL FEMUR

Position of patient

The patient is normally placed in a supine position on the table, with a sandbag under the ipsilateral buttock. If the transection point is at a suitable position, the operation is done under a tourniquet. The patient is towelled in the normal manner, the foot is preferably enclosed in a rubber glove so that the peripheral pulses can be palpated as required.

Incision

15

The proximal point of transection is marked on the skin and a medial parapatellar incision is usually made from 5 cm proximal to this point, passing distally to a level of 5 cm below the joint line. The incision on occasion is modified to encompass the biopsy scar where this is feasible, though in certain circumstances it is necessary to make a lateral parapatellar incision in order to do this.

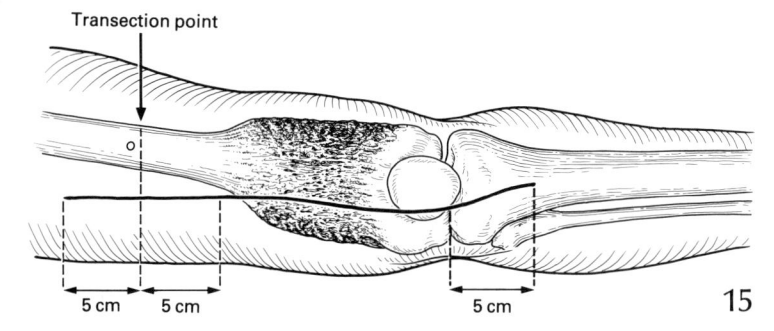

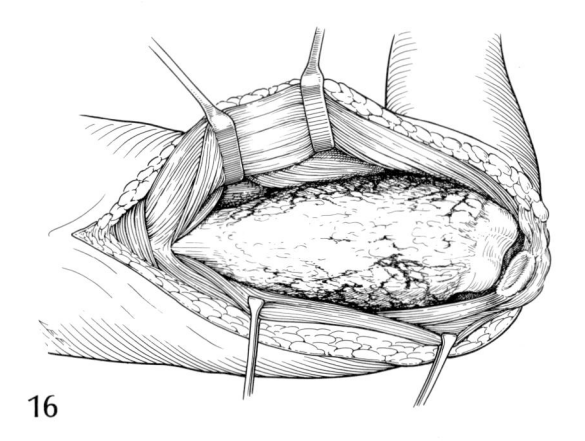

16

The incision is deepened in the midline through the tendon of the quadriceps muscle. Depending on the nature of the tumour the lesion is then marginally or widely excised, malignant tumours being resected with an adequate margin of the three vasti muscles. This resection is extended both medially and laterally.

17

At this stage the distal femur and the proximal tibia are disarticulated. This is performed by detaching the medial and lateral collateral ligaments from their tibial attachments. The patella and the quadriceps tendon are then displaced laterally. The knee is progressively flexed and the cruciate ligaments are divided. At this stage the posterior capsule is easily visualized and divided or resected at its attachment to the tibia. The manoeuvre is facilitated if preceded by gentle blunt dissection behind the capsule. The origins of popliteus and gastrocnemius are exposed and divided from their origins or resected leaving a wide margin.

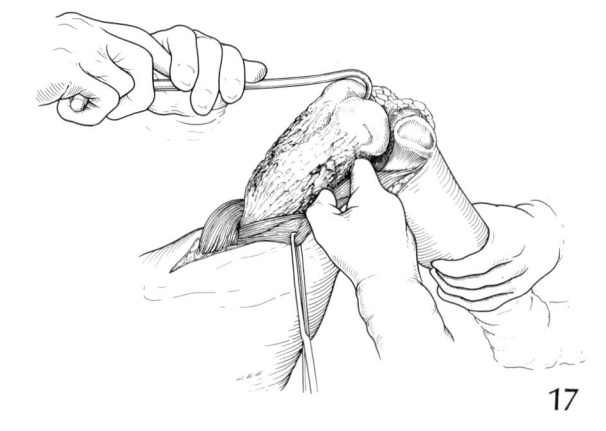

18

The dissection behind the femur is then continued in a retrograde manner. On occasion the involvement of the soft tissues is extensive and the resection can be made easier by dividing the femur and carrying the dissection distally. The neurovascular bundle is rarely involved when the tumour is otherwise removable. However, if the vessels are invaded by tumour they are resected and replaced by a graft taken from the ipsilateral saphenous vein.

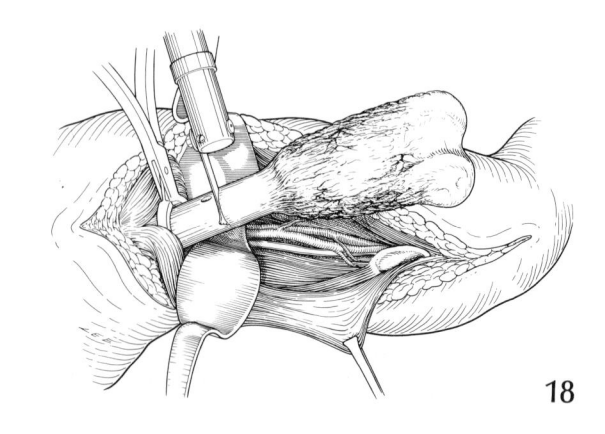

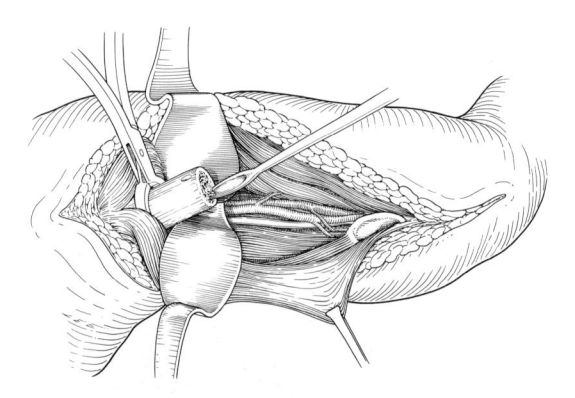

19

As with tumours of the proximal femur, marrow is removed at the time of resection and imprints made to confirm that no residual tumour is present.

Insertion of prosthesis

20

The content of the femoral canal is cleared by curettage and brushing and where necessary the canal is enlarged by the use of flexible reamers. The tibial table is prepared by removing the tibial spines so that the surface is flattened in order to receive the tibial component. Using Capener gouges, the table is breached sufficiently to accept the prosthetic stem.

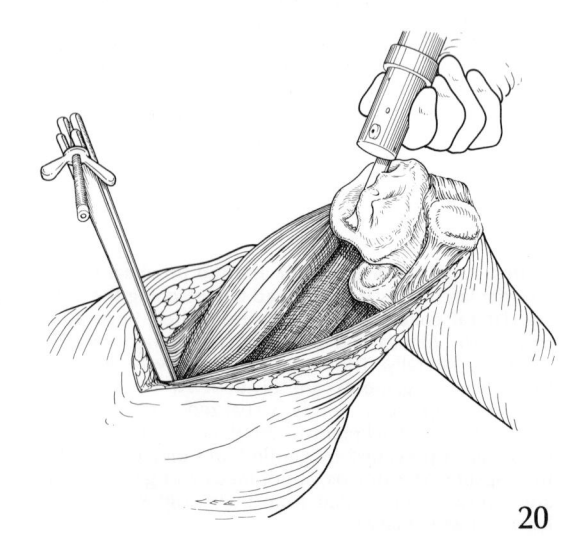

21 & 22

The medullary canal is cleared of all debris by curettage and brushing. Subsequently a cement restrictor is inserted. The two prosthetic components are then introduced and a trial reduction is made. The peripheral vessels are palpated with the knee in extension to determine that there is normal pulsation. If it is necessary to perform further resection this is normally taken from the residual femoral shaft. When a trial reduction is satisfactory, both the femoral canal and the tibia are irrigated and the two components of the prosthesis are cemented into position.

Closure

Wound repair is essentially routine though no attempt is made to close a lateral release if a lateral approach has been made. However, if a standard medial approach has been made a lateral release is performed so that subsequent subluxation of the patella does not occur. The wound is closed in layers and drained.

Postoperative management

The patient is placed on a continuous passive motion (CPM) machine as soon as drainage has ceased. The knee is then progressively passively flexed within the tolerance of the patient. The skin is carefully observed during the initial stages to confirm its viability. As soon as the patient can tolerate active movement, intensive quadriceps and hamstring exercises are instituted. Walking with crutches is begun when the wound is healed, and the crutches and sticks discontinued as muscle control is achieved.

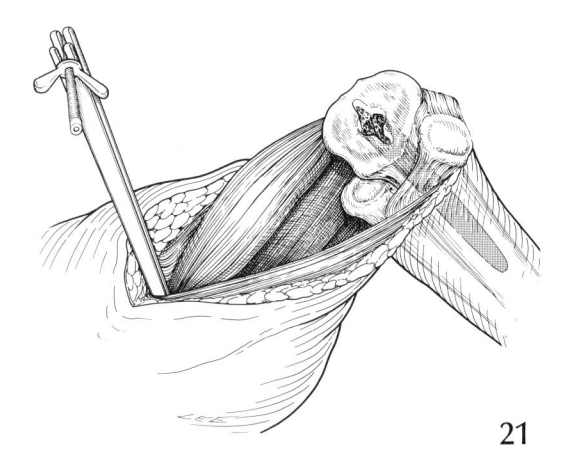

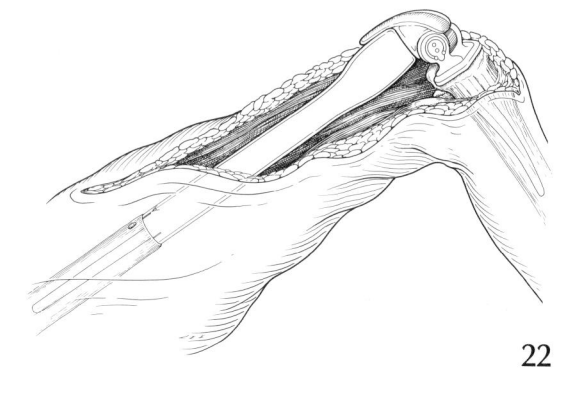

1148 Thigh and knee

REPLACEMENT OF PROXIMAL TIBIA

Position of patient

The patient is supine on the operating table and the operation is normally carried out under tourniquet control without exsanguination; towelling is performed as previously described.

Incision

23

The incision is preferably a lateral parapatellar incision though it may be modified to encompass a biopsy scar. Starting 15 cm proximal to the knee joint it runs distally to 5 cm distal to the point of transection of the tibia. The incision should avoid the crest of the tibia.

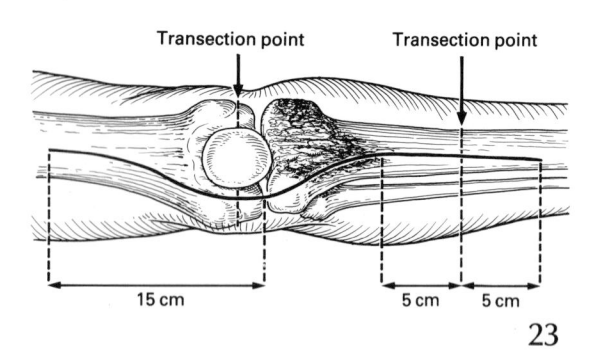

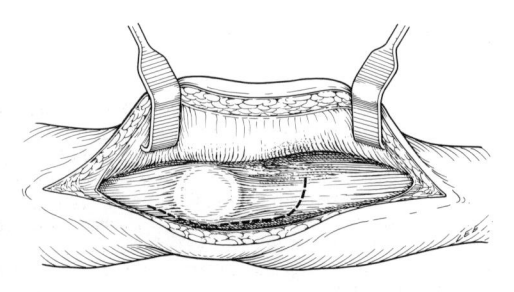

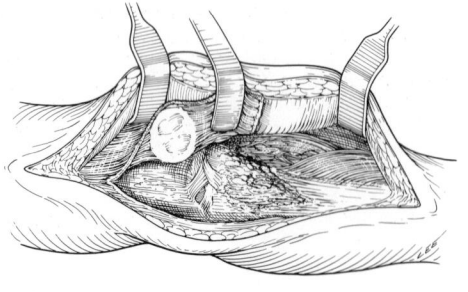

24 & 25

The affected tibia is exposed and the distance from the inferior pole of the patella to the point of transection is determined. The patellar tendon is appropriately reflected from the tibial tuberosity, preserving where possible the medial patellar expansion. The knee joint is disarticulated following the procedure described above.

The medial popliteal nerve and the associated popliteal artery and vein are identified. The origins of gastrocnemius and popliteus are defined prior to disarticulation of the knee. (The origin of soleus is identified and the muscle belly divided at a suitable distance from the tibial lesion.) The neurovascular bundle is traced distally to the point where the artery and vein enter the anterior compartment. The common peroneal nerve is only identified when the tumour encroaches or surrounds the proximal fibula, when it may be necessary to resect this portion of the fibula with the tumour. Normally, the proximal tibiofibular joint is disarticulated.

Muscles of the anterior and posterior compartments and the interosseous membrane are divided at an appropriate distance from the tumour, dissection being carried distally to the point of transection of the tibia. After transection, medullary content is removed for imprint examination. On occasion it is necessary to divide the anterior tibial artery; this can be performed without prejudicing the vascular supply.

Insertion of the prosthesis

26

The marrow cavity in the femur is opened by drilling into the intercondylar notch at the apex of the concavity. Drills of appropriate diameter are then used until the femoral canal accommodates the Stanmore femoral cutting jig (correctly adjusted for left or right knee). The condyles are marked for transection. They are excised using either a power or an amputation saw, the jig being removed at an appropriate point in the transection.

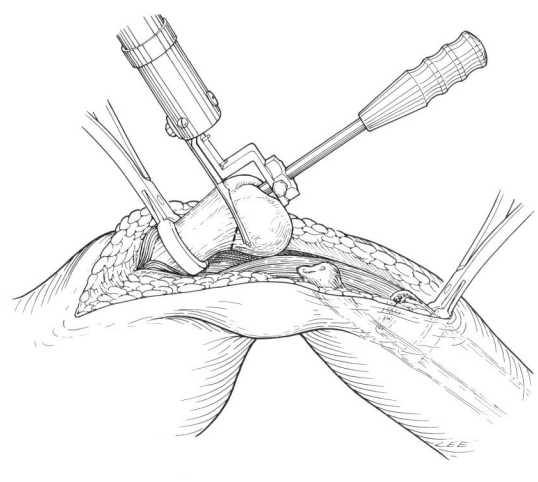

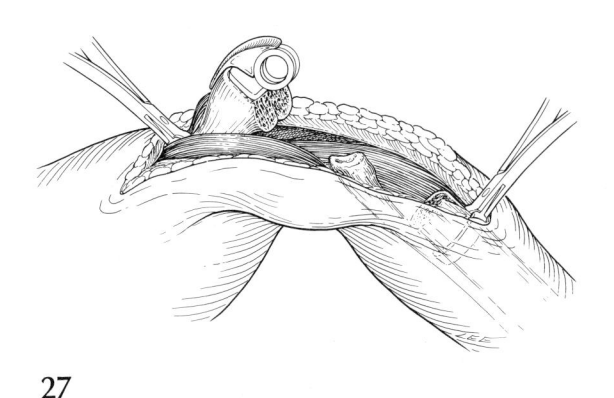

27

The femoral component is prepared, the bushes are impressed and it is inserted into the femoral shaft. Seating of the component is checked. The residual condyles are marked posteriorly and resected. The tibial component is subsequently inserted into the residual medullary cavity. Initially, it may not be accommodated, so the cavity will require reaming with flexible AO reamers until the diameter of the cavity is 1–2 mm greater than the intramedullary stem.

At this stage a trial reduction is performed and the components articulated using a test axle. It is the usual practice to employ a femoral and a tibial plateau plate so that end-bearing of the components is evenly distributed. The articulated prosthesis is extended and if there is limitation of extension it may be necessary to resect the femur further. Even when extension is free, it is essential to check for peripheral pulses and, if they are absent in extension, further resection should be performed. Occasionally the vessels will be in spasm as a sequel to surgery; if this is the case, topical lignocaine may be used. The components are removed when reduction is adequate.

1150 Thigh and knee

28

The medullary cavity is thoroughly irrigated and any residual debris removed using an intramedullary brush. A cement restrictor is inserted into the femoral medullary cavity. The femoral component is cemented into position using a cement gun containing radio-opaque antibiotic cement. While this is setting and compression is maintained by an assistant, the tibial cavity is filled using a Stanmore cement gun with an appropriate nozzle diameter. The tibial component is inserted, orientating the prosthesis in relation to the malleoli or, alternatively, the second toe. When the cement is set the tourniquet is removed and haemostasis obtained. The wound is irrigated to remove residual debris. A polythene tape is threaded into the tibial component and stitched to the patellar tendon with the correct amount of tension. The flexion of the knee is checked and should be in the region of 120°. A drain is inserted and the wound closed in layers with interrupted sutures.

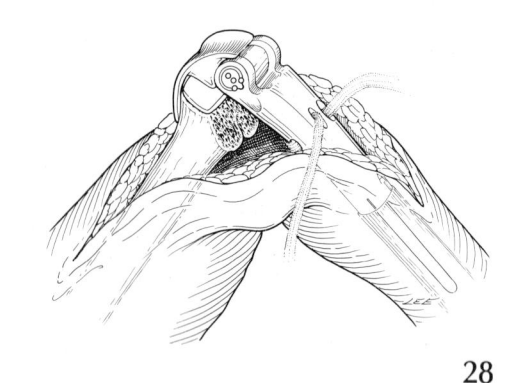

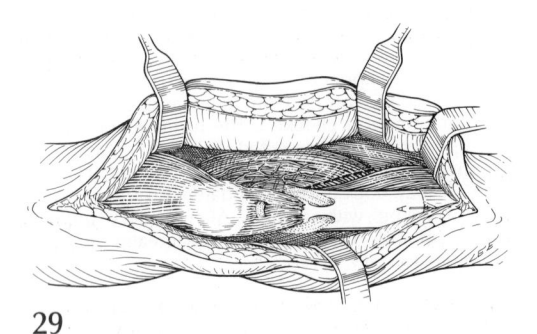

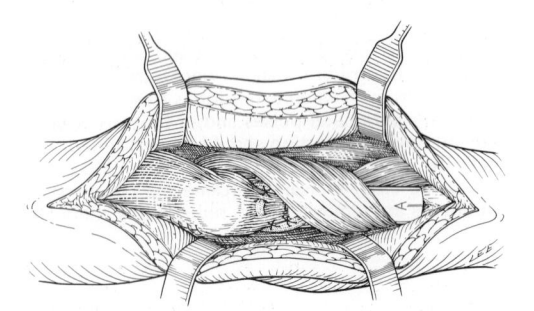

28

29

30

Closure

29 & 30

Closure following replacement of the proximal tibia may present problems. If there is a deficit in the fascia it is occasionally possible to approximate this using a polyester mesh. Alternatively, the medial belly of gastrocnemius can be turned forward as a vascularized muscle flap. Because of the tension which so frequently occurs after replacement of the proximal tibia, the skin should be closed with interrupted sutures or clips. The wound is dressed and a wool and a crêpe spica applied.

Postoperative management

The leg is placed on a supporting pillow and the pulses checked regularly. Once drainage has ceased progressive mobilization using a CPM machine is commenced. Walking starts when the wound is healed, and crutches and sticks dispensed with as muscle control is achieved.

Complications

Infections

The most serious complication of prosthetic replacement is infection. The individual who is immunologically compromised by cytotoxic drugs before operation is particularly vulnerable. Biopsy must always be performed using scrupulous surgical techniques and sources of sepsis, such as dental caries, should be treated initially.

The overall infection rate, in over 1000 cases, is approximately 5.5 per cent. This relatively high figure was initially due to the fact that some cases were operated upon when they were too advanced for conventional surgery. The majority of patients who have manifested postoperative problems have had superficial soft tissue infections that have responded to or have been controlled by long-term antibiotics. Approximately 2 per cent have manifested osteomyelitis either of early or late onset and of these 0.5 per cent have required an amputation.

Loosening

As with routine prosthetic replacements, loosening may occur with massive prosthetic replacements. The incidence, however, is surprisingly low at 2.1 per cent per decade. There are possibly two reasons why this is so. First, the patients are relatively young and, in consequence, have good bone stock. Second, the prostheses are custom-built for the individual and the medullary pin is shaped to conform to the canal.

Prosthetic fracture

Initially, when prostheses were manufactured from materials that were not of a uniform quality, the risk of fracture due to metal fatigue or excessive loading was relatively high. Now that prostheses are manufactured of materials that conform to the requirements of the British Standards Institute, the incidence of such breakages is negligible. The overall incidence in the series is 1.9 per cent, and it has been possible to revise all such cases apart from the prostheses in two patients.

Local recurrences

There are two factors responsible for local recurrences:
1. The inability to excise the primary tumour with an adequate margin of soft tissue
2. Injudicious biopsy causing soft tissue contamination.

Both factors predispose to local recurrence particularly if chemotherapy fails to control the tumour. It is frequently possible to excise such recurrences and sterilize the area with local radiotherapy. Rarely is it necessary to amputate the affected limb.

Conclusions

The management of bone tumours and, in particular, malignant bone tumours, is dependent on collective management by the radiologist, oncologist, radiotherapist, pathologist, and surgeon in conjunction with a supporting nursing and paramedical team.

As a result of adequate chemotherapy coupled with surgery, Rosen[6,7] claimed an 85 per cent survival rate for osteogenic sarcoma and a 90 per cent survival rate for Ewing's sarcoma of the appendicular skeleton. In the UK the 5-year survival for osteosarcoma would appear to be in the region of 65 per cent, whereas Ewing's sarcoma is approximately 50 per cent. Although there are obvious risks to prosthetic replacement, there are also distinct advantages over other methods of replacement. These are:

1. Early mobilization: the average time for a patient to be fully ambulant is 8 weeks postoperatively
2. Apart from the surgical scar, the body image is maintained
3. Children, adolescents and young adults in whom the prognosis is poor may be rapidly returned to a reasonably normal existence even though their life span is limited
4. Extending prostheses are the only way of combating the loss of growth potential in the lower limb of a child
5. Twenty-five years of experience in this field coupled with a probability survival of 60 per cent at 20 years suggest that massive prosthetic replacement is more successful than any other form of limb salvage surgery.

References

1. Rosen G, Suwansirikul, Kwon C. et al. High dose methotrexate with citrovorum factor rescue and adriamycin in childhood osteogenic sarcoma. *Cancer* 1974; 33: 1151–63.

2. Burrows HJ, Wilson JN, Scales JT. Excision of tumours of humerus and femur, with restoration by internal prosthesis. *J Bone Joint Surg [Br]* 1975; 57-B: 148–59.

3. Bramwell VHC. Chemotherapy of operable osteosarcoma. *Baillière's Clinical Oncology. Bone Tumours*. London: Baillière Tindall, 1989: 175–203.

4. Enneking WF, Spanier SS, Goodman MA. A system for the surgical staging of musculo-skeletal sarcoma. *Clin Orthop* 1980; 153: 106–20.

5. Westbury G. The management of soft tissue sarcomas. *J Bone Joint Surg [Br]* 1989; 71-B: 2–3.

6. Rosen G, Nirenberg A, Caparros B. et al. Osteogenic sarcoma: eight per cent, three-year, disease-free survival with combination chemotherapy (T-7). *Nat Cancer Inst Monogr* 1981; 56: 213–20.

7. Rosen G. Current management of Ewing's sarcoma. *Prog Clin Cancer* 1982; 8: 267–82.

Illustrations by Robert Lane

Treatment of leg length inequality

Andrew M. Jackson FRCS
Consultant Orthopaedic Surgeon, University College Hospital, and The Hospital for Sick Children, Great Ormond Street, London, UK

Introduction

Leg length discrepancies of less than 2 cm are commonplace, seldom cause a problem and, if they do, a small shoe-raise is the treatment. A greater difference in leg length will cause postural imbalance and an uneven gait. Patients seek primarily a cosmetic improvement and invariably reject a cumbersome shoe-raise or extension orthosis if there is a more attractive alternative. However, there are also solid orthopaedic reasons which justify the correction of significant leg length discrepancies. The avoidance of backache in later life and osteoarthritis of the hip and knee of the longer leg are obvious. Scoliosis frequently becomes fixed with age. Stiffness in the spine and major joints may make it difficult for an individual to tolerate even a minor discrepancy.

Aetiology

The discrepancies that require correction usually have a congenital basis or are caused by premature epiphyseal arrest. The congenital group includes the whole spectrum of lower limb dysplasias, hemi-atrophy and hemi-hypertrophy, vascular malformations and a variety of syndromes such as neurofibromatosis, Ollier's disease, Klippel–Trenaunay syndrome and Silver's syndrome.

Premature growth-plate arrest may be iatrogenic as happens, for example, when avascular necrosis complicates the treatment of congenital dislocation of the hip, or may be secondary to trauma, infection or radiotherapy. Both infection and trauma can also cause overgrowth of the affected limb. Rarely, midshaft fractures heal with excessive shortening, sometimes combined with angular and rotational deformities, and these need correction. Neurological disorders such as spina bifida, spinal dysraphism and cerebral palsy account for a large number of patients with limb length discrepancies but relatively few of them are candidates for equalization procedures. Leg lengthening techniques have been performed in certain types of dwarfism where short stature alone is the problem, but the advisability of this sort of surgery is debatable and the surgeon must be highly selective.

The short paralytic limb of poliomyelitis is much less common than it used to be. Two or three centimetres of shortening in a paralysed limb is advantageous if it is associated with weak hip flexors or a foot drop since it enables the foot to clear the ground easily during the swing phase of gait. In such patients larger discrepancies can be reduced but should never be totally corrected.

Preoperative

Assessment of the patient with a leg length discrepancy

True and apparent shortening

It is fundamental to distinguish between true and apparent shortening and to bear in mind that some patients have both. Fixed deformities of the hips should be corrected before considering other equalization procedures. If an upper femoral osteotomy is required to adjust the neck–shaft angle, then the true leg length may well be altered by about 1.5 cm; this must be allowed for in determining the correction required for apparent deformity. Occasionally it is appropriate to add a formal femoral shortening to such a procedure.

A special problem arises in the child with a short leg secondary to a poor outcome of treatment for congenital dislocation of the hip. Osteotomies in this instance need to be carefully planned since the future of the hip joint is of equal importance to the correction of the leg length discrepancy. A preoperative arthrogram is often helpful; an abduction osteotomy may uncover the femoral head and need to be combined with some sort of acetabular shelf procedure, and perhaps a trochanteric epiphysiodesis should be added to the operation. A Salter osteotomy may improve the cover of the femoral head and add a little to leg length. On occasion, a more ambitious trans-iliac lengthening may be contemplated.

A true leg length discrepancy associated with fixed pelvic obliquity and scoliosis needs to be regarded with caution. It may well be to the patient's advantage to have a short leg on the 'downhill' side of the pelvis. Correction of true leg length in such a patient may render it difficult for them to compensate for an unbalanced scoliosis and may interfere with walking.

Measurement of the discrepancy

By tape It is traditional to measure true leg length with a tape measure as the distance from the anterior superior iliac spine to the medial malleolus, but this can be misleading. First, pelvic asymmetry occurs if the triradiate cartilage is damaged early in life by infection or radiotherapy, and as a consequence the anterior spines are at different levels. Second, in patients treated for congenital dislocation of the hip, the anterior spine may have been removed. Third, deformities of the hindfoot can alter leg length. The distance between the medial malleolus and the sole will be increased if the hindfoot is in calcaneus or decreased if there is a congenital hindfoot coalition.

Blocks The estimation of leg length discrepancy using blocks may seem crude but in the absence of pelvic obliquity or fixed deformity of the hips it is the most accurate guide to the amount of correction required. The effect of leg length equalization on the hip joints can be studied on a standing radiograph of the pelvis taken using appropriate blocks.

Scanogram This gives a very accurate measurement from hip to ankle providing both legs will lie flat on the X-ray table. It is a useful method for monitoring limb growth and discrepancy and determining exactly how much shortening is in the femur and how much is in the tibia. In the presence of complex deformities it can be very helpful to see the whole of both lower limbs on one film. More recently CT scanograms have proved quicker to perform and easier to measure and store.

In practice all three methods of measurement are used and should there be a discrepancy in the results obtained from different methods an explanation must be sought.

Assessment of associated abnormalities

It is strongly recommended that a systematic list is made of all the features which adversely affect the patient's stance and gait (*see Table 1*). If leg length discrepancy does not stand out as being a major contributor to the problem, then an equalization procedure will not on its own result in much improvement. Furthermore, there are some specific abnormalities that will rule out one or more of the treatment options. For example, instability of the hip owing to acetabular dysplasia and instability of the knee owing to congenital ligament deficiency are both contraindications to femoral lengthening on the grounds that a major joint dislocation is liable to occur.

Patients with severe limb dysplasias will not be candidates for leg equalization procedures. If the foot is deemed to be useless an early Syme's amputation may be the correct decision; if the length at maturity will be out of range of leg lengthening techniques then there is no alternative but to treat the problem with a suitable orthosis or prosthesis.

Monitoring the patient and predicting the discrepancy

If patients are referred early, which is advisable, their maturation and leg length discrepancy can be monitored on an annual basis. The parental height is noted and the child's height standing on the normal leg is recorded on a growth chart. Skeletal age should be estimated between the age of 10 and 12 years to rule out any serious abnormality of skeletal development. Predicting the patient's overall height at maturity is necessary in choosing a sensible course of action.

An accurate prediction of the discrepancy at maturity is also fundamental if epiphysiodesis is to be performed at the correct time or if leg lengthening is to be performed much before the end of growth. In the latter instance, an over-lengthening may be indicated. The methods of prediction all assume that growth proceeds in a linear fashion. There are three main methods of prediction: (*1*) the White/Menelaus method; (*2*) the Anderson–Green method; and (*3*) Moseley's straight-line graph.

As well as monitoring growth, the annual visit allows the surgeon to check on the progress of any associated deformities, perhaps offer a shoe-raise as an interim measure, and to get to know the patient and parents. An assessment of character, emotional stability and motivation are important because leg lengthening should not easily be recommended for the faint-hearted or the uncooperative. The realistic expectations of surgery and a knowledge of the complications that can occur must be imparted to the patient.

Table 1 Associated abnormalities to be looked for in the spine and involved leg

Spine	Structural scoliosis Mobility
Pelvis	Fixed pelvic obliquity Asymmetry
Hip	Soft tissue contracture Bony deformity Dysplasia Muscle weakness (Trendelenburg-positive)
Femur	Deformity (angular or rotational)
Knee	Soft tissue contracture Bony deformity Dislocation of patella Ligamentous instability
Tibia	Deformity (angular or rotational)
Ankle	Soft tissue contracture Bony deformity Absent fibula Ball-and-socket joint
Foot	Soft tissue contracture Bony deformity Dysplasia

General	Muscle – wasting
	          – weakness
	          – fibrosis
	Neurovascular abnormalities
	Congenital fibrous bands

Possible procedures and indications

Shortening the long leg

These procedures are ideal if the long leg is the abnormal one. If the patient tends to stand and walk with the knee of the long leg slightly flexed, then procedures that shorten the long leg will not significantly reduce the effective height of the patient.

Epiphysiodesis

Permanent epiphysiodesis is preferable to stapling. Only one operation is required and the complication rate is lower. Staples can displace or break and removal of staples is not always followed by the normal resumption of growth. As already stated, the timing of epiphysiodesis is critical and depends on predictions that the short leg will continue to grow at a specific rate until maturity. The operation that is described has the advantage that it is the smallest and least disruptive of all the leg equalization procedures. It requires the shortest hospital admission and recovery should be complete in 6 weeks. It may be superseded in the future by a reliable method of performing transcutaneous epiphysiodesis.

The disadvantages are that the predictions are not always realized in practice and it is therefore the least accurate method of correcting a discrepancy. Because of this inaccuracy it is wise to aim at reducing the discrepancy to 1 cm since the patient is usually displeased if the procedure converts the longer leg into the shorter one. From a cosmetic point of view the scarring is sometimes obvious and there may be a delay between the time of operation and the cessation of growth. Parental worry occurs because the operation is usually performed on the normal leg and the surgery must be followed by careful follow-up.

The indications for epiphysiodesis follow.

1. If there is sufficient growth left to effect a correction
2. If the patient is growing on or above the 50th centile and will be taller than average height
3. If the discrepancy is 6 cm or less; with increasing discrepancy, the potential for error is magnified.

Femoral and tibial shortening

These procedures are precise if applied once skeletal maturity has been reached. Good internal fixation allows early mobilization; and using the method to be described for the femur, postoperative muscle weakness and non-union are most unlikely. Shortening necessarily leads to an increase in soft-tissue bulk, but if the femur is shortened proximally, this bulkiness and the scarring are not visible when normal clothes are worn.

Tibial shortening gives a poor cosmetic result, and the muscles may never take up the slack. If more than 2 or 3 cm are resected there is liable to be a problem with skin closure and the vascularity of the limb may be threatened. There can be few indications for this procedure and it will not be described.

The indications for femoral shortening follow.

1. If the patient is skeletally mature
2. If the discrepancy is less than 6 cm
3. If the discrepancy is principally in the femur
4. If the patient is on or above the 50th centile.

Operations on the short leg

Femoral and tibial lengthening

Many methods of leg lengthening have been described and currently there is great interest in improving the distraction techniques. Advances in the design of distraction apparatus have allowed the lengthening to be performed on an ambulatory basis. The demonstration that a bone gap can consistently be bridged with callus without the need for bone grafting, and also the development of epiphyseal distraction, have revolutionized the approach and shortened the duration of treatment. Decisions have to be made about the choice of apparatus and the technique of lengthening to be employed. It is beyond the scope of this chapter to cover all these developments but the choices will be considered briefly.

Choice of apparatus The basic choice is between a single-bar distractor such as the Wagner or Orthofix (Biomet Ltd, Bridgend, UK) devices and a frame with all-round support such as the Ilizarov or Monticelli frames. The single-bar fixators are sturdy and compact and a minimum of soft tissues are transfixed by the pins. However, they fail frequently to keep perfect alignment during the lengthening. The Monticelli frame, on the other hand, will consistently produce a beautifully straight lengthened segment but it is bulky and more easily applied to the tibia than the femur.

Choice of site Diaphyseal lengthening allows both the upper and lower pins to be placed through solid cortical bone. Should internal fixation be necessary at a later date, then there is good bone stock on either side of the lengthened segment. One should bear in mind that plating is probably the easiest way to correct significant angular deformity at the end of lengthening, if the frame itself does not possess the capability.

Metaphyseal lengthening has the advantage that the callus response is more readily achieved when the lengthening is made through cancellous bone, but the pin fixation can be less reliable. Metaphyseal lengthening is the method of choice if deformity at this site is to be corrected concurrently with lengthening.

Epiphyseal lengthening has the advantage that no osteotomy is required. The lack of incisions is cosmetically attractive but the lengthening can be unusually painful. Nevertheless, a strong and wide lengthened segment can be produced which consolidates quickly. One has to assume that even if the distraction is performed slowly, at half a millimetre a day, and the growth-plate does not rupture, it still may not function normally at the end of the procedure.

A few surgeons have gained experience in synchronous lengthening of the femur and tibia of the same leg and of epiphyseal lengthening synchronously at the upper and lower end of the tibia. We have tended to tackle the bigger discrepancies by a combination of lengthening of one leg and shortening of the other.

LEG SHORTENING

EPIPHYSIODESIS

A preoperative radiograph is necessary to check the anatomy of the physis to be fused. The growth-plates are usually slightly convex towards the joint. Image intensification enables the surgeon to make small vertical incisions, 3.5 cm in length, centred at the correct level with certainty. Each growth-plate is approached from medial and lateral aspects; if femur and tibia are to be tackled, four separate incisions will give the most satisfactory cosmetic result. With the patient supine the limb is exsanguinated, draped and positioned on a thigh rest in 30°–40° of flexion.

Surgical approach

1a & b

Lower femoral physis

The lateral incision splits the fascia lata. The vastus lateralis is retracted forwards from the lateral intermuscular septum to expose the periosteum which overlies the physis. In a similar fashion, the medial incision splits the deep fascia 1 cm in front of the adductor tubercle and the vastus medialis is retracted forward from the medial intermuscular septum to expose the relevant portion of the femur. The origin of the medial ligament lies posteriorly and must not be disturbed. On both sides the superior geniculate arteries may have to be divided.

Upper tibial physis

The lateral incision is made just in front of the fibular head and the anterior aspect of this bone is exposed. The dissection is not carried posteriorly nor are retractors placed behind the fibular head for fear of damaging the common peroneal nerve. The tibia is exposed and the origins of peroneus longus and tibialis anterior are reflected downwards for 1 cm.

The anteromedial aspect of the growth-plate lies subcutaneously and its exposure poses no problems. The pes anserinus is retracted backwards as is the anterior margin of the medial ligament.

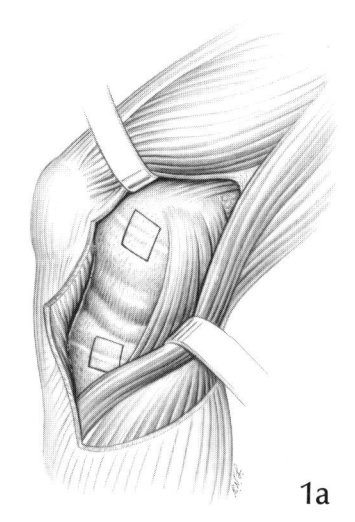

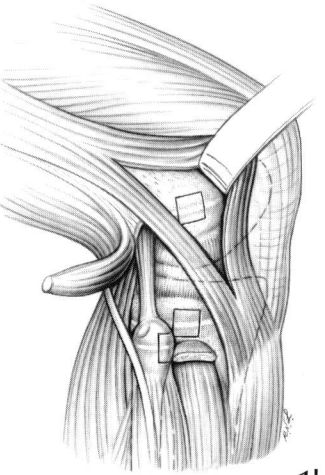

Technique

2 & 3

An I-shaped incision 2 cm long is made in the periosteum and the anterior and posterior osteoperiosteal flaps elevated with an osteotome. The physis is seen as a white line traversing the window that has been opened in the periosteum. Using a 1.5 cm osteotome, a square block of bone as deep as possible is removed with care; a curved osteotome will help to ease the block out. Then, with a small gauge or curette, as much of the growth-plate as possible is removed from the depths of the hole anteriorly, posteriorly and towards the centre of the bone. The same procedure is performed on the opposite side. The excavation of the growth-plate on medial and lateral sides should meet centrally.

When this has been achieved the bone blocks are rotated through 90° and punched back into the holes from which they were taken. The osteoperiosteal flaps are sutured back in position over the bone blocks. The skin is sutured with a subcuticular suture and for comfort the limb is immobilized in a plaster of Paris cylinder for 2 weeks.

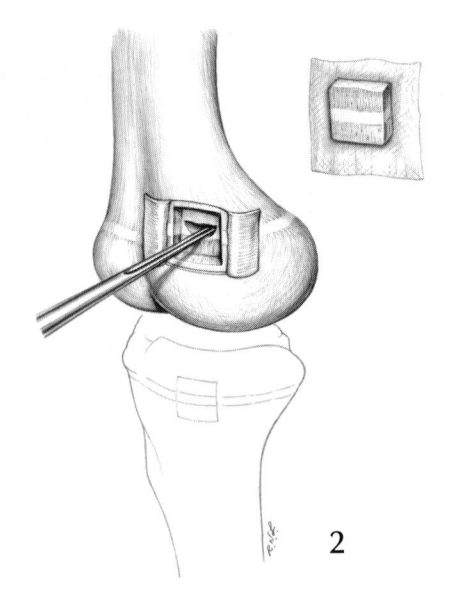

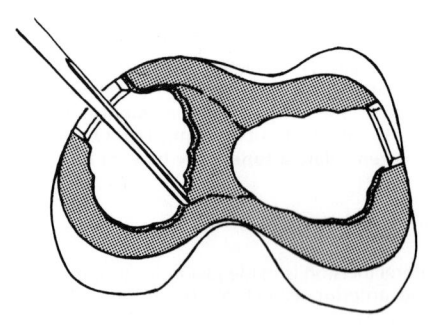

Postoperative management

Weight-bearing is allowed as comfort dictates and physiotherapy is commenced when the cast is removed. It usually takes 6 weeks for the knee to regain a full range of pain-free movement. Careful follow-up will determine if the expected correction is being achieved without the development of deformity. If only the femoral physis has been fused and the expected correction is not being achieved, fusion of the upper tibial physis may be performed at a later date.

FEMORAL SHORTENING

The patient is positioned on an orthopaedic table as for pinning of a fractured hip. The image intensifier is placed to give an anteroposterior view of the hip and the operated leg is held in neutral rotation and under slight traction.

The lateral aspect of the greater trochanter and upper femoral shaft are exposed in the standard way through a lateral incision which has to be lengthened, bearing in mind the size of the segment of femur to be removed (see chapter on 'Total hip replacement arthroplasty' pp. 943–964). The vastus lateralis is reflected off the bone anteriorly and the lesser trochanter identified. The exposure is maintained with two deep self-retaining retractors.

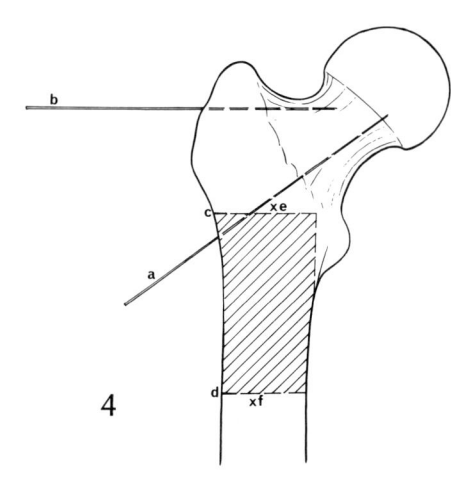

4

A guide wire (a) is inserted along the front of the femoral neck as a marker and advanced into the femoral head so that it stays in place. A second marker wire (b) is inserted in the mid-lateral line through the greater trochanter and onwards into the upper femoral neck at right angles to the femoral shaft. The bone to be resected is now marked out. The upper osteotomy is planned so that the lesser trochanter remains attached to the proximal fragment, and iliopsoas function will therefore be unimpaired. The level of the proximal osteotomy is opposite the upper margin of the lesser trochanter and a line (c) is made on the bone with an osteotome. The length of bone to be resected is measured with a ruler and the level of the lower cut (d) is marked. This length is checked. Two further longitudinal marks (e) and (f) are made so that rotational alignment (x–x) is not lost after the bone has been resected.

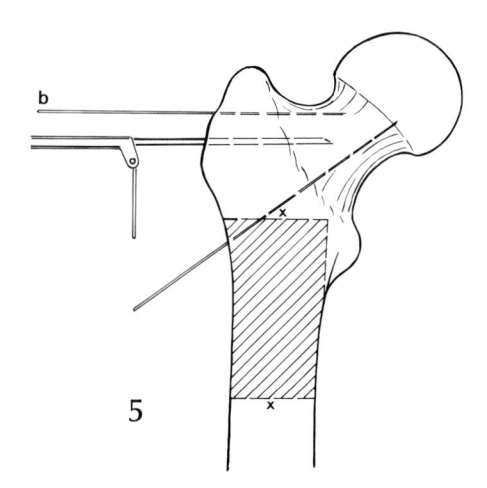

5

The seating chisel enters the greater trochanter 2 cm above the proximal osteotomy line. Its entry into the bone is facilitated by drilling the cortex with four or five small drill holes. The chisel fitted with the chisel guide is hammered into the centre of the femoral neck, parallel to and just below the guide wire (b), usually to a depth of 4–5 cm. The depth of insertion will dictate the size of the blade–plate. The seating chisel is eased back a little with the extractor to make its later removal easier but it is left in place as it will prove useful in controlling the proximal fragment, and it also gives the line of the proximal osteotomy.

6

It is important that the distal osteotomy is performed first. The cut is made at right angles to the shaft with a power saw, the blade being cooled with saline. This allows the proximal fragment to be abducted from the wound whilst the soft tissues are stripped from the medial aspect up as far as the lesser trochanter. It also makes it easier to cut the vertical limb of the proximal osteotomy. The proximal cut is made and the segment of bone removed.

7

Traction on the limb is released and the two fragments brought together with due attention to the rotational markers. The seating chisel is removed and the right-angled blade–plate held on the driving device is hammered into the channel cut by the chisel. The plate is clamped to the shaft with a bone clamp and, if the cuts have been made correctly, the osteotomy should be open a little on its lateral aspect. This gap will close as compression is applied with the tensioning device.

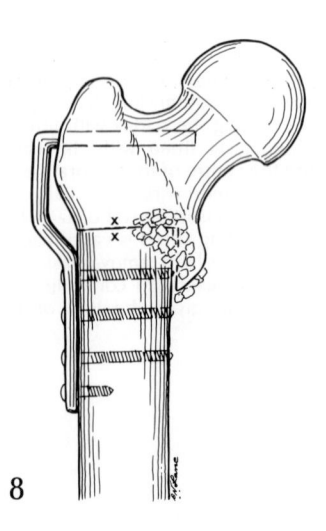

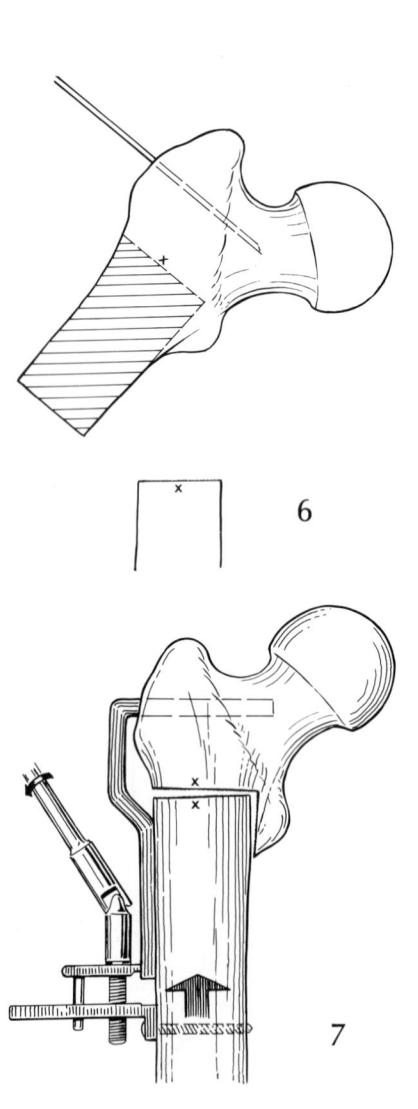

8

Once the osteotomy is compressed the plate is screwed to the bone and the tensioning device removed. Bone graft obtained from the medullary cavity of the excised segment is placed around the osteotomy. The wound is closed in layers over a suction drain.

Postoperative management

The leg is mobilized for 3 or 4 days in 'slings and springs' or on Hamilton Russell traction and the patient is then allowed partial weight-bearing on crutches. Union usually occurs by 8 weeks when full weight-bearing is allowed. The high level of bone resection should not give rise to any muscular weakness and the plate should not be removed for at least 1 year.

LEG LENGTHENING

On admission to hospital these patients should be assessed by a physiotherapist and taught shadow walking – how to walk with crutches without bearing weight. In the case of tibial lengthening, a foot-drop appliance is made which can be connected to the fixator.

FEMORAL LENGTHENING

The preferred method is a midshaft lengthening using a single-bar leg-lengthening device applied to the lateral aspect of the femur. Details specific to the type of fixator employed are not included in the description but are available from the manufacturers. The method of bone division is an oblique diaphyseal corticotomy.

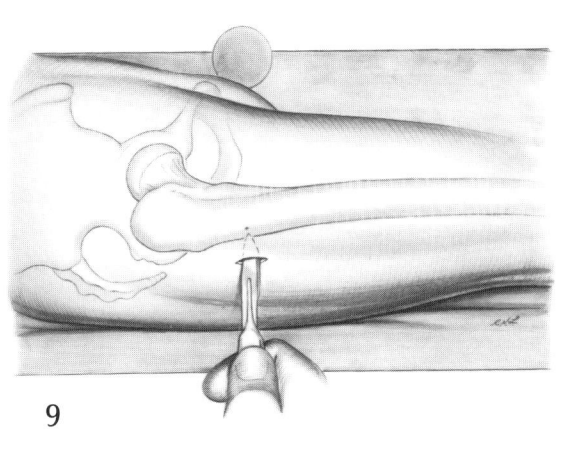

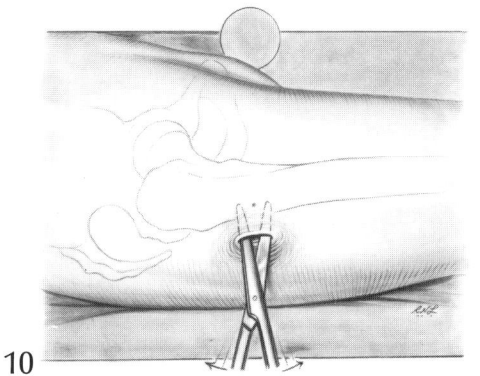

Stage 1: Application of the apparatus

The patient, under general anaesthesia, is placed in the lateral position and the leg to be operated on is separately draped. An image intensifier is arranged so that it can be moved into place during the operation: with the C-arm above the operating table a horizontal beam will give an anteroposterior view of the femur which is essential for checking the placement of the pins.

Pin insertion

The four pins are placed in line 1 cm anterior to the mid-lateral line and the upper pin is inserted first. The technique of pin insertion is important. Large 6 mm cortical threaded pins are required.

9 & 10

A deep longitudinal incision 1 cm long is made down to bone. A pair of blunt-tipped scissors are inserted into the track created and the blades opened to stretch the soft tissues.

11

A trocar and cannula are next inserted into the hole and by careful palpation the midline of the cortex is identified. This is important because the screw must pass through the middle of the bone and fix well to both cortices. The trocar must be held perpendicular to the long axis of the femur. The cannula is removed maintaining pressure on the trocar which is tapped gently with a hammer so that its teeth engage on the cortex.

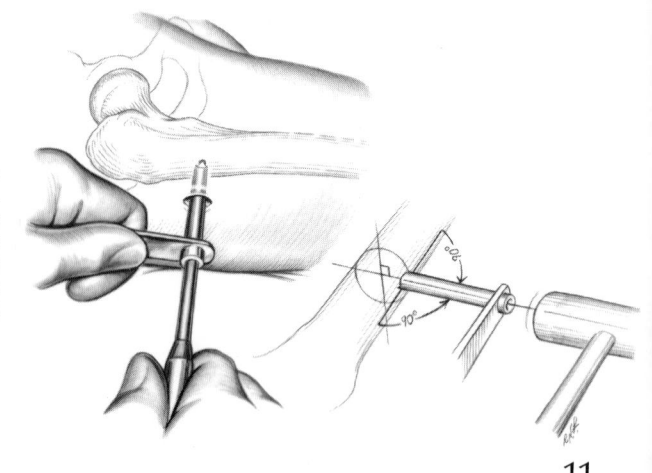

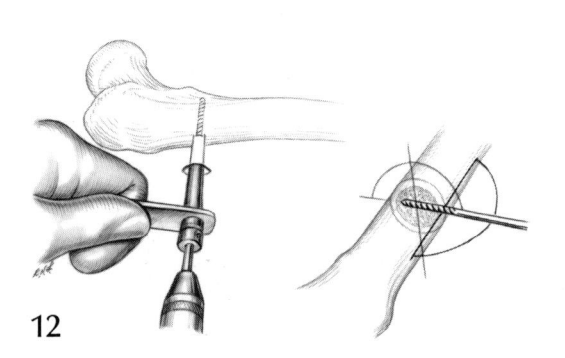

12

The femur is then drilled using the correct size drill bit. A low-speed power-drill gives good control and minimizes the risk of thermal necrosis. It is crucial that the drill is at a right angle to the long axis of the bone and this should be checked both by eye and with the image intensifier, especially when the first and most critical hole is made.

13

If the first pin is not inserted correctly then the template which is to be used next, and ultimately the external fixator, will not be parallel to the femoral shaft. It is important that the second cortex is completely penetrated. The pin of appropriate length and with a self-tapping tip is then inserted by hand. The screw should be tightened until at least two threads are seen to protrude beyond the far cortex. Should there be any heaping up of soft tissues around the pin, the skin incision must be extended to relieve this problem.

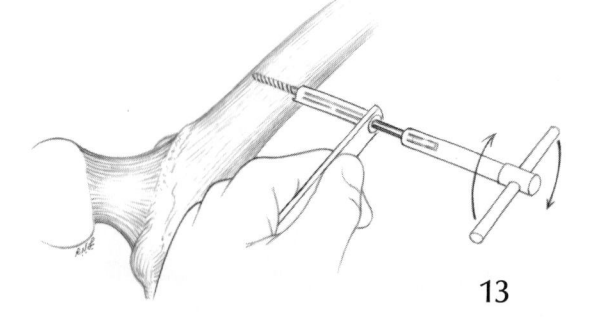

14 & 15

The template is passed over the proximal pin and if this has been correctly placed the template will lie parallel to the femoral shaft. The lowest pin is inserted next through the cortical bone that lies just above the femoral flare. The two remaining pins are now inserted and the template is removed. The knee is flexed fully to confirm that the soft tissues impaled by the pins will allow this movement. It is wise at this stage to adjust the leg-lengthening device so that it fits exactly over the pins in the position in which they have been inserted.

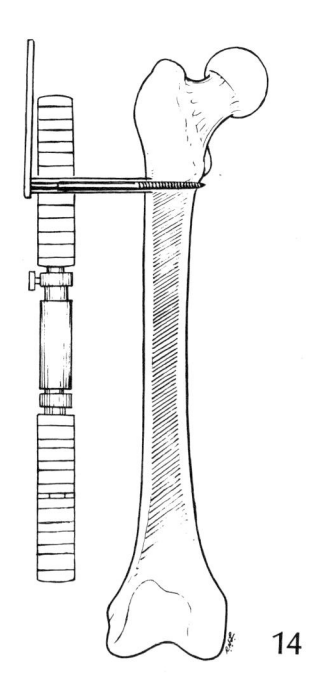

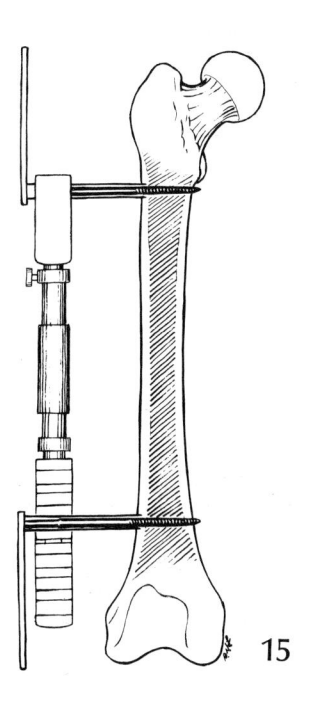

1162 Leg and foot

Stage 2: Soft tissue release and corticotomy

16

The midshaft of the femur is approached through a short posterolateral incision. The tensor fasciae latae is split longitudinally to expose the vastus lateralis. At the proximal end this split is carried anteriorly and at its distal end posteriorly, in effect forming a Z-cut in the fascia which will facilitate the lengthening.

17

The vastus lateralis is then reflected forwards and the lateral intermuscular septum is divided. A perforating branch of the femoral artery invariably needs to be secured as the femoral shaft is exposed. The periosteum must be treated with great care. It is incised longitudinally and stripped carefully off the bone. The intention is to divide the femur with a minimum of trauma and then to re-suture the periosteum. Four retractors are inserted subperiosteally to maintain the exposure.

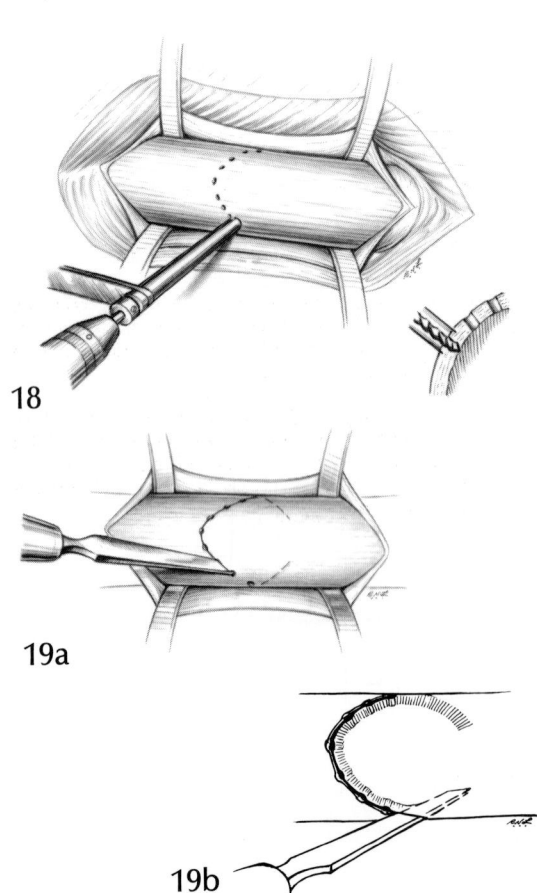

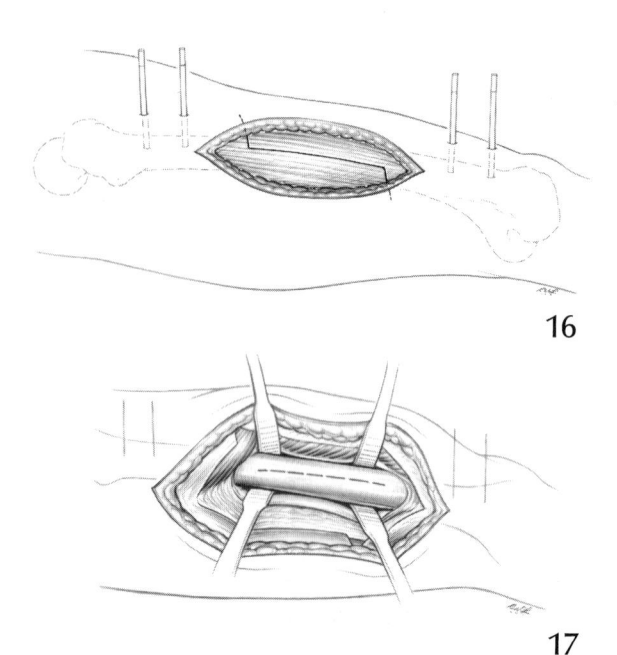

18, 19a & b

The bone is divided in an oblique fashion to present a greater surface area for callus formation. The oblique corticotomy is performed by, first, placing a small drill through a drill sleeve so that only 5 mm of the drill protrudes beyond the tip of the guide; drill holes are then made along the line of the proposed corticotomy. These are then joined together with a small osteotome without entering the medullary cavity. It is then possible to cut some way round the back of the bone beyond the limits of vision with the same instrument.

20

The osteotomy is completed by gently flexing the thigh until the far cortex cracks. The pins must not be used for leverage.

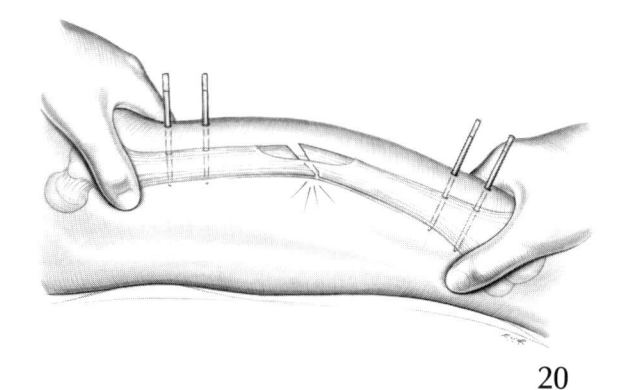

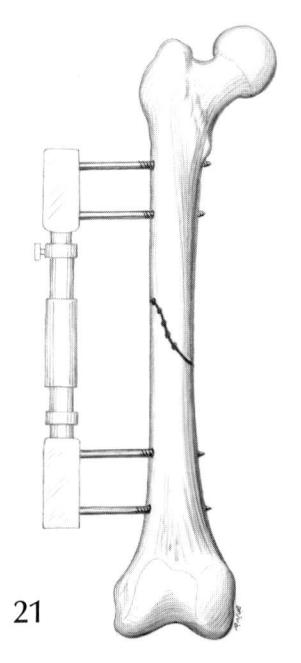

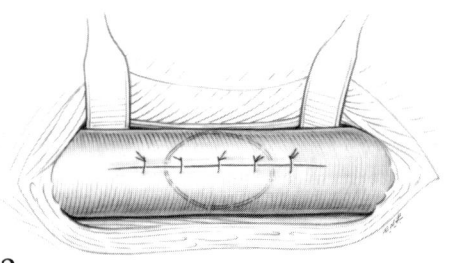

21 & 22

The leg lengthening device is then applied and the alignment at the femur checked. The periosteum is sutured back over the corticotomy and the wound closed in layers over a suction drain.

At the end of the procedure the fixator should be 2 cm clear of the skin to allow for postoperative swelling of the thigh. No distraction is performed at this stage. A Marcain (Astra Pharmaceuticals Ltd, Kings Langley, UK) femoral nerve block will reduce postoperative pain.

1164 Leg and foot

Stage 3: Distraction

A postoperative anteroposterior radiograph of the femur is taken to check the alignment and pin insertion. The drain is removed at 48 hours. Analgesia is prescribed as required and physiotherapy to encourage hip and knee flexion are commenced on day 1. As the pain subsides the patient is encouraged to shadow walk with crutches.

The lengthening device is left undisturbed for 2–3 weeks depending on the age of the patient. By then callus formation has commenced and the vascularity between the proximal and distal fragments should be re-established. The lengthening is commenced at the rate of 0.5 mm twice daily and alignment radiographs should be taken at 2-week intervals. The first film will confirm the separation at the corticotomy site and subsequent films will also show the quality of the callus response. If this response is poor the distraction should be discontinued for a week.

The pin sites are cleaned daily with an alcohol solution and redressed. Any crusts are removed. Should the skin heap up around the pins as lengthening proceeds it is a small procedure under local anaesthesia to make a relieving incision.

The distraction is continued until the desired length is achieved, but if complications intervene the distraction may have to be abandoned short of the objective. The distraction phase needs close supervision and should only be performed as an outpatient procedure if the patient is completely reliable.

Stage 4: Consolidation

Once the distraction is complete the bone must be protected from undue stress whilst the callus segment matures. Bone grafting at this stage is seldom necessary. There are three approaches to this problem (see *Illustrations 23, 24 and 25*).

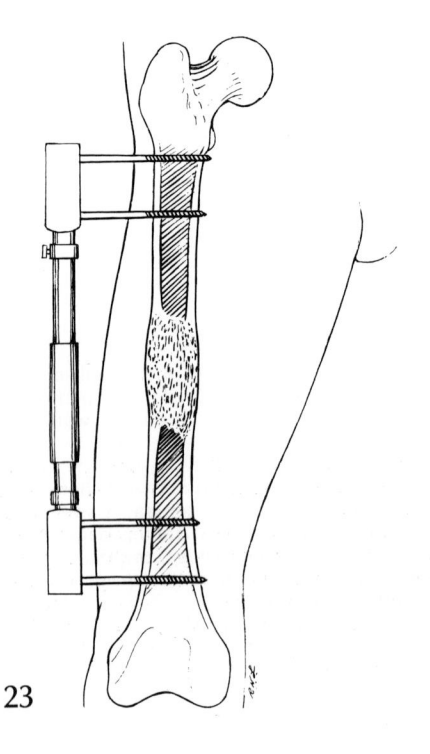

23

If the fixator is well tolerated and providing there is no angular deformity, it is preferable to leave the fixator in place for 5 or 6 weeks while the patient continues shadow walking. By then the callus will be strong enough to resist compressive forces and full weight-bearing is allowed. If the device allows the callus to be subjected to axial compression forces, the necessary adjustment to the device is made at this time. Full weight-bearing is continued until the callus begins to differentiate into cortex and medulla. It is then safe to remove the device but it is wise to revert to partial weight-bearing for 2 months and then gradually increase activities again.

Treatment of leg length inequality 1165

24

If there is significant deformity at the end of lengthening, the best way of correcting this is by plating the femur through a posterolateral approach while removing the external fixator. At least four screws are required above and below the lengthened segment together with special heavy duty bridging plates which are not weakened in their central section by screw holes.

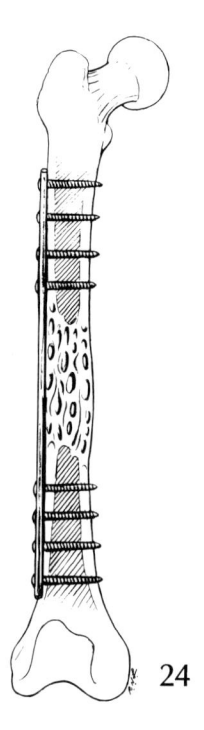

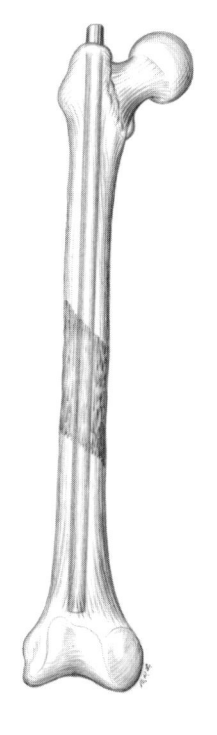

25

The third alternative is to stabilize the bone by means of closed femoral nailing. This can be performed at the stage when the callus is mature enough to resist axial compression forces. Nailing gives immediate whole-bone protection and facilitates the recovery of stiff joints as well as allowing early and safe weight-bearing. The risk is obviously that of infection and for this reason the fixator must be removed and the leg maintained on traction for 1–2 weeks so that the pin tracks are healed before closed nailing is performed.

1166 Leg and foot

TIBIAL LENGTHENING

The principles of lengthening the tibia are exactly the same as for the femur. For simplicity the diagrams are drawn with a single-bar fixator. As already stated, the Monticelli frame has the advantages of all-round support to which I have already referred.

Stages 1 and 2: Application of apparatus and corticotomy

26

The pins are inserted in the standard way through the subcutaneous border of the tibia. Under X-ray control an oblique midshaft corticotomy is made under vision exactly as for femoral lengthening.

Through a separate lateral incision at the same level 1 cm of fibula is excised and the interosseous membrane is also divided.

A third incision 1 cm long is made over the distal fibula and a diastasis screw is inserted in order to neutralize any distraction forces that may be imposed on the lateral malleolus. If the heel cord is tight preoperatively, it will have to be lengthened; and after passage of the diastasis screw, dorsiflexion of the foot is checked.

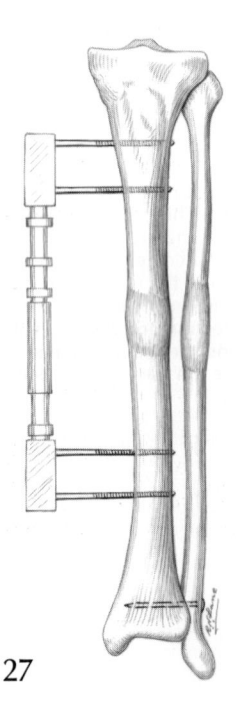

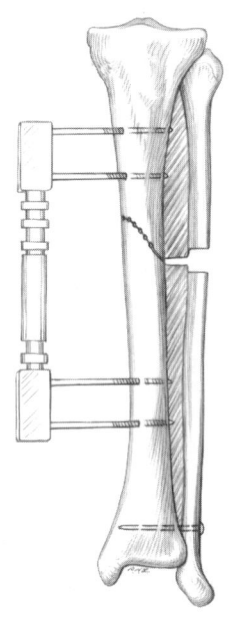

Stage 3: Distraction

The limb is elevated postoperatively and physiotherapy commenced. From day 1 the foot-drop spring-splint is worn. When pain and swelling subside the patient is allowed up on crutches, shadow walking. Lengthening is commenced at 2–3 weeks as for femoral lengthening and regular radiographs are taken to check alignment and the quality of callus formation.

Stage 4: Consolidation

27

The management during this phase depends on the callus response. It is invariably possible to maintain the fixator in place without the need for bone grafting or internal fixation. After 5–6 weeks of shadow walking, weight-bearing is increased and the lengthened segments subjected to axial compression forces if this is appropriate. As a rule of thumb, the device is left on for a further 1 week per centimetre lengthened. When this time has expired and if the radiograph shows good consolidation with the beginning of differentiation into cortex and medulla, the device is removed. Before the pins are removed it is wise to test the strength of the lengthened tibia.

The pin tracks are cleaned and a long-leg cast applied. Full weight-bearing is allowed and 2 weeks later the cast is removed. A cast-brace is applied for a further 6 weeks.

Complications

Complications are to be expected when leg lengthening is undertaken. Vigilance on the part of the surgeon will often lead to the recognition of problems as they emerge, and appropriate action at this stage will prevent serious trouble. Some of the more common complications are listed below.

Loss of patient compliance

Patients may tamper with the distraction device and make highly inappropriate adjustments. Some are unable to control their youthful exuberance for the duration of the lengthening, and foolish behaviour can result in unnecessary trauma to the limb.

Pin-track infection

This can be minimized by removal of crusts and regular cleansing of the skin around the pins with an alcoholic solution. A relieving incision is mandatory if the skin begins to heap up on one side of a pin. If there is surrounding erythema, antibiotics should be prescribed. Failure to control infection will lead to loosening of the pins and is a cause for their premature removal.

Loss of alignment

This will occur if the single-bar external fixator is not parallel to the bone, if the pins bend or if the attachment of the pin to the fixator fails. If the angulation is not corrected, further distraction tends to increase the deformity rather than increase the length.

Muscle contractures

Most of these problems are encountered in patients with congenital discrepancies. A slight preoperative contracture will become more pronounced during lengthening. Therefore prophylactic open adductor tenotomies, anterior hip releases, and lengthening of the hamstrings and heel cord are all occasionally indicated. Similar procedures are sometimes required at the end of lengthening. The importance of physiotherapy in minimizing contractures and keeping the joints as mobile as possible should not be underestimated.

Joint damage

Dislocation of the hip or knee is usually a forseeable complication and will seldom be encountered if femoral lengthening is avoided in patients who are at risk. A sudden increase in joint pain and stiffness should always arouse suspicion.

Pain

This can be a difficult problem and the cause must always be sought and not simply suppressed with analgesics. Epiphyseal lengthening is probably the most painful form of distraction, but pain is often encountered towards the end of lengthening and may be a reason to 'go slow'.

Neurovascular damage

This may complicate pin insertion but is remarkably rare during distraction performed at the correct rate.

Tibiofibular joint displacement

Downward migration of the head of the fibula will tighten up the lateral collateral ligament of the knee and cause fixed flexion deformity, whereas upward migration of the lateral malleolus will de-stabilize the ankle mortise. A correctly placed osteotomy and a diastasis screw should prevent these complications.

Complications of internal fixation

All the well-known complications can occur if internal fixation is employed. This includes infection, bent plates, screws pulling out, and fractures at one or other end of the plates.

Delayed union

If there is poor callus response, bone grafting is best performed early, using cancellous bone from the iliac crest. Non-union after leg lengthening is extremely rare.

Fractures

Fractures may occur at a variety of sites and times and include the following.

1. Early fracture at one end of the lengthened segment when the fixator is removed
2. Fracture at the level of the end of a plate
3. Fracture away from the site of lengthening related to disuse osteoporosis
4. Late stress fractures through a lengthened segment usually in the presence of a slight deformity.

Further reading

General

Symposium. Equalization of leg length. *Clin Orthop* 1978; 136: 1–312.

Coleman SS. Lower limb length discrepancy. In: Lovell WW, Winter RB, eds. *Pediatric orthopaedics*, 2nd ed. Philadelphia: Lippincott, 1986: 781–863.

Growth prediction

Anderson M, Messner MB, Green WT. Distribution of lengths of the normal femur and tibia in children from one to eighteen years of age. *J Bone Joint Surg [Am]* 1964; 46-A: 1197–1202.

Anderson M, Green WT, Messner MB. Growth and predictions of growth in the lower extremeties. *J Bone Joint Surg [Am]* 1963; 45-A: 1–14.

Menelaus MB. Correction of leg length discrepancy by epiphyseal arrest. *J Bone Joint Surg [Br]* 1966; 48-B: 336–9.

Moseley CF. A straight line graph for leg length discrepancies. *J Bone Joint Surg [Am]* 1977; 59-A: 174–9.

Leg lengthening

Armour PL, Scott JHS. Equalisation of leg length. *J Bone Joint Surg [Br]* 1981; 63-B: 587–92.

De Bastiani G, Aldegheri R, Brivio LR, Trivella G. Chondrodiatasis – controlled symmetrical distraction of the epiphyseal plate: limb lengthening in children. *J Bone Joint Surg [Br]* 1986; 68-B: 550–6.

Hood RW, Riseborough EJ. Lengthening of the lower extremity by the Wagner method: a review of the Boston children's hospital experience. *J Bone Joint Surg [Am]* 1981; 63-A: 1121–31.

Monticelli G, Spinelli R. Distraction epiphysiolysis as a method of limb lengthening. III. Clinical applications. *Clin Orthop* 1981; 154: 274–85.

Wagner H. Surgical lengthening or shortening of femur and tibia: technique and indications. In: Hungerford DS. *Progress in orthopaedic surgery*. Berlin: Springer-Verlag, 1977.

Illustrations by Peter Cox after F. Price

Distal gastrocnemius release

W. J. W. Sharrard MD, ChM, FRCS
Emeritus Consultant Orthopaedic Surgeon, Royal Hallamshire Hospital and Children's Hospital, Sheffield;
Professor of Orthopaedic Surgery, University of Sheffield, UK

Preoperative

Indications and assessment

There is a limited indication for this operation for specific shortness of the gastrocnemius muscles in cerebral palsy and occasionally in other paralytic conditions. Shortness of the gastrocnemii is assessed by determining the range of dorsiflexion of the ankle with the knee extended compared with the range with the knee flexed. If there is a full or adequate range of dorsiflexion with the knee flexed but it is less than a right angle with the knee extended, shortness of the gastrocnemii is present. The condition is particularly likely to present in diplegic cerebral palsy, when it usually develops bilaterally. Gastrocnemius release is not indicated when there is equinus deformity which does not alter when the knee is flexed.

Anaesthesia and position of patient

General anaesthesia is needed. The shortness of the gastrocnemius is confirmed with the patient anaesthetized. The limb is exsanguinated by elevation for a minute and inflation of a cuff tourniquet on the upper thigh. The patient is placed prone with a sandbag under the anterior aspect of the thigh to lift the limb away from the operating table so that the ankles can be dorsiflexed. The skin is prepared and the lower limbs are covered to the level of the mid-thigh by sterile stockinette stuck to the posterior aspect of each calf with adhesive solution, or an oval is cut out of the stockinette in the region of the calf and the operative area is covered by an adhesive transparent drape.

Operation

Incision

1

A posterior longitudinal incision 8–12 cm long is made in the midline of the calf centred half-way between the knee and the ankle. The incision is deepened through the subcutaneous fat. Immediately beneath the fat layer the sural vein and the sural nerve need to be identified and retracted medially or laterally.

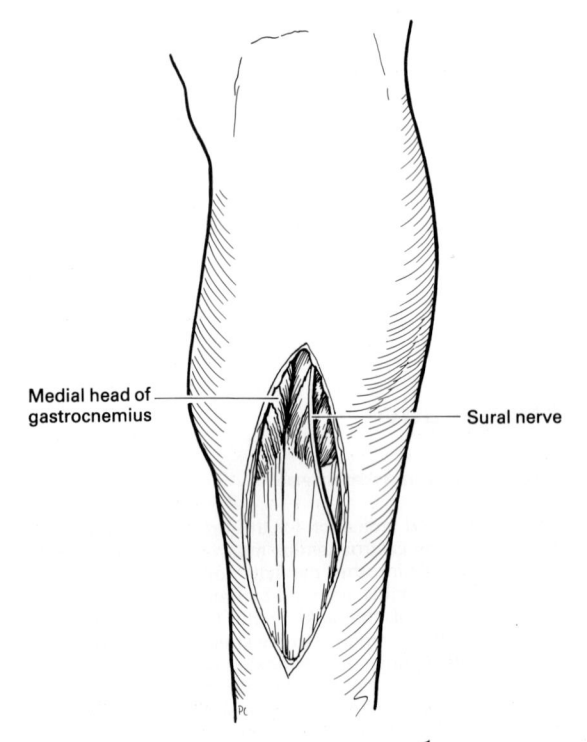

Exposure and division of the gastrocnemius tendons

2a & b

The two bellies of the gastrocnemius muscle and their flattened aponeurotic tendons are exposed by a vertical incision through the deep fascia.

The midline gap between the distal ends of the bellies of the muscle and the tendons arising from them is identified by blunt dissection. The medial side of the tendon of the medial gastrocnemius is identified by blunt dissection and a MacDonald blunt dissector passed transversely beneath the tendon to the midline. Care must be taken to separate the gastrocnemius tendon from the soleus aponeurosis deep to it, with which it blends distally. The gastrocnemius tendon is divided transversely by cutting down onto the blunt dissector. The tendon is mobilized upwards, separating some weak fascial attachments laterally.

The lateral gastrocnemius tendon is similarly identified on its lateral side, separated from the soleus by a MacDonald blunt dissector, divided and mobilized upwards. At this point, the whole of the gastrocnemius insertion should be freely mobile so that, when the ankle is dorsiflexed keeping the knee straight, the soleus aponeurosis and the distal stumps of the gastrocnemius tendon can be seen to move distally whilst the proximal tendons and muscle bellies of the gastrocnemius remain static and, in effect, retract upwards.

The proximal tendons can be sutured with one or two fine non-absorbable sutures to the underlying soleus aponeurosis but this is not strictly necessary since the tendons will remain proximally displaced when the knee is extended and the ankle dorsiflexed.

Wound closure

The wound is closed by interrupted or continuous non-absorbable sutures to the deep fascia and interrupted absorbable sutures to the subcutaneous fat. The skin is sutured by a subcuticular absorbable suture or by interrupted non-absorbable sutures.

The patient is turned into the supine position, the tourniquets removed and plaster cast applied from the groin to the toes with the knee fully extended and the ankle dorsiflexed as fully as possible. Overcorrection does not occur.

Postoperative management

The circulation to the toes needs to be observed for the first 24 hours. The patient can then return home. Plaster fixation is maintained for 3½ weeks, the patient being allowed to bear weight on the plaster after the tenth day. After the plaster is removed, physiotherapy is given to encourage activity and walking function.

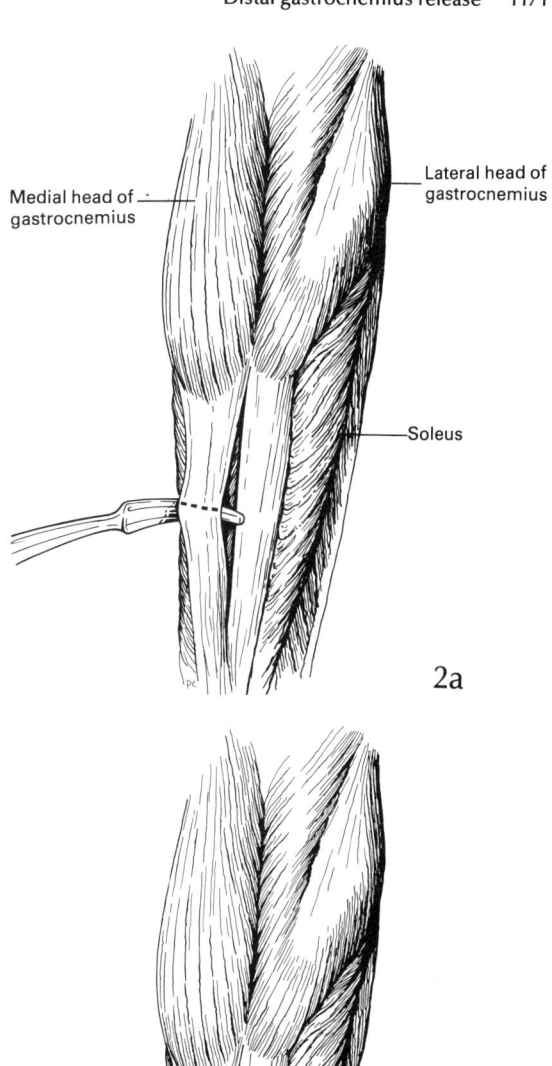

Further reading

Strayer LM. Recession of the gastrocnemius: an operation to relieve spastic contracture of the calf muscles. *J Bone Joint Surg [Am]* 1950; 32-A: 671–6.

Illustrations by Gillian Oliver after B. Hyams

Lengthening and repair of the tendo Achillis

B. Helal MChOrth, FRCS
Honorary Consultant Orthopaedic Surgeon, The Royal London Hospital and The Royal National Orthopaedic Hospital, London, and Enfield Group of Hospitals, UK

S. C. Chen FRCS
Consultant Orthopaedic Surgeon, Enfield Group of Hospitals, UK

Introduction

The tendo Achillis may be tight as a result of upper motor neurone problems or secondary to muscle contracture. Degenerative changes due to overuse, injury, or urate deposits in gout give rise to peritendinitis and possibly partial or total rupture. Injections of steroid may also cause rupture. The methods described below deal with these problems.

LENGTHENING

This procedure is used to correct an equinus deformity of the ankle which may arise from a variety of conditions such as cerebral palsy, longstanding lateral popliteal nerve injury or inadequate splintage following ankle injuries. If the equinus deformity is severe or longstanding then release of the posterior ankle joint capsule and tibialis posterior may be necessary. In addition, gastrocnemius release can be performed to achieve further lengthening.

INCOMPLETE TENOTOMY[1]

The advantage of this technique is that a large incision is avoided. It is of limited use in severe contractures as no exposure is made of other tight structures such as tibialis posterior and the posterior joint capsule.

In performing this procedure, it must be remembered that the fibres of the tendo Achillis spiral through almost 90° from their insertion to their origin. Viewed from behind, the rotation is from medial to lateral.

Lengthening and repair of the tendo Achillis 1173

Incisions

1

A tiny skin incision is made on the medial side of the tendo Achillis at its insertion. The anterior two-thirds of the tendo Achillis is cut. This is best done by inserting a tenotome into the substance of the tendo Achillis at the junction of the middle third and posterior third of the tendon and cutting forwards.

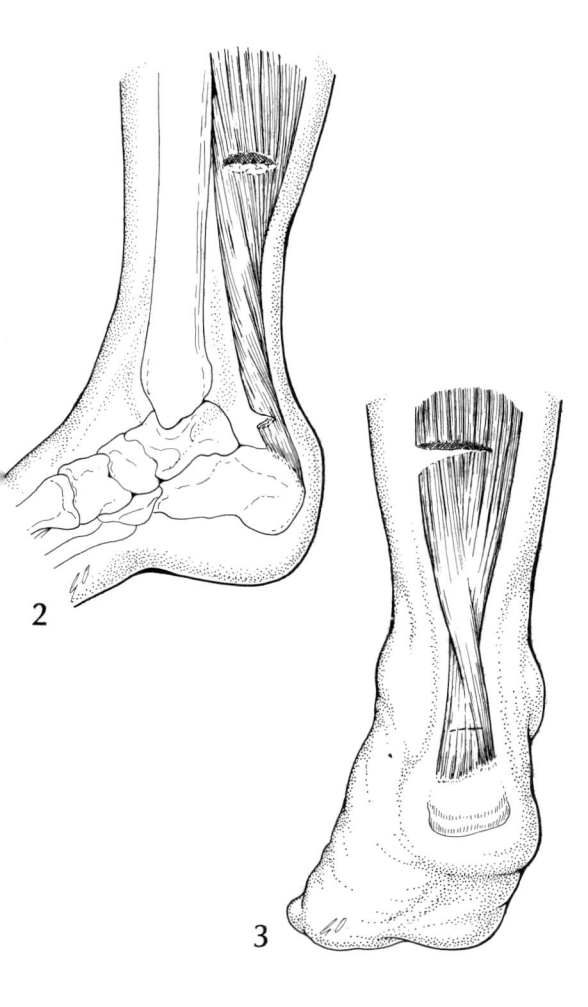

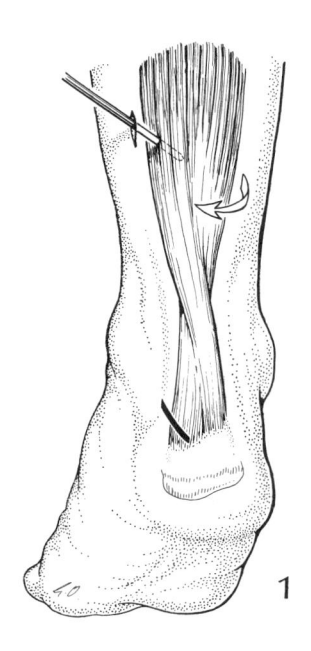

2 & 3

Another short incision is made on the medial side of the tendo Achillis at its musculotendinous junction. With the ankle in dorsiflexion the medial two-thirds of the tendon is divided at the musculotendinous junction. Dorsiflexion of the ankle lengthens the tendo Achillis and stitches are not necessary.

Postoperative management

A below-knee plaster cast is applied with the ankle in neutral position. At the end of 6 weeks the plaster is removed and ankle exercises commenced.

1174 Leg and foot

Z-PLASTY OF TENDO ACHILLIS

In severe contractures of the tendo Achillis it is necessary to lengthen it by complete division of the tendon.

Incision

4

A straight vertical incision is made down the back of the ankle. A Z-shaped incision is made in the tendo Achillis so that the lateral half of the tendon is attached to the calcaneum.

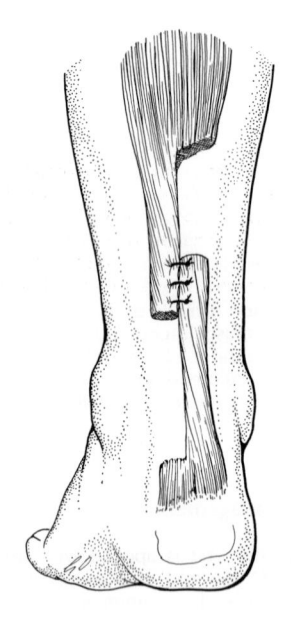

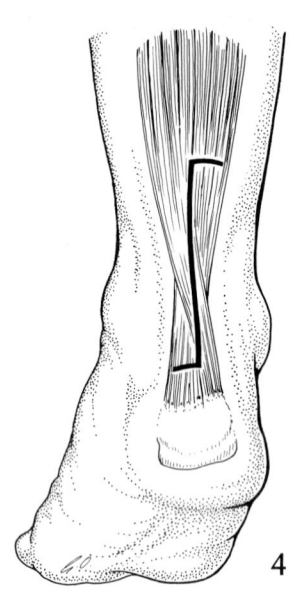

Repair

5

The foot is brought up to the neutral position and the tendo Achillis sutured together with three thick synthetic slowly absorbable sutures (polydioxanone-PDS). The deep fascia is sutured carefully and the skin wound closed.

Postoperative management

A below-knee plaster cast is applied with the ankle in neutral position. It is removed after 6 weeks and ankle exercises started.

Gastrocnemius contracture

The calf muscles consist of the gastrocnemius which arises proximal to the knee joint, and the soleus which is attached distal to the knee.

Usually both muscles contribute to the equinus deformity, but occasionally the gastrocnemius is mainly affected. It is relatively easy to distinguish between the two types. Where the gastrocnemius only is affected, the equinus deformity disappears when the knee is flexed; whereas where both muscles are affected, knee flexion does not influence the equinus deformity.

The functional result is better when the soleus is not lengthened. The gastrocnemius can be detached from its proximal attachment to the posterior part of the femoral condyles (Silfverskiöld operation) or divided distally (Strayer operation).

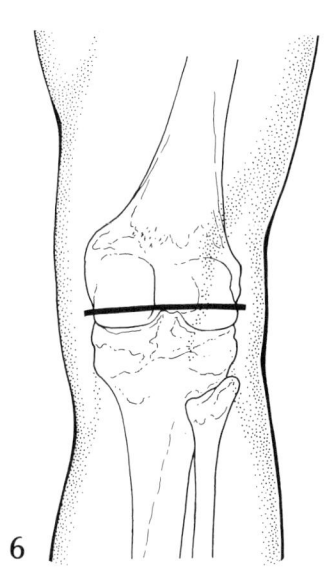

PROXIMAL DETACHMENT OF THE GASTROCNEMIUS (Silfverskiöld operation[2])

Incision

6

The patient lies prone, and the operation performed under tourniquet control. A transverse incision is made across the popliteal space along the joint crease, extending from the medial hamstring to the lateral hamstring muscles. Care must be taken not to damage the lateral popliteal nerve as well as the tibial nerves and vessels.

1176 Leg and foot

Dissection

7 & 8

The deep fascia is incised, and the two heads of gastrocnemius are identified. It may be necessary to divide the motor branches to the gastrocnemius from the tibial nerve if the gastrocnemius is grossly hypertonic. The heads of gastrocnemius are elevated from the posterior aspect of the femoral condyles by blunt dissection, and divided close to bone. The deep fascia, fat and skin are sutured in layers.

Postoperative management

An above-knee plaster cast is applied with the ankle in dorsiflexion, and the knee fully extended. The plaster cast is removed at the end of 4 weeks and physiotherapy commenced.

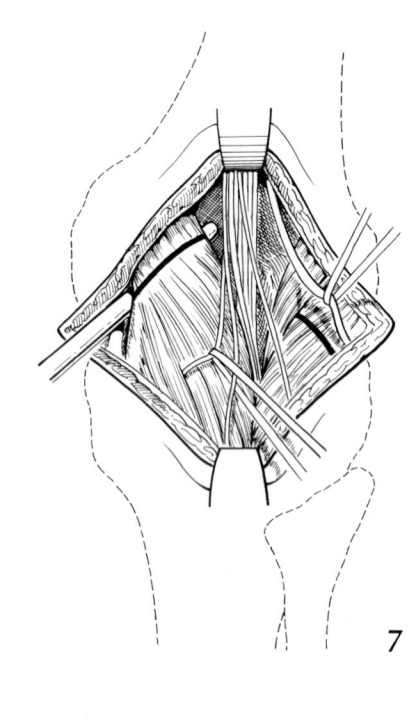

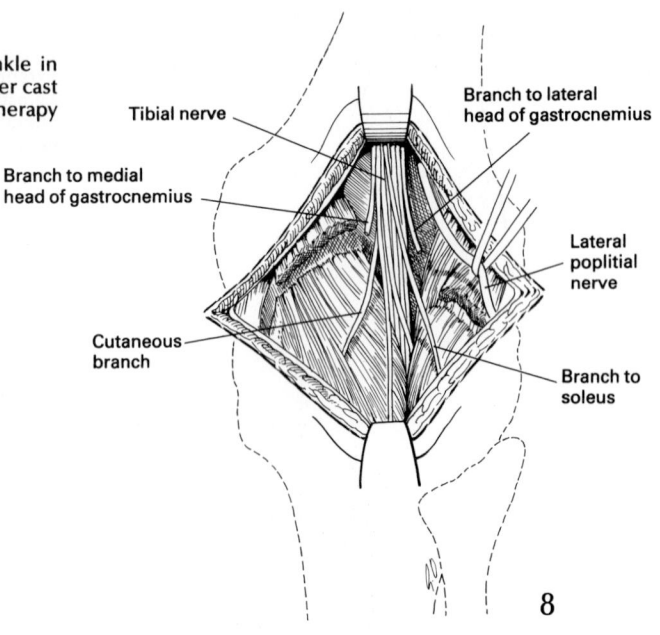

DISTAL DIVISION OF THE GASTROCNEMIUS (Strayer operation[3])

Incision

9

The patient lies prone, and the operation is performed under tourniquet control. A vertical incision is made down the middle of the calf. The sural nerve medially, and the superficial peroneal nerve laterally, are identified and protected.

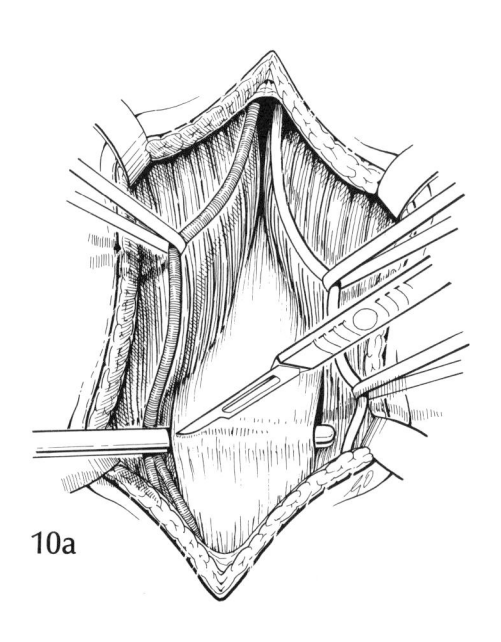

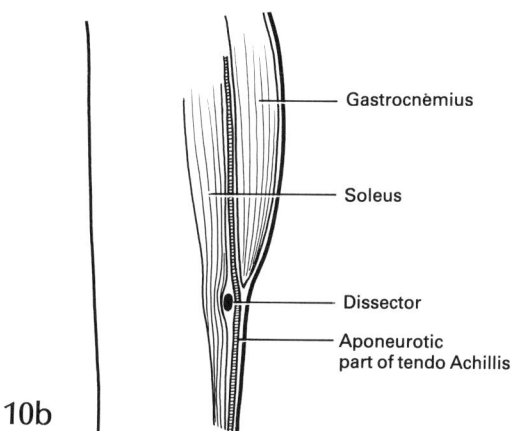

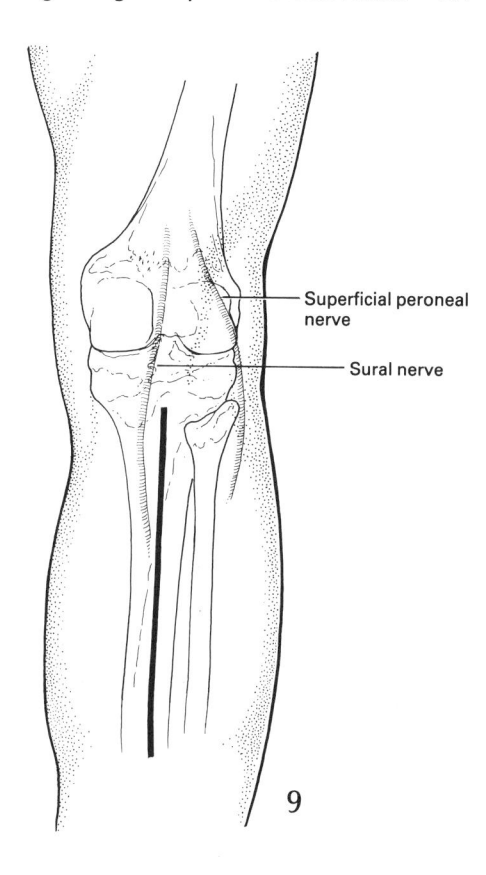

Dissection

10a & b

The deep fascia is incised in line with the skin incision, and the calf muscles exposed. The gastrocnemius is separated from the deeper soleus muscle by blunt dissection which is extended distally to the common tendo Achillis.

11

The gastrocnemius is divided at its musculotendinous junction. The ankle is dorsiflexed to separate the cut gastrocnemius. The muscle bellies of the gastrocnemius may have to be dissected off the deeper soleus to obtain adequate dorsiflexion of the ankle. Sometimes the aponeurosis of the soleus may be contracted and has to be incised, taking care not to damage the soleus muscle itself.

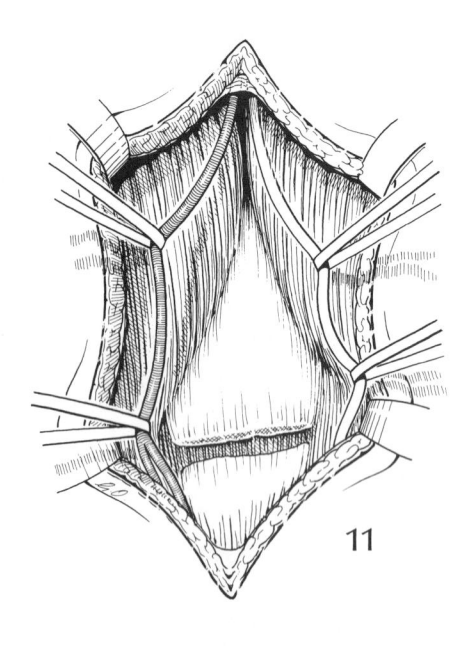

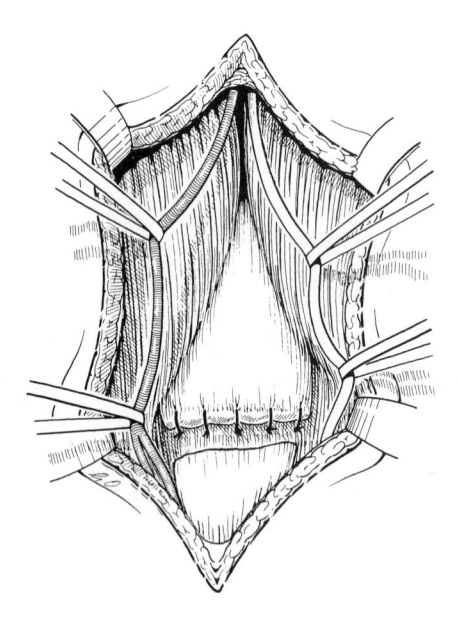

Closure

12

The proximal cut end of the gastrocnemius is sutured to the underlying aponeurosis of the soleus with interrupted sutures, whilst the ankle is kept fully dorsiflexed. The wound is closed in layers.

Postoperative management

An above-knee plaster cast is applied with the ankle in dorsiflexion, and the knee fully extended. The plaster cast is removed at the end of 4 weeks and physiotherapy started.

REPAIR

Ruptures of the tendo Achillis usually present acutely. However, the diagnosis is not always easy and some patients present with chronic ruptures weeks or months after the injury. The operative techniques will be considered separately.

Acute rupture of the tendo Achillis

This condition usually occurs following an acute injury to a degenerate tendon and is therefore most common after the age of 40 years.

The history is typical: the patient experiences sudden severe pain behind his ankle and, thinking that he has received a kick or blow, may strike out at any unfortunate individual who might happen to be behind him.

Diagnosis

Diagnosis of this condition can be difficult as the flexors of the toes can still plantarflex the ankle. Two clinical signs are very useful.

1. The patient cannot stand on tiptoe on the affected leg.
2. When the patient is lying prone with the feet over the end of the examination couch, squeezing of the relaxed calf muscles will not cause plantarflexion of the ankle if the tendo Achillis is ruptured, whereas the ankle will plantarflex if the tendo Achillis is intact (Simmonds' and Thompson's test[4, 5]).

A gap in the tendo Achillis is not always palpable due either to incomplete separation of the frayed and ruptured ends or to congealed blood in the gap.

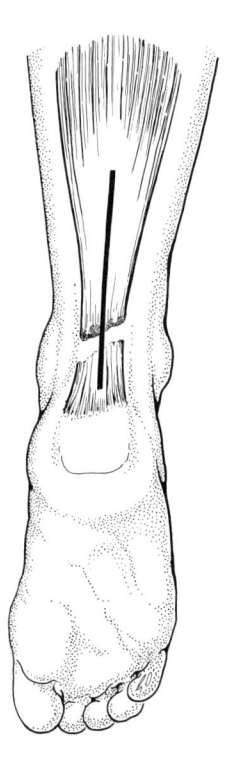

OPEN REPAIR

Incision

13

A vertical incision is made straight down the back of the lower leg, taking care not to extend down to the calcaneum. The deep fascia is divided to expose the ruptured tendo Achillis. (Skin healing is a problem and it is important not to curve the skin incision or extend it too far distally.)

Repair

14

The ruptured tendo Achillis usually frays, and it is not possible to insert any sutures which will take tension. However, by plantarflexing the ankle, the frayed ends of the tendo Achillis can be brought together with one non-absorbable suture using the Kessler technique[6]. The frayed ends are approximated as well as is possible with several chromic catgut sutures.

Closure

The deep fascia is stitched carefully and the skin closed with interrupted sutures taking care not to invert the skin edges.

Postoperative management

A below-knee plaster cast is applied from the toes to the tibial tuberosity with the foot in equinus. At the end of 3 weeks the skin sutures are removed and another plaster cast reapplied but with the foot in as near a neutral position as possible. After 6 weeks the plaster cast is removed and ankle exercises started. Full weight-bearing is started when the ankle can dorsiflex to neutral.

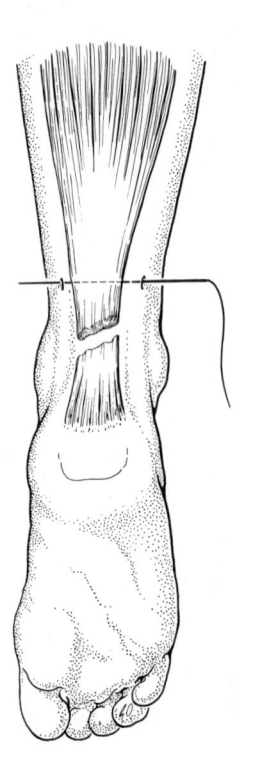

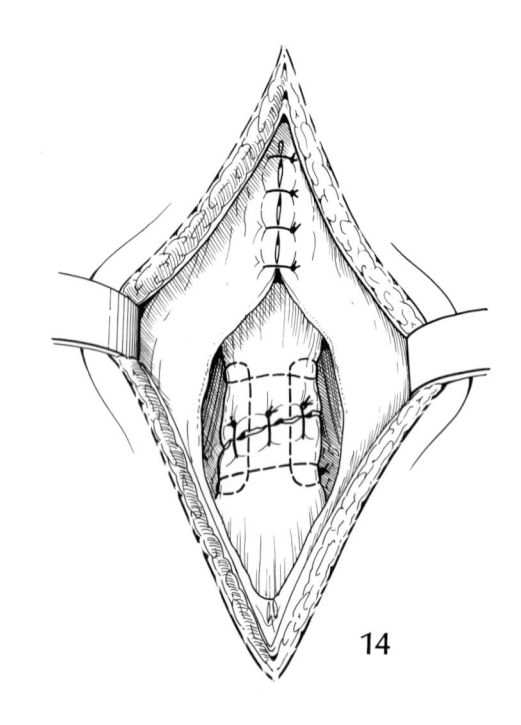

CLOSED REPAIR (Ma and Griffith[7])

The problem with open repair of an acutely ruptured tendo Achillis is skin healing. The vascularity of the skin in this area is poor, and injudicious skin incisions and rough retraction compromise an already poor blood supply.

Position of patient

The patient lies prone, and the operation is performed under tourniquet control. The gap in the tendo Achillis is assessed. The ankle is held plantarflexed throughout the procedure so that the tendon ends are approximated, and the subcutaneous tissue and skin are relaxed. This allows for the various manoeuvres to be carried out.

Stab incisions

15

A stab incision is made on the lateral side of the tendon about 3 cm proximal to the rupture. A No. 1 non-absorbable suture on a straight needle is passed transversely across in the substance of the tendon. As the tip of the needle comes out through the skin on the medial side it makes another stab wound in the skin.

16

The two ends are mounted on straight cutting needles and passed obliquely across to the other side, to come out just proximal to the ruptured end, making sure that the needles are still in the substance of the tendon. Two stab wounds are made in the skin at the point of exit on either side, distal to the other end of the rupture – that part of the tendon which is still attached to the calcaneum.

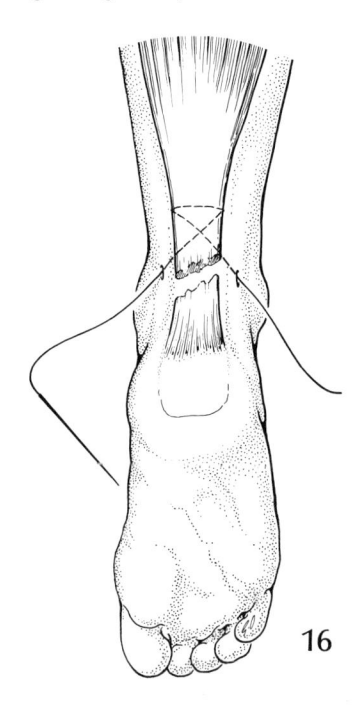

17

The straight needle on the medial side is driven transversely across the substance of the distal tendon stump about 2–3 cm away from the ruptured end. This comes out through the previously made stab wound on the lateral side.

It must be ensured that the suture is freed from the subcutaneous tissue and lying tightly within the substance of both parts of the ruptured tendon.

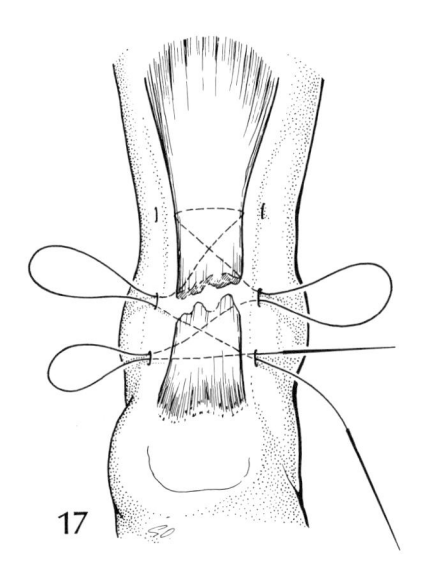

Suture of wounds

18

The suture is then knotted on the lateral side, making sure that the tendon ends are brought together. This can be observed through the medial stab wound. The several stab wounds are sutured with one stitch to each wound.

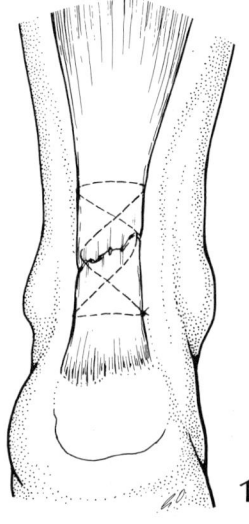

Postoperative management

A non-weight-bearing below-knee plaster cast is applied with the ankle plantarflexed for 4 weeks. This is followed by a further 4 weeks in a weight-bearing cast with the foot brought up, as near as possible without force, to a plantigrade position. Physiotherapy is then started.

1182 Leg and foot

Old ruptures

The calf muscles retract in old ruptures and a gap is almost always present in the tendo Achillis.

Incision

19

As before, a straight vertical incision is made down the back of the leg, taking care not to extend it too far distally onto the calcaneum.

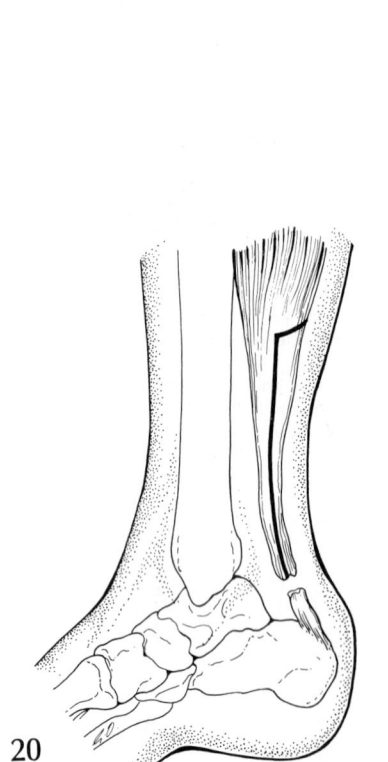

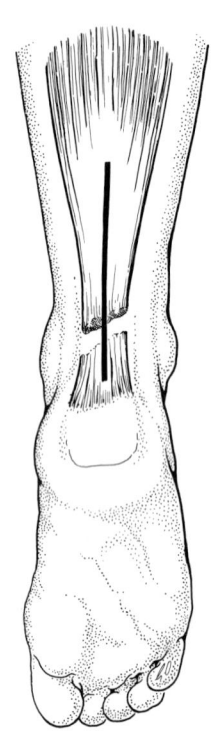

Division and slide

20

The ruptured ends of the tendo Achillis are identified – these are usually rounded off and thickened. They should be freshened.

An incision is made across the proximal segment of the tendo Achillis at the musculotendinous junction, directed downwards and forwards and cutting through the posterior half of the tendon.

21 & 22

The posterior half of the tendon is slid downwards to approximate the tendon ends. The ends are sutured together using non-absorbable suture material. A Kessler grasping stitch is inserted and supplemented with several chromic catgut sutures, with the ankle in full plantarflexion.

The tendon slide in the proximal segment of the tendo Achillis is also reinforced with chromic catgut sutures.

Postoperative management

A below-knee plaster cast is applied with the foot in equinus. The plaster cast is changed at 3 weeks, placing the ankle as near to the neutral position as possible. The plaster cast is removed at 6 weeks and passive and active exercises started.

References

1. White JW. Torsion of the Achilles tendon; its surgical significance. *Arch Surg* 1943; 46: 784–7.

2. Silfverskiöld N. Reduction of the uncrossed two-joint muscles of the leg to one-joint muscles in spastic conditions. *Acta Chir Scand* 1923; 56: 315.

3. Strayer LM. Recession of the gastrocnemius: an operation to relieve spastic contracture of the calf muscles. *J Bone Joint Surg [Am]* 1950; 32-A: 671–6; 712.

4. Simmonds FA. Test for rupture of tendo Achillis. In: Apley AG. *A system of orthopaedics and fractures*. London: Butterworths, 1959.

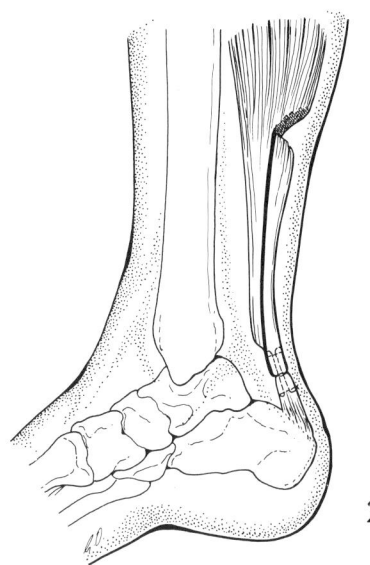

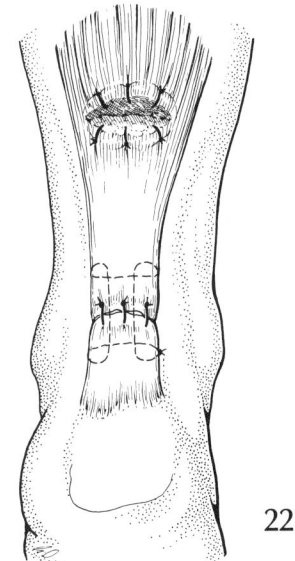

5. Thompson TC. A test for rupture of the tendon Achillis. *Acta Orthop Scand* 1962; 32: 461–5.

6. Kessler I. The "grasping" technique for tendon repair. *Hand* 1973; 5: 253–5.

7. Ma GW, Griffith TG. Percutaneous repair of acute closed ruptured Achilles tendon: a new technique. *Clin Orthop* 1977; 128: 247.

Illustrations by Gillian Oliver after B. Hyams

Transfer of tibialis posterior tendon to the dorsum of the foot

B. Helal MChOrth, FRCS
Honorary Consultant Orthopaedic Surgeon, The Royal London Hospital and The Royal National Orthopaedic Hospital, London, and Enfield Group of Hospitals, UK

S. C. Chen FRCS
Consultant Orthopaedic Surgeon, Enfield Group of Hospitals, UK

Introduction

In poliomyelitis, leprosy, peripheral neuropathy or injury to the lateral popliteal nerve, the peroneal muscles and tibialis anterior may be paralysed leading to a foot drop deformity, but the tibialis posterior muscle may be normal. The tendon of this muscle can be transferred through the interosseous space onto the dorsum of the foot to restore dorsiflexion.

Operation

1

Two small skin incisions are made on the medial aspect of the foot and ankle: (1) posterior to the medial malleolus; and (2) at the attachment of the tibialis posterior to the navicular.

2

The tibialis posterior tendon is divided as near to the navicular attachment as possible and withdrawn into the proximal skin incision by pulling on it. The lower incision is closed.

A non-absorbable suture is attached to the end of the tendon using a Kessler stitch.

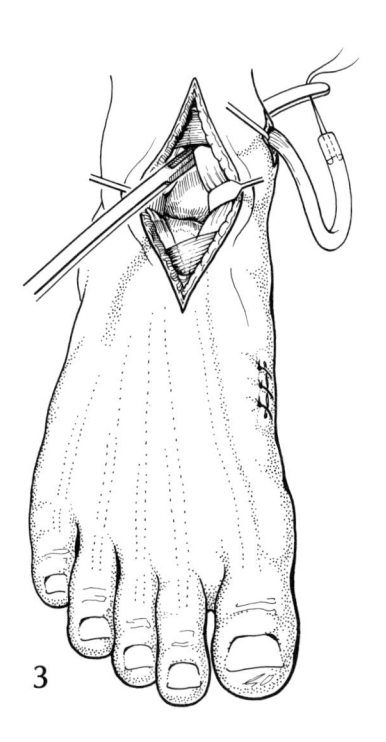

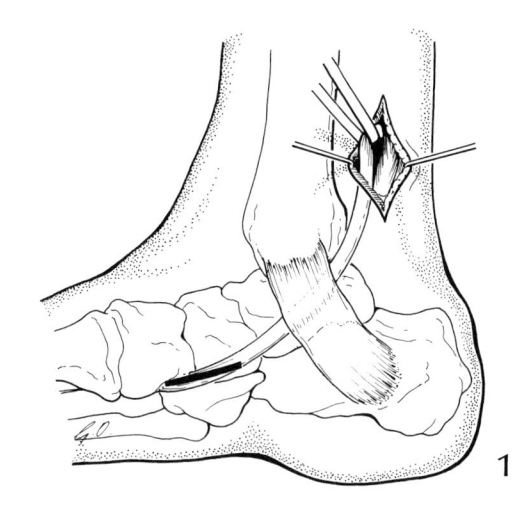

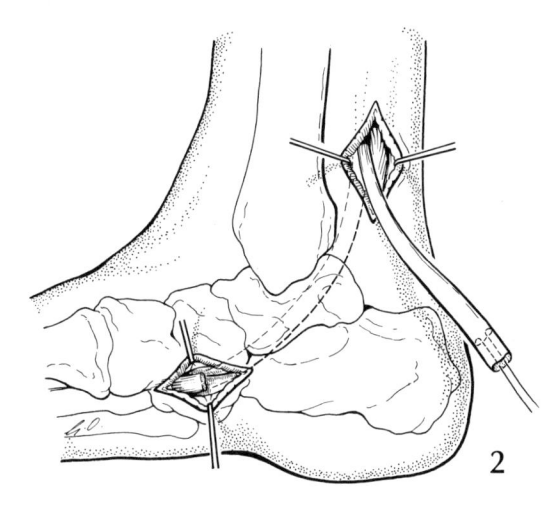

3

A third incision is then made on the front of the ankle.

The tendons and neurovascular bundle are retracted laterally and curved artery forceps are passed through the interosseous membrane. The artery forceps are opened in order to enlarge the hole in the interosseous membrane.

Next, the artery forceps are directed into the wound behind the medial malleolus. The end of the suture attached to the tibialis posterior tendon is grasped.

1186 Leg and foot

4

The tendon is pulled taut and the tibialis posterior muscle and tendon in the posterior compartment of the leg inspected to ensure that the tendon is not twisted and that the line of pull upon the intermediate cuneiform is straight. The tibialis posterior muscle is freed by blunt dissection if necessary.

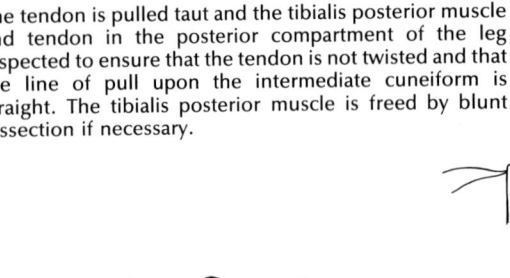

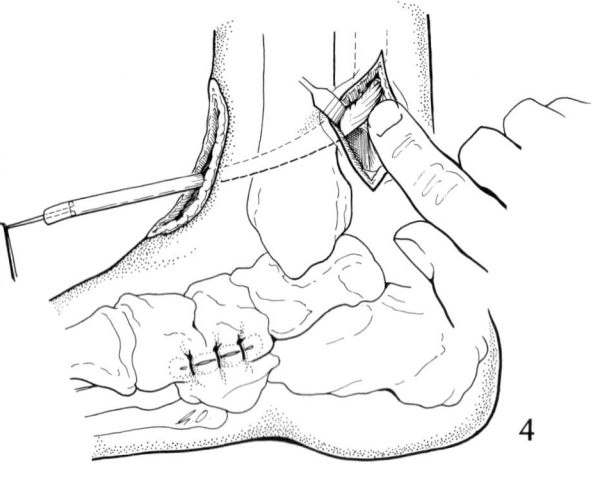

5

A final skin incision is made over the intermediate cuneiform. The bone is exposed and, with a Paton's burr, a hole is made in the centre of this bone large enough to thread the tibialis posterior tendon through.

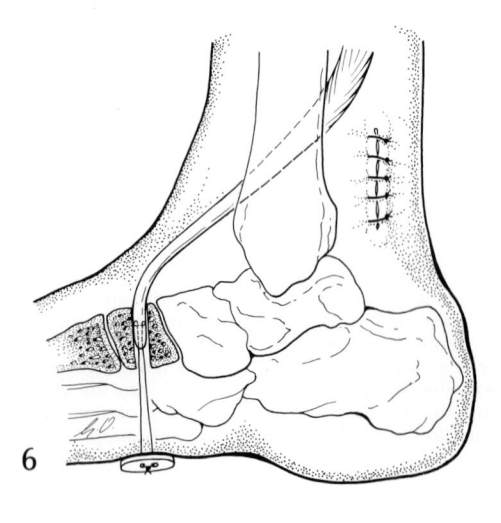

6

The sutures are threaded through a large straight needle and this is passed through the hole in the intermediate cuneiform and through the sole of the foot. There is usually just sufficient length of posterior tibial tendon to pass into the cuneiform bone. The sutures are tied over a large button on the sole of the foot with the ankle in neutral position and with the tendon taut. The remaining skin incisions are closed.

Postoperative management

A below-knee plaster cast is applied from the toes to the tibial tuberosity with the ankle in neutral position. No weight-bearing is allowed for 6 weeks. The plaster is removed at the end of 6 weeks and the sutures over the button undone. The button is removed and the sutures cut just deep to the skin. Passive and active ankle exercises are commenced.

Illustrations by Phillip Wilson after G. Lyth

Multiple tendon transfers into the heel

E. W. Somerville FRCS (Ed), FRCS
Emeritus Consultant Orthopaedic Surgeon, Nuffield Orthopaedic Centre, Oxford, UK

Introduction

Indications

This operation is performed for the correction of calcaneocavus deformity of the foot in patients between the ages of 5 and 18 years. The deformity of calcaneocavus results from a pure muscle imbalance. In young people, where there is an isolated paralysis of the muscles inserted into the tendo Achillis, with all the other muscles of the calf acting normally, this deformity will always develop. The mechanism of the deformity is shown in *Illustrations 1 and 2*.

1

Plantarflexion of the foot is achieved by: the heel being drawn up by the gastrocnemius and soleus muscles; and the forefoot being pulled down by the other muscles of the calf which pass behind the malleoli and are attached to the plantar surface of the forefoot.

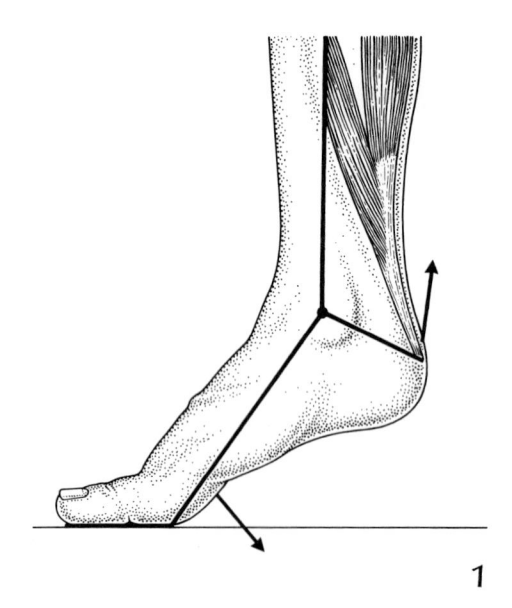

2

If the gastrocnemius and soleus muscles are paralysed or the tendon is cut and not repaired during the growth period, attempts to plantarflex the foot will result in the forefoot being pulled down without the heel being pulled up. The heel assumes an increasingly calcaneus position and the forefoot becomes increasingly plantarflexed until this position becomes fixed.

The hypertrophy of the tibialis anterior which is often seen in this condition is not related to the development of the deformity; rather, the hypertrophy results from dorsiflexion against a severe mechanical disadvantage.

Principle of treatment

The aim of surgical treatment is to remove the deforming force by taking the tendons which are inserted into the forefoot and transferring them to the heel where they will pull the tuberosity of the calcaneum upwards, thereby acting as a correcting force.

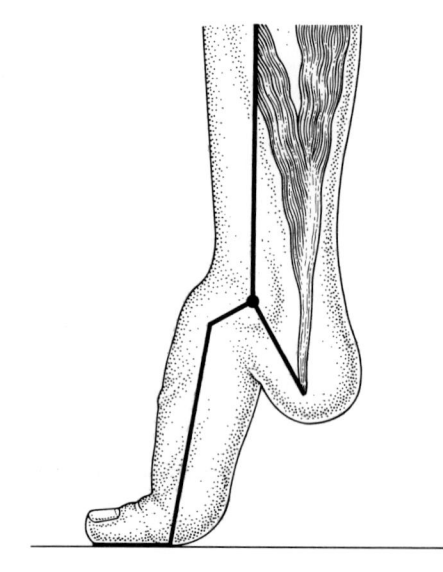

Operation

Position of patient

The patient is placed on the operating table in the prone position with a sandbag under the ankles so that the toes will not rest on the table when the foot is dorsiflexed.

Incision

3

A right-angled incision is made, the vertical limb of which extends from above and behind the medial malleolus downwards to the lower border of the calcaneum. It is situated one-third of the distance between the tendo Achillis and the medial malleolus. At the lower border of the calcaneum it turns at 90° posteriorly and laterally to pass round the back of the heel, finishing below the lateral malleolus at the level of the lower border of the calcaneum.

The skin flap, which must be kept as thick as possible, is turned up the smallest amount that will allow access to the tendons behind the medial malleolus and the peroneal tendons on the other side. The tendo Achillis is divided as its lower end is turned up, exposing the upper border of the calcaneum.

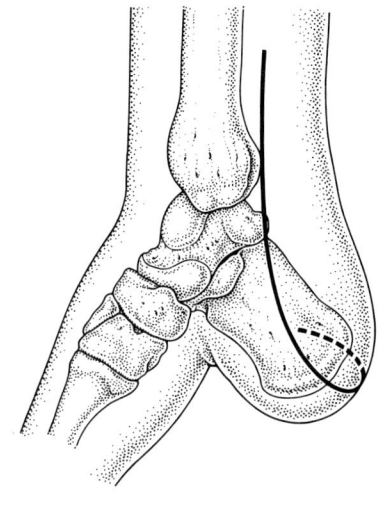

4

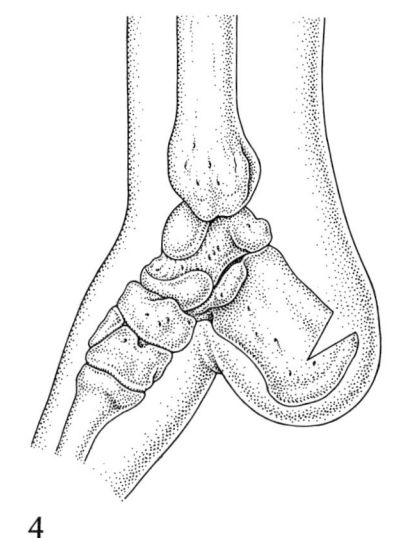

A groove is cut in the end of the calcaneum to a depth of 2.5 cm with an osteotome.

1190 Leg and foot

5a & b

The tibialis posterior, the flexor digitorum longus and the flexor hallucis longus tendons are divided behind the medial malleolus with as much length as possible and are stripped upwards so that they can be brought without kinking to the midline. The peroneal tendons are similarly treated. A strong catgut suture is introduced into each tendon, the ends being left very long. Holes of 0.8 mm (1/32 inch) are drilled from the posterior aspect of the calcaneum into the bottom of the groove. Using a Mayo trocar-ended needle each suture end is passed through one of these holes.

5a 5b

6a & b

When they have been passed through the heel is pushed upwards, which is quite different from the forefoot being pulled down, the tendons are pulled down as tightly as possible into the bottom of the groove and the sutures are tied over the bone.

Care must be taken to ensure that the tendons have been cut previously to a length which will only just allow them to reach the bottom of the groove. The skin flap is sutured back into position with as few interrupted sutures as possible.

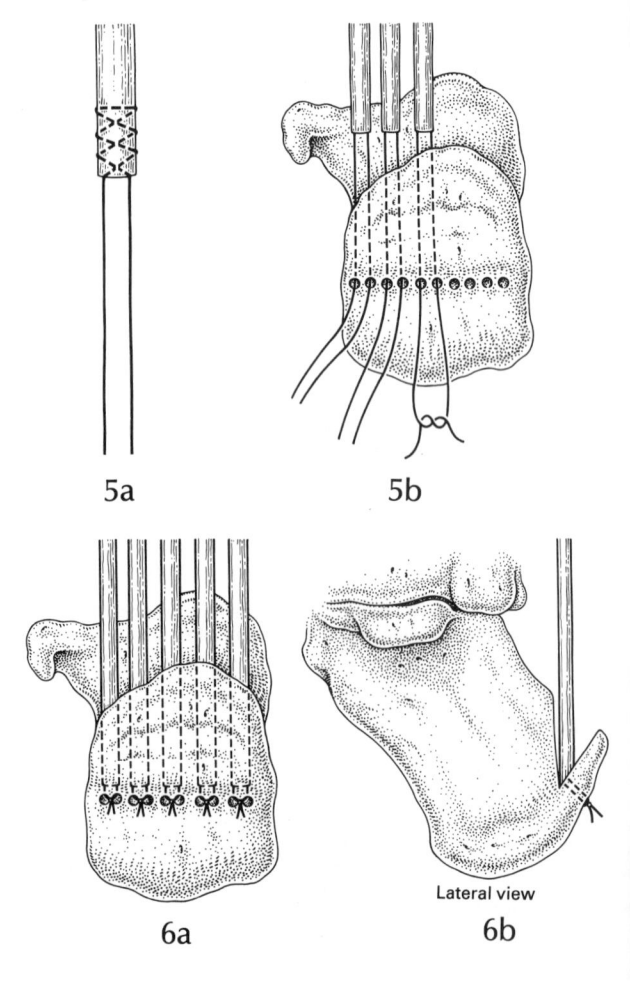

Lateral view
6a 6b

Postoperative management

A well-padded below-knee plaster cast is applied with the heel pushed well upwards and extending distally to the end of the toes.

The leg is kept elevated until the postoperative swelling has settled, which may take a week. The leg should not be lowered too soon. The patient is then allowed to walk with crutches, but weight-bearing is not allowed until the plaster is removed at 6 weeks.

Comment

This operation is really the second half of the Jones' operation in which the tendon transfers are preceded by a formal stabilization of the foot to bring the forefoot in line with the calcaneum. When bony union is established the tendon transfers are carried out. The results of the tendon transfers alone in children up to at least the age of 18 years are so good that the bone operation is contraindicated. In adults, however, in whom the operation is rarely necessary, bone resection may be required. After the tendon transfer the restoration of the foot to a normal appearance is remarkably rapid and function is also rapidly restored.

Illustrations by Philip Wilson after G. Lyth

Arthrodeses of the ankle

E. W. Somerville FRCS (Ed), FRCS
Emeritus Consultant Orthopaedic Surgeon, Nuffield Orthopaedic Centre, Oxford, UK

Introduction

Arthrodesis of the ankle provides pain relief and stability in patients with a disorganized joint following ankle fractures, fractures of the talus or infections. Deformity and weakness secondary to neuromuscular diseases can be greatly alleviated by ankle stabilization. The best results occur in the young and those with healthy subtalar and tarsal joints.

Indications

1. To relieve pain in arthritic conditions or following severe trauma.
2. To stabilize the ankle in cases of drop foot where there is no deformity in the distal joints.

This is a better operation than the Lambrinudi operation, which is described in the chapter on 'Arthrodeses of the foot' (pp. 1199–1207), because it allows greater correction and there is no tendency to relapse. However, only small degrees of varus can be corrected at the ankle joint and marked varus is better corrected by the Lambrinudi procedure.

Operations

ANKLE ARTHRODESIS BY THE ANTERIOR APPROACH (WATSON-JONES)

Position of patient

The patient is placed on the operating table in the supine position with a small flat sandbag underneath the buttock.

Incision and exposure

1a & b

An anterior incision is made 10 cm above the ankle joint extending to 5 cm below. The tibialis anterior tendon is exposed and, together with the tendon of the extensor hallucis longus, is retracted medially, the tendons of the extensor digitorum communis being retracted laterally. The tendon sheaths are preserved if possible. The dorsalis pedis artery will often have to be divided between ligatures but can sometimes be retracted out of the way. The anterior capsule of the ankle joint is then exposed.

The capsule is excised across the front of the joint to the tips of the malleoli which will allow the joint to be opened up widely with forced plantar flexion. Using a sharp chisel, rather than an osteotome, the articular surfaces are excised from the lower end of the tibia, the upper surface of the talus and from the lateral surfaces of the talus and the medial and lateral malleoli, if possible down to cancellous bone. Care must be taken to prevent the chisel from damaging important structures lying posterior to the ankle joint and the medial malleolus. The lower surface of the tibia and the upper surface of the talus are fitted together in the selected position for the foot, and the site for the graft in the talus is defined. The graft is outlined on the anterior surface of the tibia. The joint is again opened up so that the notch for the graft may be cut in the body of the talus. This notch will measure 13 mm wide, 19 mm deep and 10 mm anteroposteriorly. The bone removed is preserved for later use.

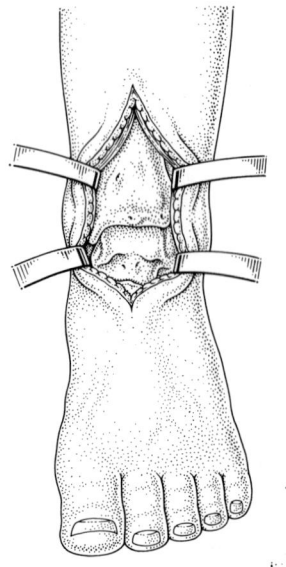

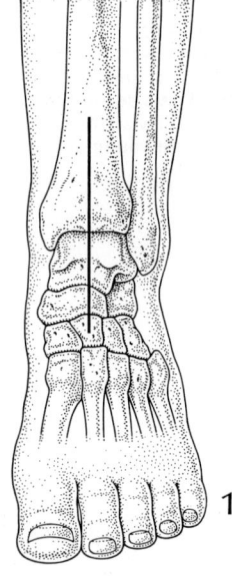

2

A graft 13 mm wide at the bottom, very slightly wider at the top and 7.5 cm in length, is cut from the anterior surface of the tibia with a circular saw and when freed is driven hard down into the talus. If it has been tapered correctly it will fit tightly into the lower part of the groove and into the notch. While the graft is being driven down heavy counterpressure must be applied to the undersurface of the heel to prevent distraction of the talus and tibia. Since excising the articular surfaces will have made the talus smaller and the joint mortise bigger there will be gaps on one or both sides which must be filled with the bone which was previously removed and with other cancellous bone from the tibia.

Wound closure

The tendons are allowed to resume their normal position and are held in place by lightly suturing the extensor retinaculum. The wound is closed in layers.

Postoperative management

A long leg plaster cast is applied with the knee slightly bent to control rotation. For this reason a short plaster must not be used. The leg is elevated for several days until the postoperative reaction is over, when the patient is allowed up on crutches without weight-bearing. A walking heel is applied at 6 weeks but the plaster should not be reduced to below-knee before 10 weeks. Union should be sound in 4 months but may sometimes be slower.

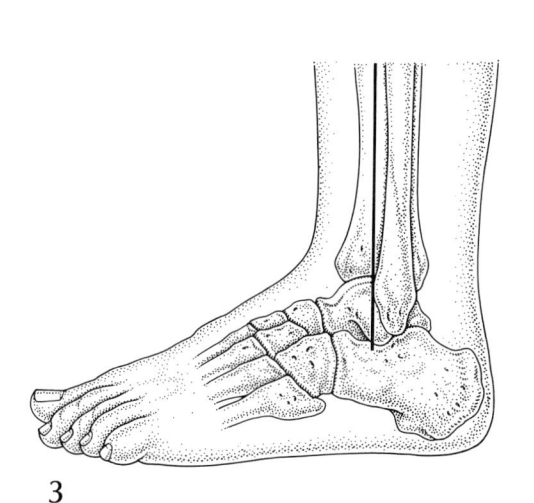

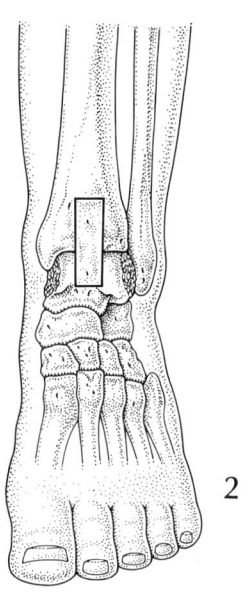

ANKLE ARTHRODESIS BY THE LATERAL APPROACH

Position of patient

The patient is placed on the operating table in the supine position with a large sandbag under the buttock on the operation side so that he is tilted into the semilateral position.

Incision and exposure

3

A straight incision 13 cm in length is made over the anterior border of the lower fibula extending to just below the tip of the lateral malleolus. The fibula is exposed subperiosteally and anteriorly and posteriorly within the limits of the incision but anteriorly the exposure is carried to the middle of the tibia.

1194 Leg and foot

4

With a small circular saw the adjacent surfaces of tibia and fibula are excised including the inferior tibiofibular joint, the articular surfaces of the lateral malleolus and the lateral side of the talus. This excision is carried 6.5 cm above the ankle joint at which level the fibula is divided. The fibula, together with the excised bone, is removed, exposing the lateral aspect of the ankle joint. A small bone lever is passed behind the joint to keep the tendons out of the way and with a sharp chisel the articular surfaces of talus and tibia are excised in parallel while the foot is held in the required position. Care must be taken not to remove too much bone from the lateral side of the joint unless it is intended to correct some varus.

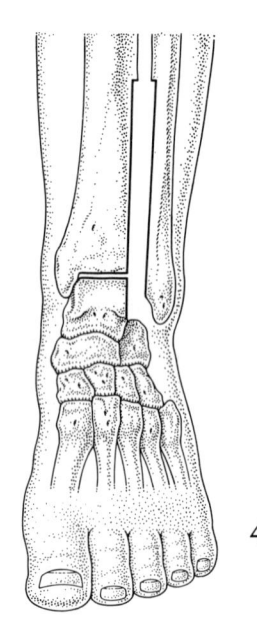

5

With the tibia and talus held in close apposition, the removed lower end of the fibula, the medial side of which will already be raw from the circular saw, is applied to the lower end of the tibia and talus, which will be similarly raw, and is fixed in position with two screws above and one screw below the joint.

Wound closure

The peroneal tendons are replaced in position behind the lateral malleolus and held there by repair of the retinaculum. The soft tissues are drawn lightly together and the skin is closed.

Postoperative management

This is as for the anterior approach.

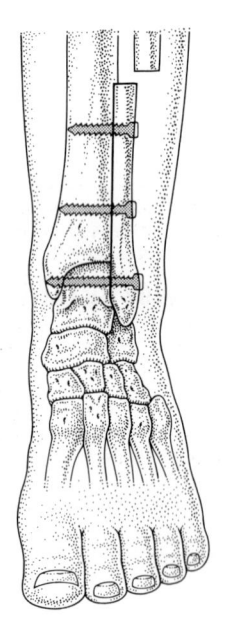

COMPRESSION ANKLE ARTHRODESIS (CHARNLEY)

The patient is placed on the operating table in the supine position.

Incision and exposure

6a

An incision is carried across the front of the ankle joint from the tip of the medial malleolus to the tip of the lateral malleolus. All the anterior tendons are divided between stay sutures and retracted and the dorsalis pedis artery is divided between ligatures. The capsule of the joint is incised in its entirety and both malleoli are osteotomized through their bases.

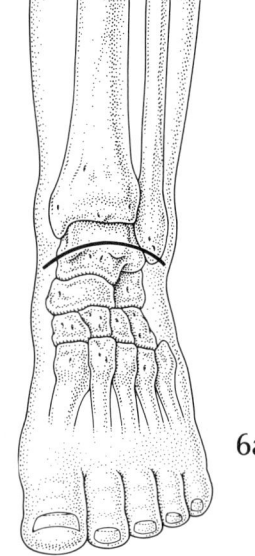

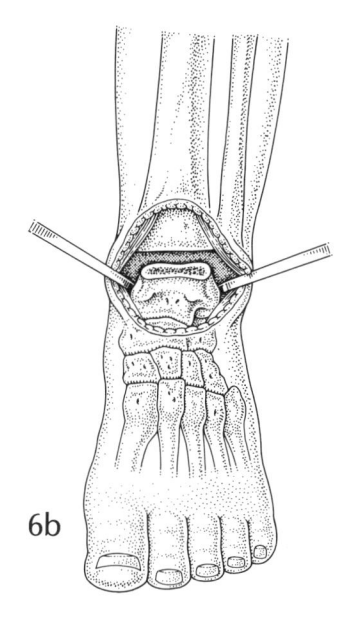

6b

The ankle joint is completely dislocated by plantarflexion of the foot and the malleoli are excised. The lower 13 mm of the tibia is cleared of soft tissue as far as possible. Two small bone levers are placed behind the lower end of the tibia, being passed through the ankle joint with the foot plantarflexed. These are to protect the posterior tibial nerve and blood vessels from damage. With soft tissue retraction the lower end of the tibia is divided with a handsaw 6 mm from the articular surface and at 90° to the long axis of the bone. The foot is lined up into the required position and a cut is made with the saw in the body of the talus parallel to the cut end of the tibia. The foot is again dislocated, the two bone levers are reversed to lie behind the talus and the excision of the upper surface of the talus is completed with the saw.

7a & b

A stout 15 cm Steinmann pin is passed through the centre of the lower end of the tibia 5 cm from the cut surface and parallel to it. The cut surfaces are placed in close apposition and a similar Steinmann pin is passed through the body of the talus parallel to the first pin. This pin should be placed so that it lies just anterior to the centre of the bone. Where the pins pass through the skin a small incision is made with a tenotomy knife so that the skin edges will not slough from pressure. While this is being done the skin edges of the main wound should be held lightly together to ensure that the wound can be closed with the pins in position. Compression clamps are applied to the pins with the butterfly nuts downwards so that they can be tightened equally until there is good compression with some bending of the pins.

Wound closure

The tendons are sutured together under slight tension, the tendon sheaths and subcutaneous tissue are sutured as a single layer over them and the skin is lightly closed.

Postoperative management

Opinions differ as to the necessity for plaster postoperatively. If the bones are porotic, plaster should always be applied to reduce the risk of the pins cutting out. The author prefers always to apply a plaster for the patient's comfort but it need only be below-knee.

The foot is kept elevated until the postoperative swelling has settled when the patient is allowed up on crutches. At 5 weeks the plaster and pins are removed and a below-knee walking plaster is applied and retained until union is sound at 8–10 weeks.

Complications

Since this operation always involves division of the dorsalis pedis artery there must be no doubt that the posterior tibial artery is patent. In post-traumatic conditions this may not always be so, in which case it is possible to perform compression arthrodesis through two lateral incisions without disturbing the dorsalis pedis artery.

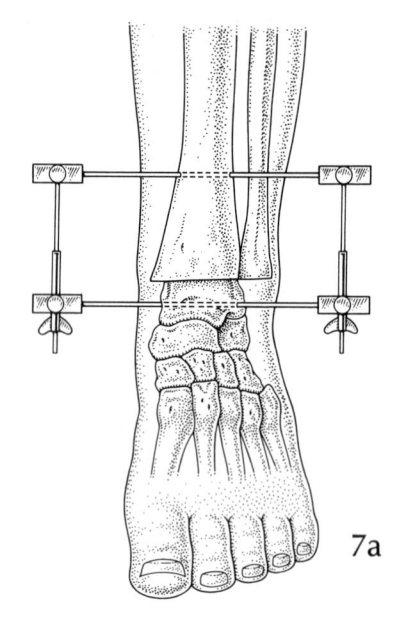

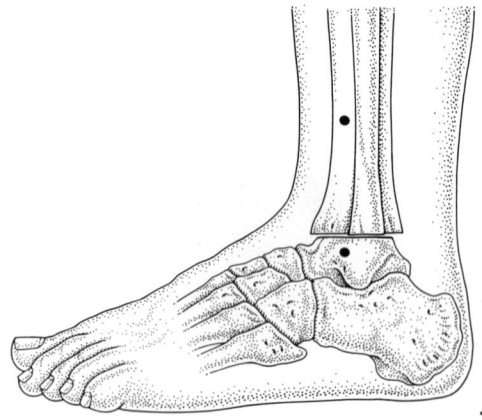

'TREPHINE' ANKLE ARTHRODESIS (THOMAS)

This is a simple, neat operation with minimal postoperative reaction but with the difficulty that if there is deformity of the joint it cannot easily be corrected. This operation is best confined to those ankles where no change of position is required.

Position of patient

The patient is placed on the operating table in the supine position.

8a

Incision and exposure

A 5 cm vertical incision is made over the medial malleolus which is then exposed subperiosteally.

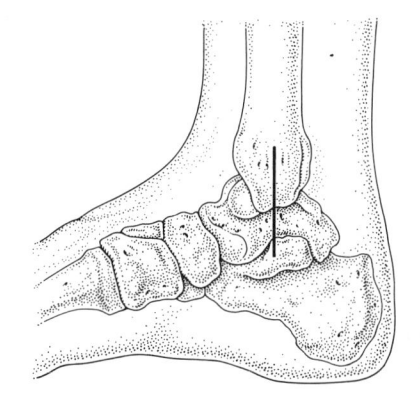

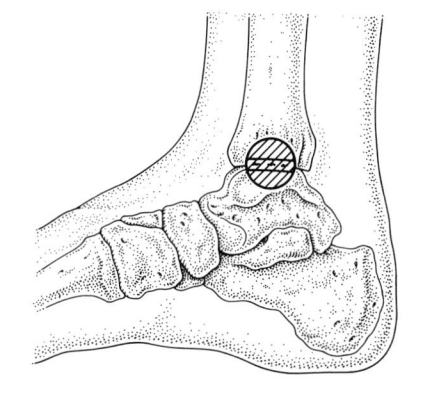

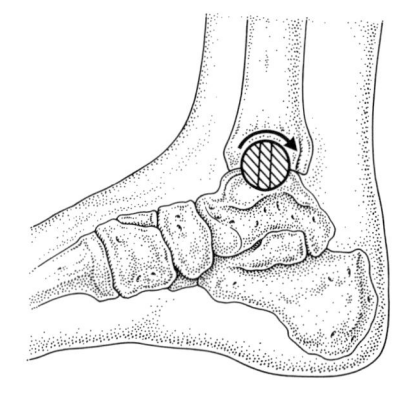

8b & c

The exact position of the ankle joint is determined by direct vision. A 19 mm trephine is centred over the joint on the medial side of the medial malleolus and is passed across the joint to the lateral side, taking out a core with the joint in the centre of it. This core is rotated through 90° and is then hammered in to make it spread. Alternatively the core may be removed completely and replaced by a piece of cancellous bone from the iliac crest which is similarly hammered in.

Wound closure

The periosteum and skin are closed with chromic catgut sutures.

Postoperative management

A below-knee walking plaster is applied. As soon as the postoperative reaction has settled the patient may start to walk with weight-bearing. Union is a little slow after this operation, usually taking 4 months.

OPTIMUM POSITION FOR ANKLE ARTHRODESIS

Opinions differ as to the position in which the foot should be placed. Some believe it should be related to the height of heel worn, particularly in women. However, this presents problems when shoes are not worn, and callosities may develop under the metatarsal heads if it is too extreme. A more sensible position for both men and women is sufficient plantarflexion, i.e. 5°–10°, to allow for a small heel and at the same time to compensate for the 13 mm shortening resulting from the excision of the joint.

A position of 5°–10° dorsiflexion is less often advocated though it has many advantages. In this position the patient stands well, has a more normal gait and will run better, which is of great importance in the younger patient. There is no risk of callosities developing on any part of the foot. Although not applicable in all cases serious consideration should be given to it when determining the position preoperatively.

In the presence of weakness or paralysis of the quadriceps, arthrodesis in dorsiflexion is absolutely contraindicated. In this condition the foot must always be placed in some equinus.

PANTALAR ARTHRODESIS

In certain patients where trauma to the ankle and foot has been extensive, resulting in painful deformity of both, it may be necessary to perform arthrodesis of the ankle, subtalar and mid-tarsal joints. This is, however, not a good operation because it leads to so much rigidity of the foot that persistent painful callosities are a not infrequent sequel. It should therefore be avoided whenever possible. For this reason the author recommends that, where there is a possibility that pantalar arthrodesis will be necessary, a subtalar stabilization of the foot with correction of the deformity should be performed. This will relieve the symptoms sufficiently often so that no further surgery will be required. However, if symptoms persist to a degree that arthrodesis of the ankle is necessary there is no difficulty in doing this as a second stage by one of the techniques already described above.

Illustrations by Philip Wilson after G. Lyth

Arthrodeses of the foot

E. W. Somerville FRCS, FRCS(Ed)
Emeritus Consultant Orthopaedic Surgeon, Nuffield Orthopaedic Centre, Oxford, UK

Introduction

Arthrodesis has been supplanted in many of the larger joints by replacement arthroplasty, but in the foot it remains an important technique.

Indications

Arthrodeses of the foot are indicated for (1) correction of valgus and varus deformity, (2) stabilization in paralytic conditions, and (3) fixation of painful and arthritic joints. Not infrequently two of these factors may be combined in the same foot.

Stabilization of the foot and the correction of varus

NAUGHTON DUNN'S OPERATION (TRIPLE ARTHRODESIS)

This was the first operation of its kind to be described. Since then there have been many modifications but the original is still the most commonly used and in the author's opinion is the one to be preferred. It consists of fusion of the subtalar, talonavicular and calcaneocuboid joints.

The operation aims to correct varus of the heel by removal of a suitable wedge from the subtalar joint, to correct adduction and varus of the forefoot by excision and fusion of the calcaneocuboid joint, which will shorten the foot, and to produce backward displacement of the foot at the talonavicular joint, which will improve stability.

Indications and contraindications

This operation is indicated for the correction of equinovarus deformity such as often follows the incomplete correction of club foot but which may also be found in paralytic conditions and as a post-traumatic lesion when it will be accompanied by osteoarthritis in one or more of the joints. This deformity is also quite commonly found in rheumatoid arthritis.

The operation should not be performed under the age of 13 years because of the risk of damaging the growth of the foot.

Position of patient

The patient is placed in the supine position on the operating table with a sandbag beneath the buttock on the operation side to give a tilt of about 30°.

Incision

1

A curved incision begins just above and behind the lateral malleolus, curving downwards and forwards to pass about 2.5 cm below the tip of the malleolus and up towards the dorsum of the foot to finish over the base of the second or third metatarsal.

Exposure and excision

2

The peroneal tendons are exposed by splitting the tendon sheaths from behind the lateral malleolus down to the calcaneocuboid joint. The belly of the extensor digitorum brevis is defined, separated from the talus and turned down to expose the sinus tarsi. The calcaneocuboid joint is excised using a 3.8 cm (1½ inch) osteotome or chisel so that the excision on each side of the joint will be clean. The two cuts should be either parallel or slightly more separated below than above, never the reverse, since this will lead to boating of the sole of the foot which will cause a painful callosity under the prominence.

A small bone lever is passed over the neck of the talus to expose the talonavicular joint. With a 3.8 cm (1½ inch) gouge the navicular is divided obliquely from above downwards and before backwards, excising the concave surface articulating with the head of the talus. The talocalcaneal ligaments are incised and the sinus tarsi cleaned of all soft tissue.

With the knee bent to 90° and controlled by an assistant the surgeon takes the heel in one hand and forcibly inverts it, dislocating all three joints. The separated fragments of bone in the mid-tarsal joints are easily excised with a scalpel. A bone lever is passed over the medial side of the calcaneus to protect the important structures there while the articular surface is being excised. A 5 cm (2 inch) chisel is used to excise the articular surface from the anterior to the posterior extremity, with care being taken to include the sustentaculum tali.

Reversing the bone lever the articular surface of the talus is similarly excised. Usually more bone will unconsciously be removed from the outer than from the inner side so that it is often unnecessary to remove a wedge consciously, but care must be taken to ensure that sufficient bone is removed so that the heel will lie in some slight degree of valgus at the end of the operation. The articular surface of the head of the talus is removed with bone cutters to the shape of the raw surface of the navicular with which it will lie in contact. The use of a chisel for this will run the risk of fracturing the neck of the talus if it is soft or brittle.

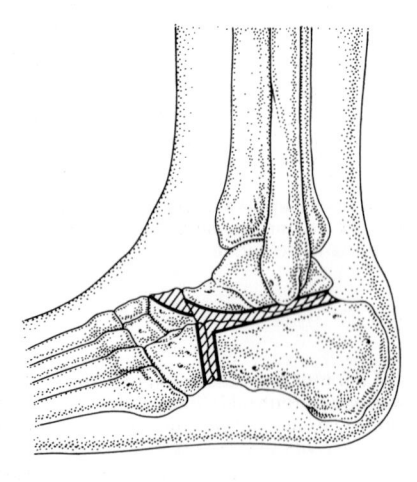

Reduction

3

When all the joint surfaces are prepared the foot is reduced. If the excision has been carried out well the surfaces will fit together accurately with the heel in slight valgus – never varus. If the operation has been correctly performed it should not be necessary to use wires or staples to hold the position. Wires and staples increase the risk of infection and the use of them is an admission of failure.

Wound closure

With the foot held in the reduced position the peroneal tendons are replaced and held in position by lightly suturing the retinaculum. The extensor digitorum brevis is reattached to the talus and the subcutaneous tissues lightly approximated. The skin closure is important. It should be done with the fewest possible everting stitches even if gaps are left between them. The skin edges of this incision are apt to slough, but this can be reduced to a minimum by very loose closure. This sloughing should not be mistaken for infection and even though it may at times be extensive it can be largely ignored, needing only to be covered with a dressing and enclosed in plaster. When the plaster is removed it will be healed.

Postoperative management

A full-length plaster cast should always be applied to control rotation for the first 6 weeks. If the plaster is carried to the tips of the toes on the dorsal and plantar surfaces so that only the tips are showing it should not be necessary to split the plaster, but this does not in any way exonerate the surgeon from ensuring that the circulation is satisfactory at all times.

The foot is kept elevated until the postoperative reaction has passed. The patient is then allowed up on crutches and at the end of 6 weeks the plaster is reduced to below-knee. If possible it is better not to remove and replace the plaster. A walking heel is applied and the patient is allowed to start weight-bearing. This plaster must be retained until 4 months after the operation. When the plaster is finally removed swelling is to be expected and this may persist for several months.

LAMBRINUDI OPERATION

Indication

This operation is a stabilization of the foot in paralytic conditions to correct drop foot where there is a varus deformity making an arthrodesis of the ankle inadvisable.

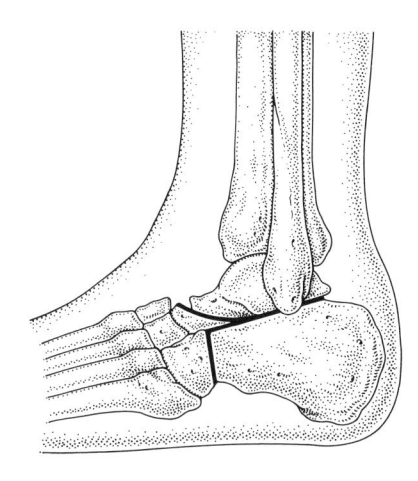

Principle

In doing the stabilization a wedge is removed with its base forward at the mid-tarsal joint so that when the wedge is closed the forefoot will be dorsiflexed about 25°, thus reducing the drop foot by this amount as well as correcting the deformity in the foot. It is not safe to try to reduce the drop foot by more than 25° because the base of the wedge would be so great that there would be a risk of non-union at the mid-tarsal joint.

Usually this operation produces an improvement rather than full correction and it will unfortunately be found that in many cases there will be a gradual recurrence of deformity due to stretching of ligaments. If it is apparent that the patient will need to wear a caliper and that this will correct the deformity, the operation should not be done; but there are occasions when it will not be possible for the patient to wear the caliper unless deformity has been corrected surgically.

The best results are in those patients in whom the paralysis is incomplete and in whom the ligaments are strong and tight.

Position of patient

The patient is placed on the operating table in the supine position with a sandbag under the buttock on the operation side to give a 30° tilt, as in the Naughton Dunn procedure.

Incision

The incision is also similar, curving below the lateral malleolus from behind and extending to the centre of the dorsum of the foot (see Illustration 1).

1202 Leg and foot

Exposure and excision

The peroneal tendons are exposed by splitting their sheaths from behind the malleolus to the calcaneocuboid joint. The belly of the extensor digitorum brevis is defined, separated from the talus and turned down.

The calcaneocuboid joint is excised, making sure that the excision is slightly wider below than above to avoid boating of the outer border of the foot which can be a problem with this operation. A small bone lever is passed over the neck of the talus to expose the talonavicular joint. The ligaments of this joint are divided, the sinus tarsi is cleared of all soft tissue, the talocalcaneal ligaments are divided and the foot is dislocated at the subtalar and mid-tarsal joints.

A small bone lever is passed across the subtalar joint and over the medial side of the calcaneum. The articular surface of the calcaneum is excised throughout its length with a very broad chisel, removing more bone anteriorly than posteriorly. Any temptation to increase the size of the wedge by taking too much bone from the anterior end must be resisted because if the contact between calcaneum and cuboid is too small non-union may result with subsequent boating, which will be very difficult to correct. Most of the wedge is obtained by excision from the talus.

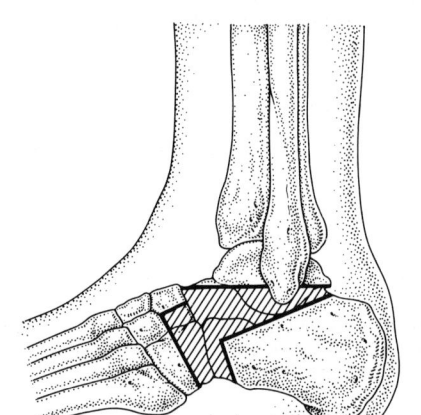

4

The line of excision for the talus should be carefully marked out, extending anteriorly from the edge of the articular cartilage of the upper part of the head of the talus and posteriorly to the posterior lip of the body of the talus. The whole of this piece of bone is excised, making due allowance for whatever lateral wedge has to be removed to give slight valgus to the heel. The navicular is then divided at the junction of its lower and middle thirds, the line of division being slightly upwards and backwards, and the lower third is removed. The upper surface of the neck of the talus is roughened.

Reduction

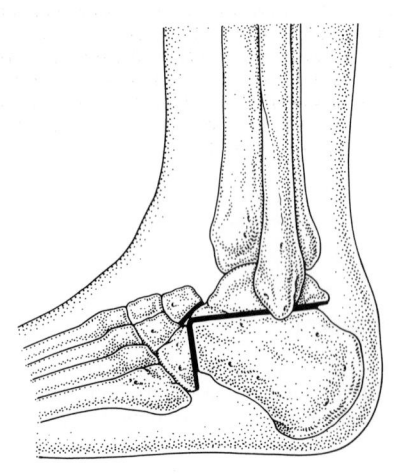

5

Any loose fragments of bone are excised and the dislocation is reduced, the upper surface of the calcaneus being pushed upwards into contact with the undersurface of the navicular. The calcaneocuboid joint is reduced, ensuring that there is no boating at this level, and the forefoot is displaced backwards so that the cut surface of the navicular is in contact with the roughened area on the superior surface of the neck of the talus. Again, the use of pins or wires to hold the position should be avoided.

Wound closure

The peroneal tendons are replaced and held in position by light suturing of the retinaculum. The belly of the extensor digitorum brevis is reattached to the talus, the subcutaneous tissues lightly approximated and the skin closed with a minimum of interrupted sutures.

Postoperative management

With the foot carefully held in the correct position a leg plaster cast is applied.

The leg is kept elevated until the postoperative swelling has settled, when the patient is allowed up on crutches. At 6 weeks the plaster is reduced to below-knee and a walking heel is applied. The plaster is retained for a minimum of 4 months.

Arthrodeses for the correction of valgus

Valgus deformity of the foot is caused by:

1. *Paralysis* – due to muscle imbalance
2. *Spasticity* – due to cerebral palsy or local lesions in the subtalar joint, e.g. spastic valgus foot
3. *Abnormal posture* – mobile flat foot where collapse of the arch in weight-bearing is closely associated with instability of the heel or valgus of the foot resulting from a tight tendo Achillis but with irreversible stretching of the medial ligaments of the foot
4. *Trauma* – fractures of the os calcis.

Operations for spastic and paralytic valgus deformities

These deformities may be corrected by a triple arthrodesis such as the Naughton Dunn operation, but this will be much more difficult than in feet with varus deformities. The dislocation of the foot and the removal of a medial wedge is always more difficult than is the removal of a lateral one. Apart from these difficulties the operation is the same.

GRICE–GREEN OPERATION

This is an extremely useful operation which can be employed any time after the age of 7 years. It can be done earlier but the small amount of bone may lead to non-union of one end of the graft, and it is better to postpone the operation. There is no upper age limit.

Indications

This operation is indicated for (1) symptomatic flat feet; (2) valgus feet due to a tight tendo Achillis; (3) the valgus of cerebral palsy, provided the heel can be manipulated to the neutral position; (4) for relieving pain due to damage to the subtalar joint by fracture of the calcaneum; and (5) for poliomyelitis.

Principle

The Grice–Green procedure is a simple operation for fusion of the subtalar joint without interference with any of the other joints. Fusion of the subtalar joint in isolation by excision will cause malalignment of the rest of the mid-tarsal mechanism, leading to degenerative changes and pain. The Grice–Green operation causes no change in the relationship between the talus and the calcaneum so there is no disorganization of the mid-tarsal mechanism.

Position of patient

The patient is placed on the operating table in the supine position with a sandbag under the buttock on the operation side.

Incision

An incision is made from the lateral aspect of the head of the talus obliquely backwards and downwards to below the tip of the lateral malleolus.

Preparation of the graft bed

The belly of the extensor digitorum brevis is identified, detached from the talus and turned down, exposing the sinus tarsi. All the soft tissue is cleared from the sinus tarsi, exposing the neck of the talus, the non-articular area on the upper surface of the calcaneum and the anterior part of the subtalar joint. A groove is cut in the undersurface of the neck of the talus as close to the articular surface as is possible.

6

An osteotome of suitable size is wedged, angled forwards, between this groove and the anterior part of the non-articular area of the calcaneum. If, when the heel is forcibly everted, the osteotome becomes wedged more tightly and does not displace then the angulation is correct. A second groove is cut in the base area where the osteotome became embedded. The appropriately sized osteotome which will hold the heel in the correct position, i.e. very slight valgus, is wedged in the grooves to assess the size of the graft required. The osteotome is removed and the wound closed with a towel clip.

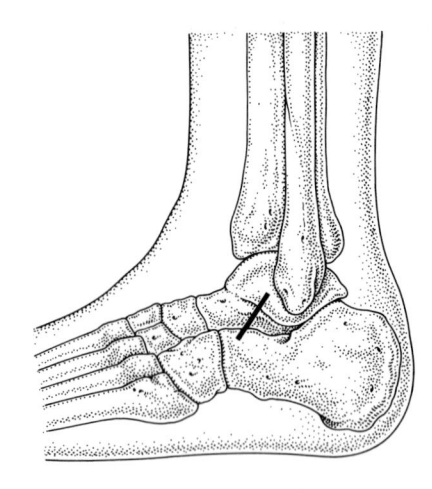

Insertion of graft

7

A second incision is made over the subcutaneous surface of the tibia in its upper third. The periosteum is split and the bone exposed. A graft, the length of which is equal to the width of the osteotome and 13 mm wide, is removed with a saw. The graft is at once introduced into the two grooves and tested to ensure it is the right length. When it is firmly jammed in position the heel should be in slight valgus. If the graft is a little too long one of the grooves is slightly deepened. This is easier than shortening the graft. Behind the graft the articular surface is removed from the calcaneum and the space between it and the graft packed with cancellous bone from the tibia.

Wound closure

The belly of the extensor digitorum brevis is reattached by sutures and the wound is loosely closed.

Postoperative management

A padded below-knee plaster is applied. The leg is kept elevated until the postoperative reaction is over when the patient is allowed up on crutches. After 2 weeks a walking heel is applied and the plaster is retained for 3 months.

MODIFICATIONS TO GRICE–GREEN OPERATION

Two useful modifications have been suggested which are worth consideration.

Fibular graft

8

A 5 cm incision is made over the neck of the talus. The extensor tendons are exposed and separated and the neck of the talus defined with a small bone lever on either side. A 6 mm (¼ inch) hole is drilled through it and this is then enlarged to 13 mm (½ inch). With the heel held in the required position the 13 mm drill is passed into the calcaneum to a depth of at least 2.5 cm. A piece of fibula is taken of the appropriate length, which will usually be about 6 cm. It is trimmed to fit the hole and driven in. Plaster immobilization is required for at least 3 months.

Because (a) the fibula, being sclerotic, is not a good bone for grafting and (b) the graft is not under compression, union may be slow or even uncertain. Also the neck of the talus is somewhat brittle and there is a risk of fracture. For these reasons this operation is best avoided.

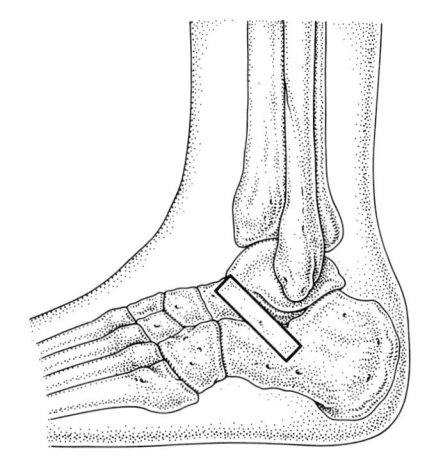

Screw fixation

9

The sinus tarsi is approached and cleared of all soft tissue. The exposed bony surfaces are decorticated. Cancellous bone is removed from the iliac crest and packed into the sinus tarsi. A second small incision is made over the upper surface of the neck of the talus and the neck is exposed and drilled for a screw. With the heel held in the correct position the screw is introduced, extending well into the calcaneum. Since the calcaneum is soft bone, it is undesirable to drill it if a firm grip with the screw is to be obtained. Plaster immobilization should be for 3 months but union may be complete before this. The fixation with this screw is poor.

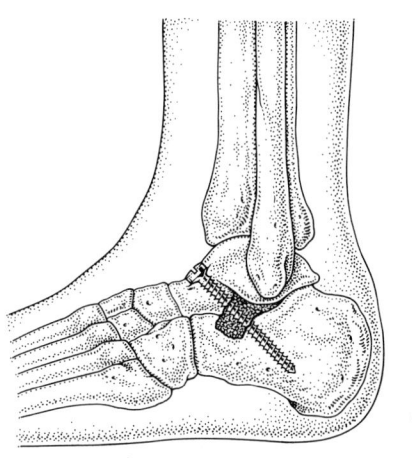

Postoperative precautions

Operations around the ankle and foot where there is little room for subcutaneous swelling are frequently very painful postoperatively when swelling takes place. For this reason the plaster, including the underlying dressing, is often split in its entire length in the anterior midline. This will involve the plaster being changed quite early which is often a disadvantage. Elevation alone is not enough to control this swelling. Two simple measures will often help greatly.

The tourniquet can be removed before the plaster is applied. This, however, may involve bleeding which will spoil the plaster and cause subsequent softening. It is usually sufficient to remove the tourniquet while the first plaster bandage is being applied. This will give time for the swelling resulting from the removal to occur before the plaster is complete.

The second measure, whose rationale is less obvious, is more effective. If the plaster is taken only to the base of the toes, even though there may be a toe platform, the toes become very swollen and cause much pain, necessitating the urgent splitting of the plaster. However, if the plaster is taken to the tips of the toes, both on the plantar and dorsal surfaces, so that only the tips are visible, swelling will not occur and pain will be greatly reduced. Splitting of the plaster will rarely be necessary and the plaster may remain intact until union is complete. This immobilization does not cause stiffness, since it is the postoperative swelling and oedema which are the cause of stiffness.

It cannot be over-emphasized that none of these measures in any way exonerates the surgeon from keeping a close watch to ensure that the circulation is satisfactory.

CALCANEONAVICULAR SYNOSTOSIS

10

This is a congenital abnormality in which the postero-inferior part of the navicular is joined to the anterosuperior part of the calcaneum by a bridge of bone. During early life this usually produces no symptoms and on examination there is a full range of movement in subtalar and midtarsal joints. Symptoms and signs of spastic flat-foot develop, usually during teenage but sometimes not until adult life. It seems that the synostosis itself is not responsible for the signs and symptoms but gives rise to arthritic changes which are responsible.

Lateral radiographs show the bar quite clearly. If the radiographs are taken before ossification is complete, the appearance will suggest a fibrous union between the two bones which, if followed up, will go on to show bony union.

Operative excision of the bar will only be successful if carried out before the rigidity has developed. Even then, results are not always satisfactory and frequently a triple arthrodesis will be necessary.

Operation

The patient lies in the supine position with a sandbag under the buttock on the affected side. A straight incision is made over the outer side of the talonavicular joint, which is then exposed. It will be found that what appeared radiologically to be a bar is in fact a sheet of bone 0.5 cm thick joining the navicular to the calcaneum across the whole width of the joint. This sheet of bone must be excised widely so that it can be clearly demonstrated that there is no contact between calcaneum and navicular in any position when the foot is put through a full range of movement. The skin of the wound is closed with interrupted polypropylene sutures.

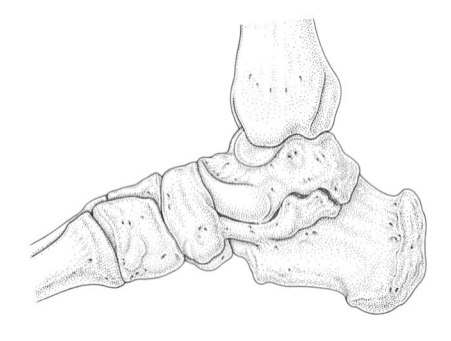

Postoperative management

A below-knee plaster is applied with the foot in the neutral position. After 10 days the plaster is removed and active movements are encouraged, but a broad heel should be worn on the shoe to prevent sudden and unexpected strains.

TALOCALCANEAL SYNOSTOSIS

11

In this condition the two bones are joined by a strong synostosis in the region of the sustentaculum tali. Symptoms rarely arise until teenage and some not until adult life. The symptoms are similar to spastic flat-foot. They arise from the development of arthritic changes in the midtarsal joint. This lesion is not visible in either lateral or anteroposterior radiological views. To see it radiologically a special view must be taken from the back with the foot in full dorsiflexion.

Excision of the bar is useless and should not be attempted. It is necessary to fuse the talonavicular and calcaneonavicular joints. The subtalar joint is already fused and nothing need be done to it.

Operation

The operation is carried out as already described.

Postoperative management

A below-knee plaster of Paris cast is applied and the foot is elevated high on two pillows for 24 hours postoperatively. The patient then walks without bearing weight with crutches for 4 weeks. Then a new well-fitting plaster is applied and weight-bearing commences. The plaster is bivalved and a radiograph taken of the foot out of plaster at 3 months from operation. If fusion has occurred the patient progresses to unprotected walking, but further protection in a cast may be necessary if fusion is not solid.

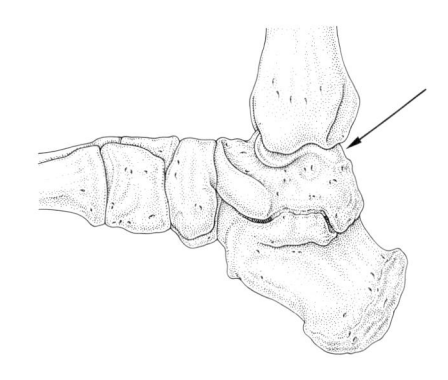

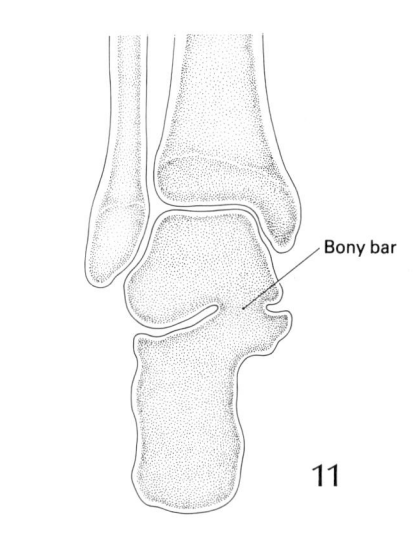

Illustrations by Philip Wilson after G. Lyth

Wedge tarsectomy

E. W. Somerville FRCS (Ed), FRCS
Emeritus Consultant Orthopaedic Surgeon, Nuffield Orthopaedic Centre, Oxford, UK

Introduction

Indications

This operation is performed in cases of pes cavus where the deformity is rigid and beyond relief by conservative measures or in which the deformity is obviously getting worse as in certain neurological conditions such as Friedreich's ataxia. When there is deterioration in the presence of neurological changes it is advisable to carry out bony correction and stabilization before the deformity is too severe. If the correction is left too late, there may be difficulty in getting the patient to walk again and he may even remain chairbound. When the deformity is a simple but severe cavus a formal foot stabilization will not be necessary. Correction can be obtained in the mid-foot by a wedge tarsectomy.

Operation

Position of patient

The patient is placed on the operating table in the supine position.

First stage

It is necessary to flatten the foot as much as possible. With the tight structures in the sole of the foot put on the stretch to the greatest extent possible, a subcutaneous tenotomy is carried out. In a line below the medial malleolus just anterior to the medial tubercle of the tuberosity of the calcaneum a short-bladed tenotomy knife is introduced through the skin with the blade parallel to the skin surface. The blade is passed between the skin and the tight plantar fascia and is then rotated with its sharp edge towards the fascia. Maintaining as much tension as possible the fascia is completely divided in its full width down to the bone. The division of the fascia must always be away from the skin. It is in such a case that the tension can be maintained by a Thomas' wrench. Tenotomy of the flexor tendons to all the toes will often improve the degree of correction.

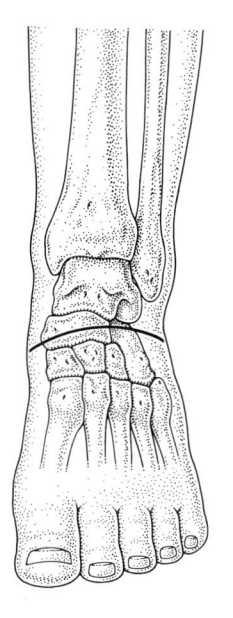

Incision

1

This is made transversely across the dorsum of the foot from one side to the other at the point where the deformity is greatest.

The tendons are exposed and divided with the exception of the tibialis anterior. Disregarding the joints, a wedge estimated to be the correct size is removed. It will usually be smaller on the lateral side of the foot than on the medial.

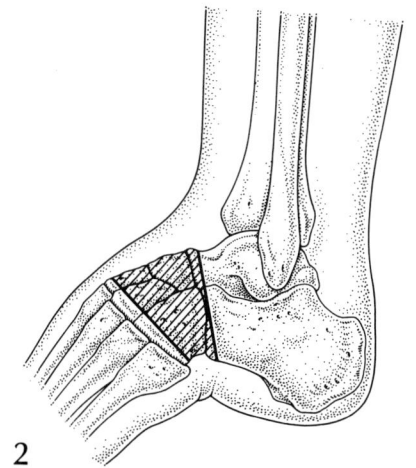

2

Depending on the success of the soft tissue release it may be necessary to remove a trapezoid, even though this will shorten the foot considerably, as otherwise the wedge will not be closed.

Wound closure

With the forefoot strongly dorsiflexed to close the gap the remains of the capsule are sutured. The tendons are left unsutured. The subcutaneous tissues are lightly sutured and the skin lightly closed with interrupted sutures. If the toes remain clawed dorsal capsulotomies are carried out to achieve extension.

Postoperative management

A moderately padded below-knee plaster of Paris cast is applied, extending to the tips of the toes on the dorsal and plantar aspects with the forefoot pushed well up into dorsiflexion.

The foot is kept elevated until postoperative swelling has settled, after which the patient may walk with crutches and at 4 weeks bear weight on a walking heel. The plaster should be retained for 4 months because union is often slow.

The neurological pes cavus is a severe problem. There is loss of soft tissue from the sole of the foot particularly under the metatarsal heads so that callosities are present. After the operation the distribution of weight will improve but the foot will still be stiff, perhaps even stiffer than before, so that callosities can still be a problem. The foot will be short, necessitating special footwear. Clawing of the toes may be such that further surgery will still be required to prevent callosities resulting from pressure on the uppers of the shoes.

Illustrations by Philip Wilson

Operations for flat foot and pes cavus

Leslie Klenerman ChM, FRCS
Professor and Head of University Department of Orthopaedic and Accident Surgery, Royal Liverpool Hospital, Liverpool, UK

Introduction

Flat foot and pes cavus are the extremes of a range which extends from a foot which is unstable because of collapse of the longitudinal arch to one which is mechanically inefficient because of an exaggerated high arch. Despite the obvious abnormal appearance of these feet, treatment must always be related to symptoms.

PES PLANUS

The hypermobile flat foot in children or adolescents may require operative correction because of difficulty in walking or, more rarely, pain. The absence of a positive great toe extension test[1], which demonstrates that the 'windlass' mechanism of the plantar fascia is ineffective, indicates the need for surgery.

In the growing child, two options are available. In the younger child (below 5 or 6 years), the treatment of choice is the reversed Dillwyn Evans procedure[2,3]. Where the heel is better developed, a medial displacement rotation osteotomy of the calcaneum will be equally effective[1]. Most flat feet are mobile. If the foot is rigid and painful, this is due to the presence of an underlying tarsal anomaly, of which the calcaneonavicular bar is the commonest variety.

Preoperative preparation

Preoperative assessment of a flat or rigid foot is made primarily on clinical grounds. Radiographs are essential for the diagnosis of tarsal anomalies. Calcaneonavicular bars are seen on oblique views of the foot but for talocalcaneal bars computed tomography is necessary. Lateral weight-bearing radiographs are useful as a record of the preoperative state of the foot. The relationship between the axis of the first metatarsal and that of the talus is used to show the extent of a flat foot, and the relationship of the axis of the first metatarsal and the axis of the calcaneum is used for the cavus foot.

General anaesthesia and a high thigh tourniquet are necessary. In operations on the dorsum of the foot, skin flaps should be kept as thick as possible. Care is necessary to avoid damage to skin nerves. The sural nerve behind the lateral malleolus and the branches of the musculocutaneous nerve on the dorsum of the foot are especially at risk of damage.

Leg and foot

REVERSED DILLWYN EVANS PROCEDURE

The principle underlying the operation is the concept that the lateral side of the longitudinal arch of the foot is too short. The operation was designed to lengthen this by the insertion of a tibial bone graft immediately proximal to the calcaneocuboid joint.

Technique

1 & 2

An oblique incision is made over the lateral surface of the calcaneum above and parallel to the peroneal tendons. The sural nerve is protected and the anterior end of the calcaneum is divided through its narrow part in front of the peroneal tubercle using an osteotome. The osteotomy is parallel with and 1.5 cm proximal to the articular surface of the calcaneocuboid joint.

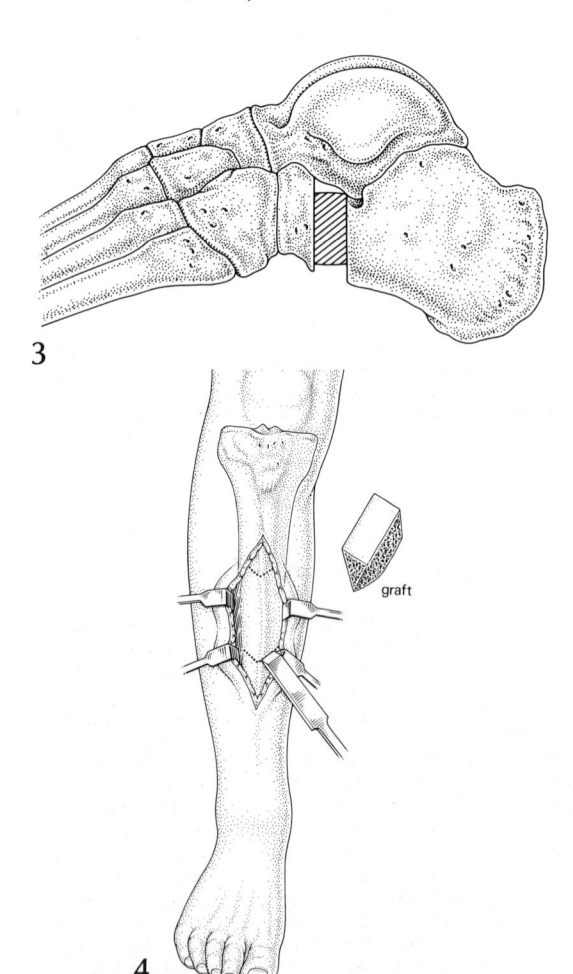

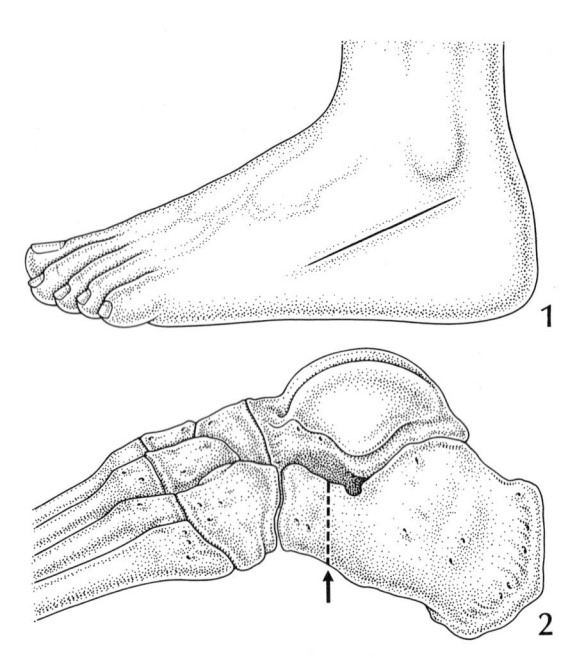

3

A graft of cortical bone is taken from the crest of the ipsilateral tibia and inserted into the osteotomy site. Further grafts are inserted above and below the first graft to ensure that the two surfaces of the calcaneum remain apart. Occasionally it may be necessary to lengthen the peroneal tendons.

4

The graft is taken from the crest of the tibia of the operated leg. A skin incision is made two fingers'-breadth distal to the tibial tuberosity, to ensure that the graft will be well clear of the epiphysis. The graft needs to be sufficiently long to extend from the superior to the inferior surface of the calcaneum. It should include the anterior third of the tibial crest. It is best to mark out the dimensions of the graft with an osteotome and then with a fine drill follow the linear markings so that the graft does not shatter when it is removed with an osteotome.

Postoperative management

At the end of the operation it is advisable to release the tourniquet and to secure haemostasis before the wound is closed. Suction drainage is helpful to reduce swelling. Wool and a crêpe bandage provide a firm dressing to reduce oozing. A second layer of wool and a plaster of Paris backslab are applied to immobilize the foot. It is unwise to use a complete plaster cast immediately after the operation because of the danger of a compartment syndrome. At the end of 2 weeks when the slab is removed a complete plaster can be applied, which is retained for 8 weeks and partial weight-bearing is allowed.

MEDIAL DISPLACEMENT ROTATION OSTEOTOMY OF CALCANEUM

The primary function of a calcaneal osteotomy is to shift the posterior weight-bearing pillar of the foot medially and, in doing so, to place the line of tibial thrust through the subtalar joint, so that there is neither a medial nor lateral moment of rotation, and to distribute the weight evenly over the support area of the sole. It modifies the action of triceps surae from eversion to inversion. A closing wedge combined with displacement is best.

Technique[1]

5

A longitudinal incision is made over the lateral aspect of the heel in the line of the peroneal tendons, which extends from the tendo Achillis to the plantar surface of the foot. The skin flaps are not undermined, but it is necessary to identify the peroneal tendons superiorly, to act as a guide for the line of the osteotomy. A bone spike is inserted anterior to the tendo Achillis at the upper end of the wound and onto the plantar surface of the calcaneum at the lower end.

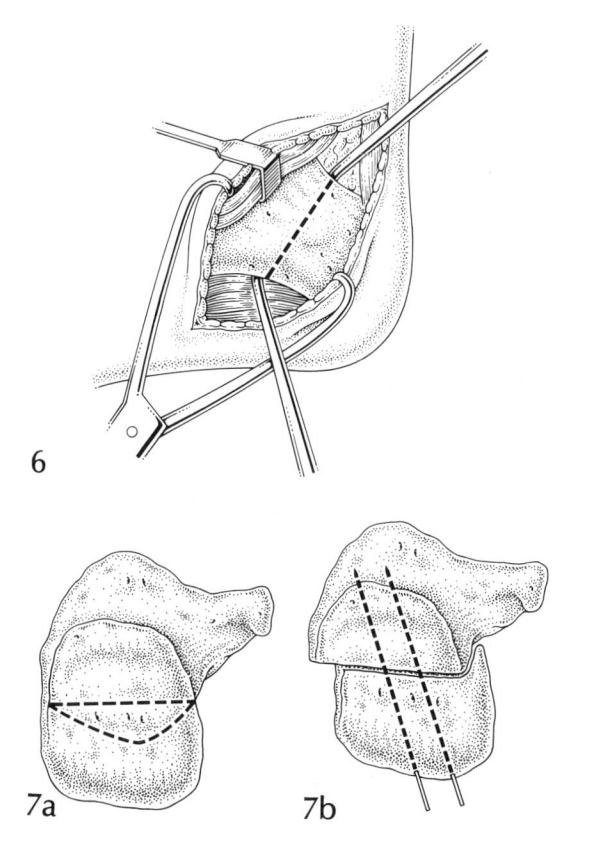

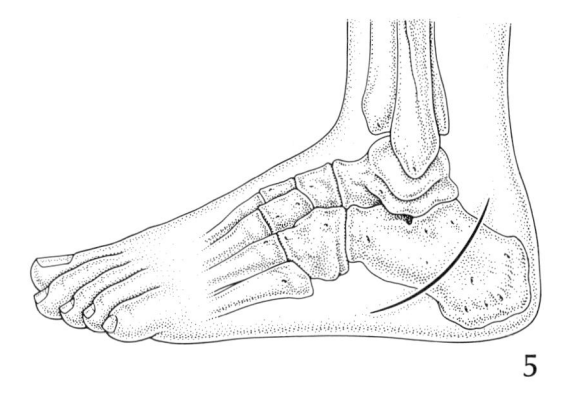

6, 7a & b

The periosteum is reflected in the line of the incision. The osteotomy is carried out as indicated in the diagram so as to produce a small medial spike, which can be used to lock the displaced posterior part of the calcaneum. Two percutaneous Kirschner wires are used to hold the posterior segment in place.

Postoperative management

The wound is closed in layers and a padded plaster of Paris backslab applied. This is converted to a full below-knee plaster after 10 days, when the operation wound is healed. The patient should remain non-weight-bearing for 4 weeks, when the Kirschner wires should be removed and a below-knee walking plaster applied for 2 weeks.

Full weight-bearing in plaster is allowed when the wound is healed and when Kirschner wires have been removed. The foot functions more effectively under load.

Once the plaster cast has been removed and although the postoperative appearances are satisfactory on radiographs, swelling of the foot may be a major problem. Encouragement to walk with a supporting elastic bandage, with instructions to elevate the leg when resting, help reduce the oedema. Physiotherapy does not play a major role in the rehabilitation of the patient after foot surgery.

EXCISION OF CALCANEONAVICULAR BAR FOR TREATMENT OF RIGID FLAT FOOT

The cause of rigidity is a tarsal anomaly, of which the most common is a calcaneonavicular bar. In children under 14 years of age, excision of the bar is a useful procedure[4]. The results are much less effective for older adolescents and adults, where it may be necessary to carry out a formal triple arthrodesis.

Technique

8

An incision is made 1 cm below the tip of the lateral malleolus, and is curved forward onto the muscle belly of the extensor digitorum brevis. The skin flaps are retracted and care is taken to avoid damage to the sural nerve.

9 & 10

Extensor digitorum brevis is divided in the line of its fibres to reveal the underlying bony bar. This is cleared of soft tissue, using a perosteal elevator. The talonavicular and calcaneocuboid joints should be opened, so that all the available landmarks are clearly defined. Using an osteotome, the bar is then removed in its entirety as a rectangle, not as a wedge. Extensor digitorum brevis is allowed to fall back into place and the skin is sutured.

The foot is immobilized in below-knee non-weight-bearing plaster until the wound is healed. At 14 days, the cast is removed and the patient is encouraged to bear weight and use the foot normally.

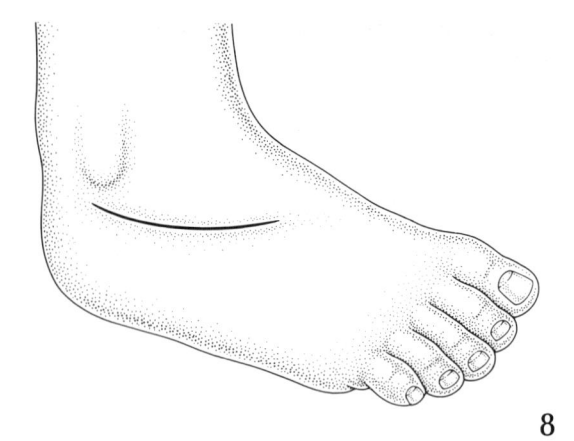

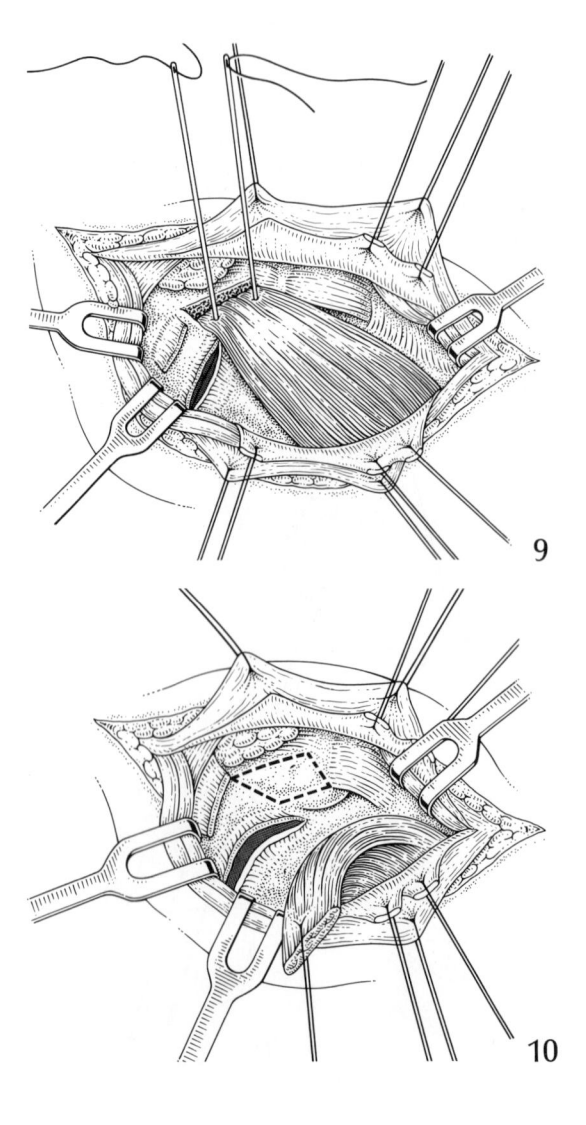

TENDON TRANSFER FOR RUPTURED TIBIALIS POSTERIOR TENDON

A grossly pronated foot may result from spontaneous rupture of the tibialis posterior tendon. In patients over 60 years of age, excellent correction of the deformity can be obtained by means of a medial displacement/rotation osteotomy of the calcaneum, as described for the idiopathic hypermobile flat foot. In the younger patient, the treatment of choice is a tendon transfer using the flexor digitorum longus as the motor power for inversion[5].

Technique

11 & 12

An incision is made on the medial side of the ankle, extending from the malleolus to the navicular. It is essential to confirm the diagnosis by opening the tendon sheath of tibialis posterior. The skin incision can then be extended proximally and distally. The abductor hallucis is reflected plantarward and the 'master knot' of Henry released, i.e. the site where flexor hallucis and flexor digitorum longus cross (with hallucis above the digitorum) and the origin of flexor hallucis brevis.

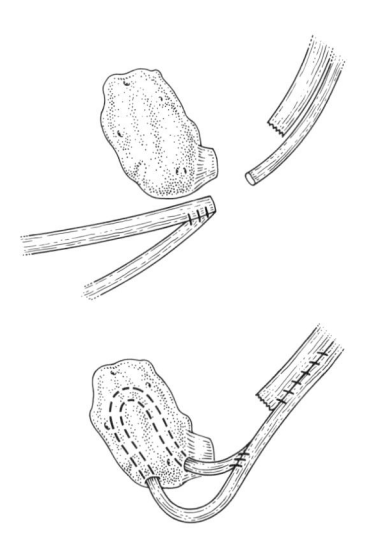

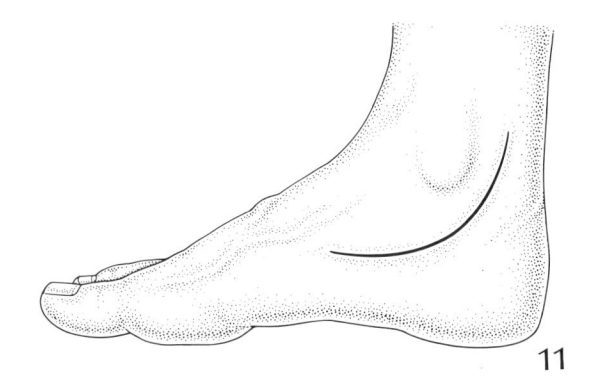

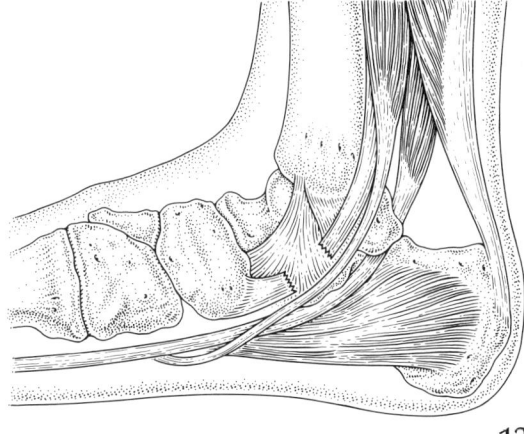

13

Flexor digitorum longus is divided at this point, and sutured distally to flexor hallucis longus. The proximal part of flexor digitorum longus is withdrawn from the site of division and rerouted through the sheath of tibialis posterior. It is attached to the navicular by passing it through a hole in the bone and tying the tendon to itself with the foot in equinus and inversion. The tendon should be sutured as tightly as possible. Side-to-side suture of flexor digitorum longus and the proximal part of the tendon of tibialis posterior should be attempted if possible. After wound closure, the foot is immobilized in a below-knee plaster in a position of equinovarus for 4 weeks and then placed in a plantigrade position in a walking cast for a further 4 weeks.

PES CAVUS

In the adult the indication for operative treatment is pain, while in the growing child the reason may be progressive deformity. The foot requires careful assessment to determine the main site of deformity which may be in the hind-, mid- or fore-foot, and these are sometimes combined.

If the heel is inverted and there is tightness of the plantar fascia, then a combination of a Steindler release and an osteotomy to remove a laterally based wedge from the calcaneum, as described by Dwyer[6], is the treatment of choice. With correctable clawing of the great toe and the lesser toes, a combination of Robert Jones' tendon transfer of extensor hallucis longus to the neck of the first metatarsal and Girdlestone's flexor to extensor tendon transfer will produce correction. When the hindfoot deformity is rigid, a triple arthrodesis is needed. On occasions, with mobile deformities, there is obvious tightness of the tendo Achillis which has to be lengthened to allow the foot to take up a plantigrade position. Very occasionally it may be thought necessary to carry out a mid-tarsal osteotomy, as described by Cole[7] and Japas[8] and, if so, then the alternative procedure of a tarsometa-tarsal truncated wedge, as described by Jahss[9], is preferable.

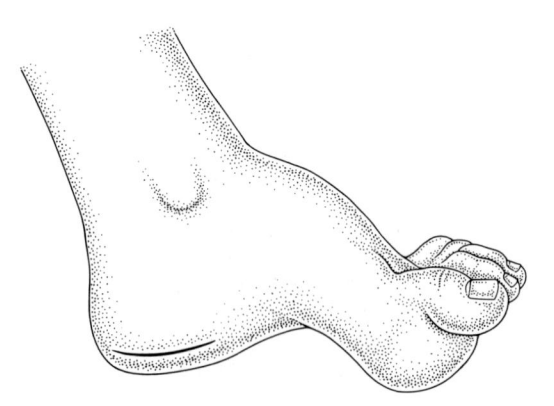

STEINDLER RELEASE OF PLANTAR FASCIA

14

This operation is usually combined with a laterally based Dwyer's osteotomy of the calcaneum. A longitudinal incision is made from the medial side of the posterior aspect of the heel to a point about 4 cm in front of the tubercle of the calcaneum.

Operations for flat foot and pes cavus 1217

15 & 16

The upper surface of the plantar fascia is then dissected from the covering fat layer of the foot and freed across the width of the foot with a blunt instrument, such as artery forceps. The fascia is then incised at its insertion into the calcaneum. A sharp periosteal elevator is then inserted and a subperiosteal stripping of all structures is carried out. By keeping close to the medial tuberosity, the dissection is a safe distance from the vessels and nerves. The wound is then closed in layers.

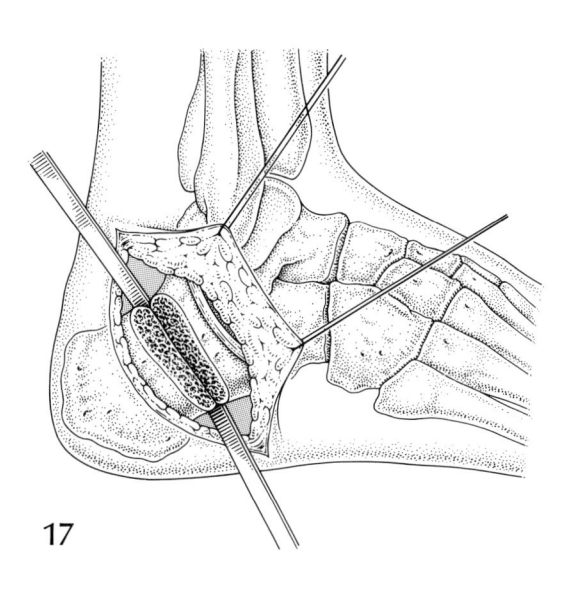

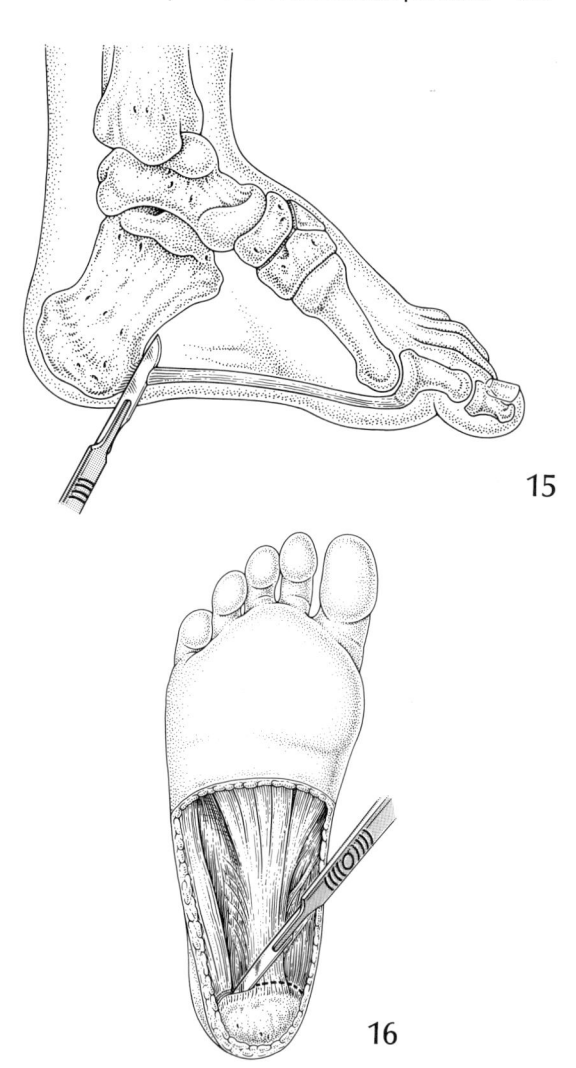

CALCANEAL OSTEOTOMY FOR PES CAVUS

17

The approach is the same as for the medial displacement/rotation osteotomy used for the correction of the valgus hindfoot. The osteotomy is again carried out in a line parallel to the peroneal tendons extending from a point immediately anterior to the insertion of the tendo Achillis, and a sufficiently large wedge of bone is excised from the lateral aspect of the heel to correct the varus inclination. In order to close the wedge, an awl passed through the posterior section of the calcaneum provides leverage to produce good bony apposition, which can be made secure by the insertion of a staple.

TARSOMETATARSAL TRUNCATED WEDGE ARTHRODESIS[9]

18

Three longitudinal dorsal incisions are used. The medial incision is made with its centre over the tarsometatarsal joint of the first ray. The underlying joint is exposed. The distal osteotomy is done first, while the first metatarsal is still fixed in position. The proximal osteotomy of the medial cuneiform is then performed so that a small, dorsally truncated wedge is removed. It is safer to be conservative, as it is always possible to resect more bone if necessary.

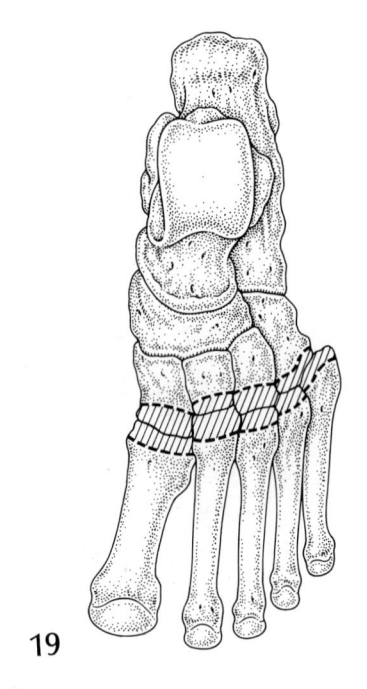

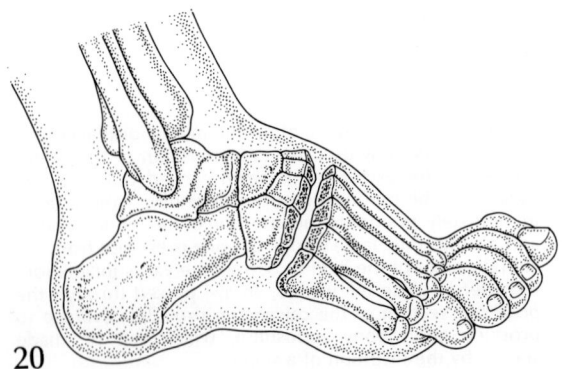

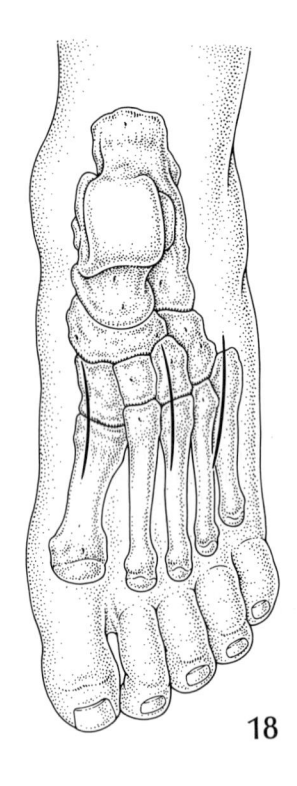

19 & 20

In a similar manner, further osteotomies of the second and third tarsometatarsal joints are made through a skin incision between the bases of the second and third metatarsals. It must be remembered that the base of the second metatarsal is more proximal than the adjacent metatarsals. The third incision is for osteotomies at the bases of the fourth and fifth metatarsal. The forefoot can then be dorsiflexed to close the wedges.

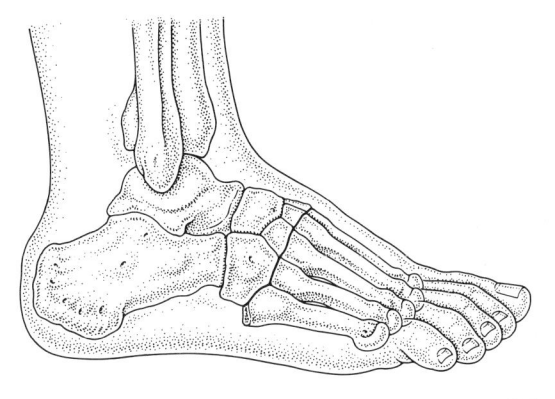

21 & 22

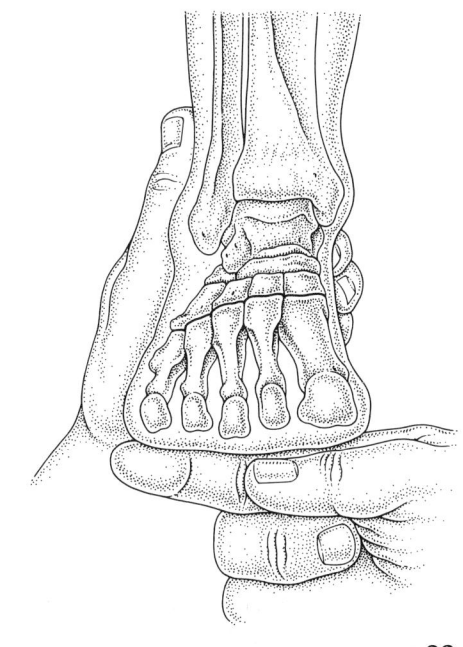

A finger is used to palpate the bone ends to check whether it is necessary to remove small segments of bone which block reduction. At the end of the operation, the forefoot should be at right angles to the tibia, and the metatarsal heads should all be level.

A padded plaster cast is applied, and the patient should not bear weight until the wound is healed. After 14 days the plaster cast is changed, and a walking plaster applied for a period of approximately 4 weeks. Provided union is sound, the plaster immobilization can be discontinued 6 weeks after the operation.

References

1. Rose GK. Pes planus. In: Jahss MH, ed. *Disorders of the foot*. Philadelphia: Saunders, 1982: 486–520.
2. Evans D. Calcaneo-valgus deformity. *J Bone Joint Surg [Br]* 1975; 57-B: 270–8.
3. Phillips GE. A review of elongation of os calcis for flat feet. *J Bone Joint Surg [Br]* 1983; 65-B: 15–8.
4. Mitchell GP, Gibson JMC. Excision of calcaneo-navicular bar for painful spasmodic flat foot. *J Bone Joint Surg [Br]* 1967; 49-B: 281–7.
5. Mann RA. Traumatic injuries to the soft tissues of the foot and ankle. In Mann RA, ed. *Surgery of the foot*. St Louis: C.V. Mosby Company, 1986; 476–80.
6. Dwyer FC. Osteotomy of the calcaneum for pes cavus. *J Bone Joint Surg [Br]* 1959; 41-B: 80–6.
7. Cole WH. The treatment of claw foot. *J Bone Joint Surg* 1940; 22: 895–908.
8. Japas LM. Surgical treatment of pes cavus by tarsal V-osteotomy. A preliminary report. *J Bone Joint Surg [Am]* 1968; 50-A: 927–44.
9. Jahss MH. Tarsometatarsal truncated wedge arthrodesis for pes cavus and equinovarus deformity of the fore part of the foot. *J Bone Joint Surg [Am]* 1980; 62-A: 713–22.

Illustrations by Peter Cox

Operations for congenital talipes equinovarus

E. H. Bates FRCS, FRACS
Chairman, Section of Orthopaedics, Prince of Wales Children's Hospital, Sydney, Australia

Introduction

Roughly 50 per cent of club feet defy adequate correction by non-operative measures.

Timing

The timing of primary surgical intervention varies widely between 3 weeks and 12 months. Most surgeons prefer to manipulate and splint club feet for at least 3 months before abandoning non-operative treatment. Very early surgery carries greater risk of overcorrection and surgical trauma to a foot whose bones are largely cartilaginous.

Indications

The choice of primary soft tissue procedure is influenced by the child's age and by the type and extent of deformity.

Feet that are almost corrected by non-operative measures require less extensive surgery. A limited posterior release may be all that is required.

In general, however, feet requiring surgery should be subjected to those soft tissue releases required to correct subtalar rotation and to reduce the talonavicular joint.

Depending on the extent and site of major deformities, combinations of medial, posteromedial, plantar-medial and lateral releases may be required. In all cases, the object is to obtain full correction of each component of the deformity.

Operative position

With babies, the prone position provides excellent access for all soft tissue releases.

Operations

POSTERIOR SOFT TISSUE RELEASE

1

A transverse incision (a) just above the insertion of the Achilles tendon, or a longitudinal incision (b) just medial to the Achilles tendon, are equally effective.

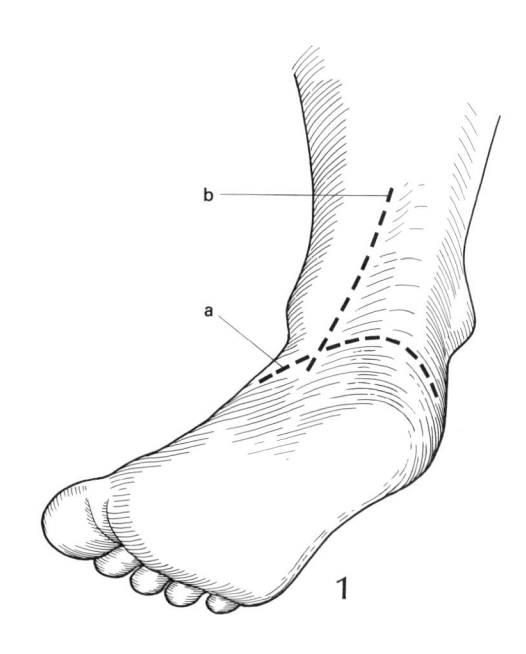

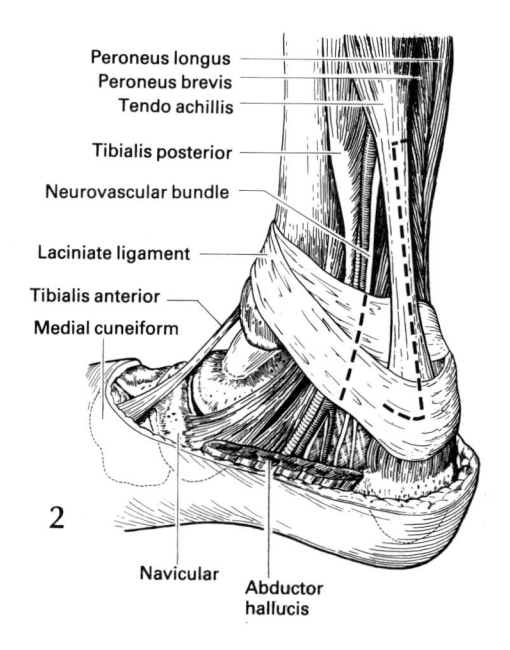

2

The Achilles tendon is elongated (Z-plasty) and the medial half of this tendon is detached from the calcaneum.

The neurovascular bundle is identified beneath the laciniate ligament between the Achilles tendon and the medial malleolus. Fine calcaneal branches may be sacrificed, but high division of the posterior tibial nerve is a common variation which should prompt careful dissection.

3

The deeper investing layer of fascia is divided in the midline and the flexor hallucis longus tendon is identified and traced downwards to the medial side of the subtalar joint. This tendon can be used to retract the neurovascular bundle medially.

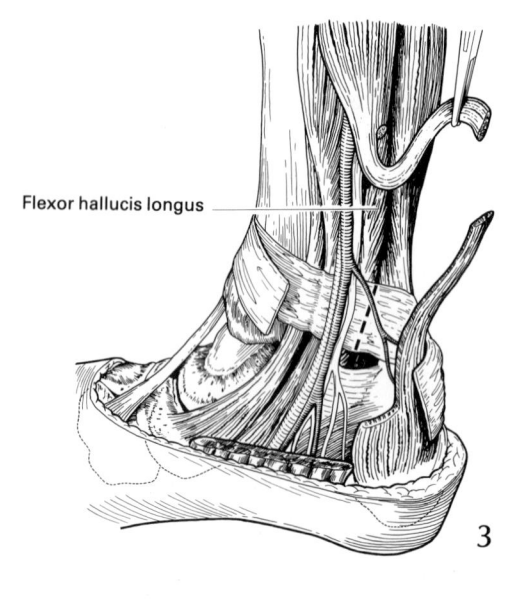

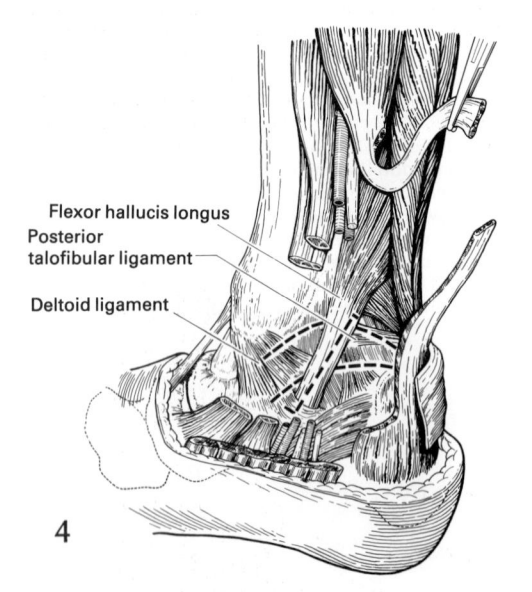

Tibialis posterior and flexor digitorum longus tendons and the neurovascular bundle are resected in this diagram for clarity.

4

The ankle capsule is incised transversely and the arthrotomy extended medially to involve no more than the posterior quarter of the deltoid ligament. It is then extended laterally to the fibula, and the posterior talofibular ligament is divided.

The subtalar joint capsule is incised transversely and this arthrotomy extended medially and forwards to the flexor hallucis longus tendon, and then laterally deep to the peroneal tendon sheath.

The flexor hallucis longus tendon is elongated by dividing it obliquely over a length of 2–3 cm.

The tendons of tibialis posterior and flexor digitorum longus are exposed above and behind the medial malleolus, just in front of the neurovascular bundle. Z-lengthening of these tendons at their musculotendinous junction completes the posterior release operation.

MEDIAL SOFT TISSUE RELEASE

5

A horizontal curvilinear incision from the neck of the first metatarsal to a point just distal to the tip of the medial malleolus is made: (*a*) to leave a skin bridge between it and the longitudinal posterior incision, this bridge covering the neurovascular bundle; (*b*) to join up with the longitudinal posterior incision; or (*c*) to be extended to a full Cincinnatti-type exposure.

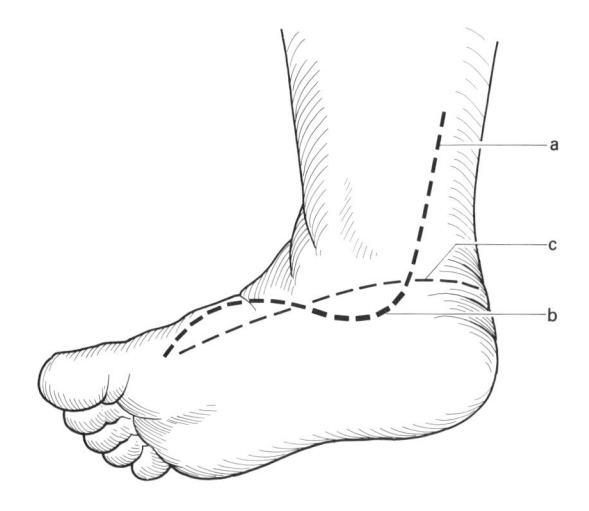

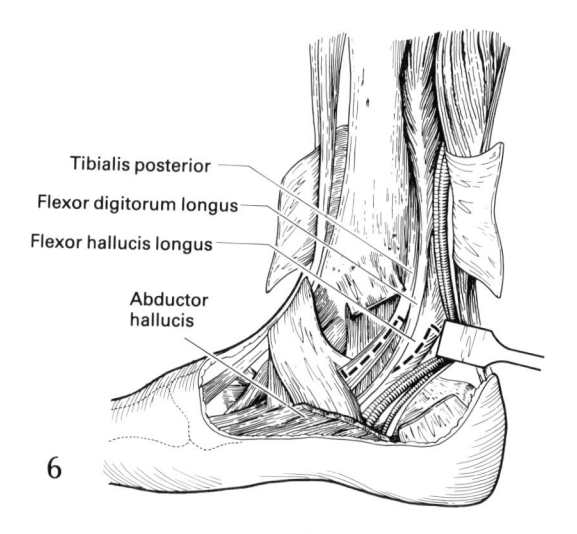

6

The neurovascular bundle is mobilized distally to ensure its protection during the medial subtalar arthrotomy. The abductor hallucis origin is detached from the flexor retinaculum. The insertion of the tibialis posterior tendon and the route of the flexor digitorum longus tendon, anterior to the neurovascular bundle, are exposed by dividing the thickened investing fascia. The tibialis posterior tendon is separated from all its insertions except that to the navicular and then it is Z-lengthened. With its division the talonavicular joint is exposed.

The flexor digitorum longus tendon is traced under the tarsus to expose Henry's knot and it is separated from the flexor hallucis longus tendon by sharp dissection.

7

The talonavicular joint is opened by medial capsulotomy and the arthrotomy extended dorsally to the lateral extent of the navicular and inferiorly to join the anterior part of the subtalar joint. The medial capsule of the subtalar joint is divided and the arthrotomy extended posteriorly, deep to the neurovascular bundle. This capsulotomy will then communicate with the posterior capsulotomy of the subtalar joint if a posterior release has been performed.

The capsule of the naviculocuneiform joint is incised medially, superiorly and inferiorly. In most cases the dissection to date will be adequate to permit easy reduction of the talonavicular joint.

Residual forefoot adduction may require a similar capsulotomy of the cuneiform–metatarsal joint. The tibialis anterior insertion should not be disturbed. In the event of persisting metatarsus varus, the tendon of abductor hallucis is identified near the neck of the first metatarsal and divided within the muscle fibres.

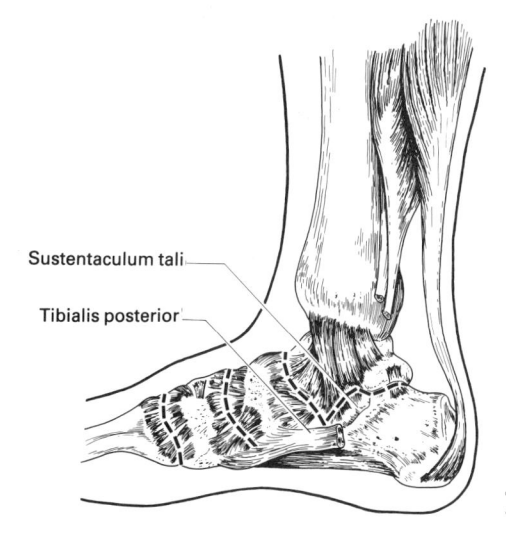

1224 Leg and foot

PLANTAR SOFT TISSUE RELEASE

8

In feet with evidence of early cavus, especially repeat soft tissue operations, division of inferior structures may be required. If planned as an isolated procedure the incision in the illustration is preferred.

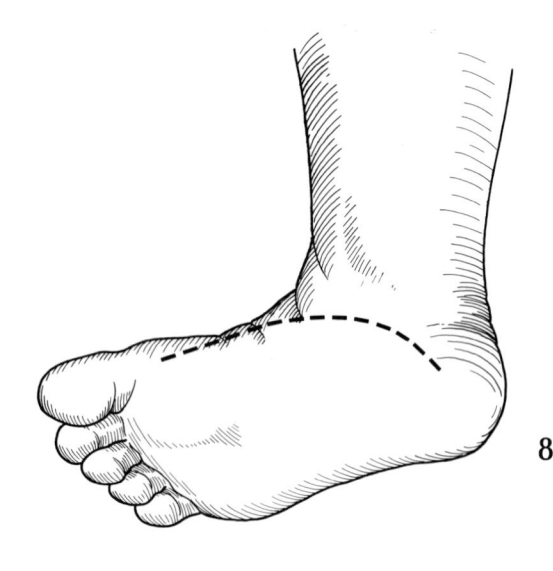

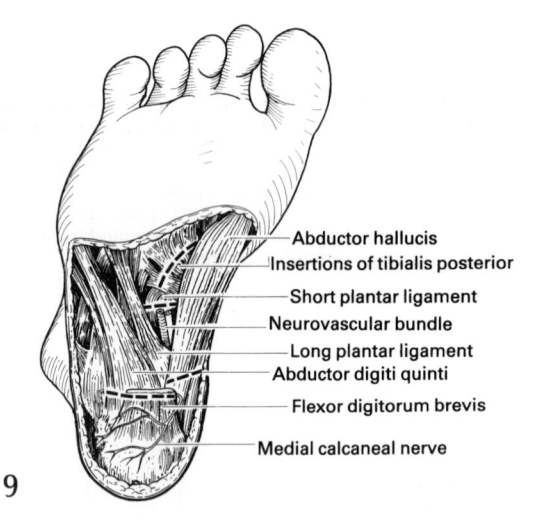

9

The origin of the abductor hallucis is mobilized from the os calcis and flexor retinaculum, allowing the muscle to retract forwards with the neurovascular bundle. Care should be taken to avoid damage to the calcaneal branch of the posterior tibial nerve.

The proximal attachments of the plantar aponeurosis, flexor digitorum brevis and a variable portion of the abductor digiti quinti are divided (Steindler's operation).

The tendinous insertions of the posterior tibial tendon to the cuneiforms and metatarsals are divided. The inferior capsules of the talonavicular and naviculo-cuneiform joints are divided laterally under full vision, which involves division of the spring and short plantar ligaments.

Operations for congenital talipes equinovarus 1225

LATERAL SOFT TISSUE RELEASE

Recent thought and writing suggests that derotation of the calcaneum beneath the talus is the prime object of club foot surgery. This subtalar mobilization involves posterior, medial and lateral releases.

10

The lateral release requires prolongation of the horizontal incision forward below the lateral malleolus toward the calcaneocuboid joint (a). If a longitudinal posterior incision has been used, then a separate lateral incision will be required (b).

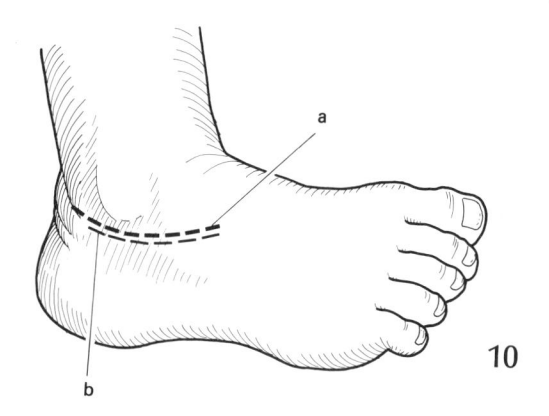

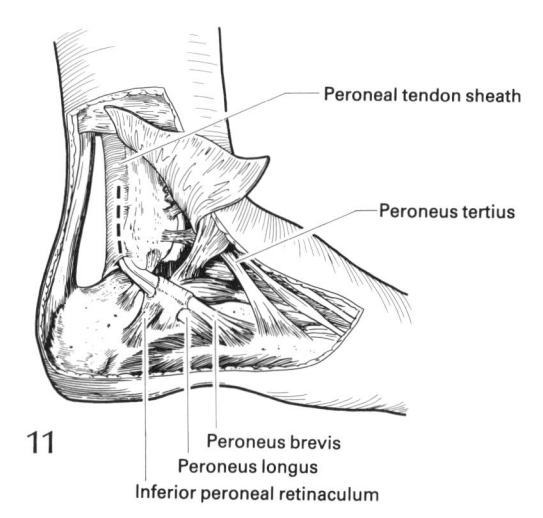

11

The peroneal tendons are mobilized to permit their retraction laterally; this is done by dividing part of their sheaths.

12

The subtalar capsulotomy is extended forwards to the sinus tarsi. The calcaneofibular ligament is divided. If the fibula remains posteriorly displaced it may be necessary to divide the posterior tibiofibular syndesmosis.

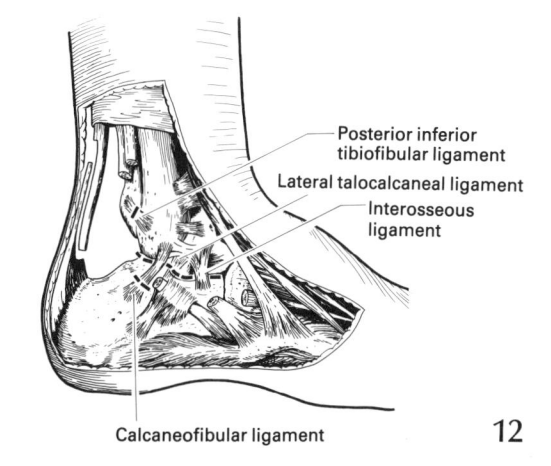

Postoperative management

Maintenance of reduction and accommodation of swelling after soft tissue correction is best achieved using a Liverpool plaster. The foot should be reviewed (under general anaesthesia) at 2 weeks and if wound healing is complete, the definitive above-knee cast is applied for an initial period of 6 weeks.

Subsequently the plaster may be changed without anaesthesia and, if correction is adequate, a below-knee cast can be used for a further 6 weeks.

By this time the foot will fall readily into a corrected position and a Denis Browne's boot and bar splint are used to maintain this correction for most of the time until the child is standing or walking. It is the author's opinion that, for the walking child, persistence with this splint at night reduces the incidence of relapse if compliance is maintained and that it should be used until the age of 5 years.

SECONDARY CLUB FOOT SURGERY

Late presenting club foot and feet relapsing or inadequately corrected by primary surgery present some of the great challenges in club foot treatment. Innumerable 'secondary' procedures have been described. These include tendon transfers, tarsal osteotomies, bone resection and the final salvage procedure, triple arthrodesis.

TENDON TRANSFER

Despite their place in foot deformity of neuromuscular origin, the principles of tendon transfer do not support their use in idiopathic talipes equinovarus.

TARSAL OSTEOTOMIES

Osteotomies have been described for the calcaneum (Dwyer and Pandy), the talus (Hjelmstedt and J. Roberts) and the metatarsals (Green and Herndon).

BONE RESECTION

Dillwyn Evans' calcaneocuboid wedge resection and arthrodesis, performed as he described in conjunction with a medial soft tissue release, is probably the most reliable operation for secondary correction.

Wedge tarsectomy may be used in the older uncorrected foot to offset the need for triple arthrodesis.

Talectomy has also been used for secondary correction but is not recommended.

TRIPLE ARTHRODESIS

As a last resort, there are few feet that will not become plantigrade and functionally acceptable if a triple arthrodesis is performed.

Acknowledgement

I wish to thank my colleague, W. K. Chung, FRACS, for his assistance.

Further reading

Attenborough CG. Severe congenital talipes equino-varus. *J Bone Joint Surg [Br]* 1966; 48-B: 31–9.

Crawford AH, Marxen JL, Osterfeld DL. The Cincinatti incision: a comprehensive approach for surgical procedures of the foot and ankle in childhood. *J Bone Joint Surg [Am]* 1982; 64-A: 1355–8.

Evans D. The relapsed club foot. *J Bone Joint Surg [Br]* 1961; 43-B: 722–33.

Green AD, Lloyd-Roberts GC. The results of early posterior release in resistant club feet: a long term review. *J Bone Joint Surg [Br]* 1985; 67-B: 588–93.

McKay DW. New concept and approach to club foot treatment: principles and morbid anatomy. *J Paediatr Orthop* 1982; 2: 347–56.

Steindler A. Stripping of the os calcis. *J Orthop Surg* 1920; 2: 8–12.

Turco VJ. Surgical correction of the resistant club foot: one stage posteromedial release with internal fixation: a preliminary report. *J Bone Joint Surg [Am]* 1971; 53-A: 477–97.

Illustrations by Gillian Oliver after B. Hyams

The Robert Jones operation for clawing of hallux

B. Helal MChOrth, FRCS
Honorary Consultant Orthopaedic Surgeon, The Royal London Hospital and The Royal National Orthopaedic Hospital, London, and Enfield Group of Hospitals, UK

S. C. Chen FRCS
Consultant Orthopaedic Surgeon, Enfield Group of Hospitals, UK

Introduction

This operation is carried out for clawing of the big toe due to paralysis of the flexor hallucis brevis and weakness of dorsiflexion of the ankle. The extensor hallucis longus overacts and causes flexion at the interphalangeal joint and dorsiflexion of the big toe. If a callosity develops over the dorsum of the interphalangeal joint or under the metatarsal head correction is necessary.

Operation

Arthrodesis of interphalangeal joint

1a & b

A transverse incision is made across the interphalangeal joint of the big toe. The extensor hallucis longus tendon is identified and detached at its insertion.

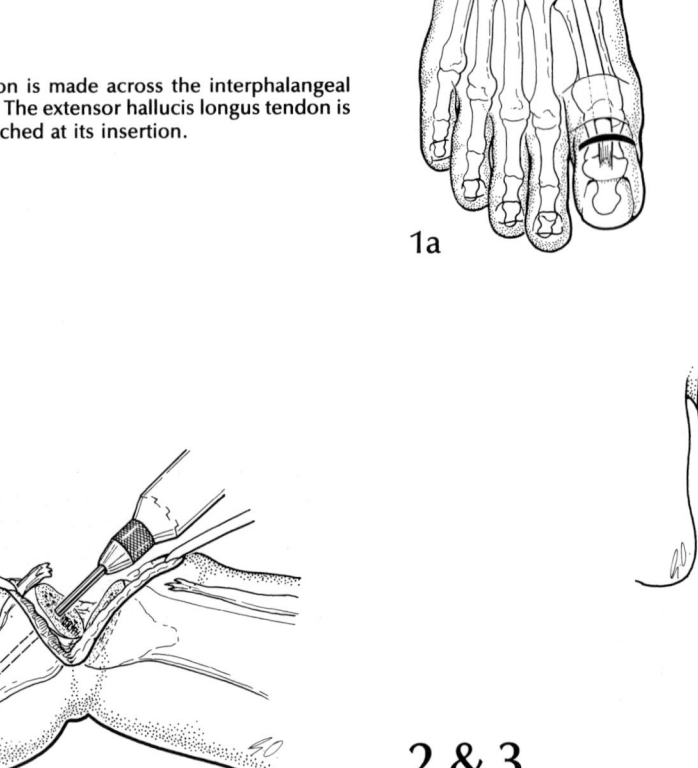

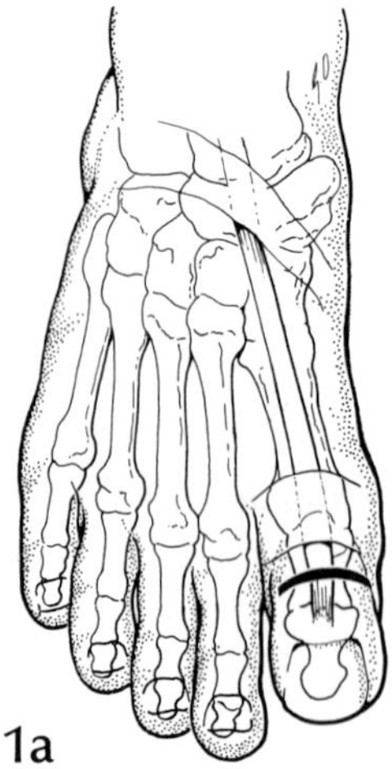

1a

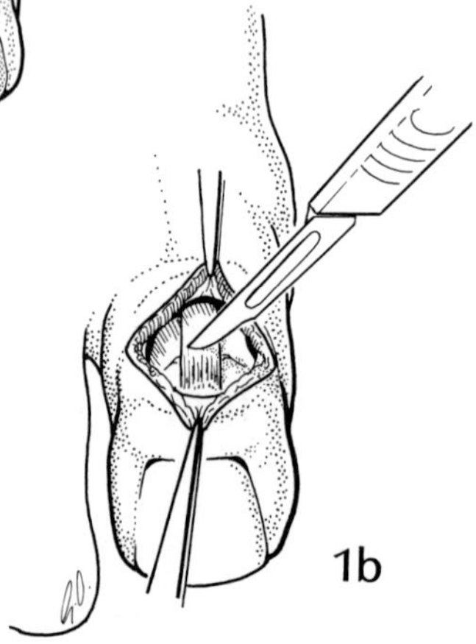

1b

2

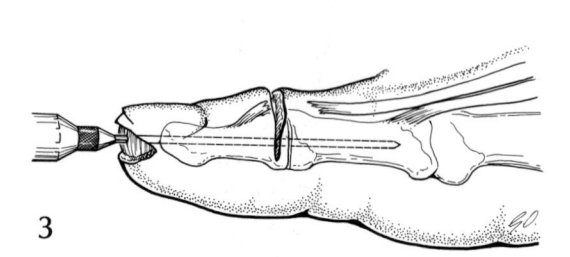

2 & 3

The interphalangeal joint is opened up and the articular cartilage removed. The distal phalanx is drilled in a retrograde manner and then the drill passed back again through the distal phalanx and the proximal phalanx drilled. The interphalangeal joint is arthrodesed using a screw.

3

Tendon transfer to metatarsal neck

4

A second incision is made along the dorsomedial side of the first metatarsal head and neck.

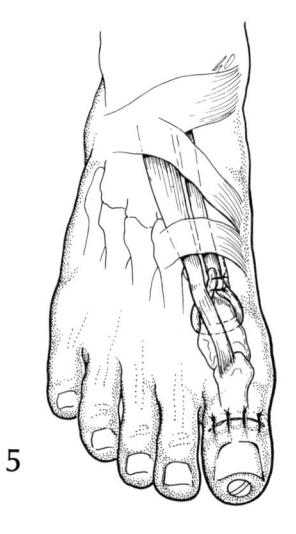

5

The neck of the first metatarsal is exposed. The surgeon drills transversely across the neck. The detached extensor hallucis longus tendon is pulled into the proximal wound and passed through the drill-hole in the neck of the first metatarsal. While an assistant pushes the head of the first metatarsal dorsally, with the tendon taut, it is sutured to itself using non-absorbable sutures.

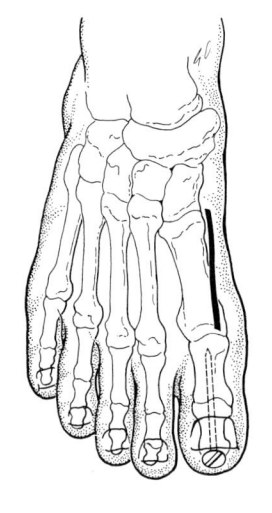

Postoperative management

6

A plaster cast is applied from the tibial tuberosity to the big toe, with the big toe and the ankle in neutral position. The plaster is removed at 3 weeks and active exercises and weight-bearing started.

Reference

Jones R. The soldier's foot and the treatment of common deformities of the foot, Part II. Claw-foot. *Br Med J* 1916; 1: 749–53.

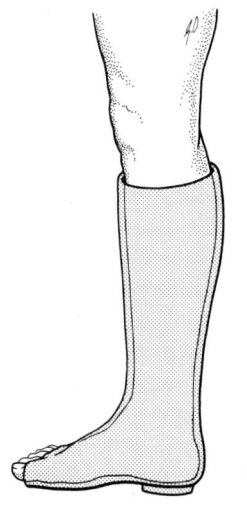

Flexor to extensor transfer for clawing of the lateral four toes (Girdlestone's operation)

B. Helal MChOrth, FRCS
Honorary Consultant Orthopaedic Surgeon, The Royal London Hospital and The Royal National Orthopaedic Hospital, London, and Enfield Group of Hospitals, UK

S. C. Chen FRCS
Consultant Orthopaedic Surgeon, Enfield Group of Hospitals, UK

Introduction

Claw toes, that is hyperextension of the metatarsophalangeal joint and flexion of the interphalangeal joints, are due either to overactivity of the toe extensors in the presence of normal toe flexors, caused by poliomyelitis or a peripheral neuropathy, or more commonly to loss of intrinsic foot muscle tone.

For the operation to be successful, the metatarsophalangeal and interphalangeal joints must be fully mobile.

Operation

Incisions

1

Dorsolateral incisions are made from the metatarsal neck to the distal interphalangeal joint of the lateral four toes. The surgeon starts on the second toe first and works laterally.

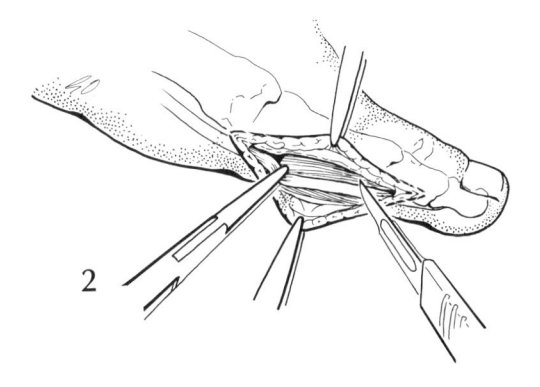

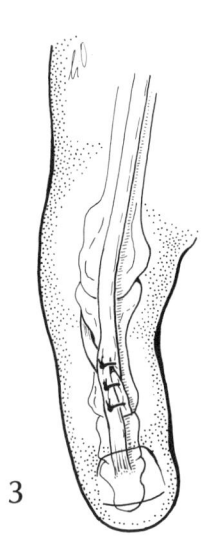

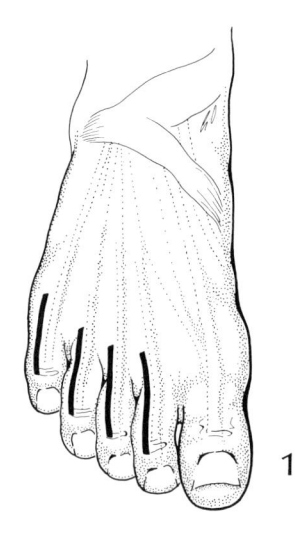

2

The lateral edge of the skin incision is retracted. The long and short flexor tendons are found and the long flexor tendon is held with artery forceps to prevent it from retreating proximally into the foot when it is divided at its insertion.

Tendon transfer[1]

3

The long flexor tendon is brought around the lateral side of the proximal phalanx well proximal and close to the bone so that the neurovascular structures are not compressed.

The extensor tendon is split and the long flexor tendon is passed through and sutured to it, proximal to the proximal interphalangeal joint and with the toe plantar-flexed at the metatarsophalangeal joint, using non-absorbable sutures.

Postoperative management

A padded crêpe bandage is applied to the foot. At the end of 2 weeks mobilizing exercises to the toes are started, and walking allowed. In older patients a below-knee plaster of Paris walking cast is necessary to hold the correction.

Reference

1. Taylor RG. The treatment of claw toes by multiple transfers of flexor into extensor tendons. *J Bone Joint Surg [Br]* 1951; 33-B: 539–42.

Illustrations by Gillian Oliver

Forefoot reconstruction

B. Helal MChOrth, FRCS
Honorary Consultant Orthopaedic Surgeon, The Royal London Hospital and The Royal National Orthopaedic Hospital, London, and Enfield Group of Hospitals, UK

S. C. Chen FRCS
Consultant Orthopaedic Surgeon, Enfield Group of Hospitals, UK

Introduction

In rheumatoid arthritis, the forefoot can be deformed by a combination of factors. There may be imbalance of muscle, as well as progressive damage to the metatarsophalangeal and interphalangeal joints of the toes, secondary to synovitis, synovial proliferation, effusion and bone erosion. These changes lead to clawing of the toes, i.e. hyperextension of the metatarsophalangeal joints and flexion of the interphalangeal joints. The metatarsophalangeal joints may be subluxated or dislocated, and the articular surfaces may be destroyed.

When the metatarsophalangeal joints only are affected and are at the subluxation stage, corrective procedures, such as the telescopic osteotomies of the second, third and fourth metatarsals can be carried out. When the metatarsophalangeal joints have dislocated but where the articular surfaces are still relatively normal, open reduction of the joints followed by telescopic osteotomies are feasible. When the articular surfaces are damaged, excision arthroplasties, such as the Fowler[1] or the Hoffmann[2] operations may be performed. The Fowler operation is technically more demanding, but it preserves more of the metatarsal bone. The Hoffmann operation is relatively easy to do, as the dislocated metatarsal heads present in the plantar wound, but more of the metatarsal bones are excised, although the proximal phalanges are not operated upon. In very severe cases, replacement of the metatarsophalangeal joints with a Silastic implant, like the Universal Small Joint Ball Spacer prosthesis (Corin Medical Ltd, Cirencester, UK) may be used.

TELESCOPIC OSTEOTOMIES OF THE SECOND, THIRD AND FOURTH METATARSALS

The objective of this operation is to redistribute the body weight from the prominent second, third and fourth metatarsal heads to all five. The principle of the technique is to perform an oblique osteotomy to the distal metatarsal shaft to allow the head and neck to rise to a more comfortable position. In addition, the oblique osteotomy allows the metatarsal shaft to shorten slightly.

Reduction of dislocated metatarsophalangeal joints

(If the joints are only subluxated, this stage is omitted.)

1a, b & c

Short incisions are made along the dorsum of the second, third and fourth metatarsophalangeal joints. The capsules are incised transversely, and the collateral ligaments released from the sides of the metatarsal heads. The extensor tendons are cut. The dislocated joints are reduced and held in place with Kirschner wires introduced obliquely across the joints in a downward and backward direction. It is important that the dislocations are reduced before proceeding to the telescopic osteotomies, as it would be difficult to reduce the dislocations after the osteotomies.

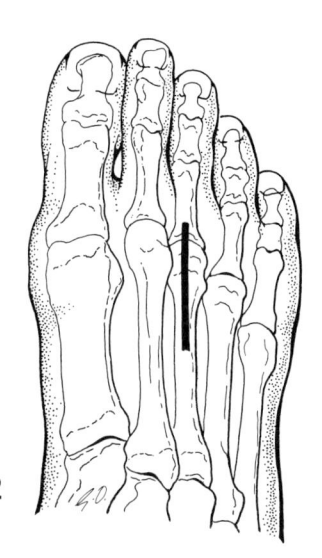

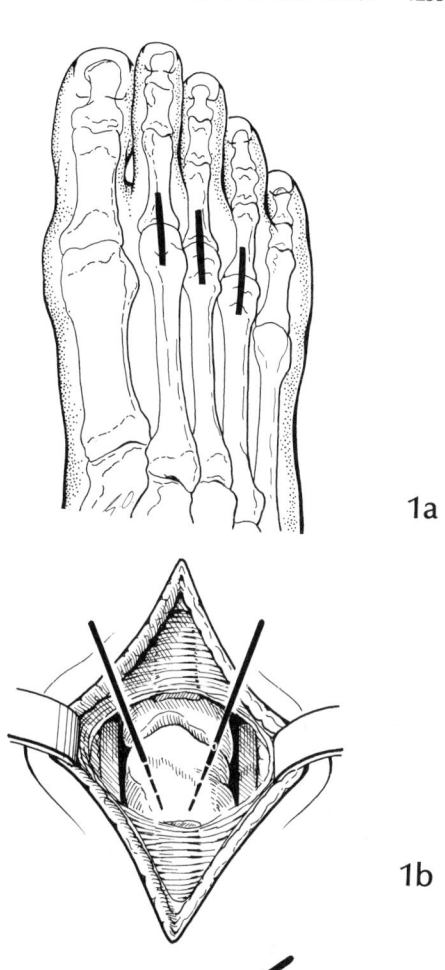

Incision for osteotomies

2

A 4 cm incision is made on the dorsum of the foot along the third metatarsal. The periosteum is incised along the shaft of the third metatarsal and stripped off the bone.

1234 Leg and foot

Siting the osteotomies

3

Retractors are placed on either side of the bone to protect the soft tissues. An oblique cut is made in the distal shaft of the metatarsal (not the neck), angled 45° downwards and forwards.

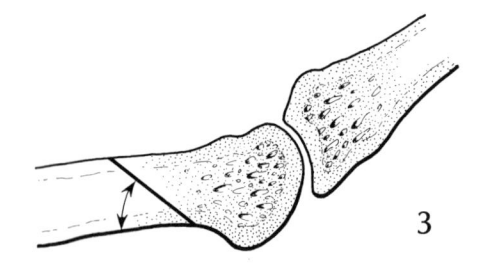

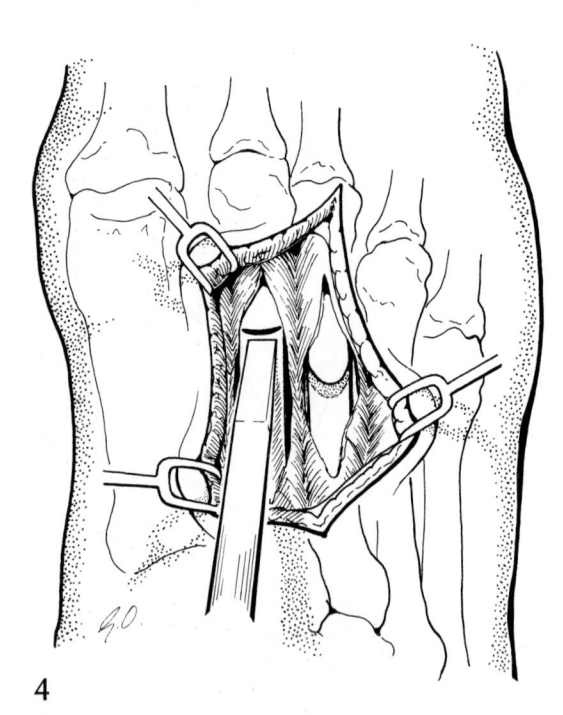

4

Through the same skin incision, the second metatarsal is exposed. The periosteum is incised along the shaft and stripped off. Trethowen ring–spike retractors are placed on either side of the bone and an oblique cut is made as described earlier.

5a & b

Through the same skin incision, the fourth metatarsal is identified, and its periosteum stripped off. The spike retractors are placed on either side of the bone. At this stage the fifth metatarsal must not be mistaken for the fourth: this mistake is easily made as the bones are close together. By palpating the fifth metatarsal through the skin, a check may be made that the last bone exposed is indeed the fourth metatarsal.

Again, an oblique cut is made as described earlier. It is important to free the incarcerated metatarsal head from the underlying soft tissue by passing an osteotome between the bone and soft tissue.

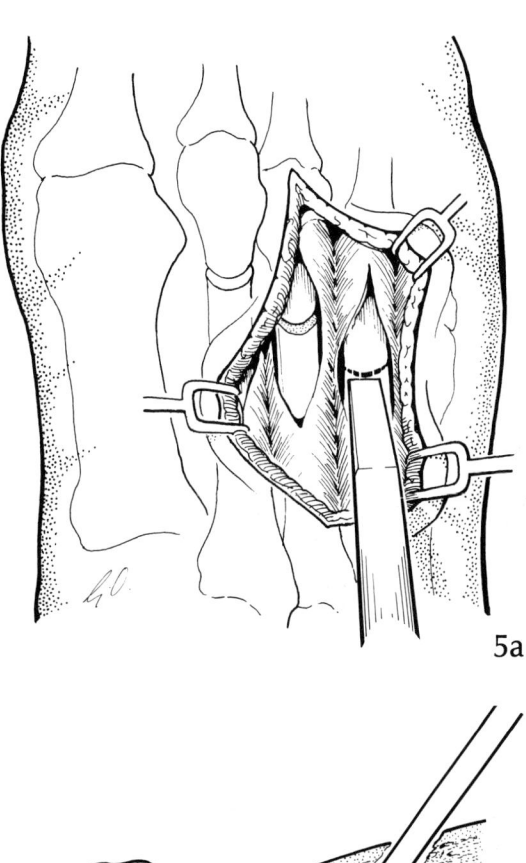

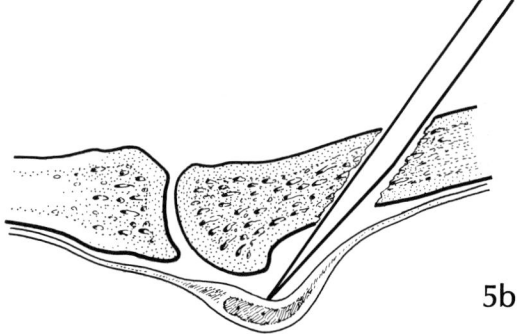

6

At the end of the procedure the three oblique osteotomies should describe a gentle curve which is convex distally. It is important that the soft tissues, especially the intrinsic muscles, are not damaged, or cross-union of the bones may occur.

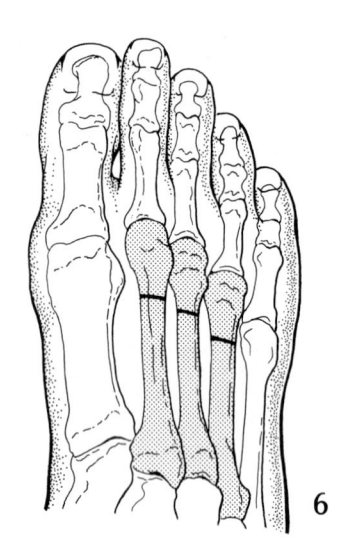

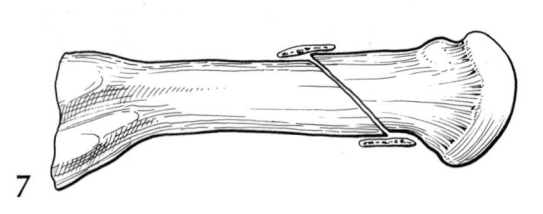

7

The sharp spikes of the distal cut ends of each metatarsal are nibbled away, and the bone chips deposited around the osteotomy sites to encourage bony union.

The skin wound is sutured, and a well padded bandage is applied to the foot and ankle.

Postoperative management

8

It is important that the middle three metatarsal heads are not raised too high, or undue pressure will fall on the first and fifth metatarsal heads, leading to painful callosities.

Early weight-bearing is desirable in the rheumatoid patient. Three days after the operation, the well-padded bandage is removed, and an adhesive dressing applied to the wound. The callosity under the middle three metatarsal heads helps elevation of the middle three metatarsal heads to the correct level. The patient is encouraged to walk, fully weight-bearing and wearing loose-fitting flat shoes for 3 months.

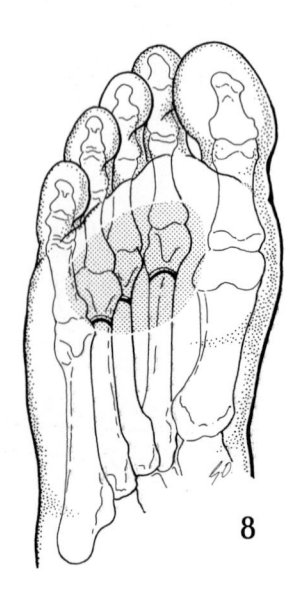

CORRECTION OF ASSOCIATED HALLUX VALGUS AND BUNIONETTE OF 5TH TOE

Once the metatarsal osteotomies have united, which usually takes about 3 months, the associated hallux valgus and bunionette, if present, are dealt with. It is important to stage these procedures to obtain optimum spread of weight when walking.

9a & b

A dorsomedial incision is made over the neck and distal shaft of the first metatarsal. An oblique osteotomy is made, directed laterally, posteriorly and inferiorly at 45°. The joint capsule is left untouched. The wound is sutured.

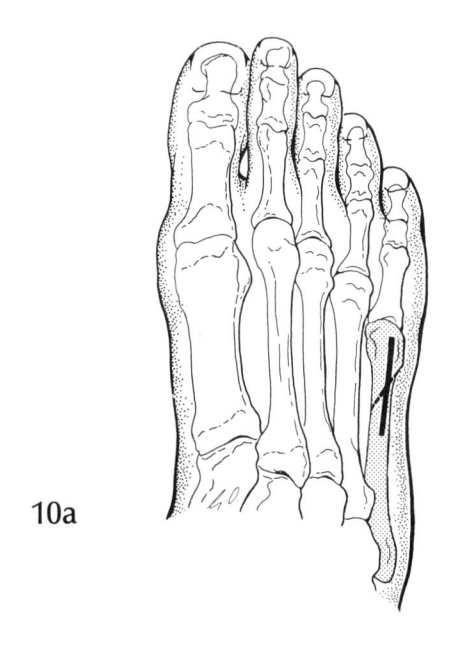

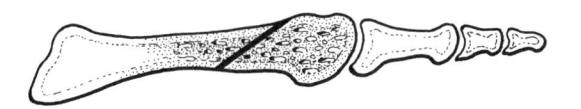

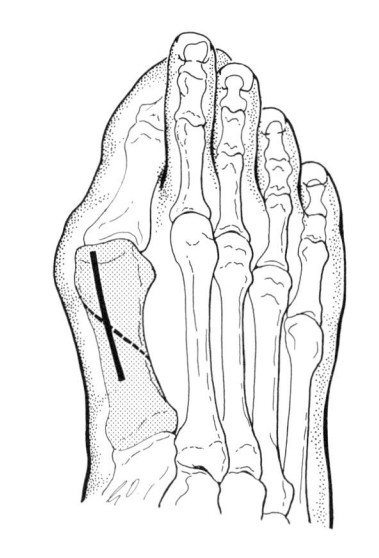

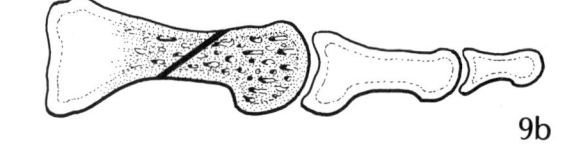

10a & b

When a bunionette is present, it is ill-advised to excise the prominence, which is the metatarsal head, as there is not an exostosis as in hallux valgus.

A dorsolateral incision is made over the neck and distal shaft of the fifth metatarsal. An oblique osteotomy is made, directed medially, posteriorly and inferiorly at 45°. A below-knee walking plaster cast is applied with the big toe immobilized in valgus.

Postoperative management

The plaster cast is removed at the end of 8 weeks. Check radiographs are taken to make sure that bony union has taken place. Active toe exercises are started.

1238 Leg and foot

FOWLER OPERATION

11

A dorsomedial incision is made over the metatarsophalangeal joint of the big toe. The joint is exposed. The proximal third of the proximal phalanx is excised. The dome of the metatarsal head is excised.

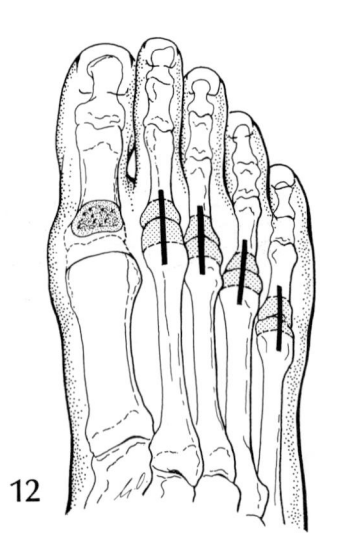

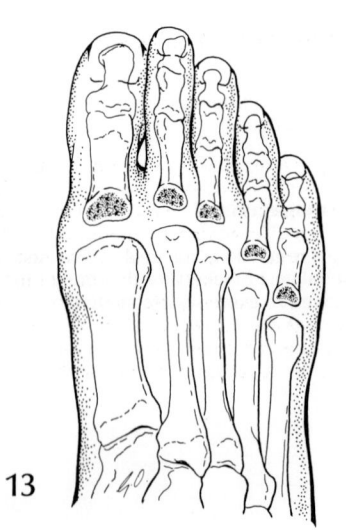

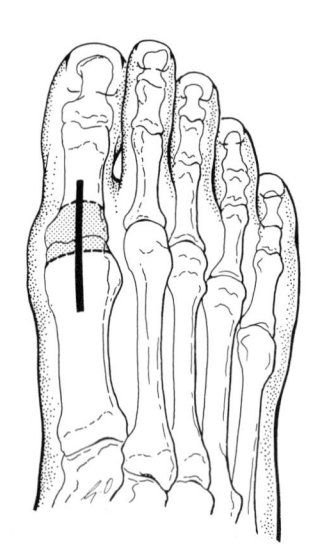

12 & 13

Longitudinal incisions are made over the metatarsophalangeal joints of the second to fifth toes. The proximal third of the proximal phalanges and the metatarsal heads are excised, leaving the flare of the necks behind. The ends of the bones are rounded off by bone nibblers. At the end of the procedure, the ends of the metatarsals describe a gentle curve, convex distally. The level of the first metatarsal is checked to make sure that it is in line with the gentle curve described by the lateral four metatarsals. Only sufficient bone is removed to align it with the other metatarsals. Ideally, the sesamoid bones should still rest on bone. Any further adjustment of the lateral four metatarsals can also be made at this stage. The several wounds on the dorsum of the foot are now sutured.

Forefoot reconstruction 1239

14 & 15

A transverse elliptical incision is made on the sole of the foot encompassing the callosities which are usually present. The undersurfaces of the second to fifth metatarsal heads are exposed by retracting the flexor tendons. The keel of each metatarsal beneath the neck is excised leaving a flat surface. The toes are brought down by suturing the elliptical skin wound with interrupted nylon sutures. A well-padded bandage is applied.

Postoperative management

The padded bandage is removed a week after surgery, and a lightly padded bandage is applied. The patient is encouraged to bear weight using a walking aid. At the end of 2 weeks, the dressings are taken down, and the skin sutures removed. Active plantarflexion exercises are started. The patient is advised to wear flat loose-fitting shoes.

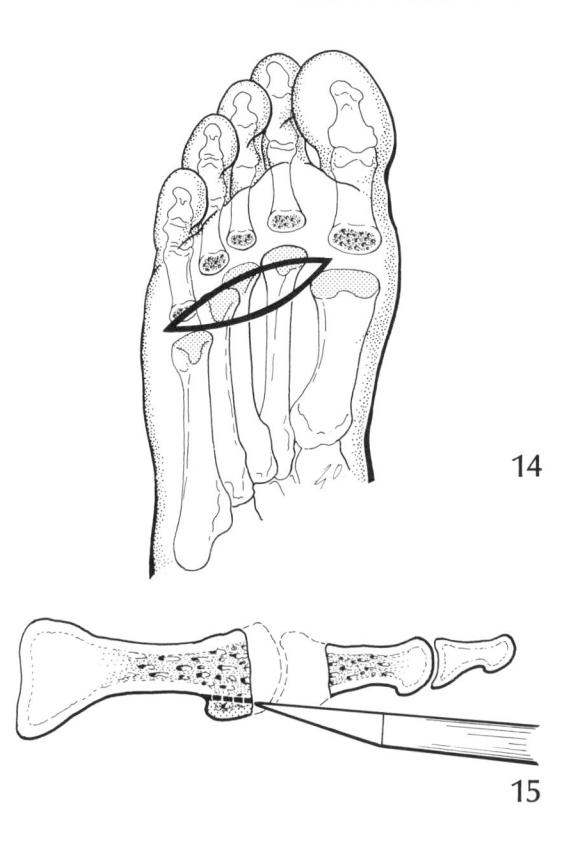

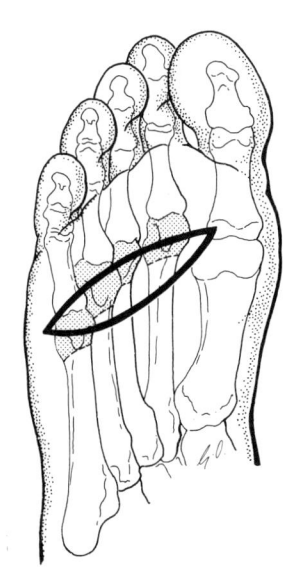

HOFFMANN OPERATION (Kates-Kessel technique[3])

16

A transverse elliptical incision is made on the sole of the foot, encompassing the callosities which are usually present. The flexor tendons are retracted, and the capsule of each joint is incised, exposing the dislocated metatarsal heads. These are excised at the level of the necks. The ends of the second to fifth metatarsals should describe a gentle curve, convex distally. (Kates and Kessel recommend removal of the first metatarsal head through the sole incision but this is technically more difficult and we recommend adherence to the Hoffmann technique.)

17 & 18

A dorsomedial incision is made over the metatarsophalangeal joint of the big toe. The first metatarsal head is excised in line with the other metatarsals. The skin incision is sutured, after repairing the joint capsule.

It is important to maintain the same relative lengths of the metatarsals to ensure a good result. Kates advised inspection by image intensifier at operation.

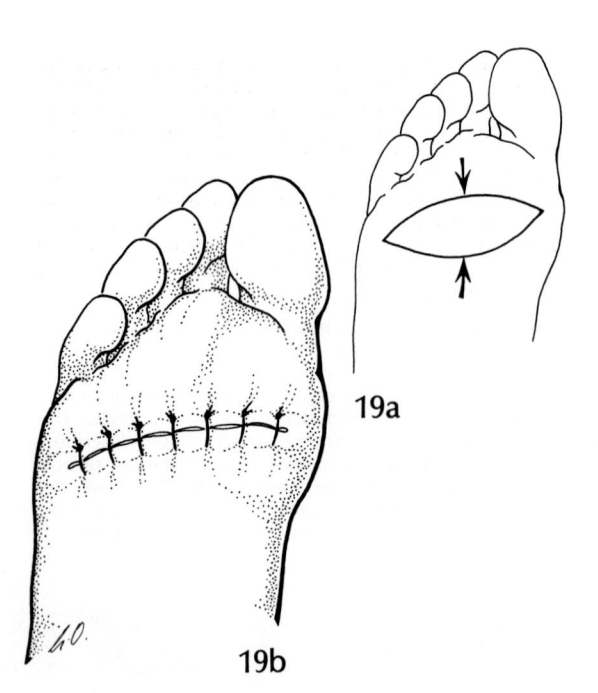

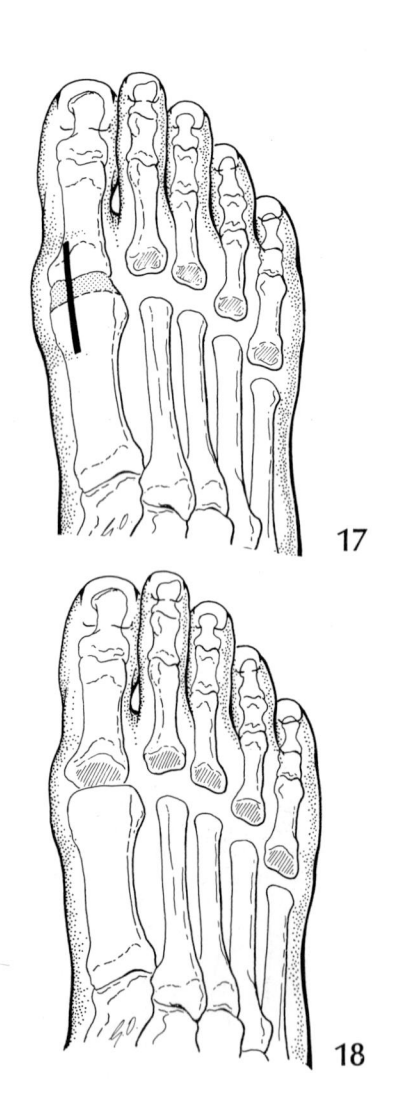

19a & b

The elliptical skin wound on the sole of the foot is now sutured with interrupted nylon stitches, bringing the toes down. A well-padded bandage is applied.

Postoperative management

A week after the operation, the well-padded bandage is taken down and the wounds inspected. A lightly padded bandage is applied, and the patient encouraged to walk using a walking aid. At the end of 2 weeks, the sutures are removed. The patient is advised to wear flat loose-fitting shoes.

PROSTHETIC REPLACEMENT OF THE METATARSOPHALANGEAL JOINTS

20

The Universal Small Joint Ball Spacer is a prosthesis made of silicone elastomer, and consists of a ball with truncated ends and two thin flexible stems, reinforced with Dacron ribbon (du Pont, UK). There are four sizes: No. 1 is 10 mm long and 15 mm wide, No. 2 is 9 × 13 mm, No. 3 is 8 × 11 mm and No. 4 is 7 × 9 mm.

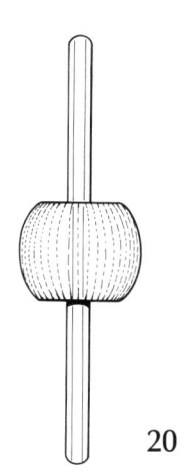

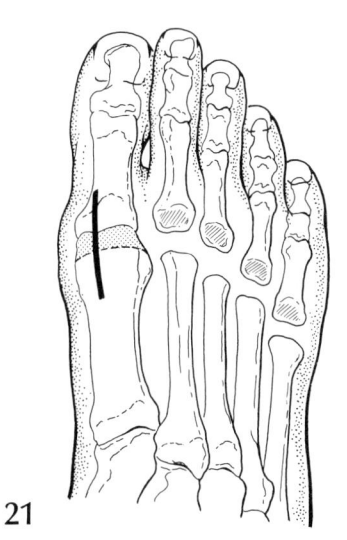

Prosthetic replacement in big toe

21

A straight dorsomedial incision is made across the metatarsophalangeal joint of the big toe. About 7.5 mm of the head is removed with a power saw, and the edges trimmed with a small bone nibbler. It is important not to remove too much of the head, otherwise the sesamoid bones will drop into the space created by the bone excision. Holes are made in the metatarsal and the proximal phalanx using a small Paton burr. It is important to site these holes in the centre of each bone and opposite each other. They should be along the longitudinal axes of the two bones.

22a & b

A drill hole is made in the medial side of the metatarsal stump. A suture of No. 1 PDS material (Ethicon, Edinburgh, UK) is placed in the capsule, either ventromedially or medially to correct any valgus with or without a rotational deformity. This suture is passed through the hole made in the medial side of the metatarsal. The correct size prosthesis (usually a No. 1) is inserted, making sure that it sits snugly in the space created. The big toe is moved up and down several times to make sure the prosthesis is well-seated.

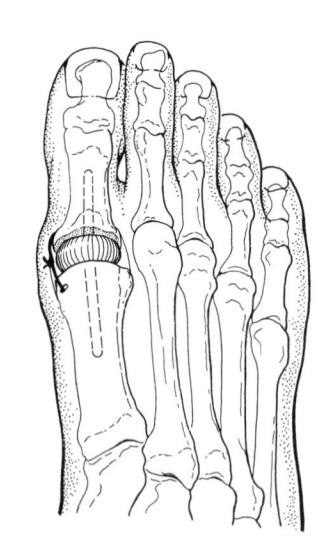

22a

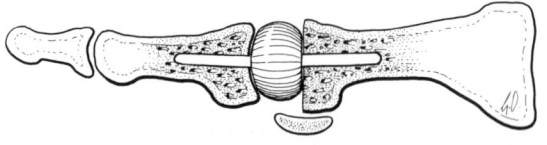

22b

22c

The capsule of the metatarsophalangeal joint of the big toe is attached to the metatarsal using the PDS suture already inserted in it. The capsules are sutured and the skin wounds closed.

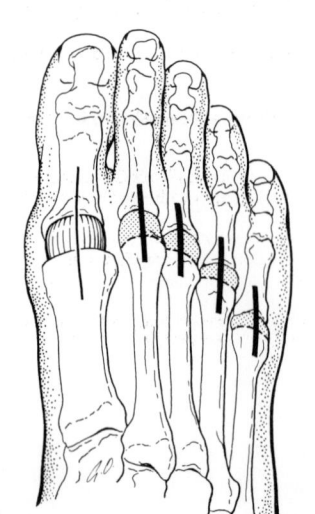

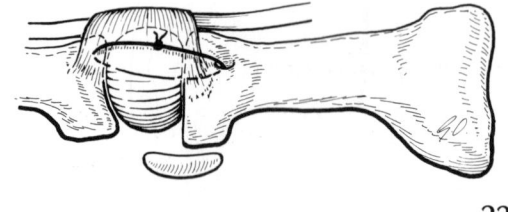

22c

Prosthetic replacement in lesser toes

23

Longitudinal incisions are made over the metatarsophalangeal joints of the lateral four toes. The metatarsal heads are excised so that they describe a gentle curve with the first metatarsal, convex distally. The proximal phalanges are brought down in line with the metatarsals. If necessary the collateral ligaments may have to be released from the sides of the metatarsals.

24

Holes are made in the metatarsals and proximal phalanges, in a similar fashion to the big toe. The correct size prostheses (usually No. 2 or 3) are inserted.

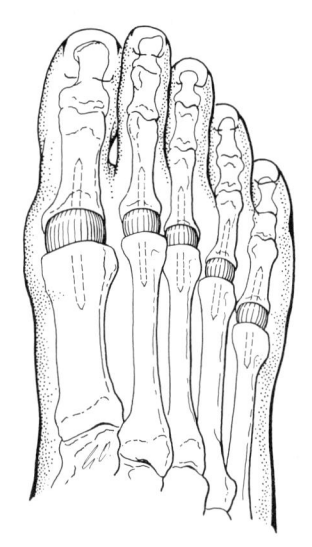

Closure

A transverse elliptical incision is made in the sole of the foot, encompassing the callosities which are usually present. The skin edges are sutured which results in the toes being brought down (see *Illustration 19a,b*). Well-padded bandages are applied.

Postoperative management

The bandages are removed a week after operation, and active and passive toe exercises are started. A lightly padded bandage is applied, and the patient is encouraged to walk. After a fortnight loose-fitting flat shoes are worn.

References

1. Fowler AW. A method of forefoot reconstruction: an operation for the relief of irreversible claw toes. *J Bone Joint Surg [Br]* 1959; 41-B: 507–13.
2. Hoffmann P. An operation for severe grades of contracted or clawed toes. *Am J Orthop Surg* 1912; 9: 441–9.
3. Kates A, Kessel L, Kay A. Arthroplasty of the forefoot. *J Bone Joint Surg [Br]* 1967; 49-B: 552–7.

Further reading

Chen SC, Ali MA. Metatarsal osteotomies: a comparison between the power saw and bone cutters. *J Bone Joint Surg [Br]* 1985; 67-B: 671.

Chen SC, Khan O. A comparative study of metatarsophalangeal osteotomies with and without open reduction of associated MTP joint dislocations. *J Bone Joint Surg [Br]* 1985; 67-B: 671.

Helal B. Metatarsal osteotomy for metatarsalgia. *J Bone Joint Surg [Br]* 1975; 57-B: 187.

Helal B. Surgery for adolescent hallux valgus. *Clin Orthop* 1981; 157: 50–63.

Helal B, Chen SC. Arthroplastik des Großzehengrundgelenks mit einer neuen Silastik – Endoprothese. *Orthopäde* 1982; 11: 200.

Helal B, Chen SC. Arthroplasty of the metatarso-phalangeal joint of the big toe using a new silicone elastomer prosthesis. *Med Chir Pied* 1986; 7: 95.

Helal B, Gupta SK, Gojaseni P. Surgery for adolescent hallux valgus. *Acta Orthop Scand* 1974; 45: 271–95.

Illustrations by Peter Cox after F. Price

Hallux valgus and hallux rigidus

H. Piggott FRCS
Consultant Orthopaedic Surgeon, United Birmingham Hospitals,
Royal Orthopaedic Hospital, Birmingham, and Warwickshire Orthopaedic Hospital, Coleshill, UK

HALLUX VALGUS

General considerations

The normal big toe is in slight valgus, determined by the shape of the metatarsal and proximal phalanx, but the articular surfaces of the metatarsophalangeal joint are everywhere in contact. Hallux valgus, by contrast, shows subluxation of the metatarsophalangeal joint, the phalanx being displaced laterally. A small intermediate group has the phalanx displaced to the lateral limit of the metatarsal head, leaving its medial border 'exposed'; this type sometimes progresses to subluxation. Although hallux valgus may develop in rheumatoid arthritis and some neurological disorders, in the great majority its cause is unknown and it starts insidiously in childhood and slowly progresses. There is a progressive buckling of the first skeletal ray, and later, presumably as a result of the altered mechanics, other forefoot changes appear, including depression of the second (and sometimes third and fourth) metatarsal head and dorsal subluxation or dislocation of the metatarsophalangeal joints, with hammer deformity of the proximal interphalangeal joints. Pes valgus is often present. Osteoarthritic changes may develop in the first metatarsophalangeal joint and a bunion forms over the medially projecting first metatarsal head, often with infective episodes.

Symptoms in this complex deformity are unpredictable and may be absent. The commonest complaints are: shoe pressure pain at the bunion, osteoarthritic symptoms in the first metatarsophalangeal joint, weight-bearing pain under the forefoot, shoe pressure on a hammer toe and a general foot ache on standing.

Choice of operation

With such a variable picture, selection of procedures must depend on overall assessment of symptoms, anatomical changes, way of life in relation to activity, shoe wear and personality. Some general guides are the following.

1. Physiological valgus is not a surgical problem; neither is a broad but otherwise normal forefoot.
2. In the early stages of deformity, when there is subluxation of the first metatarsophalangeal joint, but no secondary changes, treatment aims at permanent correction of the subluxation without damaging the joint.
3. In later stages when degenerative changes are present, surgery is determined by symptoms, and this may involve operation on the metatarsophalangeal joint or on other parts of the forefoot, or both.

This chapter considers only big toe operations.

Osteotomy

Osteotomy of the first metatarsal neck allows lateral displacement of the metatarsal head and slight shortening of the metatarsal shaft which slackens off the bowstrung long tendons so that the subluxation can be reduced without opening the joint. Division of the insertion of adductor hallucis and realignment of the tendon of extensor hallucis longus prevents recurrence of deformity. The operation is appropriate in the early stages before secondary changes have appeared.

Keller arthroplasty

The base of the proximal phalanx is excised to form a false joint and the medial prominence of the metatarsal head trimmed off. The false joint usually has enough mobility to allow a reasonable range of heel heights, but the big toe is short and push-off is weakened. This operation is suitable where symptoms arise from shoe pressure at the first metatarsal head or from degenerative changes in the first metatarsophalangeal joint, in a patient who does not need to walk long distances.

Arthrodesis

This gives a strong first ray, but the range of heel heights is limited and must be agreed preoperatively. It must *not* be done when the interphalangeal joint is stiff (unless excision arthroplasty of the latter is performed simultaneously). It is advised where symptoms arise from osteoarthritis of the joint, with or without metatarsal head pressure, in an active patient.

Exostectomy

Exostectomy has a limited place, where symptoms are restricted to shoe pressure discomfort. Postoperative recovery is more rapid than after arthroplasty or arthrodesis. It is not recommended for the younger patient with hallux valgus since it does nothing to prevent progression of the deformity.

INTERPHALANGEAL VALGUS

Valgus deformity is not uncommon at the interphalangeal joint of the big toe, and occasionally symptoms arise from shoe pressure on the prominent medial side of the joint. The deformity is due to the shape of the bones, not subluxation of the joint, and it can be corrected by osteotomy of the distal end of the proximal phalanx. Rarely, in late cases with degenerative osteoarthritis, arthrodesis is advisable.

HALLUX RIGIDUS

Hallux rigidus is a stiffening of the first metatarsophalangeal joint from arthritis, usually osteoarthritis, and may develop in quite young people. Transient episodes of pain and stiffness can occur and these should be treated conservatively, operation being reserved for persistent or frequently repeated symptoms.

The choice between arthrodesis, Keller arthroplasty and exostectomy depends on the same considerations as in hallux valgus, arthrodesis being for the vigorous who are content with a limited range of heel heights, arthroplasty for the less active and those who wish to wear high heels sometimes, while exostectomy is limited to the few whose symptoms are confined to shoe pressure on an exostosis, which in hallux rigidus is often dorsal, small and well localized.

Contraindications

1. Relative contraindications to all these procedures are severe diabetes, and arterial or venous insufficiency.
2. Stiffness of the metatarsophalangeal or the interphalangeal joint is a contraindication to arthrodesis of the other (though one of them may be arthrodesed and the other converted to a pseudarthrosis by excision of articular surfaces).
3. An infected bunion may delay surgery until it is controlled.

Preoperative

Position for operation

General anaesthesia is preferred. A pneumatic tourniquet is a great advantage but can be omitted on the rare occasions when there is circulatory doubt or any tendency to thrombosis. The patient is supine, and a slightly head-up position gives more comfortable access to the dorsum of the foot. Draping leaves the whole foot and ankle exposed; this is particularly important in assessing the position for arthrodesis. For most operations, the surgeon is more comfortable at the foot of the table facing the patient's head, but a right-handed operator may work conveniently on the left foot from that side of the table, an important point when bilateral procedures are performed simultaneously. A shelf clamped to the side of the foot of the table allows separation of the feet and further facilitates bilateral operation.

Operations

METATARSAL NECK OSTEOTOMY

Division of adductor hallucis

1

A straight dorsal incision is made from mid-phalanx to mid-metatarsal and the exposure deepened between the first and second metatarsal heads to expose the tendon of adductor hallucis at its insertion to the lateral sesamoid. This is facilitated by keeping close to the capsule of the first metatarsophalangeal joint while firm retraction is applied to the first and second metatarsals. The tendon is divided at its insertion.

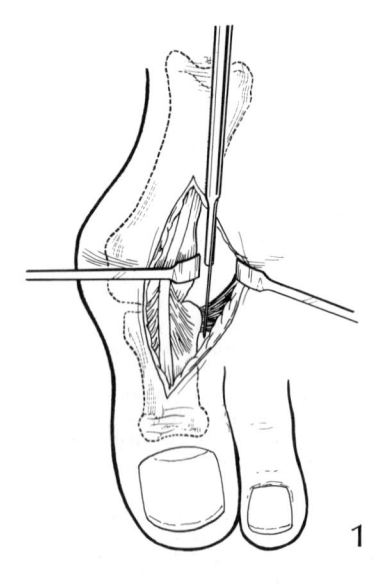

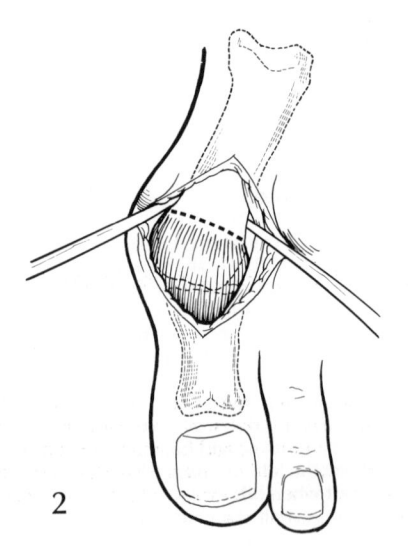

Line of osteotomy

2

The periosteum of the neck and distal shaft of the first metatarsal is approached by a longitudinal incision through the paratenon and extensor hood a few millimetres medial to the tendon of extensor hallucis longus, and the bone is then exposed subperiosteally. The neck is divided strictly transversely, immediately proximal to the joint capsule. It is essential to perform the osteotomy through this broad part of the bone to allow room for adequate lateral displacement of the head, which must be at least half its width. An oscillatory power saw is best but care must be taken to protect the extensor hallucis longus tendon. If power is not available, multiple small drill holes joined by cutting forceps are a good alternative.

Peg and socket

3a & b

The metatarsal head must be moved laterally by about half its diameter and the metatarsal shaft shortened about 8 mm to slacken off the long tendons, both flexor and extensor, which are bowstrung on the lateral side of the joint. Shortening in the long axis of the metatarsal would elevate the head slightly from the weight-bearing position and to avoid this (which would put excess strain on the lesser metatarsal heads), the head is displaced in a slightly plantar direction. To achieve this lateral and plantar displacement, the cortex of the proximal fragment is trimmed away to leave a stout projecting 8 mm lateroplantar peg. A socket is then made in the dorsomedial part of the cut surface of the head to fit the peg precisely. A small osteotome is used as a hand tool and the fit must be exact. The head is then displaced laterally and plantarwards, and peg and socket fitted and impacted. Finally, the now medially projecting distal part of the shelf is trimmed off smooth.

Fashioning and fitting the peg and socket must be precise and the immobilization is then very secure. The socket should be cut fractionally too small, 'lined up', and finally the peg trimmed to exactly the right size; a large peg should *not* be forced into a small socket – this will crush the cancellous bone of the head and result in a loose fit.

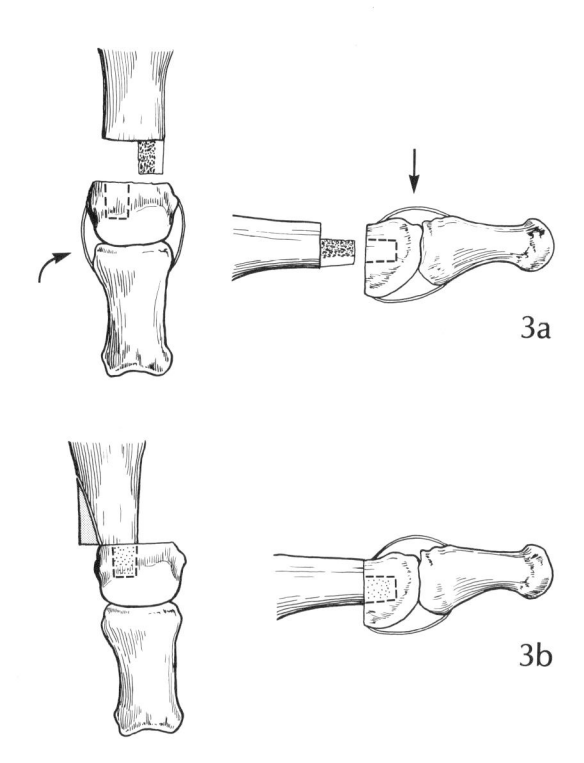

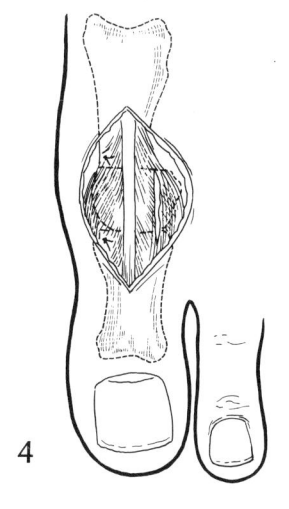

3a

3b

Realignment of extensor hallucis longus

4

The extensor hallucis longus tendon is now realigned centrally over the metatarsophalangeal joint. To do this the extensor hood is incised longitudinally on the lateral side of the tendon, and reefed medially. A plaster of Paris boot is applied with a cylindrical extension for the big toe, holding it in slight varus and flexion.

1248 Leg and foot

KELLER ARTHROPLASTY

Skin incision

5

The excision extends on the dorsum from the middle of the proximal phalanx to just proximal to the metatarsal head. The curve illustrated is a safeguard against contracture and is also concealed by the shoe. A bursa, if present, is excised at this stage, but if the overlying skin is adherent and thin, only its deep wall is removed.

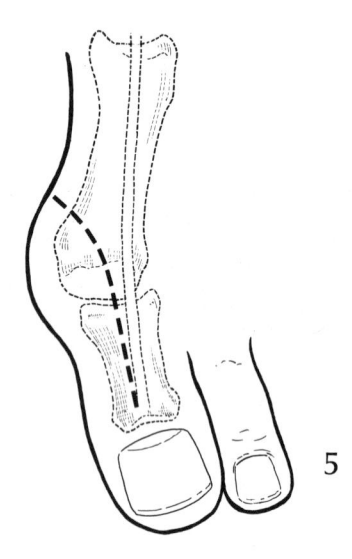

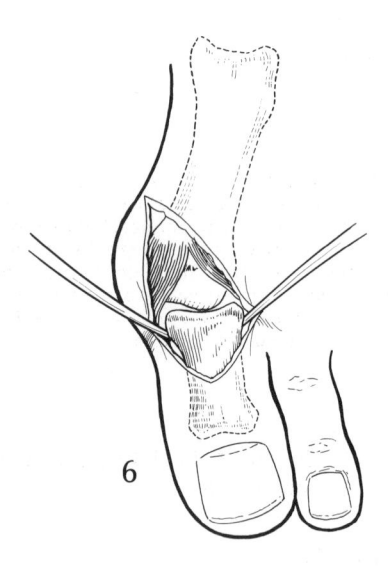

Capsular incision

6

The capsule is incised in the same line as the skin and detached with a scalpel from the sides of the base of the phalanx. Narrow spike retractors are inserted to protect the long tendons.

Dislocation of proximal phalanx

7

A sharp hook is inserted through the articular surface of the base of the phalanx and with help from the retractors serves to dislocate the joint with the phalanx in the strongly flexed position. A few touches of the knife on the plantar aspect release the phalanx from the capsule; by keeping very close to bone, the long flexor tendon is avoided.

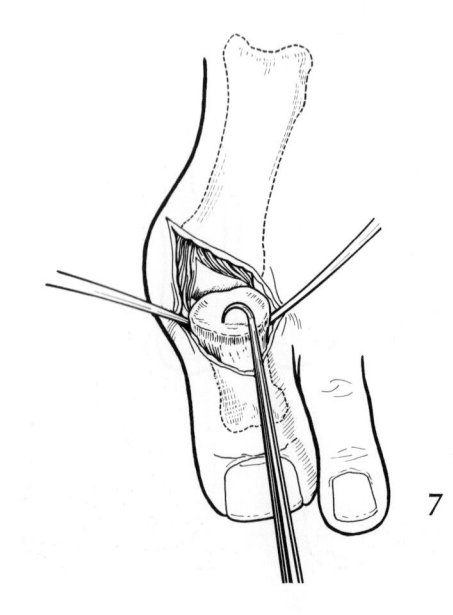

Excision of proximal phalanx

8

Approximately half the phalanx is excised. Sharp-pointed bone-cutting forceps may be used, taking small bites to avoid splintering; any rough edges are carefully smoothed off. The aim is a long fibrous joint to allow free mobility; hence adequate bony excision is essential, but removing more than half the phalanx is likely to give an obviously short toe and shoe pressure on the projecting second toe may result.

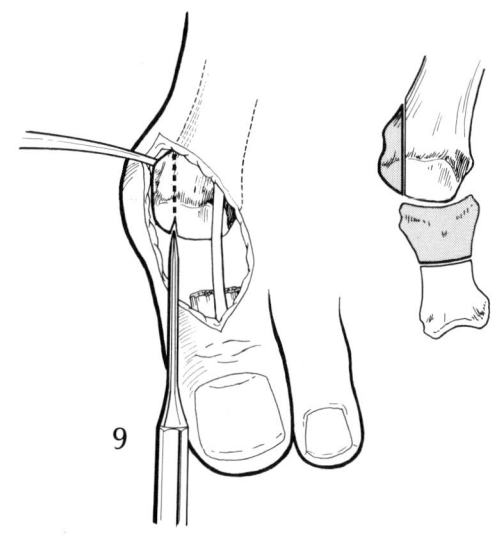

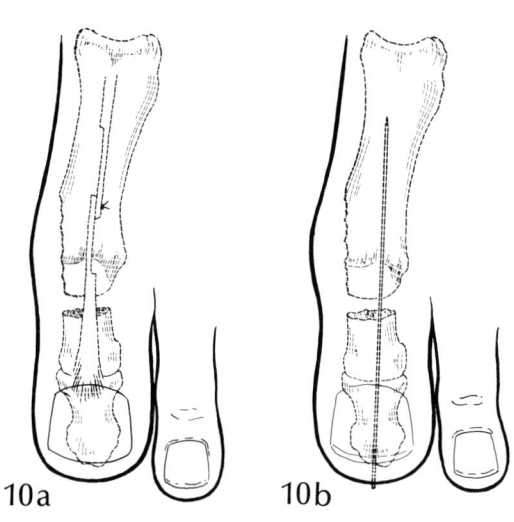

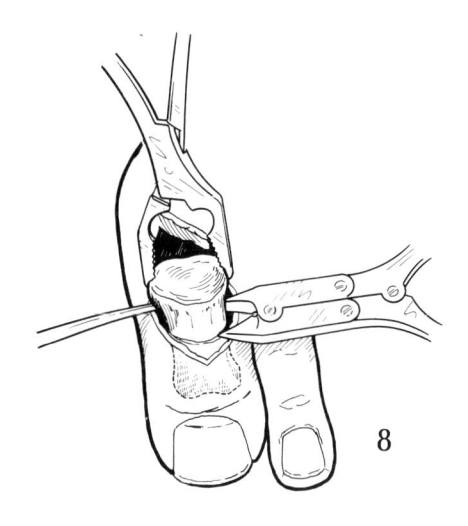

Excising exostosis

9

A narrow spike retractor under the metatarsal head holds the capsule clear and the 'exostosis' (really the non-articulating part of the metatarsal head) is removed with an osteotome, any resulting sharp edges being smoothed off with nibbling forceps. The line of osteotomy is determined by lining up the remains of the phalanx on the metatarsal head and removing enough of the latter to ensure there is no medial projection.

Elongating the extensor hallucis longus tendon or insertion of Kirschner wire

10a & b

If the big toe now lies comfortably straight, and with a gap of 4 mm or more at the pseudarthrosis, it remains only to suture the capsular incision and skin. However, sometimes the toe is found to flop into valgus, and sometimes the phalanx is held tightly against the metatarsal head by the tension of the longitudinal muscles. If the problem is valgus only, a Kirschner wire should be passed longitudinally across the pseudarthrosis. It is inserted in the cut proximal end of the phalanx and passed distally to emerge through the end of the toe, then pushed back into the first metatarsal shaft. Six millimetres are left projecting and bent plantarwards. If the pseudarthrosis is 'tight', in addition to inserting a Kirschner wire, the extensor hallucis longus tendon is lengthened by Z-plasty. The Kirschner wire is withdrawn 6 weeks later.

Wool and a firm crêpe bandage are applied with a spica configuration to hold the big toe in slight valgus.

ARTHRODESIS

Incision

11

A dorsal longitudinal incision starts at the metatarsal neck and ends at the distal end of the proximal phalanx by curving plantarwards and medially. The capsule is opened in the line of incision, and the base of the proximal phalanx delivered as in the Keller procedure (*see Illustration 7*).

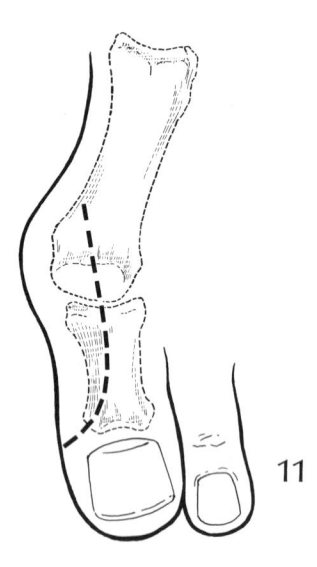

Excision of joint surfaces and alignment

12

Alignment of the phalanx is critical. Valgus should be such that the big toe lies alongside the second, nearly but not quite touching it. To determine the degree of dorsiflexion, the metatarsal is placed in the position it will take in shoes (the customary heel height having been agreed preoperatively), with the phalanx just clear of the ground.

Rotation must be avoided completely. The best way of ensuring a good fit is to remove both joint surfaces with an oscillating power saw, to leave flat cancellous surfaces fitting precisely in the desired alignment. The phalangeal surface is cut first, then the toe is lined up in the desired postoperative position and the plane of metatarsal section marked on the medial and dorsal surfaces of the head with a fine osteotome so that the two cut surfaces will be parallel. This needs much practice and a good eye, and there is no room for error. A good alternative is to remove articular cartilage and underlying cortical bone with nibbling forceps and small gouges, preserving the mutual curve of the articular surfaces, so that the phalanx may be aligned by ball and socket motion.

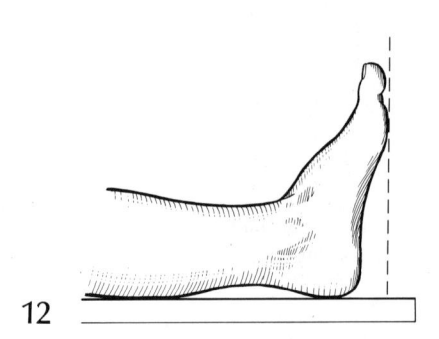

Screw fixation

13a & b

A screw is inserted obliquely as shown. To allow accurate insertion of the drill and subsequent recessing of the screw head, a small notch is cut with nibbling forceps at the point of entry to the phalanx and the screw should engage the opposite cortex of the metatarsal shaft. The screw must be tightened only enough to prevent movement at the arthrodesis. Positioning of the joint and screw is critical and if the screw is incorrectly placed it is difficult to resite – second attempts usually pass along the original track. The cautious surgeon will therefore have in reserve a miniature Charnley compression apparatus.

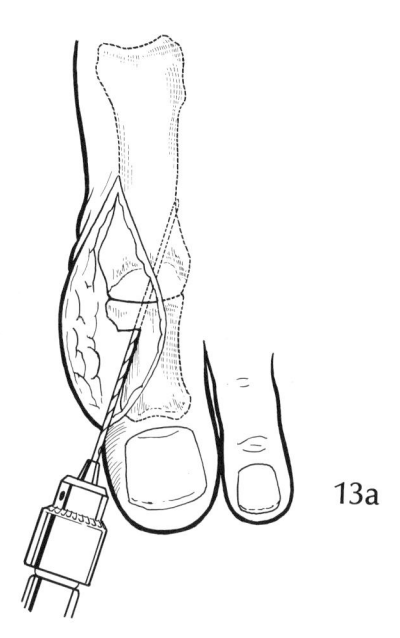

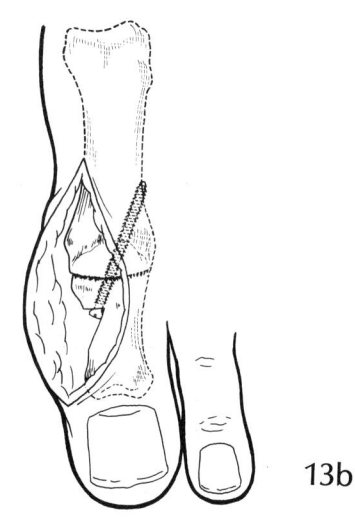

EXOSTECTOMY

Line of osteotomy

14

The skin incision is as for the Keller procedure and similarly a bursa, if present, is excised. The capsule is incised in the same line but is detached from the medial side of the phalanx only enough to allow access for the osteotome. Plantarflexion and valgus deviation of the phalanx combined with a narrow spike retractor under the metatarsal head complete the exposure. The line of bone section should ensure that there is no projection beyond the line of the phalanx. Sharp edges are rounded off with nibbling forceps.

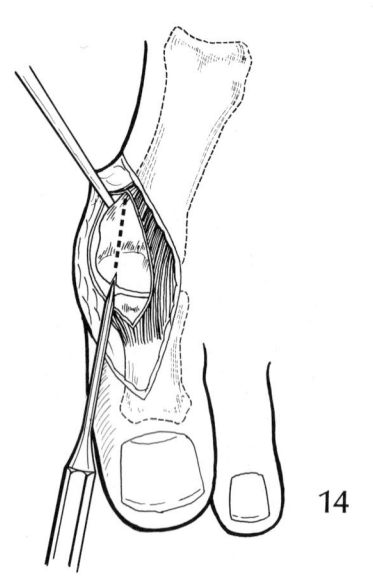

Capsular closure

15

The medial capsular flap is trimmed of any redundancy and then sutured back to effect a firm closure of the joint.

A small dorsal exostosis, most commonly seen in hallux rigidus, may be removed through a very limited curved or elliptical incision directly over it, skin and capsule being incised in the same line.

OSTEOTOMY OF NECK OF PROXIMAL PHALANX

16a & b

This is done only for interphalangeal valgus. A medial longitudinal incision extends from the base of the proximal to the middle of the distal phalanx; keeping to the 'mid-lateral' line of the toe will ensure that dissection is dorsal to the plantar digital nerve. The periosteum is incised and elevated from the distal part of the proximal phalangeal shaft, and a small wedge of bone, based medially, is excised with fine pointed bone-cutting forceps. The osteotomy is carried right through the lateral cortex, leaving only a bridge of periosteum – if the lateral cortex is left intact the wedge tends to spring open and correction is lost. It is then easy to close the wedge, and a strong catgut suture passed through small drill holes, as shown, will hold it closed. A fine Kirschner wire in a T-handle makes an excellent drill for this purpose. A padded malleable metal strip splint, curved to fit the toe, is adequate immobilization, but if there is any doubt about the stability of the suture, a Kirschner wire may be passed longitudinally from the tip of the toe across the osteotomy.

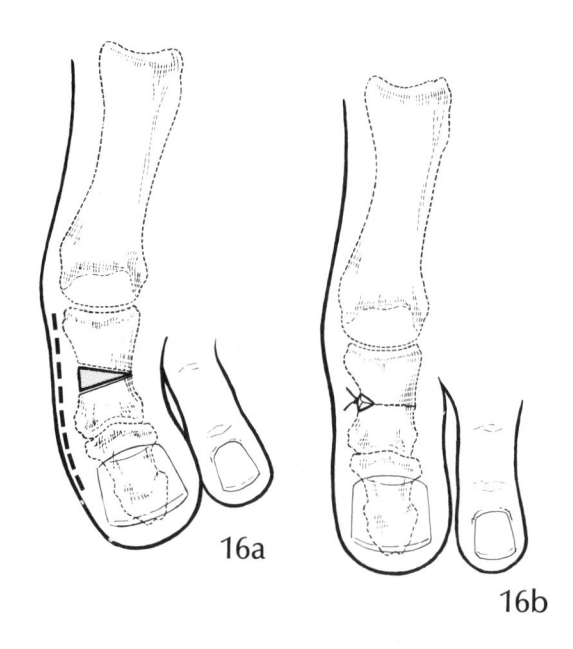

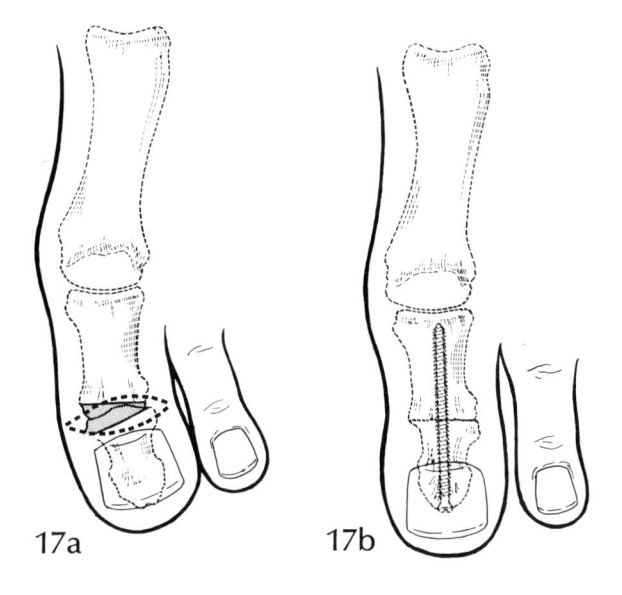

INTERPHALANGEAL ARTHRODESIS

17a & b

When osteoarthritic changes are present, with or without deformity, the interphalangeal joint may be arthrodesed, provided the metatarsophalangeal joint has full movement and is free of degenerative change. A dorsal transverse narrow elliptical incision is made, and the extensor tendon and dorsal joint capsule are incised transversely. The articular surfaces are trimmed off to expose cancellous bone and obtain a flush flat fit. Fixation may be secured by a longitudinal screw, or, if the distal phalanx is very small, by two longitudinal Kirschner wires.

Postoperative management

In all cases the foot is elevated in bed until pain and swelling have subsided, which is usually after 2–3 days. Pain may be quite severe and adequate analgesia is essential. Thereafter follows a progression from sitting out with feet elevated to crutch-walking in unilateral cases, or assisted walking in bilateral cases, to full weight-bearing and finally removal of dressings or plaster according to individual comfort and the mechanical needs of the different operations.

Metatarsal neck osteotomy and arthrodesis are immobilized immediately by a plaster of Paris boot or below-knee plaster cast with a cylindrical extension incorporating the big toe. Weight-bearing is permitted as soon as comfort permits, usually 4–5 days postoperatively, and the position is checked radiologically. Union is usually firm enough to permit removal of plaster 6 weeks after operation. If subcuticular sutures have been used, they may be left *in situ* until final removal of plaster.

At the conclusion of Keller arthroplasty or exostectomy, ample wool and a firm bandage are applied to hold the toe in slight varus and flexion. Patients are usually older than those selected for osteotomy or arthrodesis, skin quality may have been impaired by past inflammation, and after the Keller operation there is sometimes a tendency for the incision to sink a little into the gap created by the joint excision; for all these reasons interrupted skin sutures are preferred in these two operations and walking is prohibited, except for essential nursing needs, until healing is sound and sutures are removed, usually after about 2 weeks. For a Keller arthroplasty a thermoplastic splint is fitted to hold the big toe in slight overcorrection and is worn full-time for 6 weeks and at night for a further 6 weeks.

The interphalangeal operations, on the other hand, need only a malleable metal toe splint for 4 weeks, unless there is doubt about the security of fixation, in which case a plaster boot or below-knee plaster cast with a big toe spica extension is applied.

After all types of big toe operation, physiotherapy begins as soon as pain permits, usually about 24 hours postoperatively, and consists, as far as immobilization permits, of active exercises of intrinsic foot muscles, calf and dorsiflexors, and the antigravity exercises appropriate for any period of bed rest. The patient is taught these exercises *preoperatively*; he continues them through the whole period of immobilization and after that as long as any tendency to swelling remains, until full mobility is attained. Temporary elastic support of foot, ankle and leg may occasionally be necessary for swelling after removal of bandages or plaster boot.

Illustrations by Peter Cox

Dorsal nerve transfer for plantar digital neuroma (Morton's metatarsalgia)

W. N. Gilmour FRCS, FRACS
Emeritus Consultant Surgeon, Royal Perth Hospital and Princess Margaret Hospital for Children, Perth, Australia

Introduction

Morton, in his original description of pain occurring in the forefoot and radiating into the fourth toe, indicated this to be of neural origin.

Pathology

1 & 2

It has become clear that the pathology commences as an inflammation of the intermetatarsophalangeal bursa with secondary involvement of the plantar digital nerve – and also the vessel, creating an endarteritis. The nerve swelling is mostly due to oedema of the epineurium and surrounding tissue more than a true 'neuroma'. The space between the third and fourth toes is usually affected; that between the second and third less frequently. A transverse section shows the metatarsal heads with the bursa and its relationship to the plantar nerve and vessels.

Mechanics

It is postulated that the reason for this difference is the movement which goes on between the third and fourth metatarsal heads. In the forefoot the first metatarsal and the paired fourth and fifth metatarsal heads are weight-bearing with the central second and third being elevated, making up the transverse arch.

The metatarsals function as three units. The gap between the first and second metatarsals avoids the necessity for a bursa; but maximum movement occurs between the third and the fourth heads, hence the bursa and its frequent enlargement.

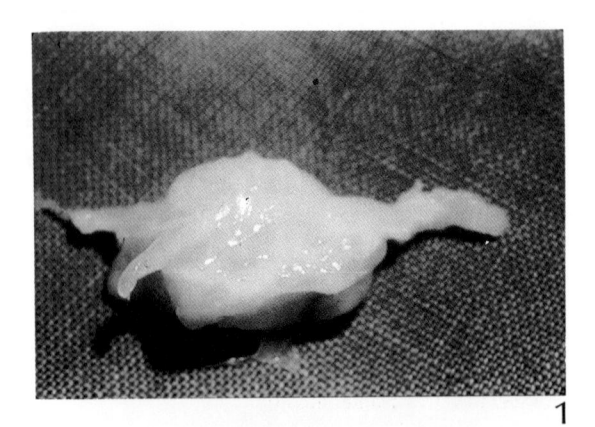

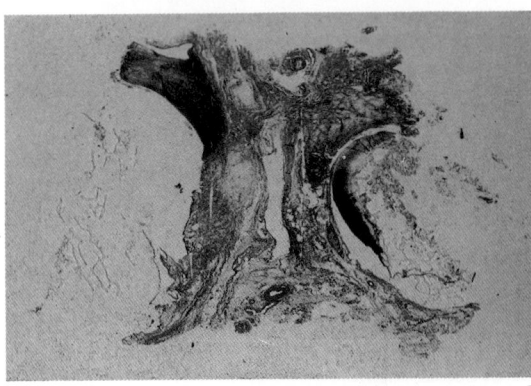

Preoperative

Diagnosis

The symptoms are of a pain which is burning and severe, radiating into the fourth or third toes and occurring at rest as well as when walking. At times it is described as knife-like.

The individual usually has a favourite pair of shoes and will be seen to remove the shoe at odd occasions.

The foot is usually architecturally normal. Some sensory loss may be determined and the 'neuroma' can be squeezed up between the metatarsal heads. Occasionally a dorsal lump will form or the toes will separate.

Principles of treatment

The bursitis and nerve involvement is reversible and may be assisted by (1) shoe selection, (2) metatarsal dome insole, and (3) infiltration with steroid. The conventional operation has been excision of the 'neuroma' through a plantar or dorsal incision. This results in the formation of a true end-neuroma which may repair distally into the weight-bearing area with the return of nerve symptoms. This may be dealt with by a second operation to dissect out the neuroma and implant it deeply in the muscles of the foot.

A more logical approach is to transfer the nerve from a plantar to a dorsal side.

Operation

The patient may select local or general anaesthesia. The operation is done in the supine position with the foot elevated.

Incision

3

A dorsal or a plantar incision may be chosen; it is remarkable how well the skin will heal without scar formation with a plantar incision.

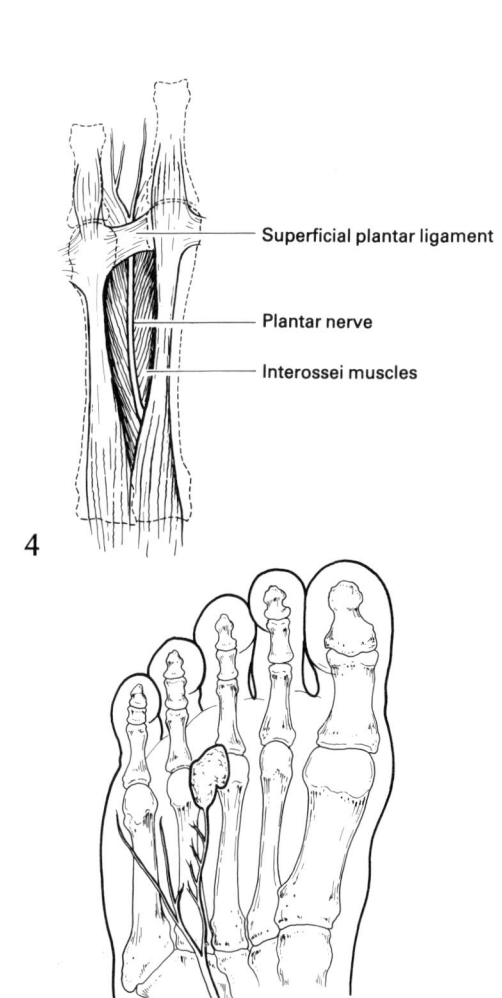

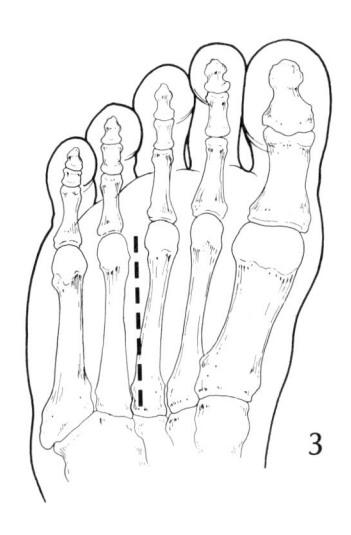

Dissection

4 & 5

The nerve is found by dividing the superficial plantar ligament (which is a portion of the plantar fascia). The bursa is opened and the 'neuroma' dissected out from the surrounding tissue between the metatarsal heads. The distal dissection is taken well into the adjoining toes and along the proximal phalanx. The proximal dissection involves splitting the lumbrical. The nerve of the 3–4 space has a contribution from the medial plantar nerve and this is preserved. Small superficial twigs to the skin of the pad must be divided.

Nerve transposition

6

The bursa is opened and the space between the third and fourth metatarsals is opened by dividing the deep plantar ligament. The nerve can now be transposed onto the dorsum and above the metatarsophalangeal joint; it lies without tension if the proximal and distal dissection is adequate.

Postoperative management

The skin is closed and the foot bandaged to keep the metatarsal heads together.

Weight-bearing is allowed after 10 days, with the removal of the sutures. The foot is kept bound with adhesive strapping for 2 weeks.

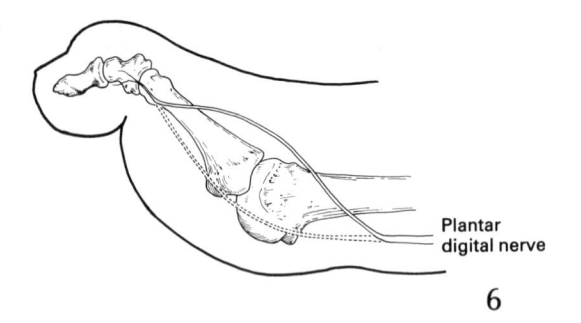

Illustrations by Peter Cox

Hammer and mallet toe

H. Piggott FRCS
Consultant Orthopaedic Surgeon, United Birmingham Hospitals,
Royal Orthopaedic Hospital, Birmingham, and Warwickshire Orthopaedic Hospital, Coleshill, UK

HAMMER TOE

Hammer toe is a flexion deformity of the proximal interphalangeal joint, most commonly affecting the second toe. Mobile at first, it later becomes fixed and may be associated with dorsal subluxation of the metatarsophalangeal joint. The distal interphalangeal joint may be normal or hyperextended; sometimes it is flexed. Hammer toe may occur in isolation or in association with hallux valgus; in the latter case, when deformity is extreme, the second toe may be so far dorsally displaced as to lie on top of the valgus big toe. Pain is caused by shoe pressure on the dorsum of the proximal interphalangeal joint, which develops a callosity and sometimes a small bursa.

Choice of operation

When the deformity and symptoms are limited to the proximal interphalangeal joint, it should be corrected by arthrodesis. *Mobile* dorsiflexion of the metatarsophalangeal joint can be treated simultaneously by subcutaneous extensor tenotomy and capsulotomy, but if this joint is subluxed, especially if irreducible, arthrodesis of the proximal interphalangeal joint is likely to result in an elevated 'anti-aircraft-gun toe' and excision of the proximal part of the proximal phalanx is preferred.

If the metatarsophalangeal joint is subluxed and the predominant symptom is weight-bearing pain under the metatarsal head, then reduction of the subluxation by metatarsal osteotomy (see p. 1264) is undertaken and the hammer toe corrected only if it still projects significantly when the metatarsal has been realigned.

Associated hallux valgus may need surgical correction at the same time as the second toe. Very occasionally, especially in the elderly, if the big toe abuts firmly on the third, if the intervening second toe, often hammered, is completely displaced dorsally and if symptoms are restricted to painful shoe pressure on that toe, surgery may be limited to amputating it.

MALLET TOE

This is a flexion deformity of the distal interphalangeal joint, most commonly affecting the second toe and usually occurring as an isolated deformity. Symptoms arise from pressure, either under the pulp from weight-bearing or on the dorsum from the shoe. Treatment is by arthrodesis of the distal interphalangeal joint.

Operations

SPIKE ARTHRODESIS

Incision

1

A dorsal ellipse of skin is excised over the apex of the deformity. The underlying extensor aponeurosis is similarly excised to open the joint.

Division of collateral ligaments

2

The key to easy access is detachment of the collateral ligaments from the head of the proximal phalanx, cutting retrograde from within the joint, which is held strongly flexed.

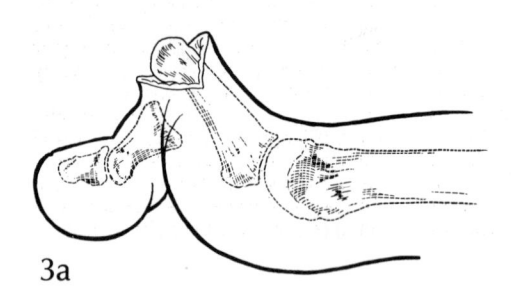

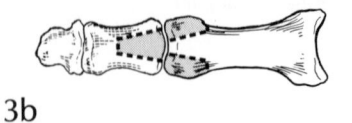

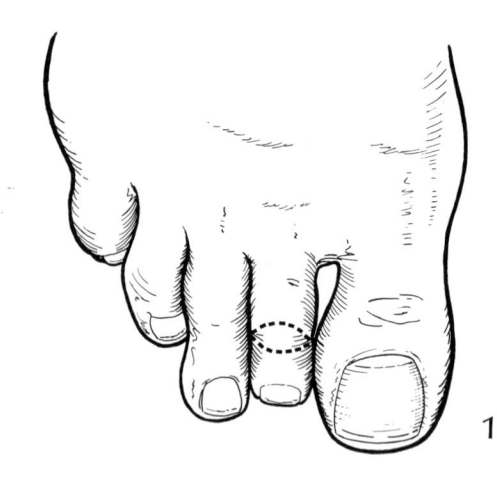

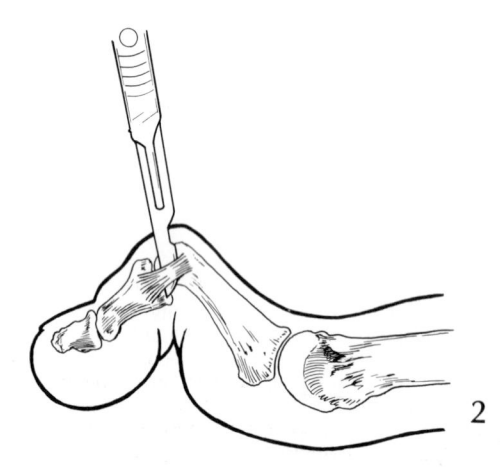

Delivery, spike and socket

3a & b

The phalangeal head is then easily delivered and trimmed to make a stout spike. Small nibbling forceps are ideal and trimming starts most easily at the plantarolateral and plantaromedial aspects of the condyles; the dorsal cortex is left intact since strength of the spike depends on it. A matching conical hole is drilled in the proximal phalanx, starting with an awl and enlarging with burrs until a firm press-fit is obtained.

Suture and splintage

4

Two or three vertical mattress sutures close the incision, and a malleable padded metal toe splint or a plaster strip is applied.

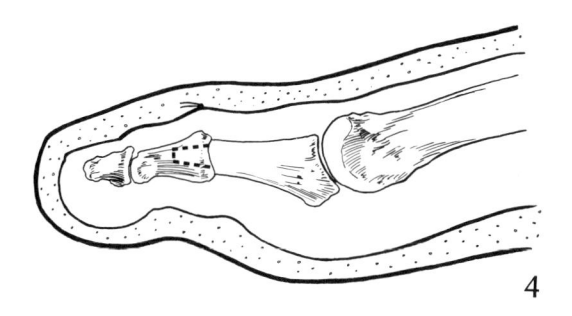

Kirschner wire method

5

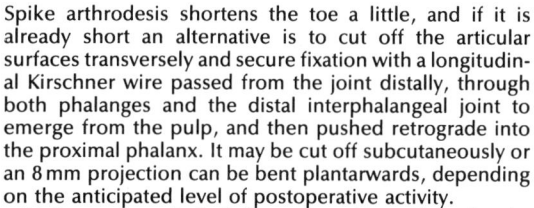

Spike arthrodesis shortens the toe a little, and if it is already short an alternative is to cut off the articular surfaces transversely and secure fixation with a longitudinal Kirschner wire passed from the joint distally, through both phalanges and the distal interphalangeal joint to emerge from the pulp, and then pushed retrograde into the proximal phalanx. It may be cut off subcutaneously or an 8 mm projection can be bent plantarwards, depending on the anticipated level of postoperative activity.

Mallet toe may similarly be corrected by spike arthrodesis of the distal interphalangeal joint, but the distal phalanx is not big enough for an adequate socket, and the Kirschner wire technique is more suitable. (When both interphalangeal joints are deformed, Kirschner wire arthrodesis of both may be performed simultaneously.)

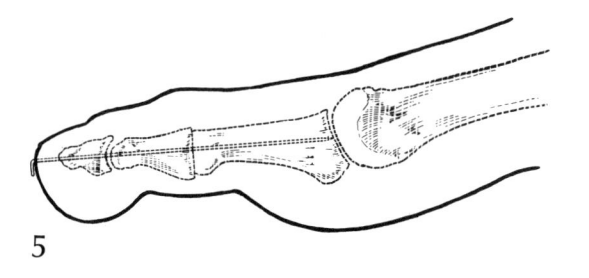

PARTIAL EXCISION OF PROXIMAL PHALANX

6a, b & c

An S-incision is made to minimize risk of contracture. The extensor tendon is split longitudinally; and traction on the base of the phalanx with a strong towel clip, combined with a few touches of the scalpel to detach the capsule, allows easy delivery into the incision. The required amount of phalanx, usually about one-half, is removed with fine-pointed, bone-cutting forceps. If the toe tends to 'cock-up' the extensor expansion is divided transversely. Skin only is sutured and the toe is bandaged in slight plantarflexion.

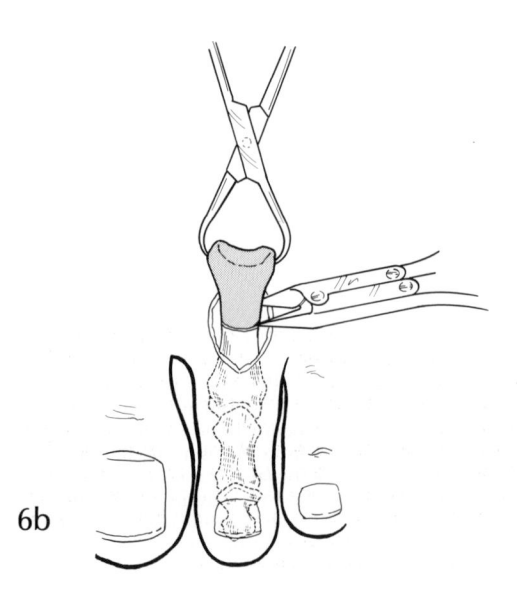

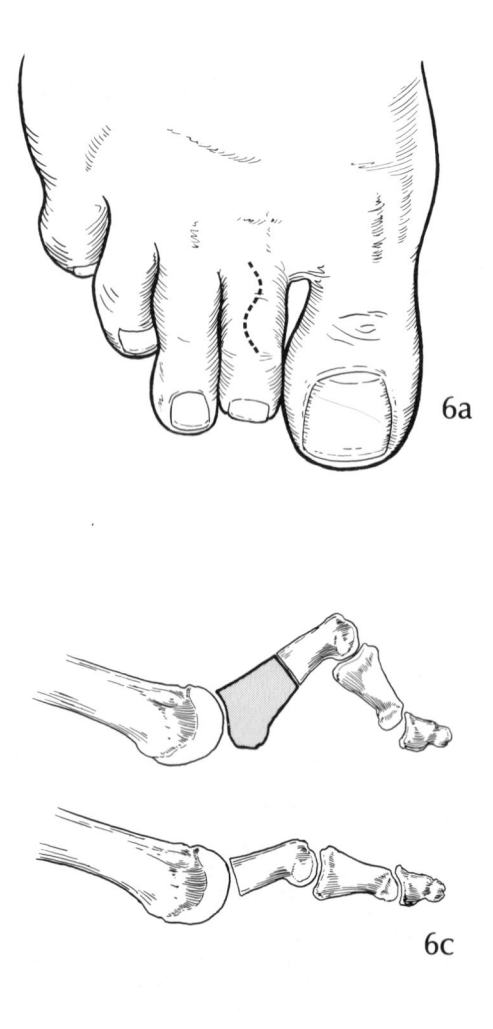

Postoperative management

The foot is elevated in bed until pain is minimal, usually 24–48 hours. Thereafter increasing walking is permitted, provided there is no pain or swelling. The position of a spike arthrodesis should be checked by X-ray at this stage. Sutures are removed after 12–14 days. Union of a spike is usually sound by 4 weeks and the splint may be removed then, but a 'flush-cut' Kirschner wire arthrodesis usually takes longer and the wire should remain *in situ* for 6–8 weeks. If the wire was cut off subcutaneously, local anaesthesia is required for its withdrawal, over the end of the wire if very superficial or as a digital block if it is more than 1–2 mm deep. Fine-pointed, short-nosed milliner's pliers facilitate withdrawal of the wire through a 4 mm stab incision which does not require suture.

Illustrations by Peter Cox after F. Price

Subluxation of the lesser metatarsophalangeal joints

H. Piggott FRCS
Consultant Orthopaedic Surgeon, United Birmingham Hospitals,
Royal Orthopaedic Hospital, Birmingham, and Warwickshire Orthopaedic Hospital, Coleshill, UK

Introduction

Some or all of the lesser metatarsophalangeal joints may become subluxed. This is most common in the second toe in association with hallux valgus, but also occurs in connection with hammer toe, while multiple subluxations may be a feature of rheumatoid arthritis or advanced pes cavus with clawing. The resulting pain on weight-bearing under the displaced metatarsal heads may demand surgical treatment and often has to be combined with correction of hallux valgus.

If only one or at the most two joints are subluxed surgery aims at correction of the displacement, but where all are affected there is little or no prospect of restoring normal anatomy, and forefoot arthroplasty by excision of all the metatarsophalangeal joints is preferred. Exceptionally, in the more active patient, and provided the interphalangeal joint of the great toe has a good range of movement, it may be preferable to combine excision arthroplasty of the second, third, fourth and fifth metatarsophalangeal joints with arthrodesis of the first.

Care must always be taken to distinguish the pressure symptoms of subluxation from intermittent claudication and Morton's metatarsalgia.

Operation is performed under general anaesthesia and with the use of a pneumatic tourniquet.

Operations

REDUCTION OF SINGLE METATARSOPHALANGEAL SUBLUXATION BY METATARSAL SHORTENING

The object is to shorten the metatarsal at the neck to allow the long toe tendons to slacken off, at the same time elevating the metatarsal head and reducing the subluxation so that the thick plantar capsule of the metatarsophalangeal joint is restored to its normal position under the head.

1a & b

Through a dorsal longitudinal S-incision, the metatarsal neck is exposed subperiosteally, divided transversely, trimmed down to a spike and impacted into a conical burr hole in the metatarsal head. The amount of shortening and elevation is determined by the extent of neck resection and should be just enough to bring the displaced metatarsal head into alignment with the others; usually it suffices to trim the neck and impact the spike without segmental resection.

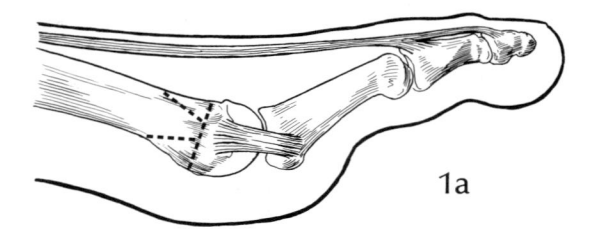

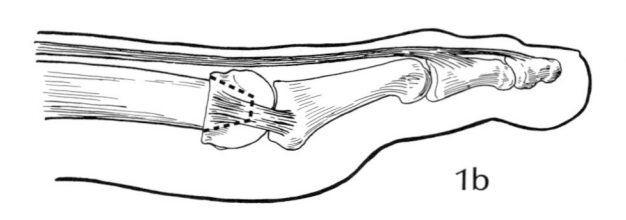

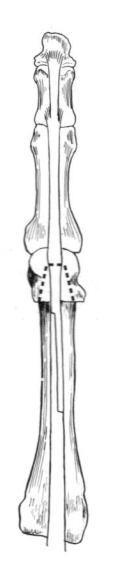

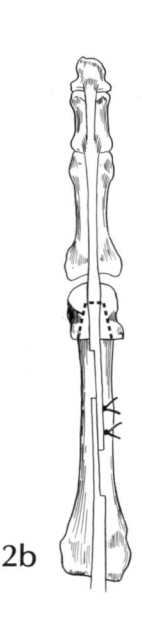

2a & b

It is often necessary to elongate the extensor tendon. If the subluxation is passively reducible preoperatively the bone shortening may be all that is required, but more commonly it is found at completion of osteotomy that some degree of subluxation remains. If it can be reduced by simple flexion, Z-elongation of the extensor tendon is performed immediately proximal to the osteotomy.

3a & b

Often the subluxation is irreducible because of capsular contracture. In these cases the initial approach to the metatarsal neck is made by centering the extensor tendon Z-lengthening over the joint. The dorsal capsule is divided transversely and the collateral ligaments are severed from the metatarsal head by cutting retrogradely from inside the joint. The plantar capsule, if adherent, is separated from the undersurface of the head with a blunt curved elevator.

Suture of the extensor tendon with fine catgut and skin closure complete the operation.

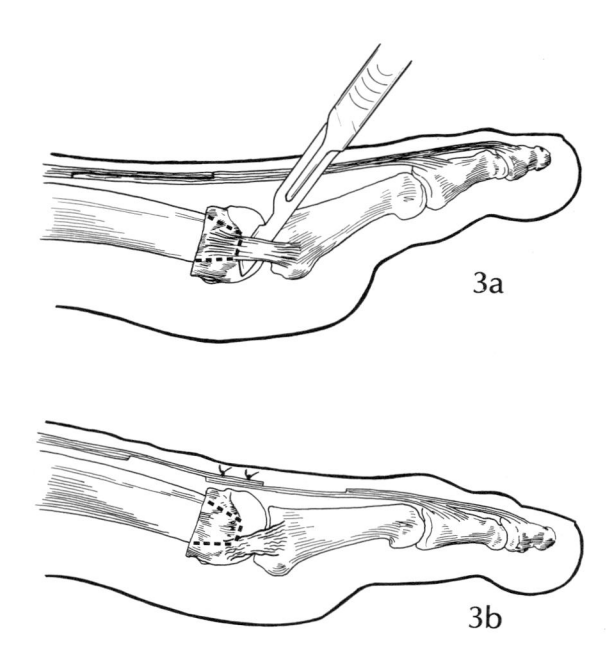

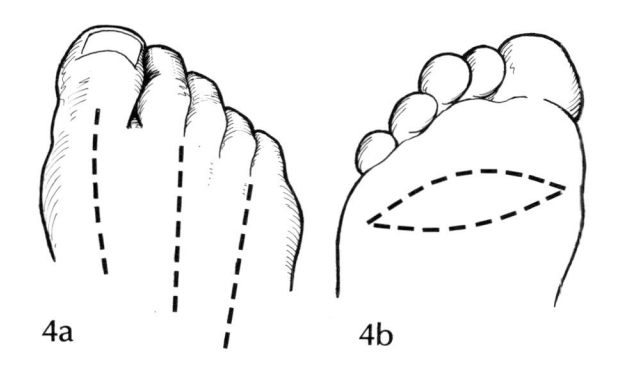

FOREFOOT ARTHROPLASTY

The incisions

4a & b

Three dorsal longitudinal incisions, each approximately 2 inches long, are made, one for the first joint and one for each pair of lesser joints. A separate elliptical incision is made in the sole 2–3 cm in width at its widest part, proximal to the weight-bearing skin.

Bone excision

5a & b

The base of each proximal phalanx is exposed by incising the dorsal joint capsule, and, using a towel clip through the bone as a retractor, pulling it dorsally. It is freed from capsular attachments with a knife and the phalanx is divided near its middle with a small bone-cutting forceps. The base of the phalanx is discarded.

The metatarsal heads are trimmed to remove all palpable plantar prominences, leaving the five metatarsal heads as a whole forming a smooth curve convex distally.

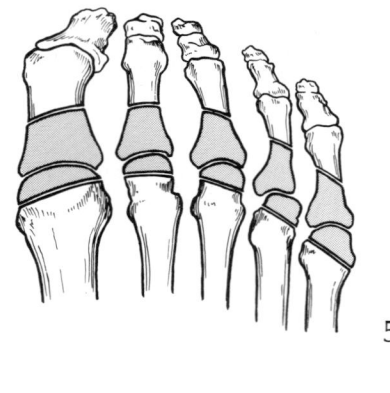

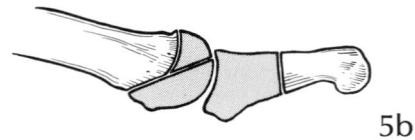

Closure

6

Attention is now turned to the plantar elliptical incision, which is sited just proximal to the metatarsal heads. The whole ellipse of skin and underlying fat is discarded, and the incision closed. This has the effect of drawing the thick plantar capsules of the metatarsophalangeal joints, which have been displaced distally by the subluxation, back to their proper position under the refashioned metatarsal heads which are then properly cushioned against weight-bearing.

Finally, the dorsal incisions are closed.

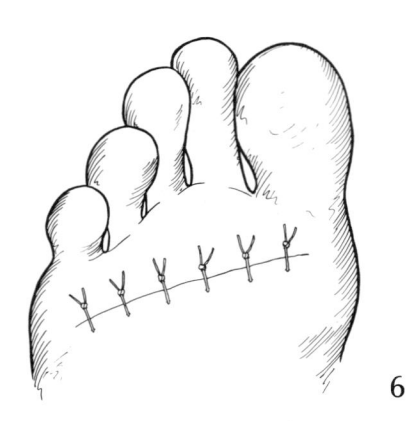

Postoperative management

This is similar for both operations described, but for single metatarsophalangeal reduction postoperative swelling is likely to be less and rehabilitation consequently faster than with forefoot arthroplasty. A well-padded plaster of Paris boot is applied, incorporating the toes in the straight position and moulded well upwards under the metatarsal heads. Considerable toe swelling may occur, so the plaster should be split and the foot well elevated. Unless other considerations prevail there should be no hurry to start weight-bearing, but usually about 2 weeks postoperatively swelling has subsided enough to allow removal of sutures and application of a close-fitting, well-moulded, plaster of Paris boot or wooden sandal in which walking may be started. This should be removed about 1 month postoperatively, and mobilizing exercises for the toes, foot and ankle are then begun.

Illustrations by Peter Cox after F. Price

Dorsally displaced fifth toe

H. Piggott FRCS
Consultant Orthopaedic Surgeon, United Birmingham Hospitals,
Royal Orthopaedic Hospital, Birmingham, and Warwickshire Orthopaedic Hospital, Coleshill, UK

Introduction

This is usually an isolated congenital anomaly, but care should be taken not to overlook clawing of all toes and early pes cavus, which require more extensive treatment. Symptoms arise from shoe pressure.

The Weedon–Butler operation described here is appropriate for most cases; but in an elderly patient with severe displacement, disarticulation through the metatarsophalangeal joint may be preferred. Lesser procedures involving skin only are not recommended since they do not correct the dorsal contracture of the deeper tissues.

Operation

(Weedon–Butler)

Incision

1a & b

An elliptical incision is made to surround the base of the toe, as for amputation, with proximal linear extensions at both ends; the plantar extension should incline slightly medially toward the centre of the sole. Dissection is deepened to expose the base of the phalanx and the joint capsule, care being taken to preserve the neurovascular bundles, which are most easily identified by blunt dissection with fine scissors.

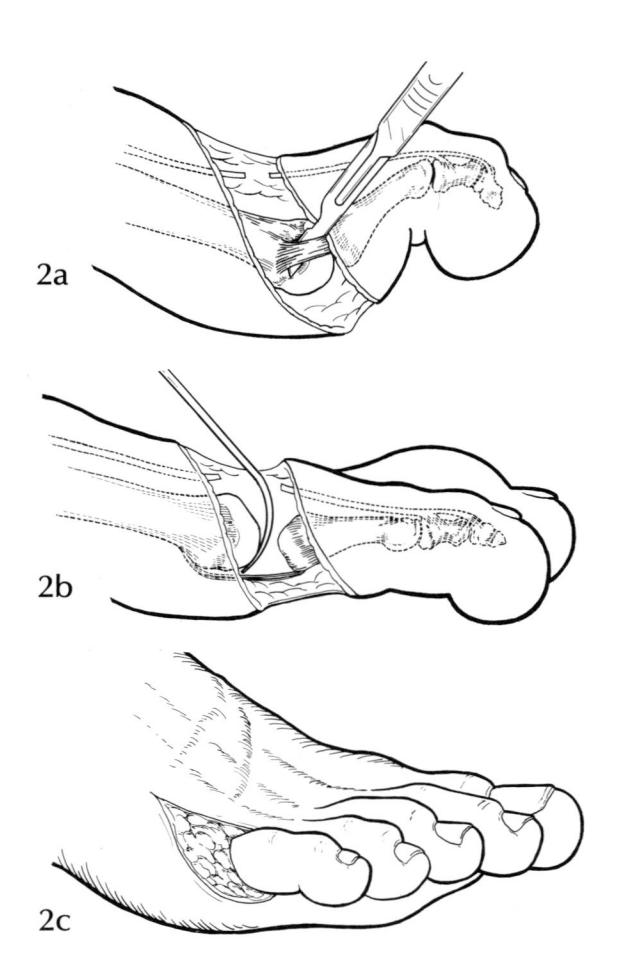

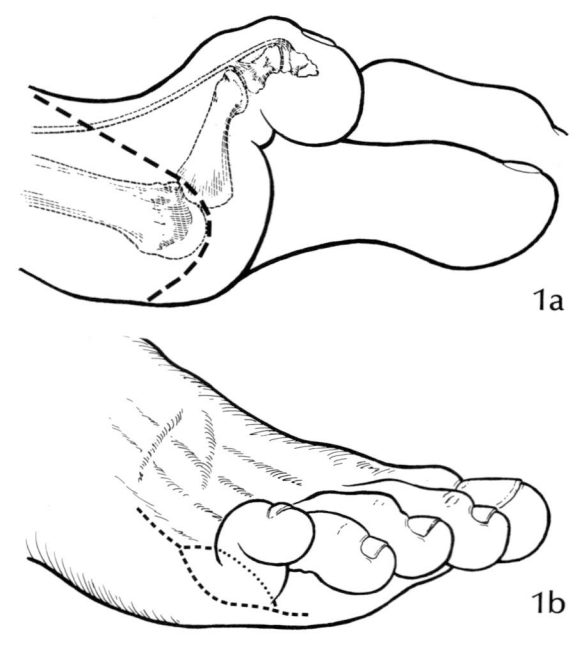

Mobilization

2a, b & c

The extensor tendon and dorsal joint capsule are incised transversely and the collateral ligaments are detached from the metatarsal head by cutting them retrograde from within the joint. In some instances the whole lateral capsule may have to be released, and in severe cases the plantar capsule may be adherent to the undersurface of the metatarsal head from which it must be separated with a fine elevator. The toe will then lie in the corrected position in line with the other toes.

Closure

3a & b

The whole mobilized toe on its pedicle, consisting of neurovascular bundles, flexor tendons and plantar joint capsule, is now anchored in its corrected position by the plantar skin suture, the plantar linear extension of the incision being opened up in a V to receive the toe, while the dorsal end is closed behind it as a Y.

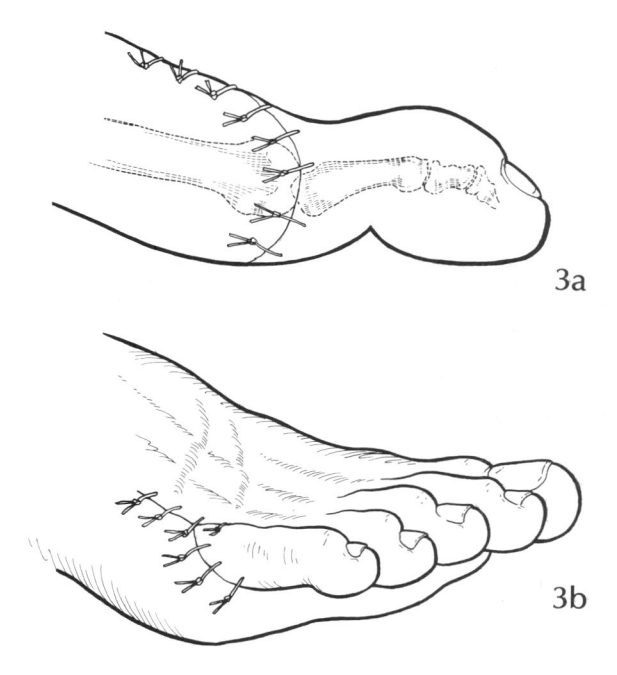

Postoperative management

The toe is carefully bandaged in the corrected position of slight plantar flexion. The circulation must be observed carefully and the bandages slackened if necessary. Elevation of the foot continues for 48–72 hours, when walking in an open-fronted shoe or sandal can begin. Sutures are removed after 14 days.

Illustrations by Peter Cox after F. Price

Ingrowing toe-nail

H. Piggott FRCS
Consultant Orthopaedic Surgeon, United Birmingham Hospitals,
Royal Orthopaedic Hospital, Birmingham, and Warwickshire Orthopaedic Hospital, Coleshill, UK

Introduction

The lateral or medial edge or both edges of the great toe-nail may be affected. The lesser toes are less commonly involved. While most cases occur in healthy individuals, the surgeon should look for neurological disease with sensory loss and for diabetes. An isolated episode may have been caused by careless nail-trimming and should be treated conservatively, but persistent or frequently repeated inflammation needs surgery. If only one edge of the nail is affected, excision of that edge and the underlying nail bed is sufficient, but involvement of both edges demands removal of the whole nail and germinal matrix to prevent regrowth. Neither operation should be performed in the presence of sepsis, which is most quickly cleared up by preliminary removal of the nail edge or whole nail, according to its extent.

For nail removal or wedge resection of matrix, a tubular tourniquet round the base of the toe suffices, but for total excision of nail and matrix a proximal pneumatic cuff is essential since a toe tourniquet prevents adequate skin mobilization.

Operations

WEDGE RESECTION

1a & b

The excision extends proximally to the base of the distal phalanx to ensure complete removal of germinal matrix within the wedge and deeply at the side to remove all epithelium and nail bed from the lateral gutter. Inadequate excision will be followed by regrowth of a troublesome nail spike.

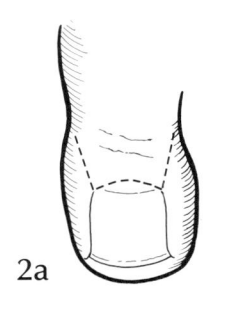

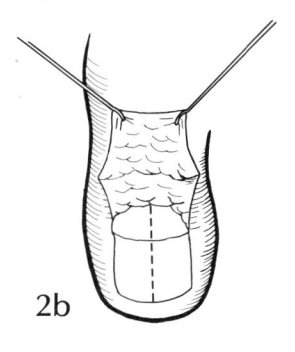

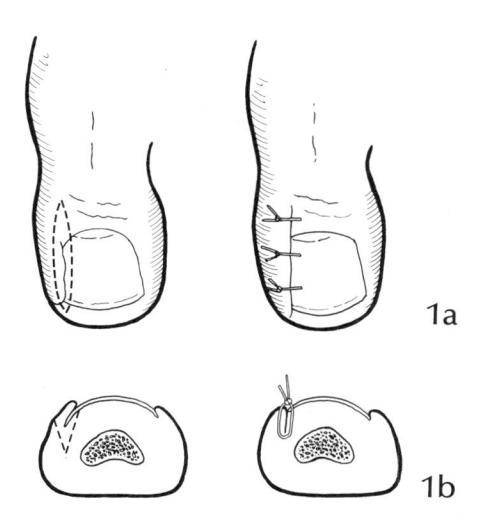

THE ZADIK PROCEDURE

Exposure

2a & b

The lateral limbs of the incision extend proximally as far as the interphalangeal joint to allow complete exposure of germinal matrix and adequate mobility of the skin flap for advancement; the transverse limb is at the distal edge of the hangnail. The skin flap is elevated, with all the scanty subcutaneous fat, and turned proximally. The nail, if not previously removed, is split longitudinally with strong pointed scissors and avulsed.

Excision of germinal matrix

3

The whole germinal matrix must be excised or a stunted deformed nail fragment will regrow. The distal limit is indicated by the lunula, and to ensure complete removal proximally all the dense white matrix tissue must be dissected out to expose the underlying extensor tendon insertion. The nail bed distal to the lunula does not generate nail tissue and postoperatively will cover itself with ordinary cornified epithelium. The lateral recesses, if deep, may be excised at this stage as illustrated in wedge resection (*see above*).

Closure

4

The skin flap, provided it has been adequately mobilized proximally, can be advanced to cover the small raw area corresponding to the lunula without tension. Fine atraumatic sutures are essential and insertion is easier if they are passed first through the skin flap, then brought out through the residual nail bed. A small longitudinal stab in the centre of the flap and a firm (but not too tight) dressing will prevent haematoma formation.

Postoperative management

After the Zadik procedure there is a risk of slow healing at the distal end and occasionally a little of the flap edge is lost. This can be minimized by elevation of the foot until pain-free, usually 48–72 hours, and avoiding weight-bearing until healing is complete, usually about 2 weeks. If this is impossible, a malleable splint or extended plaster of Paris boot should be fitted to prevent movement of the big toe.

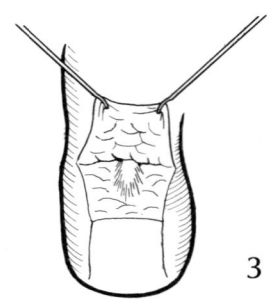

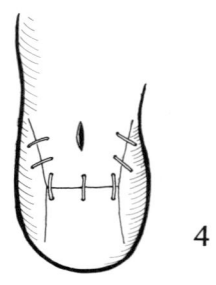

Index

Abdomen,
  vascular injury to, 52
Abdominal tube pedicle skin flap, 8
Abscess,
  Brodie's, 61, 62–63
  paraspinal, 560
  subperiosteal, 55
Acetabuloplasty,
  Pemberton, 878
Acetabulum,
  dysplasia,
    innominate osteotomy for, 893
  fracture dislocation, 339
    reduction of, 344
    with stove-in hip, 321, 328
  Kocher–Langenbeck approach to, 342
  marginal fracture, 339
  posterior wall fracture, 343
  replacement of posterior rim, 339–345
    devices for, 360
    fixation, 345
    preoperative, 339
    postoperative management, 345
    special tools required, 341
Achilles tendon *See Tendo Achillis*
Acromioclavicular joint,
  chronic dislocation, 690
  injuries to, 686–691
    classification, 686
    indications for surgery, 687
    operations for, 687
    stabilization, 689
    Weaver–Dunn technique, 690
Amputation,
  See also under limb concerned
  antibiotics in, 399
  in children, 400
  complications, 400
  for Dupytren's contracture, 856, 863
  general principles, 397–401
  fingers, 193
  indications for, 397
  management of individual tissue, 399
  phantom limb pain in, 401
  preoperative, 398
  preparations for, 399
  rehabilitation, 401
  stump oedema, 401

Aneurysm,
  false, 50
Ankle,
  arthrodesis of, 1191–1197
    by anterior approach, 1192
    by lateral approach, 1193
    in haemophiliacs, 87
    tendon transfer in, 1198
  compression arthrodesis, 1195
  equinovarus deformity, 307
  equinus deformity in, 1172
    prevention of, 131
  fractures of, 284–294
    arthrodesis following, 1191
    in children, 365
    classification of, 284
    complications, 368
    exposure of fracture, 287, 292
    indications for lateral fixation, 286
    lateral complex, 287
    medial complex, 292
    non-union, 368
    partial growth arrest complicating, 368
    postoperative management, 294
    preoperative, 286
    reduction of, 288, 293
    type A injuries, 285, 293
    type B injuries, 285, 291, 293
    type C injuries, 286, 293
  pantalar arthrodesis, 1198
  surgical approach to, 58, 60
  trephine arthrodesis, 1197
Ankylosing spondylitis,
  hip in, 965
  hip replacement in, 945
Antibiotics,
  in amputation, 399
  in fractures from metastases, 385
  in osteomyelitis, 55, 56, 63, 64, 66
  in tendon injury, 17
Aorta,
  deceleration injury, 52
Arm,
  See also Forearm, etc.
  amputation through, 402–408
    above elbow, 407, 408
    below elbow, 403, 408
    disarticulation at elbow, 405, 408

Arm (*cont.*)
  amputation through (*cont.*)
    indications, 402
    postoperative management, 408
    preoperative, 402
    prosthetics for, 408
    skin flaps and cover, 405, 406
  compartment syndromes, 303
    Volkmann's ischaemic contracture following, 307
  decompression, 304
  fracture of long bones, 153–164
  ischaemia of muscles, 141
  traction systems, 141–144
Arteries,
  bypass injury, 41
  end-to-end anastomosis, 45, 46
  injuries,
    spasm following, 47
  ligation of, 40
  patching, 44
  reconstruction, 42
  repair of, 40
    patching, 44
    suturing, 43
    vein graft, 46
  suturing of, 43
Arteriovenous fistula, 51
Arthritis,
  septic, 54
Arthrography, 1057
Arthroscopy,
  See under joint concerned
Atherosclerosis,
  amputation for, 397
Atlantoaxial fractures and dislocations, 642
Atlantoaxial fusion, 476
Atlantoaxial instability, 472
Atlantoaxial joint,
  anatomy of, 454
Atlas,
  anatomy of, 454
  fracture of ring, 472
Avascular necrosis,
  following elbow fracture, 361
  following femoral neck fracture, 364
Avulsion flaps, 3

1273

Axis,
　anatomy of, 454
Axontmesis, 295

Bankart operation, 681
Bateman's operation, 707
Bennett's fracture subluxation, 183
Berger's approach to forequarter
　amputation, 410
Biceps,
　rupture of, 709–712
　　distal tendon, 711
　　long head, 710
　　postoperative management, 710, 712
　tenodesis, 703
Biceps tendon,
　redirection of, 751
Blood vessels,
　See also Arteries, Veins, etc.
　injury and repair, 39–53
　management in amputation, 400
Bone,
　cancer of, 1141
　　biopsy in, 91
　　diagnosis, 92
　　management of, 1151
　　metastases, 92, 96, 97, 394–396
　　recurrence, 1151
　　screening, 91
　　staging, 92
　of children, 251
　healing and union, 101
　management in amputation, 400
　round cell tumours, 92, 96
Bone biopsy, 91–99
　aspiration, 94
　closed, 93
　complications, 97
　excisional, 93
　haemostasis, 97
　infection in, 98
　needles for, 94
　open, 93
　operation, 93, 94
　planning, 92
　postoperative management, 96
　trephine, 94
Bone grafting, 375–376
　for non-union, 371
　in fractures, 119
　obtaining bone for, 375
Bone infection,
　acute, 54–60
　　draining in, 56
　　pathology, 54
　　postoperative management, 56
　　principles of treatment, 55
　　surgical treatment, 56
　chronic, 61–67
　　two-stage procedure, 66
　microbiology of, 55
Bone metastases, 92, 96, 97, 394–396
　*See also under Spine, Metastatic bone
　disease*
　causing fractures, 384
　　bone grafts for, 391
　　cementing and compression fixation,
　　　386
　　indications for operation, 384
　　intramedullary nailing, 389
　　operations for, 385

Bone metastases (*cont.*)
　causing fractures (*cont.*)
　　plating for, 386
　　plating with cement, 387
　　realignment, 387
　　stabilization, 391
　halo–body casts for, 487
Boutonnière deformity of finger, 819
　repair, 827
　secondary repair, 818
Bowstringing in tendon repair, 23
Boytchev procedure, 675
Brachial plexus,
　birth palsy, 705
　iatrogenic injury, 25, 452
　injuries to, 26
　nerve grafts for, 37
Brachioradialis,
　transfer to flexor digitorum
　　profundus, 762
Bristow–Helfet procedure, 683
Brodie's abscess, 61, 62–63
Bryant's traction, 138
Buck's traction, 134
Bunnell criss-cross stitch, 812
Bunnell double right-angle stitch, 813
Bunnell withdrawal stitch, 814

Calcaneal osteotomy for pes cavus, 1217
Calcaneocavus deformity of foot, 1187
Calcaneonavicular synostosis, 1206
Calcaneonavicular bar,
　excision of, 1214
Calcaneum,
　beak fractures, 315
　correction of deformity, 316
　crush injuries, 315
　injuries to, 315
　medial displacement rotation
　　osteotomy, 1213
　removal of, 318
　traction, 126
Capitellum,
　fracture of, 173–174
Carpal scaphoid,
　AO lag screw, 799
　fractures of, 794–804
　　AO lag screw for, 799
　　Herbert bone screw for, 801
　　indications for operation, 795
　　internal fixation of, 799
　　Matte–Russe bone graft for, 796
　　non-union, 795
　　of proximal pole, 804
　　operations, 796
Carpal tunnel decompression, 788, 789
Carpus,
　Lauenstein procedure, 773
Cauda equina, 533
　complicating reduction of
　　spondylolisthesis, 558
Cerebral palsy, 512, 1152, 1169
　forearm paralysis in, 745
　hip adductors in, 926
　hip contracture in, 921
　hip extenders in, 936
　hip flexion deformity in, 931
　knee deformity in, 940, 981
　wrist and finger deformity in, 752

Cervical spine,
　anterior fusion, 463–470
　　Bailey strut graft technique, 469
　　Cloward dowel procedure, 466
　　indications for, 463, 492
　　operation, 464
　　postoperative management, 470
　　preoperative, 463
　　Robinson block graft procedure, 468
　bilateral fracture dislocation, 630, 633
　fracture dislocations, 478, 630
　　anterior stabilization, 637
　　closed reduction, 630
　　open posterior reduction, 635
　　posterior fusion with plates or wires,
　　　640
　　requiring fusion, 637
　　spinal jacket for, 667
　Hodgson approach to, 561, 563
　infections, 561
　metastatic bone disease,
　　anterior cord decompression, 575
　　anterior stabilization, 577
　　posterior decompression and
　　　stabilization, 579
　pathology of, 454
　posterior fusion, 471–481
　　atlantoaxial, 476
　　indications for, 492
　　interspinous, 478
　　occipitocervical, 472
　　operations, 472
　　postoperative management, 475, 477,
　　　479, 481
　　preoperative, 471
　posterolateral fusion, 480
　problems,
　　management of, 456
　Southwick and Robinson approach, 561–
　　562
　transoral approach to, 453–462
　　anterior, 456
　　assessment of, 456
　　operation, 457
　　position of patient, 457
　　preoperative, 455
　　surgical exposure, 458
　unilateral dislocation, 631, 634
Charnley compression arthrodesis of
　ankle, 1195
Chemonucleosis for herniated
　intervertebral disc, 530–533
Children,
　amputation in, 400
　ankle fractures in, 365
　bones of, 351
　congenital dislocation of hip,
　　operations for, 870–892
　fractures in,
　　operative treatment, 351
　fracture of femoral neck in, 362
　high femoral osteotomy in, 900
　quadriceps contracture in, 1002
　recurrent dislocation of patella in,
　　1103
　trigger finger and thumb in, 869
Chondromalacia patellae, 1032
　arthroscopic surgery for, 1030, 1039
　diagnostic arthroscopy for, 1036
Chondrosarcoma, 95
Christmas disease, 77
Claw toes, 1230

Index 1275

Club foot,
  bone resection, 1226
  lateral soft tissue release, 1225
  medial soft tissue release, 1223
  operations for, 1220–1231
    indications for, 1220
  plantar soft tissue release, 1224
  posterior soft tissue release, 1221
  postoperative management, 1226
  secondary surgery, 1226
  triple arthrodesis for, 1226
Colles' fracture, 163
  carpal tunnel compression following, 788
Common peroneal nerve,
  care of, 299
  injury to, 25
Compartment syndromes, 49, 283, 295–308
  arm, 307
  evaluation and treatment, 298
  fasciotomy for, 295
    indications for, 296
  foot, 301
  forearm, 303
  hand, 305
  leg, 298, 307
  pain in, 295
  pathogenesis of, 295
  perifibular fasciotomy, 299
  thigh, 301
  tissue pressure, 296
    measurement, 297
  Volkmann's ischaemic contracture following, 307
Congenital anomalies,
  amputation for, 398
Costotransversectomy, 614
Cotrel–Dubousset instrumentation, 491
Coxa vara, 949
  after femoral neck fracture, 364
  congenital,
    correction of, 907
    high femoral osteotomy for, 900
Craniocervical junction,
  anatomy of, 454
  development of, 453
  movement of, 454
  radiography of, 455
  stabilization of, 460
Craniocleidodystostosis, 949
Cross-leg skin flaps, 10
Cruciate ligament,
  arthroscopy, 1014
Crush injuries,
  primary care of, 3
Cutaneous axial-pattern skin flap, 11

Darrach's procedure, 769
  postoperative management, 772
Degloving injuries, 4
Deltoid paralysis, 707
Denham pin, 125
de Quervain's disease, 787
Diabetes mellitus,
  amputations in, 397
  gangrene in, 444
Digital nerve,
  injury of, 25
Dillwyn Evans procedure,
  reversed, 1212

Dorsal nerve transfer,
  for plantar digital neuroma, 1255–1258
    operation, 1257
    postoperative management, 1258
    preoperative, 1256
Duchenne's muscular dystrophy, 512
Dunn device for stabilization of spine, 665
Dupuytren's contracture, 855–864
  aetiology of, 855
  amputation for, 856
  clinical features of, 855
  dermofasciotomy, 856, 862
  extension, 864
  fasciotomy, 856, 863
  open-palm technique (McCash), 86
  operative principles, 857
    haemostasis, 862
    involving more than one ray, 860
    involving one ray, 857
  pathology of, 855
  postoperative management, 864
  preoperative, 856
  prognosis, 856
  recurrent, 862, 864
  selection of operation, 856
  Skoog technique, 860
  timing of surgery, 856
Dupuytren's diathesis, 855
Dural sac,
  care of, 528
Dynabrace Oxford Fixation System, 147

Elbow,
  amputation above, 407, 408
  amputation below, 403, 408
  arthroplasty, 729–735
    complications, 733
    indications and contraindications, 730
    infection following, 733
    insertion of prosthesis, 731
    loosening of prosthesis, 734
    postoperative management, 733
    results, 733
    skin problems following, 734
  biomechanics of joint, 730
  dislocation,
    following arthroplasty, 734
  fractures, 165–174
    in children, 354, 360
    complications of, 361
    diagnosis of, 165
    fixation, 165
    non-union, 361
    unstable, 360
  hemiarthroplasty, 729
  instability of, 76
  lateral condyle fracture in children, 354
  medial epicondyle fracture in children, 356
  prosthesis for, 730, 731
  surgical approach to, 58, 59
  synovectomy,
    for rheumatic disease, 73
    indications and contraindications, 73
    postoperative management, 75, 76
    preoperative, 73
    technique, 74
    ulnar neuritis during, 75, 76

Elbow flexion,
  restoration by tendon replacement, 736–744
    anterior transfer of triceps tendon, 740
    Bunnell's modification, 739
    Steindler's flexorplasty, 737
    transfer of pectoralis major tendon, 742
Epiphysiodesis, 1154
Epiphyses,
  fracture of, 352
  injuries to, 351
  premature union, 364
Equinus deformity, 989
Erb's palsy, 705–708
  Fairbank's operation,
    Sever's modification, 706
  postoperative management, 708
Extensor carpi radialis longus,
  transfer to flexor pollicis longus, 763
Extensor tendon repair, 21

Facial wounds, 4
Fairbank's operation,
  Sever's modification, 706
False aneurysms, 50
Fasciotomy,
  forearm, 304
  for trauma, 49
  hand, 305
  indications for, 296
  perifibular, 299
  postoperative management, 304
Femoral epiphysis,
  anatomy of, 910
  open replacement of, 914
  slipped,
    replacement of, 914
  upper, See Upper femoral epiphysis
Femoral osteotomy, 884
  for coxa vara, 888
Femur,
  avascular necrosis, 200
  biplane trochanteric osteotomy, 916
  condylar fracture, 394
  deformities, 992
  fractures of,
    bracing in, 110
    caused by metastases, 392
    in children, 136, 138
    skeletal traction for, 125, 134, 136
  fracture of neck,
    cervicotrochanteric, in children, 362
    complications, 364
    delay and non-union, 364
    hip replacement after, 950
    indication for operation, 362
    pertrochanteric, 362
    postoperative management, 364
    transcervical, 362
    transepiphyseal, 362
  geometric flexion osteotomy, 919
  high osteotomy, 900–908, 965
    postoperative management, 907, 908
  intracapsular fracture of neck, 199–208
    classification, 200
    closed reduction, 203
    fracture fixation, 205
    indications for internal fixation, 201

Index

Femur (cont.)
  intracapsular fracture of neck (cont.)
    open reduction, 204
    operative technique, 202
    postoperative management, 208
    preoperative, 202
  lateral fracture in upper end, 139
  lengthening, 1154, 1159
    soft tissue release and corticotomy, 1162
  lengthening osteotomy of, 382
  metastases in, 396
  plate removal from, 120
  preparation for knee arthroplasty, 1127
  replacement for tumour, 1142
    distal, 1145
    insertion of prosthesis, 1143, 1146
    postoperative management, 1144, 1147
    proximal, 1142
  resection of lower end, 1133
    reversed wedge osteotomy, 905
  Robert Jones valgus osteotomy, 907
  rotation osteotomy, 901
    indications for, 901
    postoperative management, 903
    prevention of complications, 903
    with varus, 904
  shaft fracture, 1003
    availability of equipment for nailing, 240
    Küntscher's nailing technique, 223–241
    Melbourne cross pinning technique, 234, 240
    oblique spiral, 137
    postoperative management, 240
    preoperative, 223
    technical requirements, 224
    traction for, 137, 226
    transverse, 137
  shortening, 380, 906, 1154, 1157
  skeletal traction, 126
  subtrochanteric fracture, 216–222
    caused by metastases, 394
    classification, 217
    complications, 222
    indications for Zickel nail fixation, 216
    postoperative management, 222
    preoperative, 218
    Zickel nail fixation, 216, 218–221
  supracondylar fractures, 242–251
    bone grafting in, 250
    caused by metastases, 394
    classification, 243
    general considerations, 242
    indications for operation, 244
    internal traction, 242
    open, 244
    operation, 246
    pathological, 244, 250
    placement of lateral condylar window, 247
    postoperative management, 251
    preoperative, 244
  trochanteric fractures, 209–215
    caused by metastases, 393
    classification, 209
    fixation, 210
    internal fixation, 210, 213
    operative details, 212
    postoperative management, 215
    preoperative, 211

Femur (cont.)
  T or Y bicondylar fractures, 244
  unicondylar fractures, 244
  wedge osteotomy, 908
Fibrin glue in nerve repair, 37
Fibula,
  compound fracture of, 14
Fibular osseocutaneous free skin grafts, 15
Fingers,
  amputation of, 193
  Boutonnière deformity, 819
    repair of, 827
    secondary repair, 818
  compartment syndrome, 305
  distal interphalangeal joint deformity, 809
  extensor tendon injury, 809
  flexor digitorum profundus injury, 810
  flexor digitorum superficialis in, 811
  flexor tendons,
    blood supply, 828
  flexor tendon division, 828–835
    delay in primary repair, 832
    delayed repair, 832
    indications for operation, 830
    postoperative management, 834
    preoperative, 830
    technique of repair, 831
    tenolysis, 835
  flexor tendon injury, 827
    primary repair, 820, 828
    tendon graft operation, 820
  fractures,
    fixation, 178
    fixation by crossed K-wires, 177
    head of proximal phalanx, 181
    Kirschner wires in, 176–180
    Lister's intraosseous wiring, 180
    postoperative management, 179
    proximal phalanx shaft, 177
    shafts of metacarpals, 185
  gliding tendon implants, 839, 852
    pulley reconstruction, 843
  mallet deformity, 809, 827
  mallet fracture, 815
  metacarpals,
    fracture, 185
  paralysis of, 759
  proximal interphalangeal joint,
    deformity, 809
    dislocation of, 196
    fracture-subluxation, 184
  replantation of, 193
  rheumatoid disease,
    Swanson arthroplasty for, 68–72
  tendon injury,
    pulley reconstruction, 843
  tendon repairs, 18, 20
  tenography technique, 832
  transfer of extensor indicis to thumb, 760
  trigger, 865–869
    in children, 869
    conservative treatment, 865
    operative details, 866
    postoperative management, 868
Fisk splint, 130
  suspension of, 133
Flat foot,
  See Pes planus
Flexor carpi ulnaris,
  transfer of, 746, 756

Flexor digitorum profundus,
  transfer of brachioradialis to, 762
Flexor pollicis longus,
  transfer of extensor carpi radialis longus to, 763
Flexor tendon repair, 21
Foot,
  amputations, 441
  arthrodesis of, 1199–1207
    Lambrinudi operation, 1201
    postoperative precautions, 1205
  calcaneocavus deformity of, 1187
  compartment syndromes in, 301
  correction of varus, 1199
  crush injury, 315, 320
  flat See pes planus
  fractures and dislocations, 309–320
    caused by metastases, 395
  Lambrinudi arthrodesis, 1191, 1201
  major disruptive lesions, 318
  pantalar arthrodesis, 1198
  reconstruction, 1232–1243
    correction of bunionette, 1237
    correction of hallux valgus, 1237
    Fowler operation, 1238
    Hoffmann operation, 1239
    osteotomies of metatarsals, 1233
    postoperative management, 1236, 1240, 1242
    prosthetic replacement of joints and toe, 1241, 1242
  sole of,
    skin cover of wounds, 4
  stabilization of, 1199
  subluxation of lesser
    metatarsophalangeal joint, 1263–1266
  surgical approach to, 58, 60, 310
  tendon transfer, 1215
  tendon transfer to heel, 1187
  transfer of tibialis posterior tendon to dorsum, 1184–1186
  triple arthrodesis, 1199
  valgus deformities, 1203
Foot drop, 307
Forearm,
  compound wound of, 15
  interosseous membrane of,
    release of, 750
  pronation deformity of, 746
  release of flexor muscles, 752
  supination deformity of, 750
  tendon reconstruction in, 745–764
    paralytic conditions, 753
    spastic conditions, 746
    triple transfer, 754
Forefoot,
  arthroplasty, 1265
  reconstruction, 1232–1343
    correction of hallux valgus, 1237
    Fowler operation, 1238
    Hoffmann operation, 1239
    osteotomies of metatarsals, 1233
    postoperative management, 1236, 1240, 1242
    prosthetic replacement of joints and toe, 1241, 1242
Forequarter amputation, 409–413
  anterior approach (Berger), 410
  indications and contraindications, 409
  operation, 470
  posterior approach to (Littlewood), 413

Forequarter amputation (*cont.*)
  postoperative management, 413
  preoperative, 410
  prosthesis for, 413
Fowler operation, 1238
Fractures,
  See also under bone concerned
  bone grafting in, 119, 391
  bone healing and union, 101, 117, 370
  callus formation, 370
  caused by metastases, 384
    bone grafts for, 391
    cementing and compression fixation, 386
    indications for operation, 384
    intramedullary nailing, 389
    operations, 385
    plating for, 386
    plating with cement, 387
    postoperative management, 395
    preoperative, 385
    prevention, 395
    realignment, 387
    stabilization, 391
  in children, 351
  complications of injury, 120
  compression, 103
  delayed union, mal- and non-union, 122, 370, 371, 377–383
    atrophic, 370
    bone grafting for, 371
    causes of, 370
    hypertrophic, 370
  diagnosis, 104
    manipulation in, 105
  diaphyseal, 145
  external bridging callus, 101
  external skeletal fixation, 145–152
    applications, 146
    choice of frame, 145, 147, 149, 150
    indications for, 145
    postoperative management, 146, 148
    rehabilitation, 146
    removal of frame, 146
  external skeletal traction, 113
  failure of consolidation, 146
  healing, 117, 370
  history and mechanism of injury, 102
  implant removal, 120
  infection in, 122
  instability in, 145
  internal fixation, 114
  intramedullary nailing, 116
  Kirschner wires in, 115
  management,
    aims of, 100
    bracing, 110
    external skeletal fixation, 145–152
    general principles, 100–122
    grafting, 119
    internal fixation, 114
    in haemophilia, 89
    intramedullary nailing, 116
    methods of holding, 108
    plaster of Paris in, 109
    plate fixation, 117
    reduction, 107
    three-point fixation, 109
    traction *See Fractures, traction*
    wire fixation, 115
  medullary callus, 101

Fractures (*cont.*)
  of long bones,
    delayed union, mal- and non-union, 369–383
  open, 120
  operative treatment,
    in children, 351–368
  pathological,
    See also Fractures, caused by metastases
    prevention of, 395
  plate fixation, 117
  primary callus response, 101
  radiology, 104
  rotational mal-union, 377
  screw fixation, 114
  self-stabilizing, 108
  skeletal traction, 111, 123, 125
    complications, 129
    sites of, 126
  skin traction, 111, 123, 124
  splints for, 129
  tendon injury and, 17
  traction, 123–144
    arm, 141
    Buck's, 134
    complications, 129
    Denham pin, 125
    duration of, 144
    external skeletal, 113
    fixed, 123
    Hamilton Russell, 135
    Kirschner wires in, 125
    leg, 134
    management of patient, 143
    ninety-ninety, 136
    Perkins', 134
    removal, 144
    skeletal, 111, 123, 124, 126, 129
    skin, 111, 124
    sliding, 123, 138
    Steinemann pin, 125
    Tulloch Brown, 135
    weights, 133
  union,
    following radiotherapy, 384
  wire fixation, 115
Fraser's approach to spine, 612

Galeazzi fracture, 160, 163
Gallé spinal fusion, 644
Gallows traction, 138
Ganglion,
  palmar, 791
  wrist, 790
Garré's sclerosing osteomyelitis, 62
Gastrocnemius,
  contracture, 1175
  distal division of, 1177
  proximal detachment of, 1175
  release, 989–992, 1169–1171
    indications and assessment, 1169
    operation, 1170
    postoperative management, 1171
    preoperative, 1169
Gastrocnemius tendon,
  exposure and division, 1171
Girdlestone's operation, 1230–1231
Girdlestone's pseudarthrosis of hip, 965–969

Glenohumeral joint,
  arthroscopic appearance of, 694, 695, 696
  dislocation of, 671
Goldthwaite–Roux operation, 1103
Grafts, skin, *See Skin grafts*
Grice–Green operation, 1203
  modification of, 1205
Growth plates,
  damage from traction, 129
  in epiphyseal fractures, 352
Gunshot injuries,
  primary care of, 3

Haemarthroses, 78, 80
Haemophilia,
  acquired, 77
  antifibrinolytic agents in, 79
  arthrodesis of hip in, 87
  arthrodesis of knee in, 83
  clinical signs, 78
  cysts and pseudotumours, 78, 89
  hip replacement in, 80
  management of fractures in, 89
  surgical procedures in, 77–90
    complications, 89
    postoperative management, 80
    preoperative, 78
    technique, 79
  synovectomy of knee in, 82
  types of, 77
Haemophilia A, 77
Haemophilia B, 77
Haemorrhage,
  control of,
    emergency, 39
    in haemophilia, 79
Hallux,
  clawing of, 1227–1229
Hallux rigidus, 1245–1254
  arthrodesis for, 1250
  exostectomy, 1252
  metatarsal neck osteotomy for, 1246
  osteotomy of neck of proximal phalanx, 1253
  postoperative management, 1254
  preoperative, 1245
Hallux valgus, 444, 1244, 1245
  interphalangeal arthrodesis for, 1253
  Keller arthroplasty for, 1248
  osteotomy for, 1244
  postoperative management, 1254
Halo–body system, 486–490
  criteria for success, 490
  design of system, 488
  indications for, 487
  postapplication management, 490
  procedure, 489
  for transoral approach to cervical spine, 460
Halofemoral traction, 482–485
  complications, 485
  application of halo, 483
  postoperative management, 485
Hamilton Russell traction, 135
Hammer toe, 1259, 1263
Hamstrings,
  transfer to quadriceps, 985–988
    complications, 988
    indications, 985
    postoperative management, 988

Index

Hamstring,
  distal release, 981–984
    operation, 982
    postoperative management, 984
Hamstring,
  proximal release, 940–942
    operation, 941
    postoperative management, 942
Hand,
  acute injuries of, 188–198
    aetiology of, 188
    in children, 198
    operative treatment, 195
    postoperative management, 198
    primary treatment, 192
    skin closure, 197
    types of, 189
  blunt injury, 189
  compartment syndromes, 305
  extensor tendon reconstruction and repair, 827, 852
  flexor pollicis longus injury, 811
  flexor tendons,
    injury, 810
    in palm, 811, 827
    methods of repair, 820
    rheumatoid tenosynovitis of, 865
  flexor tendon reconstruction, 836, 839
    See also Hand, gliding tendon implants
  fractures and dislocations, 196
    See also specific bones, etc.
    caused by metastases, 392
    indications for operation, 176
    instruments for treatment, 176
    operative treatment, 175–187
  fracture-subluxation, 183
  gliding tendon implants, 836
    active programme, 853
    care of, 837
    complications, 848, 851
    contraindications, 838
    indications for, 838
    passive programme, 839
    postoperative management, 848, 851, 854
    preoperative, 839
    pulley reconstruction, 843
    replacement of implant, 849
    selection of tendon motor, 850
    special indications, 852
    stage I, 839
    tendon grafts, 849, 850
    testing pulley system, 847
  gunshot wounds, 191
    treatment, 195
  high-pressure injuries, 190, 191, 195
  infected wounds, 195
  injuries of,
    primary care, 4
  palmar ganglion, 791
  rheumatoid arthritis, 765
  roller injury, 190
  sharp injury, 190
  tendon graft attachment, 814
  tendon injuries, 808–827
    back of hand, 819, 827
    Bunnell criss-cross stitch, 812
    Bunnell double right-angle stitch, 813
    Bunnell withdrawal stitch, 814
    indications for operation, 809
    Kessler grasping stitch, 812
    operations for, 812

Hand (*cont.*)
  tendon injuries (*cont.*)
    in palm, 811, 825
    physiotherapy, 827
    postoperative management, 826
    problems, 808
    Pulvertaft interlacing method, 813
    sutures for, 812
    tenolysis, 851
    surgery of, 812
    tenolysis, 838
Harrington instrumentation, 550
  development of, 491
Harrington–Luque instrumentation, 518
Hartshill triangle, 661
Heel,
  tendon transfer to, 1187–1198
Hepatitis B, 78
Herbert bone screw, 801
Hindquarter amputation, 414–418
  indications and contraindications, 414
  operation, 415
  postoperative management, 418
  preoperative, 415
Hip,
  adductor release, 926–930
    indications and assessment, 926
    operation, 927
    partial neurectomy of obdurator nerve in, 929
    posterior adductor transfer, 929
    postoperative management, 930
  anterior approach to, 951
  anterolateral approach to, 951, 955
  arthritis of, 965
    arthrodesis for, 971
  arthrodesis of, 970–980
    bone graft, 978
    indications and contraindications, 971
    intra-articular, 971
    ischiofemoral, 975
    postoperative management, 974, 980
    preoperative, 971, 975
    special complications, 980
  arthrodesis,
    with iliofemoral graft, 971
  assessment of stability, 875
  congenital dislocation,
    arthrodesis for, 971
    assessment of stability, 875
    Chiari operation, 879
    closed adductor tenotomy, 872
    Colonna operation, 889
    femoral osteotomy, 884
    high femoral osteotomy for, 900, 901, 904
    innominate osteotomy for, 893
    lateral shelf acetabuloplasty, 879, 882
    open reduction, 873
    operations for, 870–892
    Pemberton acetabuloplasty, 878
    replacement for, 947
    stability of, 875
  congenital dysplasia, 949
  degenerative conditions,
    replacement for, 948
  direct lateral approach to, 951, 957
  disarticulation of, 419–421
    operation for, 420
    postoperative management, 421
    preoperative, 419
    prosthetics, 421

Hip (*cont.*)
  dislocation after leg shortening, 1167
  flexion contracture, 921–925
    iliopsoas tenotomy, 923
    operations for, 922
    release of tight iliotibial tract, 922
    Soutter operation, 924
    posterior adductor transfer, 929
  flexor release,
    iliofemoral approach to, 931
    indications and assessment, 931
    operation, 932
    postoperative management, 935
    preoperative, 931
  Gibson approach, 952
  Girdlestone's pseudoarthrosis of, 965–969
    Batchelor's modification, 968
    indications and contraindications, 965
    limitations, 965
    postoperative management, 969
  infratectal or juxtatectal transverse fractures, 328, 338
  lateral approach, 951
  Moore approach to, 952
  persistent fetal alignment of, 900
  posterior column fracture, 327
  replacement arthroplasty, 943–964
    anterolateral approach, 955
    anatomy of, 952
    direct lateral approach, 957
    for failed surgery, 950
    in haemophiliacs, 80
    indications, 943
    posterior approach, 952
    postoperative management, 962
    surgical approaches, 951
  septic arthritis, 948
  stove-in, 321–338
    acetabular fracture with, 328
    equipment for operation, 325
    extended iliofemoral approach, 336
    ilioinguinal approach, 330
    indications for operation, 323
    infratectal or juxtectal transverse fracture, 328, 338
    lateral approach, 336
    posterior approach, 326
    posterior column fracture, 327
    postoperative management, 338
    preoperative, 322
    replacement and fixation of fracture, 334
    T-fractures, 329, 338
  surgical approach to, 58, 951
  T-fracture, 329, 338
  test of stability, 876
  tuberculosis of, 948
Hoffmann operation, 1239
Human immunodeficiency virus, 78
Humerus,
  See also Shoulder, etc.
  displaced fracture of greater tuberosity, 155
  fractures of,
    bracing in, 110
    caused by metastases, 391
    compartment syndromes and, 303, 307
    postoperative care, 155
    traction for, 112, 141, 142
    T–Y, 171

Humerus (cont.)
 fracture of neck,
  caused by metastases, 391
 fractures of shaft, 158
  closed intramedullary nailing, 160
  plating, 159
 metastases in, 396
 Neer hemiarthroplasty, 156
 proximal fractures, 153
  indications for operation, 153
  operation, 154
  two- and three-part, 158
 replacement of head, 716
 resection of head, 716
 supracondylar fracture, 307
  metastases causing, 392

Iliac bone for grafting, 66, 375
Iliac vein,
 injury to, 52
Iliopsoas tendon,
 anterolateral approach to, 933
 approach to, 937
 division, 934
 lengthening or recession, 936
  operation, 937
  postoperative management, 939
  preoperative, 936
Iliopsoas tenotomy, 923
Iliotibial tract,
 release of, 922
Infection,
 amputation and, 398, 400
Inferior radioulnar joint,
 capsulotomy of, 750
Infrapatellar fat pad,
 arthroscopy, 1013, 1033
Innominate osteotomy, 893–899
 indications and contraindications, 893
 operation, 894
 postoperative management, 899
 special requirements for, 893
Intercostobrachial nerve,
 damage to, 452
Interphalangeal valgus, 1245
Intervertebral disc,
 See also Lumbar disc, etc.
 degeneration, 463
 excision of, 508
 herniated, 530
 infection, 533
 resorption, 528
Ischaemia, 295
 amputation and, 398
 of limbs, 25
 signs of, 39

Jefferson fracture, 472
Jewett nail-plate, 215
Joints,
 bleeding into, 78
 contractures in amputations, 400
Joint infection,
 acute, 55
 aspiration of, 57
 chronic, 61–67
Jones operation, 1190

Kaneda device, 592
Kates–Kessel technique, 1239
Keller arthroplasty, 1248
Kessel prosthesis, 718
Kessler grasping stitch, 19, 812
Kienböck's disease of lunate, 791
Kirschner wires,
 in fractures, 115
 in traction, 125
Kleinert technique, 21
Klippel–Trenaunay syndrome, 1152
Knee,
 See also Patella
 acute osteochondral fracture, 1073
 amputation above, 398, 422
  indications and contraindications, 422
  operation, 423
  postoperative management, 426
  preoperative, 422
  prostheses, 426
 amputation below, 431
  anterior and posterior flaps, 435
  indications and contraindications, 431
  long posterior flap, 432
  postoperative management, 436
  preoperative, 431
  prosthetics, 436
 anatomy of, 1008
 anterior cavity,
  loose body removal, 1074
 anterior cruciate ligament,
  arthroscopy, 1014
  repair, 1085
 arthritis of,
  tibial osteotomy for, 1113–1118
 arthrodesis of,
  in haemophiliacs, 83
 arthroplasty of, 1119–1130
  complications, 1130
  correction of deformity, 1121
  extension gap, 1125
  flexion gap, 1123
  indications and contraindications, 1119
  operation, 1120
  postoperative management, 1130
  preoperative, 1119
  preparation of femur, tibia and patella, 1127
 articular cartilage,
  arthroscopy, 1017
  surgical arthroscopy, 1027
  avascular necrosis of, 1073
 chronic anterior cruciate deficiency, 1096
 clinical examination, 1079
 compression arthrodesis, 1131–1136
  complications, 1136
  indications and contraindications, 1131
  operation, 1132
  postoperative management, 1136
  preoperative, 1131
 deformity, 940
 diagnostic arthroscopy of, 1007–1018
  anteromedial approach, 1016
  central approach, 1016
  indications for, 1009
  operation, 1011
  pathological findings, 1017
  posteromedial approach, 1017
  postoperative management, 1015

Knee (cont.)
 diagnostic arthroscopy of (cont.)
  preoperative, 1009
  preparation and position, 1010
 disarticulation at, 427, 430
  indications and contraindications, 427
  postoperative management, 430
  preoperative, 427
  prosthetics, 430
  using lateral flaps, 428
 excessive lateral pressure syndrome, 1032
 fixed flexion deformity of, 86
 flexion contractures, 1061
 flexion deformity, 981
  correction, 984
 haemarthroses in, 82, 1112
 infrapatellar fat pad,
  diagnostic arthroscopy, 1033
 intercondylar notch
  arthroscopy, 1014
 lateral compartment,
  arthroscopy, 1015
 lateral gutter,
  arthroscopy, 1015
 ligament injury, 1079–1101
 limited flexion, 1003
 loose bodies in, 1073–1078
  arthroscopic removal, 1073
  diagnostic arthroscopy, 1035
  indications for removal, 1073
  in osteochondritis dissecans, 1077
  open removal, 1074
  posterior compartment, 1076
  suprapatellar pouch and anterior cavity, 1074
  symptoms and signs, 1073
 medial collateral ligament,
  repair of, 1080
 medial compartment,
  arthroscopy, 1013
 meniscus,
  diagnostic arthroscopy, 1033, 1034
  tears in, 1036
 open meniscectomy,
  indications, 1062
  medial, 1063
  preoperative, 1062
 osteoarthritis, 1036
  loose bodies in, 1073
 osteochondral fracture, 1073
  treatment of, 1078
 osteochondritis dissecans, 1073
  treatment, 1076
 pigmented villonodular synovitis, 1109
 posterior compartment,
  loose bodies in, 1031, 1076
 posterior cruciate ligament,
  repair of, 1083, 1093
 postoperative infection, 1061, 1112
 proximal hamstring release, 940
 rheumatoid arthritis, 1109
 suprapatellar pouch,
  loose body removal from, 1074
 surgical arthroscopy, 1019–1042
  See also Meniscectomy
  articular cartilage, 1027, 1039
  chondromalacia patellae, 1030, 1039
  division of synovial fold or shelf, 1025
  instruments, 1021
  lateral release, 1032
  removal of loose bodies, 1030, 1039

Knee (*cont.*)
  surgical arthroscopy (*cont.*)
    synovial tags, 1026, 1037, 1038
    synovium, 1023, 1037
    triangulation, 1–20
  synovectomy of, 1027, 1109–1112
    complications of, 1112
    operation, 1110
    postoperative management, 1112
    preoperative, 1109
  synovial biopsy, 1023, 1037
  synovial fold or shelf,
    division of, 1025
  synovial membrane,
    arthroscopy, 1017, 1033
  synovial osteochondromatosis, 1073
    treatment, 1078
  synovial tags,
    excision of, 1026, 1037, 1038
  tuberculosis, 1109
  valgus deformity, 1113, 1121
  varus deformity, 1121
Knee hinge, 130
Knock knee, 1113
Kocher–Langenbeck approach to acetabulum, 342
Küntscher's closed intramedullary nailing for femoral shaft fractures, 223–241
  availability of equipment, 240
  Melbourne cross pinning, 234, 240
  postoperative management, 240
  preoperative, 223
  technical requirements, 224
  traction, 226
Kyphosis,
  correction of, 662, 664

Lacerations, 2
Lambrinudi arthrodesis, 1191, 1201
Laminectomy,
  definition, 519
Lateral condyle,
  fracture of, 173
Latissimus dorsi,
  free flap from, 14
Lauenstein procedure, 773
Leg,
  amputation through, 422
    above knee, 422
    below knee, 431
    disarticulation at knee, 427
  avulsion flap, 3
  compartment syndromes in, 298
    perifibular fasciotomy for, 299
    postoperative management, 300
    Volkmann's ischaemic contracture following, 307
  diaphyseal lengthening, 1154
  epiphyseal lengthening, 1154
  insertion of Steinmann pin, 128
  lengthening, 1154, 1159–1167
    complications, 1167
    joint damage following, 1167
    muscle contractures, 1167
    pin-track infection, 1167
    soft tissue release and corticotomy, 1162
    tibiofibular joint displacement after, 1167

Leg (*cont.*)
  length inequality, 1152–1168
    aetiology of, 1152
    assessment of, 1152, 1153
    associated anomalies, 1153
    measurement, 1153
    monitoring patient, 1153
    preoperative, 1152
    procedures and indications, 1154
  massive replacement for tumours, 1137–1151
    See also specific bones
    assessment, 1138
    complications, 1151
    indications and contraindications, 1137
    operation, 1142
    preoperative, 1138
    prosthetic failure, 1151
  prostheses for tumour surgery, 1138
  short,
    true and apparent, 1152
  shortening, 1154
    epiphysiodesis, 1154, 1155
    techniques, 1155
  traction systems, 134
  tumour surgery, 1137
    recurrences, 1151
Leprosy, 1184
Ligamentum patellae,
  rupture of, 995, 996, 998
Limb,
  ischaemia, 39, 49
  replacement, 53
  revascularization, 48
Lister's intraosseous wiring, 180
Littlewood's approach to forequarter amputation, 413
Ludloff approach to iliopsoas tendon, 936, 937
Lumbar disc,
  central prolapse, 527
  extraforaminal prolapse, 528
  large subrhizal prolapse, 526
  prolapse, 519–529
    associated with special problems, 528
    preoperative, 520
    indications for operation, 520
    operation, 523
    sequestered fragments, 527
    types of, 519
  small subrhizal prolapse, 526
Lumbar spine,
  approach to, 619
  fracture dislocation,
    closed reduction, 647
    open reduction and internal fixation, 649
    spinal jacket for, 667
  infections, 568
  instability, 545
  metastatic bone disease,
    anterior decompression and stabilization, 587
    complications, 595
    posterior decompression and stabilization, 594
    posterior stabilization, 594
    supplementary instrumentation, 593
  paraspinal approach to, 622
  posterior fusion, 539–544

Lunate,
  Keinbock's disease, 791
Luque instrumentation, 491
  for neuromuscular scoliosis, 512–518
    choice of procedure, 514
    exposure of spinous process, 515
    indications for, 512
    insertion of rods, 516
    postoperative management, 518
    preoperative, 513
    technique, 514

Magnuson–Stack procedure,
  modified, 683
Malleolus,
  fracture of, 286, 289, 291
    in children, 365
Mallet deformity of finger, 809
  repair of, 827
Mallet fracture of finger, 815
Mallet toe, 1259
Maquet operation, 1107
Matte–Russe bone graft of carpal scaphoid, 796
Medial cutaneous nerve,
  as donor nerve, 34
Medial malleolus,
  fractures, 365
Median nerve,
  compression, 788
  injuries, 25, 193, 789
  paralysis,
    combined with radial nerve paralysis, 764
    combined with ulnar nerve paralysis, 764
  repair by grafting, 32
  tendon reconstruction for palsy, 759–763
Meniscectomy of knee, 1019, 1062–1072
  arthroscopic, 1040–1042, 1043–1055
    basic technique, 1044
  lateral, 1067
    postoperative management, 1069
  medial, 1063
    postoperative management, 1066
Meniscus,
  arthroscopic repair, 1056–1061
    complications, 1061
    contraindications, 1057
    indications, 1056
    inside-out technique, 1059
    investigations, 1057
    outside-in technique, 1060
    postoperative management, 1061
    technique, 1058
  bucket-handle tear, 1040, 1045
    excision, 1040, 1046
  diagnostic arthroscopy, 1033, 1034
  discoid lateral,
    arthroscopic surgery, 1054
    excision of, 1065
  excision of tag tears, 1041, 1048
  lateral,
    excision of posterior horn, 1070
    radial tears, 1042, 1052
  medial,
  medial,
    excision of retained posterior horn, 1070
  parrot-beak tears, 1042, 1053

Meniscus (cont.)
 posterior horn cleavage tears, 1042, 1051
 posterior third bucket-handle tears, 1041, 1042, 1049
 surface flap tear, 1055
 tears of,
  diagnostic arthroscopy, 1017, 1035
  torn cystic lateral, 1052
Mesh grafts, 3
Metacarpals,
 traction on, 127
Metacarpal head,
 resection of, 69
Metacarpal pin traction, 143
Metacarpophalangeal joint,
 Swanson arthroplasty, 68–72
  complications, 72
  dressings, 71
  in rheumatoid disease, 68–72
  insertion of implant, 70
  indications and contraindications, 68
  postoperative management, 72
  preoperative, 68
  technique, 69
Metaphyseal wedge osteotomy, 377
Metastatic bone disease, 92, 96, 97, 384–396, 487, 571
Monteggia fracture, 160, 163, 169
 open reduction of radial head, 170
Morton's metatarsalgia,
 dorsal nerve transfer for, 1255–1258
Muscles,
 bleeding into, 78
 injury to, 48
 ischaemic, 48
 management in amputation, 399
Muscle autografts in nerve repair, 37
Muscle skin flaps, 13
Myelitis, 533
Myocutaneous skin flap, 13

Naughton Dunn's operation, 1199
Necrosis, 400
Neer hemi-arthroplasty, 156
Neer prosthesis, 719
Nerves,
 epineural repair, 37
 management in amputation, 400
 peripheral See Peripheral nerves
Nerve grafts,
 vascularized, 37
Nerve root anomalies, 528
Nerve transfer, 37
Neurapraxia, 25
 in compartment syndromes, 295
Neurolysis, 37
Ninety-ninety traction, 136

Obturator nerve,
 partial neurectomy, 929
Occipitoatlantal joints,
 anatomy of, 454
Odontoid,
 congenital anomalies, 476
 fractures, 486
  internal fixation, 642
Oedema of amputation stump, 401
Olecranon,
 fracture of, 167
 traction, 127, 142

Ollier's disease, 1152
Os calcis,
 osteomyelitis of, 66
Osteoarthrosis,
 hip replacement for, 944
Osteochondritis dissecans, 1073
 arthroscopic surgery of, 1027, 1031, 1038
  removal of fixation devices, 1028
  removal of fragments, 1027
 diagnostic arthroscopy, 1017
 treatment of, 1076
 with loose body, 1077
Osteoid osteoma, 91
Osteomyelitis,
 amputation for, 398
 chronic, 61
 chronic suppurative, 64
  postoperative management, 66
  preoperative, 64
  surgery of, 65
 diagnosis of, 55
 drainage in, 56
 Garré sclerosing, 62
 haematogenous, 64
 pathology of, 54
 presentation, 55
 principles of treatment, 55
 purulent, 61
 surgical treatment, 56
Osteoporosis, 595

Pain,
 from traction, 143
 in compartment syndromes, 295
Palmaris longus,
 transfer of, 758
Pantalar arthrodesis, 1198
Patella,
 See also Knee
 chondromalacia, 1032
  arthroscopic surgery, 1030, 1039
  diagnostic arthroscopy, 1036
 decompression and realignment, 1107
 fat pad,
  arthroscopy, 1013, 1033
 fractures of, 252–255, 955
  exposure of fracture, 253
  indications for operation, 252
  operative details, 253
  postoperative management, 255
  preoperative, 252
  rigid internal fixation, 254
 lateral subluxation, 1102
 Maquet operation, 1107
 preparation for knee arthroplasty, 1127
 recurrent dislocation of, 1102–1108
  in children, 1103
  Goldthwaite–Roux operation, 1103
  in teenagers and adults, 1106
 recurrent subluxation, 1032
 release and repositioning, 1103
 Trillat operation, 1108
Patellofemoral joint,
 arthroscopy of, 1013, 1033
 osteoarthritis, 1107
Pectoralis major tendon,
 transfer of, 742
Pelvic osteotomy, 879
 Chiari operation, 879
 Coventry screw and plate fixation, 887
 using four-hole plate, 886

Pelvis,
 cancer of, 414
 fractures of,
  external skeletal fixation, 150
Pemberton acetabuloplasty, 878
Peripheral nerves,
 epineural repair, 37
 grafting, 24, 32, 34
  donor nerve, 34
  indications for, 34
  partial repair, 36
  postoperative management, 36
  technique, 34
 iatrogenic injury, 25
 identification, 28
 injuries of, 25
  diagnosis, 25
  findings, 31
  vascular injuries and, 25
 primary repair of, 24
  postoperative management, 30
 primary sutures, 26
 repair of divisions, 24–38
  fibrin glue in, 37
  muscle autografts in, 37
  prognosis, 38
  rehabilitation in, 38
 secondary repair, 24, 30–33
  indications and contraindications, 30
  mobilization, 32
  postoperative management, 33
  resection and biopsy, 32
  technique, 31
Perkins' traction, 134
Perthes' disease,
 arthrosis following, 949
 high femoral osteotomy for, 900, 901
 innominate osteotomy for, 893
Pes cavus, 1216–1219
 calcaneal osteotomy for, 1217
 Steindler release of plantar fascia, 1216
 tarsometatarsal truncated wedge arthrodesis for, 1218
 wedge tarsectomy for, 1208
Pes planus, 1211–1215
 excision of calcaneonavicular bar, 1214
 preoperative, 1211
 reversed Dillwyn Evans procedure, 1212
Peyronie's disease, 855
Phalen's test, 788
Phantom limb, 401
Plantar digital neuroma,
 dorsal nerve transfer for, 1255–1258
Pneumothorax, 452
Poliomyelitis, 512, 936, 981, 1152, 1184
 hip deformity in, 931
Popliteal artery,
 damage to, 1061
Popliteal nerve injury, 1184
Posterior interosseous nerve,
 injury to, 25
Presacral nerve,
 care of, 556
Pressure garments, 86
Pridie technique, 87
Pronator teres,
 redirection of, 749
 transfer of, 758
Protrusio acetabuli,
 hip replacement for, 946
Proximal phalanx,
 fracture of shaft, 177

Pubic symphysis,
  exposure and fixation, 346–350
    apparatus required, 347
    indications for, 346
    operation, 348
    postoperative management, 350
    preoperative, 347
    reduction, 349
Pulvertaft interlacing method, 813
Putti–Platt operation, 675–679

Quadricepsplasty, 1003–1006
  complications of, 1006
  indications, 1003
  operation, 1004
  postoperative management, 1006
Quadriceps,
  contracture in infancy, 1002
  rupture of, 995–1002
    old lesions, 998
    recent lesions, 996
  transfer of hamstrings to, 985–988
Quadriceps tendon,
  lengthening and repair, 1001
  rupture of, 997, 1001

Radial nerve,
  care of, 790
  iatrogenic injury, 25
  paralysis,
    combined with median nerve paralysis, 764
    combined with ulnar nerve paralysis, 764
    following synovectomy, 76
    tendon reconstruction, 753
Radial nerve repair palsy splint, 21
Radiotherapy,
  fracture union following, 384
Radius,
  deformities, 358
    of head, 358
  distal fractures, 163
    external skeletal fixation, 149
  excision of head, 166
  exposure of, 161
  fracture,
    caused by metastases, 392
    compartment syndromes and, 303
    postoperative management, 162, 164
    rigid plate fixation, 161
  fracture of head, 165–167
  fracture of neck in children, 358
  fracture of shaft, 160
  reduction of head, 170
  split head,
    reconstruction, 167
Respiratory distress syndrome, adult, 114
Reversed dynamic slings, 86
Rheumatoid arthritis, 765
  forefoot deformity, 1232
  hallux valgus, 1244
  halo–body cast in, 487
  hip replacement in, 944
  of hand and feet, 765
  of knee, 1109, 1119
  radio-ulnar joint involvement, 805
  Swanson arthroplasty for, 68–72
  synovectomy of elbow for, 73–76
  wrist arthroplasty for, 782

Robert Jones operation for clawing of hallux, 1227
Robert Jones valgus osteotomy, 907
Rotator cuff,
  repair, 697–704
    indications for, 697
    operation, 698
    postoperative management, 704
    principles of, 702
  surgical exposure of, 698

Salter–Harris classification, 352
Scaphoid,
  See Carpal scaphoid
Scoliosis,
  idiopathic, 482, 491–503
    indications for instrumentation, 491
    indications for posterior fusion, 491
    investigations, 492
    Luque instrumentation for, 512–518
      choice of procedure, 514
      exposure of spinous process, 515
      indications, 512
      insertion of rods, 516
      preoperative, 513
      technique, 514
  neuromuscular
    Luque instrumentation for, 518
  posterior procedures,
    bone grafting, 502
    excision of facet joints, 498
    exposure of laminae, 496
    insertion of Harrington hook, 497, 498
    insertion of Harrington rod, 501
    insertion of wires, 500
    operative details, 495
    planning fusion levels, 493
    postoperative management, 502
    preoperative, 492
    splitting spinous process tips, 495
    tightening of wires, 501
Semilunar cartilage
  See Meniscus
Septic arthritis, 54
Shoulder,
  See also Humerus, etc.
  arthrodesis of, 721–728
    alternative techniques, 726
    anterior operation, 721, 722, 728
    indications and contraindications, 721
    operation, 722
    posterior operation, 721, 727, 728
    postoperative management, 728
    preoperative, 721
  arthroplasty of, 713–720
    complications, 720
    excision, 713
    indications, 713
    loosening of prosthesis, 720
    Neer prosthesis, 719
    postoperative management, 720
    preoperative, 714
    total replacement, 713
    use of Kessel prosthesis, 718
    use of Stanmore prosthesis, 717, 718
  arthroscopy of, 692–696
    appearances of, 695–696
  dislocation following arthroplasty, 720
  distraction at joint, 721
  excision arthroplasty, 713
  hemiarthroplasty, 713

Shoulder (cont.)
  prosthesis for, 713
  recurrent anterior dislocation, 671–685
    aetiology, 671
    anterior apprehension test, 673
    approach to, 678
    Bankart operation, 681
    choice of operation, 675
    management of initial dislocation, 672
    modified Boytchev procedure, 684
    modified Bristow–Helfet procedure, 683
    modified Magnuson–Stack procedure, 683
    operations for, 676
    pathological, 675
    posterior stress test, 674
    postoperative management, 684
    preoperative, 673
    Putti–Platt operation, 675, 679
    structures to protect, 675
    sulcus sign, 674
    voluntary, 674
  resection of humeral head, 716
  surgical approach to, 58, 59
  tuberculosis, 721
Silfverskiöld operation, 1175
Silver's syndrome, 1152
Skeletal traction, 111, 123, 125
  complications of, 129
  sites of, 126
Skin,
  management in amputation, 399
Skin cover, 1–15
Skin flaps, 7–15
  abdominal tube pedicle, 8
  cross-leg, 10
  cutaneous axial-pattern, 11
  fasciocutaneous, 12
  free, 14
  local, 8
  muscle, 13
  principles of, 7
  regional, 8
Skin grafts,
  application of, 5
  delayed, 6
  mesh, 3, 6
  small split skin, 6
  split skin, 5
Skin loss, 5
Skoog technique, 860
Skull halo,
  preparation for, 625
  in spinal injuries, 624
Sliding traction, 123, 138
Soutter operation for hip contracture, 924
Spina bifida, 981, 1152
Spinal canal,
  opening, 524
Spinal fusion,
  vascular damage during, 53
Spinal stenosis,
  assessment, 534
  classification, 534
  lumbar disc prolapse with, 528
  posterior decompression for, 534–538
  posterior decompression,
    multiple level, 538
    postoperative management, 538
    preoperative, 534
    technique, 535
  presentation, 534

Index

Spine,
 See also Cervical spine, Lumbar spine, etc.
 abscess, 560
 anterior approaches to, 598–615
  cervicothoracic area, 603
  Fraser's muscle splitting, 612
  retroperitoneal approach to L2–5, 610
  to C1–C2, 598
  to C3–T1, 600
  to T4–11, 605
  to thoracolumbar junction, 607
  to upper thoracic spine, 603
  transperitoneal midline approach to L4–S1, 613
 anterior decompression and fixation, for kyphosis, 662
 application of plaster of Paris jacket, 667
 approaches to, 597–623
  indications, 597
 cleft cleavage fractures, 652
 costotransversectomy, 614
 deformity, 482
  anterior instrumentation, 509
  anterior procedures, 504–511
  indications for operation, 504
  operations, 506
  postoperative management, 511
  preoperative, 505
 exposure of laminae, 496
 fractures and dislocations, 487
  Hartshill triangle, 661
  internal fixators, 655
  kyphotic deformities following, 662
  posterior fusion, 660
  postural reduction, 628
  spinal jacket for, 667
  spinal plates for, 659
  traction for, 125
  with locked facets, 647
 Fraser's muscle-splitting approach, 612
 fusion of Gallé type, 644
 infection, 487
  operations for, 559–570
 injuries, 624–669
  See also under Cervical spine, Lumbar spine etc
  application of halo and caliper, 624
  postural reduction plus maintenance, 628
  preparation for halo and calipers, 625
 instability, 463, 480, 487
 intertransverse fusion, 545–548
  postoperative management, 548
  with decompression, 548
  without decompression, 546
 intracranial fragments, 662
 metastatic bone disease of, 571–596
  aims of treatment, 571, 574
  anterior cord decompression, 575
  anterior decompression, 582, 587
  anterior stabilization, 577
  basic principles of treatment, 572
  complications of treatment, 595
  decompression in, 572
  failure of stabilization, 595
  indications for treatment, 571
  investigations, 574
  Kaneda device, 592
  laminar removal and replacement, 594
  posterior decompression and stabilization, 579

Spine (*cont.*)
 metastatic bone disease of (*cont.*)
  posterior spinal fusion in, 594
  posterior stabilization, 594
  postoperative treatment, 595
  preoperative, 574
  stabilization, 572, 573
  supplementary instrumentation, 593
  timing of surgery, 574
 paraspinal approach to lumbar spine, 622
 posterior approaches, 616–623
  to C1–7, 616
  to lumbar spine, 619
  to thoracic spine, 618
 rheumatoid arthritis of, 487
 thoracic,
  approaches to, 603, 618
 thoracolumbar junction,
  approach to, 607
 tongue-splitting approach to, 600
 transoral approach to, 598
 transperitoneal midline approach to, 613
 tuberculosis of, 559
 unstable fractures, 476
Splints, 129–133
 Fisk, 130
 suspension, 133
 preparation of, 131
 Thomas's, 129
 for femoral shaft fracture, 137
Spondylitis,
 pyogenic, 559
Spondylolisthesis,
 anatomical lesions, 551
 combined traction and fusion technique, 552
 disc prolapse and, 528
 gradual reduction, 554
 indications for surgery, 552
 intertransverse fusion for, 545–548
 measurements in, 551
 surgical reduction of, 549–558
  anterior lumbosacral fusion, 556
  bone grafting, 557
  complications, 558
  gradual, 554
  historical background, 550
  neurological examination, 555
  operations, 554
  postoperative management, 557
  preoperative, 552
  skull–femoral traction, 555
Stanmore prosthesis, 717
Steindler flexorplasty, 737
 Bunnell's modification, 739
Steindler release of plantar fascia, 1216
Steinmann pin,
 in fracture traction, 125
 insertion in leg, 128
Strayer operation, 1177
Subacromial space,
 approach to, 693, 698
 arthroscopic appearances of, 694
Subperiosteal abscess, 55
Subscapularis and interspinatus tendon transplantation, 703
Subtalar joint,
 approach to, 60
Sural nerve as donor nerve, 34, 35
Suturing wounds, 2

Swanson arthroplasty,
 of metacarpophalangeal joint, 68–72
  complications, 72
  dressings, 71
  indications and contraindications, 68
  insertion of implant, 70
  postoperative management, 72
  preoperative, 68
  technique, 69
Syme's amputation, 437–440
 alternatives to, 437
 indications and contraindications, 437
 postoperative management, 440
 preoperative, 437
 prosthetics, 440
 technique, 438
Synostosis,
 after elbow fracture, 361
Synovectomy, 1027
 of elbow, 73–76
 of knee in haemophilics, 82
Synovitis from tendon implants, 848

Talipes equinovarus,
 congenital, 1220
  indications for operation, 1220
  lateral soft tissue release, 1225
  medial soft tissue release, 1223
  operations for, 1220–1231
  plantar soft tissue release, 1224
  posterior soft tissue release, 1221
  postoperative management, 1226
  secondary surgery, 1226
Talocalcaneal synostosis, 1207
Talonavicular dislocation, 319
Talonavicular fracture-subluxation, 319
Talus,
 fracture dislocation, 312
 fracture of lateral process, 314
 fracture of neck, 311
 infection, 1191
 injuries to, 311
 inversion fracture, 313
 total dislocation of, 313
Tarsal osteotomies in club foot, 1226
Tarsectomy, 1208–1210
Tarsometatarsal disruption, 318
Tarsometatarsal truncated wedge arthrodesis, 1218
Tarsus,
 disruption of, 319
 fracture caused by metastases, 395
Tendo Achillis,
 acute rupture, 1179
  closed repair, 1180
  open repair, 1179
 incomplete tenotomy, 1172
 lengthening and repair, 1172–1183
 old rupture,
  repair of, 1182
 repair of, 1179
 Z-plasty, 1174
Tendons,
 care of during surgery, 21
 sheaths and pulleys, 18
Tendon injury,
 primary care, 17
Tendon repair, 16–23
 adhesions following, 23
 anchorage to bone, 20
 apical suture, 20

1284 Index

Tendon repair (cont.)
  associated injury, 17
  bowstringing, 23
  complications, 23
  contraindications, 17
  immobilization in, 22
  indications for, 17
  of unequal girth, 20
  preoperative, 17
  primary, 17
  protection after surgery, 21
  pulley reconstruction, 23
  replacement, 18
  suture materials, 19
  technique of, 19
  tension of, 22, 23
  timing of, 17
  transfer of, 18
Tendon transfer, 18
  to foot, 1184, 1187
Tenography technique, 832
Tenolysis, 835
Tetanus, 198
Thigh,
  cancer of, 414
  compartment syndromes, 301
Thomas arthrodesis of ankle, 1197
Thomas' splint, 129
  in femoral shaft fracture, 137
Thoracic outlet syndrome,
  anterior and posterior approach to, 452
  axillary approach to, 447–452
    choice of procedure, 448
    complications, 452
    indications and contraindications, 447
    postoperative management, 451
    preoperative, 448
    transaxillary first rib resection, 448
  recurrence, 452
Thoracic spine,
  costotransversectomy approach, 566
  fracture dislocations,
    closed reduction, 647
  infections of, 566
    operations for, 564
  metastatic bone disease,
    anterior decompression for, 582
    complications, 595
    posterior decompression and
      stabilization, 594
    posterior stabilization, 594
    stabilization, 587
Thoracolumbar spine,
  transpleural approach to, 564
Thorax,
  vascular injury of, 52
Thumb,
  Bennett's fracture-subluxation, 183
  flexor pollicis longus injury, 811
  transfer of extensor indicis to, 760
  trigger, 865–869
    in children, 869
    conservative treatment, 865
    operative details, 866
    postoperative management, 868
Tibia,
  anterolateral bone grafting, 371
  compound fractures of, 14
  diaphyseal fractures, 147
  fracture,
    bracing in, 110
    caused by metastases, 395

Tibia (cont.)
  external skeletal fixation, 147
  skeletal traction, 126
  traction for, 112, 134, 138
  traction weights, 133
  fractures of shaft, 268–283
    classification of open wounds, 269
    external fixation, 272, 275
    follow-up, 283
    internal fixation by intramedullary
      nailing, 278
    internal fixation by plating, 275
    non-operative management, 270
    operative treatment, 272
    postoperative management, 278, 283
    soft tissue injury in, 268
  lengthening, 1154, 1166
  medial condyle fracture, 258
  metaphyseal wedge osteotomy, 377
  metastases in, 396
  osteotomy,
    for arthritis of knee, 1113–1118
    operation, 1115
    postoperative management, 1118
  plateau fractures, 256–267
    approach to, 262
    associated fractures, 258
    bicondylar, 258, 266
    classification, 257
    cleavage, 257, 264
    depressed, 257, 258, 265
    laterally injured, 260
    medial condyle, 258
    medial injury, 261
    operative approach, 259
    postoperative management, 267
    preoperative, 259
    reconstruction and fixation, 264
    symptoms and signs, 259
  plate removal from, 120
  posterolateral bone grafting, 373
  preparation for knee arthroplasty,
    1127
  replacement for tumour, 1148–1150
  resection of upper end, 1133
  shortening, 1154
Tibialis posterior tendon,
  ruptures, 1215
  transfer of tendon to, 1215
  transfer to dorsum of foot, 1184–1186
Tibiofibular joint displacement,
  after leg lengthening, 1167
Tibiofibular syndesmosis, 290
Tillaux fracture, 290
Tissue pressure, 296
  measurement of, 297
Toes,
  amputation of, 444–446
  claw, 1230
  crush injuries, 320
  gangrene of, 397
  hammer, 1259, 1263
  mallet, 1259
  metatarsal shortening, 1264
  open fractures, 320
  ray resection, 444
  subungual haematoma, 320
Toe, big
  clawing of, 1227
  prosthetic replacement of, 1241
Toe, fifth
  dorsally placed, 1267–1269

Toe-nail
  ingrowing, 1270–1272
Transmetatarsal amputation, 441–443
Triceps disruption, 734
Triceps tendon,
  anterior transfer, 740
Trigger finger and thumb, 865–869
  in children, 869
  treatment, 865
  operative details, 866
  postoperative management, 868
  preoperative, 866
Trillat operation, 1108
Trochanteric osteosynthesis, 951
Trochanteric osteotomy, 963
Tauge's looped suture method, 19
Tuberculosis, 948
Tulloch Brown traction, 135
Tumours,
  amputation for, 398
  replacement surgery for leg, 1137–1151

Ulna,
  Darrach's procedure, 769
  excision of, 769
  exposure of, 162
  fracture, 169
    caused by metastases, 392
    compartment syndrome and, 303
    plating of, 162
    postoperative management, 162
  fracture of shaft, 160
  Lauenstein procedure, 773
Ulnar nerve,
  decompression of, 75
  injury to, 25, 734
  paralysis,
    combined with median nerve
      paralysis, 764
    combined with radial nerve paralysis,
      764
  repair by grafting, 32
  tendon reconstruction, 764
Ulnar neuritis, 75
Upper femoral epiphysis,
  anatomy of, 910
  slipped, 909–920
    acceptable deformity, 912, 913
    arthrodesis for, 971
    biplane trochanteric osteotomy for,
      916
    choice of treatment, 912
    geometric flexion osteotomy for, 919
    growth plate and, 912
    pinning in situ, 912
    technical errors, 913
    unacceptable deformity, 913, 919

Valgus deformity, 1113
Veins,
  injuries to, 48
Vein grafts,
  for arterial repair, 46
Vena cava laceration, 52
Venous insufficiency, 397
Volkmann's ischaemic contracture, 290,
  291
Volkmann's fracture, 290, 291
Volkmann's ischaemic contracture, 25, 37,
  141
  following compartment syndromes, 307

Walton manoeuvre, 631
Watson–Jones approach to hip, 951
Watson–Jones arthrodesis of ankle, 1192
Weaver–Dunn technique, 690
Weedon–Butler operation, 1268
Whoosh test, 43
Wounds,
  closure of, 1
  debridement, 2
  drainage, 2
  management of,
    in open fractures, 120
  mesh grafts, 3, 6
  nerve inury, 25
  primary care of, 48
  skin flaps for, 7–15
  skin grafts for, 5
  suturing, 2
  treatment of, 1
Wrist,
  arthrodesis of, 779, 791
    bone graft fixation, 792, 793

Wrist (cont.)
  arthrodesis of (cont.)
    indications for, 779
    internal fixation, 781
    limited, 782
    plate fixation, 793
    postoperative management, 782, 793
  arthroplasty, 782
    indications, 782
    postoperative management, 786
    procedure, 782
  Darrach's procedure, 769
  decompression procedures, 787
  de Quervain's disease, 787
  dorsal synovectomy, 766
  flexion deformity, 752
  flexor synovectomy, 777
  flexor tendon injury, 811, 827
  fractures caused by metastases, 392
  ganglion, 790
  Lauenstein procedure, 773
  limited arthrodesis, 782

  mobile radial deviation of, 805–807
  operations on, 766
  osteoarthritis of, 791
  panarthrodesis of, 791
  paralysis of, 759
  rheumatoid arthritis of, 765
  ruptured extensor tendons, 774, 776
  surgery of, 765–804
  tendon injury at, 826
  transfer of extensor indicis proprius, 775

Yount procedure, 922

Zadik procedure for ingrowing toe-nail, 1271
Zickel nail fixation, 216–222
  complications, 222
  indications for, 216
  technique, 218